# PRESENT KNOWLEDGE IN NUTRITION

# Present Knowledge in

# Nutrition

Ninth Edition

## Volume I

**Edited by**
**Barbara A. Bowman**
**and Robert M. Russell**

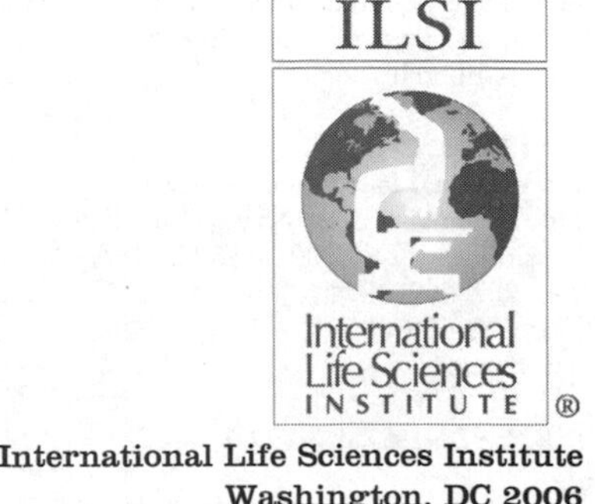


International Life Sciences Institute
Washington, DC 2006

ILSI Press
International Life Sciences Institute
One Thomas Circle, NW, Ninth Floor
Washington, DC 20005-5802, USA
Tel: 202-659-0074
Fax: 202-659-3859
www.ilsi.org

ISBN: 978-1-57881-199-1

Printed in the United States of America

# Contents

# Preface

Nutrition continues to be an evolving science, and *Present Knowledge in Nutrition* continues to be a favored ready reference—a constant companion on the professional bookshelf that is often turned to first when questions on nutrition arise, and known for its up-to-date, concise, authoritative chapters by distinguished experts. Each new edition represents tangible evidence of the growing scope and challenge of nutrition as a field, with an increasing number of chapters. Each chapter presents fresh perspectives from new disciplines as well as current research. In particular, this edition reflects the remarkable impact of genomics on the field of nutrition and growing realization of the potential for this new knowledge to transform the human condition.

The first edition of *Present Knowledge in Nutrition* was published in 1953, just a few years after the isolation of Vitamin $B_{12}$, which was the last of the vitamins to be identified. The fourth edition, edited by Dr. Mark Hegstead and published in 1976, contained 53 chapters, compared with 70 chapters in the current edition, reflecting the broad and interdisciplinary scope of nutrition science. For the first time, *Present Knowledge in Nutrition* is being published in two volumes—the first volume contains chapters on systems biology, energy physiology, and the nutrients (chapters 1-40), and the second volume contains chapters on nutrition and the life cycle, immunity, chronic diseases, diet and food, public health, and international nutrition. Volume II concludes with a section on emerging issues in nutrition, covering food-borne illness and food safety, food biotechnology, and bioactive components in food and supplements.

Collaborating as editors on this volume was a tremendous honor, but also a daunting task. Critical research questions have moved beyond the understanding of the role of inadequate nutrient intakes in deficiency to also include, often simultaneously, the role of nutrition in chronic disease prevention and the consequences of overnutrition. Most of the chapters in this edition conclude with a discussion of future directions, including research needs, to challenge and prepare the reader for developments in the years ahead.

Our task as editors was also challenged by *Present Knowledge in Nutrition*'s broad use in the field. Historically, the book has had an incredibly diverse readership including undergraduate, graduate, and post graduate students in nutrition, public heath, medicine, and related fields; dieticians, physicians, and other health professionals; and academic, industrial and government researchers. *Present Knowledge in Nutrition*'s readers range from food scientists and technologists to regulators, policy makers and members of the wider public. We expect the ninth edition to become a standard text and authoritative reference work in classrooms, libraries, laboratories, clinics, and offices around the world. We believe we have achieved a highly readable, well-organized, comprehensive, and timely summary of current nutrition science.

This edition of *Present Knowledge in Nutrition* reflects the dedication and hard work of many people. First, we want to thank our expert authors from seven countries around the world for their diligent efforts to present the essence of a topic, often condensing decades of specialized research into concise, accessible chapters with a manageable number of references. We wish to thank the members of our editorial board for their assistance in developing the framework for this book, our colleagues at the Jean Mayer USDA Human Nutrition Research Center on Aging at Tufts University and the Centers for Disease Control and Prevention, especially Sarah Peterson from Tufts. Fourth, we are indebted to Suzie Harris and the patient, professional, and dedicated staff at the International Life Sciences Institute (ILSI), especially Suzanne White and Eleanore Tapscott.

Finally, we dedicate this volume to our parents and families, mentors, colleagues and students from whom we have learned so much.

Barbara A Bowman, Atlanta, Georgia
Robert M. Russell, Boston, Massachusetts
Editors

*These findings and conclusions are those of the authors and do not necessarily represent the views of the Centers for Disease Control and Prevention.*

# Contributors


## Editors

Barbara Bowman, PhD
Centers for Disease Control and Prevention
Atlanta, Georgia, USA

Robert M. Russell, MD, PhD
Jean Mayer USDA Human Nutrition Research Center on Aging
Tufts University
Boston, Massachusetts, USA

## Editorial Advisory Board

Benjamin Caballero, MD, PhD
Center for Human Nutrition
Johns Hopkins University
Baltimore, Maryland, USA

Paul Coates, PhD
Office of Dietary Supplements
National Institutes of Health
Bethesda, Maryland, USA

Fergus Clydesdale, PhD
Department of Food Sciences
University of Massachusetts
Amherst, Massachusetts, USA

Joseph G. Hautvast, MD
International Union of Nutritional Sciences
Wageningen, Netherlands

Janet King, PhD
Children's Hospital
Oakland Research Institute
Oakland, California, USA

Alfred H. Merrill, PhD
School of Biology
Georgia Institute of Technology
Atlanta, Georgia, USA

Penelope S. Nestel, PhD
International Food Policy Research Institute
Washington, DC, USA

Irwin H. Rosenberg, MD
Friedman School of Nutrition Science & Policy
Tufts University
Boston, Massachusetts, USA

## Authors

Janice Albert, MS
Nutrition and Consumer Protection Division
Food and Agriculture Organization of the United Nations
Rome, Italy

Lindsay H. Allen, PhD
Department of Nutrition
University of California
Davis, California, USA

John J.B. Anderson, PhD
Department of Nutrition
School of Public Health and School of Medicine
University of North Carolina
Chapel Hill, North Carolina, USA

Jamy D. Ard, MD
Departments of Nutrition Sciences and Internal Medicine
University of Alabama
Birmingham, Alabama, USA

Lynn B. Bailey, PhD
Department of Food Science and Human Nutrition
University of Florida
Gainesville, Florida, USA

C.J. Bates, DPhil
Elsie Widdowson Laboratory
MRC Human Nutrition Research
Cambridge, United Kingdom

Charles Baum, MD
Department of Medicine
University of Illinois
Chicago, Illinois, USA

John Beard, PhD
Department of Nutrition
College of Health and Human Development
The Pennsylvania State University
University Park, Pennsylvania, USA

Gary R. Beecher, PhD
Food Composition Laboratory
Beltsville Human Nutrition Research Center
Agricultural Research Service
US Department of Agriculture
Beltsville, Maryland, USA

Jeffrey B. Blumberg, PhD
Antioxidants Research Laboratory
Jean Mayer USDA Human Nutrition
Research Center on Aging
Tufts University
Boston, Massachusetts, USA

Annalies Borrel, MSc
Friedman School of Nutrition Science & Policy
Tufts University
Boston, Massachusetts, USA

Ronette R. Briefel, DrPH, RD
Research Department
Mathematica Policy Research, Inc.
Washington, DC, USA

Mona S. Calvo, PhD
US Food and Drug Administration
Washington, DC, USA

Wayne W. Campbell, PhD
Department of Foods and Nutrition
Purdue University
West Lafayette, Indiana, USA

Gabriela Camporeale, PhD
Department of Nutrition and Health Sciences
University of Nebraska
Lincoln, Nebraska, USA

Robert Carter III, MD
Departments of Medicine and Microbiology
University of Alabama
Birmingham, Alabama, USA

Samuel N. Cheuvront, PhD
Thermal and Mountain Medicine Division
US Army Research Institute of Environmental Medicine
Natick, Massachusetts, USA

Paul M. Coates, PhD
Office of Dietary Supplements
National Institutes of Health
Bethesda, Maryland, USA

Robert J. Cousins, PhD
Department of Food Sciences and Human Nutrition
Center for Nutrition Sciences
University of Florida
Gainesville, Florida, USA

Sai Krupa Das, PhD
Jean Mayer USDA Human Nutrition
Research Center on Aging
Tufts University
Boston, Massachusetts, USA

Bess Dawson-Hughes, MD
Calcium and Bone Metabolism Laboratory
Jean Mayer USDA Human Nutrition
Research Center on Aging
Tufts University
Boston, Massachusetts, USA

Adam Drewnowski, PhD
Nutritional Sciences Prorgram
School of Public Health and Community Medicine
University of Washington
Seattle, Washington, USA

John W. Erdman, Jr., PhD
Department of Food Science
University of Illinois
Urbana, Illinois, USA

Guylaine Ferland, PhD
Centre de Recherche
Institut Universitaire de Géariatrie de Montréal
Montreal, Quebec, Canada

Edward A. Frongillo, Jr., PhD
Division of Nutritional Sciences
Cornell University
Ithaca, New York, USA

Daniel D. Gallaher, PhD
Department of Food Science and Nutrition
University of Minnesota
St. Paul, Minnesota, USA

Sanford C. Garner, PhD
Constella Group, Inc.
Durham, North Carolina, USA

Peter J. Gillies, PhD, FAHA
DuPont Central Research and Development and
Department of Nutrition Science
The Pennsylvania State University
University Park, Pennsylvania, USA

Amy Gorin, PhD
Department of Psychiatry and Human Behavior
Brown Medical School
Providence, Rhode Island, USA

Jesse F. Gregory III, PhD
Department of Food Science and Human Nutrition
University of Florida
Gainesville, Florida, USA

Olivier Guérin, MD
Service de Gériatrie
Hôpitaux de Nice
Nice, France

Sung Nim Han, PhD
Jean Mayer USDA Human Nutrition
Research Center on Aging
Tufts University
Boston, Massachusetts, USA

James M. Harnly, PhD
Food Composition Laboratory
Beltsville Human Nutrition Research Center
Agricultural Research Service
US Department of Agriculture
Beltsville, Maryland, USA

Susan L. Hefle, PhD
Department of Food Science and Technology
University of Nebraska
Lincoln, Nebraska, USA

William C. Heird, MD
Department of Pediatrics
Baylor College of Medicine
Houston, Texas, USA

Helen L. Henry, PhD
Department of Biochemistry
University of California, Riverside
Riverside, California, USA

Daniell B. Hill, MD
Department of Internal Medicine
University of Louisville
Louisville, Kentucky, USA

Joanne M. Holden, MS, RD
Nutrient Data Laboratory
Beltsville Human Nutrition Research Center
Agricultural Research Service
US Department of Agriculture
Beltsville, Maryland, USA

Robert A. Jacob, PhD, FACN
Grand Forks Human Nutrition Research Center
Agricultural Research Service
US Department of Agriculture
Grand Forks, North Dakota, USA

Carol S. Johnston, PhD
Department of Nutrition
Arizona State University East
Mesa, Arizona, USA

Peter J.H. Jones, PhD
School of Dietetics and Human Nutrition
Macdonald Campus of McGill University
Ste-Anne-de-Bellevue, Quebec, Canada

Heather I. Katcher,
Department of Nutrition Science
The Pennsylvania State University
University Park, Pennsylvania, USA

Young-In Kim, MD, FRCP(C)
Departments of Medicine and Nutritional Sciences
University of Toronto
Toronto, Ontario, Canada

Philip J. Klemmer, MD
School of Medicine
University of North Carolina
Durham, North Carolina, USA

Penny M. Kris-Etherton, PhD
Department of Nutrition
Pennsylvania State University
University Park, Pennsylvania, USA

Alice H. Lichtenstein, DSc
Cardiovascular Nutrition Research Program
Jean Mayer USDA Human Nutrition
Research Center on Aging
Tufts University
Boston, Massachusetts, USA

Brian L. Lindshield, BS
Division of Nutritional Sciences
University of Illinois
Urbana, Illinois, USA

Joanne R. Lupton, PhD
Department of Nutrition and Food Science
Texas A & M University
College Station, Texas, USA

Luis Marsano, MD
Department of Internal Medicine
University of Louisville
Louisville, Kentucky, USA

Reynaldo Martorell, PhD
Robert W. Woodruff Health Sciences Center
Emory University
Atlanta, Georgia, USA

Tahsin Masud, MD
Renal Division
Emory University School of Medicine
Atlanta, Georgia, USA

Craig J. McClain, MD
Department of Internal Medicine
University of Louisville
Louisville, Kentucky, USA

Donald B. McCormick, PhD
Department of Biochemistry
Emory University
Atlanta, Georgia, USA

Megan A. McCrory, PhD
School of Nutrition and Exercise Science
Bastyr University
Kenmore, Washington, USA

Heather McGuire, MD
Department of Nephrology
Billings Clinic
Billings, Montana, USA

Catherine McIsaac, MS, RD
Medical Center
University of Vermont
Burlington, Vermont, USA

Alfred H. Merrill, Jr., PhD
School of Biology
Georgia Institute of Technology
Atlanta, Georgia, USA

Simin Nikbin Meydani, DVM, PhD
Department of Pathology and Sackler
Graduate School of Biomedical Sciences
Jean Mayer USDA Human Nutrition
Research Center on Aging
Tufts University
Boston, Massachusetts, USA

Paul E. Milbury, MS, CFII
Antioxidants Research Laboratory
Jean Mayer USDA Human Nutrition
Research Center on Aging
Tufts University
Boston, Massachusetts, USA

Joshua W. Miller, PhD
Department of Medical Pathology
University of California
Davis, California, USA

John A. Milner, PhD
Nutrition Science Research Group
National Cancer Institute
National Institutes of Health
Rockville, Maryland, USA

William E. Mitch, MD
Renal Division
Emory University School of Medicine
Atlanta, Georgia, USA

Pablo Monsivais, PhD
Nutritional Sciences Program
School of Public Health and Community Medicine and
Dental Public Health Sciences
School of Dentistry
University of Washington
Seattle, Washington, USA

Scott J. Montain, PhD
Military Nutrition Division
US Army Research Institute of Environmental Medicine
Natick, Massachusetts, USA

Suzanne P. Murphy, PhD
Cancer Research Center
University of Hawaii
Honolulu, Hawaii, USA

Marguerite A. Neill, MD
Division of Infectious Diseases
Brown University Medical School
Memorial Hospital of Rhode Island
Pawtucket, Rhode Island, USA

Forrest H. Nielsen, PhD
Grand Forks Human Nutrition Research Center
Agricultural Research Service
US Department of Agriculture
Grand Forks, North Dakota, USA

Chizuru Nishida, PhD
Department of Nutrition for Health and Development
World Health Organization
Geneva, Switzerland

Anthony W. Norman, PhD
Department of Biochemistry
University of California, Riverside
Riverside, California, USA

Marga C. Ocké, PhD
Department of Chronic Diseases Epidemiology
National Institute for Public Health
and the Environment
Bilthoven, The Netherlands

Christine M. Olson, PhD
Division of Nutritional Sciences
Cornell University
Ithaca, New York, USA

Andrea A. Papamandjaris, PhD
Regulatory and Scientific Affairs
Nestlé, Inc.
North York, Ontario, Canada

David L. Pelletier, PhD
Division of Nutritional Sciences
Cornell University
Ithaca, New York, USA

Paul B. Pencharz, MD, PhD
Division of Gastroenterology/Nutrition
Hospital for Sick Children
Toronto, Ontario, Canada

Harry G. Preuss, MD
Division of Nephrology and Hypertension
Georgetown University Medical Center
Washington, DC, USA

Joseph R. Prohaska, PhD
Department of Biochemistry and Molecular Biology
University of Minnesota
Duluth, Minnesota, USA

Charles J. Rebouche, PhD
Department of Pediatrics
University of Iowa
Coralville, Iowa, USA

Patrick Ritz, MD
Service de Nutrition
Centre Hospitalier Universitaire
Angers, France

Richard S. Rivlin, MD
The American Health Foundation
New York, New York, USA

Susan B. Roberts, PhD
Jean Mayer USDA Human Nutrition
Research Center on Aging
Tufts University
Boston, Massachusetts, USA

Lisa M. Rogers, PhD
Department of Nutrition
University of California
Davis, California, USA

Robert B. Rucker, PhD
Department of Nutrition
University of California
Davis, California, USA

Edward Saltzman, MD
Jean Mayer USDA Human Nutrition
Research Center on Aging
Tufts University
Boston, Massachusetts, USA

Lisa M. Sanders, PhD
University of North Carolina
Chapel Hill, North Carolina, USA

Charles R. Santerre, PhD
Department of Foods and Nutrition
Purdue University
West Lafayette, Indiana, USA

Michael N. Sawka, PhD
Thermal and Mountain Medicine Division
US Army Research Institute of Environmental Medicine
Natick, Massachusetts, USA

Eva M. Schmelz, PhD
Department of Nutrition and Food Sciences and
Karmanos Cancer Institute
Wayne State University
Detroit, Michigan, USA

Stéphane Schneider, MD
Archet University Hospital
Nice, France

Anuraj H. Shankar, MD
Helen Keller International/Indonesia
Jakarta, Indonesia

Noel W. Solomons, MD
Center for Studies of Sensory Impairment,
Aging and Metabolism (CeSSIAM)
Guatemala City, Guatemala

Sally P. Stabler, MD
Department of Medicine
University of Colorado Health Sciences Center
Denver, Colorado, USA

Virginia A. Stallings, MD
Division of Gastroenterology and Nutrition
Children's Hospital of Philadelphia
Philadelphia, Pennsylvania, USA

Aryeh D. Stein, MPH, PhD
Rollins School of Public Health
Emory University
Atlanta, Georgia, USA

Barbara J. Stoecker, PhD
Department of Nutritional Sciences
Oklahoma State University
Stillwater, Oklahoma, USA

Roger A. Sunde, PhD
Department of Nutritional Sciences
University of Wisconsin
Madison, Wisconsin, USA

Paolo M. Suter, MD
Department of Internal Medicine
Medical Policlinic/University Hospital
Zurich, Switzerland

Deborah Tate, PhD
Department of Psychiatry and Human Behavior
Brown Medical School
Providence, Rhode Island, USA

Robert V. Tauxe, MD, MPH
Centers for Disease Control and Prevention
Atlanta, Georgia , USA

Christine L. Taylor, PhD
Science and Health Coordination
Food & Drug Administration
Rockville, Maryland, USA

Steve L. Taylor, PhD
Department of Food Science and Technology
University of Nebraska
Lincoln, Nebraska, USA

Howard C. Towle, PhD
Department of Biochemistry, Molecular Biology, and Biophysics
University of Minnesota
Minneapolis, Minnesota, USA

Maret G. Traber, PhD
Department of Nutrition and Food Management
Linus Pauling Institute
Oregon State University
Corvallis, Oregon, USA

Wija A. Van Staveren, PhD
Division of Human Nutrition and Epidemiology
Wageningen University
Wageningen, The Netherlands

Bruno J. Vellas, MD, PhD
Department of Internal Medicine and Gerontology
Centre Hospitalier Universitaire
Toulouse, France

Frank Vinicor, MD, MPH
Division of Diabetes Translation
Centers for Disease Control and Prevention
Atlanta, Georgia, USA

Stella Lucia Volpe, PhD
School of Nursing
University of Pennsylvania
Philadelphia, Pennsylvania, USA

May Dongmei Wang, PhD
The Wallace H. Coulter Department of Biomedical Engineering and The Petit Institute of Bioengineering and Bioscience
Georgia Institute of Technology
Atlanta, Georgia, USA

Mary Lee Sell Watts, MPH, RD
Legislative and Political Affairs
American Dietetic Association
Washington, DC, USA

Connie M. Weaver, PhD
Department of Foods and Nutrition
Purdue University
West Lafayette, Indiana, USA

Robert C. Weisell, PhD
Nutrition and Consumer Protection Division
Food and Agriculture Organization of the United Nations
Rome, Italy

Jonathan Wells, PhD
Lawrence Berkeley National Laboratory
Berkeley, Kitsap, California, USA

Rena R. Wing, PhD
Department of Psychiatry and Human Behavior
Brown Medical School
Providence, Rhode Island, USA

Judith Wylie-Rosett, EdD, RD
Department of Epidemiology and Social Medicine
Albert Einstein College of Medicine
Bronx, New York, USA

Helen Young, PhD
Famine Center
Friedman School of Nutrition Science & Policy
Tufts University
Medford/Somerville, Massachusetts, USA

Vernon R. Young, PhD, DSc
Laboratory of Human Nutrition
Massachusetts Institute of Technology
Cambridge, Massachusetts, USA

Steven H. Zeisel, MD, PhD
Department of Nutrition
University of North Carolina
Chapel Hill, North Carolina, USA

Janos Zempleni, PhD
Department of Nutritional Science and Dietetics
University of Nebraska
Lincoln, Nebraska, USA

Michael B. Zimmermann, MD, MSc
Laboratory for Human Nutrition
Swiss Federal Institute of Technology
Zurich, Switzerland

# I Systems Biology

# 1

# Genomics, Proteomics, Metabolomics and Systems Biology Approaches to Nutrition

Eva M. Schmelz, May Dongmei Wang, and Alfred H. Merrill, Jr.

## Introduction

Genomics (genes and expressed mRNAs), proteomics (proteins, including post-translational modifications), metabolomics (metabolites), and other "-omics" (Table 1) are new and still-evolving technologies for the acquisition of qualitative and quantitative information about all of the components of their respective subjects or at least a functional subset (e.g., all lipids for lipidomics). The rationale behind "-omics" analysis is that biological systems are so complex that limiting one's view only to a few components in isolation from a "big picture" that includes all levels of regulation (Figure 1) can lead to incorrect conclusions. With respect to nutrition, the Long Range Planning Committee of the American Society for Nutrition,[1] as well as other scientists and clinicians, have challenged nutritionists to use these new technologies to develop "individualized nutrition recommendations" because "the genetic and phenotypic variation among humans is so wide that a diet that may be optimal for one individual could predispose another to disease." The goal is to identify the "nutrition phenotype," which is a "defined and integrated set of genetic, proteomic, metabolomic, functional, and behavioral factors that, when measured, form the basis for assessment of human nutritional status."[2]

The basic requirements for "omic-" technologies are summarized in Table 2. In looking at the list, one is reminded of the common retort of analytical chemists that: "Yes, I can analyze your samples quickly, accurately, and at relatively low cost; however, at most, I can provide only two of these at the same time." These conditions are regularly encountered in genomic studies in which scientists can analyze the relative expression of thousands of genes using micro-arrays, but the methodologies are ineffective in detecting subtle changes and miss transcripts that are present in low amounts (and is often costly); therefore, individual genes of interest are still analyzed by more laborious (but sensitive and accurate) techniques such as quantitative real-time polymerase chain reaction (QRT-PCR). In addition, once the analyses have been done, handling of the very large data sets requires sophisticated bioinformatics and visualization methods to integrate and interpret the results. The combination of "-omics" technologies with bioinformatic tools for analysis and interpretation of the results for a given biologic system is often described as a "systems biology" approach.[3]

In a nutshell, systems biology seeks to understand how all of the pertinent components of a biologic system interact functionally over time and under varying conditions. The definition of a "system" is quite flexible,[3,4] and can be a family of interacting molecules such as a metabolic pathway or other functional unit (e.g., a ribosome or an organelle), cells, organs, individuals, communities, and

**Table 1.** Examples of "-omics" Technologies*

| Name (Specialization Prefix)† | What is Analyzed/Types of Applications |
|---|---|
| Genomics | |
| Nutrigenomics | Genes and expressed mRNAs in the context of nutrition |
| Pharmacogenomics | Genes and expressed mRNAs in the context of pharmacology |
| Toxicogenomics | Genes and expressed mRNAs in the context of toxicology |
| Chemical genomics | Use of small molecule compounds to study biologic function and therapeutic potential of small molecules |
| Structural genomics | Prediction of protein structure from gene homologies |
| Functional genomics | Combined approaches to link physiological functions and genomic sequence information |
| Transcriptomics | Transcription factors/gene regulation |
| Proteomics | Proteins (including post-translational modifications) |
| Interactomics | Protein-protein interactions; pathway networks |
| Toponomics | Topological position of proteins in the cell |
| Glycomics | Glycoconjugates (glycoproteins, glycolipids) |
| Metabolomics | Metabolites (all categories or subsets, such as lipidomics) |
| Fluxomics | Metabolite flux through complex pathways |
| Cytomics | Structural and functional studies of cells and cellular systems |
| Physiomics | Structural and functional studies or complex organisms |
| Populomics | Genetic and phenotypic diversity of human populations; how they interact with the environment, and how their behavior influences health and disease patterns |
| Nutridynamics | How food components are affected by the food matrix itself and what they do in the body |
| [Economics] | Not a biological omic field, but one that will need to be integrated with the other omics for systems approaches |

* This listing is not meant to include all "-omics" fields; furthermore, these definitions are not necessarily the ones used by all scientists.

† Each of the main categories in this list can theoretically be subdivided into the subspecialties listed under genomics; for example, nutrimetabolomics.

even ecosystems. The scope of the system for nutrition is immense because each person is actually a complex ecosystem of their own tissues plus associated intestinal microorganisms, and food is complex and variable in nutrient composition and bioavailability; therefore, the number of parameters is huge. Indeed, nutritionists were cognizant of the need for comprehensive approaches long before the term "systems biology" was coined, because nutritional requirements are not fixed quantities but are affected by genetics and epigenetic programming, age, physical activity and other behaviors, plus numerous (patho)physiologic and environmental factors, including the intake of other categories of nutrients.

The oft-stated promise of systems biology is that it will eventually improve "all aspects of health care, including the detection and monitoring of diseases, drug discovery, treatment evaluation, and ultimately, predictive and preventative medicine."[4] Nonetheless, systems biology is still in its infancy and, despite the tremendous power of the technologies already available, no one knows how long it will take to learn enough about the human system to predict and prevent disease that arises from multiple causes. This does not argue against starting the long journey now, because even if it takes decades to implement a comprehensive, individualized system, there will be early payoffs in the identification of new biomarkers for disease and a better understanding of disease risk factors of relevance to nutrition. Therefore, this chapter describes "-omics" technologies from the perspective of a nutritionist who wishes to build a conceptual framework to understand how systems biology approaches are evolving and changing our field.[5,6]

## Genomics

Genomics is the study of all genes, including structural genes, regulatory sequences, and noncoding DNA segments, and their expression (i.e., mRNAs) in the organism(s) of interest under the condition(s) of interest. Genomics has spawned additional gene-based "-omics,"

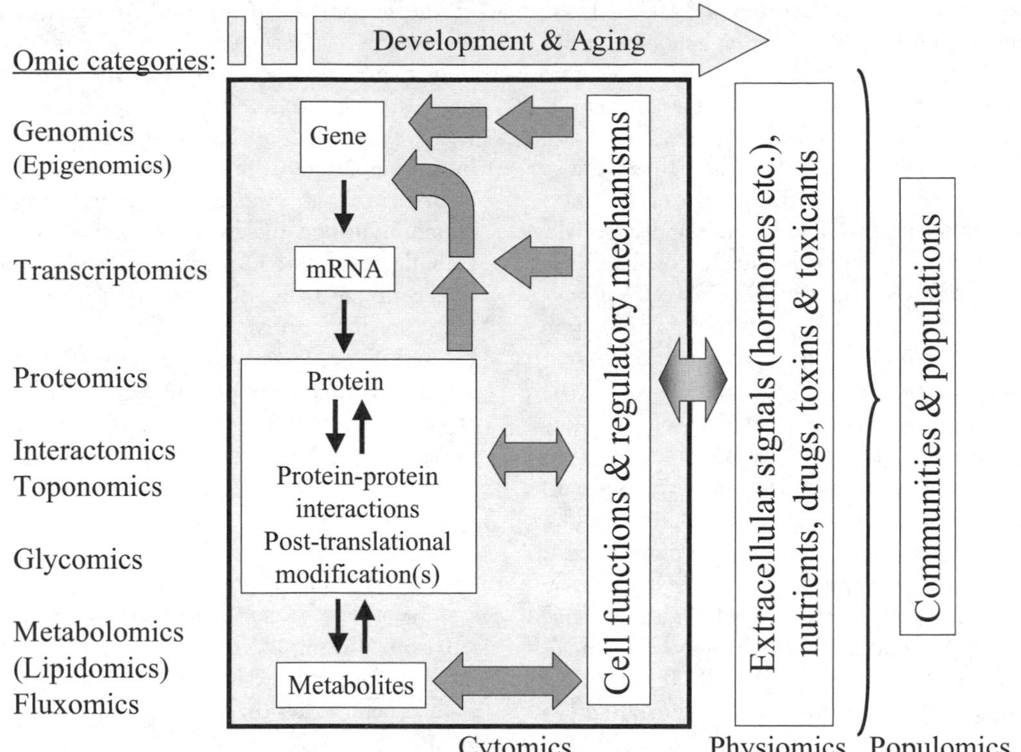


Figure 1. Summary of some of the central dogma of underlying components of biological systems and the concept that they are regulated by both intrinsic factors (the starting genome) and extrinsic factors (from cell-cell communication to nutrients, etc.). Only a few of the interaction arrows are shown, but these already illustrate the complexities that necessitate "-omics" and systems approaches.

some of which define basic cell regulatory mechanisms (transcriptomics, the complete set of RNA transcripts produced by the genome at any one time) and others that relate genomics to other scientific disciplines, such as toxicogenomics and nutrigenomics (nutritional genomics), which refers to the application of genomic approaches to nutrition to determine how genetic variation affects the utilization of single nutrients or whole foods, and how nutrients (individually or in groups) affect gene expression.[5-12]

**Table 2.** What Does One Expect to Get from "-omics" Technologies?

- Information about entire families of molecules, or at least subsets
- A high degree of certainty about the identity of the components
- Quantitative information (at least differences and changes)
- The ability to get information relatively easily and quickly
- The ability to get the information in a format that is readily used
- Availability of tools to facilitate utilization of the information
- Cross platform (genomics ⟷ proteomics ⟷ metabolomics, etc.)

The goal of nutritional genomics is to understand how diet influences the balance between health and disease during the life span of an organism and its changing needs, such as for maintenance, growth, maturation, pregnancy, aging, stress, and disease. It is an underlying assumption that an understanding of these mechanisms will lead to better—even individualized—dietary recommendations for disease prevention and management of chronic disease (with fewer adverse side effects). This may be a rather straightforward process in inherited monogenic diseases (i.e., those caused by alterations in a single gene that is transmitted through families in readily recognizable patterns), but will be more difficult in diseases such as cancer, type 2 diabetes, and other chronic diseases. This is because the latter are often multistep processes that involve genetic mutations that may be inherited or arise spontaneously in only some cells during the lifetime and (or) may involve defects in the control or function (due to genetic mutation or environmental factors) of one or more stage-specific genes. Furthermore, the gene changes may be nuclear or mitochondrial, with the latter genome being the most labile over time and implicated in many degenerative diseases and the extension of the life span by calorie restriction.[13]

## *The Human Genome and Genomic Technologies*

The human genome contains approximately 2.9 billion nucleotides that code for a still unknown number of genes, but estimated to be on the order of 30,000.[5] There is tremendous sequence variation in the genome, known as genetic polymorphisms, and these can arise from changes in a single nucleotide (called single nucleotide polymorphism, or SNP), sequence repeats, insertions, deletions, and recombination. When the polymorphism results in a functional difference in the gene of that individual versus others in the population—and especially when this results in disease—it is usually called a mutation. Changes in DNA sequence that have been confirmed to be caused by external agents such as irradiation or carcinogens are also generally called mutations rather than polymorphisms.

SNPs are the most common category of polymorphism, and occur as transition substitutions between purines (A, G) or pyrimidines (C, T) (the most common) and transversion substitutions (between a purine and a pyrimidine). Comparison of equivalent chromosomes in two individuals will reveal approximately one base difference per 1300 base pairs,[14] most of which are in noncoding regions of the genome (approximately two-thirds), where they have little or no known effect. SNPs in coding regions of the genome are about equally distributed between "silent" mutations (called synonymous codon changes), in which the substitution causes no amino acid change in the protein it codes for, and non-synonymous codon changes, in which the substitution alters the encoded amino acid (called a missense mutation) or results in premature termination of the protein (called a nonsense mutation).

Although the genotype of an individual describes his or her genetic composition with respect to a specific trait (phenotype), investigators are also collecting information about the haplotype (which involves grouping of genetic patterns found on each chromosome) because it can provide additional insight into patterns of genetic variations that contribute to human disease. Initiatives such as the International Haplotype Map Project (HapMap)[15] are using high-throughput genotyping techniques to perform genome-wide determinations of SNPs to identify and catalog genetic similarities and differences. Haplotype analysis is also very useful for identifying genetic recombinations.

Another approach is the mapping of mechanism-based candidate genes, which are specific target genes or entire known signaling pathways for which there is already a rationale for a disease link. The smaller scale of this approach makes it more practical given the large numbers of SNPs that can be found in even a small subset of the genome, and mindful of the risk that limited knowledge of disease etiology might result in investigations that may be too narrow in scope to clearly identify risk patterns. For both types of approaches, the expectation is that the identification of a large number of SNPs in the human genome will allow an association analysis of these loci with disease and complex environmental interactions using (still-evolving) mathematical models. To complicate matters further, new features of gene regulation continue to be discovered, such as polynucleotides with unconventional bases or unusual features (e.g., micro-RNAs), epigenetic control mechanisms, and new splice variations for supposedly understood genes. All in all, it will be a challenge for nutrigenomics to deal with these plus the large number of additional variables that will be imposed when nutrition is added into the equation.

## *Genomic Technologies*

Changes in the genomic sequence have classically been determined using DNA sequencing techniques, which is rapidly being replaced by higher-throughput technologies such as gene arrays that allow for the systemic analysis of variations in DNA and RNA sequence and amounts. Other assays include real-time PCR, restriction fragment length polymorphism analysis, single-strand conformation polymorphism analysis, allele-specific oligonucleotide hybridization, oligonucleotide ligation assay, and many more using radioactive, fluorescent, chemiluminescent, or enzymatic detection or by analysis of charge, size, or mass. The development of rapid detection systems for gene expression allows the evaluation of how nutrients affect the expression of a specific gene, a family of genes, complete signaling pathways, or tens of thousands of genes via DNA micro-arrays or a powerful technology called serial analysis of gene expression (SAGE). Due to the widespread use of these technologies, it is reasonable to expect that they will continue to evolve to overcome problems and limitations and reduce costs through the use of automation (e.g., robots and workstations), minimization of samples and reagents, and multiplex analysis. On the horizon are nanotechnologies (with "nano" referring to any molecular device that has a size less than 100 nm) that will enable in situ–and eventually in vivo—identification of gene polymorphisms and expression in living organisms.[16]

The results from genomic analyses are often depicted as shown in Figure 2. The upper panel shows a tabular format that is often used to show relative changes in the

Figure 2. Examples of how complex "-omics" data are displayed. The relative amounts (or change) in a component is often shown as a "hot" diagram, where the lowest amounts of a component (or -fold decrease relative to a control or other group) are shown in "cool" blue and the highest amounts (or fold increase) are shown in "hot" red, as shown in panel A. As this panel also shows, data are sometimes clustered by the type of components (genes, proteins, metabolites, or whatever species is of interest) with linkages between species depicted by interconnecting lines (as shown to the left). Panel B illustrates how data are also expressed by pathwaydiagrams (in this case, related to a KEGG pathway) (From Arakawa et al., 2005.[83]); sometimes the pathways are reorganized to reflect a biologicalfunction, as shown in panel C for inflammatory mediators in blood or lymph versus epithelial tissue (Used with permission from Lu et al., 2006.[38]). *(continues)*

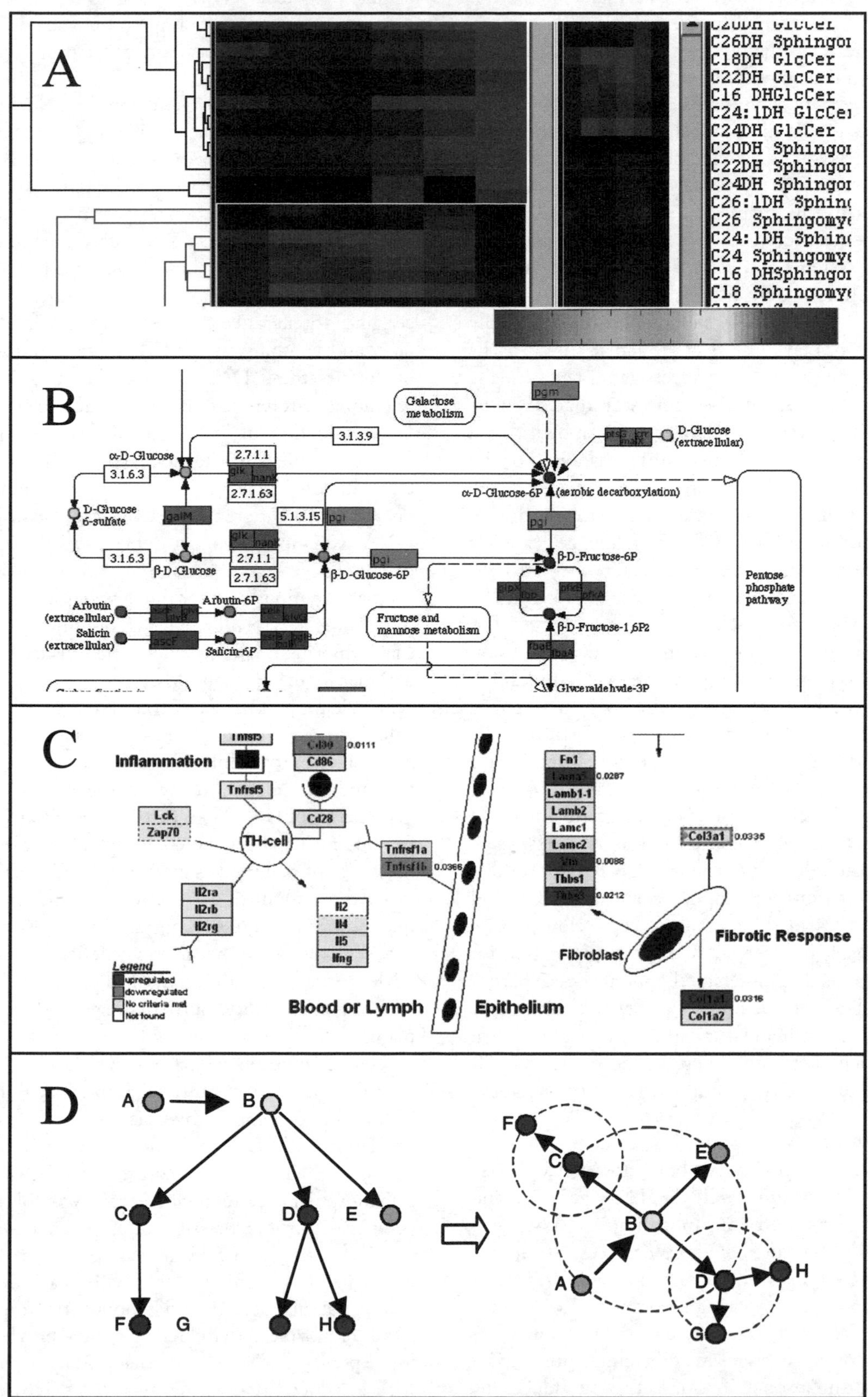


Figure 2. *(continued)* Panel D illustrates two ways to display metabolic pathway data, by nodes that represent individual metabolites and connecting lines that represent the enzyme responsible for their interconversion; a conventional pathway layout is shown on the left, and the same steps are shown on the right as in a "focus+context" format, which allows the user to highlight the specific compound of interest (compound "B" in this diagram), which results in rotation of the diagram to display that species more prominently to show the formation or removal of that species.

components of interest (with species that increase depicted in "hot" red), which is then clustered by criteria selected by the investigator, such as genes that change similarly over a time course. Because this format is difficult to interpret when hundreds or thousands of genes change, the results are often visualized by other methods, such as the overlays with cellular metabolic and regulatory pathways, as shown in Figure 2, panels B and C (and discussed later in this chapter).

Critical to the success of these analyses is the right choice of cell systems and careful control of the experimental conditions. Cell lines that are immortalized or transformed—whether spontaneously or virally induced—may or may not reflect the actual genetic background of the condition under investigation, and usually do not respond in exactly the same way that cell type would in a whole organism. The results can be affected significantly by subtle differences in the handling of the cells between different laboratories (and even within the same laboratory) due to small differences in the way investigators prepare the culture media, how long cells are left at room temperature and atmosphere, and other hard-to-control factors such as position of the Petri dish in the tissue culture incubator.

The complexity is obviously multiplied when using primary human tissues, not only with respect to the ability to obtain the desired cell type, but also to maintain a sufficient quantity and quality and to complete the process in a timely manner. A variety of primary cell types have been used to provide useful information in nutrition studies, such as hair follicle cells or exfoliated gastro-intestinal cells (including buccal cells), as well as many types of blood cells, although each of these clearly has very different biologic functions, development, and life spans, and therefore will present different gene expression profiles than other tissues of interest. A major complication for nutrition is the need to understand not only how a particular cell type behaves but how its behavior changes over the life span of the individual and under varying hormonal and environmental stimuli. There are no model systems that recapitulate all of these important *in vivo* variables.

## *Nutrigenomics*

Nutrigenomics encompasses both how nutrition affects gene expression and stability and how genetics (and epigenetics) affects nutrient utilization.[5-12] The consumption of food is an incredibly complex "stimulus," because food contains hundreds of nutrients and other bioactive compounds in varying amounts and with varying rates of uptake and clearance, plus the hormonal factors that they trigger, changes in body temperature, activity, and even the production of active substances by intestinal microflora. All of these factors can affect the short-term expression of genes that are directly or indirectly involved in health maintenance and disease, and have long-term effects on development when the presence or absence of a nutrient causes selective pressure for and against particular genotypes or activates a developmental progression or termination program. In addition, the diet can contain factors that damage or protect the stability of the genome itself.

**Nutrients Influence Gene Stability.** Nutrients are well known to affect genomic stability by regulating upstream events such as detoxification/inactivation of carcinogens or signaling events that eventually regulate gene expression. While the interactions between genotype and macronutrients have not been well established, micronutrient deficiency essentially mimics carcinogen- and radiation-induced DNA damage, thus contributing to aging, cancer, and degenerative diseases. Impaired intake of folate, zinc, and vitamins $B_{12}$ and $B_6$ induces transient single- or double-strand DNA breaks. Vitamins A, C, and E, selenium, carotenoids, lycopene, and others influence DNA oxidation at least in part due to their anti-oxidant function, while some nutrients such as iron can have one effect in deficiencies (in the case of iron, inducing DNA breaks) and a different effect (in the case of excess iron, DNA oxidation).[7] Niacin deficiency inhibits DNA repair.[17] The effects may or may not be reversible after supplementation of either the deficient nutrient alone or, often more successfully, with a combination of nutrients that exhibit additive or synergistic effects. For example, a higher intake of vitamin E, retinol, folic acid, nicotinic acid, calcium, and zinc, selenium, or epigallocatechin-3-gallate supplements has been seen to significantly increase genome stability, while a high intake of riboflavin, pantothenic acid, and biotin was associated with decreased genome stability.[18-20] To further complicate the picture, β-carotene has been noted to act in a dose-dependent manner: optimal intakes increased stability, while high or low intake had the opposite effect,[19] which illustrates how micronutrients can exhibit strict dose-dependent responses, and that either nutrient deficiency or excess can be deleterious. In addition to the direct or indirect regulation of gene stability, nutrients regulate DNA synthesis, maintenance, metabolism, and repair.

**Gene Mutations Affect Nutrient Utilization.** Genetic mutations also affect nutrient utilization. Polymorphism in the lactase-phlorizin hydrolase (LCH) gene alters the regulation of LCH and renders humans lactose tolerant throughout adulthood (in contrast to other mammals).[21] Polymorphisms in methylene-tetrahydrofolate reductase gene lead to the expression of an enzyme with reduced activity[22] and a two-fold increase of plasma homocysteine, which has been associated with heart disease, stroke and neural tube defects, and lymphocytic lymphoma. The reduced enzyme activity depletes the methyl-tetrahydrofolate pool, reduces DNA breaks, and has been associated with a reduced risk of colon cancer.[23] However, at low folate levels, this polymorphism may represent a risk factor, and higher requirements for folate intake in these circumstances have been reported.[24] A common polymorphism in manganese superoxide dismutase increases the susceptibility to oxidative stress and thereby may increase the requirement for vitamins C and E.[25] SNPs in the $O^6$-methylguanine DNA methyl-transferase (MGMT) modulate the inverse association of fruit and vegetable consumption or supplemental antioxidants and breast cancer risk in a site and haplotype-specific manner.[26]

**Nutrients Affect Gene Expression.** Reports on changes in the expression of individual genes by nutrients are too numerous to summarize here, and include instances in which the nutrient affects the gene of interest directly, by the nutrient affecting transcription, or indirectly, by nutrition affecting another regulator such as a hormone or even the nature of cell signaling machinery. From the perspective of genomics (or transcriptomics), what has been needed are annotated databases for the storage, management, and analysis of micro-array data in nutrition research (as well as for data-sharing among nutritional scientists via the Web). Saito et al.[27] have recently established a site at http://a-yo5.ch.a.u-tokyo.ac.jp/index.phtml to serve this purpose.

**Emerging Concepts in the Regulation of Gene Expression and Nutrigenomics.** Some emerging concepts about the mechanisms by which nutrients may regulate transcription are worth mentioning. First, the regulation of transcription by promoters and suppressors has become extremely complex when one considers that transcription initiation often involves the formation of multimeric "mediator" complexes that bind transcription control elements distributed across sometimes very large distances on the genome to coordinate input signals from the cell[28,29]; therefore, nutrigenomics will need to be complemented by nutritranscriptomics.

Also, many genes code for several protein isoforms that are produced by alternative splicing of the initially transcribed RNAs, and control of these occurs after transcription by modulation of the splicing machinery. If these factors are not taken into account in the design of probes to measure the mRNA of interest (e.g., if the capture nucleotides for a gene micro-array or primers for QRT-PCR do not distinguish alternative splice variants—which can sometimes vary in only a few amino acids in the final protein), this could compromise the utility of the data.

Furthermore, additional analytical tools will be needed to follow the expression and functioning of micro-RNAs (miRNAs), which are small, non-coding RNA molecules that post-transcriptionally regulate gene expression by base-pairing to mRNAs. Since the discovery a few years ago of the first miRNA gene in *Caenorhabditis elegans*, many miRNAs have been identified in multicellular organisms, and about 2% of the known human genes encode miRNAs.[30] Many miRNAs are evolutionarily conserved, and although the biological functions of most are unknown, miRNAs are essential for development and have been implicated in human disease, especially cancer.

A fourth, rapid developing area of interest is the role of nutrients in epigenetic control of genes—i.e., the regulation of gene activation and silencing via regulation of methylation of specific locations of the genome (CpG islands), a process that is potentially reversible but not usually used in normal cells to regulate gene expression. In eukaryotic cells, DNA is wrapped around core proteins (histones) with the histone N-terminal "tail" protruding from the complex, thus making it more susceptible to modification. Epigenetic gene silencing is a complex series of coordinated events that includes histone deacetylation, phosphorylation, methylation, or biotinylation, DNA hypermethylation of CpG-islands within gene promoter regions, recruitment of methyl-binding domain proteins, and other chromatin remodeling factors to suppress gene transcription. Potential targets of nutrients are therefore the enzymes that regulate DNA methylation: histone deacetylases (HDACs) that regulate the acetylation of the histone tail, DNA methyltransferases (Dnmt), kinases, or phosphatases, and enzymes that regulate histone phosphorylation, biotinylation, and methylation.

Individual patterns of CpG island methylation are maintained via Dnmt-1 activity and are highly dependent on the supply of methyl donors and cofactors via the diet (methionine, choline, folic acid, vitamin $B_{12}$, and pyridoxal phosphate[31]). Nutrient deficiencies (i.e., folate, methionine/choline, zinc, selenium, or folate) or excess of retinoic acid result in global DNA hypomethylation that is linked to increased chromosomal instability,[32] while specific genes are silenced via hypermethylation. This specific methylation pattern has also been observed in cancer cells and in aging tissue, changing cell proliferation and differentiation, predisposing the genome to further aberrant methylation, and, ultimately, increasing the cancer risk. Changes in DNA methylation can also be a result of altered Dnmt1 and demethylase activity. These enzymes are targeted by alcohol, cadmium, and nickel.[33] Supplying deficient nutrients to cells results in a restoration of the methylation status; however, maternal nutritional status modulates the fetal genome and gene expression via methylation, and this pattern may be retained throughout adulthood.[34] Maternal malnutrition may therefore lead to aberrant gene expression that could contribute to chronic disease in adults. Regulation of aberrant methylation and the reversal of altered gene expression by nutrients and other bioactive compounds in the diet would therefore be an effective disease prevention intervention.

Finally, while an ultimate goal of nutrigenomics (and the other nutri-omics) is to enable personalized dietary recommendations to minimize the deleterious consequences of aging and chronic disease, its value for some time may be to serve as a "discovery science"—that is, as a generator of new hypotheses about interrelationships between (and hence biomarkers for) diet and health. Indeed, genomic research in general has shown that while many basic structural and regulatory mechanisms have been conserved throughout evolution, they have become increasingly complex with respect to cross-talk, complementarity, and redundancy to improve the likelihood of survival (through the reproductive years) during times of environmental change and stress. Thus, dietary factors that are beneficial (or damaging) are unlikely to affect only one target (or if they do, it will be one that has a ripple effect into additional cell regulatory pathways), as has been seen, for example, in studies of:

- Long-term supplementation of the diet with vitamin E, which caused changes in an antioxidant network (down-regulation of coagulation factor IX, 5-a-steroid reductase type 1, and CD36 in rat liver, while hepatic γ-glutamyl-cysteinyl synthetase was significantly upregulated[35]), rather than only one biochemical target;
- Suppression of colon carcinogenesis by dietary sphingolipids, which induce nuclear efflux and degradation of β-catenin in mice with mutations in the APC gene (which participates in β-catenin turnover); however, micro-array analyses have revealed that sphingolipids also reduce expression of the nuclear binding partner for β-catenin, TCF4, a transcription factor that favors proliferation[36]; and
- The effect of green tea polyphenols on a wide spectrum of genes involved in nuclear and cytoplasmic transport, transformation, redox signaling, response to hypoxia, and metabolism of polycyclic aromatic hydrocarbons,[37] as well as cell cycle control and immune regulation.[38]

Likewise, if optimal benefits accrue from perhaps subtle effects on multiple targets, then foods may be associated with disease risk due to their content of an ensemble of compounds rather than an individual species. Synergy among many bioactive compounds in food may help to explain why the effective dosages for individual compounds when tested individually in model systems (cells in culture) are often higher than their concentrations in vivo.[39]

These examples illustrate the complexity of the interactions of the genome with variables in its environment—from nutrients to toxic compounds. Much is being learned, but this still gives only a partial picture because many of these factors can alter cell behavior without affecting the genome; therefore, additional technologies such as proteomics are becoming recognized as critical complements to genomic analyses.

# Proteomics

Proteomics is the characterization of all proteins in all of their forms, including post-translational modifications (for glycoproteins, this is called glycomics), protein-protein interactions (interactomics) and, in some definitions, subcellular localization (sometimes referred to as toponomics) in the organism(s) of interest under the condition(s) of interest. This information is an important partner for genomics, which only reveals what genes are present in an organism and the amounts of each mRNA, which may or may not define the amount and activity of the resulting protein. The complexity of the post-translational modifications has only begun to be addressed, because the numbers of combinations and permutations can be enormous. For example, if one considers the possibilities for a transmembrane protein, it might undergo: glycosylation; phosphorylation on multiple amino acids; covalent attachment of other peptides and/or non-covalent association with other proteins; and association with coenzymes and cofactors (including some that are covalently attached such as biotin) and with lipids via covalent (e.g., with fatty acids, isoprenes, and phosphatidylinositolglycan) and non-covalent (e.g., phospholipids, cholesterol and/or sphingolipids) interactions, the latter of which can have different degrees of structural selectivity. As already noted, some of these molecular features are so complex that they are "-omics" field themselves (e.g., glycomics and lipidomics).

## *Proteomic Technologies*

Because proteins have been studied for a long time using biochemical and immunochemical methods, there are several ways that investigators have approached proteomics, and these have been covered in several excellent reviews.[40-42]

**Mass Spectrometry.** Mass spectrometry (MS) is an especially powerful methodology for protein analysis because it is highly structure specific and sensitive, and can analyze compounds in mixtures under the appropriate conditions. Several types of MS have been applied to proteomics, but the ones most frequently used are:

- Electrospray ionization (ESI-MS), in which the compounds of interest are dissolved in solvents of choice and then sprayed into the ionization chamber of the mass spectrometer through a positively or negatively charged needle so that as the solvent evaporates (usually under vacuum), the suspended compounds retain the charge;
- Matrix-assisted laser dissociation ionization (MALDI), in which the compounds are mixed with a so-called matrix material (a compound that can be excited by laser light to ionize and transfer a charge to the analyte), dried onto a sample plate, and then illuminated with a laser to vaporize the matrix compounds and generate the charged analyte(s);
- Surface-enhanced laser desorption/ionization (SELDI) (a form of secondary ion MS, or SIMS) in which the sample is placed on a surface that is bombarded with a stream of ions to eject particles (including the biological compounds of interest) that can also be ionized. In SELDI, the proteins of interest are trapped on the surface of chips using common biochemical features of proteins (charge, hydrophobicity, recognition by antibodies, etc.); and
- Other SIMS approaches such as DIOS (direct ionization on silica) and use of new types of ion beams (such as a bismuth cluster ion source), which even

allow for direct imaging of the ions in biological samples.[43]

Once the proteins or polypeptides are ionized, they are separated using several different types of mass analyzers: a) quadrupole instruments use alternating radio frequency and DC voltage to allow only those ions with the selected mass to charge (*m/z*) to pass through the analyzer toward the next section of the instrument; b) time-of-flight (TOF) instruments in which ions are pulsed into the mass analyzer (for example, by the puff of ions from a laser burst in MALDI), and therefore reach the next section (or detector) based on their *m/z*; c) ion traps in which the ions are held in a field until the investigator wishes to release them; and d) fourier transform-ion cyclotron resonance-MS (FTMS), in which the ions are essentially trapped in the center of a field of a superconducting magnet and excited by ion cyclotron radiation. FTMS has high sensitivity and mass accuracy, but is also very expensive.

Some of these analyzers can provide information about intact proteins (which is often called "top-down" protein MS), but this may not be sufficient for identification if the protein is large or in a complex mixture. In most cases today, the proteins are enzymatically hydrolyzed to peptides that can be tentatively identified by comparison of the observed *m/z* with computer databases for known polypeptides with those characteristics, followed by a more definitive analysis of the sequence by tandem MS (described below).

In tandem MS (MS/MS), the ions are first selected in the initial mass analyzer (usually a quadrupole or TOF) and the selected "precursor" ions then enter a second field region, where they are induced to fragment (for example, by collision with a gas such as nitrogen), followed by analysis of the fragments (called the "product" ions) by another mass analyzer. Thus, a triple quadrupole mass spectrometer uses the first quadrupole to separate the precursor ions, the second for fragmentation, and the third to separate the product ions. Ion traps use a quadrupole or cyclical magnetic field to hold the ions of interest, and as they are held (or released), can be induced to fragment one or more times, thereby increasing sensitivity and allowing multiple rounds of analysis—such as MS/MS/MS (abbreviated $MS^3$) and higher ($MS^n$).

Tandem MS (MS/MS and $MS^n$) provides a high level of confidence in the identification of the compound because few compounds have identical precursor and product ions; however, in complex mixtures this possibility must be excluded. For protein sequencing, these precursor-product pairs correspond to the known *m/z* for particular amino acid sequences, and therefore they can be readily identified using free or proprietary software that also associates them with the peptide patterns of all known proteins. When there are a statistically significant number of peptides that would be produced from a given protein, the software identifies the protein that was the source of these peptides (multiple hits are usually needed because several proteins may share a common polypeptide sequence, especially if they are functionally related). The software can also identify some of the possible modifications such as acetylation at the N-terminus, methylation (which illustrates the potential for confusion because trimethylation of lysine adds the same mass as N-acetylation), phosphorylation at the serine, threonine, and tyrosine residues, and oxidation of methionine, among others. However, when post-translational modifications are analyzed using fragments of the protein produced by enzymatic hydrolysis, it is usually difficult to determine how many of the modifications are found on an individual protein molecule versus being distributed over several molecules (e.g., if the protein has two phosphorylation sites and half of the respective peptides are phosphorylated, does this mean that half of the proteins were phosphate free and the other half had both phosphorylations, or are there other combinations?). This information is more readily produced by "top-down" MS.[44]

In many cases, the samples must be processed prior to MS to enrich the proteins of interest because it is common in MS for the spectra to be dominated by a few high-abundance proteins (e.g., albumin in serum). Enrichment is usually accomplished by immunoprecipitation to recover the analyte of interest (or in some cases, to deplete the sample of the high-abundance proteins that interfere), separation of the peptides in one- and two-dimension polyacrylamide gel electrophoresis (PAGE), liquid chromatography, or other methods.

MS provides accurate information about the chemical nature of proteins, but quantitation is difficult due to differences in ionization and other factors. One way to compare the amounts of proteins in two samples of interest is to treat each protein extract with a tag (called an isotope-coded affinity tag, or ICAT) that reacts with all of the proteins. However, one sample receives a tag with an isotope (such as deuterium instead of hydrogen) that allows it to be distinguished from the tag that has been added to the other sample (which, for example, may have only the natural isotope abundance). Next, the tagged samples are mixed and analyzed by MS so that the tagged peptides are treated identically yet give two signals that differ in *m/z* by the isotope difference of the tags. Because the peptides have the same chemical composition and are in the same mixture (and therefore subject to the same factors that affect ion yield), the intensities of will be proportional to the relative amounts of the proteins in the two samples.[45] Initially, the ICAT reagents were conjugated to peptides by selective alkylation of cysteine residues with tags that either contained none or eight deuterium atoms (i.e., d0-ICAT and d8-ICAT); however, newer ICAT reagents use $^{13}C$ and $^{12}C$.

**Other Proteomic Methods.** Because antibodies have been prepared against most proteins—and companies are even making antibodies directed toward hypothetical polypeptides found in the genome—high-throughput immunochemical methods are attractive alternatives to MS analysis. With such antibodies, one can prepare micro-arrays that allow the analysis of hundreds to thousands of proteins in parallel, analogous to the types of tools that are used to measure gene expression. This approach is also attractive for post-translational modifications,[46] however, there remains the possibility that a given polypeptide may have multiple post-translational modifications (such as phosphorylation on several amino acid residues), and this will complicate the analysis. An attractive feature of an immunochemical approach is the possibility that it might be adapted to a flow-through device (such as the types used for plasmon resonance or acoustic resonance detection[47]); therefore, the device might be better able to report dynamic changes over time. These methods can also be used in conjunction with MS.[48]

### *Nutriproteomics*

There have been relatively few applications of proteomics to nutrition research thus far, but two studies illustrate the types of findings that may emerge. Mitchell et al.[49] used MALDI-TOF-MS to analyze serum samples in a randomized, controlled dietary intervention study in which participants ate a basal diet devoid of fruits and vegetables and a basal diet supplemented with cruciferous vegetables. The MALDI-TOF spectra were analyzed using peak picking algorithms and logistic regression models and identified two peaks (at *m/z* 2740 and 1847) that classified participants based on diet (basal vs. cruciferous) with 76% accuracy. The authors noted that the 2740 *m/z* species would correspond to the B-chain of alpha 2-HS glycoprotein, which has been previously found to vary with diet and to be involved in insulin resistance and immune function. In another study, Chanson et al.[50] compared liver proteins in rats pair-fed defined diets with and without folate for 4 weeks using two-dimensional electrophoresis and MALDI-TOF MS. The investigators observed changes in the apparent intensities of nine spots on the electrophoresis gels, and analysis of each spot by MS suggested that they reflected increases in glutathione peroxidase-1, peroxiredoxin 6, and MAWD-binding protein in three of the spots (interestingly, MAWD-binding protein was found both in a spot that appeared to increase and a second spot with a lower isoelectric point that decreased after folate deficiency) and decreases in cofilin 1, the GRP 75 precursor, and preproalbumin. The changes in glutathione peroxidase-1 and MAWD-binding protein were confirmed by other methods (enzymatic assay and Western blotting); therefore, they concluded that these results show that folate deficiency modifies the abundance of several liver proteins that function in adaptive tissue responses to oxidative and degenerative processes. There have been excellent reviews on the use of proteomics for nutrition studies,[5,40-42] and it is certain that this will be a growing field.

## Metabolomics

Metabolomics is the study of all metabolites—essentially all the molecules smaller than proteins and polynucleotides—in the organism(s) of interest under the condition(s) of interest. This is, in essence, what many nutritionists have been doing for a long time as they studied amino acid profiles, vitamin amounts, and such, but were limited to analysis of fewer compounds due to technical difficulties and cost. As technology has added small molecule analysis to the "-omics" repertoire, this has not only created new opportunities and challenges for nutrition,[5,51] but has also, one might say, an obligation for nutrition to fulfill its mission of deciphering the relationships between diet and health.[2]

Metabolomic approaches have, thus far, appeared in three main forms[52]:

- Use of traditional methods that are capable of profiling most or all of the members of a compound class (for example, amino acids);
- Use of "-omics" technologies (such as MS and NMR spectrometry) that are directed toward rigorously identifying and quantifying a large fraction of interrelated molecules; and
- Use of approaches in which technologies that provide a complex signal profile (such as all of the ions across a scan of different *m/z* that are detectible by MS under a given set of conditions) that can be used to look for patterns that correlate with a physiological state or disease. When the latter is used, the compounds that are the source of the signal are not usually known with certainly; however, the technique can be used as an initial screen that is followed by more rigorous identification of the peaks of interest.

Once the metabolites have been identified and quantified, the data are usually interpreted in the context of the pathway(s) in which they appear using a variety of tools that will be discussed in a separate section of this text. The goal of a metabolomic analysis is usually to identify key control points of the metabolic pathway, thus predicting which enzymes are likely to be changing, which in turn may lead to investigation of possible changes in expression of the genes that code for these proteins. The unique value of metabolomics over genomics and proteomics is that when the output of interest is a metabolite (or pathway), the method gives a direct readout of those entities rather than indirect indicators such as a gene chip that measures changes in mRNA that may or may not equate to changes in the transcribed protein, or a proteomic analysis that may give a good approximation of changes in the protein amount and post-translational modifications, but not necessarily its activity if it is subject to regulation by, say, product inhibition or allosteric modifiers.

## *Metabolomic Technologies*

Part of the challenge of metabolomics is that there are large numbers of compounds to analyze, and their chemical and physical properties vary far beyond what is encountered in genomics and proteomics.[52] In addition to the large numbers of compounds, there is tremendous variation in the amounts (which requires that the technology have a very broad dynamic range), and no single analytical methodology has been found that can analyze all low-molecular-weight metabolites.[53] Therefore, some investigators have elected to focus on methods that are applicable to subclasses of compounds, such as glycomics for carbohydrates (http://www.functionalglycomics.org/static/consortium/) and lipidomics for lipids (http://www.LipidMaps.org). This is to some degree an extension of conventional methods that have been used in clinical analysis of small molecules as indicators of specific metabolic diseases; however, in metabolomics the goal is not to focus as narrowly on the known biomarkers but to look for new or more subtle relationships among all biomolecules or a related subset. To date, two major methods have been described as metabolomic technologies, MS and NMR spectroscopy, which are described here. In practical terms, it is reasonable to use any method that generate quantitative data for all of the members of a metabolite category, such as traditional amino acid analysis—although such methods tend to be too slow and insensitive for the type of high-throughput data collection that is needed for most systems biology analyses.

**Mass Spectrometry.** Modern mass spectrometers have a combination of features that make them helpful for metabolomic analysis: sensitivities in the pmol ($10^{-12}$) to fmol ($10^{-15}$) range (and sometimes lower, depending on the instrumentation); linear dynamic ranges of $10^2$ to $10^4$ depending on the type of MS; and high mass (*m/z*) resolving power. The major disadvantage of MS is that all of the compounds of interest (i.e., the analytes) must be ionized, so it is a tremendous challenge to find conditions (solvent, pH, etc.) that produce the desired ions, and some neutral compounds are very difficult to ionize at all. A range of ionization techniques are available (as for proteomic MS), with the major ones for metabolomics being ESI, MALDI, and SIMS. Each type of ionization technique has complications and limitations. ESI is a relatively "soft" ionization technique (meaning that ionization can often be achieved with little fragmentation of the parent compound, which is good), however, it may not ionize all of the compounds of interest, and in complex mixtures, interactions between compounds may cause aggregates to form. These aggregates may either fail to enter the mass spectrometer (due to size or charge) or produce multiple species that make quantitation of the individual analytes more difficult. Both of these complications fall under the category of "ion suppression," and variation in the ionization yield from a given analyte necessitates very carefully controlled conditions and internal standards for quantitative analysis by ESI (which, however, is also the case for other MS techniques, as described below).

MALDI is also a "soft" ionization technique, and, with careful selection of the appropriate compounds to serve as the MALDI matrix, can sometimes ionize compounds that are not readily ionized by ESI. A disadvantage of MALDI is that it is a pulsed ionization technique (i.e., the ionization occurs in pulses of the laser), so the mass analyzer must be compatible with a pulsed mode of ionization (as occurs, for example, in TOF-MS), and the technique is not easily coupled with liquid chromatography, which is often used prior to MS analysis to separate compounds that have the same *m/z* and similar fragmentation profiles, such as glucosylceramide and galactosylceramide. There are, however, devices that allow the liquid chromatography eluate to be mixed with the MALDI matrix compound and spotted on MALDI plates for subsequent analysis. Because the samples and matrix compound may not mix and dry uniformly, quantitative analysis by MALDI may be more difficult. Another difficulty of MALDI is that the matrix ions are in high abundance, so if the *m/z* of the analyte is similar to that of the matrix ions, it will be difficult to detect unless it can be distinguished by an MS/MS analysis (as will be described later in this section). SIMS is the most sensitive surface analysis technique, but is more difficult to accurately quantify than the other techniques due to variation in the way the samples deposit on the surface, etc. although these limitations may be addressed with the appropriate internal standards. Once the ions are formed, they may be separated using the types of mass analyzers described under Proteomics.

**Pre-MS Separation of Samples.** The power of MS is its ability to identify compounds according to mass, however, a drawback is that some compounds have the same mass but different structure (for example, isomeric and isobaric carbohydrates and lipids) and the large numbers of compounds (and sometimes subtle differences in structure, such as a single double bond) means that there is a reasonably high probability that there will be cross contamination of the ion from a particular compound with an isotopic subspecies (for example, due to the natural abundance of $C^{13}$ vs. $C^{12}$) of another compound. In many cases, these can be distinguished by MS/MS; however, the method that is most often used to separate compounds that cannot be resolved by MS alone is a pre-MS liquid chromatographic step. Liquid chromatography is easily coupled to ESI MS/MS instruments and can also be used with MALDI if the eluant is mixed with matrix material and spotted on the MALDI plate for subsequent analysis. Companies are also developing capillary devices that will collect eluants in capillaries or chip-like devices for subsequent MS analysis.

The critical element in quantitative analysis by MS is for the ions to be definitively characterized and for there to be appropriately selected internal standards. In the ideal case, each analyte should have a matching internal standard (for example, a stable isotope version), so that the ions from the unknown and the internal standard are analyzed simultaneously; however, in many cases, there are too many subspecies for this, and investigators select internal standards that relatively accurately match the analytes under consideration. When the standard and analyte are not chemically and physically identical, all of the analytical parameters must be tested carefully to ensure that differences in the compounds, or more likely interference by other components in a complex biological extract, do not alter the relationship between the ion yields from the analyte(s) and standard(s).

**Nuclear Magnetic Resonance Spectroscopy.** NMR spectroscopy is another useful technique for analysis of large numbers of low-molecular-weight metabolites, because it not only provides structural information but the magnitude of the signal is proportional to the molar amounts, unlike MS where quantitation requires extensive use of internal standards (and can be effectively integrated with MS studies).[55] In addition, NMR spectroscopy is non-destructive, so the sample can also be analyzed by another technique. Among the limitations of NMR are its insensitivity (often requiring millimolar concentrations of the analytes of interest), which has been addressed by the development of instruments with increased field strength and highly sensitive detectors, spin sequences, and other techniques that allow analysis of complex samples in even very small sample volumes.[56,57]

**Other Metabolomic Technologies.** Just as antibodies can be used to capture proteins, antibodies have been successfully raised against many small molecules; therefore, these can be used to prepare static or flow-through chips such as those used for various categories of compounds in aqueous and gas phase, but so far mostly applied to proteins.[59] Flow-through methods are particularly likely to find applications in small-molecule analysis because the binding affinities do not need to be as high for detection as for a traditional chip, and with the appropriate bioengineering, one can theoretically generate polypeptides that bind every natural biomolecule by utilizing the substrate or product-binding sites of enzymes that metabolize that compound.

## *Nutritional Metabolomics*

There are several very interesting discussions of the concept of nutritional metabolomics but few primary research reports because this technology is still in development. Three illustrative studies are: a) a study of the effects of administration of varying levels of leucine to rats on plasma amino acids, leucine metabolites and a few other compounds (glucose, cholesterol, triglycerides, phospholipids and ions) as well as on gene expression in liver.[59] A cluster analysis of changes in gene expression related leucine feeding at 5% to the apparent up-regulation of 108 genes and down-regulation of 5 genes, and 15% supplementation up-regulated 41 genes and down-regulated 18. These included genes for amino acid and lipid metabolism as well as cell signaling and stress; b) a comparative analysis of genes and tracer metabolism in glucose metabolism[60]; and c) an analysis of the combination of genomic and metabolomics as markers of the interaction of diet and health[61] using a study of the effect of the peroxisome proliferator activated receptor-gamma (PPAR$\gamma$) agonist rosiglitazone on lipid metabolism.[62]

In addition, the equivalent of metabolomics has been practiced by metabolic physiologists and nutritionists for decades in studies of how carbohydrates are catabolized for energy, stored in glycogen, or metabolized to fat or other products, the uptake and turnover of amino acids in metabolic diseases, and lipid absorption, transport and metabolism, for examples. What has generally been lacking is the global perspective, in which the fluxes and distribution of these compounds are linked with the regulation of all of the genes, enzymes, transporters, endocrine factors, etc. Indeed, one might have thought that the endocrine research community might have been one of the first to tout the value of "endocrinomics."

## *Integration of "-omics" Technologies and a Systems Biology Approach to Nutrition*

Bioinformatics and other computational sciences are vital for the application of "-omic" technologies and systems biology approaches to nutrition. Beginning at the earliest stages of experimental design, one must make critical decisions about how the data will be collected, stored, and analyzed. Methods such as MS generate hundreds to thousands of signals per analysis (or more, if in a scanning mode where every *m/z* is being counted rather than focusing on species known to be of interest), and therefore the manual collection and analysis of the data should be minimized. In many ways, the types of decisions that are made regarding which signals are valid versus, for example, random background noise and such are analogous to the types of pattern analysis that has become a well-established field in engineering (e.g., as applied to communications) and in biomedicine (e.g., for analysis of x-ray images).[63,64] Pattern-recognition methods can be unsupervised, meaning that the programs are designed to determine pattern sets according to their properties and without prior knowledge of the sample class (this approach is often used in gene clustering, for example), or supervised, which means that the investigators have additional information that they direct the analyses to compare, for example, outcome data from clinical trials, to determine similarities and differences between the chosen groups. The application of pattern analysis to biological systems is not so simple, however, because biological researchers usually do not have the luxury of conducting very large numbers of replicates, so one must decide what criteria should be adopted in considering data to be of high-enough quality to be acceptable for databases, recognizing that if the standard is too low there will be many misleading outcomes, but if it is too high, the cost and time it would take to collect and validate the data could become prohibitive. In most laboratories, this is currently done on an empirical basis; however, as the technologies become available to larger numbers of investigators, criteria for which data are of adequate quality to be entered into globally accessible data banks will need to be standardized, whenever possible with some consensus about reference standards, such as has been done in the CDC-NHLBI Lipid Standardization program.

Once the quality of the data is certified, the next step is to annotate and store it in ways that allow ready access by investigators worldwide. This is done in a somewhat consistent way for genes and proteins, and the Lipid MAPS Consortium (www.lipidmaps.org) has proposed a nomenclature for lipids[65] that has thus far received favorable responses from other lipidomic initiatives in Japan and Europe. As noted earlier, one website has been established for the deposit of nutrigenomic datasets (http://ayo5.ch.a.u-tokyo.ac.jp/index.phtml). Once these resources are available, investigators across the world will be able to explore hypotheses without having to conduct new experiments; indeed, it will be possible to develop artificial intelligence programs that search for associations that might not be imagined by scientists who are too deeply locked in the current paradigms of their fields. The ultimate goal is to develop mathematical models for biological systems that allows one to make reasonable predictions in silico (i.e., by computer).

Data management is usually carried out through information architecture, i.e., organizational schemes (classification systems for organizing content into groups) and organizational structures (defining the relationships among the groups) that are consistent with the mental models of the users, with a combination of hierarchical, hyperlink, and database structures. In the past, some of the data management was accomplished by huge data warehousing efforts,[66] but these efforts were usually soon abandoned due to the cost of keeping the data.[67] Thus, distributed solutions were proposed with advanced computing technology such as "Web Services," which enable distributed computing with standard communication protocols and data formats (World Wide Consortium: http://www.w3.org/2002/ws/), and are based on open standards and ubiquitous Internet protocols.

Currently, the Web Services technology framework uses open protocols for description, usage and discovery of Web Services. Extensible Markup Language (XML; http://www.xml.com/) is the standard data and message formatting language. Simple Object Access Protocol (SOAP) specifies the messaging mechanism and how Web Services are used. Web Services Description Language (WSDL) is an XML-based language that is used to describe Web Services. Universal Description, Discovery, and Integration Service (UDDI) is a directory service used to list available Web Services and can automatically search and locate Web Services.

Just like the Internet, which revolutionized the computing world via its open and simple protocols (HTTP and the simple document formatting language HTML), SOAP/XML-based Web Services are widely accepted open standards provided by the World Wide Web Consortium (www.w3.org) and other standardization organizations. To facilitate the distributed data query, standardization is usually needed; it is critical to have a comprehensive suite of parsing and validation, data storage, design, and simulation tools around a single standard. The current example standardization system includes MathML (www.w3.org/Math/) for describing mathematical equations; SBML[68] for systems biology modeling, and MAGE-ML[69] for gene expression studies using high-throughput micro-arrays. The next revolution in standardization would be Resource Description Framework (RDF),[70] where information in the data can be intelligently navigated.

The analysis and interpretation of the results is often the most vexing and time-consuming task, because the genes and pathways are not only complex, but they are also unfamiliar to most investigators (very few investigators memorize all of the metabolic pathways these days, and even if they did, the obscure nomenclatures that are used for most genes—not to mention those involved in signaling instead of metabolism per se—is extremely confusing). Internet-based tools to allow searches of pathways and genes are being established, such as the Gene Ontology (GO) Consortium (http://www.geneontology.org/) and the Kyoto Encyclopedia of Genes and Genomes (KEGG) (http://www.genome.ad.jp/kegg/), which organize genes into hierarchical categories such as organisms, pathways, biological process, molecular function, and subcellular localization.

While these are useful resources, additional tools are usually needed to organize datasets in ways that are easier for the viewer to see the interrelationships that have been uncovered by the experiment. Some programs that have been developed for this purpose are MAPPFinder, FatiGO, Onto-Express, GoSurfer and GoMiner, BioPAX, Taverna, and CellDesigner. FatiGO and Onto-Express are Web applications, with the latter being the more flexible, although it is largely limited to a flat view of the biological world. GoSurfer is implemented as a Windows application and therefore lacks platform independence. MAPPFinder is a pioneering project that integrates GO analysis and biological pathway maps and provides the fundamental tree representation of the GO hierarchy, with summary and statistical data in line with each category. GoMiner,[71] which can be downloaded free of charge, also allows this type of integration, since each gene in the GoMiner tree classification is dynamically linked to the corresponding set of BioCarta and KEGG biological pathway maps, and provides integration with chromosomal information via dynamic linking to the chromosome viewer in LocusLink, which also allows dynamic linking to SNPs and MGC databases. GoMiner also uses a directed acyclic graph (DAG) view to provide a qualitative and quantitative picture of the often-complex, multiple parenthood of some categories, and has a command-line interface (through the companion program MatchMiner) that allows it to input data organized on the basis of "-omic" identifiers other than the HUGO names (i.e., it resolves IMAGE clone ids, UniGene clusters, GenBank accession numbers, Affymetrix ids, chromosome locations, gene common names, FISH clone ids, etc.), which greatly facilitates the preparation of data for analysis. In our opinion, this type of visualization allows easier appreciation of the complex, highly nonlinear relationships within biological systems and gene networks.

Even with such tools, visualization of pathways can be difficult due to the large size of the dataset. To visualize large amounts of information in a limited display, researchers have studied different techniques such as "overview-and-detail," in which the "overview" provides the overall pattern of the data, and "detail" displays the detailed information. One of the overview-and-detail methods is called a "focus + context" technique, which shows the region of interest in detail, with the remaining area shown in less detail (Figure 2D). This way, both the area of interest and the overall structure can be illustrated in the same view. Other visualization tools use techniques such as a "fisheye lens," in which the focused region of interest can be zoomed in for display with high resolution and large fonts, while the remainder of the graph is shown in low resolution and small fonts. Another tool is a focus and context view that displays the large hierarchical (tree) structure as a hyperbolic plane, and as the user focuses on a particular area, it is brought into the center of view through smooth animation. Another is a rooted tree using a circular layout, which arranges the focus by assigning a scaling factor to each node. For each of these methods, the program may use two or more viewing panels: one to show overall information and the other to display detailed information. The next wave in visualizing the information for interpretation is to link the visualization with ontology databases such as Gene Ontology,[72] Systems Biology Ontology, and naming unique identifier such as Life Science Identifier (LSID),[73] so that visual information can be linked to a public knowledge source for display.

## Challenges and Perspectives for the Future

Most of the methods that have been described here give snapshots of genes, proteins, and biomolecules, but life occurs in all three physical dimensions as well as the fourth dimension of time. Very little has been done to place "-omic" data in a subcellular, cellular, or physiologic context, and this will not be easy to do technologically; however, one hopes that developments in imaging technologies, such as MS analysis of cells and tissues[74] and nanotechnologies,[16,75] will begin to allow organisms to be understood as integrated systems. The dynamics of metabolic pathways (e.g., protein synthesis versus turnover) are also highly complex, and mathematical models to estimate metabolic pools and flux are becoming available for studies using stable isotopes,[76] as well as noninvasive methods such as magnetic resonance imaging and positron emission tomography.[77,78]

As was stated in the introduction to this chapter, a comprehensive systems analysis of all of these variables will not be completed any time soon; however, in the course of these investigations, there will undoubtedly be new discoveries that are of practical use—especially in the area of biomarkers and identification of intervention targets, such as in cancer.[79,80] To illustrate the likely usefulness of discovering additional biomarkers for disease risk, an analogy has been made[2] with improvements in the prediction of cardiovascular disease risk after the initial association with total cholesterol was refined by analysis of specific lipoprotein subclasses (LDL followed by HDL), an understanding of genetic defects in lipoproteins and lipoprotein receptors, and identification of other biomarkers (homocysteine, fibrinogen, lipoprotein(a), LDL particle size, C-reactive protein, and others). Some have referred to "-omics" as discovery science because "we are like naturalists discovering a new continent, enthralled with the diversity itself,"[81] and others have been more disparaging, referring to it as a "fishing expedition." Which is more valid will depend on the quality of the data that is collected so it can deliver its promised benefits. As said by John Weinstein[82]: "If one is going to fish, it is best to do so in teeming waters with the finest equipment and flawless technique."

## Acknowledgements

The authors acknowledge the following sources of support for their research pertinent to this review: for EMS, NIH grant CA109019; for MDW, a Georgia Cancer Coalition Distinguished Cancer Scholar Award, a Seed Grant from Institute of Bioengineering and Bioscience of Georgia Tech, NIH grants CA108468 and CA119338; and for AHM, NIH grants GM069338 (Lipid MAPS) and PA-02–132. The authors thank Mr. Geoffrey Wang and Mr. Todd Stokes for help in GoMiner and caBIG, and appreciate the help and patience of the editors of this edition of ***Present Knowledge in Nutrition.***

## References

1. German JB, Bauman DE, Burrin DG, et al. Metabolomics in the opening decade of the 21st century: Building the roads to individualized health. J Nutr. 2004;134:2729–2732.
2. Zeisel SH, Freake HC, Bauman DE, et al. The nutritional phenotype in the age of metabolomics. J Nutr. 2005;135:1613–1616.

3. Aderem A. Systems biology: Its practice and challenges. Cell. 2005;121:511–513.
4. Weston AD, Hood L. Systems biology, proteomics, and the future of health care: Toward predictive, preventative, and personalized medicine. J Proteome Res. 2004;3:179–196.
5. Trujillo E, Davis C, Milner J. Nutrigenomics, proteomics, metabolomics, and the practice of dietetics. J Am Diet Assoc. 2006;106:403–413.
6. de Vos WM, Castenmiller JJ, Hamer RJ, Brummer RJ. Nutridynamics - studying the dynamics of food components in products and in the consumer. Curr Opin Biotechnol. 2006 Mar 6; [Epub ahead of print].
7. Kaput, J, Rodriguez, RL (2004) Nutritional genomics: the next frontier in the postgenomic era. Physiol Genomics. 2004;16:166–177.
8. van Ommen B. Nutrigenomics: exploiting systems biology in the nutrition and health arenas. Nutrition. 2004;20:4–8.
9. Stover PJ. Nutritional genomics. Physiol Genomics. 2004;16:161–165.
10. Ordovas JM, Corella D. Nutritional genomics. Annu Rev Genomics Hum Genet. 2004;5:71–118.
11. Kaput J. Decoding the pyramid: A systems-biological approach to nutrigenomics. Ann N Y Acad Sci. 2005; 1055:64–79.
12. Mutch DM, Wahli W, Williamson G. Nutrigenomics and nutrigenetics: the emerging faces of nutrition. FASEB J. 2005;19:1602–1616.
13. Nisoli E, Tonello C, Cardile A, et al. Calorie restriction promotes mitochondrial biogenesis by inducing the expression of eNOS. Science. 2005;310: 314–317.
14. The International SNP MAP Working Group. Nature. 2001; 409:928–32
15. The International HapMap Consortium. The International HapMap Project. Nature. 2003;426:789–796.
16. Smith AM, Dave S, Nie S, True L, Gao X. Multicolor quantum dots for molecular diagnostics of cancer. Expert Rev Mol Diagn. 2006;6:231–244.
17. Fenech M. Nutritional treatment of genome instability: a paradigm shift in disease prevention and in the setting of recommended dietary allowances. Nutr Res Rev. 2003;16:109–122.
18. Anderson RF, Fisher LJ, Hara Y, Harris T, Mak WB, Melton LD, Packer JE. Green tea catechins partially protect DNA from (·)OH radical-induced strand breaks and base damage through fast chemical repair of DNA radicals. Carcinogenesis. 2001;22: 1189–1193.
19. Fenech M, Baghurst P, Luderer W, Turner J, Record S, Ceppi M, Bonassi S. Low intake of calcium, folate, nicotinic acid, vitamin E, retinol, beta-carotene and high intake of pantothenic acid, biotin and riboflavin are significantly associated with increased genome instability—results from a dietary intake and micronucleus index survey in South Australia. Carcinogenesis. 2005;26:991–999.
20. Kowalska E, Narod SA, Huzarski T, Zajaczek S, Huzarska J, Gorski B, Lubinski J. Increased rates of chromosome breakage in BRCA1 carriers are normalized by oral selenium supplementation. Cancer Epidemiol Biomarkers Prev. 2004;14:1302–1306.
21. Hollox EJ, Poulter M, Wang Y, Krause A, Swallow DM. Common polymorphism in a highly variable region upstream of the human lactase gene affects DNA-protein interactions. Eur J Hum Genet. 1999; 7:791–800.
22. Chango A, Boisson F, Barbe F, et al. The effect of 677C→T and 1298A→C mutations on plasma homocysteine and 5,10-methylenetetrahydrofolate reductase activity in healthy subjects. Br J Nutr. 2000; 83:593–596.
23. Chen J, Giovannucci E, Kelsey K, et al. A methylenetetrahydrofolate reductase polymorphism and the risk of colorectal cancer. Cancer Res. 1996;56: 4862–4864.
24. Davis SR, Quinlivan EP, Shelnutt KP, et al. Homocysteine synthesis is elevated but total remethylation is unchanged by the methylenetetrahydrofolate reductase 677C→T polymorphism and by dietary folate restriction in young women. J Nutr. 2005;135: 1045–50
25. Ambrosone CB, Freudenheim JL, Thompson PA, Bowman E, Vena JE, Marshall JR, Graham S, Laughlin R, Nemoto T, Shields PG. Manganese superoxide dismutase (MnSOD) genetic polymorphisms, dietary antioxidants, and risk of breast cancer. Cancer Res. 1999;59:602–606.
26. Shen J, Terry MB, Gammon MD, et al. MGMT genotype modulates the associations between cigarette smoking, dietary antioxidants and breast cancer risk. Carcinogenesis. 2005;26:2131–2137.
27. Saito K, Arai S, Kato H. A nutrigenomics database—integrated repository for publications and associated microarray data in nutrigenomics research. Br J Nutr. 2005;94:493–495.
28. Bar-Joseph Z, Gerber GK, Lee TI, et al. Computational discovery of gene modules and regulatory networks. Nat Biotechnol. 2003;21:1337–1342.
29. Sellick CA, Reece RJ. Eukaryotic transcription factors as direct nutrient sensors. Trends Biochem Sci. 2005;30:405–412.
30. Alvarez-Garcia I, Miska EA. MicroRNA functions in animal development and human disease. Development. 2005;132:4653–4662.
31. Waterland RA, Garza C. Potential mechanisms of metabolic imprinting that lead to chronic disease. Am J Clin Nutr. 1999;69:179–197.
32. Chen RZ, Pettersson U, Beard C, Jackson-Grusby L, Jaenisch R. DNA hypomethylation leads to elevated mutation rates. Nature. 1998;395:89–93.
33. Liu L, Wylie RC, Andrews LG, Tollefsbol TO.

Aging, cancer and nutrition: the DNA methylation connection. Mech Ageing Dev. 2003;124:989–998.
34. Waterland RA, Jirtle RL. Early nutrition, epigenetic changes at transposons and imprinted genes, and enhanced susceptibility to adult chronic diseases. Nutrition. 2004;20:63–68.
35. Rimbach G, Fischer A, Stoecklin E, Barella L. Modulation of hepatic gene expression by alpha-tocopherol in cultured cells and in vivo. Ann N Y Acad Sci. 2004;1031:102–108.
36. Symolon H, Schmelz EM, Dillehay DL, Merrill AH Jr. Dietary soy sphingolipids suppress tumorigenesis and gene expression in 1,2-dimethylhydrazine-treated CF1 mice and ApcMin/+ mice. J Nutr. 2004;134:1157–1161.
37. Guo S, Yang S, Taylor C, Sonenshein GE., Green tea polyphenol epigallocatechin-3 gallate (EGCG) affects gene expression of breast cancer cells transformed by the carcinogen 7,12-dimethylbenz[a]anthracene. J Nutr. 2005;135(12 suppl): 2978S–2986S.
38. Lu Y, Yao R, Yan Y, Wang Y, Hara Y, Lubet RA, You M. A gene expression sigNature. that can predict green tea exposure and chemopreventive efficacy of lung cancer in mice. Cancer Res. 2006;66: 1956–1963.
39. Gescher AJ, Steward WP. Relationship between mechanisms, bioavailibility, and preclinical chemopreventive efficacy of resveratrol: a conundrum. Cancer Epidemiol Biomarkers Prev. 2003;12:953–957.
40. Barnes S, Kim H. Nutriproteomics: identifying the molecular targets of nutritive and non-nutritive components of the diet. J Biochem Mol Biol. 2004;37: 59–74.
41. Kim H, Page GP, Barnes S. Proteomics and mass spectrometry in nutrition research. Nutrition. 2004; 20:155–165.
42. Kussmann M, Affolter M, Fay LB. Proteomics in Nutrition. and health. Comb Chem High Throughput Screen. 2005;8:679–696.
43. Touboul D, Kollmer F, Niehuis E, Brunelle A, Laprevote O. Improvement of biological time-of-flight-secondary ion mass spectrometry imaging with a bismuth cluster ion source. J Am Soc Mass Spectrom. 2005;16:1608–1618.
44. Bogdanov B, Smith RD., Proteomics by FTICR mass spectrometry: top down and bottom up. Mass Spectrom Rev. 2005;24:168–200.
45. Yi EC, Li XJ, Cooke K, et al. Increased quantitative proteome coverage with $(^{13})C/(^{12})C$-based, acid-cleavable isotope-coded affinity tag reagent and modified data acquisition scheme. Proteomics. 2005; 5:380–387.
46. Beernink HT, Nock S. Challenges facing the development and use of protein chips to analyze the phosphoproteome. Expert Rev Proteomics. 2005;2: 487–497.
47. Usui-Aoki K, Shimada K, Nagano M, Kawai M, Koga H. A novel approach to protein expression profiling using antibody microarrays combined with surface plasmon resonance technology. Proteomics. 2005;5:2396–2401.
48. Buijs J, Franklin GC. SPR-MS in functional proteomics. Brief Funct Genomic Proteomic. 2005;4: 39–47.
49. Mitchell BL, Yasui Y, Lampe JW, Gafken PR, Lampe PD. Evaluation of matrix-assisted laser desorption/ionization-time of flight mass spectrometry proteomic profiling: identification of alpha 2-HS glycoprotein B-chain as a biomarker of diet. Proteomics. 2005;5:2238–2246.
50. Chanson A, Sayd T, Rock E, et al. Proteomic analysis reveals changes in the liver protein pattern of rats exposed to dietary folate deficiency. J Nutr. 2005; 135:2524–2529.
51. Gibney MJ, Walsh M, Brennan L, Roche HM, German B, van Ommen B. Metabolomics in human nutrition: opportunities and challenges. Am J Clin Nutr. 2005;82:497–503.
52. Weckwerth W, Morgenthal K. Metabolomics: from pattern recognition to biological interpretation. Drug Discov Today. 2005;10:1551–1558.
53. Glassbrook N, Ryals J. A systematic approach to biochemical profiling. Curr Opin Plant Biol. 2001;4: 186–190.
54. Gavaghan McKee CL, Wilson ID, Nicholson JK Metabolic phenotyping of nude and normal (Alpk: ApfCD, C57BL10J) mice. J Proteome Res. 2006;5: 378–384.
55. Crockford DJ, Holmes E, Lindon JC, et al. Statistical heterospectroscopy, an approach to the integrated analysis of NMR and UPLC-MS data sets: application in metabonomic toxicology studies. Anal Chem. 2006;78:363–371.
56. Griffin JL. Metabolic profiles to define the genome: can we hear the phenotypes? Philos Trans R Soc Lond B Biol Sci. 2004;359:857–871.
57. Veshtort M, Griffin RG. SPINEVOLUTION: a powerful tool for the simulation of solid and liquid state NMR experiments. J Magn Reson. 2006;178: 248–282.
58. Corso CD, Stubbs DD, Sang-Hun L, Goggins M, Hruban RH, Hunt WD. Real-time detection of mesothelin in pancreatic cancer cell line supernatant using an acoustic wave immunosensor. Cancer Detect Prevent. 2006; In press.
59. Matsuzaki K, Kato H, Sakai R, Toue S, Amao M, Kimura T. Transcriptomics and metabolomics of dietary leucine excess. J Nutr. 2005;135(6 suppl): 1571S–1575S.
60. Lee WN, Go VL. Nutrient-gene interaction: tracer-based metabolomics. J Nutr. 2005;135:3027S–3032S.
61. German JB, Roberts MA, Watkins SM. Genomics

and metabolomics as markers for the interaction of diet and health: lessons from lipids. J Nutr. 2003;6: 2078S–2083S.

62. Watkins SM, Reifsnyder PR, Pan HJ, German JB, Leiter EH. Lipid metabolome-wide effects of the PPARgamma agonist rosiglitazone. J Lipid Res. 2002;43:1809–1817.
63. Duda RO, Hart PE, Stork DG, eds. *Pattern Classification.* New York: Wiley-Interscience; 2000.
64. Meyer-Baese A, ed. *Pattern Recognition in Medical Imaging*. New York: Academic Press; 2003.
65. Fahy E, Subramaniam S, Brown HA, et al. A comprehensive classification system for lipids. J Lipid Res. 2005;46:839–861.
66. Ritter O, Kocab P, Senger M, Wolf W Suhai S. Prototype implementation of the integrated genomic database. Comput Biomed Res. 1994;27:97–115
67. Stein LD. Integrating biological databases. Nat Rev Genet. 2003;4:337–345.
68. Hucka M, Finney A. The systems biology markup language (SBML): a medium for representation and exchange of biochemical network models. Bioinformatics. 2003;19:524–531.
69. Spellman PT, Miller M, Stewart J, et al. Design and implementation of microarray gene expression markup language (MAGE-ML), Genome Biol 2002;3(9):RESEARCH0046 (Epub 2002 Aug 23).
70. Wang XS, Gorlitsky R, Almeida JS. From XML to RDF: how semantic web technologies will change the design of 'omic' standards. Nat Biotechnol. 2005; 23:1099–1103.
71. Zeeberg BR, Feng MW, Wang G, et al. GoMiner: a resource for biological interpretation of genomic and proteomic data. Genome Biology. 2003;4:R28.
72. Ashburner M, Ball CA, Blake JA, et al. Gene ontology: tool for the unification of biology. The Gene Ontology Consortium. Nat Genet. 2000;25:25–29.
73. Clark T, Martin S, Liefeld T. Globally distributed object identification for biological knowledgebases. Brief Bioinform. 2004;5:59–70.
74. Caldwell RL, Caprioli RM. Tissue profiling by mass spectrometry: a review of methodology and applications. Mol Cell Proteomics. 2005;4:394–401.
75. Smith AM, Nie S., Chemical analysis and cellular imaging with quantum dots. Analyst. 2004;129: 672–677.
76. Hellerstein MK. New stable isotope-mass spectrometric techniques for measuring fluxes through intact metabolic pathways in mammalian systems: introduction of moving pictures into functional genomics and biochemical phenotyping. Metab Eng. 2004;6: 85–100.
77. Lanao JM, Fraile MA. Drug tissue distribution: study methods and therapeutic implications. Curr Pharm Des. 2005;11:3829–3845.
78. de Graaf C, Blom WA, Smeets PA, Stafleu A, Hendriks HF. Biomarkers of satiation and satiety. Am J Clin Nutr. 2004;79:946–961.
79. Milner JA. Molecular targets for bioactive food components. J Nutr. 2004;134:2492S–2498S.
80. Go VL, Wong DA, Wang Y, Butrum RR, Norman HA, Wilkerson L. Diet and cancer prevention: evidence-based medicine to genomic medicine. J Nutr. 2004;134:3513S–3516S.
81. Krischner MW. The meaning of systems biology. Cell. 2005;121:503–504.
82. Weinstein JN. Fishing expeditions. Science. 1998; 282:628.
83. Arakawa K, Kono N, Yamada Y, Mori H, Tomita M., KEGG-based pathway visualization tool for complex omics data. In Silico Biol. 2005;5:419–423.

# II Energy Physiology

# 2
# Lessons from Body Composition Analysis

Jonathan C.K. Wells

## Introduction

During the 20th century, scientists made major progress in developing the capacity to measure human body composition in vivo. Such progress has always been constrained by the difficulty that body composition is an internal aspect of phenotype. Whereas cadaver analysis remains the ultimate reference method, in vivo studies clearly require indirect methods, which measure body properties and combine this information with theoretical assumptions to predict actual body composition outcomes. Historically, most interest has been directed toward the fat and fat-free components of weight, although there is now increasing interest in quantifying both the regional distribution of these tissues and the chemical or functional composition of fat-free tissue.

The earliest work was conducted using simple anthropometric proxies for body composition, in particular body mass index (BMI), calculated as weight in kilograms divided by the square of height in meters. Due to the ease and low cost with which BMI can be measured, it has comprised the primary outcome in both clinical research and clinical practice. Unfortunately, the use of BMI as a proxy for body composition often leads to erroneous assumptions concerning the effects of diseases or their management, and a new evidence base derived from more sophisticated measurements is now emerging. Other long-standing and simple techniques include skin-fold thickness measurements, which provide relatively robust data on body fat stores, but offer little information about the fat-free component of weight.

In the second half of the 20th century, a variety of two-component techniques were developed, including densitometry, hydrometry, dual-energy X-ray absorptiometry (DEXA), magnetic resonance imaging (MRI), and computed tomography (CT). The application of such techniques initiated the measurement of body composition itself, although individual techniques vary in the validity of their underlying theoretical assumptions. In the last decades of the 20th century, further advances in body composition theory led to the derivation of "multi-component models" whereby data from several different techniques are combined to reduce the reliance on theoretical assumptions. These techniques and their theoretical models have been described elsewhere,[1,2] and it is sufficient to state here that it is now possible to make highly sophisticated measurements, dividing the body into sub-compartments based either on physical or chemical properties or on their regional anatomical location. It should be noted that such capability remains concentrated in a relatively small number of specialized research centers, and that the scientific quality of body composition research is variable. This review summarizes work conducted wherever possible using multi-component models or the optimum techniques for regional analyses.

The previous and current decades have seen, arguably for the first time, body composition researchers sufficiently well-armed to address a wide spectrum of issues. There is a rapidly growing body of work exploring how environmental factors, diseases, and their treatment impact on body composition. This chapter will consider the lessons from body composition analysis in diverse areas, but will begin by reviewing briefly the way in which data are expressed.

## Expressing Body Composition Data

Traditionally, data on fat mass (FM) and fat-free mass (FFM) have been treated in different ways. Typically, FM has been expressed as a proportion of weight, i.e.

percentage fat (%fat), whereas FFM has not been adjusted for size. This approach may be criticized on two counts: first, it is appropriate to adjust both components for body size before comparing individuals and groups, and second, it is more appropriate to adjust for height rather than weight, otherwise indices of relative FM and relative FFM are not independent of each other.[3,4] Similar problems relate to other indices based on convenience rather than allometric adjustment, such as limb-to-trunk skin-fold ratios for the evaluation of fat distribution.[4]

Whole-body data are now increasingly expressed in the format proposed by Van Itallie et al.,[3] whereby both FM and FFM in kilograms are divided by the square of height in meters, to give the FM index (FMI) and the FFM index (FFMI). These indices have the benefit that they are expressed in the same units as BMI (kg/m$^2$). A graph plotting these indices against each other was proposed by Hattori,[5] as shown in Figure 1. Increasing relative FM is shown vertically, increasing relative FFM is shown horizontally, and increasing BMI is shown in the positive diagonal direction. Because in each individual FFMI and FMI add up to BMI, the graph also includes negative diagonal lines with constant BMI values, and positive diagonal lines with constant values for percentage fat. Thus, these graphs allow the composition of differences or changes in body weight to be displayed, while incorporating adjustment for body size, and are used below to illustrate the changes in body composition that occur during growth.

As body composition measurements become more sophisticated by, for example, addressing specific regions of the body, adjustment for variability in body size will necessarily become more complex, but it is essential for meaningful comparisons.

# Body Composition in Healthy Individuals

As with height or weight, humans vary markedly within and between populations in body composition, and also change considerably within their lifetimes as they grow and mature. Large numbers of subjects are required to develop an understanding of such normal variability, against which other states such as specific diseases can be compared. Despite this need, there are currently inadequate body composition reference data, and many researchers continue to rely on BMI as a proxy for body fatness despite increasing evidence of its limitations.

For infants, children, and adolescents, population-specific BMI centile charts similar to growth charts have been produced. In view of the differences between populations, an international reference was derived for the purpose of defining overweight and obesity on common grounds, hence facilitating between-population comparisons.[6] These reference data have proved particularly important in monitoring secular trends in the prevalence of childhood obesity. Recent studies, however, have illustrated the inadequacy of BMI as a proxy for body fat in individuals. Statistically, BMI is designed to adjust weight for height, and the index performs this role satisfactorily for all age groups from infancy on. However, the assumption that variability in weight represents variability in FM has poor validity, and this is relevant to our understanding both of the ontogenetic development of body composition and of its variability at any one time point.

Figure 2 shows data from Fomon et al.[7] plotted on a Hattori chart.[8] Between 1 and 10 years, both boys and girls decline in relative FM, but increase in relative FFM. Thus, children of different ages can have the same BMI

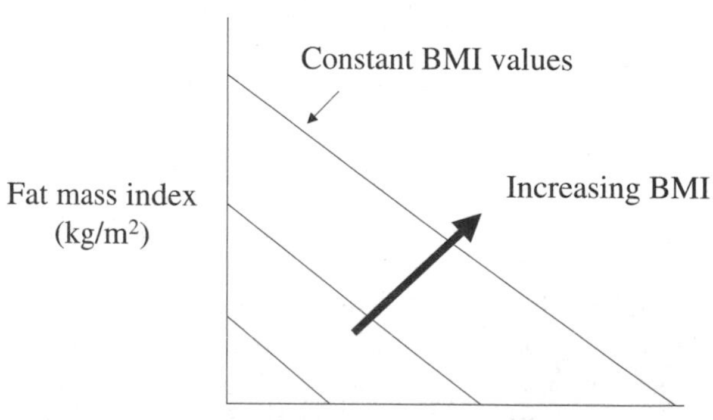


Figure 1. A Hattori graph showing the relationships between body mass index (BMI), fat-free mass index (FFMI) and fat mass index (FMI), each of which is expressed in common units of kilograms per meter squared (kg/m$^2$). The graph separates BMI into its fat and fat-free components, each of them adjusted for height. By plotting FMI on the y-axis against FFMI on the x-axis, increases in relative fatness are shown vertically and increases in relative lean mass horizontally. Since FFMI + FMI = BMI, the diagonal lines represent constant BMI values, or relatively greater weight, increasing upwards and across the graph.

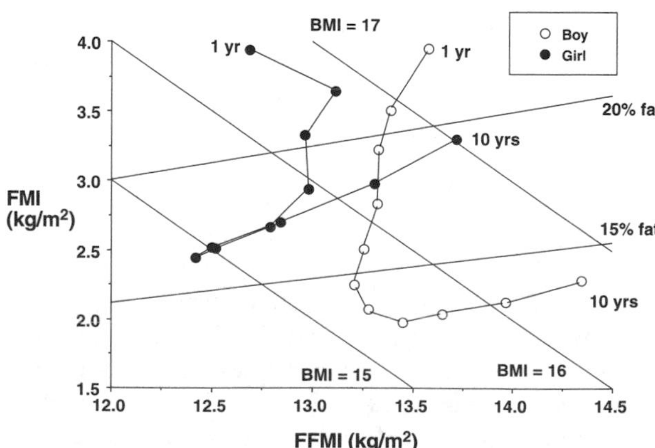


Figure 2. A Hattori graph showing changes in the relative proportions of fat and fat-free mass, adjusted for height, in the period of 1 to 10 years of age in boys and girls. The x-axis shows fat-free mass index (FFMI), the y axis fat mass index (FMI). Data points are sequentially joined up, representing each year of age, with an additional data point at 18 months. Both sexes lose fat mass relative to height from 1 to 6 years of age; however, whereas the girls subsequently regain both fat and lean, the boys gain primarily fat-free mass only from 6 years. (Used with permission from Wells, 2000.[8])

value but differ significantly in the underlying body composition. Traditionally, the increase in BMI that tends to occur in mid-childhood has been termed the "adiposity rebound," however, the data in Figure 2 show that increases in weight from mid-childhood are primarily FFM rather than FM, and this continues through adolescence.

On a similar theme, Figure 3 illustrates data from a sample of children 8 years of age. Here, the chart shows that two children of the same age and sex can have the same BMI value, and yet one can have more than double the FMI of the other. Again, therefore, BMI acts as a very poor proxy for fatness in individual children. Finally, even the use of BMI to define overweight and obesity is problematic, as there is now evidence that secular trends in weight do not match perfectly with secular trends in fatness. Thus, while secular trends in total and central fatness are well established,[9,10] it has also been hypothesized that FFM may also be decreasing, possibly due to reduced activity levels.[9] This hypothesis requires further evaluation in other populations.

Our understanding of the ontogenetic development of body composition has relied heavily on the "reference child" of Fomon et al.[7] This widely cited paper summarized data from several pediatric studies conducted in the 1960s and 1970s, primarily on infants or children 9 to 10 years of age. These data were then extrapolated to intervening age periods, and then mapped onto the US growth curves for weight and height. Recent studies of infants and children have shown relatively good agreement with the reference child, and (making allowance for the contemporary increase in childhood obesity) it seems that this model has provided a reasonable picture of the development of body composition between birth and 10 years of age. A similar dataset exists for adolescents,[11] but

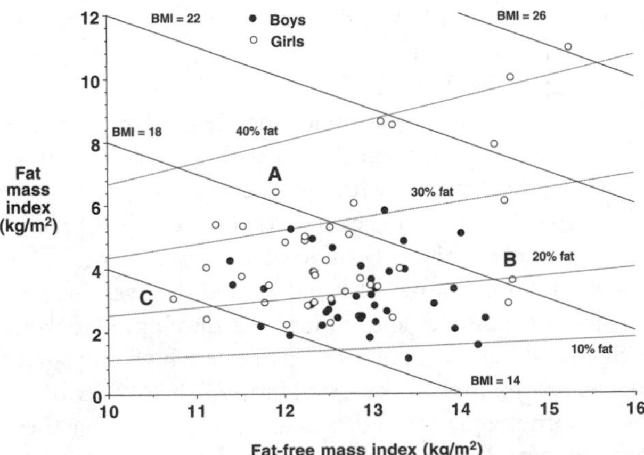


Figure 3. A Hattori graph showing the variability in fat mass index and fat-free mass index in a sample of 75 children 8 years of age. There is a wide range of fatness for a given body-mass index (BMI) value, and a wide range of BMI for a given percentage of fat (%fat). For example, children A and B both have BMI of approximately 18 kg/m$^2$, but differ in %fat by approximately 15%, while children B and C are both approximately 20% fat, but differ in BMI by approximately 4 kg/m$^2$. (Updated from data in Probst et al., 2001.[47])

is not in the mainstream scientific literature and remains relatively unknown. Newer studies are thus updating the parameters of the reference child and providing much-needed data on between-individual variability, but are not in general challenging the broader concepts, such as the chemical maturation of FFM and the developmental profile of FM.

The reference child highlights several interesting features in the development of body composition. First, humans have quite high FM at birth compared with other mammals, and then increase further during early infancy. From late infancy through to mid-childhood, relative fatness is lost while FFM is gained. With puberty, the two sexes follow markedly different trajectories: boys maintain their fatness proportional to their size and acquire considerable FFM, whereas girls gain less FFM but increase significantly in FM.[11] Data from individual studies are broadly consistent with this pattern; however, at any age, both sexes show major variability, and this is particularly the case during puberty.

These developmental patterns thus lead to the well-established sexual dimorphism in adult body composition, with women (after adjusting for their shorter stature) having more FM and less FFM than men.[12] The distribution of weight also varies between the sexes, with men having proportionally more limb muscle mass, and women having a more gynoid distribution (breasts, buttocks, and thighs) of fat than men, who have a central abdominal distribution.[12] These sex-differences in fat distribution, linked to differences in reproductive strategy, have important functional implications. Essential fat, located in bone marrow, the heart, lungs, liver, kidneys, intestines, muscles, and central nervous system, has been quantified as around 3% of body weight in men and 9% in women, while storage fat comprises around 12% and 15%, respectively.[12] The greater fatness of women confers on them a greater ability to endure conditions of famine, while the central distribution of fat in men means that they have a higher risk of cardiovascular disease despite lower total body fatness. However, because of this sex difference in fat distribution, the classification of healthy weight is similar between the sexes. Thus, conventional BMI cutoffs define normal weight in adults of either sex as 20 to 25 kg/m$^2$, overweight as 25 to 30 kg/m$^2$, and obese as >30 kg/m$^2$.

Body composition in adulthood is not constant but varies with age. In Europeans, FFM in both sexes tends to decline from around 50 years of age, whereas FM tends to increase, especially in women. Therefore, for a given BMI value, fatness tends to increase with age in Western populations[13] (Figure 4). Equivalent data from non-Western populations are not available; however, if assessed by BMI, the elderly are often relatively malnourished. Regardless of changes in total FM, its distribution also becomes more central with increasing age.[14] The significance of these age-related changes in fatness for health

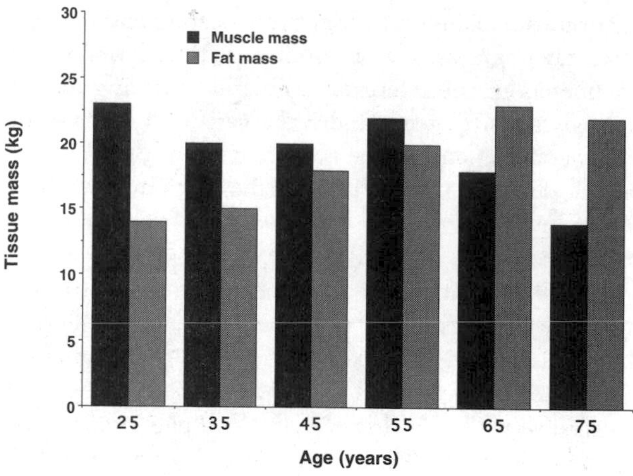


Figure 4. The relationship between age and the proportion of body weight as muscle or fat in adult healthy men. Even if body weight is maintained over time, there is a steady increase in the contribution of fat, accompanied by an equivalent loss of muscle mass. (From Cohn et al., 1987.[13] Used with kind permission from Springer Science and Business Media.)

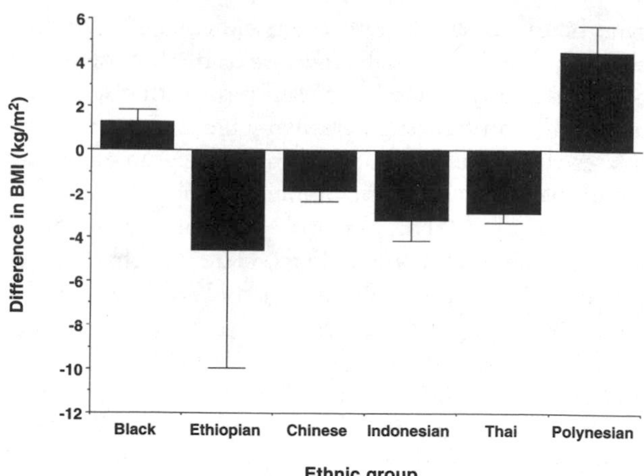


Figure 6. Adjustment in body-mass index (BMI) for various ethnic groups, required to reflect equivalent levels of percent fat (%fat) compared with Caucasians of the same sex and age (means and 95% confidence interval). Those groups above the line tend to have less fat for a given BMI value, while those below the line tend to have more. (Adapted with permission from Deurenberg et al., 1998.[16])

remains unclear, and it is not yet known if the healthy range of BMI should be redefined according to age.

Anthropologists have long recognized the marked variability in physique that exists between human populations. While all ethnic groups show a broadly similar pattern of ontogenetic development, studies now show that differences in body composition between populations are also apparent from birth. For example, low-birth-weight neonates born in India have similar fatness but reduced FFM compared with "normal" weight neonates born in the United Kingdom, as shown in Figure 5.[15] It is not yet established whether this represents a genetic trait characteristic of Asian populations, or whether it is a response to environmental factors, such as maternal physiology or nutrition, during pregnancy. During childhood, ethnic groups continue to show differences in the relative degree of adiposity for a given BMI value, and by adulthood these are seen as significant differences in the mean BMI for a given mean fat content[16] (Figure 6). Recognition of variability in the BMI-fatness relationship has led to the derivation of population-specific cutoffs for the categorization of adult overweight and obesity.[17]

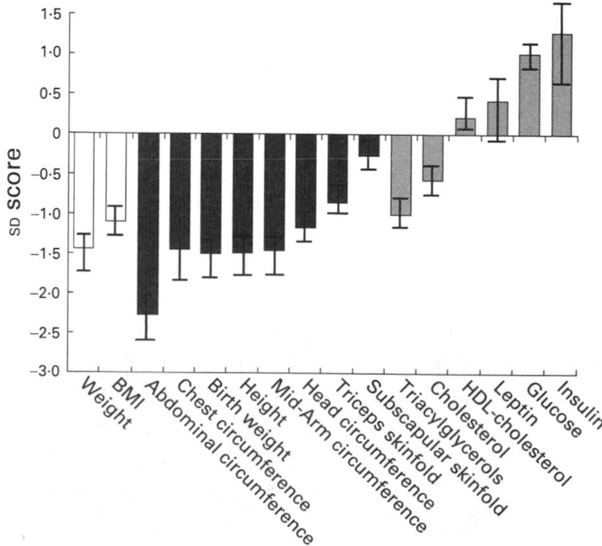


Figure 5. Differences in outcome between low birth-weight Indian neonates and normal birth-weight neonates from the UK. The Indian neonates have deficits in all anthropometric outcomes, but those for adiposity indices are smaller then those for lean mass indices. These body composition differences are associated with metabolic differences. (Used with permission from Yajnik, 2004.[15])

The significance of variability in body composition for health remains controversial, due to the lack of large, prospective studies. In cross-sectional studies, adiposity is positively associated (more so than BMI) with risk factors for cardiovascular disease, such as high blood pressure and plasma levels of cholesterol and glucose.[18] In a longitudinal study commencing at 60 years, BMI showed a U-shaped relationship with subsequent total mortality, whereas FM showed a linear relationship.[19] These findings suggest that low FFM is an independent risk factor for mortality, while also implicating fat as a "toxic" tissue with a dose-response association with adverse outcome. However, the difficulty with interpretation of such studies is that risk factors measured at earlier time points predict adverse outcome better than do current risk factors. This suggests that cardiovascular and related diseases have an "incubation period," and commence development from early in childhood.[20] Thus, the extent to which fat is toxic per se, as opposed to the extent to which it contributes disproportionately to adult diseases by influencing their development during childhood and adolescence, remains the subject of continued research.

What is clear is that central abdominal fat, in particular visceral fat, is most strongly implicated in poor health. Increases in waist circumference, which has been shown to be a good proxy for total abdominal FM, are associated with increased risk of premature death[21] and of increases in morbidity, especially the components of the metabolic syndrome.[22] Research in such areas is a major priority in the effort to reduce morbidity and mortality from the common lifestyle diseases. Lean mass has received less attention than fatness as a specific health outcome, but low levels of FFM have recently been shown to predict length of hospital stay in adults.[23]

# Programming of Body Composition

While much interest continues to be directed at factors long known to influence body composition (reviewed below), a relatively new research area is that of the developmental origins of adult diseases. A large volume of research on animals, supported increasingly by epidemiological and experimental work on humans, has demonstrated that environmental factors acting in early life exert long-term effects on many aspects of phenotype, particularly those relating to metabolism. Such associations are now investigated using the general concept of "programming" of phenotype during early "critical windows," with phenotypic variability that emerges during these windows then persisting or "tracking" subsequently. Fetal life and/or early infancy have been identified as important critical windows for many metabolic outcomes (such as blood pressure) and the risk of many diseases (such as hypertension), though the exact mechanisms whereby adult diseases are programmed remain unclear. For example, the relative importance of small size at birth versus postnatal growth rate (which is often greatest in those born small) for later disease risk is currently an area of controversy.

Body composition has particular importance for the concept of programming. First, body composition itself, including the likelihood of developing obesity, may be programmed during early critical windows. Second, the early development of body composition (during fetal life and infancy) may comprise a crucial component of the mechanism by which adult diseases are programmed. Our understanding of the programming of adult body composition has improved markedly now that outcomes more sophisticated than BMI are used. Many studies have reported positive associations between BMI at birth and in adolescence or adulthood,[24] which have often been interpreted as implying that fatter babies become fatter adults. Conversely, more recent studies have demonstrated clearly that variability in birth weight predicts variability in physique (size and regional or total FFM), but not in total FM, in later life.[25-27] Thus, it is now appreciated that bigger babies become adults with a relatively heavier physique.

It is less clear how early infant growth is related to later body composition. Several studies have found associations between rapid weight gain in the postnatal period and the subsequent likelihood of being categorized as obese.[28,29] Since most of these studies have used BMI as the outcome, it is possible once again that physique rather than fatness itself is being programmed. For example, in a study of Brazilian boys, weight gain in the first 6 months after birth was associated again with later FFM rather than FM, whereas from 1 year of age, weight gain was associated with later FM as well as FFM.[26] This study suggests that the period during which FFM is programmed by early growth extends beyond birth into early infancy, but the data require confirmation in other populations. However, these findings have major significance for our understanding of the early development of late-onset diseases. Whereas much attention has focused on the adverse effects of body fat for immediate and long-term health, the research on programming suggests that the ontogenetic development of FFM is also a critical component of the process by which such diseases develop.

Paradoxically, the above findings do not negate a relationship between fetal development and later adiposity. Whereas, overall, variability in birth weight is associated with variability in later physique, several studies have shown that low birth weight is associated with a greater tendency to central fat in later life.[30,31] It remains unclear how this association develops, but one study suggests that it may already be present at birth. In low-birth-weight Indian neonates, both central fatness and a reduction in FFM were apparent in the neonatal period,[15] and may simply track subsequently (Figure 5).

Studies increasingly demonstrate the tendency of body composition to track from infancy into early childhood[32] and from early to mid-childhood[33] and adulthood.[27] For example, Figure 7 illustrates the relationship between baseline and subsequent gain in FM in children over the period 4 to 9 years of age.[33] Those fattest at baseline gain substantially more fat in the following 5 years. However, while BMI continues to track into adolescence and adulthood, such associations may reflect the tracking of physique as well as, or instead of, FM. The onset of puberty reduces the strength of tracking in indices of fatness, espe-

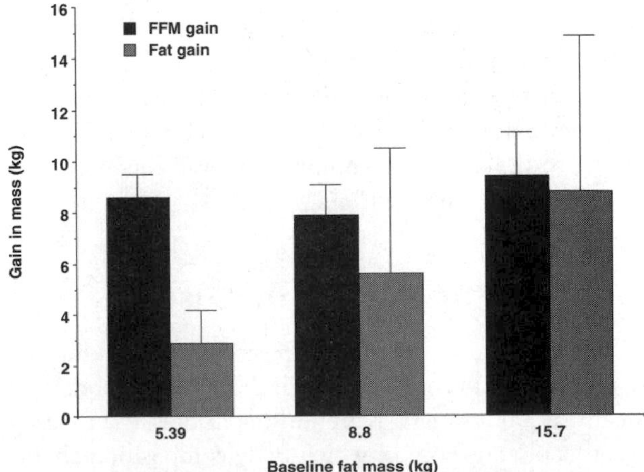


Figure 7. Relationship between fat mass at baseline and subsequent 5-year changes in both fat mass and fat-free mass in children initially 4 years of age. Whereas changes in fat-free mass are similar between the groups, those with highest baseline fatness gain three times the mass of fat as those with lowest baseline fatness. (Adapted from daa in Goulding et al., 2003.[33])

cially in boys. Although those with high BMI at 7 years are significantly more likely than their low-BMI peers to have high BMI in adulthood, there is a poorer relationship between childhood BMI and adult percentage fat.[34] Further studies are required to address this in greater detail, focusing on specific time periods, but will necessarily take time to come to maturity.

The early development of body composition has traditionally been one of the hardest issues to address, due to the lack of appropriate techniques and the vulnerability of the neonatal population. New data from MRI imaging studies show consistency with earlier cadaver analyses suggesting that neonates average around 17% adipose tissue at birth,[35] of which almost 90% is subcutaneous rather than internal. Of significance to the programming hypothesis, growth-retarded neonates have less subcutaneous fat, but similar intra-abdominal fat, as appropriately sized neonates,[36] while infants born preterm continue to have reduced total FM later in childhood.[37] These findings suggest that late gestation is an important window during which both total FM and its distribution are programmed, with potential implications for the subsequent risk of, and metabolic load exerted by, obesity.

Such research has renewed interest in the long-term significance of infant nutrition for later health, particularly in relationship to the development of obesity. Several studies, for example, have suggested that being breastfed has a protective effect against the risk of becoming obese in later life, although this relationship remains subject to debate. Research has also focused on how babies are fed, as well as what they are fed. The dynamics of infant feeding have been modeled as a signaling system operating under tension, whereby the infant signals its demand and the caregiver responds.[38] The interaction between signals and responses then determines net energy transfer to the infant, and hence weight gain. Consistent with this model, one study found that maternal rating of infant temperament at 12 weeks postpartum was strongly predictive of the child's fatness 3 years later.[39] More generally, there is increasing interest in the components of behavior that are associated with variability in infant and child growth and body composition, and therefore may be amenable to intervention.

## Body Composition in Disease

In the context of body composition, diseases may be divided for convenience into those in which abnormal weight is the primary symptom (as in obesity or eating disorders), and those in which body composition alterations, while being secondary to other symptoms, are nevertheless important for clinical outcome. While the first of these categories has been investigated for several decades, our understanding of the effects of most diseases and their treatment on body composition remains a relatively unexplored area. This area of research has long been hindered by the lack of access to technology appropriate for vulnerable patients yet sophisticated enough to address the marked changes that diseases often invoke in body properties and tissues.

Excess gain or loss of body weight influences both FM and FFM. Figure 8 illustrates the effect of increasing BMI on FM and its distribution in 47 adults; lean mass also increases.[40] Webster et al.[41] suggested as a rule of thumb that 75% of excess weight is fat, and the remainder FFM. In terms of overnutrition, this rule is relatively robust, such that the absolute mass of fat increases faster than that of lean mass with increasing weight gain. Paradoxically, this effect is typically concealed by expressing data in the form %fat, which increases much more slowly than FM.[4] Diet-induced weight loss is also broadly consistent with this rule, which allows equations based on weight and height to make reasonable predictions of the change in fatness during weight loss programs.[42] However, the addition of exercise to treatment alters the composition of weight loss due to its tendency to preserve or even increase lean mass.

Recent research has emphasized that obesity is associated with many more effects on body composition than increases in total tissue masses alone. First, the composition of FFM has been found to differ between obese and non-obese individuals.[43] Such differences include an increased hydration of FFM, generally attributed to expansion of the extracellular water pool, and a reduction in relative mineral mass. As absolute mineral mass is greater in the obese, it remains unclear as to whether there is simply a time lag in relative mineral mass catching up with the increased body weight. Second, obesity exerts

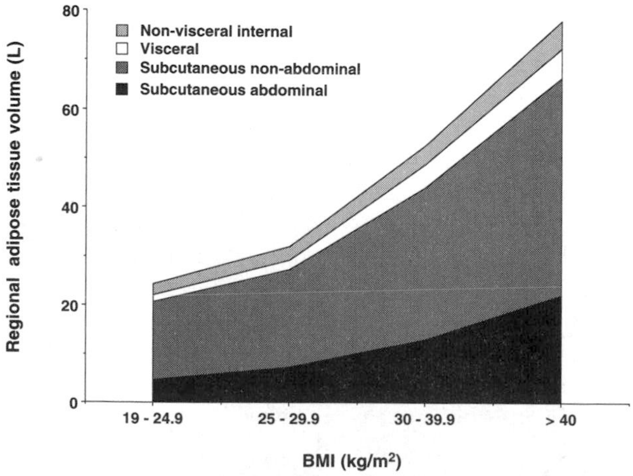


Figure 8. Relationship between body-mass index (BMI) and regional volumes of adipose tissue measured by magnetic resonance imaging (MRI) in 47 adults divided into four categories of BMI. Although in absolute terms, excess fat is disproportionately gained as subcutaneous fat, visceral fat is over three times greater in those fattest. Lean mass also increases with BMI, estimated at 40, 44, 46, and 50 kg in the four BMI groups. (Used with permission from Thomas et al., 1998.[40])

differential effects on body composition according to anatomical region. For example, a recent case-controlled study of childhood obesity suggested that, while excess FM was located disproportionately in the abdomen (similar to the data on adults shown in Figure 8), increased FFM was located in both the abdomen and the leg.[44] These findings demonstrate more generally that considerable caution is required when selecting techniques for measuring body composition in patients. All simpler approaches make assumptions about the composition or distribution of tissues on the basis of measurements in healthy subjects. Many diseases invoke changes in some tissue characteristics, thus negating the validity of these simpler approaches.

The effect of weight loss on regional adiposity can be demonstrated beneficially in the clinic using measurement of waist circumference, but more sophisticated methods such as MRI and CT scanners are required for differentiating between visceral and other depots of abdominal fat. Figure 9 shows regional changes in central FM and abdominal adipose tissue volumes during 6 months of weight loss invoked by a combination of dietary restriction and administration of the drug sibutramine.[45] Weight loss was substantially attributable to central fat depots, those most strongly associated with adverse health outcomes.

The effect of severe weight loss on body composition is more complex. Traditionally, clinicians have focused on low levels of body fat, due to the role of fat stores

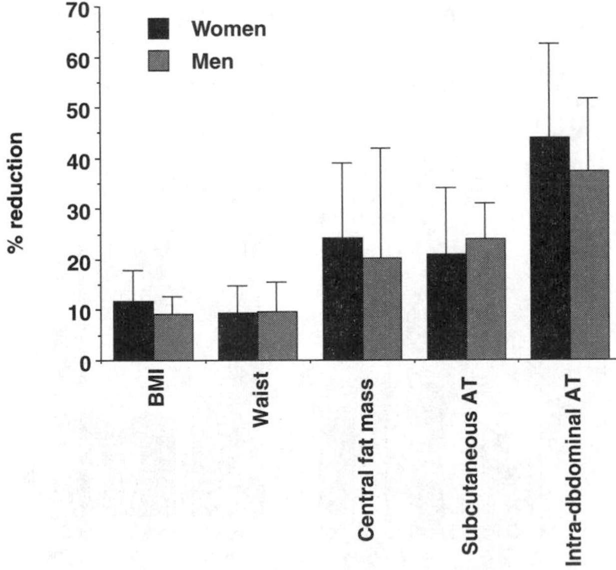


Figure 9. Regional changes in adipose tissue volume during 6 months of weight loss in 36 obese adults, measured by magnetic resonance imaging (MRI). Weight loss was invoked by a combination of dietary restriction and administration of the drug sibutramine. Central fat mass was measured by dual-energy X-ray absorptiometry (DEXA), and abdominal adipose tissue (subcutaneous and intra-abdominal) by MRI. The weight loss was dominated by loss of central fat, with visceral fat showing the greatest relative reduction. (Adapted from data in Kamel et al., 2000.[45])

in restoring reproductive function. However, a study of prepubertal children with eating disorders suggested that, expressed in standard deviation score format, loss of FFM was of the same magnitude as loss of FM.[46] Further studies on adults have estimated that when adolescent and young adult women with anorexia nervosa undergo refeeding, more than half of the weight gained is fat.[47] Both of these studies require confirmation using multicomponent models more capable of addressing the altered body properties in such patients, but they suggest that even in individuals with depleted FFM, rapid weight gain is dominated by increases in FM.

The effect of excess weight gain or loss on body composition is best quantified through measurements, but at least the broad trend is readily apparent to the clinician through measurement of body weight alone. In other disease states, unhealthy body composition may be concealed by apparently normal weight. For example, some patients of relatively normal weight may have high body fat content that is concealed by a low FFM. In an extreme case, two infants with congenital myasthenia had highly negative BMI standard deviation scores, but were around 40% fat. Conversely, a study of children with cancer showed that although they were malnourished according to measurements of arm anthropometry, this was concealed by their apparently normal weight, which could in turn be attributed to the contribution of solid tumors. Such findings are increasingly demonstrating the value to dietitians and clinicians of measuring body composition directly, and tailoring dietary requirements more appropriately.[48] As research emphasizes the importance of the childhood incubation period in the later development of lifestyle-caused diseases, it has become clear that body composition in young patients, even when not the primary disease symptom, does matter.

The most profound effects of illness on body composition, often involving perturbations of lean mass composition, are unfortunately those most difficult to study. Using a combination of methods, Plank et al.[49] were able to discern the changes in body water, protein, and FM that occurred in patients with peritonitis who developed major sepsis. While there was little change in FM, both body water and protein mass decreased substantially, including a 15% reduction in skeletal muscle mass but also a loss of visceral lean mass (Figure 10). This study highlights the limitation of crude approaches for detecting the effects of illness, and reinforces the need for continued development of methodologies appropriate for clinical care.

## Exercise and Body Composition

The reduced ratio of fat to lean in physically fit athletes is well established, although this relationship varies between different sports, especially in women. A related

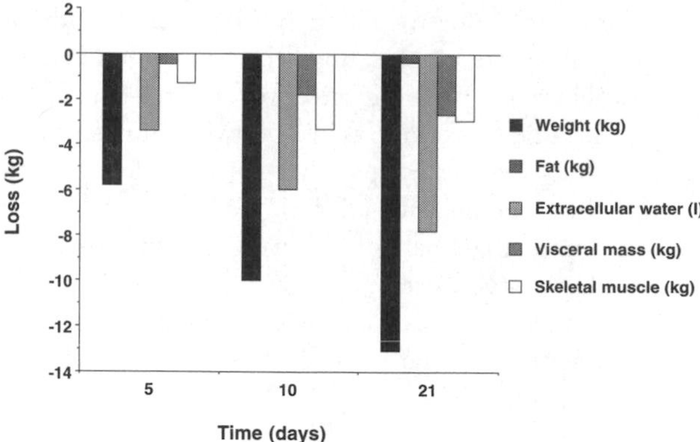


Figure 10. Changes in body weight, and various components, over 21 days in patients with peritonitis who developed secondary sepsis. Whereas fat stores declined negligibly on average (although variably between individuals), there was a major loss of protein from both skeletal muscle and visceral tissue masses. Extracellular water also decreased substantially over the same period in absolute terms, though the hydration of fat-free mass increased. (Used with permission from Plank et al., 1998.[49])

issue is that of somatotype, a categorization of both body composition and physique, which may influence the type of exercise or sport chosen by different individuals in the first place. Variation in the fat-to-lean ratio clearly reduces the capacity of BMI to discern cross-sectional variability, or longitudinal changes, in body composition in relation to exercise. In addition to its effects on body composition, exercise has been shown to reduce blood pressure, improve insulin sensitivity, and ameliorate dyslipidemia.[50] These changes in turn reduce the risk of many chronic diseases. However, it remains unclear whether such beneficial metabolic effects occur because of, or independently of, alterations in body composition.

The tendency of exercise to reduce body fat levels could imply that low physical activity levels are an important risk factor for the development of obesity. Such a relationship would have particular significance for children, given the difficulty in treating obesity once it has developed. However, the hypothesis that children are now less active than in previous generations has proven surprisingly difficult to confirm. Numerous studies have reported cross-sectional relationships between indices of physical activity and indices of body fatness, but cannot in themselves show whether those most inactive subsequently gain more fat. Furthermore, it is important to identify which factor affects the other. In a provocative study, Li et al.[51] showed that activity and body fatness were inversely related at each of three time points in infancy. However, whereas activity level at baseline did not predict subsequent fatness, baseline fatness did predict reduced activity level subsequently. The hypothesis that activity levels may be a function of body composition rather than vice versa requires confirmation in older populations. It might explain the tendency of body fat levels to track over time[27,32,33] in the absence of specific exercise interventions.

# Body Composition in Pregnancy

Interest in the changes in body composition occurring during pregnancy have long been of interest in relation to the energy requirements of pregnant women, but are now also attracting attention in the context of effects on offspring body composition and growth, and the programming of adult-onset diseases.

Until recently, World Health Organization (WHO) recommendations for energy requirements in pregnancy were based on an assumed average weight gain of 12.5 kg, including 925 g protein accretion and 3825 g fat accretion.[52] Such estimations involved many assumptions concerning the properties of body tissues during pregnancy, such as the hydration of FFM. New data, obtained with the more robust four-component model, show these previous calculations to have overestimated the proportions of protein and fat in weight gain and to have underestimated the proportion of water. Such research has led to a downward revision of the calculated energy requirements.[52]

With increasing interest in the early life programming of adult diseases, the body composition changes of pregnancy are also investigated in relation to offspring birth weight. Maternal gains in body water and FFM are related to birth weight, whereas maternal gain in FM is not.[53] The ideal weight gain has been revised slightly downwards, to 12 kg (range 10–14 kg), at which fetal and maternal complications appear to be minimized.[52]

Poor fetal growth is associated with inadequate expansion of maternal plasma volume. In this context, body composition analyses are beginning to contribute in a different way, by helping monitor hydration and appropriate expansion of plasma volume. Figure 11 shows a compari-

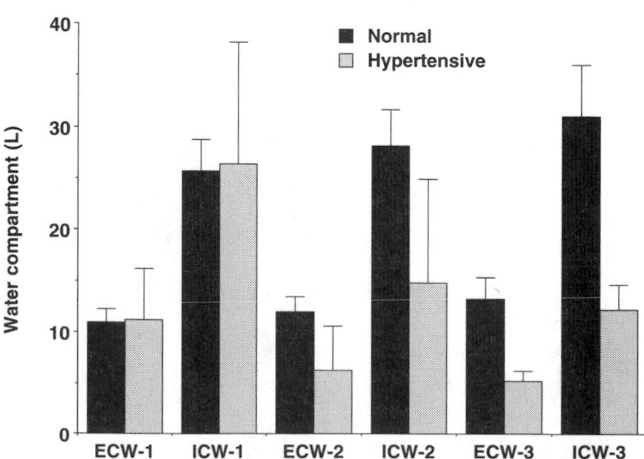


Figure 11. Changes in intracellular and extracellular water in groups of women with or without gestational hypertension in all three trimesters, estimated using multi-frequency bioelectrical impedance analysis. Whereas the healthy women retained significant water in both intracellular and extracellular compartments as pregnancy progressed, those with hypertension lost water from both compartments and failed to achieve expansion of plasma volume, which is required for optimal fetal growth. (Data from Valensise et al., 2000.[54])

son of changes in intracellular and extracellular water between groups of women with or without gestational hypertension.[54] The data show that both water pools steadily decreased through the three trimesters in the hypertensive mothers, suggesting a lack of plasma volume expansion due to insufficient fluid retention.

## Conclusion

Historically, much scientific interest in human body composition has been directed at the difficulty of measuring it. The most consistent interest from other scientific disciplines has come from those working on energetics, addressing both energy consumption (proportional to FFM) and energy stores (FM). Both of these research areas remain active, demonstrated, for example, by the continued development of methodologies able to probe ever more specific outcomes, and the exploration of the contribution of specific organs to total energy utilization. However, body composition is increasingly seen as an important health outcome in its own right. Research has demonstrated that from early life on, body composition has a significant impact on immediate and long-term health, and that it responds sensitively to environmental factors such as diet, exercise regime, and disease load. Furthermore, few metabolic outcomes can be interpreted meaningfully without taking body composition into account. Perhaps most importantly, we are finally seeing that body composition during childhood deserves particular attention in the drive to reduce the burden of adult diseases.

## References


1. Jebb SA, Elia M. Techniques for the measurement of body composition: a practical guide. Int J Obes Relat Metab Disord. 1993;17:611–621.
2. Heymsfield SB, Wang Z, Baumgartner RN, Ross R. Human body composition: advances in models and methods. Annu Rev Nutr. 1997;17:527–558.
3. Van Itallie TB, Yang M, Heymsfield SB, Funk RC, Boileau RA. Height-normalized indices of the body's fat-free and fat mass: potentially useful indicators of nutritional status. Am J Clin Nutr. 1990;52: 953–959.
4. Wells JCK, Victora CG. Indices of whole-body and central adiposity for evaluating the metabolic load of obesity. Int J Obes. 2005;29:483–489.
5. Hattori K, Tatsumi N, Tanaka S. Assessment of body composition by using a new chart method. Am J Hum Biol. 1997;9:573–578.
6. Cole TJ, Bellizzi MC, Flegal KM, Dietz WH. Establishing a standard definition for child overweight and obesity worldwide: international survey. BMJ. 2000;320:1240–1243.
7. Fomon SJ, Haschke F, Ziegler EE, Nelson SE. Body composition of reference children from birth to age 10 years. Am J Clin Nutr. 1982;35:1169–1175.
8. Wells JCK. A Hattori chart analysis of body mass index in infants and children. Int J Obes. 2000;24: 325–329.
9. Wells JCK, Coward WA, Cole TJ, Davies PSW. The contribution of fat and fat-free tissue to body mass index in contemporary children and the reference child. Int J Obes. 2002;26:1323–1328.
10. Moreno LA, Fleta J, Sarria A, Rodriguez G, Gil C, Bueno M. Secular changes in body fat patterning in children and adolescents of Zaragoza (Spain), 1980–1995. Int J Obes. 2001;25:1656–1660.
11. Haschke F. Body composition during adolescence. In: *98th Ross Conference on Pediatric Research, Body Composition in Infants and Children*. Columbus, OH: Ross Laboratories; 1989; 76–83.
12. Norgan NG. The beneficial effects of body fat and adipose tissue in humans. Int J Obes. 1997;21: 738–746.
13. Cohn SH. New concepts of body composition. In: Ellis KJ, Yasumura S, Morgan WD, eds. *In vivo Body Composition Studies*. New York: Plenum Press; 1987; 1–14.
14. Beaufrère B, Morio, B. fat and protein redistribution with aging: metabolic considerations. Eur J Clin Nutr. 2000;54(suppl 3):S48–S53.
15. Yajnik CS. Obesity epidemic in India: intrauterine origins? Proc Nutr Soc. 2004;63:387–396.
16. Deurenberg P, Yap M, van Staveren WA. Body mass index and percent body fat: a meta-analysis among different ethnic groups. Int J Obes. 1998;22: 1164–1171.
17. Wang J, Thornton JC, Russell M, et al. Asians have lower body mass index (BMI) but higher percent body fat than do whites: comparisons of anthropometric measurements. Am J Clin Nutr. 1994;60: 23–28.
18. Segal KR, Dunaif A, Gutin B, et al. Body composition, not body weight, is related to cardiovascular disease risk factors and sex hormones in men. J Clin Invest. 1987;80:1050–1055.
19. Heitmann BL, Erikson H, Ellsinger BM, et al. Mortality associated with body fat, fat-free mass and body mass index among 60 year old Swedish men: a 22 year follow-up study. Int J Obes. 2000;24:33–37.
20. Rose G. Incubation period of coronary heart disease. Int J Epidemiol. 2005;34:242–244.
21. Seidell JC, Andres R, Sorkin JD, Muller DC. The sagittal waist diameter and mortality in men: the Baltimore Longitudinal Study on Aging. Int J Obes. 1994;18:61–67.
22. Carey VJ, Walters EE, Colditz GA, et al. Body fat distribution and risk of non-insulin-dependent diabetes mellitus in women: The Nurses Health Study. Am J Epidemiol. 1997;145:614–619.
23. Pichard C, Kyle UG, Morabia A, Perrier A, Vermeu-

len B, Unger P. Nutritional assessment: lean body mass depletion at hospital admission is associated with an increased length of stay. Am J Clin Nutr. 2004;79:613–618.

24. Parsons TJ, Power C, Logan S, Summerbell CD. Childhood predictors of adult obesity: a systematic review. Int J Obes. 1999;23(suppl 8):S1–S107.
25. Hediger ML, Overpeck MD, Kuczmarski RJ, McGlynn A, Maurer KR, Davis WW. Muscularity and fatness of infants and young children born small- or large-for-gestational-age. Pediatrics. 1998;102: E60.
26. Wells JC, Hallal PC, Wright A, Singhal A, Victora CG. Fetal, infant and childhood growth: relationships with body composition in Brazilian boys aged 9 years. Int J Obes (Lond). 2005;29:1192–1198.
27. Sayer AA, Syddall HE, Dennison EM, Gilbody HJ, Duggleby SL, Cooper C, Barker DJ, Phillips DI. Birth weight, weight at 1 y of age, and body composition in older men: findings from the Hertfordshire Cohort Study. Am J Clin Nutr. 2004;80:199–203.
28. Stettler N, Zemel BS, Kumanyika S, Stallings VA. Infant weight gain and childhood overweight status in a multicenter, cohort study. Pediatrics. 2002;109: 194–199.
29. Ong KK, Ahmed ML, Emmett PM, Preece MA, Dunger DB. Association between postnatal catch-up growth and obesity in childhood: prospective cohort study. BMJ. 2000;320:967–971.
30. Malina RM, Katzmarzyk PT, Beuen G. Birth weight and its relationship to size attained and relative fat distribution at 7 to 12 years of age. Obes Res. 1996; 4:385–390.
31. Barker M, Robinson S, Osmond C, Barker DJ. Birth weight and body fat distribution in adolescent girls. Arch Dis Child. 1997;77:381–383.
32. Wells JCK, Stanley M, Laidlaw AS, Day JME, Davies PSW. The relationship between components of infant energy expenditure and childhood body fatness. Int J Obes. 1996;20:848–853.
33. Goulding A, Taylor RW, Jones IE, Lewis-Barned NJ, Williams SM Body composition of 4- and 5-year-old New Zealand girls: a DXA study of initial adiposity and subsequent 4-year fat change. Int J Obes. 2003;27:410–415.
34. Wright CM, Parker L, Lamont D, Craft AW. Implications of childhood obesity for adult health: findings from thousand families cohort study. BMJ. 2001;323:1280–1284.
35. Harrington TA, Thomas EL, Modi N, Frost G, Coutts GA, Bell JD. Fast and reproducible method for the direct quantitation of adipose tissue in newborn infants. Lipids. 2002;37:95–100.
36. Harrington TAM, Thomas EL, Frost G, Modi N, Bell JD. Distribution of adipose tissue in the newborn. Pediatr Res. 2004;55:437–441.
37. Fewtrell MS, Lucas A, Cole TJ, Wells JCK. Body composition of 8–12 year old children born preterm or term. Am J Clin Nutr. 2004;80:436–440.
38. Wells JCK. Parent-offspring conflict theory, signaling of need, and weight gain in early life. Q Rev Biol. 2003;78:169–202.
39. Wells JCK, Stanley M, Laidlaw AS, Day JME, Stafford M, Davies PS. Investigation of the relationship between infant temperament and later body composition. Int J Obes. 1997;21:400–406.
40. Thomas EL, Saeed N, Hajnal JV, Brynes A, Goldstone AP, Frost G, Bell JD. Magnetic resonance imaging of total body fat. J Appl Physiol. 1998;85: 1778–1785.
41. Webster J, Hesp R, Garrow J. The composition of excess weight in obese women estimated by body density, total body water and total body potassium. Hum Nutr Clin Nutr. 1984;38C:299–306.
42. Garrow JS, Summerbell CD. Meta-analysis: effect of exercise, with or without dieting, on the body composition of overweight subjects. Eur J Clin Nutr. 1995;49:1–10.
43. Haroun D, Wells JC, Williams JE, Fuller NJ, Fewtrell MS, Lawson MS. Composition of the fat-free mass in obese and nonobese children: matched case-control analyses. Int J Obes. 2005;29:29–36.
44. Wells JCK, Fewtrell MS, William JE, Haroun D, Lawson MS, Cole TJ. Body composition in normal weight, overweight and obese children: matched case-control analyses of total and regional tissue masses, and body composition trade in relation to relative weight. Int J Obes. 2006-in press.
45. Kamel EG, McNeill G, Van Wijk MC. Change in intra-abdominal adipose tissue volume during weight loss in obese men and women: correlation between magnetic resonance imaging and anthropometric measurements. Int J Obes. 2000;24:607–613.
46. Nicholls D, Wells JC, Singhal A, Stanhope R. Body composition in early onset eating disorders. Eur J Clin Nutr. 2000;56:857–865.
47. Probst M, Goris M, Vandereycken W, Van Coppenolle H. Body composition of anorexia nervosa patients assessed by underwater weighing and skinfold-thickness measurements before and after weight gain. Am J Clin Nutr. 2001;73:190–197.
48. Wells JCK. Body composition in childhood: effects of normal growth and disease. Proc Nutr Soc. 2003; 62:521–528.
49. Plank LD, Connolly AB, Hill GL. Sequential changes in the metabolic response in severely septic patients during the first 23 days after the onset of peritonitis. Ann Surg. 1998;228:146–158.
50. Eriksson J, Taimela S, Koivisto VA. Exercise and the metabolic syndrome. Diabetologia. 1997;40: 125–135.

51. Li R, O'Connor L, Buckley D, Specker B. Relation of activity levels to body fat in infants 6 to 12 months of age. J Pediatr. 1995;126:353–357.
52. Food and Agriculture Organization of the United Nations. *Human Energy Requirements. Report of a Joint FAO/WHO/UNU Expert Consultation. FAO Food and Nutrition Technical Report Series 1*. Rome: United Nations University, World Health Organization; 2004.
53. Butte NF, Ellis KJ, Wong WW, Hopkinson JM, Smith EO. Composition of gestational weight gain impacts maternal fat retention and infant birth weight. Am J Obstet Gynecol. 2003;189:1423–1432.
54. Valensise H, Andreloi A, Lello S, Magnani F, Romanini C, De Lorenzo A. Multifrequency bioelectrical impedance analysis in women with a normal and hypertensive pregnancy. Am J Clin Nutr. 2000;72:780–783.

# 3 Exercise

Wayne W. Campbell

## Introduction

From a developing fetus, to a growing child building strong muscles and bones, to an elite athlete rigorously training for competition, to a middle-aged person working to prevent or treat obesity, to an elderly person attempting to cope with physical frailty, exercise and nutrition may be used as tools to independently and interactively impact how the human body functions and maintains health. The potential topics within the scope of nutrition and exercise are vast. Resources such as the July/August 2004 issue of the journal *Nutrition*, which captured the spirit of the 2004 Olympics in Athens by publishing articles on nutritional supplements (e.g., substrates, vitamins, mineral, other substances, and fluids) and nutritional concerns of selected groups of active people (older competitors, children, adolescents, and athletes with anorexia athletica) are timely and may be of interest to readers. This brief, non-comprehensive review is written to highlight the integration of nutrition and exercise on energy balance and weight control, especially with regard to how much exercise is needed to help people sustain a desirable body weight and whether exercise affects appetite and food intake. The potential impact of diet on nutrient intakes and physical performance is also presented, using vegetarian versus omnivorous diets as the example.

## Energy Balance

Energy balance is the equilibrium between total energy intake (TEI) and total energy expenditure (TEE) that is necessary to maintain constant body weight. On a daily basis, differences between TEI and TEE may be several hundred kcal; however, over weeks or months, most adults balance TEI and TEE within a 2% cumulative error and maintain body weight (fat mass) within ±1 to 2 kg per year.[1] A person's TEE is the sum of the basal/resting energy expenditure (BEE and REE, respectively), the thermic effect of feeding, the energy expenditure of physical activity, and the non-exercise activity thermogenesis.[1] The terms "basal" and "resting" are often used interchangeably to describe a person's energy expenditure at rest, but there are important distinctions between the two terms. BEE describes a person's energy expenditure during standardized conditions that minimize the effects of sleep, food, and physical activity (12- to 14-h overnight fast, awake, early morning, resting supine, thermo-neutral environment). Resting energy expenditure is a broader term that applies to any "resting" state. Compared with BEE, a person's REE may be lower (e.g., during sleep), the same, or higher (e.g., after eating, after exercise, or in the afternoon or evening hours). The thermic effect of feeding is the postprandial energy expenditure necessary to digest, absorb, utilize, and store macronutrients. It is estimated to be about 10% of energy intake for mixed meals (0%–5% for fat, 5%–10% for carbohydrate, and 20%–30% for protein). Energy expenditure of physical activity is the amount of energy expended above REE during purposeful physical activities or exercise. The initiation of an intensive exercise program[2] and habitual exercise training[3,4] are known to increase a person's TEE. Non-exercise activity thermogenesis is the energy expenditure beyond BEE, thermic effect of feeding, and energy expenditure of physical activity. It includes the energy expended to perform daily activities (getting out of bed, rising from a chair, walking from room to room, etc.) and random motions (fidgeting)—basically, the energy expenditure of activities other than purposeful exercise.[5]

The Food and Nutrition Board of the National Institute of Medicine (FNB-IOM) defines the Estimated Energy Requirement as "the dietary energy intake that is predicted to maintain energy balance in a healthy adult of a defined age, gender, weight, height, and level of physical activity consistent with good health."[1] This definition applies to the general population and athletes alike, with the understanding that a highly physically active person is likely to need to consume more dietary energy than a less active or sedentary person. For many athletes who participate in intensive training, adequate dietary energy must be consumed to offset high levels of exercise-induced energy expenditure, maintain body weight and health, and maximize training effects.[6] The inability of athletes to consume adequate energy might increase the risks of fatigue, injury, and illness, result in bone and muscle losses, and cause young women to experience menstrual dysfunction.[6] The FNB-IOM report[1] on human energy requirements provides a comprehensive description of the impact of physical activity and exercise on energy expenditure. Physical activity may be defined as muscle contraction-induced movement of the body that significantly increases energy expenditure. Exercise (exercise training) is purposeful, structured physical activity performed to maintain or improve some component of health and (or) physical fitness. The energy expenditure of physical activity is the most variable component of a person's TEE and a component that can be purposefully manipulated. It is estimated to account for about 10%, 25%, 33%, and 42% of TEE for adults who are sedentary, low active, active, and very active, respectively.[1] These percentages are comparable for adult men and women who are normal weight and those who are overweight.

Similar to younger athletes, the energy requirement of older athletes is determined by several factors, including exercise mode, intensity, and duration, and body composition. While older athletes may require less dietary energy than younger athletes, their energy needs are higher than age-matched sedentary persons.[3] The decreased dietary energy needs of older versus younger athletes might be attributed to age-associated declines in the volume of training, non-exercise activity thermogenesis, fat-free mass, and REE.[7,8] Declines in REE and dietary energy requirements were not reported for older athletes whose exercise training volumes were comparable to younger athletes.[8] The initiation of endurance[3,9] or resistance[10] training programs did not increase the energy requirement of previously sedentary older people during the first few months of training. These findings suggest that older people who begin a training program may adopt more sedentary behaviors during the rest of the day; the initiation of an exercise program is not a license for older persons to increase their energy intake without monitoring body weight.

For most adults, the challenge is to effectively balance energy intake and energy expenditure to avoid weight gain and obesity. Unfortunately, a majority of people in the United States have not successfully achieved a healthy weight. Among adults ≥20 years of age in the years 1999 to 2002, 65.1% were overweight or obese with a body mass index (BMI) ≥ 25.0 kg/m$^2$, 30.4% were obese (BMI ≥ 30.0 kg/m$^2$), and 4.9% were extremely obese (BMI ≥ 40 kg/m$^2$).[11] The prevalence of overweight or obesity exceeded 50% for almost every age and racial/ethnic group (20- to 39-year-old non-Hispanic white women were the lone exception, at 49.0%). Only 33.0% of adults had a healthy weight (BMI 18.5–24.9 kg/m$^2$).

## How Much Exercise Is Needed?

Table 1 presents a listing of recommended levels of physical activity and exercise from various US government and national organizations during the past decade. This list is provided to underscore the importance of exercise for health and to highlight the rapid and profound increase in the amount of exercise recommended for people to regularly perform.

In 1996, the US Surgeon General's report on physical activity and health[12] provided a foundation for the understanding that regular, preferably daily, performance of moderate-level endurance-type physical activity would reduce the risks of developing chronic diseases for most adults. The recommendation for a minimum of 30 min/d of moderate physical activity was made with the explicit recognition that greater amounts of physical activity (increased intensity and duration) could result in greater health benefits, and that strength or resistance exercise also promotes health. People were encouraged to accumulate at least 30 minutes of physical activities into their daily lives by whatever means possible (e.g., walking, gardening, team sports). The health benefits of adopting a more physically active lifestyle include reduced risks of cardiovascular disease, coronary heart disease, hypertension, certain types of cancer, type 2 diabetes mellitus, osteoarthritis, osteoporosis, falling, depression, anxiety, poor psychological well-being, and mortality.

Unfortunately, the majority of the United States population over the age of 18 years living in the 50 states, the District of Columbia, Guam, Puerto Rico, and the US Virgin Islands do not engage in sufficient physical activities to meet this minimum goal. Results from the 2003 Behavioral Risk Factor Surveillance System telephone survey indicated that, nationwide, 24.5% of the population performed no leisure-time physical activity (e.g. running, calisthenics, golf, gardening, or walking), 15.6% were inactive (less than 10 min/week of moderate or vigorous-intensity activities), and 38.4% performed insufficient physical activities (over 10 min/week, but less than recommended amounts of moderate- or vigorous-intensity activities).[13] Only 45.9% of the population performed the recommended levels of physical activities (at least 30 min/d of moderate-intensity activities at least 5 d/week or at least ≥20 min/d of vigorous activities at least 3 d/week). The prevalence of recommended physical activity was highest (>55%) in the northwest (Alaska, Idaho, Montana, Utah, and Wyoming) and northeast (Vermont), and lowest (<40%) in the southeast (Kentucky, Louisiana, North Carolina, and Tennessee), Puerto Rico, and the Virgin Islands.

The 1996 Surgeon General's report[12] also acknowledged that low levels of physical activity may contribute

**Table 1.** Exercise Recommendations for Adults

| Year | Agency | Health Focus | Activity/Exercise Recommendation |
|---|---|---|---|
| 1996 | US Department of Health and Human Services, Centers for Disease Control and Prevention, National Center for Chronic Disease Prevention and Health Promotion[12] | Health promotion and disease prevention: *Physical Activity and Health: A Report of the Surgeon General* | 30–45 min/d of moderate intensity aerobic physical activity, preferably daily; longer exercise duration and greater intensity may increase health benefits |
| 2000 | US Department of Agriculture and US Department of Health and Human Services[15] | Health promotion and disease prevention: *2000 Dietary Guidelines for Americans* | At least 30 min/d of moderate-intensity aerobic and strength/flexibility physical activity, preferably daily |
| 2001 | US Department of Health and Human Services, Public Health Service, Office of the Surgeon General[14] | Prevention and treatment of overweight and obesity: *The Surgeon General's Call to Action to Prevent and Decrease Overweight and Obesity* | 30–45 min/d of moderate intensity aerobic and strength/flexibility physical activity, preferably daily; longer exercise duration and greater intensity may increase health benefits |
| 2002 | Food and Nutrition Board of the Institute of Medicine[1] | Health promotion, disease prevention, and weight control: *Dietary Reference Intakes for Energy, Carbohydrate, Fiber, Fat, Fatty Acids, Cholesterol, Protein, and Amino Acids (Macronutrients)* | 60 min/d of moderate-intensity physical activity and exercise |
| 2005 | U.S. Department of Agriculture, Agriculture Research Service, Dietary Guidelines Advisory Committee[17] | Health promotion, disease prevention, and weight control: *2005 Dietary Guidelines for Americans* | At least 30 min/d of moderate-intensity aerobic and strength/flexibility physical activity, preferably daily for health promotion; 60 min/d moderate- to vigorous-intensity activity for prevention of weight gain; 60–90 min/d moderate-intensity activity for prevention of weight regain after weight loss |

to an imbalance between energy expenditure and intake, resulting in increased body fat, body weight, and the prevalence of obesity. The Surgeon General's 2001 "Call to Action to Prevent and Decrease Overweight and Obesity"[14] identified the obesity epidemic as a major national health challenge, and strongly encouraged individuals, families, communities, schools, workplaces, organizations, and the media to work together to identify, promote, adopt, and sustain healthy lifestyles. This "call to action" emphasized that obesity prevention and treatment programs should include the habitual consumption of a healthy diet and regular physical activity, consistent with the 2000 Dietary Guidelines for Americans.[15] The physical activity recommendations set forth by the 2000 Dietary Guidelines for Americans[15] were consistent with the 1996 Surgeon General recommendations[12] for adults and children to strive to accumulate at least 30 and 60 minutes, respectively, of moderate physical activity on most, preferably all, days of the week. The 2000 Dietary Guidelines for Americans recommendations for physical activity underscored the benefits of including both aerobic and strength/flexibility activities for overall health. Regarding weight control, the 2000 Dietary Guidelines for Americans noted that physical activity may help people who have lost weight maintain the weight loss. However, it was acknowledged that the minimum recommendation of 30 minutes of daily activity might be insufficient to promote weight loss or prevent weight regain. The apparent inconsistency of the 2001 Surgeon General's call to action[14] on obesity to encourage people to follow the 2000 Dietary Guidelines for Americans[15] recommendations for physical activity when this amount of activity was likely inadequate to positively impact weight control is striking.

The 2002 FNB-IOM panel on energy, macronutrients, and physical activity[1] suggested that both adults and children should obtain 60 min/d of physical activity and exercise for health promotion, disease prevention, and body weight control. This report identified several issues that warrant emphasis. An individual's attainment of an "active" lifestyle, which corresponds to a physical activity level (the ratio of TEE to BEE) over 1.6, will very likely require both physical activity and exercise. Exercise was defined as a "planned, structured, and repetitive bodily movement done to promote or maintain one or more components of physical fitness," with physical fitness defined as "a set of attributes that people have that relates to the ability to perform physical activity."[1] Walking briskly for 60 minutes at 4 miles per hour, the criterion for moderate-intensity activity, would theoretically raise an otherwise sedentary person's level of activity from the sedentary category (physical activity level 1.0–1.4) to the low-activity category (physical activity level 1.4–1.6), while extending the brisk walk for more than one hour would raise the person's level of activity into the active category (physical activity level 1.6–1.9). Similar to previous exercise recommendations,[12,14,15] the FNB-IOM panel[1] emphasized that the concept of "accumulated" or "intermittent" physical activity (i.e., a combination of low, moderate, and vigorous physical activities performed throughout the day) determines a person's overall activity level. This concept is central to providing reasonable, achievable, and sustainable exercise recommendations, especially with regard to weight control.[16]

The 2005 Dietary Guidelines for Americans[17] reinforces the health benefits of at least 30 min/d of moderate physical activity and the need for many adults to exercise up to 60 min/d on most days of the week and to include vigorous physical activity (e.g., jogging and other aerobic exercise) and resistance exercise training for fitness and body weight control. The 2005 Dietary Guidelines Advisory Committee also recommended that to avoid weight regain, adults who achieved weight loss might need to accumulate 60 to 90 min/d of moderate-intensity physical activity. This recommendation is supported by cross-sectional data from the National Weight Control Registry (NWCR)[18,19] and results from observational studies and randomized clinical interventions.[20] It is also fully consistent with the consensus statement of The International Association for the Study of Obesity 1$^{st}$ Stock Conference.[21]

The NWCR is a longitudinal prospective study of men and women ages 18 years and older who have achieved over a 30-pound weight loss and maintained the loss for over one year. As of August 2005, the registry included approximately 4500 individuals. While the approaches used by the NWCR subjects to achieve weight loss varied widely, the vast majority of individuals (89%) modified both diet and exercise practices.[18] Successful weight loss maintenance, defined as maintaining an intentional 10% weight loss for at least one year, typically included eating a lower-fat, higher-carbohydrate diet, frequent self-monitoring, and regular physical activity. Walking was the most common form of exercise performed (77% of NWCR subjects), followed by cycling (21%), weight lifting (20%), aerobics (18%), running (11%), and stair climbing (9%) (18). Only 9% of NWCR registrants reported successful weight loss maintenance without regular physical activity. The average energy expenditure of physical activity was 2545 kcal/week for women and 3293 kcal/week for men,[19] which is consistent with performing moderate-intensity physical activity for 60 to 90 min/d.[17,18]

Data from a 12-month diet and exercise intervention study highlight the challenges to accurately identify the amount of exercise needed for weight control. To examine the effects of the duration and intensity of aerobic exercise on weight loss, 196 young, overweight and obese women (age range 21–40 years; body mass index range 27–40 kg/m$^2$) were randomly assigned to one of four groups.[22] The women in the four groups were instructed to exercise 5 d/week at intensities/durations that were classified as vigorous/high, moderate/high, vigorous/moderate, and moderate/moderate. The exercise sessions were not supervised, but each participant was provided a motorized treadmill and walking was the primary mode of exercise (~88% of exercise sessions). All women also participated in a social cognitive theory-based behavioral change program and a semi-controlled diet program (meal plans provided and weekly food diaries recorded) with recommended energy intakes of 1200 to 1500 kcal/d and fat intakes of 20% to 30% of TEI. All four groups of women lost weight during the first 6 months of the intervention and sustained the weight loss during the next 6 months. From baseline to month 12, mean weight losses of the vigorous intensity/high duration, moderate intensity/high duration, vigorous intensity/moderate duration, and moderate intensity/moderate duration groups were 8.9 ± 7.3 kg (mean ± SD; 10.0%), 8.2 ± 7.6 kg, (9.4%), 7.0 ± 6.4 kg (7.8%), and 6.3 ± 5.6 kg (7.3%), respectively. While all four groups lost weight, there was no statistically significant difference in response among groups, suggesting that neither the intensity nor the duration of exercise was an influence. All four groups achieved comparable reduced energy intake during the 12-month intervention period (range of group means: baseline = 2022 – 2200 kcal/d; 6-month = 1438 – 1533 kcal/d; and 12-month = 1350 – 1557 kcal/d). The authors commented that the apparent lack of effects of exercise intensity and duration on weight loss may relate to these factors not resulting in differences in TEE, as well as the strong influence of diet (TEI) on body weight control. While not directly addressed by the authors, the lack of continued weight loss from months 6 to 12, despite continued exercise and dietary energy restriction, suggests that other unmeasured factors influenced the control of body weight. It is important to note that while these subjects did not continue to lose weight from 6 to 12 months, weight was not regained.

After the clinical phase of the study was completed, the body weight change data were analyzed based on the amount of moderate or higher activity each subject reported completing.[22] The groupings were as follows: 1) <150 min/week at 6 and 12 months; 2) ≥150 min/week at month 6 and <150 min/week at month 12; 3) ≥150 min/week at 6 and 12 months; and 4) ≥200 min/week at 6 and 12 months. At month 12, weight loss was greater for group 4, compared with groups 1 and 2, with the weight loss of group 3 not different than any of the other groups. Collectively, these results support that overweight and obese women can successfully lose about 10% of their body weight during a year-long program that combines behavior-change strategies and moderate dietary energy restriction with 150 min/week or more moderate to vigorous exercise. Further, the performance of ≥200 min/week of moderate-intensity exercise, consistent with the FNB-IOM recommendation of 60 min/d,[1] will enhance weight loss over 12 months.

# Exercise and Appetite

Energy balance and the maintenance of body weight are simplistically described as the matching of TEI and TEE. It could be presumed then, that an exercise-induced increase in energy expenditure would stimulate a compensatory increase in energy intake, which would promote body weight stability. If true, this would limit the usefulness of exercise as a tool for weight loss. However, the majority of research does not support this paradigm. In a 1999 review, Blundell and King[23] noted that among 27 short-term (1 to 10 d), 6 medium-term (2 to 8 weeks), and 15 longer-term (2 to 12 months) studies in which energy expenditure was purposefully raised by increasing physical activity in lean, overweight, and obese subjects, the authors of 31 studies (64%) reported no change in energy intake, 9 (19%) reported an increase, and 8 (17%) reported a decrease. Among 27 correlation studies, the authors of 15 studies (56%) reported a positive relationship between energy expenditure and energy intake, and 12 studies (44%) showed no relationship. Collectively, these results support that there is a "rather weak coupling between activity-induced [energy expenditure] and [energy intake]."[23] The authors further speculated that this weak coupling may result in part because eating is a behavior-driven event that is maintained by well-established, long-term environmental factors (i.e., eating patterns), and postprandial physiological responses that are not easily changed by short-term adjustments in energy expenditure.

The lack of strong coupling between energy expenditure and energy intake may be important for people who want to lose or maintain body weight. Indeed, exercise may provide a more effective means of inducing a short-term energy deficit than acutely limiting food intake (e.g., eating a very low-energy meal or skipping a meal). This point is demonstrated in a study designed to assess the effects of acute energy deficits induced by exercise or reduced energy intake on appetite and subsequent food intake.[24] Eleven healthy, lean, young adult women who exercised regularly, did not smoke, and were unrestrained eaters, participated in a four-trial, repeated-measures design protocol. On four occasions, each woman came to the lab in a fasting state, completed a 40-minute period of exercise (cycling at 70% $VO_{2max}$) or rest, and then consumed a high-energy (500 kcal) or low-energy (64 kcal) breakfast meal. Thus, the four trials were: 1) exercise, high-energy breakfast; 2) exercise, low-energy breakfast; 3) rest, high-energy breakfast; and 4) rest, low-energy breakfast. The mean energy expenditure due to exercise was 317 kcal. Energy intake at the next eating occasion (lunch provided ad libitum 4 hours later) was about 120 kcal (20%) higher on the days the women consumed the low-energy breakfast, a finding consistent with a partial dietary compensation response. The performance of exercise did not influence lunchtime energy intake during either the low-energy or high-energy breakfast days (dinner-time energy intake was not measured). Consumption of the low-energy breakfast significantly increased perceptions of hunger during the morning, as well as hunger, preoccupation with food, and the frequency and strength of cravings to eat particular foods during the late afternoon hours. Exercise did not influence these responses. These results show an apparent lack of short-term coupling between exercise-induced energy expenditure and energy intake, and suggest that exercise may be used as an effective tool for body weight reduction and control.

The intensity of exercise may impact a person's perceived appetite and food intake, and thus may be an important factor to consider when incorporating exercise into a body weight control program. Very intense exercise is documented to decrease hunger for up to one hour immediately after exercise, a phenomena termed the "anorexia of exercise." Speculation exists that the anorexia of exercise is somehow related to the re-distribution of blood flow towards the muscles and away from the splanchnic (viscera) region.[25] Low- and moderate-intensity exercises do not elicit this transient appetite suppression response. Recent research also supports that the intensity of exercise might influence short-term energy intake and energy balance. For example, research with 13 healthy, physically active, young adult women showed that the women consumed 127 kcal (17%) more energy at lunch on a day they performed high-intensity exercise (treadmill walking for 37 minutes at ~70% of $VO_{2peak}$) than when they remained sedentary (i.e., rested for the same amount of time they performed exercise).[26] In contrast, energy intake at lunch was not significantly different (+68 kcal, 9%) when the women performed low-intensity exercise (treadmill walking for 65 minutes at ~40% of $VO_{2peak}$). The finding of increased energy intake after the high-intensity exercise contrasted with their expectation to observe an acute anorexia of exercise. It may be important that the subjects were provided lunch one hour after finishing exercise, a period of time beyond which the anorexia of exercise typically occurs. Potential differences in post-exercise appetite responses between women and men (the subjects originally used to establish the anorexia of exercise phenomena) cannot be ruled out.

While TEI at lunch was higher after high-intensity exercise, the net energy intake (post-exercise energy intake corrected for energy expenditure of physical activity) was lower after both high-intensity (a decrease of 186 kcal or 25%) and low-intensity (a decrease of 220 kcal or 29%) exercise, findings that are consistent with an incomplete short-term dietary compensation to exercise. However, during the afternoon, the women tended to consume more snacks on the high-intensity exercise day (an increase of 174 kcal or 20%) compared with the rest day, and total and net daily energy intakes were not significantly different among the trials. Indeed, daily TEI tended to be higher on the high-intensity exercise day than on the sedentary day (an increase of 295 kcal or 13%). Indices of appetite (hunger, fullness, desire to eat, and prospective food consumption) measured periodically throughout the day were not influenced by either high or low-intensity exercise. Collectively, these data suggest that young women may experience dietary compensation to offset an acute exercise-induced energy deficit, especially after high-intensity exercise. The authors[26] emphasized the need for more research to document potential sex-related differences in appetite and longer-term energy balance and body weight responses to variable intensity exercise programs. This need is underscored by recent observations that dietary compensation responses to different intensities of exercise by men and women are variable, and that some people are "compensators" (they increase energy intake with exercise) and others "non-compensators" (they do not change energy intake with exercise).[25] It has been speculated that the extent of dietary compensation to exercise (i.e., the lack of or delayed compensation) may relate to the more immediate need to consume fluids to offset dehydration and maintain fluid balance, which is more tightly controlled than energy balance.[25] The potential for a preferential drive to consume fluids post-exercise to influence dietary compensation raises intriguing questions regarding the use of sports beverages with and without energy. More broadly, it also brings into question how the physical form of a post-exercise snack or meal influences dietary compensation. Foods consumed as fluids are documented to elicit a weaker dietary compensation response than foods consumed as solids.[27] The interactions among exercise, the physical form of food, and dietary compensation are undocumented.

Given that the majority of adults in the United States do not perform the minimal recommended amount of exercise and that about 65% are overweight or obese, it is important to understand the influence of decreased physical activity on appetite, energy balance, and body weight control. To address the question of whether difference levels of physical activity (within the normal range for Western adults) affect appetite and energy balance, a strictly controlled energy balance experiment was conducted in six young, healthy, normal-weight men who were willing to be housed continuously in a whole-body indirect calorimeter for two 7-d periods.[28] During one period, TEE was maintained at 1.4 times REE (sedentary) and during the other period at 1.8 times REE (active). The different levels of TEE (sedentary = 2330 kcal/d, 1.4 ± 0.1 times REE; active = 3052 kcal/d, 1.8 ± 0.2 times REE) were achieved by having the subjects exercise for different amounts of time and intensities on a cycle ergometer placed inside the calorimeter chamber. While inside the chamber, the subjects were allowed to consume ad libitum foods that had overall energy and macronutrient contents of 131 kcal/100 g wet weight, and 40%, 13%, and 47% of energy from carbohydrate, protein, and fat, respectively. TEIs were not different between groups (sedentary = 3227 kcal/d, 2.0 ± 0.1 times REE; active = 3442 kcal/d, 2.1 ± 0.5 times REE), were higher then TEE, and resulted in a progressively more positive energy balance (TEI minus TEE) during the 7-d periods inside the chamber. The 7-d cumulative positive energy balance was significantly greater for the sedentary versus active periods, and was primarily due to a greater positive fat balance during the sedentary period. During the active period, 11%, 12%, and 7% of the energy, fat, and carbohydrate ingested, respectively, were retained in the body. In contrast, 28%, 50%, and 5% of energy, fat, and carbohydrate ingested were retained during the sedentary period. Changes in body weight from d 1 to d 7 were 0.90 and 0.66 kg for the sedentary and active periods, respectively (no significant difference between periods), values that were very close to the expected weight changes based on measured positive energy balances (approximately 1.0 and 0.4 kg, respectively). No differences in daily appetite perceptions (hunger, fullness, desire to eat, prospective consumption, preoccupation with thoughts of food, and urge to eat) were reported between the sedentary and active periods. These data show that differences in energy expenditure do not result in short-term adjustments in appetite and energy intake. The increased positive energy balance achieved during the sedentary period implicates a sedentary lifestyle as an import factor contributing to weight gain among Western adults. The authors acknowledge that results from studies performed in calorimeter chambers should be translated to free-living conditions with caution and these findings may not be applicable to groups of people who are not young, healthy, normal-weight men.

While in the short term, energy intake and energy expenditure are not closely coupled, and an increase in energy expenditure will promote weight loss, this negative energy balance cannot be sustained indefinitely. There are likely a number of behavioral and physiological factors that adjust to allow a person's body to re-establish "steady-state" at a different body weight (and body composition).[23] The physiological factors might include a weight-loss-induced decline in REE and a training-induced increase in maximal oxygen consumption (which would decrease the energy expenditure associated with performing exercise at a given intensity and duration). Behavioral factors might include gradually altering the amounts of exercise performed and (or) energy consumed, and becoming more sedentary when not purposefully exercising.

## Macronutrient Intakes

A person's energy needs are met by consuming carbohydrates, proteins, fats, and possibly alcohol: the macronutrients. The FNB-IOM used different criteria to establish the recommendations for energy versus macronutrient intakes. For most nutrients the recommended intake to meet the needs of virtually all healthy persons, i.e., the Recommended Dietary Allowance (RDA) or Adequate Intake, is set as the Estimated Average Requirement (based on the designated criteria) plus two standard deviations. In contrast, the Estimated Energy Requirement does not include a two-standard deviation adjustment because undesirable and potentially unhealthy weight gain would be expected to occur. There is no RDA or Tolerable Upper Intake Level for dietary energy. The FNB-IOM has set an acceptable macronutrient distribution range for diets to be 45% to 65% carbohydrates, 10% to 35% proteins, and 20% to 35% fats.[1] These recommended macronutrient intakes were established for healthy persons to maintain health and to reduce the risk of chronic disease. For athletes, the American College of Sports Medicine (ACSM), American Dietetic Association (ADA), and the Dietitians of Canada (DC) Joint Position Statement indicated that athletes should consume diets that contain 55% to 58% carbohydrates, 12% to 15% proteins, and 25% to 30% fats.[6] These suggested intakes for athletes are within the broader Dietary Reference Intake ranges set by the FNB-IOM.

It is important to recognize that while consumption of the required amount of energy from macronutrients within the acceptable macronutrient distribution range will likely insure adequate carbohydrate, protein, and fat intakes for most weight-stable adults, this may not be the case for persons who consume low energy intakes. Overweight or obese individuals[1] and athletes (e.g., gymnasts, wrestlers, and dancers)[6] who restrict energy intake, and older persons (including athletes)[7] who require less energy may be at risk of not meeting their carbohydrate and protein needs. This issue may be further complicated if an individual's macronutrient intakes are based on recommendations for athletic performance[6] instead of the RDAs.[1] For example, older endurance-trained women (age range 67–85 years; mean body weight 56 kg) were reported to consume an average of 2077 kcal/d of energy, with a macronutrient distribution of 56% carbohydrate, 16% protein, and 31% fat.[3] Thus, the carbohydrate intake of these women was about 290 g/d or 5.2 g carbohydrate/(kg·d). While this carbohydrate intake was 2.2-fold higher than the RDA of 130 g/d, it was below the 6 to 10 g carbohydrate/(kg·d) intake recommended for athletes to achieve optimal carbohydrate stores.[6] These older female athletes needed to consume 338 g/d of carbohydrates, or 65% of energy as carbohydrate, to reach the 6 g carbohydrate/(kg·d) suggested minimum intake. Careful consideration of carbohydrate intakes among older athletes is warranted because these individuals retain the capacity to store ingested carbohydrate in muscle and liver tissues before and after exercise, and utilize glycogen for energy production during sub-maximum endurance exercise.[29,30]

## Dietary Protein

The FNB-IOM has set the RDA for protein at 0.8 g/(kg·d) for all adults, independent of age or physical activity status.[1] In contrast, the ACSM, ADA, and DC committee[6] concluded that athletes required more protein to offset increased protein use for energy production during exercise, to repair muscle damage post-exercise, and for skeletal muscle hypertrophy. The ACSM, ADA, and DC committee recommended that endurance athletes consume 1.2 to 1.4 g protein/(kg·d), and strength-trained athletes consume 1.6 to 1.7 g protein/(kg·d). Regarding the protein requirement of endurance athletes, it has been appropriately emphasized that multiple factors, including exercise intensity and duration, nutrition and hydration status before and during exercise, and training status impact an individual's need for protein.[31] Based on a comprehensive evaluation of nitrogen-balance-based protein requirement studies in sedentary subjects, recreational exercisers, and highly fit athletes, Tarnopolsky[31] concluded that adults who perform low- to moderate-intensity recreational endurance exercises do not require more dietary protein than the general population; moderate-intensity endurance athletes (training 4–5 d/week for over 1 hour) require about 25% more protein (~1.1 g/(kg·d); and elite endurance athletes (training for 8–40 h/week at intensities of 60% to 85% of maximum oxygen uptake capacity) require protein intakes not to exceed 1.6 g/(kg·d). Regarding resistance training, while a consensus is lacking, it appears that lower- to moderate-intensity resistance training may improve amino acid utilization (i.e., protein use) and not alter protein need, and higher-intensity training by strength and power athletes increases the need for protein to 1.33 g/(kg·d).[32] Most athletes generally consume sufficient protein to meet their needs, especially when their diets include complete sources of protein (e.g., meats, fish, dairy, and eggs).[33] Between 10% and 20% of male and female endurance athletes are estimated to consume less than the RDA for protein, and there is a need to closely monitor the protein intakes of athletes who consume low energy intakes or increase the rigors of training.[31] The fact that most athletes consume adequate protein, even when their requirement is increased due to training, does not provide a foundation to discount or disregard the impact of exercise on protein requirements.[31]

The protein needs of older athletes are not known with confidence. Body composition changes, especially the loss of skeletal muscle mass, and declines in the intensity and volume of training might contribute to a lower protein need for older versus younger athletes. A strictly controlled diet study was conducted to evaluate the effect of resistance training on amino acid utilization and nitrogen balance in older men and women who were sedentary or performed lower-body or whole-body resistance exercise 3 d/week for 12 weeks.[34] All of the subjects in the study consumed the RDA of 0.8 g protein/(kg·d) throughout the study period. From baseline to training week 6, urinary nitrogen excretion decreased and nitrogen balance increased, which is consistent with an increased efficiency of nitrogen retention and amino acid utilization. The lack of a differential response of urinary nitrogen excretion between the sedentary and resistance training groups suggests that the shifts were attributable to a prolonged metabolic response to altered protein intake. From training weeks 6 to 12, urinary nitrogen excretion increased modestly in the two resistance training groups only, an observation that might reflect an increased protein requirement for older people who perform resistance training. Caution is warranted to not over-interpret these findings; for example, it would be inappropriate to use these data to recommend protein supplementation for older persons who perform resistance exercise.

The results from one study documented that mid-thigh muscle size (measured using a computed tomography scanner) decreased significantly in the older men and women who consumed the protein RDA for 14 weeks and remained sedentary.[34] Older subjects who performed concurrent resistance training achieved modest (~2%) hypertrophy in the exercised muscles, but the training did not prevent a decline in whole body fat-free mass.[34] In a separate study, older men who consumed the RDA for protein and a lacto-ovo-vegetarian meal plan for 12 weeks experienced an apparent loss of fat-free mass, despite performing resistance exercise 2 d/week.[35] In contrast, men who consumed 125% of the RDA for protein and included meat (omnivorous diet) experienced an increase in fat-free mass and a trend for greater hypertrophy (16% versus 7%; $P < 0.1$) of the type 2 muscle fibers in the vastus lateralis. In another study,[36] it was reported that the muscle hypertrophy response (~5% increase in mid-thigh cross-sectional muscle area) was not different between groups of older men who consumed 129% of the protein RDA with beef as the primary protein source (omnivorous diet), versus 144% of the RDA and soy (lacto-ovo-vegetarian). Collectively, the results from these studies indicate that the RDA is a marginal protein intake, and that intakes moderately above the RDA (1.2 to 1.4 g protein/(kg·d) may promote muscle hypertrophy in older persons who perform resistance training. This suggested range of protein intake should be restricted to "healthy" older persons.[7] Older persons with chronic or acute diseases that require therapeutic diets, such as people with impaired renal function, should consult a physician and registered dietitian.

## Vegetarian Diets and Exercise

The studies comparing whether omnivorous versus vegetarian diets differentially affect exercise-induced changes in indexes of physical performance[35,36] draw attention to the issue of whether the type of diet that a person habitually consumes can influence the acute and chronic responses to exercise and health. This section will briefly discuss the nutritional considerations for vegetarian athletes and the potential impact of vegetarian diets on athletic performance. There have been several more detailed reviews published elsewhere.[37-39]

A vegetarian diet is a plant-based diet that primarily includes grains, legumes, fruits, vegetables, nuts and seeds, and excludes beef, pork, poultry, and fish. A vegan diet excludes all animal products, while lacto- and ovo-vegetarian diets include milk and other dairy products, and eggs, respectively. Some people have adopted the term "semi-vegetarian" to describe a pattern of eating that limits, but does not eliminate, the consumption of animal-based foods, especially red meats. This term is ambiguous and should not be used, since the consumption of even a small amount of meat is a carnivorous diet. The ADA and DC joint position statement[40] emphasizes the general understanding that well-planned vegetarian diets are nutritionally complete and can provide health benefits to help prevent and treat certain diseases, including heart disease, diabetes, obesity, hypertension, and some types of cancers. Vegetarian diets tend to be lower in saturated fat and cholesterol, and higher in complex carbohydrates, fiber, fruits, vegetables, phytochemicals, and antioxidants than omnivorous diets. This contrasts with the concerns among some trainers and coaches that a vegetarian diet may not provide adequate nutrition for an athlete to meet their needs and to promote optimum performance.[38]

Energy intakes among vegetarians are typically lower than non-vegetarians, in part because vegetarian foods tend to have lower energy density (lower fat and higher fiber). Athletes who expend large amounts of energy during intense training and consume a vegetarian diet, especially a vegan diet, may be challenged to consume enough food to meet their energy needs. The ACSM, ADA, and DC joint position statement on nutrition and athletic performance[6] appropriately emphasizes that both vegetarian and non-vegetarian athletes must consume sufficient energy to support maintenance of lean tissue, immune and reproductive functions, and optimal performance. While an athlete's energy needs can be met by a vegetarian diet, trainers and coaches are encouraged to measure body weight periodically as one marker of the adequacy of energy intake.

The macronutrient contents of a vegetarian athlete's diet should follow the guidelines for the general public and non-vegetarian athletes (45% to 65% carbohydrate, 20% to 35% fat, and 10% to 35% protein), with the understanding that a modest 10% increase in protein intake is recommended to adjust for the incomplete digestion of plant proteins.[6] The suggestion to increase protein intake by 10% is different than increasing the energy intake from protein by 10%. For example, consider a 60-kg endurance athlete who requires 3000 kcal/d energy and consumes a vegetarian diet than contains 10% of energy from protein (300 kcal/d, 75 g protein/d, 1.25 g protein/(kg·d). To increase protein intake by 10%, the athlete would need to consume 7.5 g/d more protein, which represents about 30 kcal/d energy and would increase total protein intake to 1.38 g protein/(kg·d). In contrast, a 10% increase in energy intake as protein would double total protein intake to 20% of energy intake (150 g protein/d, 2.5 g protein/(kg·d), which would greatly exceeds the athlete's protein needs.

Regarding vegetarian diets and physical performance, summarizing the results from eight cross-sectional and short-term intervention studies from the 1970s to early 1990s, Nieman concluded that " a vegetarian diet, even when practiced for several decades, is neither beneficial nor detrimental to cardio-respiratory endurance, especially when carbohydrate intake, age, training status, body weight, and other confounders are controlled for."[38] Among these studies, it was reported that the habitual consumption of a vegan diet by sedentary women did not impair the physiological and cardiovascular responses to sub-maximal exercise.[41] Also, whether the consumption of a lacto-ovo-vegetarian diet versus a mixed diet with meat affected endurance performance of aerobically trained males (mean $VO_{2max}$ 67 mL/(kg·min) was evaluated.[42] The eight athletes consumed the vegetarian diet for 6 weeks and the mixed diet for 6 weeks using a randomized, crossover experimental design. Maximal oxygen consumption was measured using a cycle ergometer or treadmill after 0, 3, and 6 weeks of consuming each diet. The lack of differences in maximal oxygen consumption among the testing times and between the two dietary periods suggest that the consumption of a lacto-ovo-vegetarian diet does not affect endurance performance. Much of the research from the 1970s to early 1990s may be scrutinized for study design flaws, poor or undocumented dietary control, and inadequate sample size (limited statistical power). Unfortunately, additional research from higher-quality and larger studies has not been conducted more recently,[37] nor has research addressed whether the consumption of a vegetarian diet influences muscle strength, muscle hypertrophy, and whole-body composition responses in strength-trained athletes. As described earlier, research in older men suggest that the amount of protein consumed, not whether it is provided as part of a vegetarian or omnivorous diet, contributed to variations in muscle hypertrophy and body composition responses to the initiation of a strength training program.[35,36,43,44]

The discussion above regarding nutritional considerations of vegetarian versus omnivorous athletes highlights the fact that all athletes should use careful diet planning to insure that adequate energy and nutrients are consumed to fully support training and competition. Sufficient evidence is available to conclude that well-planned vegetarian diets can meet an athlete's energy and nutrient needs. While limited data are available to assess the effect of a vegetarian diet on exercise performance, it appears that athletes and others striving to improve physical functioning (e.g. older adults) may consume either a vegetarian or omnivorous diet to promote maximum performance with training.

## Summary

Exercise and nutrition are two very important factors that are capable of impacting the physical well-being and health of all humans. Research has clearly established that the performance of at least 30 minutes of moderate-intensity exercise per day contributes to an improved health profile for adults and that for some people exercising for 60 min/d or more may be necessary for weight control and the prevention of weight gain (or regain). Regarding weight control, changes in energy intake (over- or under-consumption of dietary energy) and energy expenditure (sedentary or active lifestyle) are both capable of influencing energy balance, but the short-term links between the two are limited. The apparent lack of tight control between changes in energy expenditure and energy intake is important for people who choose to use exercise to assist with weight control, because an increase in energy expenditure via exercise is not likely to be completely compensated for by increased appetite and energy intake. The obesity epidemic underscores the importance and need for more research to improve our understanding of how nutrition (e.g., the sources and quantities of macronutrients) and exercise (e.g., the type, intensity, quantity, and frequency of training) affect appetite, energy balance, body composition, and body weight control.

## References

1. Food and Nutrition Board, Institute of Medicine. Dietary Reference Intakes for Energy, Carbohydrate, Fiber, Fat, Fatty Acids, Cholesterol, Protein, and Amino Acids (Macronutrients). Washington, DC: National Academies Press; 2005. Available online at: http://www.nap.edu/books/0309085373/html.
2. Goran MI, Calles-Escandon J, Poehlman ET, O'Connell M, Danforth E Jr. Effects of increased energy intake and/or physical activity on energy expenditure in young healthy men. J Appl Physiol. 1994;77:366–372.

3. Butterworth DE, Nieman DC, Perkins R, Warren BJ, Dotson RG. Exercise training and nutrient intake in elderly women. J Am Diet Assoc. 1993;93: 653–657.
4. Withers RT, Smith DA, Tucker RC, Brinkman M, Clark DG. Energy metabolism in sedentary and active 49- to 70-yr-old women. J Appl Physiol. 1998; 84:1333–1340.
5. Levine JA, Kotz CM. non-exercise activity thermogenesis—non-exercise activity thermogenesis—egocentric & geocentric environmental factors vs. biological regulation. Acta Physiol Scand. 2005;184: 309–318.
6. Joint Position Statement: nutrition and athletic performance. American College of Sports Medicine, American Dietetic Association, and Dietitians of Canada. Med Sci Sports Exerc. 2000;32:2130–2145.
7. Campbell WW, Geik RA. Nutritional considerations for the older athlete. Nutrition. 2004;20: 603–608.
8. van Pelt RE, Dinneno FA, Seals DR, Jones PP. Age-related decline in RMR in physically active men: relation to exercise volume and energy intake. Am J Physiol Endocrinol Metab. 2001;281:E633–E639.
9. Keytel LR, Lambert MI, Johnson J, Noakes TD, Lambert EV. Free living energy expenditure in post menopausal women before and after exercise training. Int J Sport Nutr Exerc Metab. 2001;11: 226–237.
10. Campbell WW, Kruskall LJ, Evans WJ. Lower body versus whole body resistive exercise training and energy requirements of older men and women. Metabolism. 2002;51:989–997.
11. Hedley AA, Ogden CL, Johnson CL, Carroll MD, Curtin LR, Flegal KM. Prevalence of overweight and obesity among US children, adolescents, and adults, 1999–2002. JAMA. 2004;291:2847–2850.
12. US Department of Health and Human Services, Centers for Disease Control and Prevention, National Center for Chronic Disease Prevention and Health Promotion. *Physical Activity and Health: A Report of the Surgeon General.* Atlanta, GA: CDC; 1996.
13. US Department of Health and Human Services, Centers for Disease Control and Prevention, National Center for Chronic Disease Prevention and Health Promotion. US Physical Activity Statistics: 2003 State Summary Data. Available at: http://apps-.nccd.cdc.gov/PASurveillance/StateSumV.asp. Accessed February 14, 2006.
14. US Department of Health and Human Services, Public Health Service, Office of the Surgeon General. *The Surgeon General's Call to Action to Prevent and Decrease Overweight and Obesity.* Rockville, MD: US Department of Health and Human Services; 2001.
15. US Department of Agriculture and US Department of Health and Human Services. *Nutrition and Your Health: Dietary Guidelines for Americans.* 5th ed. Home and Garden Bulletin. 2000: 232.
16. Jakicic JM, Winters C, Lang W, Wing RR. Effects of intermittent exercise and use of home exercise equipment on adherence, weight loss, and fitness in overweight women: a randomized trial. JAMA. 1999;282:1554–1560.
17. U.S. Department of Agriculture, Agriculture Research Service, Dietary Guidelines Advisory Committee. *2005 Dietary Guidelines Advisory Committee Report.* Available at: www.health.gov/dietaryguidelines/dga2005/report. Accessed February 14, 2006.
18. Wing RR, Hill JO. Successful weight loss maintenance. Annu Rev Nutr. 2001;21:323–341.
19. McGuire MT, Wing RR, Klem ML, Hill JO. Behavioral strategies of individuals who have maintained long-term weight losses. Obes Res. 1999;7: 334–341.
20. Fogelholm M, Kukkonen-Harjula K. Does physical activity prevent weight gain–a systematic review. Obes Rev. 2000;1:95–111.
21. Saris WH, Blair SN, van Baak MA, et al. How much physical activity is enough to prevent unhealthy weight gain? Outcome of the IASO 1st Stock Conference and consensus statement. Obes Rev. 2003;4: 101–114.
22. Jakicic JM, Marcus BH, Gallagher KI, Napolitano M, Lang W. Effect of exercise duration and intensity on weight loss in overweight, sedentary women: a randomized trial. JAMA. 2003;290:1323–1330.
23. Blundell JE, King NA. Physical activity and regulation of food intake: current evidence. Med Sci Sports Exerc. 1999;31:S573–S583.
24. Hubert P, King NA, Blundell JE. Uncoupling the effects of energy expenditure and energy intake: appetite response to short-term energy deficit induced by meal omission and physical activity. Appetite. 1998;31:9–19.
25. Blundell JE, Stubbs RJ, Hughes DA, Whybrow S, King NA. Cross talk between physical activity and appetite control: does physical activity stimulate appetite? Proc Nutr Soc. 2003;62:651–661.
26. Pomerleau M, Imbeault P, Parker T, Doucet E. Effects of exercise intensity on food intake and appetite in women. Am J Clin Nutr. 2004;80:1230–1236.
27. Mattes RD. Dietary compensation by humans for supplemental energy provided as ethanol or carbohydrate in fluids. Physiol Behav. 1996;59:179–187.
28. Stubbs RJ, Hughes DA, Johnstone AM, Horgan GW, King N, Blundell JE. A decrease in physical activity affects appetite, energy, and nutrient balance in lean men feeding ad libitum. Am J Clin Nutr. 2004;79:62–69.
29. Cartee GD. Aging skeletal muscle: response to exercise. Exerc Sport Sci Rev. 1994;22:91–120.

30. Tarnopolsky MA, Bosman M, Macdonald JR, Vandeputte D, Martin J, Roy BD. Postexercise protein-carbohydrate and carbohydrate supplements increase muscle glycogen in men and women. J Appl Physiol. 1997;83:1877–1883.
31. Tarnopolsky M. Protein requirements for endurance athletes. Nutrition. 2004;20:662–668.
32. Phillips SM. Protein requirements and supplementation in strength sports. Nutrition. 2004;20:689–695.
33. Lemon PW. Beyond the zone: protein needs of active individuals. J Am Coll Nutr. 2000;19:513S–521S.
34. Campbell WW, Trappe TA, Jozsi AC, Kruskall LJ, Wolfe RR, Evans WJ. Dietary protein adequacy and lower body versus whole body resistive training in older humans. J Physiol. 2002;542(part 2):631–642.
35. Campbell WW, Barton ML Jr, Cyr-Campbell D, et al. Effects of an omnivorous diet compared with a lactoovovegetarian diet on resistance-training-induced changes in body composition and skeletal muscle in older men. Am J Clin Nutr. 1999;70: 1032–1039.
36. Haub MD, Wells AM, Tarnopolsky MA, Campbell WW. Effect of protein source on resistive-training-induced changes in body composition and muscle size in older men. Am J Clin Nutr. 2002;76:511–517.
37. Barr SI, Rideout CA. Nutritional considerations for vegetarian athletes. Nutrition. 2004;20:696–703.
38. Nieman DC. Physical fitness and vegetarian diets: is there a relation? Am J Clin Nutr. 1999;70: 570S–575S.
39. Fogelholm M. Dairy products, meat and sports performance. Sports Med. 2003;33:615–631.
40. Position of the American Dietetic Association and Dietitians of Canada: Vegetarian diets. J Am Diet Assoc. 2003;103:748–765.
41. Cotes JE, Dabbs JM, Hall AM, et al. Possible effect of a vegan diet upon lung function and the cardiorespiratory response to submaximal exercise in healthy women. J Physiol. 1970;209(suppl):30.
42. Raben A, Kiens B, Richter EA, et al. Serum sex hormones and endurance performance after a lacto-ovo vegetarian and a mixed diet. Med Sci Sports Exerc. 1992;24:1290–1297.
43. Campbell WW, Crim MC, Young VR, Joseph LJ, Evans WJ. Effects of resistance training and dietary protein intake on protein metabolism in older adults. Am J Physiol. 1995;268:E1143–E1153.
44. Haub MD, Wells AM, Campbell WW. Beef and soy-based food supplements differentially affect serum lipoprotein-lipid profiles because of changes in carbohydrate intake and novel nutrient intake ratios in older men who resistive-train. Metabolism. 2005;54:769–774.

# 4 Energy Metabolism

Sai Krupa Das and Susan B. Roberts

Energy is expended by the body to maintain electrochemical gradients, transport molecules, support biosynthetic processes, produce the mechanical work required for respiration and blood circulation, and generate muscle contraction. Most of these biological processes cannot directly harness energy from the oxidation of energy-containing substrates (primarily carbohydrate and fat from food and body energy stores). Instead, the resulting energy from the oxidation of metabolic fuels is captured by adenosine triphosphate (ATP) in the form of high-energy bonds. ATP is the major energy carrier to body sites, and releases the energy required for chemical and mechanical work. Use of that energy results in the production of heat, carbon dioxide, and water, which are eliminated from the body. Definitions of terms related to energy metabolism are found in Table 1.

Nutrient degradation pathways (including the Krebs cycle and the β-oxidation of fatty acids) are linked to the formation of ATP from adenosine diphosphate (ADP) and inorganic phosphate (Pi), and are often referred to as ATP generation or energy generation pathways. Likewise, the term "energy expenditure" is used to describe the degradation of ATP to ADP and Pi. In a resting adult, approximately 25 to 35 g of ATP are used every minute to drive the life-sustaining processes, and this is approximately the total amount contained in the body at any one time. During vigorous exercise, when several hundred grams of ATP are required per minute, the rate of ATP generation is adjusted rapidly to match ATP utilization. The enzymatic machinery in the body, which under resting conditions operates much below its maximal capacity, is poised to effectively maintain a high ratio of ATP to ADP. Thus, when ATP levels decrease because of increased use, the synthesis of ATP is accelerated.

The circulating levels of energy substrates needed for ATP production are kept relatively constant despite wide variations in the availability of nutrients from the gastrointestinal tract by the balance of insulin and counter-regulatory hormones such as glucagon, glucocorticoids, adrenaline, and growth hormone. These hormones jointly serve to facilitate the rapid storage of incoming nutrients from the gastrointestinal tract (carbohydrate in the form of glycogen in the liver and muscle, and fat as triacylglycerol in adipose tissue) and maintain circulating levels in the fasting state by mobilization of body stores.

The close relationship between energy metabolism and oxygen consumption stems from the fact that oxygen is required to transform food to a usable source of energy. One liter of oxygen consumed generates approximately 5 kcal (20.92 kJ). Given that there is proportionality between the volume of oxygen ($VO_2$) and ATP synthesis, and because each mole of ATP synthesized is accompanied by a given amount of heat, it would be possible to calculate heat production from $VO_2$ measurements alone. However, the heat produced by the utilization of 1 L of oxygen varies somewhat with the foodstuff consumed (Tables 2 and 3). The combustion of 1 L of oxygen during fat oxidation yields 5.682 kcal (23.77 kJ), whereas protein alone yields 4.655 kcal (19.48 kJ) and carbohydrate starch alone yields 5.048 kcal (21.12 kJ).[1] Moreover, the amount of carbon dioxide produced also varies with nutrient type, with the amount of carbon dioxide produced per mole of oxygen consumed during oxidation of fat, protein, and carbohydrate being 0.710, 0.835, and 1.00 mol, respectively. Thus, for precise conversion of oxygen utilization to energy expenditure, the balance of metabolic fuels being oxidized or carbon dioxide production must be known.

Because the ratio of carbon dioxide produced to oxygen consumed (i.e., the respiratory quotient) varies with nutrient type, it can be used to predict the ratio of metabolic fuels being oxidized if additional information on urinary nitrogen excretion is also available. The first step in this calculation is to determine protein oxidation, with the assumption that urinary nitrogen reflects protein oxi-

**Table 1.** Definitions in Energy Metabolism

Calorie and joule: A calorie is the amount of heat required to raise the temperature of 1 g $H_2O$ from 14.5 to 15.5°C. One kilocalorie (1 kcal) is 1000 times greater than 1 calorie (1 cal). One calorie is equivalent to 4.184 joules (J), and 1 kcal is equivalent to 4.184 kJ.

Energy balance: Attained when energy intake equals total energy expenditure (TEE) and body stores are stable. An individual is said to be in positive energy balance when energy intake exceeds TEE (and consequently body energy stores increase). Negative energy balance occurs when energy intake is less than TEE and body energy stores decrease.

Energy expenditure: The amount of energy used by the body, equivalent to the heat released by hydrolysis of adenosine triphosphate (ATP) to adenosine diphosphate (ADP) or adenosine monophosphate (AMP) and inorganic phosphate (Pi).

Energy metabolism: The general term used to collectively describe the multiple biochemical pathways that govern the production and use of ATP and the reducing equivalents.

Energy regulation: The process by which energy intake and energy expenditure are balanced.

Malnutrition: The general term that denotes both undernutrition and overnutrition.

Overnutrition: Occurs when energy intake exceeds energy expenditure and results in excess body fat accumulation. Several levels of overnutrition are defined in adults using the body mass index (BMI; weight in kilograms divided by height in meters squared, $kg/m^2$) (3). Overweight BMI = 25–29.9, class I obesity = 30–34.9, class II obesity = 35–39.9, class III obesity 39.99–40.0. In children BMI changes with development, and BMI definitions of overweight and obesity at different ages are now available (78, 79).

Undernutrition: Occurs when energy intake is less than TEE over a considerable period of time, resulting in clinically significant weight loss. In adults undernutrition is classified using BMI (3). A BMI of 18.5–24.9 is considered normal, a BMI of 17–18.49 is mild undernutrition, a BMI of 16–16.99 is moderate undernutrition, and a BMI $<16$ is severe undernutrition. In children, undernutrition is classified using the weight-for-height (or length) index and the height-for-age index with reference values derived from World Health Organization data (3). Wasting is defined as low weight for height, with $< -1$ standard deviation (SD) (i.e., $-1$ z-score) being mild, $< -2$ SD being moderate, and $< -3$ SD being severely wasted relative to reference values from the National Center for Health Statistics and the World Health Organization. Similarly, stunting is associated with a low height for age, with $< -1$ SD being mild, $< -2$ SD being moderate, and $< -3$ SD of the reference values being severely stunted.

dation and 1 g of urinary nitrogen is equivalent to 6.25 g of protein. $VO_2$ and volume of carbon dioxide ($VCO_2$) not from protein (non-protein $VO_2$ and $VCO_2$) are then calculated by subtracting the amount of oxygen and carbon dioxide equivalent to protein oxidation using the values in Table 2. After this, the non-protein respiratory quotient is used to calculate the ratio of fat to carbohydrate oxidation using the values shown in Table 2 for the respiratory quotient of carbohydrate and fat.

Simple equations can also be used to predict energy expenditure from oxygen consumption and carbon dioxide production; de Weir's is probably the most widely used today.[2] When 24-hour urine collections are made on the day of measurement of $VO_2$ and $VCO_2$, the complete de Weir equation, which includes an adjustment for energy expenditure for protein oxidation, is used. However, because of the difficulties of obtaining complete 24-hour urine nitrogen measurements and because of the difference between correcting for urinary nitrogen and not correcting for nitrogen is $<2\%$, the abbreviated de Weir equation is often used. The complete de Weir equation is:

$$\text{RMR (kcal/d)} = 1.44(3.941 \cdot VO_2 + 1.106 \cdot VCO_2) - 2.17 \cdot UN.$$

The abbreviated de Weir equation is:

$$\text{RMR (kcal/d)} = 1.44(3.941 \cdot VO_2 + 1.106 \cdot VCO_2).$$

$VO_2$ and VCO2 are measured in milliliters per minute and urinary nitrogen (UN) is measured in grams per day.

# Energy Requirements

The Food and Agriculture Organization of the United Nations (FAO) defines energy requirement as "the amount of food energy needed to balance energy expenditure in order to maintain body size, body composition and a level of necessary and desirable physical activity consistent with long-term good health. This includes the energy needed for the optimal growth and development of children, for the deposition of tissues during pregnancy, and for the secretion of milk during lactation consistent with the good health of mother and child."[3]

Requirement refers to habitual or usual intake over a period of time, because many human beings (especially adults) do not maintain energy balance from one day to the next but do so over a period of several days. The energy intake referred to in the FAO's definition of energy requirements[3] is the metabolizable energy intake, which is the energy that is metabolically available to the body after obligatory losses in urine and feces. Approximate metabolizable energy contents of fat, protein, and carbohydrate are 9 kcal (37.66 kJ/g), 4 kcal/g (16.74 kJ/g), and 4 kcal/g (16.74 kJ/g), respectively.

Currently, most energy requirement estimations worldwide, including the recent FAO publication,[3] are based on estimates of components of energy expenditure

**Table 2.** Relationships Among $VO_2$, $VCO_2$, and Energy Expenditure for Fat, Protein, and Carbohydrate*

| Oxidation of 1 g | $O_2$ required (L) | $CO_2$ produced (L) | Respiration quotient | Energy expended, kJ (kcal)/g | Energy equivalent, L $O_2$, kJ (kcal)/L |
|---|---|---|---|---|---|
| Carbohydrate | 827.7 | 827.7 | 1.000 | 17.5 (4.18) | 21.1 (5.048) |
| Protein | 1010.3 | 843.6 | 0.835 | 19.7 (4.70) | 19.5 (4.655) |
| Fat | 2018.9 | 1435.4 | 0.710 | 39.5 (9.45) | 19.6 (4.682) |
| Ethanol | 1459.4 | 977.8 | 0.670 | 29.7 (7.09) | 20.3 (4.86) |

* Carbohydrate is assumed to be starch; protein and fat are assumed to be mixed values found in typical human diets.
From Livesey and Elia, 1988.[1] Reproduced with permission by *The American Journal of Clinical Nutrition.* 

summed together into 24-hour values. This method (the so-called factorial approach, which is equivalent to a time and motion study; see below) is recognized as relatively imprecise (future recommendations may use energy determinations based on the doubly labeled water method described below). It is preferred over measurement of energy intake during weight stability, because energy intake is highly variable and most individuals underreport habitual intake by 25% to 50%, depending on their body fatness.[4] Doubly labeled water measurements of total energy expenditure (TEE) may ultimately replace the factorial method as a basis for all estimates of energy requirements, as they have currently for requirements in infants and children by the FAO[3] and the recent US recommendations for adults and children.[5] However, due to the relative lack of data on representative populations, the general use of TEE data is not broadly accepted at the current time.

For estimation of TEE by the more usual factorial approach, 3 major components of energy expenditure are considered: basal metabolic rate (BMR) or resting metabolic rate (RMR), thermic effect of feeding (TEF), and energy expenditure for physical activity and arousal (EEPAA).

**Table 3.** Stoichiometry of Oxidation of Specific Nutrients and High-Energy Bond Production*

| | | | ATP yield |
|---|---|---|---|
| $C_{16}H_{32}O_2$ + 23 $O_2$ (palmitate) | → | 16 $CO_2$ + 16 $H_2O$ + 10,033 kJ (2398 kcal) | 129 |
| $C_{4.6}H_{8.4}O_{1.8}N_{1.25}$ + 9.6 $O_2$ (protein) | → | 0.6 Urea + 4.0 $CO_2$ + 2.9 $H_2O$ + 2176 kJ (520 kcal) | 23 |
| $C_6H_{12}O_6$ + 6.0 $O_2$ (glucose) | → | 6.0 $CO_2$ + 6.0 $H_2O$ + 2803 kJ (670 kcal) | 36 |

* Values are in moles.
Adapted with permission from Kinney and Tucker, 1992.[80]

BMR accounts for 60% to 70% of TEE on average, and is defined as the rate of energy expenditure while lying in bed at physical and mental rest 12 to 14 hours after the last meal (i.e., in the post-absorptive state) and under thermoneutral conditions. RMR is similar to BMR except that the conditions are less rigid for the duration of the overnight fast, and thermoneutrality is not guaranteed. BMR and RMR are often used interchangeably. Both BMR and RMR are highly correlated with lean body mass, more commonly known as fat-free mass (FFM), and, to a lesser extent, with fat mass. Note that there is a positive intercept in the relationship between BMR/RMR and FFM, which is thought to result from the fact that organ sizes are relatively constant between individuals and that the FFM of larger subjects contains disproportionately more muscle than organ tissue. One consequence of the non-zero intercept is that BMR per kilogram FFM is lower for higher levels of FFM than for lower ones. Thus, differences in BMR between groups of individuals should always be assessed using regression analysis to test the group effects in a model incorporating FFM and fat mass; otherwise, heavy individuals (such as the obese) may falsely appear to have a low BMR relative to their body size.

There is also some variability in BMR because of age (elderly individuals have lower BMR after adjusting for differences in FFM between young and old groups)[6], and women may have lower adjusted BMR values than men.[7] Among young women, BMR variations on the order of 6% to 10% have been reported to occur in the course of the menstrual cycle, with luteal-phase values tending to be higher than follicular phase ones.[8] Factors such as exercise and conditions such as hyperthyroidism, catecholamine release, fever, stress, cold exposure, and burns increase BMR. There is also a hereditary component to BMR seen in the fact that variations in FFM-adjusted metabolic rate are smaller among members of the same family than between unrelated individuals.[9]

Several equations have been developed to predict BMR from weight, height, and other simple measures. The Schofield equations[10] were derived from an analysis of the world literature on BMR. They consist of a series of simple linear regression equations predicting BMR in different gender and age categories from either weight alone or weight and height. These equations have an uncertainty of prediction of only ±7% to 10% for individual values, and are used in the most recent publications of the World Health Organization.[3] Although such equations may not be suitable for unusual populations such as the extremely obese or very old, they do provide a basis for predicting energy requirements in the general population (Table 4).

TEF is the energy expenditure associated with the ingestion, digestion, absorption, transport, storage, and utilization of food, and is measurable for 12 to 18 hours after food ingestion. A significant component of the TEF (estimated at 50%–75%) is directed toward regenerating the ATP used in the processing and storage of ingested nutrients.[11] This is often referred to as the obligatory component of TEF. The increased activity of the sympathetic nervous system resulting from the sensory and metabolic stimulation resulting from food probably accounts for the remainder of TEF, and is referred to as the facultative component of TEF. TEF typically accounts for 7% to 13% of energy intake, and is directly proportional to the size of the meal consumed.[12] TEF appears to be reduced in obese individuals,[13] but the question of whether this is a cause or consequence of excess weight has not been resolved.[14,15] A separate estimate of the energy needed for TEF is not usually shown in predictions of energy requirements, because the postprandial measurements of energy expenditure for different listed activities in EEPAA (see below) include a component of energy expenditure from TEF.

EEPAA is the energy expenditure for physical activity and/or arousal. This component is highly variable and will account for an increasing proportion of TEE as individuals become more physically active. In sedentary persons, EEPAA may be only 30% of TEE, whereas it may be 60% to 70% in highly active individuals. The difficulty of measuring EEPAA using traditional methods for determining energy expenditure has made this the least accurately measured component of TEE. Energy needs for occupational activity vary widely (Table 5) and are typi-

**Table 5.** Approximate Energy Expenditure For Individual Activities Expressed as a Multiple of the Resting Metabolic Rate*

| Physical Activity Level Range | Examples |
|---|---|
| Resting 1–1.5 | Sleeping, lying down, sitting quietly, standing |
| Very Light 1.5–2.5 | Dressing, personal hygiene, slow walking, child care, driving car |
| Light to Moderate 2.5–5.0 | Fast walking, farming activities, housework |
| Moderate to Heavy 5.0–7.0 | Climbing stairs, cycling, walking with heavy load, dancing, jogging |
| Very Strenuous 7.0+ | Walking uphill, sprinting, soccer, high-intensity aerobics, swimming |

* When reported as multiples of basal needs, the energy expenditures of males and females are similar.
Adapted with permission from the Food and Agriculture Organization of the United Nations, 2001.[3]

**Table 4.** Equations to Predict Basal Metabolic Rate from Body Weight

| | | Basal metabolic rate | |
|---|---|---|---|
| | Age range (years) | kcal/day | MJ/day |
| Males | | | |
| | 0–3 | 60.9 W − 54 | 0.255 W − 0.226 |
| | 3–10 | 22.7 W +495 | 0.0949 W +2.07 |
| | 10–18 | 17.5 W +651 | 0.0732 W +2.72 |
| | 18–30 | 15.3 W +679 | 0.0640 W +2.84 |
| | 30–60 | 11.6 W +879 | 0.0485 W +3.67 |
| | >60 | 13.5 W +487 | 0.0565 W +2.04 |
| Females | | | |
| | 0–3 | 61.0 W − 51 | 0.255 W − 0.214 |
| | 3–10 | 22.5 W +499 | 0.0941 W +2.09 |
| | 10–18 | 12.2 W +746 | 0.0510 W +3.12 |
| | 18–30 | 14.7 W +496 | 0.0615 W +2.08 |
| | 30–60 | 8.7 W +829 | 0.0364 W +3.47 |
| | >60 | 10.5 W +596 | 0.0439 W +2.49 |

W, body weight in kilograms.
Adapted with permission from Shills et al., 1994.[81]

**Table 6.** Factors for Estimating Total Energy Expenditure at Different Physical Activity Levels in Men and Women 19 to 50 Years of Age

| | | Total Energy Expenditure | |
|---|---|---|---|
| Level of Activity | Activity Factor (× RMR) | 70-kg Man (RMR = 1750 kcal) | 60-kg Woman (RMR 1380 = kcal) |
| Sedentary or light | 1.40–1.69 | 2450–2958 | 1932–2333 |
| Active or moderately active | 1.70–1.99 | 2975–3483 | 2346–2746 |
| Vigorous or vigorously active | 2.00–2.40 | 3500–4200 | 2760–3312 |

RMR = Resting metabolic rate.
Adapted with permission from the Food and Agriculture Organization of the United Nations, 2001[3].

cally defined by the type (light, moderate, or heavy) and duration of work.[16] Leisure activities include all socially desirable tasks and household chores or exercises for fitness. The residual daytime for which there is no clear definition of activity is usually called non-accountable activity, and includes the energy expenditure for arousal, fidgeting, and other activities that cannot be defined specifically. EEPAA is the sum of all EEPAA components.

Energy requirements are the sum of BMR and EEPAA (which includes TEF when measurements of EEPAA are made in the postprandial state). In both current US[5] and international[3] recommendations on energy needs, TEE values are expressed as a ratio of BMR, with group mean values ranging from 1.3 to 2.4, as shown in Table 6. Current research suggests that this range may somewhat underestimate the usual activity of adults in affluent societies,[17] and future recommendations may change as doubly labeled water data are incorporated into the available data on energy needs.

# Energy Expenditure Methods

Energy metabolism research has been taking place for at least 200 years. In the late 18th century, Lavoisier made the important discovery that respiration was the basis of all life- sustaining processes, and that it was a form of chemical combustion that could be measured. By the end of the 19th century, Rubner[18] was measuring the excretion rates of urinary nitrogen, oxygen consumption, and carbon dioxide production in humans, and Atwater and Benedict[19] laid the groundwork for most modern methods of energy expenditure by building the first calorimetry chamber.

## *Calorimetry Chambers*

Energy expenditure can be measured by two methods. Direct calorimetry measures energy expenditure as the rate at which heat is lost from the body to the environment. Heat loss from the body includes non-evaporative heat losses (conduction, convection, and radiation) and evaporative heat losses in the form of water vapor. Direct calorimetry usually involves whole-body measurements in an enclosed chamber.[20] Non-evaporative heat loss is calculated by measuring the temperature gradient across the walls of the insulated chamber or by measuring the rate of heat removal before it is lost from the walls of the chamber. Evaporative heat loss is measured by condensing the water appearing in the chamber and measuring the latent heat of condensation or by measuring the increase in water content of the air in the chamber and calculating its latent heat of condensation. Heat loss is estimated from the sum of evaporative and non-evaporative loss. Today, very few calorimetric chambers work on the principle of direct calorimetry, because it is technically much more difficult than indirect calorimetry, as described below.

Indirect calorimetry predicts heat production (energy expenditure) from the rates of respiratory gas exchange: oxygen consumption and carbon dioxide production. In the simplest form of indirect calorimetry, the subject is kept in a sealed room or a canopy is placed over the subject's head, and this chamber or canopy is ventilated with a constant supply of fresh air. The subject's respiratory gas exchange is measured by comparing the composition of well-mixed air in the chamber with the composition of air entering the chamber, together with the flow rate of air. Most chamber calorimeters are furnished and include television, radio, telephone, some exercise equipment, and toilet and washing facilities, thus permitting measurements that approximate sedentary existence with tight control on intake and activity. Careful monitoring of the chamber and gases is required to ensure accurate measurements. However, indirect calorimetry is still technically much easier than direct calorimetry, and has become the method of choice for measurements of 24-hour sedentary energy expenditure, BMR, and TEF.

## *Doubly Labeled Water Method*

The doubly labeled water method is a newer technique that is considered a form of indirect calorimetry because it measures carbon dioxide production, from which energy expenditure can be calculated if information is available on the balance of metabolic fuels being oxidized.[21,22] The balance of metabolic fuels is approximately equal to the average 24-hour respiratory quotient in this case, and is called the food quotient. The food quotient can be calculated from dietary intake records for subjects in energy balance using the values shown in Table 2 to compute the oxygen and carbon dioxide equivalents of dietary macronutrient intakes. Originally developed for use in small animals,[23] the doubly labeled water method involves ingesting water containing small known amounts of the stable (i.e., non-radioactive) isotopes $^2H_2O$ and $H_2{}^{18}O$ and measuring their disappearance rates over time by collecting individual urine or saliva samples to measure their concentration changes. The labeled hydrogen leaves the body as water (in urine, respiratory water vapor, sweat, and trans-epidermal water loss), whereas labeled oxygen leaves the body as water and carbon dioxide. The latter occurs because $^{18}O$ is in equilibrium between body water pools and body bicarbonate pools through the action of the enzyme carbonic anhydrase, and bicarbonate is the precursor of expired carbon dioxide. The difference between the elimination rates of the two isotopes reflects carbon dioxide production. The doubly labeled water method is an excellent field technique if mass spectrometry facilities are available to measure isotopic concentrations, because validation studies have shown that it is accurate to ±3% to 5%[21] and allows measurements of free-living energy expenditure over 1 to 3 weeks while subjects are leading normal lives.

### *Simple Field Techniques*

A variety of simple field techniques are also available to predict the energy expenditures of free-living subjects. Although recognized as less accurate and precise than the doubly labeled water method, these techniques are widely available and can provide information that the doubly labeled water method does not (e.g., on types of activities being performed). One example is the Douglas bag method, which measures the energy costs of specific activities. With this technique, the subject wears a nose clip and a mouthpiece fitted with valves so that all expired air is collected in a bag and transported to the field laboratory for gas analysis using oxygen and carbon dioxide analyzers. Several bags (from multiple subjects or multiple measurements) can be analyzed using one set of gas analyzers, which is highly practical in field situations.

Time and motion studies, despite being one of the oldest approaches, are still used to assess physical activity in a wide variety of field studies. A record-keeper observes and records information on the subject, including behavioral variables and type, frequency, and duration of each activity. Using either the estimated energy cost of each activity or direct measurements (e.g., determined using a Douglas bag) and multiplying the energy cost of each activity with its duration, one can estimate TEE. The weakness of this method is that it is highly labor intensive and, because of the difficulty of obtaining accurate information on the energy cost of each different activity performed by each subject, gives a relatively imprecise measurement of TEE for individual subjects. Nevertheless, it is often the only method available for field studies, and also provides important information on activity types that is missing from doubly labeled water determinations of TEE.

Activity questionnaires are designed to obtain information about self-reported habitual physical activity. In some cases, questionnaires are specifically designed to determine work-related or leisure activities only. The time period in question may vary from the previous 24 hours to a week or the previous year, whereas other questionnaires attempt to categorize all forms of activity.[24] As with the simpler time and motion studies, it is necessary to use published information on the energy costs of different activities to convert activity durations to estimates of TEE. One of the concerns with the questionnaire method is that there is a wide range in the energy cost of a specific activity. The ability of subjects to accurately recall activity patterns is also subject to significant error. Evidence suggests that strenuous activity is better recalled than mild or moderate activity.[25]

Movement assessment devices such as pedometers, which are either clipped to a belt or worn on an ankle, are designed primarily to count specific movements such as steps while walking or running. Some pedometers adjust for stride length to estimate the distance walked, and the sophisticated battery-operated models also have a sensitivity adjustment. Portable accelerometers work on the principle that when an individual moves, the limbs and body accelerate, theoretically in proportion to the muscular forces responsible for the accelerations, and thus in proportion to energy expenditure.

Physiological measurements such as heart rate are easy to measure in the field and may be a practical and satisfactory method for measuring metabolism in some situations. Heart rate can be measured using monitors that allow continuous monitoring with little interference with the subject's activity. Comparison of heart rate measurements with simultaneous measurements of TEE using doubly labeled water in free-living adults has shown that the heart rate method can provide a good estimation of TEE in groups of subjects if the relationship between activity and heart rate is tested in individual subjects using a range of activities spanning the range performed in daily life. In one recent study,[26] the estimate of TEE from heart rate (3105 ± 915 kcal/d, 12.99 ± 3.83 MJ/d) was very similar to that from doubly labeled water (3080 ± 908 kcal/d, 12.89 ± 3.80 MJ/d).

## Regulation of Energy Balance

Human body weight is regulated by remarkably sensitive biological mechanisms that balance energy intake with energy expenditure (see also the chapters "Changing Dietary Behavior" and "Appetite and Hunger"). This is illustrated by the fact that only a 3% imbalance between energy intake and energy expenditure (approximately 75 kcal, or 300 kJ) will, if persistent, lead to nearly a 45.5-kg (100-pound) weight change per decade in adults. Even unmeasurable imbalances of only 1% to 2% (25–50 kcal/d, or 100–200 kJ/d) will cause considerable weight gain (13.6–27.27 kg/decade, or 30–60 lb/decade) if unchecked. The energy-regulating mechanisms that prevent such extreme weight gain in most individuals involve complex, overlapping processes at the biochemical, endocrinological, physiological, neural, and behavioral levels, all of which are functionally interdependent.

The relative importance of the specific mechanisms that cause us to start and stop eating and that determine why some people are lean and others are overweight remains uncertain. Nevertheless, there is a wealth of information from studies of both animal models and humans on the multiple overlapping mechanisms that are likely to play significant roles in short-term and long-term energy regulation. The following sections summarize some of the major factors that play an important role in energy regulation.

Information about consumed food and the immediate need for food is conveyed to the brain via neural, gastrointestinal, circulating, metabolic, and nutrient storage signals. Afferent somatosensory signals resulting from the sight, smell, and initial taste of food are transmitted to the brain via the autonomic nervous system. These signals initiate the so-called cephalic phase of digestion,[27] which causes an increase in saliva production, gastric acid production, gastric motility, and insulin secretion.[28,29] These cephalic-phase responses prepare the body to receive food, which may even include increasing the sensation of hunger, because the increase in circulating insulin causes blood glucose to decrease transiently, a phenomenon linked to the increased perception of hunger in both animals and humans.[30]

Several chemoreceptors and mechanoreceptors in the intestinal wall and their neural afferents relay information to the brain as food enters the stomach, and may provide early signals that indicate satiety.[27] Gastrointestinal processing and meal termination may be initiated by hormones, some of which also act as neuropeptides. These include cholecystokinin, pancreatic glucagon, bombesin, and somatostatin, which act on their receptors in the vagus nerve to provide sensory information to the brain that causes meal termination.[31,32] As a hormone, cholecystokinin gets released into circulation upon ingestion of a meal, stimulates pancreatic secretion and gall bladder contraction, and regulates gastric emptying and induction of satiety. Glucagon-like peptide-1 secreted from the intestinal cells of the ileum and colon is also released into the circulation after food intake. Glucagon-like peptide-1 is implicated in the short-term regulation of appetite by decreasing the feeling of hunger and suppressing energy intake by delaying gastric emptying and increasing the duration of postprandial satiety. The roles of insulin and glucagon in the control of food intake have long been suspected to be important as well, since secretion of these hormones is primarily controlled by incoming nutrients. These hormones in turn control the level of glucose and other metabolic fuels in the blood.[33,34]

Circulating nutrients may also be important both for signaling satiety after food consumption and for signaling hunger in the post-absorptive period. As suggested by Mayer almost 50 years ago,[35] low blood glucose in particular may result in a signal for hunger and high blood glucose may signal satiety. Many, but not all, studies have supported this hypothesis,[36] and there is also evidence that changes (in particular, transient declines) in blood glucose may signal hunger independent of whether blood glucose is normal or low.[37] Signaling by glucose may potentially take place either through afferent vagal signals (affected by hepatic glucose receptors signaling liver glycogen changes resulting from alterations in blood glucose) or through circulating glucose levels and their impact on brain glucose levels.

The availability of fatty acids and their metabolites may also result in afferent signals that modulate food intake,[27] as proposed by Friedman's nutrient sufficiency model of energy regulation.[38] In support of this theory, blood glucose and free fatty acids combined explained a remarkable 71% of within-subject variability in food intake in a recent crossover study designed to assess the effects of three different meal types on hunger and energy intake.[36] A central and major role for circulating glucose and fatty acids in signaling hunger and satiety may help explain the fact that delayed gastric emptying (which prolongs the postprandial period over which circulating metabolites are elevated) is consistently associated with prolonged satiety.[39,40] Moreover, dietary factors that delay nutrient digestion and absorption, including high levels of fat and low glycemic index, are also associated with prolonged satiety between meals.[36]

In addition to these short-term signals for food sufficiency and insufficiency, several hormones, peptides, and neurotransmitters are involved in the regulation of energy balance over the long term. Leptin, the product of the ob gene, is a circulating hormone produced and secreted primarily by the white adipose tissue that appears to have multiple functions in the inhibition of food intake and stimulation/maintenance of energy expenditure. In both rats and humans, circulating leptin increases with increasing body fat and decreases with fasting and body fat loss.[41,42] Once it is secreted, leptin enters the brain either by saturable transport or by diffusion into the hypothalamic structures that lack a blood-brain barrier.[43]

The administration of exogenous leptin results in significant suppression of food intake in rats,[44] whereas in humans a dose-response relationship with weight and fat loss has been observed.[45] Leptin acts as a metabolic hormone influencing a range of processes, such as insulin secretion, lipolysis, and glucose transport. Leptin may also influence the activity of a variety of neurotransmitter systems in the brain and peptides, such as catecholamines, corticosteroids, insulin, sex hormone, and growth hormone, that are involved in the control of food intake and in regulating body weight.[46,47] Experimental studies have also shown that, after a meal, the action of leptin in suppressing food intake is potentiated by the release of cholecystokinin from the intestine.[48,49]

Serotonin (5-hydroxy-tryptophan) is another neurotransmitter that, like leptin, appears to have a suppressive effect on food intake and body weight. However, it has been suggested that the suppressive effect is preferential to carbohydrates, and animal studies suggest the existence of a negative feedback loop, with carbohydrate ingestion enhancing the release of serotonin, which in turn limits the amount of the macronutrient ingested.[50]

One of the newer physiologic factors[51] reported to play a role in regulating energy homeostasis is ghrelin. Ghrelin is an orexigenic hormone secreted primarily in the stomach and duodenum, which is reported to regulate mealtime hunger, appetite, and long-term body weight.[52] In humans, plasma ghrelin levels have been shown to rise shortly before and decrease shortly after every meal, a pattern that is consistent with the hypothesis that ghrelin is a physiological meal initiator.[52] Likewise, plasma ghrelin levels are also suppressed in the obese, and diet-induced weight loss is known to cause an increase in ghrelin secretion in response to the energy deficit.[53] Although ghrelin levels are reciprocal to glucose and insulin in the fasted and postprandial states, it is unclear if the meal-related suppression of ghrelin is directly regulated by glucose or insulin.[54-56] Ghrelin is also reported to antagonize the action of leptin, and the between-meal levels of leptin and ghrelin display diurnal rhythms that are in phase with one another, suggesting that the two hormones may be counter-regulated. Future studies are needed to confirm the role of ghrelin in meal initiation and overall energy intake, and to determine whether it significantly influences other hormones involved in energy balance.

The interlinked nature of the central nervous system's control of food intake suggests that changes in one may influence the activity of many others. Achieving energy balance is therefore a product of complex interactions of several peripheral hormones and their effector systems in the central nervous system that work together to regulate food intake and energy expenditure.

# Energy Imbalance

Perturbations in energy balance underlie the most common public health nutrition problems today (see the chapters on obesity). In the United States, 65.2% of adults over 20 years of age, 16.1% of teenagers between 12 and 19 years of age, and 15.8% of children between 6 and 12 years of age are now considered overweight or obese.[57] The prevalence of obesity is also increasing in developing countries, where undernutrition has traditionally been the primary nutrition concern. For example, the prevalence of obesity has increased recently in both Brazil and China, especially in urban areas but also in very low-income families such as those living in shantytowns.[58-60] In addition to being associated with increased risks of type 2 diabetes, osteoarthritis, angina, and hypertension, obesity is also associated with premature death and increased health care costs. The estimated number of deaths attributable to obesity in the United States alone is about 300,000 per year.

The excess weight gain that accumulates in obesity results from energy intake exceeding energy expenditure over a considerable period of time, and has both genetic and environmental origins. This positive energy balance can occur because energy expenditure is low or energy intake is high, or a combination of these two factors. The importance of physical activity is suggested by several,[61-64] but not all,[65] prospective studies showing that low energy expenditure is a risk factor for excess weight gain, and mechanistically may result from the effects of energy expenditure on both energy requirements and insulin sensitivity.[61,66] In addition, the fact that excess energy intake is important, at least in the United States, is suggested by national survey statistics showing that per capita energy availability (adjusted for spoilage and waste) has increased by 400 kcal/d (1678 kJ/d) over the past 20 years.[67]

In apparent conflict with the suggestion that overeating is a common cause of overweight, some studies suggest that humans possess a considerable capacity to increase energy expenditure (for RMR and TEF) during overfeeding, with the result that weight gain is minimized in individuals with a genetic resistance to positive energy balance.[68,69] However, even in studies that showed a significant capacity for energy dissipation during overeating, weight gain still occurred. Furthermore, other overfeeding studies suggest a somewhat lower capacity for energy dissipation in normal volunteers.[70,71] Thus, although increased energy dissipation appears to occur during overeating, it is concomitant with positive energy balance and does not entirely prevent weight gain in most people.

Concerning negative energy balance, experimental underfeeding studies show a reduction in energy expenditure during weight loss (loss of both fat mass and FFM) that is disproportionate to the amount of weight lost.[72] It is also important to note that the capacity for adaptive variations in energy expenditure appears to be greater in response to undereating than to overeating.[72] This implies that there is a greater metabolic priority in preventing weight loss than in preventing weight gain, a suggestion consistent with the presumption that food shortages were more common than food abundance during early human evolution. The question of whether energy expenditure remains depressed if weight is stabilized at a lower weight remains controversial,[72] with different study approaches yielding different experimental findings.

Prolonged negative energy balance, particularly in infants and children, leads to undernutrition, also called malnutrition. Occurring most frequently (but not exclusively) in developing countries, undernutrition is usually associated with a complex mixture of multiple nutrient deficiencies (macro- and micronutrients), infections, and clinical complications. In the short term, undernutrition causes a loss of body energy stores and of FFM, and the duration and severity of undernutrition determine the magnitude of change. Reductions in absolute metabolic rate, physical activity, and TEE are commonly observed changes in most undernourished children.[73] There are also long-term energy regulation consequences of undernutrition in childhood; in particular, chronically undernourished children become stunted. Recent studies also suggest that stunted children have impaired fat oxidation[74] and impaired regulation of food intake, which would predict an increased susceptibility to obesity.[75,76] This finding may help to explain the observation[59,77] that in developing countries, stunted adults have an increased risk of overweight. Further work is needed on the mechanisms by which childhood undernutrition alters obesity risk factors.

## Future Directions

Energy balance is regulated by remarkably sensitive mechanisms that are being characterized in ongoing research. Problems with energy balance stem from both genetic and environmental causes and underlie many of the common health problems today in both developed and developing countries. Further research is needed to accurately quantify the relative importance of genetic inheritance, early life influences, and current environmental factors in the prevention, development, and treatment of obesity.

## Acknowledgment

Preparation of this chapter was supported in part by US Department of Agriculture contract 53 -3K06-5-10.

## References

1. Livesey G, Elia M. Estimation of energy expenditure, net carbohydrate utilization: and net fat oxidation and synthesis by indirect calorimetry: Evaluation of errors with special reference to the detailed compostion of fuels. Am J Clin Nutr. 1988;47:608–628.
2. de Weir JB. New methods for calculating metabolic rate with special reference to protein. J Physiol. 1949; 109:1–9.
3. Food and Agriculture Organization of the United Nations, World Health Organization, United Nations University. *Report of a Joint FAO/WHO/UNU Expert Consultation. Human Energy Requirements.* Geneva: World Health Organization; 2001.
4. Schoeller DA. How accurate is self-reported dietary energy intake? Nutr Rev 1990;48:373–379
5. Food and Nutrition Board, Institute of Medicine. Dietary Reference Intakes for Energy, Carbohydrate, Fiber, Fat, Fatty Acids, Cholesterol, Protein, and Amino Acids (Macronutrients). Washington, DC: National Academies Press; 2002. Available online at: http://www.nap.edu/books/0309085373/html.
6. Roberts SB. Influence of age on energy requirements. Am J Clin Nutr. 1995;62(suppl):1053A–1058A.
7. Ferraro R, Lillioja S, Fontvielle AM, et al. Lower sedentary metabolic rate in women compared with men. J Clin Invest. 1992;90:780–784.
8. Solomon SJ, Kurzer MS, Calloway DH. Menstrual cycle and basal metabolic rate in women. Am J Clin Nutr. 1982;36:611–616.
9. Bogardus C, Lillioja S, Ravussin E, et al. Familial dependence of the resting metabolic rate. N Eng J Med. 1986;315:96–100.
10. Schofield WN, Schofield EC, James WP. Basal metabolic rate-review and prediction, together with an annotated bibliography of source material. Hum Nutr Clin Nutr. 1985;39C:1–96.
11. Flatt JP. The biochemistry of energy expenditure. In: Bray GA, ed. *Recent Advances in Obesity Research. II. Proceedings of the 2nd International Congress on Obesity.* Westport, CT: Food and Nutrition Press; 1978.
12. Schutz Y, Bessard T, Jequier E. Diet-induced thermogenesis measured over a whole day in obese and nonobese women. Am J Clin Nutr. 1984;40: 542–552.
13. Segal KR, Gutin B, Albu J. Thermic effects of food and exercise in lean and obese men of similar lean body mass. Am J Physiol. 1987;252:E110–E117.
14. Golay A, Schutz Y, Felber JP, et al. Blunted glucose-induced thermogenesis in 'overweight patients': A factor contributing to relapse obesity. Int J Obes. 1989;13:767–775.
15. Segal KR, Edano A, Blando L, Pi-Sunyer FX. Comparison of thermic effects of constant and relative caloric loads in lean and obese men. Am J Clin Nutr. 1990;51:14–21.
16. Durnin JVGA, Passamore R. *Energy, Work and Leisure.* London: Heinemann Educational Books; 1967.
17. Black AE, Coward WA, Cole TJ, Prentice AM. Human energy expenditure in affluent societies: an analysis of 574 doubly-labelled water measurements. Eur J Clin Nutr. 1996;50:72–92.
18. Rubner M. Die Gesetze des Energieverbrauchs bei der Ern'hrung. Leipzig, 1902.
19. Atwater WO, Benedict FG. A Respiration Calorimeter with Appliances for the Direct Determination of Oxygen. Washington, DC: Carnegie Institution of Washington; 1905.
20. Murgatroyd PR. A 30 m3 direct and indirect calorimeter. In: Van Es AJH, ed. *Human Energy Metabolism: Physical Activity and Energy Expenditure Measurements in Epidemiological Research Based Upon Direct and Indirect Calorimetry.* Wageningen, The Netherlands: Euro-Nut; 1984.
21. Schoeller DA. Measurement of energy expenditure in free-living humans by using doubly labeled water. J Nutr. 1988;118:1278–1289.
22. Roberts SB. Use of the doubly labeled water method for measurement of energy expenditure, total body water, water intake, and metabolizable energy intake in humans and small animals. Can J Physiol Pharm. 1989;67:1190–1198.
23. Lifson N, Gordon GB, McClintock R. Measure-

ment of total carbon dioxide production by means of D218O. J Appl Physiol. 1955;7:704–710.
24. Jacobs DR, Ainsworth BE, Hartman TJ, Leon AS. A simultaneous evaluation of 10 commonly used physical activity questionnaires. Med Sci Sports Exerc. 1993;25:81–91.
25. Taylor CB, Coffey T, Bera K, et al. Seven-day activity and self-report compared to a direct measure of physical activity. Am J Epidemiol. 1984;120: 818–824.
26. Livingstone MB, Prentice AM, Coward WA, et al. Simultaneous measurement of free-living energy expenditure by the doubly labeled water method and heart-rate monitoring. Am J Clin Nutr. 1990;52: 59–65.
27. Fernstrom JD, Miller GD, eds. *Appetite and Body Weight Regulation: Cephalic Phase Insulin Release in Humans: Mechanism and Functions*. Boca Raton, FL: CRC Press; 1994.
28. Berthoud HR, Bereiter DA, Trimble ER, et al. Cephalic phase, reflex insulin secretion. Diabetologia. 1981;20:393.
29. Feldman M, Richardson CT. Role of thought, sight, smell and taste of food in the cephalic phase of gastric acid secretion in humans. Gastroenterology. 1986; 90:428.
30. Sawaya AL, Fuss PJ, Dallal GE, Roberts SB. Meal palatability, substrate oxidation and blood glucose in young and older men. J Physiol Behav. 2001;70:1–8.
31. Gibbs J, Young RC, Smith GP. Cholecystokinin decreases food intake in rat. J Comp Physiol Psychol. 1973;84:488–495.
32. Smith GP, Gibbs J. Satiating effect of cholecystokinin. Ann N Y Acad Sci. 1994;713:236–241.
33. Geary N. Pancreatic glucagon signals postprandial satiety. Neurosci Biobehav Rev. 1990;14:323–338.
34. Chapman IM, Goble EA, Wittert GA, et al. Effect of intravenous glucose and euglycemic insulin infusions on short-term appetite and food intake. Am J Physiol. 1998;274:R596–R603.
35. Mayer J. Glucostatic mechanisms of the regulation of food intake. N Engl J Med. 1953;249:13–16.
36. Roberts SB. High glycemic index foods, hunger and obesity: Is there a connection? Nutr Rev. 2000;58: 163–169.
37. Campfield LA, Smith FJ, Rosenbaum M, Hirsch J. Human eating: evidence for a physiological basis using a modified paradigm. Neurosci Behav Rev. 1996;20:133–137.
38. Friedman MI. Control of energy intake by energy metabolism. Am J Clin Nutr. 1995;62: 1096S–1100S.
39. Bergmann JF, Chassany O, Petit A, et al. Correlation between echographic gastric emptying and appetite: influence of psyllium. Gut. 1992;33:1042–1043.
40. Horowitz M, Maddern GJ, Chatterton BE, et al. Changes in gastric emptying rates with age. Clin Sci. 1984;67:213–218.
41. Maffei M, Halaas J, Ravussin E, et al. Leptin levels in human and rodent: measurement of plasma leptin and ob RNA in obese and weight-reduced subjects. Nature Med. 1995;1:1155–1161.
42. Considine RV, Sinha MK, Heiman ML, et al. Serum innumoreactive-leptin concentrations in normal-weight and obese humans. N Engl J Med. 1996;334: 292–295.
43. Banks WA, Kastin AJ, Huang W, et al. Leptin enters the brain by a saturable system independent of insulin. Peptides. 1996;17:305–311.
44. Hallas JL, Boozer C, Blair WJ, et al. Physiological response to long-term peripheral and central leptin infusion in lean and obese mice. Proc Natl Acad Sci U S A. 1997;94:8878–8883.
45. Heymsfield SB, Greenberg AS, Fujioka K, et al. Recombinant leptin for weight loss in obese and lean adults. JAMA. 1999;282:1568–1575.
46. Weigle DS, Duell PB, Connor WE, et al. Effect of fasting, refeeding, and dietary fat restriction on plasma leptin levels. J Clin Endocrinol Metab. 1997; 82:561–565.
47. Brunner L, Levens N. The regulatory role of leptin in food intake. Curr Opin Clin Nutr Metab Care. 1998;1:565–571.
48. Matson CA, Wiater MF, Kuijper JL, Weigle DS. Synergy between leptin and cholecystokinin (CCK) to control daily caloric intake. Peptides. 1997;18: 1275–1278.
49. Barrachina MD, Martinez V, Wang L, et al. Synergistic interaction between leptin and cholecystokinin to reduce short-term food intake in lean mice. Proc Natl Acad Sci U S A. 1997;94:10455–10460.
50. Leibowitz SF. Brain neurotransmitters and eating behavior in the elderly. Neurobiol Aging. 1988;9: 20–22.
51. Kojima M, Hosoda H, Date Y, et al. Ghrelin is a growth-hormone-releasing acylated peptide from stomach. Nature. 1999;402:656–660.
52. Cummings DE, Purnell JQ, Frayo RS, et al. A preprandial rise in plasma ghrelin levels suggests a role in meal initiation in humans. Diabetes. 2001;50: 1714–1719.
53. Cummings DE, Weigle DS, Frayo RS, et al. Plasma ghrelin levels after diet-induced weight loss or gastric bypass surgery. N Engl J Med. 2002;346:1623–1630.
54. Schaller G, Schmidt A, Pleiner J, et al. Plasma ghrelin concentrations are not regulated by glucose or insulin: a double-blind, placebo-controlled crossover clamp study. Diabetes. 2003;52:16–20.
55. Saad MF, Bernaba B, Hwu CM, et al. Insulin regulates plasma ghrelin concentration. J Clin Endocrinol Metab.2002;87:3997–4000.
56. Nakagawa E, Nagaya N, Okumura H, et al. Hyperglycaemia suppresses the secretion of ghrelin, a novel

growth-hormone-releasing peptide: responses to the intravenous and oral administration of glucose. Clin Sci. 2002;103:325–328.

57. National Center for Health Statistics. *Health, United States, 2004. With Chartbook on Trends in the Health of Americans*. Hyattsville, MD: Centers for Disease Control and Prevention; 2004. Available online at: http://www.cdc.gov/nchs/data/hus/hus04.pdf. Accessed March 2, 2006.
58. Monteiro CA, Conde WL, Popkin BM. The burden of disease from undernutrition and overnutrition in countries undergoing rapid nutrition transition: a view from Brazil. Am J Public Health. 2004;94: 433–434.
59. Sawaya AL, Dallal G, Solymos G, et al. Obesity and malnutrition in a Shantytown population in the city of Sao Paulo, Brazil. Obes Res. 1995;3:107S–115S.
60. Popkin BM, Gordon-Larsen P. The nutrition transition: worldwide obesity dynamics and their determinants. Int J Obes Relat Metab Disord. 2004;28: S2–S9.
61. Ravussin E, Lillioja S, Knowler W. Reduced rate of energy expenditure as a risk factor for body-weight gain. N Engl J Med. 1988;318:467–472.
62. Roberts SB, Savage J, Coward WA, et al. Energy expenditure and energy intake in infants born to lean and overweight mothers. N Engl J Med. 1988;318: 461–466.
63. Goran M, Shewchuk R, Gower B, et al. Longitudinal changes in fatness in white children: no effect of childhood on energy expenditure. Am J Clin Nutr. 1998;67:309–316.
64. DeLany JP. Role of energy expenditure in the development of pediatric obesity. Am J Clin Nutr. 1998; 68:950S–955S.
65. Stunkard AJ, Berkowitz RI, Stallings VA, Schoeller DA. Energy intake, not energy output, is a determinant of body size in infants. Am J Clin Nutr. 1999; 69:524–530.
66. Sigal RJ, El-Hashimy M, Martin BC, et al. Acute postchallenge hyperinsulinemia predicts weight gain. Diabetes. 1997;46:1025–1029.
67. Putnam J. U.S. food supply providing more food and calories. Food Rev. 1999;22:2–12.
68. Bouchard C, Tremblay A, Despres JP, et al. The response to long-term overfeeding in identical twins. N Engl J Med. 1990;322:1477–1482.
69. Levine JA, Eberhardt NL, Jensen MD. Role of non-exercise activity thermogenesis in resistance to fat gain in humans. Science. 1999;283:212–214.
70. Ravussin E, Schutz Y, Acheson KJ, et al. Short-term, mixed-diet overfeeding in man: no evidence for "luxuskonsumption". Am J Physiol (Endocrinol Metab). 1985;249:E470–E477.
71. Roberts SB, Young VR, Fuss P, et al. Energy expenditure and subsequent nutrient intakes in overfed young men. Am J Physiol. 1990;259:R461–R469.
72. Saltzman E, Roberts SB. The role of energy expenditure in energy regulation: findings from a decade of research. Nutr Rev. 1995;53:209–220.
73. Shetty PS. Adaptation to low energy intakes: the responses and limits to low intakes in infants, children and adults. Eur J Clin Nutr. 1999;53:S14–S33.
74. Hoffman DJ, Sawaya AL, Verreschi I, et al. Why are nutritionally stunted children at increased risk of obesity? Studies of metabolic rate and fat oxidation in shantytown children from Sao Paulo, Brazil. Am J Clin Nutr. 2000;72:702–707.
75. Hoffman DJ, Roberts SB, Verreschi I, et al. Regulation of energy intake may be impaired in nutritionally stunted children from the shantytowns of Sao Paulo, Brazil. J Nutr. 2000;130:2265–2270.
76. Martins PA, Hoffman DJ, Fernandes MT, et al. Stunted children gain less lean body mass and more fat mass than their non-stunted counterparts: a prospective study. Br J Nutr. 2004;92:819–825.
77. Popkin BM, Richards MK, Monteiro CA. Stunting is associated with overweight in children of four nations that are undergoing the nutrition transition. J Nutr. 1996;126:3009–3016.
78. Cole TJ, Bellizzi MC, Flegal KM, Dietz WH. Establishing a standard definition for child overweight and obesity worldwide: international survey. *Brit Med J* 2000;320:1240–3.
79. Roberts SB, Dallal GE. The new childhood growth charts. *Nutr Rev* 2001;59:31–6.
80. Kinney JM, Tucker HN. *Energy Metabolism: Tissue Determinants and Cellular Corollaries.* New York: Raven Press, 1992.
81. Shills ME, Olson JA, Shike M. *Modern Nutrition in Health and Disease.* Philadelphia: Lea and Febiger; 1994.

# III Energy and Macronutrients

# 5

# Protein and Amino Acids

Paul B. Pencharz and Vernon R. Young

Jac Berzelius invented the term "protein," which was accepted by the Dutch chemist Geradus J. Mulder in the "Bulletin des Sciences Physiques et Naturelles en Neerlande" in 1838.[1] A readable account of the history behind the development and understanding of protein and amino acid nutrition has been published,[2] and the earlier practical recommendations about dietary intakes for protein have been summarized by Munro.[3] This chapter will be confined to a discussion of selected, more recent developments in the general area of protein and amino acid metabolism and its nutritional corollaries, with particular emphasis on relevance to human protein and amino acid nutrition.

## The Currency of Protein Metabolism and Nutrition—Amino Acid Functions

Proteins comprise one of the five classes of complex biomolecules found in cells and tissues, the others being DNA, RNA, polysaccharides, and lipids. The building blocks of proteins are amino acids and, as such, they are the currency of protein nutrition and metabolism.

Although there are hundreds of amino acids in nature, only about 20 of these commonly appear in proteins via charging by their cognate tRNAs and subsequent recognition of a codon on the mRNA. In the special case of certain selenoproteins, such as glutathione peroxidase and type 2 iodothreonine 5′-deiodinase, there is a formation and incorporation of selenocysteine into these proteins, which involves a complex process including conversion of a seryl-tRNA to selenocysteinyl-tRNA, which is then recognized by a UGA codon.[4] Selenomethionine is also present in body proteins, but this is derived from ingestion of this amino acid in plant foods or supplements such as yeasts.[5] Finally, other amino acids, such as hydroxyproline or $N^{\tau}$-methylhistidine, are also present in proteins. These arise via a post-transitional modification of specific amino acids residues, which gives particular structural and functional properties to proteins; a good example of this relates to the vitamin K-dependent carboxylation of glutamic acid residues in a number of proteins involved in blood coagulation and bone matrix deposition.[6] However, the common 20 amino acids, along with a few others not in peptide-bound form, such as ornithine and taurine, are of more immediate interest in discussions of the nitrogen economy of the body and protein and amino acid nutritional status of the human subject.

In addition to their role as substrates for polypeptide chain formation, amino acids serve other diverse roles. Some of these are listed in Table 1. Many of these roles have been recognized for some time, but an important new development relates to an increased understanding of the mechanisms that account for the stimulation of specific or global protein synthesis by amino acids. It is now clear that amino acids, especially the branched-chain amino acid leucine, can affect the initiation of mRNA translation. This is a complex process requiring multiple steps and more than a dozen eukaryotic initiation factors (eIF).[7] Two steps in this pathway are subject to regulation: the binding of initiator methionyl-tRNA to the 40S ribosomal subunit and the binding of mRNA to the 43S pre-initiation complex. Leucine appears to increase the availability of the mRNA cap-binding protein eIF4F,[8] and regulates translation through activation of the ribosomal protein S6 kinase ($p70^{S6k}$) pathway. Oral leucine may activate the kinase, the mammalian target of rapamycin (mTOR), which phosphorylates ($p70^{S6k}$).[9] The point, however, is that leucine and perhaps other amino acids can activate signaling pathways and so alter the rates of initiation of specific and global protein synthesis. Nevertheless, much more research will be needed before the mechanisms underlying amino acid-induced changes in protein synthesis in different cells and their roles in normal physiology are fully and suitably understood and established.

**Table 1.** Some Functions of Amino Acids

| Function | Example* |
|---|---|
| Substrates for protein synthesis | Those for which there is a codon |
| Regulators of protein turnover | Leucine, glutamine |
| Regulators of enzyme activity | Arginine and *N*-acetyl glutamate synthesis |
| | Phenylalanine and phenylalanine dehydroxylase activation |
| Precursor of signal transducer | Arginine, nitric oxide |
| Neurotransmitter | Tryptophan, glutamate |
| Ion fluxes | Taurine, glutamate, oxoproline |
| Precursor of nitrogen compounds | Nucleic acid, creatinine |
| Transporter of nitrogen | Glutamine, alanine, leucine (in the brain) |
| Translational regulator | Leucine [4E-BP1 and P70(s6k) via MTOR-dependent pathway] |
| Transcriptional regulator | Leucine limitation induces CHOP expression |

* MTOR, mammalian target of ripamycin; CHOP, CCAAT/enhancer binding protein(C/EBP) homologous protein.

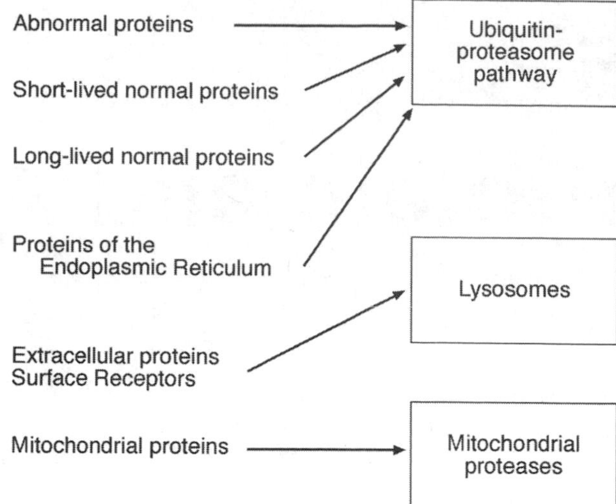


Figure 1. Substrates of different proteolytic pathway in mammalian cells. (From Locker et al.[12] Used with permission from the American Society for Nutrition.)

Evidence is accumulating that amino acids can regulate protein synthesis at the transcriptional level.[10] Because genome-wide surveys are now possible with array technology,[11] within a relatively short time a torrent of data will likely become available, giving a far more complete picture of the regulatory role played by amino acids alone and in combination with other amino acids and nutrients on the expression of genes, their protein products, and the functional interactions among these.

Tissue and organ protein content is also determined by the rate at which proteins are degraded. This overall process of protein degradation or breakdown plays many essential roles in the functioning of organisms, including, for example, cell growth, adaptation to different physiological conditions, elimination of abnormal or damaged proteins, and normal functioning of the immune system.[12] Multiple pathways for protein breakdown occur in all cells (Figure 1), with the bulk of intracellular protein being degraded via the energy-dependent, ubiquitin-proteasome pathway. Here the proteins are digested to small peptides and amino acids within a multi-subunit 20S proteasome, which, in association with a large 19S regulatory particle, forms the 26S complex. The proteasome may account for up to 1% of cellular proteins. This powerful proteolytic enzyme system cleaves peptide bonds in a unique way involving an ordered, cyclical bite-chew mechanism. This ubiquitin-proteasome pathway is activated under a number of conditions, including fasting.[12]

Studies of whole-body protein turnover have shown that protein degradation is inhibited with feeding and with increased protein intakes,[13] although it remains unclear which organs and tissues contribute most to this decline, and the relative effect of the amino acids versus carbohydrate and other energy-yielding sources still is not entirely determined. For example, oral amino acids alone do not appear to alter the rate of protein breakdown in the vastus lateralis,[14] whereas a mixed meal was shown to inhibit forearm muscle protein breakdown.[15] Thus, it is possible, at least in muscle, that amino acids enhance the inhibitory effect of proteolysis because of a carbohydrate-induced rise in insulin availability.[16] In turn, insulin reduces proteolysis, possibly by decreasing ubiquitin-mediated proteasomal activity.[17] The gut may be an important site of the meal-induced decline in whole-body protein breakdown.[18] In addition, the balance of amino acids or protein quality may influence whole-body protein breakdown. In low-birth-weight infants, it has been shown that a higher-quality amino acid mixture enhanced growth and amino nitrogen utilization by reducing whole-body protein breakdown and not by enhancing protein synthesis.[19]

The other multiple functions of the different amino acids and their putative mechanisms of action will not be elaborated here because other accounts are available.[20,21] Two further points need be made here. First, the functions of some of the amino acids can be varied and extensive, as indicated by the multiple functions played by glutamine (Table 2). These non-proteinogenic functions are relevant to dietary intake and requirement considerations, as suggested from the analysis made by Reeds[22] and presented in Table 3. Some of the pathways of end-product production can substantially affect the overall utilization of the amino acid precursor (e.g., creatinine synthesis, glycine or glutathione synthesis, cysteine or glycine utilization). Second, from a nutritional perspective, in carrying out their roles as substrates in protein synthesis (e.g.,

**Table 2.** Functions of Glutamine

| |
|---|
| Substrate of protein synthesis (codons; CAA, CAG) |
| Anabolic and trophic substance for muscle, intestine (competence factor) |
| Control for acid-base balance (renal ammoniagenesis) |
| Substrate for hepatic ureagenesis |
| Substrate for hepatic and renal gluconeogenesis |
| Fuel for intestinal enteroctyes |
| Fuel and nucleic acid precursor and important for generation of cytotoxic products in immunocompetent cells |
| Ammonia scavenger |
| Possible substrate for citrulline and arginine synthesis, although *in vivo* proline appears to be used instead of glutamine/glutamate |
| Nitrogen donor (nucleotides, amino sugars, coenzymes) |
| Nitrogen transport, 1/3 circulating nitrogen (muscle, lung) |
| Precursor of $\gamma$-aminobutyric acid (via glutamate) |
| Shuttle for glutamate (central nervous system) |
| Preferential substrate for glutathione peroxidase production? |
| Osmotic signaling mechanism in regulation of protein synthesis? |
| Stimulator of glycogen synthesis |
| Metabolism of L-arginine–nitric oxide |

for neurotransmitter signaling and detoxification functions) the amino acids turn over, and part of their nitrogen and carbon is removed from the body via catabolic and excretory pathways. Thus, the maintenance of an adequate body protein and amino acid status requires a sufficient intake of some preformed amino acids together with a utilizable source of nitrogen for the synthesis of the other amino acids and for production of physiologically important nitrogen-containing compounds.

# Nutritional Corollaries of the Amino Acids

It is no longer thought useful to classify the amino acids into two groups: those that are nutritionally indispensable (essential) and those that are dispensable (nonessential), as was done originally by Rose[23] based on a series of now-classical qualitative nitrogen balance experiments in adult men. Instead it is better to classify amino acids into three groups: the original two plus a third that is intermediate and is called "conditionally indispensable.[24] An obligatory dietary requirement exists for tryptophan, leucine, isoleucine, valine, phenylalanine, methionine, lysine, threonine, and histidine, or more specifically, for the ketoacid derivatives of the first five of these. The last three of this indispensable group of amino acids cannot be transaminated and so must be supplied in the diet. The other common amino acids in proteins can be synthesized from carbon and nitrogen donors: transamination of $\alpha$-ketoisocaproate, oxaloacetic acid, and pyruvate for glutamate, aspartic acid, and alanine, respectively; glycine from serine via serine hydroxymethlytransferase and serine from pyruvic acid; arginine and proline from glutamate; and asparagine from glutamine and aspartate. Tyrosine and cyst(e)ine are synthesized from their parent indispensable amino acids, phenylalanine and methionine, respectively. These two later amino acids, tyrosine and cysteine, are included in the conditionally indispensable amino acid group together with glutamine, arginine, and perhaps glycine and proline, because each does not appear to be synthesized at a rate sufficient to meet cellular needs under certain physiological or pathological conditions.[25,26] Thus, in severe burn injury, metabolic studies indicate that a dietary source of arginine is needed to maintain arginine homeostasis; low-birth-weight infants are unable to synthesize cysteine, proline, and possibly glycine in sufficient quantities.[24]

**Table 3.** Potential Contribution of Functionally Important End-product Synthesis to Amino Acid Needs in Adult Humans

| | Glutamate | Glycine | Cysteine<br>*µmol/kg/d* | Arginine | Methionine |
|---|---|---|---|---|---|
| Precursor kinetics | | | | | |
| Plasma flux | 4200 | 3960 | 1320 | 1800 | 528 |
| Net synthesis | 358 | 2730 | 96 | 180 | 168 |
| End-product production | | | | | |
| Creatine | | 170 | | 170 | 170 |
| Taurine | | | 7 | | |
| Nitric oxide | | | | 15 | |
| Glutathione | 550 | 550 | 550 | | |

From Table 7 in Reeds 2000,[22] where original references for these values are given.

A more recent development concerns the possible need for a preformed source of α-amino nitrogen. Previously, it had been thought that if intake of the indispensable amino acids was sufficient, only a source of nonspecific nitrogen—which might be in the form of a simple mixture such as urea and diammonium citrate—would be needed in addition.[27] However, this may not be a sufficient description of what is actually required to sustain an adequate state of protein nutriture for several reasons. The first relates to the utilization of urea nitrogen. Thus, recent emphasis has been given to a potentially key role played by the hydrolysis of urea nitrogen within the intestinal lumen (assumed to be largely a function of the activity of a microflora in the large bowel) and the significant contribution made by this liberated nitrogen to the nitrogen homeostasis of the host.[28] However, this concept has been questioned,[29] because in other studies the production of urea has been shown to increase linearly with increased protein intake, and the nitrogen released from urea via hydrolysis appears to have been rechanneled into pathways of urea formation. Thus, the extent to which urea nitrogen might be a net source of utilizable nitrogen, even under conditions of a low protein intake, remains unclear. Furthermore, as clearly outlined by Waterlow,[30] a great deal of uncertainty still exists about in vivo mechanisms responsible for both short- and longer-term regulation of urea production and therefore about the mechanisms responsible for maintenance of body protein balance.

Second, some organisms can fix atmospheric nitrogen into ammonia, and plants are able to use either the ammonia or soluble nitrates (that are reduced to ammonia) produced by nitrifying bacteria. However, vertebrates, including humans, must obtain nitrogen in the form of amino acids or other organic compounds. Glutamate and glutamine provide a critical entry of the ammonia from the nitrogen cycle[31] into other amino acids, and it is pertinent to examine briefly how the human body may obtain this nonspecific nitrogen to maintain the nitrogen economy of the individual.

Ammonia can be introduced into amino acids by ubiquitous glutamate ammonia ligase (glutamine synthetase) that catalyzes the following reaction:

$$\text{Glutamate} + NH^{+}{}_{4} + \text{ATP} \rightarrow \text{glutamine} + \text{ADP} + P_i + H^{+}$$

and by the glutamate dehydrogenase reaction:

$$\alpha\text{-Ketoglutarate} + NH^{+}{}_{4} + \text{NADPH} \leftrightarrow \text{L-glutamate} + \text{NADP} + H^{+}$$

However, because the $K_m$ for $NH^{+}{}_{4}$ in this reaction is high (>1 mmol/L), this reaction is thought to make only a modest contribution to net ammonia assimilation in mammals.[32] Furthermore, glutamate synthase is not present in animal tissues, and so a net gain of ammonia nitrogen could only occur via the glutamine synthetase retention if glutamate or possibly alanine or aspartate was already present.

A net incorporation of ammonia into glycine might also be achieved via the glycine synthase (glycine cleavage) reaction as follows:

$$CO_2 + NH^{+}{}_{4}\,H^{+} + \text{NAD} + N^5,N^{10}\text{-methylenetetrahydrofolate} \leftrightarrow \text{glycine} + \text{NAD}^{+} + \text{tetrahydrofolate}$$

The glycine might then be incorporated into proteins and such compounds as glutathione, creatine, and the porphyrins, or it can be converted to serine. The nitrogen of serine would then either be available for cysteine (and taurine) synthesis or released as ammonia via the serine dehydratase reaction. However, the glycine cleavage reaction appears to be more important in glycine catabolism[33] than in synthesis, and so the glycine-serine pathway of ammonia incorporation into the amino acid economy of the organism would appear to have only a limited effect on a net nitrogen input into the amino acid economy of the body.

The above suggests the possibility that glutamate is a key amino acid in making net amino nitrogen available to the mammalian organism; this glutamate would be derived ultimately from plant protein. Despite the significant role of glutamate as a nitrogen portal, it remains unclear whether a specific dietary need for glutamate exists if a sufficient amount of α-amino nitrogen is supplied, for example, as alanine and for aspartate. This question cannot be answered unequivocally at present, but it is clear that indispensable amino acids alone or in high concentrations relative to the dispensable amino acids will not support adequate growth in experimental animals. In sum, a source of preformed α-amino nitrogen from other than the indispensable amino acids and glycine appears to be required, but whether glutamate is needed specifically or would be a more efficient source of this α-amino nitrogen than its homologs,[34] for example, remains to be determined. Reeds[22] reviewed a number of findings revealing that diets completely devoid of glutamine and glutamate result in poorer growth in the otherwise healthy rat and pig, suggesting the possibility of a specific need for glutamate.

If the foregoing argument is correct, it introduces a new perspective on the nonspecific nitrogen component of the total protein requirement. In 1965, a Food and Agriculture Organization of the United Nations and the World Health Organization (FAO/WHO) Expert Group stated: 'The proportion of non-essential amino acid nitrogen, and hence the E/T [g total essential amino acids to total nitrogen] ratio of the diet, has an obvious influence on essential amino acid requirements. To make the best use of the available food supplies there is an obvious need to determine the minimum E/T ratios for different physiological states. Finally, the question arises whether there is an optimal pattern of non-essential amino acids."[35] This statement can just as well be repeated today, but recent studies are beginning to provide deeper insight into the nature of the nonspecific nitrogen needs of the human body. Not only is there an optimal E/T, as noted above, but it now seems likely that there is a desirable qualitative character to the nonspecific nitrogen supply—which raises the issue of the optimal sources and levels of α-amino nitrogen compounds in enteral formulations. This issue, for example, includes considerations of glutamate-proline-arginine interrelations,[36] not only in terms of the nitrogen economy of the host but also with respect to specific functions such as the capacity to maintain or stimulate the immune system and promote wound and tissue repair, and the effect that nonspecific nitrogen may have on polyamine and hormonal balance. The effect of a relatively high arginine intake in healthy subjects on arginine-citrulline-ornithine kinetics[37] has been examined. Although changes were not observed in the activity of the whole-body L-arginine–nitric oxide pathway, the generous level of arginine supplementation reduced rates of urea production and excretion and increased circulating insulin concentrations. How this apparent protein anabolic effect of high arginine supplementation is brought about (perhaps enhanced by insulin action) and what significance it has for the immune system are not known. Also, in light of current interest in immune-enhancing diets and the role arginine plays in aggravating or attenuating renal injury,[38,39] there are many unresolved questions about the quantitative role played by the nonspecific nitrogen component in supporting protein metabolism and function in the host.

## Postprandial Nitrogen and Amino Acid Utilization

The daily maintenance of body protein content is achieved through a complex set of integrated changes in rates of whole-body protein turnover, amino acid oxidation, urea production, and nitrogen excretion that occur at different rates during the postabsorptive, prandial, and postprandial periods of the 24-hour day.[40] Depending on diet composition, smaller or larger gains and losses of body proteins occur during the diurnal cycle of feeding and fasting. Amino acid and nitrogen requirements are met normally via ingestion of food proteins that undergo sequential metabolic and physiological processes. These processes include gastrointestinal digestion, peptide and amino acid absorption, transfer of amino acids into and among organs, and entry of the amino acids into metabolic pathways. Because of the recent research effort focused on the prandial-postprandial phase of protein and amino acid metabolism and utilization, this topic will be considered further here.

### *Dietary Protein Nitrogen Distribution after Protein Ingestion*

$^{15}$N-Labeled proteins have been used to follow the metabolic fate of dietary nitrogen after the ingestion of

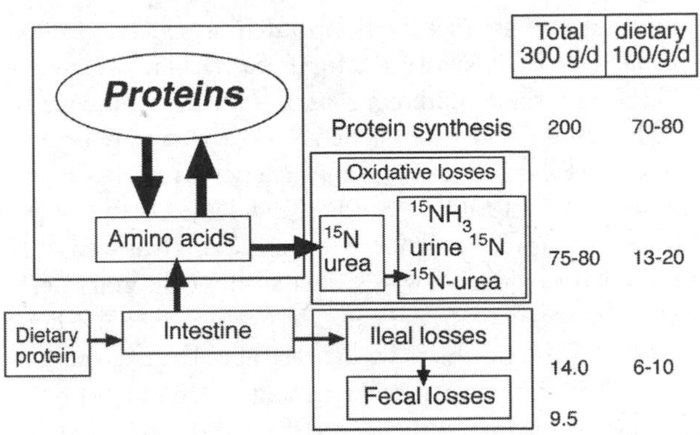


Figure 2. Contribution of dietary protein to the principal pathways of protein metabolism. (From Tomo and Bos.[41] Used with permission from the American Society for Nutrition.)

protein, and a number of these studies were summarized by Tomé and Bos.[41] As summarized in Figure 2, for approximately 100 g intake of well-balanced protein in the adult human, the fate of the dietary nitrogen is about 30% to 40% directed to anabolism, with a 17% to 25% loss via oxidative metabolism. A detailed model—based on data for [$^{15}$N]nitrogen kinetics determined in the intestine blood and urine after ingestion of $^{15}$N-labeled milk protein in humans—developed by Fouillet et al.[42] predicted that 8 hours after a meal, about 28% of the nitrogen is retained as free amino acids and 72% as protein. Approximately 30% of this protein retention occurred in the splanchnic region and 70% in peripheral tissues. This type of approach involving the use of intrinsically labeled proteins will continue to help define the factors, the mechanisms, and their quantitative significance that affect the postprandial utilization of ingested protein.

The extent and regulation of postprandial protein utilization has also been studied by acute $^{13}$C-leucine balance studies.[43] Although postprandial protein utilization is not influenced by adult age in a healthy population, it is affected by the quality of protein and the size of meals.[43] This tracer-based approach also has the potential for assessing efficacy of enteral formulations (e.g., in the nutritional support of institutionalized subjects and sick patients).

Among the additional factors that can influence the postprandial utilization of proteins is the time course of release and absorption of peptides and amino acids. This has led to the concept of slow and fast dietary proteins based on studies using $^{13}$C-leucine-labeled whey and caseins. Beaufrere et al.[44] showed that postprandial whole-body leucine oxidation over 7 hours was lower with casein than with whey protein despite a similar leucine intake (i.e., the postprandial protein utilization for casein was higher than for whey). Both of these protein sources are of high quality in adult human nutrition. Therefore, a difference in postprandial protein utilization under some circumstances might give a false indication of the comparative nutritional value of different formulations. Clearly, this new tracer-based metabolic paradigm requires further definition and standardization, but in a general context promises to be a valuable tool for understanding the metabolic basis of the requirement for protein and amino acids.

The temporal nature of the amino acid supply or pattern of feeding influences the efficiency of nitrogen and amino acid utilization. Studies involving 24-hour [1-$^{13}$C]leucine tracer balance determinations showed that daily leucine oxidation is lower when three discrete meals versus 10 small hourly meals are given over a 12-hour period.[45] This appears to be the case at both generous and limiting intakes of leucine, suggesting a better retention of oral amino acids with a less-frequent meal intake. Whether this phenomenon might be explained by the so-called anabolic drive of amino acids[40] cannot be determined yet, but it is evident that the pattern of protein and amino acid ingestion is a determinant of the efficiency of postprandial utilization. Furthermore, Arnal et al.[46] showed in studies with elderly subjects that protein retention was higher when 80% of the daily intake was consumed at midday compared with the daily protein supply given in four meals over 12 hours.

## Amino Acid Utilization by the Splanchnic Bed and the Gut

The intestines and liver modify the profile and amount of amino acids that disappear from the intestinal lumen and enter the portal and peripheral blood circulation. Although this has been known for some time, in recent years a more elaborate account of the quantitative removal and metabolic transformations of amino acids by the splanchnic region after their uptake from the lumen has been developed in humans and animal models, particularly those involving the use of different isotope tracer paradigms. For example, the combined use of tracers given orally and intravenously showed that the extent of uptake by the splanchnic region in adults differs among amino acids (Table 4),[47] and that this might also depend on the level of amino acid intake. The uptake of cystine shown here is very high, which is consistent with the data obtained in the pig.[48] The high uptake might also explain why the concentration of cysteine in the circulation shows little postprandial response to a wide range of cystine intakes.[49]

**Table 4.** Dual Isotope Tracer Model Estimates of Splanchnic Uptake of Amino Acids: Fed State in Healthy Adults*

| Amino Acid (Intake) | Uptake *% of intake* |
|---|---|
| Leucine (adequate) | 21 ± 6 |
| Leucine (flow) | 37 ± 5 |
| Leucine (adequate) | 10 ± 6 |
| Phenylalanine (adequate) | 25 |
| Phenylalanine (low) | 58 ± 4 |
| Tyrosine (adequate) | 37 |
| Arginine (adequate) | 34 ± 8 |
| Methionine (adequate) | 23 ± 2 |
| Cystine | >50 |

Taken from Young et al., 2000,[47] where references to original studies are cited.

Two important issues emerge from this rather global description of splanchnic amino acid metabolism, namely the relative importance of the gut versus the liver and the metabolic fate of the amino acids with these organ systems. This is a nutritionally important topic for several reasons. First, for example, Bertolo et al.[50] have concluded that the threonine requirement of neonatal piglets during parenteral nutrition is 45% of the mean oral requirement. This could be a result of one or a combination of factors, including a lower rate of threonine oxidation by intestinal tissues when threonine is given intravenously, and also reduced loses of threonine by the gastrointestinal tract because of reduced mucin production, these glycoproteins being rich in threonine. Second, Boirie et al.[51] reported that the splanchnic extraction of dietary leucine was twice as high in elderly men (50% ± 11%) as it was in young men (23% ± 3%), although whole-body leucine oxidation was similar for the two age groups. These investigators concluded that this difference in splanchnic uptake might limit the availability of leucine for peripheral tissue metabolism. On the other hand, Volpi et al.,[14] while also observing that the splanchnic extraction of oral phenylalanine was significantly higher in the elderly (47% ± 3%) than in the young (29% ± 5%), found that after an oral amino acid mixture was given, muscle protein synthesis was stimulated similarly in the young and the elderly.

Our understanding of the role of the gut and liver as the components of the splanchnic bed have been advanced by work from the laboratories of Reeds et al.[53] and Ball et al.[54] From this work it is now apparent that the small intestinal enterocyte plays an active role in amino acid metabolism, including the biosynthesis of arginine.[55] Arteriovenous differences and tracer studies have focused recently on the immediate fate of absorbed amino acids.[52,53] From studies of the portal availability of amino acids in pigs (summarized in Figure 3), Reeds

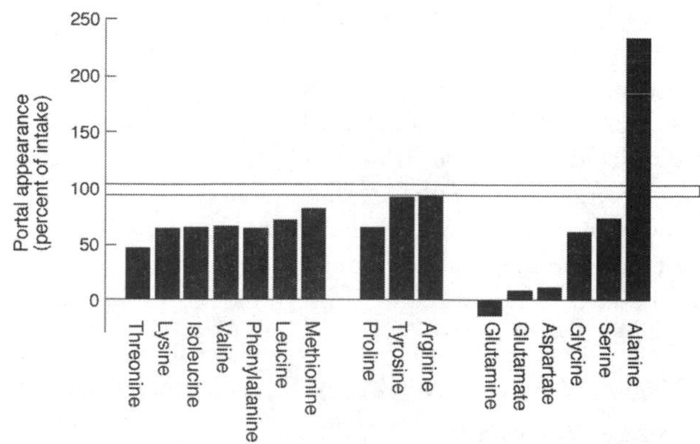


Figure 3. Portal availability of amino acids in pigs. (Used with permission from Reeds et al., 2000.[53])

et al.[53] concluded that the portal outflow varies widely among amino acids, with the portal balance of dietary threonine being consistently lower than that of other essential amino acids; nutritionally significant quantities of dietary glutamate and aspartate rarely appear in the portal blood (also, a net extraction of glutamine occurs across the gut and systemic glutamate, aspartate, and glutamine are derived almost exclusively from synthesis within the body); and some amino acids either appear in quantities similar to those ingested in dietary protein (arginine and tyrosine) or greatly exceed them (alanine).

Further details concerning the relative contributions of the arterial and dietary sources of amino acids to amino acid utilization by the intestine are given by Reeds et al.[53] Particularly important are the observations that the total utilization of lysine, leucine, and phenylalanine by the portal drained viscera might account for over 40% of the whole-body flux; the utilization of dietary glutamate, aspartate, and glutamine is considerable, and these amino acids contribute significantly to intestinal energy transformation; intestinal oxidation of leucine and lysine in milk-fed piglets accounts for about one-fifth to one-third of whole-body oxidation; with protein restriction the intestine continues to use a disproportionately large amount of indispensable amino acids[56]; the gut is an important site for synthesis of citrulline[52] that is then used for arginine synthesis, especially the kidney[57]; and mucosal glutathione is synthesized mainly from enteral precursor amino acids.[53]

In summary, beyond doubt the intestine plays a quantitatively and qualitatively crucial role in determining the amino acid needs of the individual and the availability of amino acids for the support of the body's physiological and organ systems.

## Intestinal Amino Acid Synthesis

As reviewed recently by Metges,[58] the gastrointestinal microflora make an important contribution to the status of nitrogen metabolism in the host. Considerable recent interest has focused on the possible role played by the microbial synthesis of amino acids to the amino acid economy of the host. It is important, therefore, to consider briefly whether amino acids synthesized de novo by the gastrointestinal microflora are absorbed and whether they contribute significantly to the amino acid economy of the host. On the basis of the interpretation of urinary $^{15}$N urea excretion after the administration of labeled urea, it has been suggested that the urea nitrogen liberated by urea hydrolysis in the colon can be incorporated by the intestinal microflora into amino acids and that these are subsequently absorbed the host. Although in the pig, colonic absorption of amino acids is possible, much of the experimental evidence in non-ruminant animals does not suggest quantitatively important amino acid absorption from the colon. Nevertheless, amino acids synthesized by the microflora in the pig can be absorbed, supposedly in the small intestine, and used for tissue protein synthesis. Tracer studies in animals and humans have shown a transfer of nonspecific nitrogen (ammonia, urea nitrogen, glutamate, etc.) into dispensable and indispensable amino acids.[59] For most amino acids, this input of $^{15}$N from urea may reflect nitrogen exchange or reversible transamination. However, lysine and threonine do not undergo transamination in mammalian tissues, so the appearance of $^{15}$N-labeled lysine or threonine in body proteins and plasma amino acids must reflect de novo synthesis of lysine and threonine by the intestinal microflora and the subsequent absorption of the labeled amino acids from the gastrointestinal tract. Comparative experiments with germ-free and conventional rats have confirmed that de novo synthesis of lysine is due to the activity of the indigenous microflora in the gastrointestinal tract.

Although in uremic patients and human subjects consuming a low-protein diet it had been shown that microbial lysine can be made available to the human host,[58] only recently have there been detailed attempts to quantify the significance of this source of lysine and threonine (or other amino acids) for host metabolism. Metges et al.[60] attempted to determine in healthy adults whether there is a net contribution to the lysine and threonine synthesized de novo by the gastrointestinal tract to lysine and threonine homeostasis. These experiments involved giving healthy adults either $^{15}$N-urea or $^{15}$N-ammonium chloride and monitoring the appearance of $^{15}$N in the plasma free lysine and threonine pools and in the amino acids of bacterial protein extracted from feces. Their findings confirmed the presence of microbially derived amino acids in host tissues, and it was suggested that a significant proportion of the circulating lysine and threonine in plasma might be derived from this intestinal source. However, insofar as microbial amino acid synthesis and absorption are accompanied by microbial breakdown of endogenous amino acids and oxidation of ingested and endogenous amino acids by intestinal tissues, these new data may not necessarily reflect a significant net increase in the daily availability of lysine or threonine through absorption from this microbial source. Similar findings have been made in male infants treated for severe undernutrition and given oral doses of $^{15}$N-urea.[61] It was concluded that a minimum of 4.7 mg lysine/kg body weight was made available by de novo synthesis and that urea hydrolysis can improve the quality of the dietary protein supply by enabling an increased supply of lysine and other indispensable amino acids.[61] However, a more cautious conclusion is possibly warranted. Although these recent studies[60,61] establish the significant presence of lysine and threonine of microbial origin in the plasma free amino acid pool, the quantitative significance of this source of amino acids is still unknown. Further, these new studies raise the question as to how various clinical states and diseases might affect the nutritional and metabolic interrelationships between the microbial flora of the intestine and the amino acid economy of host tissues.

## Nitrogen (Protein) Requirements

The generally accepted estimates of requirements for total nitrogen (protein) for humans are based internationally on estimates by the 1985 FAO/WHO/United Nations University (UNU) expert group,[62] and the recommendations emerging from these estimates (Table 5). The essential features of the approach to estimate protein requirement values in infants, children, and adolescents were reviewed and summarized.[63] For infants under 6 months of age, the recommendation is derived from data on breast-milk protein intake. For infants ≥6 months of age and for children and adolescents, a modified factorial approach was used, where the maintenance requirement at 6 months was taken to be 120 mg nitrogen/kg/d, declining to 103 mg nitrogen/kg/d by age 18; a growth component was estimated and 50% was added to provide a margin of safety, because growth rates vary from day to day and because protein is not stored in times of a relative excess in intake; the fractional efficiency of nitrogen utilization from high-quality protein sources for both maintenance and growth was taken to be 0.7; and the coefficients of variation for maintenance and growth were taken to be 12.5% and 35%, respectively, for calculating the total coefficient of variation and a recommended safe protein intake level.

**Table 5.** 1985 Food and Agriculture Organization of the United Nations, World Health Organization, and United Nations University (FAO/WHO/UNU) Safe Protein Intakes for Selected Age Groups and Physiological States*

| Group | Safe Protein Level g/kg/d |
|---|---|
| Infants | |
| 0.3–0.5 years | 1.47 |
| 0.75–1.0 years | 1.15 |
| Children | |
| 3–4 years | 1.09 |
| 9–10 years | 0.99 |
| Adolescents | |
| 13–14 years (girls) | 0.94 |
| 13–14 years (boys) | 0.97 |
| Young adults, 19+ years | 0.75 |
| Elderly | 0.75 |
| Women, pregnant | |
| 2nd trimester | + 6 g daily |
| 3rd trimester | + 11 g daily |
| Women, lactating | |
| 0–6 months | + ≈16 g daily |
| 6–12 months | + 1 g daily |

* Values are for proteins such as those of quality equal to hen egg, cow milk, meat, or fish.
Data summarized from FAO/WHO/UNU, 1985.[62]

The protein requirements in adult men and women, including the elderly, were derived from both short-term and long-term nitrogen balance studies with a mean requirement being set for high-quality protein at 0.6 g/kd/d for men. From this a safe protein intake level of 0.75 g/kg/d was proposed for men, women, and the elderly (Table 5). Additional estimates were included to arrive at the recommendations for pregnant and lactating women.

Currently, protein and amino acids requirement estimates are being reassessed by both the Institute of Medicine (IOM), National Academy of Sciences,[104] and an expert panel assembled by the WHO, which is yet to report on their findings. A draft version of the Dietary Reference Intake IOM report is available on the Web.[104]

### *Current Estimates for Infants and Children*

In 1996, the International Dietary Energy Consultancy Group (IDECG)[64] reevaluated the approach earlier used to derive the 1985 FAO/WHO/UNU recommendations for protein intakes in infants, and in doing so, took into account new data for estimates of the intake of breast milk, the content of protein nitrogen and non-protein nitrogen, and the efficiency of retention of non-protein nitrogen, which the group took to be 46% to 61% rather than the assumed value of 100% used by the 1985 consultation,[62] and used body weights of breast-fed rather than bottle-fed babies. These revised IDECG protein intake estimates by breast-fed infants were, depending on age, about 10% to 26% lower than the 1985 FAO/WHO/UNU values.

For infants over 6 months of age and for young children, the IDECG group[64] used the factorial approach but with some important differences from the 1985 recommendations: the 1985 maintenance requirement of 120 mg nitrogen/kg/d was revised downward to 90 mg nitrogen/kg/d; the 50% addition to account for day-to-day variation in growth was discarded; new estimates were made of the coefficient of variation for inter-individual variability in requirements for infants. However, the IDECG group retained the 70% (0.7 fraction) retention efficiency value. Thus, the more recent estimates of safe levels of protein intake are about 25% to 30% lower than those made in the 1985 FAO/WHO/UNU report[58] (Table 6).

### *Adults and the Elderly*

The 1985 FAO/WHO/UNU protein requirements and recommendations for dietary protein intakes in adults have not yet been revisited. However, in view of the rapidly growing number of elderly people in both the developed and developing regions of the world, it is important that increased attention be given to the nitrogen and amino acid needs of this sector of the population. The 1985 FAO/WHO/UNU group[62] concluded that the safe intake of protein should not be lower than 0.7 g/kg/d for

**Table 6.** International Dietary Energy Consultancy Group (IDECG)[60] Revised Estimates for the Average Requirements and Safe Level of Protein Intakes for Infants

| | Average Protein Requirement | | |
|---|---|---|---|
| Age *months* | IDECG[64] | FAO/WHO/ UNU, 1985[62] *g protein/kg/d* | IDECG Safe Protein Intake[64]* |
| 0–1 | 1.99 | — | 2.69 |
| 1–2 | 1.54 | 2.25 | 2.04 |
| 2–3 | 1.19 | 1.82 | 1.53 |
| 3–4 | 1.06 | 1.47 | 1.37 |
| 4–5 | 0.98 | 1.34 | 1.25 |
| 5–6 | 0.92 | 1.30 | 1.19 |
| 6–9 | 0.85 | 1.25 | 1.09 |
| 9–12 | 0.78 | 1.15 | 1.02 |

* Includes separate variations for maintenance (12.5% coefficient of variation) and growth, as described in Table 5 of IDECG.[64]

older adults and the elderly. There has been some limited additional study on the protein requirements of the elderly since that recommendation was made. Campbell and Evans[65] proposed a higher safe protein intake of 1 to 1.25 g/kg/d based on their own investigations and a reassessment of the literature. In contrast, Millward and Roberts,[66] in their review of the published literature, concluded that it has not been demonstrated unequivocally that the mean protein requirement increases with age. On the basis of body weight as well as fat-free mass, a group at the University of Surrey concluded from [$^{13}$C]leucine tracer studies that the apparent daily protein requirement is lower in the elderly.[67] However, the experimental approach used by these investigators has its inherent limitations and, in particular, their study subjects had not been adjusted to a standard diet before the tracer studies. Kurpad and Vaz[68] concluded that the protein requirement of the elderly is no less than in young adults, and earlier Young et al.[69] proposed, because of the increased morbidity and disease burden in the elderly, that a rational and sound recommendation for good-quality protein would be about 1 g/kg/d for this age group.

Clearly, further research into the protein requirements in the elderly would be highly desirable, although the topic of the nitrogen requirements at various stages in the life of generally healthy individuals is not currently a particularly active focus of investigation or one that is open to major controversy. This differentiates it from the requirements for indispensable amino acids, which we will be considered below.

# Requirements for Indispensable Amino Acids

## *1985 FAO/WHO/UNU Values and Those for Infants*

The state of the art with respect to the definition and determination of the quantitative needs for the specific indispensable amino acids has been reviewed by various investigators.[63,70-74,114] The 1985 FAO/WHO/UNU[62] recommendations for four separate age groups indicated that the requirements, per unit body weight, decline substantially between infancy and adulthood, falling from about 714 mg/kg/d in infants ages 3 to 4 months to about 84 mg/kg/d in adults (Table 7). When recommendations are expressed per unit of safe protein intake (less histidine), the pattern of change with growth development is also marked in that there is a fall in the ratio of total indispensable amino acids to protein—434 mg/g protein for infants and 111 mg/g protein for adults. The biological basis for this dramatic change remains unclear, particularly because daily protein maintenance accounts for a very high proportion of the total requirement, even in the young. Thus, it has been estimated that for the child 2 years of age, maintenance accounts for 80% to 90% of the total protein requirement.[73,75] The present international values (Table 7) may be confounded by the limitations of the experimental approaches used for determining requirements rather than reflecting the true requirements. In addition, the requirements for infants were derived from a combination of the lowest intakes found to be adequate for all infants tested in the studies by Holt and Snyderman[76] or those calculated by Fomon and Filer,[77] which were the lowest intakes of amino acids by infants fed a variety of formulas at levels that maintained adequate growth. The values for preschool children were obtained from studies carried out at the Institute of Nutrition for Central America and Panama (Guatemala), the data of which have only been presented in summary form in a conference proceedings[78,79]; the values for school-age children are limited to a series of studies carried out by Nakagawa et al.[80] in Japan; and the adult values are based on the studies by Rose[81] in men and from similar investigations by others in women.[82] Thus, the adult values given in this 1985 report (Table 7) are no longer considered to be acceptable or nutritionally relevant.[83]

The amino acid requirements in infants also were reassessed using a factorial approach.[64] The derived values (expressed per kilogram of body weight) for infants ages 3 to 6 months are substantially lower than those proposed in the 1985 FAO/WHO/UNU report. This is also true for the amino acid requirement values, when expressed per unit of protein, because the United Nations values were based on the amino acid composition of breast milk protein rather on experimentally derived requirement values.

**Table 7.** 1985 FAO/WHO/UNU[58] Estimates of Amino Acid Requirements* at Different Ages

| Amino acid | Infants, (3–4 mo) | Children (2 yrs) | School Boys (10–12 yrs) | Adults |
|---|---|---|---|---|
| | | mg/kg/d | | |
| Histidine | 28 | ? | ? | 8–12 |
| Isoleucine | 70 | 31 | 28 | 10 |
| Leucine | 161 | 73 | 44 | 14 |
| Lysine | 103 | 64 | 44 | 12 |
| Methionine and cystine | 58 | 27 | 22 | 13 |
| Phenylalanine and tyrosine | 125 | 69 | 22 | 14 |
| Threonine | 87 | 37 | 28 | 7 |
| Tryptophan | 17 | 12.5 | 3.3 | 3.5 |
| Valine | 93 | 38 | 25 | 10 |
| Total | 714 | 352 | 216 | 84 |
| Total expressed per gram protein (mg/g crude protein)* | 434 | 320 | 222 | 111 |

*Milligrams per gram crude protein.
From Table 38 in WHO, 1985, based on all amino acids minus histidine.

## *Adult Amino Acid Requirement Values*

The amino acid requirement estimates for adults, summarized by the 1981 United Nations consultation (Table 7) and reported by FAO/WHO/UNU in 1985, have been widely used internationally, and were based on nitrogen balance studies by Rose and others in the 1950s and 1960s.[81,82] Because the validity of these earlier nitrogen balance studies and the interpretations drawn from them were seriously questioned and debated, new approaches were undertaken to reassess the amino acid requirements for adults.[70,71,84] A detailed review of all aspects of nitrogen balance measurements is well worth consulting.[85] It is not feasible to review and comment in detail here on all of the approaches that have been used in attempts to derive quantitative values for the amino acid requirements in healthy adults. However, because of their contemporary significance, mention should be made of the tracer techniques that have now replaced or at least sidelined extensive use of earlier approaches, including nitrogen balance and response of plasma amino acid concentration to amino acid intake.

With advances in the measurement of stable isotope enrichment in biological matrices and the expanded use of tracers enriched with these isotopes in human metabolic research, a series of tracer studies were begun in the early 1980s to determine amino acid requirements in adults.[84,86,87] Since then a number of different paradigms have been used in tracer-based studies of human amino acid requirements, which are distinguished by tracer choice and protocol design. Some studies used a tracer of the test amino acid to assess the rate of the amino acid's oxidation at various test intake levels (the direct amino acid oxidation [DAAO] approach) or to determine the body $^{13}$C-amino acid balance (the direct amino acid balance [DAAB] technique). These techniques have been used to assess the requirements for leucine, valine, lysine, threonine, and phenylalanine. Some studies used an indicator tracer to assess the status of indicator amino acid oxidation (IAAO) or indicator amino acid balance (IAAB) with various levels of a test amino acid. An example of the IAAO approach is seen in the study by Zello et al.[88] on the rate of [$^{13}$C]phenylalanine oxidation at various levels of lysine intake. Kinetic studies designed to assess the retention of protein during the postprandial phase of amino acid metabolism used [$^{13}$C]leucine as a tracer.[89] Studies using these methods have been conducted by Young et al.[90-97] and by Pencharz et al.[98-101] There is also a recent review comparing the different isotope methods.[74] The current consensus is that IAAO and 24-hour IAAB are the preferred methods.

**IAAO.** This method was applied initially in studies of amino acid requirements in young growing pigs and validated against traditional approaches based on criteria of growth, nitrogen balance, and body composition.[93] The underlying concept of this technique is illustrated in Figure 4 and was discussed in detail by Zello et al.[98] Thus, the requirement for an indispensable amino acid (e.g., lysine) is determined from the pattern or rate of oxidation of another (indicator) amino acid (e.g., [$^{13}$C]phenylalanine). This approach was first applied in adults by Zello et al.[88] in a study designed to determine the dietary requirement for lysine. Pencharz et al. extended this approach to estimate the tryptophan[99] and threonine[100] requirements of healthy adults and to follow-up on the study of lysine requirements of adults.[101] A recent review is available.[74]

The experimental approach followed by the Toronto group (Pencharz, Ball, and colleagues) involved giving

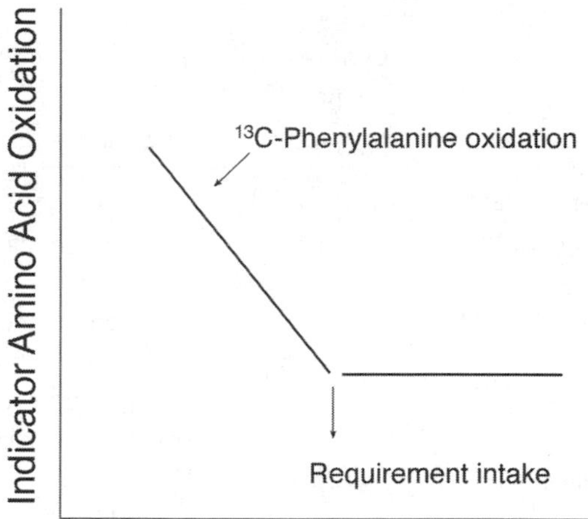


Figure 4. A schematic presentation of the indicator amino acid oxidation approach for estimating the requirements for specific indispensable amino acids. The indicator used is [$^{13}$C]phenylalanine.[98]

subjects an adequate, constant diet for a few days, followed by [$^{13}$C]phenylalanine tracer study at a test intake level of the amino acid being studied. During the tracer protocol, subjects are given small hourly meals for 7 hours, beginning 3 hours before the infusion of labeled indicator tracer. Isotope data for the last 2 hours of the 4-hour tracer period are then used to estimate the indicator amino acid oxidation rate.

The IAAO approach has a number of advantages: it is possible to carry out a relatively large number of relatively short-term tracer studies within the same subject; problems arising from changes in pool sizes and kinetics that might affect the behavior of a direct tracer and interpretation of the isotope data obtained are, presumably, obviated or largely avoided when an indicator amino acid tracer is used; and no a priori reason exists for determining the actual rate of indicator amino acid oxidation because the pattern of release of the $^{13}$C label in expired air can provide the basis for the breakpoint analysis on the intake-oxidation response curve. This pattern of $^{13}$C appearance should, in theory, parallel that for the actual oxidation rate of the indicator. However, this was not found in a study by Duncan et al.[101] of the lysine requirement for adult males; although the absolute rate of phenylalanine oxidation showed a generally similar pattern to that of $^{13}CO_2$ release, the variation precluded use of the oxidation to estimate the requirement for lysine.

The disadvantages of the IAAO method include the fact that it has been based essentially on a short-term, fed-state model. Therefore, there is uncertainty as to whether the same pattern of change or at least breakpoint in IAAO response would apply similarly to a later (or earlier) period within the 12-hour fed phase as compared with the specific 2-hour period used to date to elaborate the relationship among amino acid intake, oxidation, and requirements. The 24-hour tracer studies showed that the rate of amino acid oxidation changes throughout a constant-fed period in a complex way depending on the adequacy of amino acid intake. In summary, it is not certain whether the time frame chosen for detailed study in the investigations by the Toronto group are optimal, although they have given results generally consistent with those obtained using the 24-hour DAAO and 24-hour DAAB approaches.

Zello et al.[98] state that the IAAO technique has the advantage of permitting oxidation measurements to be taken with no prior adaptation to the level of the test amino acid in contrast to the DAAO and DAAB studies, where adaptation periods of approximately 6 to 7 days are included in the study design. This is not necessarily an advantage of the IAAO technique for two reasons. First, the DAAO procedure could be similarly applied without a period of dietary adaptation, just as is the case of the Toronto studies. Second and more important, the lack of a period of dietary adaptation to a test amino acid intake level is potentially a serious design limitation, at least in terms of how the Toronto group has applied the IAAO approach. Millward[70] argued that without a suitable adaptation period to a specific and lower test lysine intake, the IAAO approach effectively would give a higher value than the minimum physiological requirements for lysine. Young[84] offered an opposite view, namely that the minimum requirement might, in theory, be underestimated when applying the IAAO approach under conditions in which there is no adaptation to a lower than usual intake. Recent studies by Millward et al.[89] on the postprandial utilization of milk and wheat proteins support the latter view; their estimate of the nutritional quality of wheat protein was higher than they had predicted, presumably because of the buffering effect of a significant and replete free tissue (possibly muscle) lysine pool over the course of their short-term tracer study. Nevertheless, there is a need to directly establish whether and, if so, for how long an adaptation period should be included in studies involving the fed state and the IAAO technique.

Another limitation of the short-term, fed-state IAAO method is that the approach has not been validated directly or in detail in healthy adults. Support for the concept is based essentially on studies in piglets whose growth rate and intensity of protein metabolism is profoundly different from those in human adults.[73] The question to be raised is whether the breakpoint (Figure 4) in the relationship between indicator amino acid oxidation and test amino acid intake response as applied in adult humans is actually the intake level that just meets the maintenance requirement. Clearly, from the aggregate of a large number of nitrogen balance studies in adults, there is a decline in the efficiency of dietary nitrogen utilization before the minimum requirement for maintenance is reached.[62] If this curvilinear response also applies to the utilization of a limiting indispensable amino acid, it could be argued that the minimum intake required to just meet the requirement for maintenance is somewhat higher than that indicated by the breakpoint derived from short-term, fed-state, tracer IAAO studies

**24-Hour IAAO and 24-Hour IAAB.** To circumvent the various limitations of the short-term IAAO technique, a 24-hour indicator amino acid oxidation balance approach has been developed and applied in [$^{13}$C]leucine tracer studies of the lysine requirement of adult Indian subjects and more recently in studies of the threonine requirement in adults.[102-103] The approach is similar in concept to that of IAAO technique, but is based on a 24-hour indicator amino acid oxidation-daily balance protocol. The 24-hour IAAB can be regarded as a functional criterion of dietary amino acid adequacy, in contrast to a measure of the short-term, fed-state indicator amino acid oxidation rate that is a surrogate marker of adequacy. The disadvantage relates to the complexity of the 24-hour tracer study and the stringent demands and restraints that it places on the experimental subject. Further, the validity of leucine as an indicator amino acid has not been experimentally demonstrated, unlike phenylalanine and lysine.[74] It is also open to the criticism that it may not be entirely physiological in construct. However, at present, the 24-hour IAAB technique represents the state of the art. Therefore, wherever possible, it should be used as the gold standard on which to validate or compare other and possibly less complex tracer approaches. Having said this, the estimates of dietary indispensable amino acid requirements which have been determined by IAAO and 24-h IAAO/IAAB are very similar; currently these are for lysine, methionine and threonine.[74]

**Use of IAAO to Determine Amino Acid Requirements in Children.** Using IAAO and 24-h IAAO/IAAB, a complete picture of the dietary essential amino acid requirements has been obtained for adults (except for histidine[74,122]). Given the generally unsatisfactory nature of the nitrogen balance of amino acid requirement estimates in childhood (outlined above), the current view is to use a factorial approach to calculate amino acid requirements in children[104]: the adult estimate, representing the maintenance value, to which is added an estimate for growth. For the branched-chain amino acids there are paired studies using IAAO in adults and in school aged children (6–10 years) that support using the factorial method.[105,106]

**Some Estimates of Adult Human Amino Acid Requirements.** The precise, quantitative requirements for the indispensable amino acids in adults, as indicated earlier, are still a matter of debate and uncertainty because of the different methods and criteria used and differences in the interpretations of data. For illustrative purposes, the results from major studies concerned with estimation of the mean requirement for lysine in adults are summarized in Table 8. As for the other amino acids, available

**Table 8.** Estimates of Mean Requirement for Lysine: Nitrogen Balance and Tracer Studies

| Major Procedure | Mean Lysine Requirement *mg/kg/d* | Comments |
|---|---|---|
| Nitrogen Balance | | |
| Rose et al.[107] | 8.8 | Nitrogen balance; multiple levels |
| Jones et al.[110] | 6.5–8 | Nitrogen balance; multiple levels |
| Fisher et al.[121] | <1 | Nitrogen balance; variable intakes |
| Hegsted et al.[111] | 29.2 | Regression by regression |
| Millward[75] | 18.6 | Reevaluation by curvilinear regression and +0.3gN on data from Jones et al.[101] |
| Rand and Young[112] | 30.6 | Reevaluation by nonlinear regression + 0.5 g nitrogen on data from Jones et al.[101] |
| Tracer Approaches | | |
| Meredith et al.[87] | ≈30 | Fed state: multiple level, DAAO |
| Meredith et al.[87] | >20<30 | Estimated DAAB |
| El-Khoury et al.[97,112] | ≈30 | Three levels: 24-hour DAAB |
| Kurpad et al.[115] | 29 | 24-hour DAAB; four levels, IAAB |
| Zello et al.[88] | 37 | IAAO; multiple levels |
| Duncan et al.[101] | 45 | IAAO; multiple levels |
| Kriengsinyos[108] | 35 | IAAO, multiple levels |
| Kriengsinyos[109] | 35(38) | IAAO, multiple levels* |
| Millward et al.[89] | 23 | Leucine retention (PPU) |
| Millward[43] | 23–27 | Leucine retention (PPU) |

DAAO, direct amino acid oxidation; DAAB, direct amino acid balance; IAAB, indicator amino acid balance; IAAO, indicator amino acid oxidation; PPU, postprandial utilization.*Only study in women during both phases of menstrual cycle (see text).

data do not indicate any major quantitative differences between the lysine requirement in men and women. Recent IAAO studies confirm that gender differences in lysine (Table 8) are small.[108,109] However, lysine requirements in the luteal phase (38 mg/kg/d) were significantly higher than during the follicular phase (35 mg/kg/d).[109] Data from the earlier balance studies in men[107] and women[82] indicated a mean requirement of approximately 8 mg/kg/d. The short-term nitrogen balance studies by Fisher et al.[121] suggested an even lower mean requirement (<1 mg/kg/d). The latter estimate is probably complicated by an inadequate experimental design involving consecutive short nitrogen balance periods, including some with lysine and total nitrogen intake levels changing simultaneously.

Three mathematical analyses of the original nitrogen balance data led to much higher requirements after accounting for unmeasured miscellaneous nitrogen losses (Table 8). The analyses by Hegsted[111] and Rand and Young[112] of the nitrogen balance data of Jones et al.[110] gave a mean lysine requirement of about 30 mg/kg/d; the analysis by Millward[75] gave a mean requirement of 18.6 mg/kg/d, because the assumed allowance for unmeasured nitrogen losses were somewhat lower than that used in the analyses by Hegsted[111] and Rand and Young.[112]

Results from series of different tracer studies—despite their individual limitations and different designs—have yielded mean requirement values ranging from >20 to 45 mg/kg/d, with a number of studies indicating a mean value of 30 to 35 mg/kg/d (Table 8).

The studies by Meredith et al.[87] used the short-term DAAB and DAAO approaches. Also, those by Zello et al.,[88] Duncan et al.,[101] and Millward et al.[43,89] were all based on short-term, fed-state tracer paradigms. The 24-hour DAAB studies by El-Khoury et al.[97,113] included three test lysine levels: one was at a slightly higher level (15 mg/kg/d) than the FAO/WHO/UNU[62] proposed upper requirement of 12 mg/kg/d; another was at 30 mg/kg/d, which was predicted earlier to be close to the mean minimum requirement[114]; and the third was at a generous 77 mg/kg/d. Estimated mean whole body [$^{13}$C]lysine balance was negative at the 15 mg/kg/d intake and at equilibrium when the intake was 30 mg/kg/d. Because not all subjects were at equilibrium at the latter intake, it is reasonable to conclude that the minimum requirement is higher than the FAO/WHO/UNU[62] value and apparently close to the 29 mg/kg/d value obtained by Kurpad et al.[115] using the 24-hour IAAB approach. The findings from the short-term, fed-state tracer studies are consistent with this interpretation.

This mean requirement value of about 30 mg/kg/d is consistent with the requirement estimates for lysine intake that were judged by Young and El-Khoury,[116] from considerations of the prandial retention of lysine, necessary to balance the postabsorptive losses of lysine and requirement estimates based on the data of Price et al.[117] Furthermore, this author's reinterpretation of the curve of lysine intake versus plasma lysine response[87,116] leads to a breakpoint at a lysine intake of approximately 30 mg/kg/d.

A comparable summary of the available data for all of the other indispensable amino acids would be beyond the scope of this chapter. Therefore, for summary purposes, two amino acid requirement patterns for adults, expressed per body weight and per unit of protein requirement, that have been proposed more recently, together with the 1985 FAO/WHO/UNU[62] adult amino acid requirement pattern, are given in Table 9.

The requirement value presented in Table 9 of most importance and open, therefore, to scrutiny and debate is that for lysine, because it is the most likely first limiting amino acid in diets that are based predominantly on cereal staples, particularly wheat.[118] This means that it is of potential public health significance in the developing regions of the world. However, the value represented by the MIT pattern and the higher figure given in the Millward[75] pattern are supported by nitrogen balance data on the nutritional quality of whole-wheat proteins[119] and by the predicted protein nutritional value of wheat protein based on its amino acid content.[62,120] This suggests that, at least

**Table 9.** Three Proposed Patterns of Amino Acid Requirements in Healthy Adults

| Amino Acid | FAO/WHO/UNU, 1985[62] | Millward, 1999[72] | Young & Borgonha, 2000[63] |
|---|---|---|---|
| Isoleucine | 10* (13)† | 18‡ (30) | 23 (35) |
| Leucine | 14 (19) | 26 (44) | 40 (65) |
| Lysine | 12 (16) | 19 (31) | 30 (50) |
| Methionine + cystine | 13 (17) | 16 (27) | 13 (25) |
| Phenylalanine + tyrosine | 14 (19) | 20 (33) | 39 (65) |
| Threonine | 7 (9) | 16 (26) | 15 (25) |
| Tryptophan | 3.5 (5) | 4 (6) | 6 (10) |
| Valine | 10 (13) | 14 (23) | 20 (35) |

* Values expressed as mg/kg/d.
† Values expressed as mg/g protein.
‡ Present and higher estimates by Millward et al.[89,43] are now 23 and 27 mg/kg/d, respectively.

for lysine, the higher values proposed by Millward[43] and those advanced by the MIT group[63,94] are probably reasonable approximations of the actual requirement and clearly distinct from the far lower value proposed by the 1985 FAO/WHO/UNU group.[61]

## Excessive Intakes of Protein and of Amino Acids

The upper limit of protein intake in adults has been set at no more than 30% of total energy intake.[104] Briefly, consideration of maximal urea synthesis rates and observations of explorers who lived on exclusively animal-based diets provided the basis for this recommendation. For example, early American explorers in the winter suffered from "rabbit starvation" when they subsisted on a diet of rabbit meat, which contains very little fat,[104] resulting in protein intakes greater than 30% of total energy intake.

Data on excessive intakes of individual amino acids are limited except for phenylalanine, for which most of the data are centered on brain damage in persons with phenylketonuria. A recent review of available information on this topic, which systematically considers all amino acids, can be found in the IOM report.[104]

## Protein Malnutrition

Protein is the fundamental component for cellular and organ function.[104] The diet must contain not only enough protein and amino acids but also enough non-protein energy to permit optimal utilization of dietary protein.[19] Protein energy malnutrition (PEM) is quite common in the world as a whole and has been reported by the FAO in 2000 to be associated with 6 million deaths in children.[123] In the industrialized world, PEM is seen predominantly in hospitals and in association with disease.[104,124,125]

Protein deficiency has adverse effects on all organs,[126] and of particular concern in infants and young children PEM may have long-term adverse effects on brain function.[127] Patients with PEM have reduced immune function are therefore more susceptible to infection.[125] Total starvation will result in death in an initially normal weight adult in 70 days,[128] and since these persons still had some adipose tissue reserves, their deaths can be regarded as primarily being due to protein deprivation. By way of contrast, protein and energy reserves are much lower in very-low-birth-weight premature infants, and with total starvation the survival of 1000-g neonates has been calculated to be only 5 days.[129]

## Summary and Conclusions

Knowledge continues to expand about the physiology of protein and amino acid metabolism in the mammalian organism, especially in relation to human protein and amino acid nutrition. This chapter focuses attention on recent advances in relation to amino acid function and protein and amino acid utilization during the prandial and postprandial period of amino acid metabolism. The importance of the gut and the splanchnic region as a whole in the regulation of whole-body amino acid metabolism has become better appreciated and understood. Now that the post-genome era has begun, the mechanisms underlying the effect of amino acids on physiological functions and metabolic processes—including transport, catabolism, and anabolic processes—will soon be more completely described. There remains uncertainty about quantitative aspects of amino acid nutrition, especially in healthy adults, but there is now a consensus that the current international requirement estimates for adults are far too low. This has potentially important implications for the evaluation of dietary protein quality and for the planning—now and in the future—of food protein supplies for population groups. Improved in vivo metabolic tools, combined with molecular and cellular techniques, appear to offer great promise for resolving some of the outstanding issues that limit our ability to predict precisely the effect of the dietary protein and amino acid component on function and the quantitative and qualitative character of intake that optimizes development and health maintenance.

## Acknowledgements

The authors acknowledge the work of the late Dr. Vernon Young (the former author of this chapter) for his stimulation and encouragement, as well as the Canadian Institutes for Health Research for their support of our work in the areas of protein and amino acid metabolism and requirements.

## References

1. Korpes JE. *Jac Berzelius. His Life and Work.* Stockholm: Almqvist & Wiksell; 1970.
2. Carpenter KJ. Protein and Energy. A study of changing ideas of nutrition. Cambridge: Cambridge University Press; 1994.
3. Munro HN. Historical perspective on protein requirements: objectives for the future. In: Blaxter K, Waterlow JC, eds. *Nutritional Adaptation in Man.* London: John Libbey; 1985; 155–167.
4. Burke RF, Hill KE. Regulation of selenoproteins. Annu Rev Nutr. 1993;13:65–81.
5. Schrauzer GN. Selenomethionine: a review of its nutritional significance, metabolism and toxicity. J Nutr. 2000;130:1653–1656.
6. Ferland G. The vitamin K-dependent proteins: an update. Nutr Rev. 1998;56:223–230.
7. Pain VM. Initiation of protein synthesis in eukaryotic cells. Eur J Biochem. 1996;236:747–771.
8. Anthony JC, Anthony TG, Kimball SR, et al. Or-

ally administered leucine stimulates protein synthesis in skeletal muscle of postabsorptive rats in association with increased eIF4F formation. J Nutr. 2000; 130:139–145.

9. Lynch CJ, Fox HL, Vary TC, et al. Regulation of amino acid-sensitive TOR signaling by leucine analogues in adipocytes. J Cell Biochem. 2000;77: 235–251.
10. Jousse C, Bruhat A, Fafournoux P. Amino acid regulation of gene expression. Curr Opin Clin Nutr Metab Care. 1999;2:297–301.
11. Vishwannath RI, Eisen MB, Ross, DT, et al. The transcriptional program in the response of human fibroblasts to serum. Science. 1999;283:83–87.
12. Lecker SH, Solomon V, Mitch WE, Goldberg AL. Muscle protein breakdown and the critical role of the ubiquitin-proteasome pathway in normal and diseased states. J Nutr. 1999;129:227S–2237S.
13. Waterlow JC. Whole-body protein turnover in humans—past, present and future. Annu Rev Nutr. 1995;15:57–92.
14. Volpi E, Mittendorfer B, Wolf SE, Wolfe RR. Oral amino acids stimulate muscle protein anabolism in the elderly despite higher first-pass splanchnic extraction. Am J Physiol. 1999;277:E513–E520.
15. Tessari P, Zanetti M, Barazzoni R. et al. Mechanisms of postprandial protein accretion in human skeletal muscle. Insight from leucine and phenylalanine forearm kinetics. J Clin Invest. 1996;98: 1361–1372.
16. Flakoll PJ, Kulaylot M, Frexes--Steed M, et al. Amino acids augment insulin's suppression of whole body proteolysis. Am J Physiol. 1989;257: E839–E847.
17. Bennett RG, Hamel FG, Duckworth WC. Insulin inhibits the ubiquitin-dependent degrading activity of the 26S proteasome. Endocrinology. 2000;141: 2508–2517.
18. Tessari P. Regulation of splanchnic protein synthesis by enteral feeding. In: Fürst P, Young VR, eds. *Proteins, Peptides and Amino Acids in Enteral Nutrition*. Basel: Nestec Ltd/Vevey & S Karger AG; 2000; 47–61.
19. Duffy B, Gunn T, Collinge J, Pencharz PB: The effect of varying protein quality and energy intake on the nitrogen metabolism of parenterally fed very low birthweight (<1600 g) infants. Pediatr Res. 1981;15:1040–1044.
20. Cynober LA, ed. *Amino Acid Metabolism and Therapy in Health and Nutritional Disease*. Boca Raton: CRC Press, 1995
21. Fürst P, Young V, eds. Proteins, peptides and amino acids in enteral nutrition. Basel: Nestec Ltd/ Vevey & S Karger AG; 2000.
22. Reeds PJ. Dispensable and indispensable amino acids for humans. J Nutr. 2000;130(suppl): 1835S–1840.
23. Rose WC. Amino acid requirements of man. Fed Proc. 1948;8:546–552.
24. Pencharz PB, House JD, Wykes LJ, Ball RO. What are the essential amino acids for the preterm and term infant? 10th Nutricia Symposium. Dordrecht: Kluwer Academic Publishers; 1996; 278–296.
25. Reeds PJ, Burrin DG, Davis TA, et al. Protein nutrition of the neonate. Proc Nutr Soc. 2000;59: 87–97.
26. Jaksic T, Wagner DA, Burke JF, Young VR. Proline metabolism in adult male burned patients and healthy control subjects. Am J Clin Nutr. 1991;54: 408–413.
27. Williams HH, Harper AE, Hegsted DM, et al. Nitrogen and amino acid requirements. In: National Research Council. Improvement in Protein Nutriture. Washington, DC: National Academy of Sciences; 1974; 23–63.
28. Jackson AA. Nitrogen trafficking and recycling through the human bowel. In: Fürst P, Young V, eds. *Proteins, Peptides and Amino Acids in Enteral Nutrition*. Basel: Nestec Ltd/Vevey & S Karger AG; 2000; 89–108.
29. Young VR, El-Khoury AE, Raguso CA, et al. Rates of urea production and hydrolysis and leucine oxidation change linearly over widely varying protein intakes in healthy adults. J Nutr. 2000;130:761–766.
30. Waterlow JC. The mysteries of nitrogen balance. Nutr Res Rev. 1999;12:25–54.
31. Lehninger AL, Nelson DL, Cox MM. *Principles of Biochemistry*. 2nd ed. New York: Worth Publishers; 1993; 688–734.
32. Kitagiri M, Nakamura M. Is there really any evidence indicating that animals synthesize glutamate? Biochem Educ. 199;27:83–85.
33. Kikuchi G. The glycine cleavage system: composition, reaction mechanism and physiological significance. Mol Cell Biochem. 1973;1:169–187.
34. Young VR, Ajami AM. Glutamate: an amino acid of particular distinction. J Nutr. 2000;130: 892S–900S.
35. Food and Agriculture Organization of the United Nations, World Health Organization. FAO/WHO protein requirements. FAO nutritional studies no. 16. Rome: FAO; 1965.
36. Wu G, Morris SM. Arginine metabolism: nitric oxide and beyond. Biochem J. 1998;336:1–17.
37. Beaumier L, Castillo L, Ajami AM, Young VR. Urea cycle intermediate kinetics and nitrate excretion at normal and "therapeutic" intakes of arginine in humans. Am J Physiol. 1995;269:E884–E896.
38. Narita I, Border WA, Ketteler M, et al. L-arginine may mediate the therapeutic effects of low protein diets. Proc Natl Acad Sci U S A. 1995;92: 4552–4556.
39. Reckelhoff JF, Kellum JA, Racusen I, Hilderbrandt DA. Long-term dietary supplementation with

L-arginine prevents age-related reduction in renal function. Am J Physiol. 1997;272:R1768–R1774.

40. Millward DJ, Pacy PJ. Postprandial protein utilization and protein quality assessment in man. Clin Sci. 1995;88:597–606.
41. Tomé D, Bos C. Dietary protein and nitrogen utilization. J Nutr. 2000;130:1868S–1873S.
42. Fouillet H, Gaudichon C, Mariotti F, et al. Compartmental modeling of postprandial dietary nitrogen distribution in humans. Am J Physiol. 2000; 279:E161–E175.
43. Millward DJ. Postprandial protein utilization: implications for clinical nutrition. In: Fürst P, Young VR, eds. *Proteins, Peptides and Amino Acids in Enteral Nutrition.* Basel: Nestec Ltd/Vevey 7 S Karger, AG; 2000; 135–155.
44. Beaufrere B, Dangin M, Boirie Y. The 'fast' and 'slow' protein concept. In: Fürst P, Young V, eds. *Proteins, Peptides and Amino Acids in Enteral Nutrition.* Basel: Nestec Ltd/Vevey & S Karger, AG; 2000; 121–133.
45. El-Khoury AE, Sánchez M, Fukagawa NK, et al. The 24 hour kinetics of leucine oxidation in healthy adults receiving a generous leucine intake via three discrete meals. Am J Clin Nutr. 1995;62:579–590.
46. Arnal MA, Mosoni L, Boirie Y, et al. Protein pulse feeding improves protein retention in elderly women. Am J Clin Nutr. 1999;69:1202–1208.
47. Young VR, Yu Y-M, Borgonha S. Proteins, peptides and amino acids in enteral nutrition: overview and some research challenges. In: Fürst P, Young V, eds. *Proteins, Peptides and Amino Acids in Enteral Nutrition.* Basel, Nestec Ltd./Vevey and S. Karger AG; 2000; 1–23.
48. Rerat A, Simoes-Nunes C, Mendy F, et al. Splanchnic fluxes of amino acids after duodenal infusion of carbohydrate solutions containing free amino acids or oligopeptides in the non-anaesthetized pig. Br J Nutr. 1992;68:111–138.
49. Raguso CA, Ajami AM, Gleason R, Young VR. Effect of cystine intake on methionine kinetics and oxidation determined with oral tracers of methionine and cysteine in healthy adults. Am J Clin Nutr. 1997;66:283–292.
50. Bertolo RFP, Chen CAL, Law G, et al. Threonine requirement of neonatal piglets receiving an identical diet intragastrically. J Nutr. 1998;122:1752–1759.
51. Boirie Y, Gachon P, Beaufrére B. Splanchnic and whole body leucine kinetics in young and elderly men. Am J Clin Nutr. 1997;65:489–495.
52. Wu G. Intestinal mucosal amino acid catabolism. J Nutr. 1998;128:1249–1252.
53. Reeds PJ, Burrin DG, Stoll B, van Goudoever JB. Role of the gut in the amino acid economy of the host. In: Fürst P, Young V, eds. *Proteins, Peptides and Amino Acids in Enteral Nutrition.* Nestec Ltd/Vevey (Switzerland) & S. Karger, AG Basel (Switzerland); 2000; 25–46.
54. Brunton JA, Ball RO, Pencharz PB. Current total parenteral nutrition solutions for the neonate are inadequate. Curr Opin Clin Nutr Metabol Care. 2000;3:299–304.
55. Wilkinson DL, Bertolo RFP, Brunton JA, Shoveller AK, Pencharz PB, Ball RO. Arginine synthesis is regulated by dietary arginine intake in the enterally fed neonatal piglet. Am J Physiol. 2004;287: E454–E462.
56. Van Goudoever JB, Stoll B, Henry JF, et al. Adaptive regulation of intestinal lysine metabolism. Proc Natl Acad Sci U S A. 2000;97:11620–11625.
57. Young VR, El-Khoury AE. The notion of the nutritional essentiality of amino acids, revisited, with a note on the indispensable amino acid requirements in adults. In: Cynober LA, ed. *Amino Acid Metabolism and Therapy in Health and Nutritional Disease.* Boca Raton: CRC Press; 1995; 191–232.
58. Metges CC. Contribution of microbial amino acids to amino acid homeostasis of the host. J Nutr. 2000; 130:1857S–1864S.
59. Metges CC, Petzke KJ, El-Khoury AE, et al. Incorporation of urea and ammonia nitrogen into ileal and fecal microbial proteins and plasma free amino acids in normal men and ileostomates. Am J Clin Nutr. 1999;70:1046–1058.
60. Metges CC, El-Khoury AE, Henneman L, et al. Availability of intestinal microbial lysine for whole-body lysine homeostasis in human subjects. Am J Physiol. 1999;277:E597–E607.
61. Millward DJ, Forrester T, Al-Sing E, et al. The transfer of $^{15}N$ from urea to lysine in the human infant. Br J Nutr. 2000;83:505–512.
62. Food and Agriculture Organization of the United Nations, World Health Organization, United Nations University. Energy and protein requirements. Report of a Joint Expert Consultation. WHO technical report series no. 724. Geneva: WHO; 1985.
63. Young VR, Borgonha S. Nitrogen and amino acid requirements: the Massachusetts Institute of Technology amino acid requirement pattern. J Nutr. 2000;130:1841S–1849S.
64. Dewey KG, Beaton G, Fjeld C, et al. Protein requirements of infants and children. Eur J Clin Nutr. 1996;50(suppl 1):S119–S150.
65. Campbell WW, Evans WJ. Protein requirements of elderly people. Eur J Clin Nutr. 1996;50(suppl 1):S180–S185.
66. Millward DJ, Roberts SB. Protein requirements of older individuals. Nutr Res Rev. 1996;9:67–87.
67. Millward DJ, Fereday A, Gibson N, Pacy PJ. Aging protein requirements and protein turnover. Am J Clin Nutr. 1997;66:774–786.
68. Kurpad AV, Vaz M. Protein and amino acid re-

quirements in the elderly. Eur J Clin Nutr. 2000; 54(suppl 3):S131–S142.

69. Young VR, Gersovitz M, Munro HN. Human aging: protein and amino acid metabolism and implications for protein and amino acid requirements. In: Moment GB, ed. *Nutritional Approaches to Aging Research*. Boca Raton: CRC Press; 1982; 47–81.
70. Millward DJ. Metabolic demands for amino acids and the human dietary requirement: Millward and Rivers (1998) revisited. J Nutr. 1998;128: 2563S–2576S.
71. Waterlow JC. The requirements of adult man for indispensable amino acids. Eur J Clin Nutr. 1996; 50(suppl 1):5152–5179.
72. Fuller MF, Garlick PJ. Human amino acid requirements: can the controversy be resolved? Annu Rev Nutr. 1994;14:217–241.
73. Young VR. Nutrient interactions with reference to amino acid and protein metabolism in non-ruminants; particular emphasis on protein-energy relations in man. Z Ernährungwiss. 1991;30:239–267.
74. Pencharz PB, Ball RO. Different approaches to define individual amino acid requirements. Annu Rev Nutr. 2003;23:101–116.
75. Millward DJ. The nutritional value of plant-based diets in relation to human acid and protein requirements. Proc Nutr Soc. 1999;58:249–260.
76. Holt LE Jr, Snyderman SE. Protein and amino acid requirements of infants and children. Nutr Abstr Rev. 1965;37:1–13.
77. Fomon SJ, Filer LT Jr. Amino acid requirements for normal growth. In: Nyhan WL, ed. *Amino Acid Metabolism and Genetic Variation*. New York: McGraw-Hill; 1967; 391–402.
78. Pineda O, Torun B, Viteri FE, Arroyave G. Protein quality in relation to estimates of essential amino acid requirements. In: Bodwell CE, Adkins JS, Hopkins DT, eds. *Protein Quality in Humans: Assessment and in Vitro Estimation*. Westport, CT: AVI Publishing; 1981; 29–42.
79. Torun B, Pineda O, Viteri FE, Arroyave G. Use of amino acid composition data to predict protein nutritive value for children with specific reference to new estimates of their essential amino acid requirements. In: Bodwell CE, Adkins JS, Hopkins DT, eds. *Protein Quality in Humans: Assessment and in Vitro Estimations*. Westport, CT: AVI Publishing; 374–393.
80. Nakagawa I, Takahaski T, Suzuki T, Kobayashi K. Amino acid requirements of children. Nitrogen balance at the minimal level of essential amino acids. J Nutr. 1964;83:115–118.
81. Rose WC. The amino acid requirements of adult man. Nutr Abstr Rev. 1957;27:631–667.
82. Irwin MI, Hegsted DM. A conspectus of research on amino acid requirements of man. J Nutr. 1971; 101:539–566.
83. Clugston G, Dewey KC, Fjeld C, et al. Report of a working group on protein amino acid requirements. Eur J Clin Nutr. 1996;50(suppl 1):S193–S195.
84. Young VR. Amino acid flux and requirements: counterpoint: tentative estimates are feasible and necessary. In: *Food and Nutrition Board. The Role of Protein and Amino Acids in Sustaining and Enhancing Performance*. Washington, DC: National Academies Press; 1999; 217–242.
85. Manatt MW, Garcia PA. Nitrogen balance: concepts and techniques. In: Nissen S, ed. *Modern Methods in Protein Nutrition and Metabolism*. San Diego: Academic Press; 1992; 9–66.
86. Meguid MM, Matthews DE, Bier DM, et al. Leucine kinetics at graded leucine intakes in young men. Am J Clin Nutr. 1986;43:770–780.
87. Meredith CN, Wen Z-M, Bier DM, et al. Lysine kinetics at graded lysine intakes in young men. Am J Clin Nutr. 1986;43:787–794.
88. Zello GA, Pencharz PB, Ball RO. Dietary lysine requirement of young adult males determined by oxidation of L-[1ms$^{13}$C]phenylalanine. Am J Physiol. 1993;264:E677–E685.
89. Millward DJ, Fereday A, Gibson NR, Pacy PJ. Human adult amino acid requirements: [1-$^{13}$C]leucine balance evaluation of the efficiency of utilization and apparent requirements for wheat protein and lysine compared with those for milk protein in healthy adults. Am J Clin Nutr. 2000;72:112–121.
90. Bookes IM, Owen FN, Garrigus OS. Influence of amino acid level in the diet upon amino acid oxidation by the rat. J Nutr. 1972;102:27–36.
91. El-Khoury AE, Fukagawa NK, Sánchez M, et al. Validation of the Tracer-Balance Concept with Reference to leucine: 24 El-Khoury hour intravenous tracer studies with L-(1-$^{13}$C)leucine and ($^{15}$N-$^{15}$N)urea. Am J Clin Nutr. 1994;59:1000–1011.
92. MacCoss MJ, Fukagawa NK, Matthews DE. Measurement of homocysteine concentrations and stable isotope tracer enrichments in human plasma. Anal Chem. 1999;71:4527–4533.
93. Raguso C, Pereira P, Young VR. A tracer investigation of the obligatory oxidative amino acid losses in healthy, young adults. Am J Clin Nutr. 1999;70: 474–483.
94. Young VR, Bier DM, Pellett PL. A threoretical basis for increasing estimations of the amino acid requirements in adult man, with experimental support. Am J Clin Nutr. 1989;20:80–92.
95. Sánchez M, El-Khoury AE, Castillo L, et al. Phenylalanine and tyrosine kinetics in young men throughout a continuous 24-h period, at a low phenylalanine intake. Am J Clin Nutr. 1995;61: 555–570.
96. El-Khoury AE, Sánchez M, Fukagawa NK, et al. The 24 hour kinetics of leucine oxidation in healthy

adults receiving a generous leucine intake via three discrete meals. Am J Clin Nutr. 1995;62:579–590.

97. El-Khoury AE, Basile A, Beaumier L, et al. Twenty-four hour intravenous and oral tracer studies with L-[1-$^{13}$C]-2-aminoadipic acid and L-(1-$^{13}$C)lysine as tracers at generous nitrogen and lysine intakes in healthy adults. Am J Clin Nutr. 1998;68:827–839.
98. Zello GA, Wykes LJ, Ball RO, Pencharz PB. Recent advances in method of assessing dietary amino acid requirements for adult humans. J Nutr. 1985; 125:2907–2915.
99. Lazaris-Brunner G, Rafii M, Ball RO, Pencharz PB. Tryptophan requirement in young adult women as determined by indicator amino acid oxidation with L-[$^{13}$C]phenylalanine. Am J Clin Nutr. 1998;68:303–310.
100. Wilson DC, Rafii M, Ball RO, Pencharz PB. Threonine requirement of young men determined by indicator amino acid oxidation with use of L-[1-$^{13}$C]phenylalanine. Am J Clin. 2000;71:757–764.
101. Duncan AM, Ball RO, Pencharz PB. Lysine requirement of adult males is not affected by decreasing dietary protein. Am J Clin Nutr. 1996;64: 718–725.
102. Borgonha S, Regan MM, Oh S-H, Condon M, Young VR. Threonine requirement of healthy adults, derived with a 24-h indicator amino acid balance technique. Am J Clin Nutr. 2002;75: 698–704.
103. Kurpad AV, Raj T, Regan MM, Vasudevan J, Caszo B et al. Threonine requirements of healthy Indian adults, measured by a 24h indicator amino acid oxidation and balance technique. Am J Clin Nutr. 2002;76:789–797.
104. Food and Nutrition Board, Institute of Medicine. Dietary Reference Intakes for Energy, Carbohydrate, Fiber, Fat, Fatty Acids, Cholesterol, Protein, and Amino Acids (Macronutrients). Washington, DC: National Academies Press; 2002. Available online at: http://www.nap.edu/books/0309085373/html. Accessed February 16, 2006.
105. Riazi R, Wykes LJ, Ball RO, Pencharz PB. Requirement of total branched chain amino acids determined by indicator amino acid oxidation using L-[1-$^{13}$C]phenylalanine. J Nutr. 2003;133: 1383–1389.
106. Mager DR, Wykes LJ, Ball RO, Pencharz PB. Branched chain amino acid requirements in school aged children determined by indicator amino acid oxidation (IAAO). J Nutr. 2003;133:3540–3545.
107. Rose WC, Wixom RL, Lockhart HB, Lambert GF. The amino acid requirements of man. XV. The valine requirement; summary and final observations. J Biol Chem. 1995;217:987–995.
108. Kriengsinyos W, Wykes LJ, Ball RO, Pencharz PB. Oral and intravenous tracer protocols of the indicator amino acid oxidation method provide the same estimate of the lysine requirement in healthy men. J Nutr. 2002;132:2251–2257.
109. Kriengsinyos W, Wykes LJ, Goonewardene L, Ball RO, Pencharz PB. Phase of menstrual cycle affects lysine requirement in healthy women. Am J Physiol. 2004;287:E489–E496.
110. Jones EM, Bauman CA, Reynolds MS. Nitrogen balances of women maintained on various levels of lysine. J Nutr. 1956;60:549–559.
111. Hegsted DM. Variation in requirements of nutrients—amino acids. Fed Proc. 1963;22: 1424–1430.
112. Rand WM, Young VR. Statistical analysis of N balance data with reference to the lysine requirement in adults. J Nutr. 1999;129:1920–1926.
113. El-Khoury AE, Pereira PCM, Borgonha S, et al. Twenty-four hour oral tracer studies with L-[1-$^{13}$C]lysine at low (15 $mg \cdot kg^{-1} \cdot day^{-1}$) and intermediate (29 $mg \cdot kg^{-1} \cdot day^{-1}$) lysine intake in healthy adults. Am J Clin Nutr. 2000;72:122–130.
114. Young VR, El-Khoury AE. Can amino acid requirements for nutritional maintenance in adult humans be approximated from the amino acid composition of body mixed proteins? Proc Natl Acad Sci U S A. 1995;92:300–304.
115. Kurpad AV, Regan MM, Raj T, et al. Lysine requirement of healthy adult Indian subjects receiving longer term feeding, measured with a 24h indicator amino acid oxidation and balance technique. Am J Clin Nutr 2002;76:404–12
116. Young VR, El-Khoury AE. Human amino acid requirements: A reevaluation. Food Nutr Bull. 1996; 17:191–203.
117. Price GM, Halliday D, Pacy PJ, et al. Nitrogen homeostasis in man: influence of protein intake on the amplitude of diurnal cycling of body nitrogen. Clin Sci. 1985;86:91–102.
118. Pellett PL, Young VR. Role of meat as a source of protein and essential amino acids in human protein nutrition. In: Pearson AM, Dutson TR, eds. *Meat and Health. Advances in Meat Research*. Vol. 6. New York: Elsevier Applied Science; 1990; 329–370.
119. Young VR, Fajardo L, Murray E, et al. Protein requirements of man: comparative nitrogen balance response within the submaintenance-to-maintenance range of intake of wheat and beef proteins. J Nutr. 1975;105:534–552.
120. Sikka KC, Johari RP, Duggan SK. Comparative nutritive value and amino acid content of different extractions of wheat. Agric Food Chem. 1975;23: 24–26.
121. Fisher H, Brush MK, Griminger P. Reassessment of amino acid requirements of young women on low nitrogen diets. 1. Lysine and tryptophan. Am J Clin Nutr. 1969;22:1190–1196.
122. Kriengsinyos W, Wykes LJ, Ball RO, Pencharz PB. Is Histidine an indispensable amino acid in healthy adults. J Nutr. 2002;132:3340–3348.

123. Food and Agriculture Organization of the United Nations. *The State of Food and Agriculture 2000.* Rome: FAO; 2000.
124. Wilson DC, Pencharz PB. Nutritional care of the chronically ill. In: Tsang RC, Zlotkin SH, Nichols BL, Hansen JW, eds. *Nutrition During Infancy: Birth to 2 Years.* Digital Educational Publishing, Inc.; 1997; 37–56.
125. Bistrian BR. Recent advances in parenteral and enteral nutrition. A personal perspective. JPEN. 1990; 14:329–334.
126. Cornish CA, Kennedy NP. Protein-energy undernutrition in hospital in-patients. Br J Nutr. 2000; 83:575–591.
127. Pollitt E. Developmental sequel from early nutritional deficiencies: Conclusive and probability judgments. J Nutr. 2000;130:350S–353S.
128. Allison SP. The uses and limitations of nutrition support. Clin Nutr. 1992;11:319–330.
129. Heird WC, Discoll JM, Schullinger JN, Grebin B, Winters RW. Intravenous alimentation in pediatric patients. J Pediatr. 1972;80:351–372.

# 6 Carbohydrates

Lisa M. Sanders and Joanne R. Lupton

Carbohydrates, which are found in fruits, vegetables, grains, and dairy products, are the major source of energy for most of the world's population. However, the role of carbohydrates in human health extends beyond their importance as an energy source. Carbohydrates vary tremendously in structure and physiological function, and much of the recent carbohydrate research has focused on these differences and their impact on chronic diseases such as diabetes and heart disease. Within the past three years, this research has led to the development of significant nutrition public policy recommendations regarding carbohydrate intake for optimal health.

## Carbohydrates in the Food Supply

Carbohydrates have traditionally been accepted as compounds containing carbon, hydrogen, and oxygen in a molar ratio of 1:2:1. As this definition is not universal for all carbohydrates (e.g., sugar alcohols and some polysaccharides), it is more precise to define carbohydrates as polyhydroxy aldehydes, ketones, alcohols, and acids that exist as monomeric units or as polymers. The degree of polymerization is frequently used as a system by which to classify carbohydrates, with the major classes being monosaccharides and disaccharides (commonly referred to as sugars), oligosaccharides, and polysaccharides.

### *Sugars*

**Monosaccharides.** According to Food and Agriculture Organization (FAO) of the World Health Organization (WHO),[1] the term "sugars" refers collectively to monosaccharides, disaccharides, and sugar alcohols. Monosaccharides include glucose, fructose, and galactose, which are found naturally in small amounts in fruits, vegetables, and honey. However, over the past 30 years, corn syrups and high-fructose corn syrup (HFCS) have replaced refined sugars (such as sucrose) as a major source of monosaccharides in the American diet due to their increased use by the food industry as a low-cost sweetener.[2] Corn syrups contain only individual glucose units. The term "high-fructose corn syrup" is accurate, but in some ways it is misleading, since many interpret this to mean that there is more fructose than would be in an equivalent amount of table sugar (sucrose). The reason for the word "high" is that it contains more fructose than corn syrup, which is only glucose. However, compared with sucrose, which is 50% glucose and 50% fructose, it is not high. HFCS is made by hydrolyzing corn starch to individual glucose units and then using enzymes to convert glucose to fructose. The final corn syrup is made up of either 42% or 55% fructose, with the remaining sugars being glucose and higher sugars. HFCS-55 is predominant in carbonated soft drinks, whereas HFCS-42 is found in canned fruits, baked goods, flavored milks, yogurt, and ice cream.[3, 4] While the consumption of HFCS has increased over the past few decades, the overall intake of caloric sweeteners has changed only slightly, thus reflecting the replacement of refined sugars with HFCS (Figure 1).

**Disaccharides.** Disaccharides consist of two monosaccharides covalently linked by a glycosidic bond. The major dietary disaccharides include sucrose (glucose + fructose) and lactose (glucose + galactose). Sucrose occurs naturally in plants, but most often is consumed as an extract of sugarcane or beet. Sucrose is widely used as a sweetener and preservative. Milk and other dairy products are the only source of lactose. Maltose and trehalose, both disaccharides of glucose (differing only in the configuration of the glycosidic bond), are also present in small amounts in the food supply. Maltose is found in wheat and barley, and is also a product of starch hydrolysis. Trehalose is found in yeast products, mushrooms, and crustacean seafood.

**Sugar Alcohols.** Also commonly referred to as polyols, sugar alcohols are derived from the hydrogenation of mono- and disaccharides, and include sorbitol, mannitol, xylitol, isomalt, lactitol, maltitol, and erythritol. Polyols are not as easily digested as other sugars, so they produce

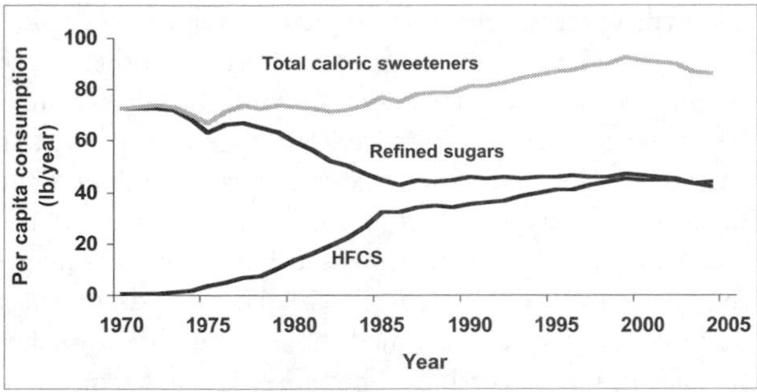


Figure 1. Changes in the US per capita consumption of refined sugars and high-fructose corn syrup (HFCS) over time (US Department of Agriculture, 2003[5]). Consumption of refined sugars (e.g., sucrose) has been replaced by HFCS over the past several decades, yet overall intake of caloric sweeteners has changed only slightly. Also, since HFCS and sucrose have nearly the same ratio of fructose and glucose, the increase in HFCS consumption has not increased the amount of fructose in the diet.

a lower glycemic response and a reduced caloric value. Additionally, sugar alcohols are less cariogenic than other carbohydrates.[6] As a result, the food industry often uses sugar alcohols as bulk sweeteners to produce low-calorie or sugar-free candies, chewing gum, baked goods, sauces, jams, jellies, beverages, and frozen desserts.

### *Oligosaccharides*

Carbohydrates with three to nine degrees of polymerization (i.e., three to nine monosaccharide units) are classified as oligosaccharides. Some oligosaccharides occur naturally in plants: stachyose and raffinose in soybeans and other legumes and fructooligosaccharides in fruits, vegetables, and grains (e.g., wheat, rye, onions, bananas, and garlic). However, because of their usefulness as food ingredients and their possible health benefits, an increasing number of oligosaccharides are now synthesized from sugars or obtained through extraction and/or partial hydrolysis of longer-chain plant polysaccharides. These manufactured oligosaccharides, such as inulin extracted from chicory root, can be found in a number of food items such as dairy products (e.g., yogurt), breads, beverages, and dessert foods. Being fairly resistant to digestion in the small intestine, oligosaccharides display physiological effects similar to fiber, and some appear to promote the growth of beneficial colonic microflora. Additionally, as a food additive, they do not change the texture or taste of the product significantly, making them ideal for creating healthier products with limited alteration in taste or mouth feel.[7]

### *Polysaccharides*

The majority of carbohydrates consumed in the food supply are polysaccharides. As the name implies, these carbohydrates have a high degree of polymerization, ranging from 10 sugar units to several thousand. Polysaccharides can be subdivided into starch and non-starch polysaccharides.

**Starch.** Starch is a polymer of glucose units covalently bound by either α-(1,4) or α-(1–6) linkages. Amylose contains only α-(1,4) bonds and thus maintains a constant linear form. Amylopectin contains α-(1,6) bonds in addition to α-(1,4) bonds, allowing for a highly branched structure. Starch is the primary storage form of carbohydrate in plants, but is found primarily in grains and grain products (e.g., cereals, corn, flour, and rice) and in some root vegetables (e.g., potatoes and beets) and legumes. Most other vegetables and fruits contain very little starch.

**Resistant Starch.** While most starch is digested and absorbed in the small intestine, a small portion escapes digestive enzymes and passes into the colon, where it may be fermented. This is referred to as resistant starch. There are four types of resistant starch, which either occur naturally or are a consequence of food processing. Resistant starch-1 (RS1) is present in the cell walls of plants, but is physically inaccessible to digestive enzymes such as α-amylase. These are most frequently found in whole grains, whole-grain products (e.g., breads and cereals), seeds, and legumes. The amount of RS1 in a food is decreased by processing techniques such as milling and refining. Raw starch granules that are resistant to digestive enzymes due to their crystalline structure and size are classified as RS2. These can be found in raw potatoes and green bananas. Food processing, particularly gelatinization (making starch more soluble using heat, water, and/or enzymes), increases the accessibility of starch to digestive enzymes, thereby decreasing the amount of RS2. Because RS1 and RS2 occur naturally in plants, they are considered dietary fiber by some. RS3 and RS4 are both formed during food processing and do not occur naturally. RS3, also called retrograded starch, is formed during the cooking and cooling or extrusion process of starchy foods such as potatoes, rice, and cereals. RS4 is chemically modified starch, such as starch esters, starch ethers, and cross-linked starches, which are manufactured by the food industry to impart desired characteristics to food products such as color, temperature stability, and altered viscosity.[8]

**Non-Starch Polysaccharides.** Similar to resistant starch, non-starch polysaccharides also escape digestion and absorption in the small intestine and are fermented in the colon. However, their resistance to digestion is not due to physical or structural barriers to digestive enzymes, but rather to the lack of enzymes capable of breaking the glycosidic bonds between the monomeric units. As a result of their indigestibility, non-starch polysaccharides are considered dietary fiber and include cellulose, hemicelluloses (e.g., β-glucans), gums and mucilages, and pectins. For more detailed information, see the chapter on dietary fiber elsewhere in this book.

### *Other Classifications of Carbohydrates*

One of the difficulties in the classification of carbohydrates is reconciling their chemical composition with their physiological functions. Each of the chemical classes described above contains carbohydrates with varying physiological effects, some of which overlap among the categories (e.g., the indigestibility and colonic fermentation of oligosaccharides and non-starch polysaccharides). This can create confusion for the consumer and the food industry with regard to dietary guidelines, labeling guidelines, and health claims, and has therefore resulted in new terminology and classifications for dietary carbohydrates.

**Extrinsic and Intrinsic Sugars.** The terms "extrinsic sugars" and "intrinsic sugars" were first used in the United Kingdom in 1989 to help consumers differentiate between sugars that were intrinsic in plant-based foods (contained in the cell wall) and sugars that were added to foods. Since lactose is not plant based and was considered an extrinsic sugar, an additional phrase, "non-milk extrinsic sugar," was developed. These terms were never widely accepted outside of the United Kingdom, and as a result are very infrequently used today.

**Added Sugars.** Added sugars are sugars and syrups that are added to foods during processing or preparation.[9] This does not include sugars that occur naturally in the food, such as lactose in milk or fructose in fruits. Added sugars are typically in the form of white table sugar, brown sugar, corn syrup, HFCS, molasses, honey, pancake syrups, fruit-juice concentrates, and dextrose. The major sources of these sugars include soft drinks, fruit beverages, dessert items, and candy. In fact, non-diet soft drinks account for 33% of added sugars in the American diet.[10] Most of these food items also have lower micronutrient densities than foods and beverages with naturally occurring sugars. Therefore, beginning in 2000, the Dietary Guidelines for Americans included the term "added sugars" to assist consumers in identifying foods that are high in added sugars. Currently, US food labels are not required to distinguish between naturally occurring sugars and those that are added to the food.

**Glycemic and Non-Glycemic Carbohydrates.** This classification system is based on the digestibility of carbohydrates and thus their ability to provide glucose to the body for metabolism. Glycemic carbohydrates are digested and absorbed in the small intestine, thereby increasing blood glucose for metabolism by tissues, while non-glycemic carbohydrates remain undigested and pass into the colon, where they can be fermented. Non-glycemic carbohydrates may still provide energy through fermentation; however, this energy is not in carbohydrate form such that it would alter blood glucose levels. Sugars and starches make up most of the glycemic carbohydrates, while oligosaccharides, resistant starches, and non-digestible polysaccharides (fiber) constitute the non-glycemic carbohydrates. The rate at which different glycemic carbohydrates are absorbed can also be measured and will be discussed further in the following section.

## Digestion and Absorption of Carbohydrates

### *Digestion*

Enzymatic digestion of carbohydrates begins immediately when food is placed in the mouth. Salivary α-amylase hydrolyzes the glycosidic bonds between glucose moieties in starches to yield glucose, maltose, and other starch fragments. Once food enters the stomach, salivary amylase is inactivated and carbohydrate digestion pauses. In the small intestine, pancreatic α-amylase completes the digestion of starch to glucose, maltose, maltotriose (a trisaccharide), and dextrins, oligosaccharide units containing one or more α-(1,6) linkages. All carbohydrates must be broken down to individual monosaccharide units before absorption is possible. Therefore, bound to the brush border of the small intestine are enzymes that hydrolyze dextrins, trisaccharides, and disaccharides to their respective monosaccharides for absorption. These enzymes include glucoamylase, maltase, lactase, and sucrase, which hydrolyze dextrins, maltose, lactose, and sucrose, respectively. A deficiency of disaccharidases in the intestine can occur in rare genetic disorders such as sucrase-maltase deficiency and alactasia (absence of lactase). These deficiencies typically result in diarrhea, abdominal pain, and/or gas following the consumption of sucrose or lactose, and the condition can generally be controlled by removing the indigestible disaccharides from the diet or by predigestion of the sugars with commercially available enzymes (e.g., lactase). Additionally, the expression of the lactase enzyme decreases in most humans following weaning, allowing undigested lactose to reach the colon, where it is fermented. This fermentation can result in the generation of gases, causing abdominal discomfort and possibly diarrhea. However, not all lactase activity is lost, as in the case of alactasia, and small amounts of milk products can be tolerated without adverse side effects.[11]

Any carbohydrates that are not digested (e.g., resistant starches and fiber) pass into the colon, where they can be fermented by the colonic microflora to short-chain fatty acids and gases such as hydrogen, carbon dioxide, and methane. Again, more information can be found on this process in the chapter on dietary fiber.

### *Absorption*

Monosaccharide absorption occurs in the small intestine by one of two mechanisms: active transport and facilitated diffusion. At the brush border surface, glucose and galactose are actively transported from the lumen into the enterocyte by a sodium/glucose co-transporter, SGLT1. In this process, glucose and galactose move against a concentration gradient, while sodium moves down a concentration gradient. The sodium gradient is maintained by pumping sodium out of the enterocyte at the basolateral membrane, a process requiring energy in the form of ATP. Fructose absorption at the brush border occurs passively and is facilitated by one of the GLUT family of glucose transporters, GLUT5. The GLUT5 uniporter has a high affinity for fructose and appears to move glucose very poorly. Once inside the enterocyte, movement of monosaccharides across the basolateral membrane and into the bloodstream is a passive process and is facilitated by GLUT2 and GLUT5 uniporters.[12] GLUT2 facilitates the movement of all three monosaccharides into the bloodstream, while GLUT5 appears to again be specific to fructose.

Mutations in these monosaccharide transporters, while rare, can lead to clinical disorders such as glucose-galactose malabsorption and Fanconi-Bickel syndrome. Glucose-galactose malabsorption, a congenital disorder, occurs when a defective SGLT1 transporter prevents the absorption of glucose and galactose, resulting in severe diarrhea when sugars and starches containing these monosaccharides are consumed. Treatment of this condition requires the removal of glucose and galactose from the diet, but fructose consumption may continue because there is no impairment of fructose absorption in this disorder. Fanconi-Bickel syndrome results from a congenital defect in the GLUT2 transporter. In addition to the intestine, GLUT2 is also expressed in the liver, kidney, and pancreas. Therefore, loss of function of this transporter not only results in monosaccharide malabsorption, but also widespread systemic effects such as tubular nephropathy, hepatomegaly, and rickets.[12]

## *Glycemic Index and Response*

As mentioned previously, glycemic carbohydrates are those that stimulate an increase in blood glucose levels after their digestion and absorption. This change in blood glucose over time is called the "glycemic response." A number of factors can influence the glycemic response to foods, including the nature of the carbohydrate consumed, the rate of digestion and absorption, the rate of clearance from the bloodstream, and the presence of other food components (e.g., fiber, fat, and protein). In an effort to better understand how different foods impact the glycemic response, Jenkins et al.[13] proposed the use of the glycemic index (GI) as a relative indicator of blood glucose response to the carbohydrate contained in a particular food. The GI is determined by comparing the blood glucose response (area under the curve) of a test food containing a specified amount of available carbohydrate to a standard food containing the same amount of carbohydrate (e.g., glucose or white bread). The response to the test food is then expressed as a percentage of the response to the standard to give the GI. High-GI foods generally include items with easily digested starches (e.g., refined grains and potatoes), free glucose, or large amounts of disaccharides rapidly hydrolyzed to glucose. Alternatively, low-GI foods (e.g., unprocessed grains, non-starchy fruits, and vegetables) contain more slowly digested or resistant starches, higher fiber content, or are rich in free fructose. Low-GI foods may also be high in fat, which slows carbohydrate digestion and absorption. The GI has been determined for a number of foods,[14] and has become more frequently used in studies relating carbohydrate intake with chronic disease, as will be discussed later in this chapter.

The GI can also be calculated for mixed meals by multiplying the grams of carbohydrate consumed in each food item by the GI for that particular food and dividing by the total grams of carbohydrate consumed in all of the foods. These values can then be added to generate the meal GI. This calculation was established initially due to concerns that the presence of other macronutrients (e.g., fat and protein) in a mixed meal may invalidate the use of individual food GIs as indicators of glycemic response.[15,16] A number of investigations[17] have shown the meal GI to be a useful indicator of the glycemic response to mixed meals, although debate over its accuracy continues.[18]

Since the GI is a reference value, it reflects the glycemic response to the same amount of carbohydrate from each food (50 g). However, the proportion of carbohydrate contained in foods varies tremendously. Glycemic load, which multiplies the GI by the amount of carbohydrate consumed, is a more accurate indicator of glycemic response because it takes into account the quantity of carbohydrate consumed. For example, as seen in Table 1, chocolate cake

**Table 1.** Glycemic Index Based on Glucose as Index Food and Glycemic Load*

| Food | Glycemic Index | Glycemic Load |
|---|---|---|
| Apple | 38 ± 2 | 6 |
| Banana | 51 | 13 |
| Carrot | 47 ± 16 | 3 |
| Cheese pizza | 60 | 16 |
| Chocolate cake | 38 ± 3 | 20 |
| Kidney beans | 28 ± 4 | 7 |
| Lentils | 29 ± 1 | 5 |
| Macaroni and cheese | 64 | 32 |
| Oatmeal | 69 | 24 |
| Orange juice | 50 ± 4 | 13 |
| Peaches, canned in natural juice | 38 ± 8 | 4 |
| Peanuts | 14 ± 8 | 1 |
| Popcorn, plain | 72 ± 17 | 8 |
| Potato, baked | 85 ± 12 | 26 |
| Raisin Bran® | 61 ± 5 | 12 |
| Rice, long-grain | 75 ± 7 | 28 |
| Soda, non-diet | 58 ± 5 | 16 |
| Spaghetti | 58 | 28 |
| White bread | 70 | 10 |
| Whole milk | 27 ± 4 | 3 |

* Glycemic load is calculated as the glycemic index multiplied by the grams of carbohydrate per serving and divided by 100. Data from Foster-Powell and Miller 1995[14] and Foster-Powell K, Holt SH, Brand-Miller JC. International table of glycemic index and glycemic load values: 2002. Am J Clin Nutr. 2002; 76:5-56.

actually has a lower GI than carrots, but the proportion of carbohydrate in a serving of chocolate cake (52 g) is significantly greater than that in a serving of carrots (6 g). Therefore, eating a serving of chocolate cake will have a greater effect on blood glucose than eating a serving of carrots, even though the GI for chocolate cake is less. In this case, glycemic load, which is much lower for the carrots, would be a more accurate indicator of glycemic response. The glycemic load for a meal or for diets can also be determined by simply adding the glycemic load of each food item.

## Metabolism of Carbohydrates

### *Energy Value of Carbohydrates*

Traditionally, carbohydrates have been assigned an energy value of 4 kcal/g (17 kJ/g). This value is derived from Atwater's calculations of the heat of combustion of carbohydrates from various food commodities.[19] However, the actual caloric values of carbohydrates can vary from practically zero in the case of some fibers (e.g., gums and cellulose) to 4.2 kcal/g for most digestible starches. Most sugars have a lower caloric value than starches, ranging from 3.75 to 3.95 kcal/g. The greatest difficulty has come in assigning caloric values to non-digestible polysaccharides and oligosaccharides, which are primarily fermented in the colon. Short-chain fatty acids produced by fermentation (e.g., acetate, propionate, and butyrate) are quickly metabolized and therefore provide a source of energy. However, the amount of energy varies with the degree of fermentability. Smith et al.[20] determined metabolizable energy values for several non-starch polysaccharides with values ranging from 0 to 2.3 kcal/g. The FAO/WHO consultation on carbohydrates recommended that the energy value for carbohydrates that enter the colon be set at 2 kcal/g.[1] Polyols are also incompletely absorbed and thus provide less calories than most other digestible carbohydrates. The caloric values of polyols range from 0.2 to 3 kcal/g;[21] however, for labeling purposes, the European Union has established a standard value of 2.3 kcal/g for sugar alcohols, while the United States assigns values on an individual case basis.[22] The American Diabetes Association advises health professionals to use a value of 2 kcal/g for sugar alcohols.[23]

### *Fate of Absorbed Monosaccharides*

Absorbed monosaccharides are transported through the bloodstream to tissues, where they are used as an energy source. Cellular uptake is achieved by GLUT transporters. Galactose and fructose are taken up primarily in the liver by the GLUT2 transporter(24). Galactose is phosphorylated and converted to glucose-1-phosphate, the precursor for glycogen synthesis. Fructose is phosphorylated to an intermediate in the glycolytic pathway (fructose-1-phosphate). As it continues through the glycolytic pathway, it will be cleaved to form dihydroxyacetone phosphate and glyceraldehyde. These intermediates can then continue through glycolysis or, under certain conditions, serve as precursors for glycogen and triglyceride synthesis. Glucose is used by most cells in the body for energy. A number of tissue-specific isoforms of GLUT transporters are responsible for glucose uptake, including: GLUT2 in the liver, pancreas, kidney and small intestine; GLUT3, primarily in the brain; GLUT4, in insulin-sensitive tissues such as adipose and skeletal muscle; and GLUT1, which is ubiquitously expressed but predominates in erythrocytes and the brain. Many other glucose transporters have been identified and are more thoroughly discussed in Scheepers et al.[24]

### *Glycolysis*

The initial steps in the metabolism of glucose, which occurs in the cytoplasm of all cells, is called glycolysis, and results in the generation of ATP and two three-carbon molecules of pyruvate. If the cell is under anaerobic conditions (or lacks mitochondria in the case of erythrocytes), pyruvate will be reduced to lactate and exported to the liver for gluconeogenesis (the Cori cycle). Under aerobic conditions, pyruvate can enter the mitochondria and be decarboxylated to acetyl coenzyme A, which then enters the citric acid cycle. This cycle completes the catabolism of glucose to carbon dioxide and water, accompanied by the oxidation of coenzymes ($NAD^+$ and FAD), which can then pass off their electrons in the electron transport system to generate large amounts of ATP.

### *Gluconeogenesis*

Because glucose is the primary energy source for the body, it is critical that blood glucose levels are maintained (70–100 mg/dL or 3.9 to 5.5 mmol/L) to supply tissues with needed fuel. Glucose can be generated from a number of precursors, including pyruvate, lactate, glycerol, and most amino acids. The synthesis of glucose is basically a reversal of glycolysis, with many of the same enzymes utilized; however, gluconeogenesis occurs only in the liver and kidney. The glucose produced is then released into the bloodstream for use by all tissues.

### *Regulation of Glycolysis and Gluconeogenesis*

A number of controls are present in the glycolytic and gluconeogenic pathways to insure that adequate energy is supplied to cells and that blood glucose levels are maintained. These controls include allosteric and/or covalent modification of key enzymes, alterations in the expression of enzymes, and hormonal regulation. The three key regulatory enzymes in the glycolytic pathway are glucokinase/hexokinase, phosphofructokinase-1, and pyruvate kinase. Because these steps in glycolysis are irreversible, the gluconeogenic pathway utilizes four corresponding enzymes (glucose 6-phosphatase, fructose 1,6-bisphosphatase, phosphoenolpyruvate carboxykinase, and pyruvate carboxylase), which are also irreversible in the pathway of glucose generation. These "paired" enzymes are regulated such that the stimulation of one coordinates

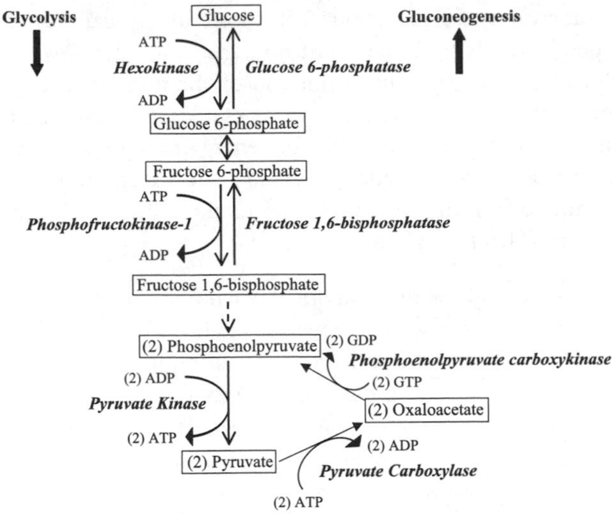


Figure 2. Glycolysis and gluconeogenesis pathways. Left side of the diagram represents glycolysis, while the right side represents gluconeogenesis. Dashed arrow represents steps that were left out of the diagram.

with the inhibition of the other (Figure 2). For example, elevated blood glucose levels will positively affect the glycolytic enzyme glucokinase/hexokinase, while simultaneously inhibiting the activity of glucose 6-phosphatase, the corresponding gluconeogenic enzyme.

These enzymes are also subject to hormonal regulation by insulin, glucagon, epinephrine, and glucocorticoids. Insulin, an anabolic hormone, is secreted by the β-cells of the pancreas in response to an increase in blood glucose, such as that which follows a carbohydrate-containing meal. Insulin acts to decrease blood glucose levels by increasing glucose uptake by tissues and by decreasing gluconeogensis by the liver. To increase tissue uptake, insulin triggers the translocation of GLUT4 receptors to the cell surface in skeletal muscle and adipose tissue. Insulin also stimulates each of the regulatory enzymes in the glycolytic pathway, while also inhibiting the key enzymes of gluconeogenesis. An increase in glucose storage in the form of glycogen is also stimulated by insulin. Glucagon, epinephrine, and glucocorticoids are counter-regulatory hormones to insulin, and are released when blood glucose levels are low, such as during fasting or starvation. Glucagon, produced by the α-cells of the pancreas, and epinephrine and glucocorticoids, produced by the adrenal gland, enhance gluconeogenesis and glycogenolysis (release of glucose from glycogen storage) and inhibit glycolysis. Epinephrine also increases lipolysis during fasting.[25]

### *Storage of Glucose*

The liver and skeletal muscle are able to store excess glucose in the form of glycogen, a branched-chain glucose polymer. The liver is able to store 10% of its weight as glycogen, while skeletal muscle stores approximately 1%.[25] When blood glucose levels fall, the breakdown of liver glycogen is triggered and the glucose released is used to maintain blood glucose levels. During continued fasting, the liver will be depleted of its glycogen stores within 24 hours. Skeletal muscle glycogen can be broken down and used as fuel by the skeletal muscle, which occurs primarily during exercise. Skeletal muscle glycogen is not as effective as liver glycogen at normalizing blood glucose levels during fasting; however, lactate generated in the muscle can be circulated to the liver for gluconeogenesis. Glycogen synthesis and degradation is regulated by hormones, as described in the previous section.

### *Contribution to Amino Acid and Triglyceride Synthesis*

Some metabolites of glucose, such as pyruvate and intermediates in the citric acid cycle, can be used in the synthesis of certain amino acids. Additionally, fatty acids can be formed from oxaloacetic acid and acetyl-coenzyme A (cleavage products of the tricarboxylic acid cycle intermediate citrate). Intermediates in the glycolysis pathway can be modified to serve as the glycerol backbone for triglycerides. However, the contribution of carbohydrates to these processes is considered minimal, especially lipogenesis, which occurs to a very limited extent.[26]

### *Inborn Errors in Metabolism*

A number of disease states associated with deficiencies or genetic defects in certain key enzymes responsible for carbohydrate metabolism have been characterized. Some errors in metabolism, such as those involved in fructose or galactose metabolism, are discovered early and are easily treated by removal of those monosaccharides from the diet. However, genetic defects in enzymes involved in gluconeogenesis or glycogenolysis are much more life-threatening because individuals with these diseases suffer from frequent hypoglycemia, hepatomegaly, and acidosis. Treatment typically involves small, frequent feedings of carbohydrate to prevent hypoglycemia and acidosis.

## Dietary Requirements and Carbohydrate Quality

### *Established Requirements and Recommendations*

For the first time, there is a Dietary Reference Intake (DRI) value for carbohydrates, established by the US Institute of Medicine. The Recommended Dietary Allowance (RDA) is set at 130 g/d for adults and children and is based on the average minimum amount of glucose used by the brain.[27] This recommendation was based on human studies in which arteriovenous gradients of glucose were measured with estimates of brain blood flow. Although there is not an absolute requirement for glucose, since the brain can switch to using ketone bodies (primarily from fat metabolism), the 130 g/d represents a recommendation that would not require the brain to resort to the use of ketone bodies. This RDA is not the recommendation for overall carbohydrate intake, but rather, the recommendation for what is needed by the brain. Most people consume well over the RDA for carbohydrate.

A second recommendation for carbohydrate is the newly coined AMDR (acceptable macronutrient distribution range) value of 45% to 65% of total calories in the form of carbohydrate.[27] The low end of the range was set to allow for sufficient intake of dietary fiber, which would be very difficult to obtain from foods below a level of 45% of calories coming from carbohydrate, since all fiber (with the exception of lignin) is carbohydrate. Also, as the intake of one macronutrient gets too low, another macronutrient (either fat or protein in this case) could become too high. There was concern that less than 45% of calories from carbohydrate could result in the intake of excess fat, which in turn could contribute to obesity. At the higher end of the range (65% of calories from carbohydrate), the concern was hypertriglyceridemia and the concern that intakes of fat or protein could be too low.

There is also an adequate intake (AI) value for total fiber of 14 g/1000 calories, which equates to 38 g/d for men under 50 and 25 g/d for women under 50. The fiber recommendation was based on decreased risk of coronary heart disease with higher-fiber diets.

The DRI macronutrient report[27] made a recommendation that added sugar intake should not exceed 25% of total calories. This recommendation was based on diminishing intake of micronutrients as the percent of calories from added sugars increased. Although the significant "drop-off" in micronutrient intake was not always at the 25% added sugar intake level for each age and gender group, the overall pattern showed a decline at the 25% intake level. Since the release of the macronutrient report in 2002, the 2005 US Dietary Guidelines Advisory Committee (DGAC)[9] did a complete evidence-based review of human studies on added sugar intake and human health. In addition to the impact of added sugar intake on micronutrient intake, the DGAC reviewed longitudinal studies on added sugar intake and weight gain that were not available to the DRI macronutrient panel. Although not definitive, these studies suggest that the intake of added sugars in the form of sugar-sweetened beverages over time contribute to weight gain. The DGAC also developed a concept they termed "discretionary calories," which are defined as the difference between one's energy requirement and one's requirement for nutrients from foods. The idea is that all of the nutrient requirements should come from appropriate food pattern choices, and this comes at a calorie cost. The DGAC report lists values for "discretionary calories" that can then be spent on added sugars, or added fat, alcohol, or larger portions of foods. It is clear from the analysis of eating patterns in the United States today that many people have no "discretionary calories" to spend on non-nutrient-dense foods, and most have not many. For example, a sedentary woman over 50 has about 150 discretionary calories to spend, which could be spent on a glass of wine, low-fat forms for dairy products (instead of the nonfat variety), or some butter or margarine on vegetables or bread. Thus, the inability to stay within one's energy requirement and still meet nutrient needs appears to be the most significant factor to limiting "added sugar" intake. The conclusion of the 2005 DGAC was:

> Compared with individuals who consume small amounts of foods and beverages that are high in added sugars, those who consume large amounts tend to consume more calories but smaller amounts of micronutrients. Although more research is needed, available prospective studies suggest a positive association between the consumption of sugar-sweetened beverages and weight gain. A reduced intake of added sugars (especially sugar-sweetened beverages) can lower calorie intake, and may be helpful in achieving recommended intakes of nutrients and in weight control.

The 2005 Dietary Guidelines also recommend to increase the intake of whole grains (three servings per day) at the expense of refined grains.[9] What constitutes a whole grain as opposed to a refined grain? Whole grains consist of the entire kernel or seed of the grain, which consists of three components: the bran layer (which contains most of the fiber), the endosperm (which is primarily starch), and the germ (which contains some fat and other nutrients). When whole grains are refined, most of the bran and germ are lost, leaving the endosperm. Refined grains are then enriched with thiamin, riboflavin, iron, and niacin, fortified with folic acid, and are called "enriched grains." Whole grains do not have to be intact in the food product to be called "whole grains" but they do have to have the same ratio of bran to endosperm to germ as they had in the intact kernel. Whole grains have been shown to decrease the risk of coronary heart disease and type 2 diabetes, and there is growing evidence that they can protect against weight gain.[9] This is independent of their fiber content and the health benefits attributed to fiber. Not all whole grains are high in fiber. For example, wheat has a substantial bran layer containing fiber, but rice does not. Consumers would benefit from choosing whole-grain products that are also high in dietary fiber, as they would then benefit from both the whole grain and the fiber effects. Whole grains should be substituted for refined grains rather than added "on top" of the diet, since modeling of the USDA database showed that adding three servings of whole grains to the typical diet would exceed energy requirements.[9] A summary of the new requirements and recommendations can be found in Table 2.

## *Current Intakes*

According to FAO/WHO statistics,[1] carbohydrate consumption worldwide ranges from 40% to 80% of en-

**Table 2.** Summary of US Recommendations and Requirements for Carbohydrate Intake

| 2005 Dietary Guidelines Advisory Committee[9] | Institute of Medicine Dietary Reference Intakes[27] |
|---|---|
| • Added sugars should not exceed 25% of total calories<br>• Three servings/d of whole grains | • RDA for carbohydrate set at 130 g/d for adults and children<br>• AMDR for carbohydrate set at 45%–65% of total calories<br>• AI for fiber of 14g/1000 calories |

AI = Adequate Intake; AMDR = acceptable macronutrient distribution range; RDA = recommended dietary allowance.

ergy intake. Most industrialized countries fall at the bottom of this range, while underdeveloped countries fall closer to the top of the range. Approximately 50% of carbohydrates consumed are in the form of starch, but this number is higher in countries where starches and grains are staple food items. Industrialized nations have shown an increase in sugar intake to 20% to 25% of calories from sugars, and a substantial portion of these calories are from added sugars such as corn syrups and sucrose.

Whole-grain consumption varies worldwide. Food consumption data from the United States and the United Kingdom report very low intakes at less than one serving of whole grains each day. However, studies in Scandinavian populations show consumption of whole-grain foods to be almost four times the amount consumed in the United States.[28]

### *Quality of Carbohydrate*

It is becoming increasingly obvious that the effects of carbohydrates on health extend beyond their ability to provide the body with energy. The type and amount, as well as the quality, of carbohydrate can make a significant impact on health. As discussed previously, carbohydrate sources can vary greatly in their ability to alter blood glucose levels. This effect on glycemic response has stimulated investigation into the role of glycemic and nonglycemic carbohydrates in the development of chronic diseases such as diabetes and obesity. There is also a difference in carbohydrate quality between whole and refined grains. While the starch component of the grain remains the same, the refining process removes the fiber, vitamins, minerals, and other bioactive components. The presence of these other components can dramatically change the physiological response (e.g., the glycemic response) to the starch contained in the grain. The same is often true for naturally occurring and added sugars. While these sugars do not differ chemically, added sugars are often found in foods with low micronutrient density compared with the naturally occurring sugars often found in fruits with an abundance of micronutrients.

Carbohydrate quality is an important factor in the relationship of carbohydrates to health. As described in the following section, it is often the quality rather than the amount of carbohydrate that makes the biggest impact on health and the development of chronic diseases.

## Carbohydrates in Chronic Disease

### *Energy Balance and Obesity*

A number of epidemiological studies have shown that an increased intake of added sugars is associated with an increase in overall energy intake.[9] However, there is inconsistency regarding the relationship of added sugars to weight gain. Several studies in children and adults have found a negative relationship between the intake of added sugars and body-mass index (BMI),[29-31] while other prospective studies report an increase in BMI or weight gain with increased intake of added sugars.[32-34] It is suggested that the variability of these findings may be due to underreporting of food intake, especially among obese individuals, as well as inadequate adjustments for physical activity.[9,27] Many of these studies are in populations of children and adolescents, as childhood obesity has become more prevalent over recent decades.[35] Furthermore, non-diet soft drinks are the largest source of added sugars in the US and consumption by adolescents is increasing;[36] therefore, many of the previously mentioned investigations have focused on added sugars from sweetened beverages. A recent school-based intervention targeted at reducing soft drink intake found a decrease in the number of overweight and obese children when consumption of soft drinks was reduced even modestly.[37] Based on many of these investigations, the Dietary Guidelines for Americans reported in 2005 that "the preponderance of prospective data available suggests that added sugars (particularly in beverages) are associated with an increase in energy intake. As a result, decreasing the intake of added sugars (particularly in beverages) may help prevent weight gain and may aid in weight loss".[9]

A few short-term studies have suggested a strong positive relationship between high-GI meals and increased energy intake.[27] However, the long-term effects of GI on intake has not been investigated. Furthermore, epidemiological studies have reported no association between GI and BMI.[38-40] Long-term clinical trials are needed before a link between GI and obesity or energy intake over time can be determined.

There has been much debate surrounding the ratio of carbohydrate to fat in the diet and its impact on weight maintenance and weight loss. This is evidenced by the popularity of diet plans ranging from very low in carbohydrate (and high in fat) to very high in carbohydrate (and low in fat). The primary concern over these diets is their long-term efficacy and safety, as they have not been adequately tested for periods of longer than 12 to 18 months. The theory behind the low-carbohydrate/high-fat diet is that extremely low intakes of carbohydrate (sometimes less than 20 g/d) will prevent elevations in insulin such that lipolysis and fat oxidation are increased. Along with this comes an increase in ketone production and appetite suppression. A number of short-term (6- to 12-month) clinical trials have evaluated the efficacy of a low-carbohydrate diet compared with a more balanced macronutrient diet (60% kcal from carbohydrate, 25%–30% kcal from fat, 15% kcal from protein) (27). All of these investigations found that initial weight loss was greater with the low-carbohydrate diet, but after 12 to 18 months, there was little to no difference in weight loss between the diets. Some of the long-term health concerns with a low-carbohydrate diet include the increased intake of saturated fat and cholesterol, increased urinary calcium loss,[41] micronutrient deficiency due to decreased fruit and vegetable intake, and decreased fiber intake.[42] While high-carbohydrate/low-fat diets may provide more fruit, vegetable, and fiber intake, the dramatic decrease in fat intake (≤10% kcal) can contribute to essential fatty acid deficiency, poor absorption of fat-soluble vitamins, and decreased intake of micronutrients such as vitamin $B_{12}$ and zinc.[27,42] An increase in carbohydrate intake has also been shown in a number of clinical trials to elevate blood triglycerides and decrease HDL cholesterol.[27] After a review of the literature on different ratios of carbohydrate to fat to protein and weight maintenance, the DGAC concluded that the ratio is not as important as the total calories consumed over time.[9] Future research should focus on the effects of long-term changes in macronutrient composition in the diet. This includes not only risk of chronic disease, but also physiological effects on the kidney, bone, liver, gastrointestinal system, and other organ systems.

Ultimately, the issue of greater importance than the carbohydrate to fat distribution in the diet is the total energy provided. It has been shown that isocaloric diets do not alter energy expenditure or weight change regardless of the ratio of carbohydrate to fat in the diet.[27] Thus, energy intake has to be restricted for weight loss to occur, and low-fat and low-carbohydrate diets will not result in weight loss if they are isocaloric.

## Diabetes and Insulin Sensitivity

Diabetes is a disorder of carbohydrate metabolism characterized primarily by hyperglycemia resulting from ineffective uptake of glucose by tissues. Type 1 diabetes is an autoimmune disease that typically occurs early in life and results in a total loss of insulin production, while type 2 diabetes develops over time as tissues develop a resistance to insulin and insulin release from the pancreas slowly diminishes. Because carbohydrates have the greatest effect on blood glucose of all of the macronutrients, their role in the development of diabetes has been closely examined. Evidence from prospective studies with follow-up periods as long as 16 years have shown no relationship between the amount of carbohydrate in the diet and the development of diabetes. There also is no apparent association between sugar consumption and the development of type 2 diabetes.[9]

However, whole grains and dietary fiber, particularly cereal fiber, have been shown in a number of epidemiological studies to be inversely associated with the risk of type 2 diabetes.[43] In fact, it appears that the risk reduction due to whole grains may be attributed to the fiber content of the whole grain. Additionally, a recent meta-analysis[44] concluded that a high-carbohydrate/high-fiber diet appears to be the most effective diet for controlling blood glucose levels and serum lipoproteins. More information can be found in the chapters on fiber and diabetes.

A number of randomized, controlled trials have investigated the effect of a low-GI diet compared with a high-GI diet in patients with diabetes.[44] While these studies are short-term (1–2 months), taken together, they show that low-GI diets appear to improve blood glucose control as well as blood lipid profiles. Most long-term prospective studies have supported the relationship between GI and diabetes incidence,[39,40,45,46] but not all studies have found a relationship.[47] Interestingly, in the Nurses' Health Study, the risk of type 2 diabetes was greatest in individuals with a high glycemic load and low cereal fiber intake,[40] suggesting an interaction between glycemic load and fiber intake.

## Cardiovascular Disease and Blood Lipids

Several epidemiological studies have found a consistent relationship between increased intake of whole grains and reduced risk of coronary heart disease.[9] Many of these same studies report an inverse relationship between cereal fiber intake and coronary heart disease, suggesting that the fiber content of the whole grain may play an important role in coronary heart disease prevention. However, findings by Liu et al.[48] suggest that there may be a synergistic protective effect of all components of the whole grain (e.g., vitamin B6, vitamin E, folate, and fiber) and not a protective effect of fiber alone. A recent review of the literature reports that whole grains may protect against cardiovascular disease by favorably altering blood lipids, decreasing blood pressure, providing antioxidant protection, and decreasing inflammatory responses.[49]

There have been no well-established associations discovered between sugar intake and coronary heart disease, and only a few studies have shown an inverse association between overall carbohydrate intake and coronary heart disease. However, a more consistent positive relationship between sugar intake and low-density lipoprotein (LDL) levels has been reported.[27] Sugar intake has also been associated with increases in plasma triacylglycerol concentrations; however, these findings are not as consistent as with LDL levels.[26] Epidemiological studies generally report an inverse relationship between sugar intake and high-density lipoprotein (HDL) levels, yet intervention studies have shown mixed results with either no effect or a decrease in HDL with increased sugar intake.[27]

### *Cancer*

Carbohydrate intake has not been shown to be strongly linked to cancer incidence, with the exception of colorectal cancer. Generally, diets high in refined carbohydrates and sugars appear to increase the risk of colon cancer, while diets high in whole grains appear to be protective.[9] While some of the benefit of whole grains may be due to fiber content, there continues to be debate with regard to the protective effect of fiber on colon cancer.[50] See the fiber chapter for more information.

## Future Directions

A major area to follow in terms of future carbohydrate research is the relationship between the glycemic load of the diet (over time) and health. Studies required to address this important issue will target human clinical intervention trials with high- and low-glycemic load diets and appropriate end points such as hemoglobin A1C, insulin resistance, and blood glucose levels. Type 2 diabetes is on the rise, and its relationship with carbohydrate intake is an important area for future consideration. Also, the difference in health-protective effects from consuming dietary fiber per se and high-fiber diets is very important. High-fiber diets may be a proxy for a healthy diet, since if one meets the AI for dietary fiber without exceeding one's energy requirement, this will be (by definition) a healthy diet.

## References


1. Food and Agriculture Organization/World Health Organization Expert Consultation on Carbohydrates in Human Nutrition. *Carbohydrates in Human Nutrition: A Report of a Joint FAO/WHO Expert Consultation*. FAO Food and Nutrition Paper no. 66. Rome: FAO; 1998.
2. Bray GA, Nielsen SJ, Popkin BM. Consumption of high-fructose corn syrup in beverages may play a role in the epidemic of obesity. Am J Clin Nutr. 2004; 79:537–543.
3. White, J. Fructose syrup: production, properties and applications. In: Shenck F, Hebeda R, eds. *Starch Hydrolysis Products - Worldwide Technology, Production, and Applications*. New York: VCH Publishers; 1992; 177–200.
4. Hanover L, White J. Manufacturing, composition, and applications of fructose. Am J Clin Nutr. 1993; 58:724S–732S.
5. US Department of Agriculture. Economic Research Service. *Sugar and Sweetener Situation and Outlook Yearbook 2003*. Available at: http://usda.mannlib.cornell.edu/reports/erssor/specialty/sss-bb/2003/sss2003.pdf.
6. Food and Drug Administration. Rules and regulations - food labeling: health claims, dietary sugar alcohols and dental caries. Federal Regist. 1997: 63653–63655.
7. Meyer PD. Nondigestible oligosaccharides as dietary fiber. J AOAC Int. 2004;87:718–726.
8. Tungland BC, Meyer D. Nondigestible oligo- and polysaccharides (dietary fiber): their physiology and role in human health and food. Comp Rev Food Sci Food Safe. 2002;1:73–92.
9. US Department of Agriculture. Dietary Guidelines Advisory Committee. *2005 Dietary Guidelines Advisory Committee Report*. Available at: http://www.health.gov/dietaryguidelines/dga2005/report.
10. Guthrie JF, Morton JF. Food sources of added sweeteners in the diets of Americans. J Am Diet Assoc. 2000;100:43–51.
11. Swallow DM. Genetics of lactase persistence and lactose intolerance. Annu Rev Genet. 2003;37: 197–219.
12. Wright EM, Martin MG, Turk E. Intestinal absorption in health and disease—sugars. Best Pract Res Clin Gastroenterol. 2003;17:943–956.
13. Jenkins DJ, Wolever TM, Taylor RH, et al. Glycemic index of foods: a physiological basis for carbohydrate exchange. Am J Clin Nutr. 1981;34: 362–366.
14. Foster-Powell K, Miller JB. International tables of glycemic index. Am J Clin Nutr. 1995;62: 871S–890S.
15. Coulston AM, Hollenbeck CB, Swislocki AL, Reaven GM. Effect of source of dietary carbohydrate on plasma glucose and insulin responses to mixed meals in subjects with NIDDM. Diabetes Care. 1987;10:395–400.
16. Hollenbeck CB, Coulston AM, Reaven GM. Comparison of plasma glucose and insulin responses to mixed meals of high-, intermediate-, and low-glycemic potential. Diabetes Care. 1988;11:323–329.
17. Willett W, Manson J, Liu S. Glycemic index, glycemic load, and risk of type 2 diabetes. Am J Clin Nutr. 2002;76:274S–280S.
18. Pi-Sunyer FX. Glycemic index and disease. Am J Clin Nutr. 2002;76:290S–298S.
19. Merrill AL, Watt BK. *Energy Value of Foods: Basis and Derivitization. Agriculture Handbook No. 74*. Washington, DC: US Government Printing Office; 1973; 2–3.
20. Smith T, Brown JC, Livesey G. Energy balance and thermogenesis in rats consuming nonstarch polysaccharides of various fermentabilities. Am J Clin Nutr. 1998;68:802–819.
21. Warshaw HS, Powers MA. A search for answers about foods with polyols (sugar alcohols). Diabetes Educ. 1999;25:307–321.
22. Zumbe A, Lee A, Storey D. Polyols in confectionery:

the route to sugar-free, reduced sugar and reduced calorie confectionery. Br J Nutr. 2001;85:S31–S45.

23. American Diabetes Association. Nutrition recommendations and principles for people with diabetes mellitus. Diabetes Care. 2000;23:S43–S46.
24. Scheepers A, Joost HG, Schurmann A. The glucose transporter families SGLT and GLUT: molecular basis of normal and aberrant function. JPEN J Parenter Enteral Nutr. 2004;28:364–371.
25. McGrane MM. Carbohydrate metabolism - synthesis and oxidation. In: Stipanuk MH, ed. *Biochemical and Physiological Aspects of Human Nutrition*. Philadelphia: WB Saunders; 2000; 158–205.
26. Parks EJ, Hellerstein MK. Carbohydrate-induced hypertriacylglycerolemia: historical perspective and review of biological mechanisms. Am J Clin Nutr. 2000;71:412–433.
27. Food and Nutrition Board, Institute of Medicine. Dietary Reference Intakes for Energy, Carbohydrate, Fiber, Fat, Fatty Acids, Cholesterol, Protein, and Amino Acids (Macronutrients). Washington, DC: National Academies Press; 2002. Available online at: http://www.nap.edu/books/0309085373/html.
28. Lang R, Jebb SA. Who consumes whole grains, and how much? Proc Nutr Soc. 2003;62:123–127.
29. Lewis CJ, Park YK, Dexter PB, Yetley EA. Nutrient intakes and body weights of persons consuming high and moderate levels of added sugars. J Am Diet Assoc. 1992;92:708–713.
30. Gibson SA. Are diets high in non-milk extrinsic sugars conducive to obesity? An analysis from the Dietary and Nutritional Survey of British Adults. J Hum Nutr Diet. 1996;9:283–292.
31. Bolton-Smith C, Woodward M. Dietary composition and fat to sugar ratios in relation to obesity. Int J Obes Relat Metab Disord. 1994;18:820–828.
32. Ludwig DS, Peterson KE, Gortmaker SL. Relation between consumption of sugar-sweetened drinks and childhood obesity: a prospective, observational analysis. Lancet. 2001;357:505–508.
33. Berkey CS, Rockett HR, Field AE, et al. Sugar-added beverages and adolescent weight change. Obes Res. 2004;12:778–788.
34. Mrdjenovic G, Levitsky DA. Nutritional and energetic consequences of sweetened drink consumption in 6- to 13-year-old children. J Pediatr. 2003;142: 604–610.
35. Troiano, RP and Flegal, KM. Overweight children and adolescents: description, epidemiology, and demographics. Pediatrics. 1998;101:497–504.
36. Cavadini C, Siega-Riz AM, Popkin BM. US adolescent food intake trends from 1965 to 1996. Arch Dis Child. 2000;83:18–24.
37. James J, Thomas P, Cavan D, Kerr D. Preventing childhood obesity by reducing consumption of carbonated drinks: cluster randomised controlled trial. BMJ. 2004;328:1237.
38. Liu S, Willett WC, Stampfer MJ, et al. A prospective study of dietary glycemic load, carbohydrate intake, and risk of coronary heart disease in US women. Am J Clin Nutr. 2000;71:1455–1461.
39. Salmeron J, Ascherio A, Rimm EB, et al. Dietary fiber, glycemic load, and risk of NIDDM in men. Diabetes Care. 1997;20:545–550.
40. Salmeron J, Manson JE, Stampfer MJ, et al. Dietary fiber, glycemic load, and risk of non-insulin-dependent diabetes mellitus in women. JAMA. 1997;277: 472–477.
41. Reddy ST, Wang CY, Sakhaee K, et al. Effect of low-carbohydrate high-protein diets on acid-base balance, stone-forming propensity, and calcium metabolism. Am J Kidney Dis. 2002;40:265–274.
42. Freedman MR, King J, Kennedy E. Popular diets: a scientific review. Obes Res. 2001;9:1S–40S.
43. Murtaugh MA, Jacobs DR Jr, Jacob B, et al. Epidemiological support for the protection of whole grains against diabetes. Proc Nutr Soc. 2003;62:143–149.
44. Anderson JW, Randles KM, Kendall CW, Jenkins DJ. Carbohydrate and fiber recommendations for individuals with diabetes: a quantitative assessment and meta-analysis of the evidence. J Am Coll Nutr. 2004; 23:5–17.
45. Buyken AE, Toeller M, Heitkamp G, et al. Glycemic index in the diet of European outpatients with type 1 diabetes: relations to glycated hemoglobin and serum lipids. Am J Clin Nutr. 2001;73:574–581.
46. Hu FB, van Dam RM, Liu S. Diet and risk of Type II diabetes: the role of types of fat and carbohydrate. Diabetologia. 2001;44:805–817.
47. Meyer KA, Kushi LH, Jacobs DR Jr, et al. Carbohydrates, dietary fiber, and incident type 2 diabetes in older women. Am J Clin Nutr. 2000;71:921–930.
48. Liu S, Stampfer MJ, Hu FB, et al. Whole-grain consumption and risk of coronary heart disease: results from the Nurses' Health Study. Am J Clin Nutr. 1999;70:412–419.
49. Anderson JW. Whole grains protect against atherosclerotic cardiovascular disease. Proc Nutr Soc. 2003; 62:135–142.
50. Lupton JR. Microbial degradation products influence colon cancer risk: the butyrate controversy. J Nutr. 2004;134:479–482.

# 7

# Nutrients and Gene Expression

Howard C. Towle

The essential role of macronutrients as oxidative substrates for generating energy and providing building blocks for the biosynthesis of cellular components has been understood for many decades. Recently, a new and exciting role for macronutrients as regulators of cell function has emerged. All classes of macronutrients—carbohydrates, lipids and proteins—contain components that can function as signaling molecules to alter cell physiology. One of the major pathways by which these signaling molecules affect cell function is to change the pattern of gene expression in the tissues responsible for fuel storage and utilization. This chapter will review current knowledge and recent advances in our understanding of how nutrients control gene expression. In particular, the role of carbohydrates in modulating expression of genes in the liver will be described in some detail. The effects of nutrient-genome interactions on processes related to energy balance provide insights into the potential importance of this regulation in human health and disease.

## Dietary Carbohydrates and Hepatic Lipogenesis

When mammals are fed a high-carbohydrate diet, much of the excess carbohydrates are converted to the preferred energy storage form of triglycerides. This process, termed de novo lipogenesis, occurs in adipose tissue and liver to varying extents depending on the species. The ability to effectively perform lipogenesis is promoted at two distinct levels in response to dietary carbohydrates. The first involves the rapid activation of key enzymatic steps in the pathway. These enzymes generally catalyze irreversible steps in the pathways of glycolysis and fatty acid biosynthesis that are rate-determining in the overall process. For example, the activities of the glycolytic enzyme phosphofructo-1-kinase and the enzyme catalyzing the first committed step in fatty biosynthesis, acetyl coenzyme (CoA) carboxylase, are activated in response to a high-carbohydrate diet.[1] The regulation of enzyme activities involves both covalent modification and allosteric effectors such as fructose-2,6-bisphosphate. These changes occur within minutes and provide acute regulation of the metabolic pathways of fuel oxidation.

A second level of response to carbohydrate feeding involves the induction of the mass of key enzymes and proteins in the lipogenic pathway.[1-3] This induction takes hours, and therefore is thought to be an adaptive response. Increasing the lipogenic potential via induction of these key rate-determining enzymes allows the organism to more effectively convert dietary carbohydrates to triglycerides. In earlier times, when simple carbohydrates were relatively scarce in the environment, the presence of this adaptive mechanism may have provided a significant evolutionary advantage. Needless to say, in the present-day world of high-fructose corn syrup and sucrose-laden sweets, promotion of lipogenesis may be a contributory factor in the development of liver steatosis and obesity in humans.

Enzymes that have been shown to be induced by feeding a high-carbohydrate diet to rodents include: those involved in glycolysis, such as pyruvate kinase; those involved in fatty acid biosynthesis, such as acetyl CoA carboxylase and fatty acid synthase; and those involved in NADPH generation, such as malic enzyme (Table 1). The latter are critical because of the need for NADPH reducing power to drive the process of fatty acid synthesis. In addition, enzymes of fatty acid maturation and triglyceride formation are subject to induction by this dietary regime. In the liver, the products of lipogenesis are predominantly packaged to form very-low-density lipoproteins (VLDL), and are transported to other tissues to

**Table 1.** Enzymes and Proteins Induced in Liver by Feeding of a High-Carbohydrate Diet*

| |
|---|
| Glycolytic |
| GLUT2 glucose transporter |
| Glucokinase |
| Phosphofructo-1-kinase |
| Aldolase |
| Pyruvate kinase |
| Fatty Acid Biosynthesis |
| ATP-citrate lyase |
| Acetyl CoA-carboxylase |
| Fatty acid synthase |
| NADPH-Generating |
| Malic enzyme |
| Glucose-6-phosphate dehydrogenase |
| 6-Phosphogluconate dehydrogenase |
| Fatty Acid Maturation and Packaging |
| Stearoyl-CoA desaturase |
| Glycerol-P-acyltransferase |
| Acyl coenzyme A synthetase (long chain) |
| Apolipoprotein E |
| S14 |

* All of the proteins and enzymes shown have been found to be induced by feeding of a high carbohydrate, fat-free diet to rats or mice. In every case, induction occurs at the level of mRNA levels. For references, see Towle et al., 1997.[2]

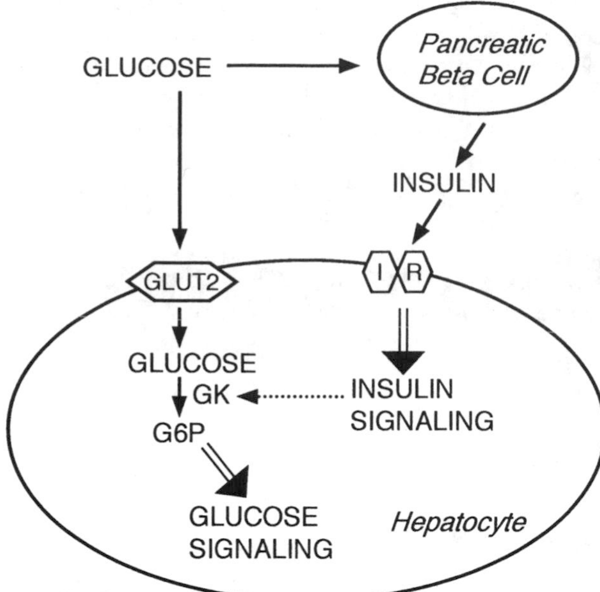


Figure 1. Dual role of glucose and insulin in cell signaling in the hepatocyte. Increased plasma glucose levels following a meal lead to the secretion of insulin from the pancreatic beta cell. Insulin acts through the membrane-bound insulin receptor (IR) to stimulate many processes in the cell, including the expression of the glucokinase (GK) gene. Increased glucose levels reaching the hepatocyte result in the rapid uptake of glucose through the actions of the glucose transporter GLUT2 and its conversion to glucose-6-phosphate (G6P) by GK. Both increased glucose metabolism and insulin can act as signaling events to initiate changes in the hepatocyte, including the induction of lipogenic enzymes.

provide energy or to adipose tissue for storage. Formation of VLDL is mainly driven by substrate availability, so that increased lipogenesis leads to secretion of triglyceride-laden VLDL particles. VLDL is also the critical transport vehicle for hepatic cholesterol and, as will be discussed later, the production of enzymes involved in cholesterol and triglyceride biosynthesis are mechanistically linked in the liver.

## Roles of Insulin and Carbohydrates in Hepatic Lipogenesis

When mammals consume a meal high in simple carbohydrates, plasma glucose levels rapidly rise. Increased plasma glucose levels in the endocrine pancreas trigger increased insulin secretion (Figure 1). Insulin acts on the hepatocyte, and thus provides one signal input that can alter hepatic function. For example, insulin increases the intracellular levels of fructose-2,6-bisphosphate in the hepatocyte, an important allosteric activator of the phosphofructo-1-kinase enzyme activity.[4] Insulin is also an important regulator of gene expression and provides one means of controlling enzyme induction following a high-carbohydrate meal.[5] In addition to insulin, hepatocytes are also presented with increased availability of monosaccharide substrate for oxidation following a high-carbohydrate meal. Increased uptake and metabolism of carbohydrates has been found to initiate a second signaling pathway that can influence lipogenic enzyme genes. The distinct roles of insulin and carbohydrates in mediating induction were elucidated from studies on isolated hepatocytes in culture.[2] Primary hepatocytes that are maintained in 5.5 mM glucose (to approximate fasting plasma glucose levels) without insulin express very low levels of the enzymes necessary for lipogenesis. Switching the medium to one with elevated glucose levels (e.g., 25 mM) and insulin leads to an induction of lipogenic enzyme genes that closely mimics the situation in intact animals fed a high-carbohydrate diet. Using cultured hepatocytes, it has been possible to resolve to some degree the respective roles of insulin and glucose.

When insulin is added to cells that have been maintained in 5.5 mM glucose, only glucokinase of the lipogenic enzyme genes shown in Table 1 is induced.[6] This observation suggests that glucokinase production is directly affected by an insulin receptor-driven signaling pathway. For the other lipogenic enzyme genes, however, the addition of insulin alone is insufficient to cause induction and elevated glucose must also be added. Non-metabolizable analogs of glucose do not support this response; however, other carbohydrates (such as fructose) do. These observations led to the hypothesis that some metabolite generated from glucose metabolism acts as an intracellular signal that alters lipogenic enzyme gene expression.

The essential role of the glucose transporter GLUT2 and glucokinase in promoting glycolysis in the liver is worthy of note. These two proteins function in high Michaelis-Menten constant ($K_m$) glucose transport and glucose phosphorylation in the liver. Consequently, rates of glucose uptake and phosphorylation are proportional to plasma blood glucose levels over the critical range of 5.5 to 20 mM that is encountered post-prandially. These two isozymes are also co-expressed in the beta cell of the pancreas and certain neuroendocrine cells of the medial hypothalamus and intestine.[7] The beta cell shares the capability of the hepatocyte to respond to increased plasma glucose by secreting and increasing the production of insulin. Although not rigorously proven, the neuroendocrine cells expressing these two high $K_m$ isozymes might also be expected to respond to glucose metabolism.

The regulatory pathway controlling lipogenic enzyme genes in adipocytes differs in its initial stages from that in the hepatocyte.[8] The adipocyte does not express either GLUT2 or glucokinase; instead, glucose transport is largely dependent on the glucose transporter GLUT4. The activity of this transporter is regulated by insulin. In low-insulin conditions, GLUT4 is sequestered in an internal membrane compartment and is not available for glucose transport. When insulin levels rise, GLUT4 is translocated to the plasma membrane and helps to reduce plasma glucose levels by importing glucose for triglyceride formation. Therefore, the response of the adipocyte is indirectly coupled to glucose through glucose-regulated insulin secretion of the beta cell. In the adipocyte, hexokinase II is the primary glucose-phosphorylating enzyme. This enzyme has a low $K_m$ for glucose and therefore is poised to convert all incoming glucose to glucose-6-phosphate. Thus, in the adipocyte, the rate-determining step in glycolysis is at the level of glucose uptake and not its phosphorylation.

In addition to being regulated by insulin and glucose, the production of the enzymes of the lipogenic pathway are regulated by a number of other physiological factors in a similar manner. Thyroid hormones are capable of stimulating expression of many or most of the genes of lipogenesis.[9] Thyroid hormones signal energy sufficiency. In most cases, the effects of thyroid hormones and glucose/insulin are synergistic. In contrast, glucagon acts as one of the key hormones of the fasting state to repress expression of all of the lipogenic enzyme genes. Thus, in times of need, energy is directed to hepatic production, rather than storage, of glucose. Dietary fatty acids have also been shown to repress expression of many of the enzymes of lipogenesis.[10,11] This effect is restricted to polyunsaturated fatty acids (PUFAs) and acts to counterregulate the effects of glucose/insulin. Therefore, the production of enzymes critical to lipogenesis is coordinated to respond to several physiological cues of energy status.

## Cellular Sites for Controlling Gene Expression

The induction of lipogenic enzymes following a high-carbohydrate meal could potentially be mediated at any step in the pathway leading from gene transcription to protein synthesis. In every study to date, changes in lipogenic enzyme production have correlated with proportional changes in mRNA levels, indicating that translational regulation is not a major site of control. Alterations in mRNA levels occur predominantly via changes in rates of transcriptional initiation or mRNA stability. The transcription rates of a number of lipogenic enzyme genes have been shown to be elevated in response to a high-carbohydrate diet.[2] Evidence for regulation at the level of mRNA stability for lipogenic enzymes genes has come from direct measurements of RNA turnover. For example, fatty acid synthase mRNA is stabilized by treatment of HepG2 hepatoma cells with glucose.[12] Similarly, alterations in glucose-6-phosphate dehydrogenase RNA levels have been shown to reflect differences in RNA stability rather than transcription.[13] In this case, the changes in RNA stability occur in the nucleus rather than in the cytoplasm. It is likely that for many genes, transcription and mRNA stability are both controlled to provide induction of lipogenic enzymes. In this manner, transcriptional changes could account for early responses within the first few hours, and mRNA stabilization could account for increased production if the carbohydrate stimulatory signal persists. At present, very little is known about the molecular mechanisms involved in mRNA turnover or its regulation in mammalian cells. However, we have learned a great deal about the pathways involved in transcriptional regulation, and this review will focus on these mechanisms.

## Transcriptional Control and the Identification of DNA Regulatory Sequences

Regulation of transcriptional initiation in mammals is dependent on the actions of sequence-specific transcription factors. These factors consist of several discrete functional domains. The DNA-binding domain recognizes a unique DNA sequence of approximately 8 to 12 base pairs and serves to localize the specific factor to the group of genes that it will control. Any particular gene may contain from a few to more than a dozen regulatory sequences recognizing distinct sets of transcription factors. Thus, control of gene transcription is multifactorial and combinatorial. The transactivation domain is involved in mediating the process of transcriptional activation, either by altering chromatin structure or directly by recruiting the basal transcriptional machinery. The third functional domain of the transcription factor is a regulatory domain that serves to link its activity to a specific signaling cascade within the cell. The human genome encodes as many as 2000 distinct transcription factors, providing a complex array of protein to tightly regulate the level of transcription.[14] Consequently, the sequence-specific transcription factors are key elements in the process of controlling gene transcription. Identifying the nature of these factors is critical to developing an understanding of the nutrient-regulated signaling cascades. In addition, these proteins serve as logical targets for the development of drugs to control aspects of metabolic function and obesity. One approach to identifying nutrient-regulated transcription factors is to first identify the key DNA regulatory site to which the factor binds; this site can then be used to help detect and purify the sequence-specific DNA-binding protein of interest.

Mapping of the critical regulatory sequences for mediating control by carbohydrates has been undertaken using the reporter gene assay. In this approach, the 5′-flanking region of the gene of interest containing the transcriptional promoter is cloned upstream of a reporter gene, such as luciferase, in a plasmid vector. The plasmid DNA is then transfected into a cell of interest, such as a primary hepatocyte. The promoter sequences will be recognized by the cellular transcriptional machinery and transcribed into RNA and protein. In this manner, reporter enzyme levels provide a measure of promoter activity under various conditions of cell incubation.

Using this assay, the 5′-flanking promoter regions of several lipogenic enzyme genes have been shown to be more active in cells incubated with glucose and insulin than in cells incubated in basal conditions.[15,16] By making deletion and point mutations in the 5′-flanking regions of these genes, the key regulatory sites critical for glucose or insulin regulation have been mapped. Regulatory sequences that are responsible for glucose regulation of gene transcription have now been defined for four of the lipogenic enzyme genes: the L-type pyruvate kinase gene, the S14 gene, the fatty acid synthase gene, and the acetyl-CoA carboxylase gene.[15-18]

Pyruvate kinase catalyzes the conversion of phosphoenolpyruvate to pyruvate, the final step in glycolysis. This reaction is the third "irreversible" step in glycolysis and is subject to control at both the level of enzyme activity and the level of gene expression. The S14 gene encodes a 17-kD polypeptide involved in some as-yet-unidentified aspect of lipid metabolism.[19] Fatty acid synthase and acetyl-CoA carboxylase catalyze the essential reactions of palmitate biosynthesis from acetyl-CoA precursors. The regulatory sequences found in these four genes are called carbohydrate response elements (ChoREs). The ChoRE can confer glucose responsiveness when it is linked synthetically to a heterologous promoter not normally regulated by glucose. Therefore, this element is necessary and sufficient to confer the carbohydrate response.

A comparison of the ChoREs from these four genes reveals some interesting features (Figure 2). First, when compared with each other, sequence similarities are apparent, allowing the development of a "consensus" sequence. This conservation implies that these four genes are regulated by a common transcription factor that recognizes the ChoRE in each. Differences in the sequences of individual ChoREs presumably result in variations in the binding of the glucose-regulated transcription factor, and therefore differential extents of induction in response to glucose. Second, each of the elements contains two motifs related to the sequence (5′)CACGTG. This motif is known as an E box element, and it is the core recognition site for a family of transcription factors containing linked basic, helix-loop-helix, and leucine zipper (bHLH/LZ) domains.[20] In this family, the basic amino

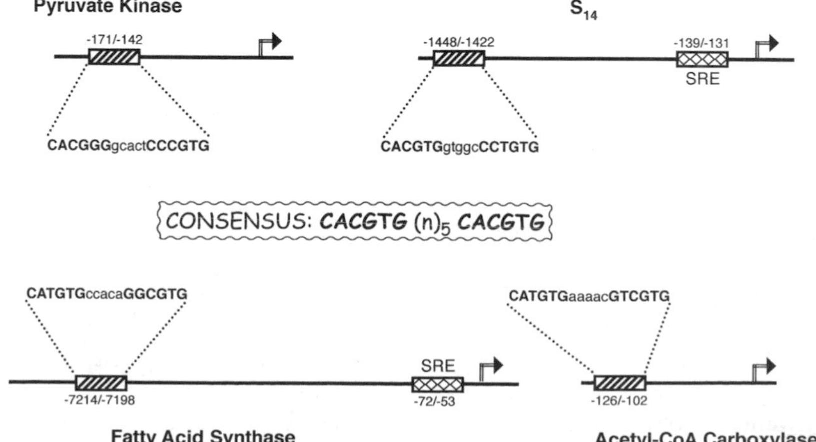


Figure 2. Organization of DNA sequences of several lipogenic genes involved in regulation by carbohydrate. Location of the binding sites for the carbohydrate response elements (ChoREs) in each gene is indicated. Sequence similarities in the ChoREs are shown in the consensus sequence. E box motifs are indicated by capital letters. Location of the sterol regulatory element (SRE) for those genes in which it is known is indicated. Numbers refer to positions of the regulatory sequences relative to the transcriptional initiation site.

acid residues make specific contacts with the bases of the E box. This occurs only in the context of a dimer formed by interactions in the helix-loop-helix and leucine zipper regions. Therefore, the glucose-regulated transcription factor was predicted to be a member of the bHLH/LZ protein family. Third, in all of the ChoREs characterized to date, the two E box motifs are separated by five base pairs of DNA that are not conserved in sequence. Experiments have shown that synthetically changing this spacing to either six base pairs or four base pairs results in a significant or complete loss of the ability to support a glucose response, respectively.[16] This observation implies that two E box-binding dimers may recognize the ChoRE and be positioned at a critical distance to interact with each other or with a third component to form a glucose-responsive complex.

## ChREBP: The Carbohydrate-responsive Transcription Factor

Using the ChoRE from the pyruvate kinase gene as an affinity reagent, a candidate transcription factor for mediating the glucose response was isolated from rat liver.[21] This transcription factor was designated ChoRE-binding protein (ChREBP), and had several features that supported its role in mediating the glucose response. First, ChREBP is a member of the bHLH/LZ family that recognizes E box sites. Second, ChREBP is most abundantly expressed in liver and in brown and white adipose tissue, all sites of active lipogenesis. Third, when introduced into hepatocytes, ChREBP was found to increase the activity of a co-transfected, ChoRE-containing promoter under high- but not low-glucose conditions. Fourth, ChREBP was found to shuttle between the cytoplasm and nucleus in a glucose-dependent fashion.[22] ChREBP is mainly nuclear in conditions when lipogenesis is active, but predominantly cytoplasmic in conditions not favoring fatty acid biosynthesis.

Despite this evidence supporting a role for ChREBP, efforts to demonstrate its direct binding to the ChoRE sequence in vitro were unsuccessful. Since all bHLH/LZ proteins bind to DNA as dimers, this observation suggested that ChREBP might function as a heterodimer with another family member. Protein interaction screening in yeast revealed that ChREBP forms heterodimers with a partner known as Max-like factor X (Mlx),[23,24] a member of the Myc/Max family of bHLH/LZ proteins.[25] Like Max, it has been found to be capable of heterodimerizing with a number of other family members, including Mad1, Mnt, Mad4, and MondoA. In some cases, the resulting heterodimers are repressors of transcription, whereas with other partners an activator is formed. However, no target genes have been identified for Mlx complexed with any of these heterodimeric partners. ChREBP was found to bind to ChoREs in vitro in the presence of Mlx.[24] This binding was observed for ChoREs from several lipogenic enzyme genes. However, binding was lost when the spacing between the E box elements was changed from the natural spacing of five base pairs. Furthermore, the ability of ChREBP to activate promoter activity was dependent on the presence of Mlx. The correlation between in vitro binding and activation supported the ChREBP/Mlx heteromer as the functional glucose-responsive transcription factor.

Physiological support for the role of ChREBP in mediating the glucose response of lipogenic enzyme genes has come from two kinds of experiments. In one, knockout mice were developed in which the gene for ChREBP was deleted from the chromosome.[26] These mice are viable, but display a complex pattern of metabolic abnormalities. The ChREBP-deleted mice are mildly hyperglycemic and insulin-resistant and have greatly elevated hepatic glycogen stores. This phenotype is consistent with a defect in glycolysis in these animals, perhaps due to reduced pyruvate kinase gene expression. In animals fed a high-starch diet, the mRNA levels for several glycolytic and lipogenic enzymes were reduced in the liver, rates of lipogenesis were reduced by greater than 50%, and both the brown and white adipose fat pad weights were reduced. The phenotype of the ChREBP-deleted mice supports a critical physiological role of ChREBP in glucose utilization and lipogenesis.

One limitation in interpreting the phenotype of knockout mice is that the effects observed in the liver could be due to indirect effects of altering metabolism in extra-hepatic tissues. An alternate approach to evaluating the role of ChREBP in hepatocytes has been to transiently inhibit ChREBP activity. This has been accomplished by two techniques: 1) introducing dominant-negative mutants that inhibit ChREBP activity and 2) using small interfering RNAs to reduce ChREBP expression.[27,28] Dominant-negative forms for ChREBP were made by introducing mutations into the basic region of Mlx that contacts the DNA. These mutant forms are still capable of heterodimerizing with ChREBP, but block its binding to ChoRE sites. When introduced into cultured hepatocytes, the dominant-negative Mlx forms blocked the glucose induction of several lipogenic enzyme genes examined. However, no effects were seen on insulin induction of gene expression. Similar observations were made using small interfering RNA to inhibit ChREBP expression. These data support the direct role of ChREBP in the glucose-signaling pathway and validate the role of Mlx as a partner in the process.

How do changes in glucose metabolism in the hepatocyte result in alterations in ChREBP activity? The current model suggests that under low-glucose conditions, cAMP levels rise in the hepatocyte, thereby activating the cAMP-dependent protein kinase (PKA) (Figure 3). Three sites of phosphorylation by PKA were predicted in ChREBP.[22] One of these sites (serine 196) is located adjacent to the nuclear localization signal required for nuclear import of the protein. Mutation of this residue

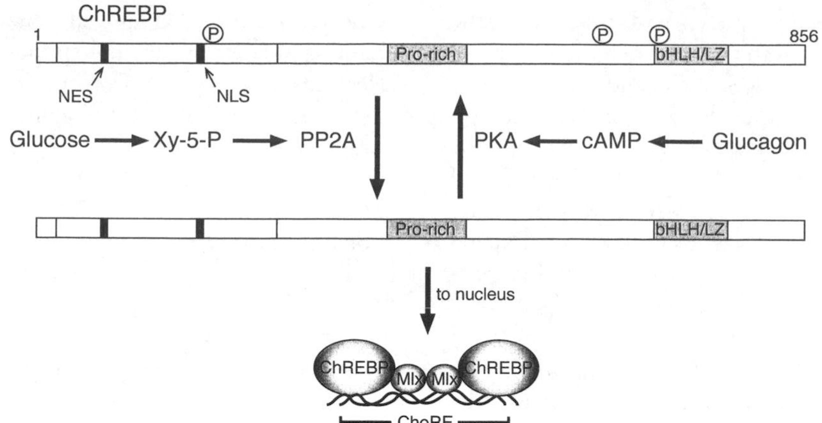


Figure 3. Model for the regulation of carbohydrate response element (ChoRE) binding protein (ChREBP) in response to glucose and cAMP. ChREBP is indicated as a linear sequence showing the relative location of the transcriptional activation domain (Pro-rich), the DNA-binding domain (bHLH/LZ), the nuclear localization signal (NLS) and the nuclear export signal (NES). The positions of three residues (serine-196, serone-626 and threonine-666) that are potential phosphorylation sites for cAMP-dependent protein kinase (PKA) are shown. PKA is activated in response to elevated cAMP levels following the interaction of glucagon with its hepatic receptor under fasting conditions. Phosphorylation of these residues causes cytoplasmic localization of ChREBP. When glucose levels are elevated, increase in xylulose-5-phosphate (Xu-5-P) levels are postulated to activate a protein phosphatase 2A (PP2A) isoform to desphosphorylate these critical sites and activate nuclear localization and DNA binding of ChREBP with its heterodimer partner Max-like factor X (Mlx) to the ChoRE element.

to an alanine residue resulted in ChREBP localized to the nucleus independent of glucose, whereas mutation to an aspartate residue to mimic the phosphorylated state resulted in a constitutively cytoplasmic form. Therefore, PKA phosphorylation of this residue in low-glucose conditions sequesters ChREBP in the cytoplasm, where it cannot stimulate transcription.

In addition, two residues (serine 626 and threonine 666) were found to be important for controlling DNA-binding activity of ChREBP. Again, the phosphorylated forms were less active with significantly reduced DNA binding, suggesting that PKA inhibits any nuclear ChREBP from binding to the ChoRE. When glucose levels are high, cAMP levels are reduced and PKA activity is inhibited. It has been postulated that a specific isoform of protein phosphatase 2a (PP2a) acts to remove the inhibitory phosphates from ChREBP. This PP2A form is activated by xylulose-5-phosphate, an intermediate in the pentose phosphate shunt that rapidly increases when glucose levels are elevated.[29] Removal of the inhibitory phosphates results in nuclear import and DNA binding by ChREBP.

It is interesting that the pentose phosphate shunt plays a role in generating a metabolic regulator of lipogenesis. The first two enzymes in the shunt (glucose-6-phosphate dehydrogenase and 6-phosphogluconate dehydrogenase) produce NADPH, which is needed to drive fatty acid biosynthesis. This situation provides a potential couple between increased utilization of NADPH for supporting triglyceride formation and the formation of the active intermediate involved in stimulating lipogenic enzyme production. Furthermore, the same PP2A isoform that dephosphorylates ChREBP also activates the bifunctional enzyme responsible for generation of the allosteric effector fructose-2,6-bisphosphate.[21] Fructose-2,6-bisphosphate is an activator of the glycolytic enzyme phosphofructo-1-kinase, a rate-determining step in glycolysis. In this manner, changes in metabolic flux and transcription of metabolically important genes can be coupled in the cell.

## SREBP: The Insulin-responsive Transcription Factor

As indicated above, both glucose and insulin activate signaling pathways required for the induction of lipogenic enzyme genes. Insight into the insulin-signaling pathway required for lipogenic enzyme induction has come from the study of a second transcription factor, sterol response element binding protein (SREBP). SREBP was first characterized as a transcription factor that binds to the sterol regulatory element (SRE).[30,31] This element is found within the promoter sequences of a set of genes regulated in response to cholesterol. When cellular cholesterol levels are low, transcription of genes involved in cholesterol biosynthesis and uptake are increased. SREBP is synthesized in a precursor form of approximately 125 kD, and resides in the endoplasmic reticulum (Figure 4). Low sterol levels lead to the proteolytic cleavage of the cytosolic amino-terminal domain of the precursor, which subsequently translocates to the nucleus to bind to the SRE and activate transcription.[32] This negative feedback control ensures that cells will have adequate supplies of cholesterol for membrane biosynthesis and other cellular needs.

SREBP occurs in three forms: SREBP-1a, SREBP-1c, and SREBP-2. SREBP-1a and 1c are products of the same gene that is transcribed from two promoters to produce alternate first exons. SREBP-1c is the predomi-

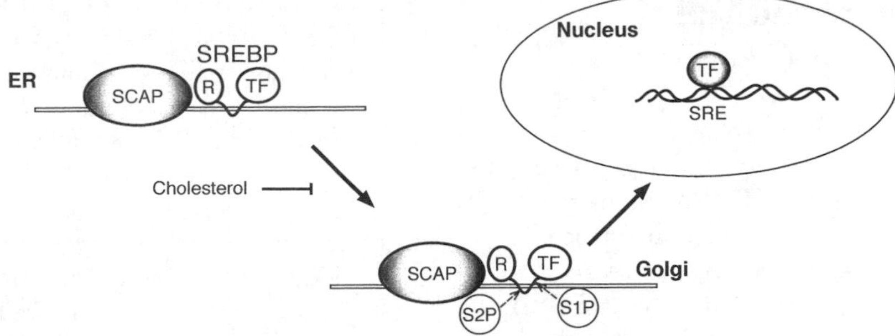


Figure 4. Model for sterol response element binding protein (SREBP) control by cholesterol. SREBP is synthesized as a large molecular weight precursor that resides in the endoplasmic reticulum in association with sterol cleavage activating protein (SCAP). SCAP senses low cellular cholesterol levels in the membrane and activates translocation of SREBP to the Golgi apparatus. Two site-specific proteases (S1P and S2P) cleave the SREBP precursor near its site of membrane attachment to release the amino-terminal transcriptionally active fragment (TF). This fragment translocates to the nucleus and binds to regulatory sequences (SRE) located within genes that are responsible for increased cholesterol uptake and biosynthesis. As cellular levels of cholesterol increase, the translocation of the SREBP precursor to the Golgi apparatus is inhibited and SREBP levels fall to inactivate the pathway.

nant form in liver and adipose tissue. SREBP-2 is the product of a distinct gene that shares a high degree of homology in the DNA-binding domain with SREBP-1 and significantly less similarity outside of this region. In whole animals, SREBP-2 levels in the nucleus are increased under conditions favoring cholesterol biosynthesis, indicating a role of this factor in cholesterol homeostasis. However, nuclear levels of SREBP-1 were not altered in these conditions, suggesting that it may play a different role in the animal.

Several observations have suggested a role for SREBP in regulating the process of lipogenesis. SREBP was shown to bind to the promoter regions of many lipogenic enzyme genes, such as fatty acid synthase.[33] When transgenic mice were made that overexpressed the nuclear form of SREBP-1, thus bypassing the normal endoplasmic reticulum cleavage event for activation, an interesting phenotype was observed: these animals had greatly enlarged livers due to a deposition of triglycerides and cholesterol.[34] In association with this lipid accumulation, the mRNA levels for many of the lipogenic enzyme genes were dramatically elevated. Therefore, at least when overexpressed, SREBP-1 is capable of promoting lipogenic enzyme gene expression.

Further evidence supporting a role for SREBP in regulating the lipogenic gene family has emerged from two studies. In one, mice were generated with a homozygous deletion of the SREBP-1 gene.[35] Although these mice had normal levels of lipogenic enzymes on standard chow, they were significantly aberrant in their ability to induce these enzymes in response to a high-carbohydrate diet. The induction of virtually all enzymes in the lipogenic pathway, including S14, L-PK, and fatty acid synthase (FAS), were either completely or largely blocked in the liver. Interestingly, cholesterol responses in these animals were normal, supporting the distinct role of SREBP-2 in cholesterol regulation. In a complementary study, cultured hepatocytes expressing a dominant negative form of SREBP were blocked in the normal glucose-mediated induction of lipogenesis and lipogenic gene induction.[36] Based on these two results, SREBP is certainly required for maintaining a normal carbohydrate response in the liver and may serve to coordinate fatty acid and cholesterol biosynthesis.

SREBP-1c mRNA and protein were found to be induced by feeding a high-carbohydrate diet to fasted animals.[37] When examined in cultured hepatocytes or adipocytes, this regulation was specific for insulin and was not dependent on the glucose concentration. SREBP-1c thus joined glucokinase as a direct insulin-regulated gene product. Regulation of SREBP-1c gene expression by insulin occurs at the level of transcription. However, this raises an interesting question. If insulin induces SREBP-1c transcription, what transcription factor is responsible for mediating this effect? One possible candidate is SREBP-1c itself; that is, SREBP-1c may be autogenously regulated.

The activity of SREBP-1c appears to be regulated by the insulin-signaling pathway involving phosphatidylinositol 3-kinase and protein kinase B (Akt).[38,39] One downstream target of this pathway is glycogen synthase kinase 3 (GSK3). GSK3 phosphorylates and inhibits glycogen synthase in the absence of insulin. Upon insulin activation of the phosphatidylinositol 3-kinase pathway, GSK3 is phosphorylated and inactivated, allowing for increased glycogen synthase activity and glycogen deposition. Recent data suggest that SREBP-1c may also be a target of GSK3, and that its phosphorylation by this kinase inhibits its transcriptional activity.[39] Therefore, initial insulin signaling would activate basal SREBP-1c in the cell, which would increase transcription of lipogenic enzyme genes—as well as SREBP-1c itself. This would result in a feed-forward mechanism to further enhance lipogenesis in the presence of insulin. It is interesting that controlling the activity of a common downstream regulator, GSK3, could coordinately regulate intracellular metabolism and transcription by insulin, as noted earlier for PP2A.

## PUFAs and Repression of Lipogenic Enzyme Gene Expression

Dietary PUFAs suppress the expression of lipogenic enzyme genes.[10,11] The effects of PUFAs occur rapidly (within a few hours of feeding) and affect many or most of the lipogenic enzyme genes. Neither unsaturated or monounsaturated fatty acids are effective. Since PUFAs represent one of the major products of the pathway, suppression by PUFAs can be viewed as a form of end-product inhibition. SREBPs have been implicated in the suppression of lipogenic enzyme gene expression by PUFAs.[10,40] Supplementing a high-carbohydrate diet with PUFAs was shown to decrease both the precursor and nuclear forms of SREBP-1c, but not SREBP-2, in liver. Likewise, treatment of cultured hepatocytes with PUFAs also decreased the nuclear content of SREBP-1c. The changes in SREBP mediated by PUFA treatment result from effects at several different levels. PUFAs have been found to inhibit transcription of the SREBP-1c gene, as well as to enhance the turnover of SREBP-1c mRNA. In addition, the proteolytic release of active SREBP-1c from its membrane-anchored precursor is inhibited by PUFAs. The molecular mechanisms responsible for these changes have not been elucidated, but the effects of PUFAs on SREBP-1c appear to be indirect, as no evidence of direct binding has been observed. The important role of SREBP-1c in mediating the effects of PUFAs has been substantiated in mouse models. Neither transgenic mice overexpressing SREBP1 or mice in which the SREBP-1 gene has been deleted suppress the lipogenic enzyme gene in response to PUFAs. Consequently, SREBP functions to integrate signals from both insulin (glucose) and PUFAs to regulate lipogenic enzyme production.

## PPARs: Receptors for Fatty Acids and Fatty Acids Derivatives

In addition to their suppressive effects on lipogenic enzyme gene expression, dietary fatty acids influence the expression of a wide variety of other genes.[41] In many cases, fatty acids act in a positive fashion to increase expression of genes. For example, in liver, acyl-CoA oxidase, L-type fatty acid-binding protein, and carnitine palmitoyltransferase-1 are induced by dietary fatty acids. These gene products are all involved in different aspects of fatty metabolism, and their induction is presumably an adaptive response of the tissue or cell to increased delivery of fatty acids. In this case, both saturated and unsaturated fatty acids can act as inducers, indicating that a distinct mechanism is involved.

A critical component in the pathway by which fatty acids can regulate gene expression was identified as the peroxisome proliferator-activator receptor (PPAR).[42,43] PPARs are members of the nuclear receptor family of ligand-activated transcription factors. The first members of this family to be characterized were receptors for the steroid hormones, thyroid hormones, and vitamin D3. These receptors share structurally related DNA-binding, transactivation, and ligand-binding domains. A family of related genes that were predicted to have similar functions, but for which ligands were not known, were found in the human genome and were termed "orphan receptors." What has become clear in the past decade is that most of these orphan receptors are in fact receptors that have evolved to recognize specific metabolic intermediates in the pathways they control.[44] These receptors provide a direct means for controlling transcription rates of specific genes in response to changing levels of a critical ligand (Figure 5).

The PPARs were first discovered as receptors for a class of hypolipidemic agents, including fibrates, that promote peroxisome proliferation in rodent models. Subsequently, it was shown that fatty acids could serve as direct ligands for the PPARs.[45] However, the situation is complicated by the presence of multiple classes of PPARs that differ in their tissue distribution and ligand specificity. Furthermore, these receptors can bind to specific prostaglandin and leukotriene metabolites derived from fatty acids. Therefore, it has been difficult to pinpoint the actual intracellular ligand responsible for activating PPARs in various tissues. However, the structure of PPAR bound to arachidonic acid has been determined, demonstrating that fatty acids can certainly bind in the ligand-binding domain of the PPARs.[46] This structural analysis suggested that 18- and 20-carbon fatty acids are likely the preferred ligands for PPAR activation.

Genes that respond to the PPARs contain a DNA-binding motif known as the peroxisome proliferator response element (PPRE).[42] These motifs consist of a direct repeat of the consensus sequence (5′)AGGTCA separated by one base pair. Interestingly, other members of the nuclear receptor family also recognize repeats of the

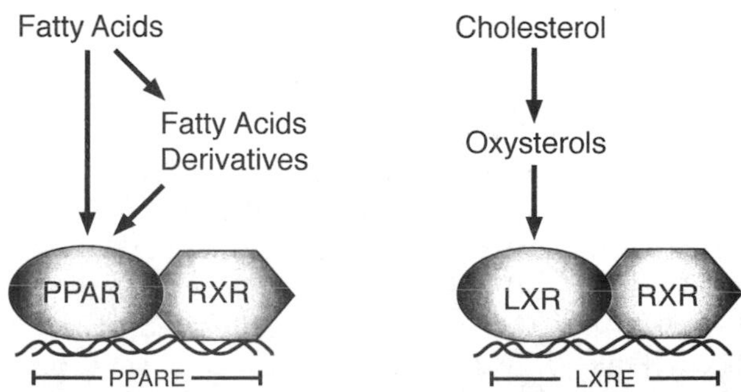


Figure 5. Nuclear receptors act as ligand-mediated transcription factors in response to nutrients and their metabolites. Nuclear receptors related to the steroid hormone receptor family bind to DNA as heterodimers with retinoid X receptor (RXR). Peroxisome proliferator-activator receptors (PPARs) are receptors that are activated by directly binding to fatty acids or to metabolites of fatty acids. This binding triggers activation of genes containing the PPARE regulatory site. Similarly, liver-X receptor (LXR) functions as a receptor for oxysterols derived from cholesterol. Genes containing the LXRE regulatory site respond to increased oxysterols levels by increasing their transcription.

AGGTCA motif; however, spacing between the repeated motifs determines to a large extent binding specificity. PPARs bind to this sequence as heterodimers with another nuclear receptor, retinoid X receptor (RXR). While RXR can function as a receptor for certain retinoids, it also turns out to be a common heterodimeric partner for a wide number of nuclear receptors. The physiological advantage of this system is not immediately apparent, except for those genes in which both retinoids and other ligands can work together to control expression. Genes that respond positively to dietary fatty acids contain PPREs and mutations in this sequence ablate the response of these genes to fatty acids.

Three different genes encode PPARs in the human genome: PPARα, PPARδ, and PPARγ. PPARδ is ubiquitously expressed and little is yet known about its physiological functions. PPARα is the predominant PPAR isoform expressed in liver. It plays a major role in the control of genes involved in lipid metabolism, including fatty acid oxidation in mitochondrial and peroxisomal compartments, ketogenesis, fatty acid binding, and fatty acid transport. Therefore, PPARα ligands promote lipolysis under conditions of increased fatty acid uptake in the liver. This occurs during fasting periods, when enhanced lipolysis of triglyceride stores in adipose provides substrate for oxidation. Experiments with mice lacking the PPARα gene have been instrumental in demonstrating the role of this receptor during the fasting response.[47]

The PPARγ isoform was originally thought to be an adipose-specific form. It promotes adipogenesis from precursor cells, and therefore is thought to play an important role in the development of adipose tissue.[48] It is also the target of the thiazolidinedione class of type 2 antidiabetic drugs. These drugs increase insulin sensitivity and glucose homeostasis through activation of gene transcription in the major organs involved in glucose disposal. Recently, PPARγ isoforms have been found to also be expressed in muscle and liver, indicating that the action of these drugs could occur through these tissues as well. However, adipose tissue is thought to be the major site of action. The insulin-sensitizing actions of the thiazolidinediones could occur based on the ability of PPARγ to alter synthesis and secretion of adipocyte hormones such as adiponectin and TNFα.[49] However, further work is necessary to substantiate this hypothesis.

## LXR: A Nuclear Receptor Regulating Cholesterol Homeostasis

Although PPARs were among the first of the orphan receptors to be "adopted" by an endogenous ligand, the physiological roles of several more have now been elucidated. Among these is the liver-X receptor (LXR), which plays a critical role in regulating cholesterol homeostasis. Understanding the mechanisms for regulating cholesterol metabolism is of significance, since large variations can occur in both metabolic demand and dietary intake for this key cellular nutrient. It is extremely important for cholesterol levels to be tightly regulated, as there is no enzymatic pathway in humans for recovery of the carbon and chemical energy invested in synthesizing the cholesterol molecule. The most fundamental role of cholesterol in mammals is to provide structural support and hydrophobic character to cellular membranes. Its unique physical properties make it ideal to provide rigidity and selective permeability to the lipid bilayer. However, the same chemical properties that are advantageous in membrane function make it a potentially harmful compound when it accumulates in atherosclerotic plaques.

As explained above, SREBP-2 plays an essential role in increasing cholesterol levels in a cell when more cholesterol is needed. This is accomplished by increasing the transcription of genes encoding proteins involved in cholesterol uptake and biosynthesis. But what happens when cholesterol levels in a cell are too high? In this case, it is necessary first to transport that cholesterol to the liver. Then, in the liver, cholesterol is excreted either as cholesterol or as bile acids. The two orphan receptors, LXR and the farnesoid X receptor (FXR), are directly involved in these latter processes and are controlled in this regard by binding to cholesterol derivatives that signal excess cholesterol to the cell.

LXR was first discovered as an orphan nuclear receptor, and is encoded by two different genes[50]: the LXRα gene is expressed predominantly in liver, intestine, adipose tissue, kidney, and macrophages, while the LXRβ gene is expressed in all tissues. Ligands for LXRs were identified from small molecule screens that found certain oxysterols, such as 22(R)-hydroxycholesterol and 27-hydroxycholesterol, as ligands for the receptor.[51,51] Like PPARs, LXRs bind to specific sites in the DNA as heterodimers with RXR. They recognize a direct repeat of the consensus motif (5′)AGGTCA separated by four base pairs.

The physiology of LXR receptors has been dissected through the study of mice carrying disruption of the LXR genes, as well as the treatment of mice with LXR-specific pharmacologic ligands. On a high-cholesterol diet, LXRα null mice exhibit dramatically increased plasma LDL cholesterol and decreased HDL cholesterol levels, a status associated with increased risk for cardiovascular disease in humans.[53] Conversely, administration of a synthetic LXR agonist to mice results in increased excretion of cholesterol and bile acids. In explaining these effects, particular interest has been generated by the role of the ATP-binding cassette (ABC) transporter family of proteins.[54]

ABC transporters are integral membrane proteins that couple the hydrolysis of ATP with the transport of various substances across the membrane. The ABCA1 protein is critical for the efflux of cellular cholesterol to form HDL cholesterol in the first step of reverse cholesterol transport. The ABCA1 gene contains an LXR response element in the promoter and is a direct target for LXRs.

Another potentially important target gene for LXR in this process encodes apolipoprotein E (ApoE). ApoE is a component of the LDL particle that is recognized by liver cells in clearing LDL from circulation. Regulation of ApoE expression by LXRs in adipose and macrophages (but not liver) results in enhanced liver uptake of these cholesterol-laden particles. Therefore, the activation of LXRs by oxysterols that occurs under high-cholesterol conditions leads to a concerted activation of genes that promote cholesterol transport from peripheral tissues to the liver. Consequently, LXR is considered to be a key receptor of cholesterol homeostasis.

Metabolism of cholesterol and fatty acids are inextricably linked in humans, so it was not surprising to discover that LXR also played a role in control of fatty acid metabolism. Mice disrupted for the LXRα gene were noted to be deficient in the expression of the SREBP-1c gene.[55] As a consequence, the expression of many lipogenic enzyme genes, including acetyl CoA-carboxylase and fatty acid synthase, were reduced in these animals. Conversely, administration of synthetic LXR ligands to mice triggers induction of the lipogenic pathway and leads to elevated plasma triglycerides. This action is mediated by an LXR response element in the promoter of the SREBP-1c gene that activates its transcription.[55] Why would mammals want to increase fatty acid synthesis in conditions of elevated cholesterol? Free cholesterol is highly toxic to cells, so esterification with fatty acids is an important mechanism to control these toxic effects. Increasing fatty acid production may provide a substrate for this esterification. Therefore, these actions are consistent with the role of LXR in overall cholesterol homeostasis in the organism.

In addition to PPARs and LXRs, the endogenous ligands for several other orphan receptors have been identified.[56] These include FXR, which functions in the control of bile acid synthesis. FXR is activated by binding of bile acids and serves to promote cholesterol excretion by stimulating transcription of the rate-limiting enzyme in bile acid synthesis, Cyp7A1. Therefore, FXR and LXR work in conjunction with each other as general sterol regulators in the body. The steroid and xenobiotic receptor (SXR) and the coxsackievirus and adenovirus receptor (CAR) are orphan receptors that bind to a range of chemically and structurally diverse ligands. These ligands include a large number of xenobiotic compounds that are found in food and serve to coordinate metabolism and elimination of various xenobiotics through regulation of target genes of the cytochrome P450 family. This process occurs in the liver, and functions physiologically to detoxify these compounds and promote their excretion. Many drugs used for the treatment of common illnesses can also bind to and activate these receptors, so there is great interest in their role in controlling effective treatment. Finally, a number of orphan nuclear receptors remain without identified ligands. While it is not certain that a ligand will exist for every member, there is still much room for discovery of important regulators of metabolism in this class of transcription factors.

## mTOR: Sensor of Amino Acids and Energy Status

Mammalian target of rapamycin (mTOR) has recently emerged as a central component of a signaling pathway that senses energy status and controls cell growth.[57,58] Cell growth is defined as an increase in cell mass and size due to macromolecular biosynthesis. Since cell proliferation is intimately linked to cell growth, the TOR pathway plays a crucial role in controlling decisions in the cell that trigger progression through the cell cycle. This pathway can be influenced by specific nutrients such as amino acids or by growth factors and cytokines.

mTOR was discovered and named based on its interaction with the immunosuppressant drug rapamycin.[58] Rapamycin acts in the cell by interacting with its intracellular receptor, FKBP12. This complex in turn binds to the C-terminal region of mTOR. Identification of mTOR revealed that it is an extremely large protein containing 2549 amino acids with several distinct structural domains. Among these was a protein kinase domain in the C-terminal region of mTOR. Binding of rapamycin-FKBP12 to mTOR inhibits its protein kinase activity and blocks the biosynthetic pathways stimulated by mTOR. The immunosuppressive effects of rapamycin stem from its ability to inhibit cell proliferation in B and T cells; however, mTOR is expressed widely and influences cell growth in all tissues. In fact, rapamycin was discovered based on its antifungal activity, and yeast contains two orthologous TOR genes. In yeast, TOR is sensitive to changes in amino acid, nitrogen, and glucose levels, and inhibition of TOR with rapamycin triggers a response program similar to nutrient starvation. Therefore, the function of TOR is highly conserved evolutionarily.

The search for targets of the mTOR protein kinase activity revealed two important control proteins in the protein translational machinery.[59,60] One of these is the translational inhibitory protein 4E-BP1. The initiation step in the translational process involves binding of the mRNA by a complex of three initiation factors collectively referred to as eIF4F. This complex then promotes binding of the ribosome to the mRNA. 4E-BP1 acts by binding to one of the components of the eIF-4F complex (eIF4E) and blocking its participation in the initiation process. The interaction of 4E-BP1 with eIF4E is regulated by the phosphorylation of 4E-BP1. When unphosphorylated or hypophosphorylated, 4E-BP1 binds to eIF4E and thereby inhibits translation. However, the hyperphosphorylated form of 4E-BP1 cannot interact with eIF4E and translation can then proceed. mTOR is capable of phosphorylating 4E-BP1 on multiple residues and thus promotes translation when it is active.

A second target of mTOR is another protein kinase that phosphorylates one of the ribosomal proteins known as S6. The S6 kinase is activated by protein phosphorylation by mTOR. The consequence of this phosphorylation is to promote the translation of a set of mRNAs that possess a specific signal (5′-oligopyrimidine tract). This set of mRNAs encodes ribosomal proteins and other translation factors that can lead to increased cellular capacity for protein synthesis. In addition to direct effects on the translational process, mTOR also controls transcription of many genes involved in protein synthesis, including ribosomal RNAs, transfer RNAs, and ribosomal proteins. Although these pathways are not yet as well characterized, it is clear that mTOR stimulates a program in the cells that elevates its capacity to carry out protein synthesis, thus stimulating cell growth.

Amino acid availability is one of the major nutrient signals controlling the activity of mTOR. Switching cultured mammalian cells from their normal medium containing amino acids to one that does not results in reduced signaling through the mTOR pathway. Amino acids are thus positive regulators of mTOR signaling. Leucine has proven to be the most effective of the various amino acids when given alone, although several other amino acids can also effect the response. Other nutrients, such as carbohydrates, can influence signaling through the mTOR pathway, although these have not been studied to the same extent. Generally, this pathway appears to respond to energy status from many different inputs. One of the major questions is how so many different inputs can funnel into the common regulation of the central mTOR component.

While the mechanism by which mTOR is regulated in response to nutrient signaling is not yet known, it is clear that mTOR functions as part of large, multi-protein complex. The first of the proteins that was shown to interact with mTOR was termed Raptor (regulatory-associated protein of TOR).[61,62] Raptor binds to the N-terminal region of mTOR and is required for mTOR signaling; it also binds to both S6 kinase and 4E-BP1, downstream effectors of mTOR, and thus may be important for target selection. The strength of binding between Raptor and mTOR is altered in response to nutrient starvation, suggesting that signaling may involve changes in this protein-protein interaction. A second component that associates with mTOR is a G protein β-subunit-like protein (GβL).[63] GβL interacts specifically with the kinase domain of mTOR and plays a positive role in mTOR activation by nutrients. Thus, these three components (and possibly others) comprise a nutrient-sensitive mTOR complex. While much remains to be learned about the mTOR pathway, it is already clear that this pathway is of fundamental importance in regulating energy homeostasis in the cell.

## Conclusions

Over the past decade, nutrient control of gene expression has emerged as a major topic of importance in human nutrition. The idea that nutrients and metabolites derived from nutrients can serve as important intracellular signals controlling the expression of genes involved in metabolic pathways is now strongly established. In a number of cases, the critical components in the nutrient-controlled signaling pathways have been identified. Many of these components have turned out to be transcription factors that function to activate sets of genes encoding key enzymes in the metabolic pathways. The consequence of these signaling pathways is to change the protein and enzyme armament of the cell to one more readily suited for the nutrient state. Coupled with hormonal cues, the integration of information from metabolic signals determines the state of energy utilization versus energy storage in key tissues such as the liver.

Tissue-specific effects of energy nutrients such as glucose clearly play a major role as intracellular determinants of cell physiology. The impact of this pathway on human health and disease needs to be further analyzed. Obesity is a highly complex disorder that involves an imbalance between energy intake and expenditure. Under normal circumstances, the rate of synthesis of fatty acids in humans is low due to the high percentage of fats in our diets. As a result, the de novo synthesis of fatty acids is usually ignored as a significant contributory factor in human obesity. However, this low rate of lipogenesis is due to the effective regulatory circuit that allows dietary fatty acids to inhibit lipogenesis. If that regulatory circuit were defective due to genetic or environmental factors, even a small increase in fatty synthesis could make a significant contribution to an undesired increase in body weight. Furthermore, altering the activity of critical components in the nutrient signaling pathways provides a potential means of intervention for treating metabolic disorders. The next decade should prove an informative one for furthering our understanding in this area, leading to new insights into the role of macronutrient signaling in human health and disease.

## References

1. Hillgartner FB, Salati LM, Goodridge AG. Physiological and molecular mechanisms involved in nutritional regulation of fatty acid synthesis. Physiol Rev. 1995;75:47–76.
2. Towle HC, Kaytor EN, Shih HM. Regulation of the expression of lipogenic enzyme genes by carbohydrate. Annu Rev Nutr. 1997;17:405–433.
3. Vaulont S, Vasseur-Cognet M, Kahn A. Glucose regulation of gene transcription. J Biol Chem. 2000; 275:31555–31558.
4. Pilkis SJ, Claus TH, Kurland IJ, Lange AJ. 6-Phosphofructo-2-kinase/fructose-2,6-bisphosphatase: a metabolic signaling enzyme. Annu Rev Biochem. 1995;64:799–835.
5. O'Brien RM, Granner DK. Regulation of gene expression by insulin. Physiol Rev. 1996;76: 1109–1161.
6. Iynedjian PB. Mammalian glucokinase and its gene. Biochem J. 1993;293(part 1):1–13.
7. Jetton TL, Liang Y, Pettepher CC, et al. Analysis of upstream glucokinase promoter activity in transgenic

mice and identification of glucokinase in rare neuroendocrine cells in the brain and gut. J Biol Chem. 1994;269:3641–3654.
8. Girard J, Ferre P, Foufelle F. Mechanisms by which carbohydrates regulate expression of genes for glycolytic and lipogenic enzymes. Annu Rev Nutr. 1997; 17:325–352.
9. Yen PM. Physiological and molecular basis of thyroid hormone action. Physiol Rev. 2001;81: 1097–1142.
10. Jump DB. Dietary polyunsaturated fatty acids and regulation of gene transcription. Curr Opin Lipidol. 2002;13:155–164.
11. Sampath H, Ntambi JM. Polyunsaturated fatty acid regulation of gene expression. Nutr Rev. 2004;62: 333–339.
12. Semenkovich CF. Regulation of fatty acid synthase (FAS). Prog Lipid Res. 1997;36:43–53.
13. Salati LM, Szeszel-Fedorowicz W, Tao H, et al. Nutritional regulation of mRNA processing. J Nutr. 2004;134:2437S–2443S.
14. Tupler R, Perini G, Green MR. Expressing the human genome. Nature. 2001;409:832–833.
15. Bergot MO, Diaz-Guerra MJ, Puzenat N, Raymondjean M, Kahn A. Cis-regulation of the L-type pyruvate kinase gene promoter by glucose, insulin and cyclic AMP. Nucleic Acids Res. 1992;20: 1871–1877.
16. Shih HM, Liu Z, Towle HC. Two CACGTG motifs with proper spacing dictate the carbohydrate regulation of hepatic gene transcription. J Biol Chem. 1995;270:21991–21997.
17. O'Callaghan BL, Koo SH, Wu Y, Freake HC, Towle HC. Glucose regulation of the acetyl-CoA carboxylase promoter PI in rat hepatocytes. J Biol Chem. 2001;276:16033–16039.
18. Rufo C, Gasperikova D, Clarke SD, Teran-Garcia M, Nakamura MT. Identification of a novel enhancer sequence in the distal promoter of the rat fatty acid synthase gene. Biochem Biophys Res Commun. 1999;261:400–405.
19. Cunningham BA, Moncur JT, Huntington JT, Kinlaw WB. "Spot 14" protein: a metabolic integrator in normal and neoplastic cells. Thyroid. 1998;8: 815–825.
20. Atchley WR, Fitch WM. A natural classification of the basic helix-loop-helix class of transcription factors. Proc Natl Acad Sci U S A. 1997;94:5172–5176.
21. Uyeda K, Yamashita H, Kawaguchi T. Carbohydrate responsive element-binding protein (ChREBP): a key regulator of glucose metabolism and fat storage. Biochem Pharmacol. 2002;63:2075–2080.
22. Kawaguchi T, Takenoshita M, Kabashima T, Uyeda K. Glucose and cAMP regulate the L-type pyruvate kinase gene by phosphorylation/dephosphorylation of the carbohydrate response element binding protein. Proc Natl Acad Sci U S A. 2001;98: 13710–13715.
23. Cairo S, Merla G, Urbinati F, Ballabio A, Reymond A. WBSCR14, a gene mapping to the Williams-Beuren syndrome deleted region, is a new member of the Mlx transcription factor network. Hum Mol Genet. 2001;10:617–627.
24. Stoeckman AK, Ma L, Towle HC. Mlx is the functional heteromeric partner of the carbohydrate response element-binding protein in glucose regulation of lipogenic enzyme genes. J Biol Chem. 2004;279: 15662–15669.
25. Billin AN, Eilers AL, Queva C, Ayer DE. Mlx, a novel Max-like BHLHZip protein that interacts with the Max network of transcription factors. J Biol Chem. 1999;274:36344–36350.
26. Iizuka K, Bruick RK, Liang G, Horton JD, Uyeda K. Deficiency of carbohydrate response element-binding protein (ChREBP) reduces lipogenesis as well as glycolysis. Proc Natl Acad Sci U S A. 2004; 101:7281–7286.
27. Dentin R, Pegorier JP, Benhamed F, et al. Hepatic glucokinase is required for the synergistic action of ChREBP and SREBP-1c on glycolytic and lipogenic gene expression. J Biol Chem. 2004;279: 20314–20326.
28. Ma L, Tsatsos NG, Towle HC. Direct role of ChREBP/Mlx in regulating hepatic glucose-responsive genes. J Biol Chem. 2005;280:12019–12027.
29. Kabashima T, Kawaguchi T, Wadzinski BE, Uyeda K. Xylulose 5-phosphate mediates glucose-induced lipogenesis by xylulose 5-phosphate-activated protein phosphatase in rat liver. Proc Natl Acad Sci U S A. 2003;100:5107–5112.
30. Brown MS, Goldstein JL The SREBP pathway: regulation of cholesterol metabolism by proteolysis of a membrane-bound transcription factor. Cell. 1997; 89:331–340.
31. Osborne TF. Sterol regulatory element-binding proteins (SREBPs): key regulators of nutritional homeostasis and insulin action. J Biol Chem. 2000;275: 32379–32382.
32. Brown MS, Goldstein JL. A proteolytic pathway that controls the cholesterol content of membranes, cells, and blood. Proc Natl Acad Sci U S A. 1999;96: 11041–11048.
33. Magana MM, Osborne TF. Two tandem binding sites for sterol regulatory element binding proteins are required for sterol regulation of fatty-acid synthase promoter. J Biol Chem. 1996;271:32689–32694.
34. Shimano H, Horton JD, Hammer RE, Shimomura I, Brown MS, Goldstein JL. Overproduction of cholesterol and fatty acids causes massive liver enlargement in transgenic mice expressing truncated SREBP-1a. J Clin Invest. 1996;98:1575–1584.
35. Shimano H, Yahagi N, Amemiya-Kudo M, et al. Sterol regulatory element-binding protein-1 as a key transcription factor for nutritional induction of

lipogenic enzyme genes. J Biol Chem. 1999;274: 35832–35839.
36. Foretz M, Guichard C, Ferre P, Foufelle F. Sterol regulatory element binding protein-1c is a major mediator of insulin action on the hepatic expression of glucokinase and lipogenesis-related genes. Proc Natl Acad Sci U S A. 1999;96:12737–12742.
37. Horton JD, Bashmakov Y, Shimomura I, Shimano H. Regulation of sterol regulatory element binding proteins in livers of fasted and refed mice. Proc Natl Acad Sci U S A. 1998;95:5987–5992.
38. Ribaux PG, Iynedjian PB. Analysis of the role of protein kinase B (cAKT) in insulin-dependent induction of glucokinase and sterol regulatory element-binding protein 1 (SREBP1) mRNAs in hepatocytes. Biochem J. 2003;376:697–705.
39. Kim KH, Song MJ, Yoo EJ, Choe SS, Park SD, Kim JB. Regulatory role of glycogen synthase kinase 3 for transcriptional activity of ADD1/SREBP1c. J Biol Chem. 2004;279:51999–52006.
40. Clarke SD. Polyunsaturated fatty acid regulation of gene transcription: a molecular mechanism to improve the metabolic syndrome. J Nutr. 2001;131: 1129–1132.
41. Duplus E, Glorian M, Forest C. Fatty acid regulation of gene transcription. J Biol Chem. 2000;275: 30749–30752.
42. Desvergne B, Wahli W. Peroxisome proliferator-activated receptors: nuclear control of metabolism. Endocr Rev. 1999;20:649–688.
43. Kliewer SA, Lehmann JM, Milburn MV, Willson TM. The PPARs and PXRs: nuclear xenobiotic receptors that define novel hormone signaling pathways. Recent Prog Horm Res. 1999;54:345–368.
44. Sladek R, Giguere V. Orphan nuclear receptors: an emerging family of metabolic regulators. Adv Pharmacol. 2000;47:23–87.
45. Gottlicher M, Widmark E, Li Q, Gustafsson JA. Fatty acids activate a chimera of the clofibric acid-activated receptor and the glucocorticoid receptor. Proc Natl Acad Sci U S A. 1992;89:4653–4657.
46. Xu HE, Lambert MH, Montana VG, et al. Molecular recognition of fatty acids by peroxisome proliferator-activated receptors. Mol Cell. 1999;3:397–403.
47. Aoyama T, Peters JM, Iritani N, et al. Altered constitutive expression of fatty acid-metabolizing enzymes in mice lacking the peroxisome proliferator-activated receptor alpha (PPARα). J Biol Chem. 1998;273: 5678–5684.
48. Spiegelman BM. PPARγ: adipogenic regulator and thiazolidinedione receptor. Diabetes. 1998;47:507–514.
49. Rangwala SM, Lazar MA. Peroxisome proliferator-activated receptor gamma in diabetes and metabolism. Trends Pharmacol Sci. 2004;25:331–336.
50. Repa JJ, Mangelsdorf DJ. Nuclear receptor regulation of cholesterol and bile acid metabolism. Curr Opin Biotechnol. 1999;10:557–563.
51. Janowski BA, Willy PJ, Devi TR, Falck JR, Mangelsdorf DJ. An oxysterol signalling pathway mediated by the nuclear receptor LXRα. Nature. 1996; 383:728–731.
52. Lehmann JM, Kliewer SA, Moore LB, et al. Activation of the nuclear receptor LXR by oxysterols defines a new hormone response pathway. J Biol Chem. 1997;272:3137–3140.
53. Peet DJ, Turley SD, Ma W, et al. Cholesterol and bile acid metabolism are impaired in mice lacking the nuclear oxysterol receptor LXRα. Cell 1998;93: 693–704
54. Tontonoz P, Mangelsdorf DJ. Liver X receptor signaling pathways in cardiovascular disease. Mol Endocrinol. 2003;17:985–993.
55. Repa JJ, Liang G, Ou J, et al. Regulation of mouse sterol regulatory element-binding protein-1c gene (SREBP-1c) by oxysterol receptors, LXRα and LXRβ. Genes Dev. 2000;14:2819–2830.
56. Mohan R, Heyman RA. Orphan nuclear receptor modulators. Curr Top Med Chem. 2003;3: 1637–1647.
57. Hay N, Sonenberg N. Upstream and downstream of mTOR. Genes Dev. 2004;18:1926–1945.
58. Fingar DC, Blenis J. Target of rapamycin (TOR): an integrator of nutrient and growth factor signals and coordinator of cell growth and cell cycle progression. Oncogene. 2004;23:3151–3171.
59. Proud CG. mTOR-mediated regulation of translation factors by amino acids. Biochem Biophys Res Commun. 2004;313:429–436.
60. Kimball SR, Jefferson LS. Regulation of global and specific mRNA translation by oral administration of branched-chain amino acids. Biochem Biophys Res Commun. 2004;313:423–427.
61. Kim DH, Sarbassov DD, Ali SM, et al. mTOR interacts with raptor to form a nutrient-sensitive complex that signals to the cell growth machinery. Cell. 2002;110:163–175.
62. Hara K, Maruki Y, Long X, et al. Raptor, a binding partner of target of rapamycin (TOR), mediates TOR action. Cell. 2002;110:177–189.
63. Kim DH, Sarbassov DD, Ali SM, et al. GβL, a positive regulator of the rapamycin-sensitive pathway required for the nutrient-sensitive interaction between raptor and mTOR. Mol Cell. 2003;11:895–904.

# 8

# Dietary Fiber

Daniel D. Gallaher

## Introduction and Definition of Dietary Fiber

Dietary fiber is the term applied to a heterogeneous mixture of plant materials that have in common a resistance to hydrolysis by the enzymes of the mammalian digestive system. It includes both plant cell wall material, such as cellulose, hemicelluloses, pectin, and lignin, and intracellular polysaccharides, such as gums and mucilages. However, the term "dietary fiber" has sometimes been applied more broadly to include other components of foods that are non-digestible, primarily carbohydrate, and typically from plant sources. Examples include waxes, cutins, and indigestible cell wall proteins that are associated with the plant cell wall. Other non-cell wall compounds include resistant starch (starch that is resistant to digestion by mammalian enzymes), Maillard reaction products, oligosaccharides, and animal-derived materials that resist digestion (e.g., aminopolysaccharides such as chitosan). Although these are minor components of most foods, they may have physiological activities that are difficult to separate from those traditionally attributed to dietary fiber, thus making it difficult separate the responses due to fiber from those due to other materials found in fiber-rich foods. Although many studies have been conducted on purified fibers to isolate the effect of dietary fiber from fiber-rich foods, this approach can be problematic, as purification may alter the physical form and properties of the fiber and therefore its physiological effect. For example, fermentation of plant cell wall material differs from that of the same fibers in purified form.[1] In recognition of these issues and others, a Panel on the Definition of Dietary Fiber was convened by the Food and Nutrition Board of the US Institute of Medicine to propose a new definition for dietary fiber. The recommendations that were developed are as follows[2]:

- Dietary fiber consists of non-digestible carbohydrates and lignin that are intrinsic and intact in plants.
- Functional fiber consists of isolated, non-digestible carbohydrates that have beneficial physiological effects in humans.
- Total fiber is the sum of dietary fiber and functional fiber.

To maintain consistency with the recommendations, these definitions will be employed in the following discussion where appropriate.

The major components of dietary fiber include cellulose, mixed linkage β-glucans, hemicelluloses, pectins, and gums. These are characterized by their sugar residues and the linkages among them. Cellulose and mixed-linkage β-glucans are glucose polymers with β 1→4 linkages; in the mixed linkage β-glucans, these linkages are interspersed with β 1→3 bonds. Cellulose is found in all plant cell walls, whereas mixed-linkage β-glucans exist in significant concentration in only a few cereals, particularly oats and barley. The hemicelluloses are a diverse group of polysaccharides with varying degrees of branching. The major backbone sugar for pectins is galacturonic acid, and side chains typically include galactose and arabinose. The degree of methoxylation on the uronic acid residues varies. The structural features of gums vary according to the source. Typically, these are a minor polysaccharide constituent in most foods. However, certain gums are used frequently in research studies (e.g., guar gum and locust bean gum, which are galactomannans). The structures of amylose and several types of non-digestible carbohydrates are shown in Figure 1. Most non-digestible carbohydrates are polysaccharides of ten units or more. However, oligosaccharides that have beta linkages, such as oligofructose, are also included in the definition of dietary fiber because they are naturally present in certain foods and are likewise non-digestible carbohydrates. Lignin is a non-carbohydrate component that is included in the definition of dietary fiber. It has a highly complex, three-dimensional structure and contains phenylpropane units. Lignin is usually not an important component of human foods,

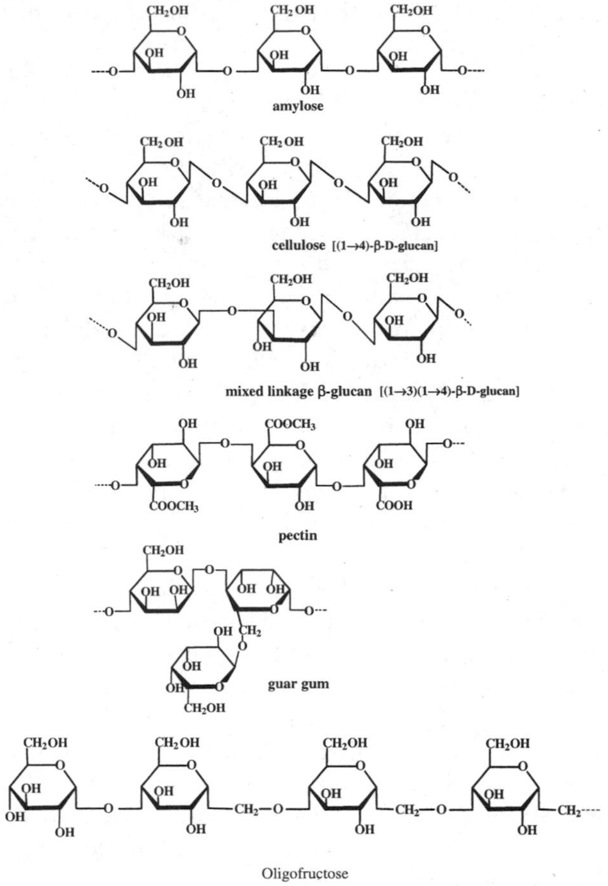

Figure 1. Structure of starch and several types of dietary fiber.

because it is generally associated with tough or woody tissue. The one exception is foods that contain intact seeds consumed with the food.

Dietary fiber has often been classified in the past as soluble or insoluble. The reference to solubility is not quite correct, as it simply indicates those fibers that are dispersible in water. Originally it was believed that this categorization might provide a simple way to predict physiological function, but this has not been the case. For example, it was originally considered that insoluble fiber produced fecal bulking and that soluble fiber lowered cholesterol concentrations. However, certain sources of soluble fiber can increase stool weight as effectively as insoluble fibers. Likewise, not all soluble fibers lower cholesterol. It has been recommend that the classification of dietary fiber as soluble or insoluble fiber be discontinued, as it does not predict physiologic function.[2] Given the diversity in chemical and physical properties among fiber sources, it is unlikely that a single property of fiber will predict the range of physiological effects of a particular fiber.

# Methods of Analysis

Given the heterogeneous nature of dietary fiber, it is not surprising that the development of methods to measure dietary fiber has been challenging and has led to several different approaches. Current methods of analysis fall into one of two categories: gravimetric and component (or chemical) analysis. Gravimetric methods are simpler and faster, and therefore more suitable for routine analysis. The most commonly used method of dietary fiber analysis is the gravimetric method, which results in what is commonly referred to as Total Dietary Fiber (TDF).[3] This and similar gravimetric procedures that measure total fiber can be modified to give estimates of soluble and insoluble fiber.[4] A modification has been developed that allows for the measurement of fructose-containing compounds of less than 10 units.[5] Component analysis involves hydrolyzing the fiber residue to monomeric sugars,[6] which are then measured by high-performance liquid chromatography, colorimetrically, or, more commonly, by gas chromatography after derivitization. Summation of the monomeric sugars then yields a value for total dietary fiber. When desired, lignin can be estimated separately and added to the sum of the individual sugars. A number of methods of analysis are summarized in Table 1.

Some foods, particularly thermally processed foods, contain starch that escapes digestion within the small intestine. This so-called resistant starch is formed during

**Table 1.** Methods of Analysis for Dietary Fiber

| Method | Components measured | Comments |
|---|---|---|
| Neutral detergent fiber | Cellulose, insoluble hemicelluloses, lignins | Soluble fibers are lost |
| Acid detergent fiber | Cellulose and lignin | Soluble fibers are lost |
| Gravimetric procedures | Non-starch polysaccharides, lignin, some retrograded starch, Maillard reaction products | AOAC-approved method (as Total Dietary Fiber); can be modified to give soluble and insoluble fiber |
| Component analysis procedures | Non-starch polysaccharides | Can be modified to give cellulose and non-cellulose polysaccharides separately |
| Inulin and oligofructose | Fructans | Allows for determination of fructose polymers, including those with less than 10 units |

retrogradation of amylose, and consequently is formed in large amounts in high-amylose foods such as potatoes.[7] Resistant starch is not removed in enzymatic-gravimetric procedures such as the gravimetric method, and consequently is measured as dietary fiber in these procedures.

# Physical Properties of Dietary Fiber

The monomeric sugar content of a fiber provides little insight into its physiological effects. For example, as shown in Figure 1, amylose, cellulose, and beta-glucans are all glucose polymers; however, the nature of the linkages in the polymers result in drastically different physical properties and hence different physiological responses when these polymers are consumed in the diet. Understanding the physiological actions of different types of dietary fiber has come about primarily from the knowledge of their physical, not chemical, properties. These properties include water-holding capacity, viscosity, susceptibility to fermentation, inhibition of digestive enzymes, bile acid-binding capacity, and cation exchange capacity. Although each of these physical properties has been suggested to be responsible for one or more of the physiological actions of dietary fiber, it is now clear that two of them, viscosity and susceptibility to fermentation, are the most important in understanding these actions. Table 2 shows these properties for a number of different types of dietary fiber.

### *Viscosity*

Certain types of dietary fiber can form highly viscous solutions. These include pectins, various gums, mixed linkage beta-glucans, and algal polysaccharides such as agar and carrageenan. The viscosity achieved within the small intestine is influenced by the concentration of fiber in the meal, the hydration rate of the fiber, and the rate of stomach emptying. For example, a slow rate of hydration appears to explain why some guar gum preparations are ineffective in improving blood glucose control.[8] A slower rate of stomach emptying would likely lead to a lower concentration of fiber within the intestinal contents, thus decreasing viscosity.

### *Susceptibility to Fermentation*

Dietary fibers vary in the degree to which they are fermented by large intestinal microflora. The degree and rate of fermentation will be influenced by the type of fiber, the physical form or context (e.g., within a food vs. isolated; particle size), and the microflora present in the host. In general, soluble fibers are fermented to a greater extent than insoluble fibers, but there are notable exceptions to this. For example, psyllium, xanthan gum, and synthetically modified celluloses, all of which are classified as soluble, are highly resistant to fermentation. Isolated fibers are fermented more readily than those found within a food. Fiber sources fed as a large particle size are less completely fermented than the same sources fed in a small particle size.[9] Cellulose is quite resistant to fermentation, whereas fibers such as pectins and guar gum are completely fermented. Fermentation of dietary fiber by the colonic microflora produces short-chain fatty acids (SCFA), primarily acetate, propionate, and butyrate and gases ($CO_2$, $H_2$, and, in some individuals, $CH_4$). The relative order of concentration of the SCFA in fecal material is generally acetate $>$ propionate $\geq$ butyrate. The effect of purified fiber or fiber-rich sources on fecal SCFA concentrations in humans has been inconsistent, with some studies showing no effect[10] and others an increase.[11] However, SCFA are avidly taken up by the large intestine, such that concentrations in the large intestinal lumen progressively decreases from the cecum to the sigmoid colon/rectum.[12] Thus, fecal concentration may not accurately reflect actual production of SCFA.

SCFA can be utilized by the colonic epithelial cells as an energy source. These cells utilize most of the butyrate that is produced in the large bowel, but only some of the propionate and acetate. Propionate is cleared by the liver so that only acetate appears in peripheral tissue in significant quantities. Due to the production of SCFA, fiber is a source of energy in the diet. Estimates are that it contributes 1.5 to 2.5 kcal/g of fiber.[13]

**Table 2.** Viscosity and Susceptibility to Fermentation of Selected Dietary Fibers

| | | Viscosity | |
|---|---|---|---|
| | | **High** | **Low** |
| Fermentability | High | • Guar gum<br>• β-glucans<br>• Glucomannan<br>• Pectins | • Gum acacia<br>• Oligofructose<br>• Inulin |
| | Low or None | • Modified celluloses (e.g., methylcellulose)<br>• Psyllium | • Cellulose<br>• Hemicelluloses |

In animal models, fermentable fibers cause significant enlargement of the cecum, with little or no effect on the colon, whereas non-fermentable fibers appear to have the opposite effect.[14] This is likely due to the higher concentration of SCFA achieved in the cecum with fermentable fibers and the greater colonic effort to propel non-fermentable fibers through the colon.

Most efforts examining the physiological effects of fermentation have focused on the generation of SCFA. In experimental animal models, the presence of SCFA has been shown to promote wound healing in the intestine, leading to the hypothesis that these compounds are important for maintaining the health of the gastrointestinal mucosa.[15] There is also a large body of evidence demonstrating that butyrate decreases the growth of human colon cancer cell lines. However, animal studies have not indicated a reduction in colon cancer risk using various methods of introduction of butyrate.[16] Certainly, the production of SCFAs in the large intestine is an important consequence of consuming fermentable fiber sources; however, the metabolic consequences of their production remain incompletely understood.

# Physiological Response to Sources of Dietary Fiber

A large number of physiological responses to consuming fiber, either as dietary fiber or functional fiber, have been studied. To date, only three of these, lowering of plasma cholesterol levels, modification of the glycemic response, and improving large bowel function, are widely accepted responses to fiber consumption. These physiological responses are most easily understood in the context of the physical properties of dietary fiber and the effects on gastrointestinal function. Numerous studies have also examined the effect of fiber on nutrient availability. However, in general, physiologically important reductions in nutrient absorption by fiber have not been established.

## *Plasma Cholesterol Lowering*

Many studies in both humans and animal models have shown that certain types of dietary fiber lower plasma cholesterol concentrations. In humans, these reductions occur in the LDL fraction, with little or no change in HDL cholesterol. These studies have been done with foods rich in dietary fiber (dietary fiber), fractions from food that are fiber-enriched (i.e., brans), and isolated polysaccharides (functional fiber). Many of these studies have been conducted with a relatively high intake of the fiber source. However, a meta-analysis of human studies examining cholesterol lowering by fiber indicated that consumption of 2 to 10 g of fiber is associated with significant plasma cholesterol-lowering.[17] These studies indicate that viscosity is a property consistently associated with cholesterol lowering. Most, if not all, isolated fibers that are viscous will lower plasma cholesterol in humans and plasma and liver cholesterol in animals. These include pectins, psyllium, and various gums such as guar gum, locust bean gum, and modified celluloses such as hydroxypropyl methylcellulose. In contrast, isolated fibers or fiber sources that are not viscous, such as cellulose, lignin, corn bran, and wheat bran, have rarely been found to alter plasma cholesterol. In addition, reducing the viscosity of a viscous fiber also reduces its cholesterol-lowering ability.[18] Finally, the consumption of fiber-rich sources containing viscous polysaccharides, such as oat bran and barley (sources of mixed linkage beta-glucans), and legumes usually results in a lowering of plasma cholesterol.

The role of fermentation of dietary fiber in cholesterol lowering has been controversial. The first report linking fermentation with cholesterol lowering found that the SCFA propionate, a product of large intestinal fermentation, reduced liver cholesterol in cholesterol-fed rats[19] and reduced cholesterol synthesis in cultured hepatocytes.[20] Although others reported no inhibition of cholesterol synthesis in hepatocytes by propionate,[21] animal feeding studies of a mixture of SCFAs found reduced plasma cholesterol and a lower rate of liver cholesterol synthesis.[22] However, animal feeding studies of fermentable fibers find increased 3-hydroxy-3-methylglutaryl coenzyme A reductase activity, the rate-limiting enzyme for cholesterol synthesis.[23] Finally, reduced liver cholesterol was found in germ-free rats fed viscous but fermentable fibers,[24] indicating that cholesterol lowering occurs in the absence of fermentation. At this point, it is clear that fermentation of a fiber is not a necessary condition for cholesterol lowering. What role it plays in cholesterol lowering, if any, remains uncertain.

How dietary fibers lower cholesterol remains a subject of investigation. Over the years, a number of hypotheses have been put forth, which are summarized in Table 3. These hypotheses postulate either increased steroid excretion as bile acids or cholesterol, decreased cholesterol synthesis, or an increased rate of removal of cholesterol from the plasma. Although several properties of fiber may be involved with several of these hypotheses, only viscosity is common to them all.

Various cholesterol-lowering fibers increase the excretion of bile acids and/or neutral sterols (cholesterol and its bacterial metabolites), supporting the role of enhanced steroid excretion. Oat bran and psyllium are examples of dietary fiber sources demonstrated to increase bile acid excretion.[25,26] A fiber-induced increase in bile acid excretion is believed to lower cholesterol by increasing bile acid synthesis, resulting in an increased conversion of cholesterol to bile acids. If cholesterol synthesis rates do not increase sufficiently to compensate for the increased conversion of cholesterol to bile acids or the loss of cholesterol itself, then cholesterol concentrations will decrease. However, not all fibers that lower cholesterol increase bile acid excretion.[27] Hydroxypropyl methylcellulose, a synthetically modified cellulose that is highly viscous decreases cholesterol absorption, and does so proportionally to its viscosity.[28]

**Table 3.** Possible Mechanisms of Cholesterol Lowering by Dietary Fiber

| Effect | Possible Mechanism(s) | Possible Characteristic(s) |
|---|---|---|
| Increased bile acid excretion | Reduced reabsorption in the small intestine; decreased solubility in the colon | Bile acid binding; fermentation; viscosity |
| Decreased cholesterol absorption | Decreased micellar diffusion; delayed triacylglycerol digestion | Viscosity |
| Reduced hepatic cholesterol synthesis | Inhibition of hydroxy-methylglutaryl-coenzyme A reductase by propionate or hydrophobic bile acids; reduced insulin stimulation of cholesterol synthesis | Fermentation; viscosity |

Viscous fibers slow lipid digestion and absorption, which can prolong the presence of intestinal triacylglyceride-rich lipoproteins in plasma. Because cholesterol transferred to intestinal triacylglyceride-rich lipoproteins is cleared by the liver, reverse cholesterol transport may be enhanced during the postprandial period.[29]

Overall, the evidence indicates that more than one mechanism contributes to the cholesterol-lowering effects of dietary fiber, but that viscosity is a key property responsible for the effect.

## *Modification of the Glycemic Response*

Consumption of viscous fibers will reduce the postprandial glycemic and insulinemic responses. Figure 2 illustrates this phenomenon for a hypothetical viscous fiber. Fibers such as wheat bran or cellulose, which are insoluble and therefore have no viscosity, produce either a modest or undetectable effect on the postprandial blood glucose or insulin curves. This modified glycemic response occurs when viscous fiber is either co-administered with a glucose load or as part of a meal in both normal and diabetic individuals. Long-term blood glucose control, as measured by glycated hemoglobin, is also improved with feeding guar, a highly viscous fiber.[30] A delayed rate of stomach emptying, delayed starch digestion within, or a slowing of glucose absorption from the small intestine could explain this effect. Studies examining the effect of viscous fibers on the rate of glucose absorption within the small intestine have been contradictory, with evidence both for[31] and against[32] a slowing of absorption. Likewise, studies examining the effect of viscous fibers on the rate of gastric emptying have been inconsistent, with both no effect[33] and a slowing reported.[32] Consequently, the mechanism by which viscous fibers improve the glycemic response to a meal remains to be established.

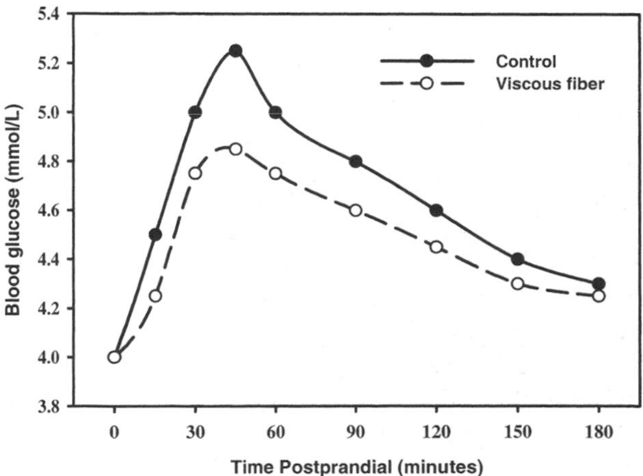


Figure 2. Typical effect of viscous fiber on postprandial blood glucose response.

## *Improving Large Bowel Function*

Fiber in the diet can influence large bowel function by reducing transit time, increasing stool weight and frequency, diluting large intestinal contents, and providing fermentable substrate for the colonic microflora. These factors are influenced by the source and amount of fiber in the diet. Transit time decreases with wheat bran supplementation and the addition of fruits and vegetables to the diet. However, results with other fiber sources have not consistently shown this effect.

Stool weight is increased by fiber sources in a dose-related manner.[34] Generally, fiber sources that are resistant to fermentation, such as wheat bran, produce the greatest increase in stool weight. More fermentable fiber sources, such as fruits and vegetables, produce a moderate increase in fecal output, whereas legumes and pectin increase stool weight only slightly. The increase in stool weight is mainly due to an increase in the microbial cell mass or unfermented fiber. Which mechanism predominates depends on the degree of fermentation of the fiber. For example, wheat bran is more effective in increasing the amount of undigested residue, whereas the fiber in fruits and vegetables or oat bran can be fermented extensively and thereby causes an increase in stool weight by increasing the microbial cell mass in the feces.

## *Lowering Nutrient Availability*

In vitro, various fiber sources can inhibit the activity of pancreatic enzymes that digest carbohydrates, lipids, and proteins.[35] How fiber inhibits digestive enzyme activity is not clear, but in some non-purified fiber sources, specific enzyme inhibitors exist.[36] How important this inhibition is remains unclear, as an excess of digestive enzymes is secreted in response to a meal. In addition to direct inhibition of digestive enzyme activity, the presence of plant cell walls in a food provides a physical barrier to digestion,[37] slowing the penetration of digestive enzymes into plant foods. Consequently, grinding of the fiber source to a fine particle size may disrupt the cell wall structure sufficiently to allow a more rapid digestion.

The effect of dietary fiber on vitamin absorption has been studied for most vitamins, and it appears that fiber generally has little if any effect on vitamin absorption.[38] The effect of fiber on mineral absorption is less clear. Natural sources of fiber, such as cereals and fruits, generally depress absorption of minerals such as calcium, iron, zinc, and copper.[39] However, at least part of this effect is likely due to the presence of phytic acid or other chelators in these foods, which are known to interfere with mineral absorption.[40] There is convincing evidence indicating that no dietary fiber has a detrimental effect on mineral balance or absorption.[41] Indeed, inulin-type fructans appear to enhance intestinal magnesium[42] and possibly calcium absorption.[43]

## Dietary Fiber and the Prevention of Disease

Numerous epidemiological studies have examined whether dietary fiber intake is associated with a lower incidence of certain chronic disorders such as cardiovascular disease and large bowel cancer. These studies have been inconsistent in demonstrating such a relationship. However, in such studies it is impossible to distinguish between the effects of dietary fiber per se and fiber-rich foods, which contain a rich assortment of phytochemicals that may also affect disease risk. Such foods may also change the overall macronutrient composition, since foods high in fiber are typically low in fat, saturated fatty acids, and cholesterol. Perhaps as an illustration of this, in a recent pooled analysis of 13 prospective cohort studies, a statistically significant inverse correlation was found between dietary fiber and colorectal cancer. However, once the results were corrected for other colon cancer risk factors, the correlation lost statistically significance, suggesting that dietary fiber was not protective against colon cancer.[44] In contrast, data analysis from 10 prospective cohort studies did yield a statistically significant inverse relationship between dietary fiber intake and risk of coronary heart disease.[45]

Unfortunately, the clinical trials needed to confirm the epidemiological associations (or lack of them) are few, due to the expense and difficulty of conducting such trials. There are no clinical studies that directly examine the effect of dietary fiber supplementation on disease end points such as the incidence of diabetic complications, development of atherosclerosis, or cancer. The studies that most directly examine the effect of dietary fiber on cancer risk are those using colonic polyp or adenoma recurrence as an end point. Colonic polyps and adenomas are considered precursors to the development of tumors, and therefore their recurrence after removal is considered a marker of risk of tumor development. MacLennan et al.[46] examined the effect of either a low fat diet, high fiber diet, or the combination of the two on recurrence of adenomatous colonic polyps. Although neither dietary fat reduction nor increased dietary fiber alone significantly reduced polyp recurrence, the combination of the two resulted in a statistically significant reduction in recurrence. However, in 2000, two randomized trials[47,48] examined the effect of diets high in fiber on recurrence of colorectal adenomas, and found no significant reduction in recurrence with diets high in fiber after 4 years. In one study,[47] fiber intake was elevated by providing foods supplemented with wheat bran. However, those in the high-fiber groups consumed less of the cereal supplement, which may complicate interpretation. The mean total intake of fiber was 18.1 g/d in the low-fiber group and 27.5 g/d in the supplemented group. The second study[48] provided subjects with a diet low in fat and high in fruits and vegetables. Although there was no difference in the recurrence of polyps, the authors suggest that although fiber may not be protective in the prevention of recurrence, but may be important at other stages in the development of colorectal neoplasia. Thus, evidence from human trials for a protective effect of fiber on colon cancer risk is lacking.

Presently, there is no compelling evidence from trials with disease end points that increased dietary fiber consumption reduces the incidence of chronic disease in humans. Nonetheless, results from epidemiological studies, studies of the physiological effects relevant to disease conditions (e.g., cholesterol lowering), and animal studies do suggest an important role of dietary fiber in disease prevention. However, the associations between disease risk and dietary factors are multifactorial, and our present knowledge indicates that fiber cannot be isolated as a single factor but must be evaluated in the context of the total dietary pattern.

## Dietary Fiber Intake

Intake data from the Continuing Survey of Food Intakes by Individuals (CSFII) have estimated dietary fiber consumption in the United States from 16.5 to 17.9 g/d for men and 12.1 to 13.8 g/d for women. These values do not include intake of inulin or oligofructose, as the dietary fiber values in the food databases used to calculate these values for fiber consumption were generated before methods were established for their measurement. It is estimated that the American diet supplies an average of

2.6 g/d of inulin and 2.5 g/d of oligofructose, primarily from wheat and onions.[49]

It is widely viewed that the intake of dietary fiber is below what is desirable for optimal health. However, determining what the dietary intake should be is problematic, as it is not obvious how to determine the optimal intake. Suggestions have been made that stool weight and transit time, as indicators of large bowel function, may be useful in assessing the adequacy of fiber intake.[50] Cummings et al.[51] demonstrated that stool weight increases in a dose-response relationship for dietary fiber intake up to 32 g/d. They reported that a dietary fiber intake of 18 g/d was associated with a stool weight of 150 g/d, which was associated with a lower risk of colon cancer. This is similar to the estimate of 10 g/1000 kcal of dietary fiber recommended by the Life Sciences Research Office Expert Panel, which also used stool weight as a physiological predictor of adequacy of fiber intake.[52] More recently, an adequate intake (AI) for fiber has been set based on epidemiological associations between dietary fiber intake and risk of coronary heart disease.[53] The AI of 14 g/1000 kcal is for total fiber and translates to a recommended AI of 38 g/d for men and 25 g/d for women 19 to 50 years of age.

For consumers, it is important that recommendations on fiber intake be expressed in terms of foods that provide dietary fiber, because some benefits associated with fiber are likely due to components in foods other than the fiber. Food selection should be guided to meet the recommendations for the consumption of fruits, grains, vegetables, and beans suggested in the Food Guide Pyramid and the Dietary Guidelines. Meeting these recommendations and selecting items higher in fiber (e.g., fruit vs. fruit juice, whole-grain vs. milled grains) encourages the use of fiber-containing foods in the diet.[54]

## Future Directions

The effects of dietary fiber on cholesterol metabolism and on the postprandial glucose response have been thoroughly examined, and the phenomena of cholesterol lowering and attenuated glucose response are well established. What remains uncertain, in spite of considerable study, is the mechanism(s) behind the phenomena. Determining the relative contributions of increased cholesterol and/or bile acid excretion and altered cholesterol synthesis to the reduction in plasma cholesterol by dietary fiber has been a challenging and an incompletely realized objective. Likewise, the role of delayed stomach emptying and slowed intestinal absorption of glucose in understanding the effect of dietary fiber on the postprandial glucose response remains to be clarified.

Understanding the influence of dietary fiber on the microbial populations of the large intestine is an area worth revisiting. Studies done years ago suggested that dietary fiber had at best minor influences on the microbial populations. However, molecular biology techniques now exist that allow determination of changes in the colonic microbiota and the effect of other dietary fiber types with far greater sensitivity than in the past. Using such techniques, it is now clear that fructans such as inulin act as prebiotics, stimulating the growth of beneficial bacteria such as bifidobacteria in the large intestine. These techniques allow us to answer the question of whether all fermentable dietary fibers act as prebiotics or only specific types.

There is highly suggestive evidence from animal studies that certain dietary fiber types, such as β-glucans and fructans, are immunostimulatory. Understanding whether this results in a physiologically important immune response, what part of the molecule is responsible for the effect, and to what degree these effects occur in humans with fiber feeding are likely to be important avenues for further research.

Finally, given the growing prevalence of obesity in populations worldwide, as well as the suggestion by some studies of increased satiety with dietary fiber consumption, the role of dietary fiber in weight management, if any, deserves continued investigation.

## References

1. Bourquin LD, Titgemeyer EC, Garleb KA, et al. Short-chain fatty acid production and fiber degradation by human colonic bacteria: effects of substrate and cell wall fractionation procedures. J Nutr. 1992; 122:1508–1520.
2. Food and Nutrition Board, Institute of Medicine, Panel on the Definition of Dietary Fiber, Standing Committee on the Scientific Evaluation of Dietary Reference Intakes. Dietary Reference Intakes: Dietary Reference Intakes: Proposed Definition of Dietary Fiber. Washington, DC: National Academies Press; 2001. Available online at: http://darwin.nap.edu/books/0309075645/html. Accessed February 22, 2006.
3. Prosky L, Asp NG, Furda I, et al. Determination of total dietary fiber in foods and food products: collaborative study. J Assoc Off Anal Chem. 1985;68: 677–679.
4. Marlett JA: Analysis of dietary fiber in human foods. In: Kritchevsky D, Anderson JW, Bonfield C, eds. *Dietary Fiber: Chemistry, Physiology, and Health Effects.* New York: Plenum Press; 1990; 31–48.
5. Prosky L, Hoebregs H. Methods to determine food inulin and oligofructose. J Nutr. 1999;129:1418S–1423S.
6. Englyst HN, Quigley ME, Hudson GJ. Determination of dietary fibre as non-starch polysaccharides with gas-liquid chromatographic, high-performance liquid chromatographic or spectrophotometric measurement of constituent sugars. Analyst. 1994;119: 1497–1509.
7. Berry CS. Resistant starch: formation and measure-

ment of starch that survives exhaustive digestion with amylolytic enzymes during the determination of dietary fibre. J Cereal Sci. 1986;4:301–314.

8. Ellis PR, Morris ER. Importance of the rate of hydration of pharmaceutical preparations of guar gum; a new in vitro monitoring method. Diabet Med. 1991;8:378–381.
9. Heller SN, Hackler LR, Rivers JM, et al. Dietary fiber: the effect of particle size of wheat bran on colonic function in young adult men. Am J Clin Nutr. 1980;33:1734–1744.
10. Noakes M, Clifton PM, Nestel PJ, et al. Effect of high-amylose starch and oat bran on metabolic variables and bowel function in subjects with hypertriglyceridemia. Am J Clin Nutr. 1996;64:944–951.
11. Takahashi H, Yang SI, Hayashi C, et al. Effect of partially hydrolyzed guar gum on fecal output in human volunteers. Nutr Res. 1993;13:649–657.
12. Macfarlane GT, Gibson GR, Cummings JH. Comparison of fermentation reactions in different regions of the human colon. J Appl Bacteriol. 1992;72: 57–64.
13. Smith T, Brown JC, Livesey G. Energy balance and thermogenesis in rats consuming nonstarch polysaccharides of various fermentabilities. Am J Clin Nutr. 1998;68:802–819.
14. Elsenhans B, Blume R, Caspary WF. Long-term feeding of unavailable carbohydrate gelling agents. Influence of dietary concentration and microbiological degradation on adaptive responses in the rat. Am J Clin Nutr. 1981;34:1837–1848.
15. Velazquez OC, Lederer HM, Rombeau JL. Butyrate and the colonocyte. Production, absorption, metabolism, and therapeutic implications. Adv Exp Med Biol. 1997;427:123–134.
16. Lupton JR. Microbial degradation products influence colon cancer risk: the butyrate controversy. J Nutr. 2004;134:479–482.
17. Brown L, Rosner B, Willett WW, et al. Cholesterol-lowering effects of dietary fiber: a meta-analysis. Am J Clin Nutr. 1999;69:30–42.
18. Gallaher DD, Hassel CA, Lee KJ. Relationships between viscosity of hydroxypropyl methylcellulose and plasma cholesterol in hamsters. J Nutr. 1993;123: 1732–1738.
19. Chen WJ, Anderson JW, Jennings D. Propionate may mediate the hypocholesterolemic effects of certain soluble plant fibers in cholesterol-fed rats. Proc Soc Exp Biol Med. 1984;175:215–218.
20. Wright RS, Anderson JW, Bridges SR. Propionate inhibits hepatocyte lipid synthesis. Proc Soc Exp Biol Med. 1990;195:26–29.
21. Nishina PM, Freedland RA. Effects of propionate on lipid biosynthesis in isolated rat hepatocytes. J Nutr. 1990;120:668–673.
22. Hara H, Haga S, Aoyama Y, et al. Short-chain fatty acids suppress cholesterol synthesis in rat liver and intestine. J Nutr. 1999;129:942–948.
23. Nishina PM, Schneeman BO, Freedland RA. Effects of dietary fibers on nonfasting plasma lipoprotein and apolipoprotein levels in rats. J Nutr. 1991; 121:431–437.
24. Alvarez-Leite JI, Andrieux C, Forezou J, et al. Evidence for the absence of participation of the microbial flora in the hypocholesterolemic effect of guar gum in gnotobiotic rats. Comp Biochem Physiol Physiol. 1994;109:503–510.
25. Marlett JA, Hosig KB, Vollendorf NW, et al. Mechanism of serum cholesterol reduction by oat bran. Hepatology. 1994;20:1450–1457.
26. Trautwein EA, Kunath-Rau A, Erbersdobler HF. Increased fecal bile acid excretion and changes in the circulating bile acid pool are involved in the hypocholesterolemic and gallstone-preventive actions of psyllium in hamsters. J Nutr. 1999;129:896–902.
27. Carr TP, Wood KJ, Hassel CA, et al. Raising intestinal contents viscosity leads to greater excretion of neutral sterols but not bile acids in hamsters and rats. Nutr Res. 2003;23:91–102.
28. Carr TP, Gallaher DD, Yang CH, et al. Increased intestinal contents viscosity reduces cholesterol absorption efficiency in hamsters fed hydroxypropyl methylcellulose. J Nutr. 1996;126:1463–1469.
29. Bourdon I, Yokoyama W, Davis P, et al. Postprandial lipid, glucose, insulin, and cholecystokinin responses in men fed barley pasta enriched with beta-glucan. Am J Clin Nutr. 1999;69:55–63.
30. Gallaher DD, Olson JM, Larntz K. Dietary guar gum halts further renal enlargement in rats with established diabetes. J Nutr. 1992;122:2391–2397.
31. Blackburn NA, Redfern JS, Jarjis H, et al. The mechanism of action of guar gum in improving glucose tolerance in man. Clin Sci (Lond). 1984;66:329–336.
32. Leclere CJ, Champ M, Boillot J, et al. Role of viscous guar gums in lowering the glycemic response after a solid meal. Am J Clin Nutr. 1994;59:914–921.
33. Bianchi M, Capurso L. Effects of guar gum, ispaghula and microcrystalline cellulose on abdominal symptoms, gastric emptying, orocaecal transit time and gas production in healthy volunteers. Dig Liver Dis. 2002;34(suppl 2):S129–S133.
34. Cummings JH. The effect of dietary fiber on fecal weight and composition. In: Spiller GA, ed. *Dietary Fiber in Human Nutrition.* 2nd ed. Boca Raton, FL: CRC Press; 1993; 263–349.
35. Schneeman BO, Gallaher DD. Effects of dietary fiber on digestive enzymes. In: Spiller GA, ed. *Dietary Fiber in Human Nutrition.* 2nd ed. Boca Raton, FL: CRC Press; 1993; 377–385.
36. Gallaher DD, Schneeman BO: Nutritional and metabolic response to plant inhibitors of digestive enzymes. In: Friedman M, ed. *Advances in Experimental*

*Medicine and Biology.* Vol. 199. New York: Plenum Press; 1986; 167–184.

37. Snow P, O'Dea K. Factors affecting the rate of hydrolysis of starch in food. Am J Clin Nutr. 1981;34: 2721–2727.
38. Kasper H. Effects of dietary fiber on vitamin metabolism. In: Spiller GA, ed. *Dietary Fiber in Human Nutrition.* Boca Raton, FL: CRC Press; 1993; 253–260.
39. Sandstrom B, Almgren A, Kivisto B, et al. Zinc absorption in humans from meals based on rye, barley, oatmeal, triticale and whole wheat. J Nutr. 1987;117: 1898–1902.
40. Torre M, Rodriguez AR, Saura-Calixto F. Effects of dietary fiber and phytic acid on mineral availability. Crit Rev Food Sci Nutr. 1991;30:1–22.
41. Gordon DT, Stoops D, Ratliff V: Dietary fiber and mineral nutrition. In: Kritchevsky D, Bonfield C, eds. *Dietary Fiber in Health and Disease.* St. Paul, MN: Eagan Press; 1995; 267–293.
42. Coudray C, Demigne C, Rayssiguier Y. Effects of dietary fibers on magnesium absorption in animals and humans. J Nutr. 2003;133:1–4.
43. Weaver CM. Inulin, oligofructose and bone health: experimental approaches and mechanisms. Br J Nutr. 2005;93(suppl 1):S99–S103.
44. Park Y, Hunter DJ, Spiegelman D, et al. Dietary fiber intake and risk of colorectal cancer: a pooled analysis of prospective cohort studies. JAMA. 2005; 294:2849–2857.
45. Pereira MA, O'Reilly E, Augustsson K, et al. Dietary fiber and risk of coronary heart disease: a pooled analysis of cohort studies. Arch Intern Med. 2004;164: 370–376.
46. MacLennan R, Macrae F, Bain C, et al. Randomized trial of intake of fat, fiber, and beta carotene to prevent colorectal adenomas. J Natl Cancer Inst. 1995; 87:1760–1766.
47. Alberts DS, Martinez ME, Roe DJ, et al. Lack of effect of a high-fiber cereal supplement on the recurrence of colorectal adenomas. Phoenix Colon Cancer Prevention Physicians' Network. N Engl J Med. 2000;342:1156–1162.
48. Schatzkin A, Lanza E, Corle D, et al. Lack of effect of a low-fat, high-fiber diet on the recurrence of colorectal adenomas. Polyp Prevention Trial Study Group. N Engl J Med. 2000;342:1149–1155.
49. Moshfegh AJ, Friday JE, Goldman JP, et al. Presence of inulin and oligofructose in the diets of Americans. J Nutr. 1999;129:1407S–1411S.
50. Cummings JH, Englyst HN. Gastrointestinal effects of food carbohydrate. Am J Clin Nutr. 1995;61: 938S–945S.
51. Cummings JH, Bingham SA, Heaton KW, et al. Fecal weight, colon cancer risk, and dietary intake of nonstarch polysaccharides (dietary fiber). Gastroenterology. 1992;103:1783–1789.
52. Pilch S. *Physiological Effects and Health Consequences of Dietary Fiber.* Bethesda, MD: Life Sciences Research Office; 1987.
53. Food and Nutrition Board, Institute of Medicine. Dietary Reference Intakes for Energy, Carbohydrate, Fiber, Fat, Fatty Acids, Cholesterol, Protein, and Amino Acids (Macronutrients). Washington, DC: National Academies Press; 2005. Available online at: http://darwin.nap.edu/books/0309085373/html/. Accessed February 22, 2006.
54. Gambera PJ, Schneeman BO, Davis PA. Use of the Food Guide Pyramid and US Dietary Guidelines to improve dietary intake and reduce cardiovascular risk in active-duty Air Force members. J Am Diet Assoc. 1995;95:1268–1273.

# 9

# Lipids: Absorption and Transport

Alice H. Lichtenstein and Peter J.H. Jones

Fat has long been recognized as an essential component of the diet. It contributes a concentrated source of energy and essential fatty acids, and serves as a carrier for other nutrients such as the fat-soluble vitamins A, D, E, and K. The bioavailability of lipid-soluble compounds in the diet is dependent on fat absorption.

## Chemistry

### *Fatty Acids*

Fatty acids are hydrocarbon chains with a methyl and carboxyl end. Most fatty acids have an even number of carbon atoms that are arranged in a straight chain. The majority of dietary fatty acids vary in chain length from 4 to 22 carbons (Table 1). Although by no means the most metabolically active, those with 16 and 18 carbons comprise the bulk of the fatty acids in both the diet and the human body. Individual fatty acids are distinguished from each other not only by chain length, but also by degree of saturation, conformation, and location of double bonds. Fatty acids with no double bonds are referred to as saturated. Those with a single double bond are monounsaturated, and fatty acids with multiple double bonds are polyunsaturated (Figure 1). The double bonds within unsaturated fatty acids can appear in the more common *cis* configuration, in which hydrogen atoms are on the same side of the carbon chain, or in the *trans* configuration, in which hydrogen atoms are on opposite sides of the carbon chain (Figure 2). The presence of double bonds, per se, and their number, position, and conformation allows for fatty acids to occur as multiple isomers.

Geometric isomers of fatty acids result from differences in the conformation (spatial orientation) of the double bond (s). In practical terms, the presence of a *cis* relative to a *trans* double bond results in a greater bend or kink in the carbon atom chain (Figure 2). This kink impedes the fatty acids from aligning or packing together, thereby lowering the melting point of the fat. The presence of a *trans* double bond reduces the internal rotational mobility of carbon atoms, and this type of bond is less reactive to chemical change than a *cis* double bond.

Positional isomers of fatty acids are defined by differences in the location of double bonds within the acyl chain. These differences result in small alterations to the melting point of the fatty acid, but large differences in the way the fatty acids are metabolized. The most common distinction made among potential isomers of fatty acids is the location of the first double bond from the methyl end of the acyl chain. Fatty acids in which the first double bond occurs 3 carbons from the methyl end are called omega-3 fatty acids, frequently denoted ω-3 or n-3 fatty acids. Major dietary sources of ω-3 fatty acids include soybean (7% of total fatty acids) and canola (10% of total fatty acids) oils, which are rich in α-linolenic acid (18:3 ω-3), and fish, especially fatty fish, which is high in eicosapentaenoic acid (EPA, 20:5 ω-3) and docosahexaenoic acid (DHA, 22:6 ω-3). The class of fatty acids in which the first double bond occurs 6 carbons from the methyl end is termed ω-6 fatty acids. Major dietary sources of ω-6 fatty acids include corn, safflower, soybean, and sunflower oils, which are rich in linoleic acid (18:2 ω-6). Enzymes that metabolize fatty acids to bioactive compounds distinguish among positional isomers. The metabolic products of the different positional isomers of fatty acids have different and at times opposite physiological effects.[1,2]

Most double bonds occur in a non-conjugated sequence—that is, they are separated by a carbon atom not involved in a double bond. Some of these occur in the conjugated form, which means they do not have an intervening carbon atom separating the double bonds

**Table 1.** Common Fatty Acids

| Code | Common Name | Formula |
|---|---|---|
| **Saturated** | | |
| 4:0 | butyric acid | $CH_3\ (CH_2)_2COOH$ |
| 6:0 | caproic acid | $CH_3\ (CH_2)_4COOH$ |
| 8:0 | caprylic acid | $CH_3\ (CH_2)_6COOH$ |
| 10:0 | capric acid | $CH_3\ (CH_2)_8COOH$ |
| 12:0 | lauric acid | $CH_3\ (CH_2)_{10}COOH$ |
| 14:0 | myristic acid | $CH_3\ (CH_2)_{12}COOH$ |
| 16:0 | palmitic acid | $CH_3\ (CH_2)_{14}COOH$ |
| 18:0 | stearic acid | $CH_3\ (CH_2)_{16}COOH$ |
| **Monounsaturated** | | |
| 16:1n-7 *cis* | palmitoleic acid | $CH_3\ (CH_2)_5CH=$ (c) $CH\ (CH_2)_7COOH$ |
| 18:1n-9 *cis* | oleic acid | $CH_3\ (CH_2)_7CH=$ (c) $CH\ (CH_2)_7COOH$ |
| 18:1n-9 *trans* | elaidic acid | $CH_3\ (CH_2)_7CH=$ (t) $CH\ (CH_2)_7COOH$ |
| **Polyunsaturated** | | |
| 18:2n-6,9 all cis | linoleic acid | $CH_3\ (CH_2)_4CH=$ (c) $CHCH_2CH=$ (c) $CH\ (CH_2)_7COOH$ |
| 18:3n-3,6,9 all *cis* | α-linolenic acid | $CH_3CH_2CH=$ (c) $CHCH_2CH=$ (c)$CHCH_2CH=$ (c) $CH\ (CH_2)_7COOH$ |
| 18:3n-6,9,12 all *cis* | γ-linolenic acid | $CH_3\ (CH_2)_4CH=$ (c) $CHCH_2CH=$ (c) $CHCH_2CH=$ (c) $CH\ (CH_2)_4COOH$ |
| 20:4n-6,9,12, 15 all *cis* | arachidonic acid | $CH_3\ (CH_2)_4CH=$ (c) $CHCH_2CH=$ (c) $CHCH_2CH=$ (c) $CHCH_2CH=$ (c) $CH\ (CH_2)_3COOH$ |
| 20:5n-3,6,9, 12,15 all *cis* | eicosapentaenoic acid | $CH_3\ (CH_2CH=$ (c)$CH)_5\ (CH_2)_3COOH$ |
| 22:6n-3,6,9, 12,15,18 all cis | docosahexaenoic acid | $CH_3\ (CH_2CH=$ (c) $CH)_6\ (CH_2)_2COOH$ |

(Figure 3). Conjugated double bonds tend to be more reactive chemically; for example, they may be more likely oxidized.[3] Although there is considerable speculation regarding their role in disease progression, the current state of knowledge is insufficient to make any firm conclusions.[4,5]

## *Triacylglycerol*

Triacylglycerol, commonly referred to as triglyceride, is composed of three fatty acids esterified to a glycerol molecule (Figure 4). Each position of the three carbons

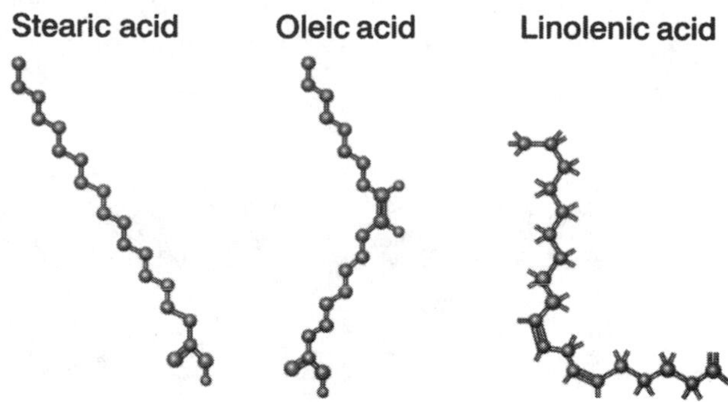


Figure 1. Examples of fatty acids: a saturated fatty acid (stearic acid), a monounsaturated fatty acid containing a *cis* double bond (oleic acid), and a polyunsaturated fatty acid containing a *trans* double (linoleic acid).

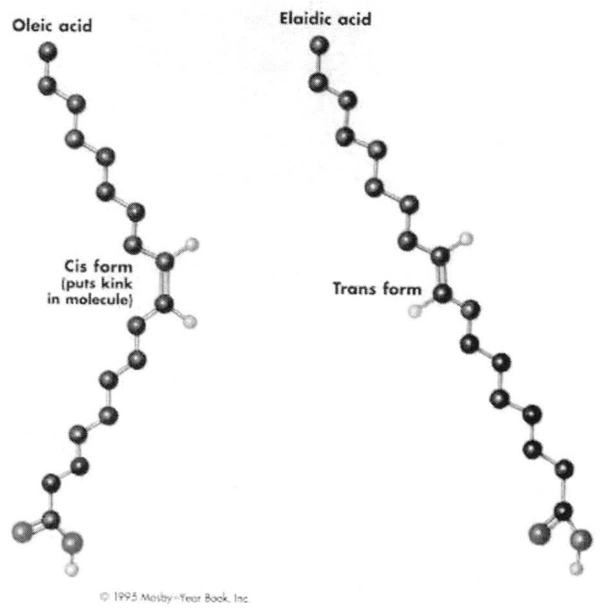


Figure 2. Conformational difference between *cis* (oleic acid) and *trans* (elaidic acid) double bond containing fatty acids.

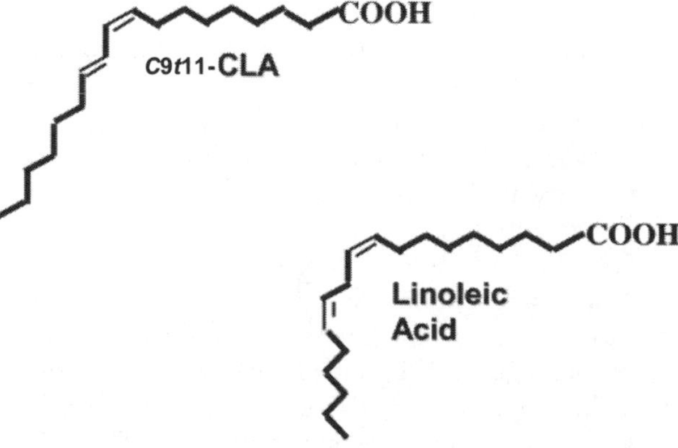


Figure 3. Structures of *c9t11*-conjugated linoleic acid (CLA) and linoleic acid [18:2 (n-6]. (Adapted with permission from Belury MA. Inhibition of carcinogenesis by conjugated linoleic acid: potential mechanisms of action. J Nutr. 2002 Oct;132 (10):2995-2998.)

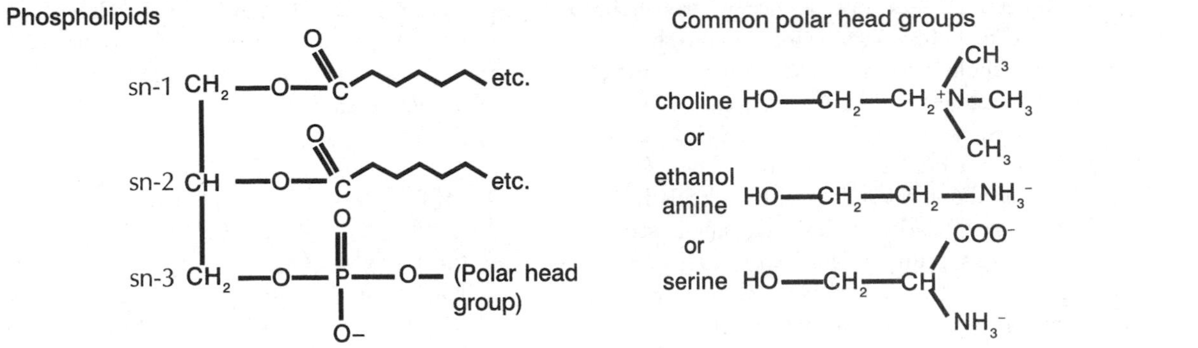

Phospholipids

sn-1 $CH_2$—O—C(=O)—etc.

sn-2 CH —O—C(=O)—etc.

sn-3 $CH_2$—O—P(=O)(O−)—O— (Polar head group)

Common polar head groups

choline HO—$CH_2$—$CH_2$—$N^+$($CH_3$)$_3$

or

ethanol amine HO—$CH_2$—$CH_2$—$NH_3^-$

or

serine HO—$CH_2$—CH($COO^-$)($NH_3^-$)

Figure 4. Common lipids: Cholesterol (cholesteryl ester), triacylglycerol, phospholipids, and common polar head groups.

comprising the glycerol molecule allows for a stereochemically distinct fatty acid bond position: sn-1, sn-2, and sn-3. The fatty acid moieties of the triacylglycerol molecule account for about 90% of its weight, depending on the length of the constituent fatty acids. A simple triacylglycerol contains three identical fatty acids and is exceedingly rare in nature. A triacylglycerol with two or three different fatty acids is called a mixed triacylglycerol, and comprises the bulk of the lipids in both the diet and the body. The melting point of a triacylglycerol is determined by the specific fatty acids esterified to glycerol moiety: chain length; number, position and conformation of the double bonds; and the stereochemical position of the fatty acids. In vivo, triacylglycerol serves as a storage form of energy and as a reservoir for fatty acids that can be used as a substrate for the synthesis of bioactive compounds.

Mono- and diacylglycerides have one and two fatty acids, respectively, esterified to glycerol. Rarely present in nature, they are intermediate products formed during triacylglycerol digestion and are frequently added to processed foods for their ability to act as emulsifiers. Recently, a cooking oil composed solely of diacylglycerides has been introduced into the market and some health benefits have been attributed to it.[6] Limited experience and scientific literature make it difficult to determine at this time whether there is an advantage to diacylglycerols compared with traditional cooking oils composed of predominantly triacylglycerols.[7]

## *Phospholipids*

A phospholipid is composed of two fatty acids esterified to a glycerol molecule and one polar head group attached via a phosphate linkage (Figure 4). Phospholipid molecules are amphipathic. The fatty acids confer hydrophobic properties and the polar head group hydrophilic properties. Long-chain fatty acids are preferentially esterified to the number 2 position of the glycerol backbone of the phospholipid molecule. The most predominant polar head groups of phospholipids, choline, serine, inositol, or ethanolamine, vary in size and charge. In vivo, due to their amphipathic nature, phospholipids serve as the major structural components of cellular membranes and are critical constituents of lipoprotein particles necessary for the transport of lipids in the bloodstream. The fluidity of cell membranes is determined in part by the fatty acid profile of the constituent phospholipids. Cell membrane-associated phosphatidylinositol, although a minor constituent quantitatively, is the predominant source of arachidonic acid. Arachidonic acid is a substrate for cyclooxygenase and 5-lipoxygenase, resulting in the formation of postiglandin. Other phosphatidylinositol-derived compounds, such as inositol$^{1,4,5}$ triphosphate and diacylglycerol, play important roles in cell signal transduction pathways as components of second messenger cascades.[8] Signaling through various phosphoinositides have a role in mediating cell growth and differentiation, apoptosis, intracellular vesicle trafficking, ion channel activation, insulin action, cytoskeletal changes, and motility.

## *Cholesterol and Cholesteryl Esters*

Cholesterol is an amphipathic molecule that is composed of a steroid nucleus and branched hydrocarbon tail. Its occurrence in the food supply is for the most part restricted to fats of animal origin. About 40% to 60% of dietary cholesterol is absorbed.

Cholesterol occurs naturally in two forms, either free or esterified to a fatty acid at carbon number 3 (Figure 4). Free cholesterol is a critical component of cell membranes and, along with the phospholipid fatty acid profile, influence fluidity. Intracellularly, free cholesterol is an important mediator of cholesterol homeostasis. It inhibits the activity of 3-hydroxy 3-methylglutaryl coenzyme A (HMG CoA) reductase, the rate-limiting enzyme in de novo cholesterol biosynthesis, thereby minimizing intracellular cholesterol accumulation. It increases the activity of acyl-CoA cholesterol acyltransferase (ACAT), the intracellular enzyme that esterifies free cholesterol, thereby lowering intracellular concentrations. It decreases the synthesis of low-density lipoprotein (LDL) cell surface receptors, thereby diminishing the uptake of additional cholesterol from plasma. It is critical for all these factors to work in concert to allow for adequate free cholesterol for optimal cellular functioning while limiting the buildup of free intracellular cholesterol due to its cytotoxic nature.

An ester of cholesterol is formed when a fatty acid is esterified to cholesterol. Cholesteryl esters are less polar than free cholesterol. As a consequence, whereas lipoprotein-associated free cholesterol is localized to the surface of the particle, cholesteryl ester is sequestered in the core. The majority of cholesterol in plasma is carried on LDL. Cholesteryl esters are formed in plasma as a result of the activity of lecithin cholesterol acyltransferase (LCAT) and account for about two-thirds of the circulating cholesterol.[9,10] Intracellularly, cholesteryl ester is stored in lipid droplets and accounts for a major portion of atherosclerotic plaque. In the arterial wall, cholesteryl ester is either derived from lipoprotein particles or is synthesized endogenously as a result of the activity of ACAT.[11-13]

### *Plant Sterols*

Fats derived from plant materials contain phytosterols, compounds structurally related to cholesterol, commonly referred to as plant sterols. Cholesterol and phytosterols differ chemically with regard to their side-chain configuration and steroid-ring-bonding patterns. The most common dietary phytosterols are β-sitosterol, campesterol, and stigmasterol (Figure 5).[14,15] In contrast to cholesterol, phytosterols are poorly absorbed and levels in plasma tend to be low. Because of their ability to displace cholesterol from intestinal micelles, they can reduce the absorption efficiency of cholesterol.

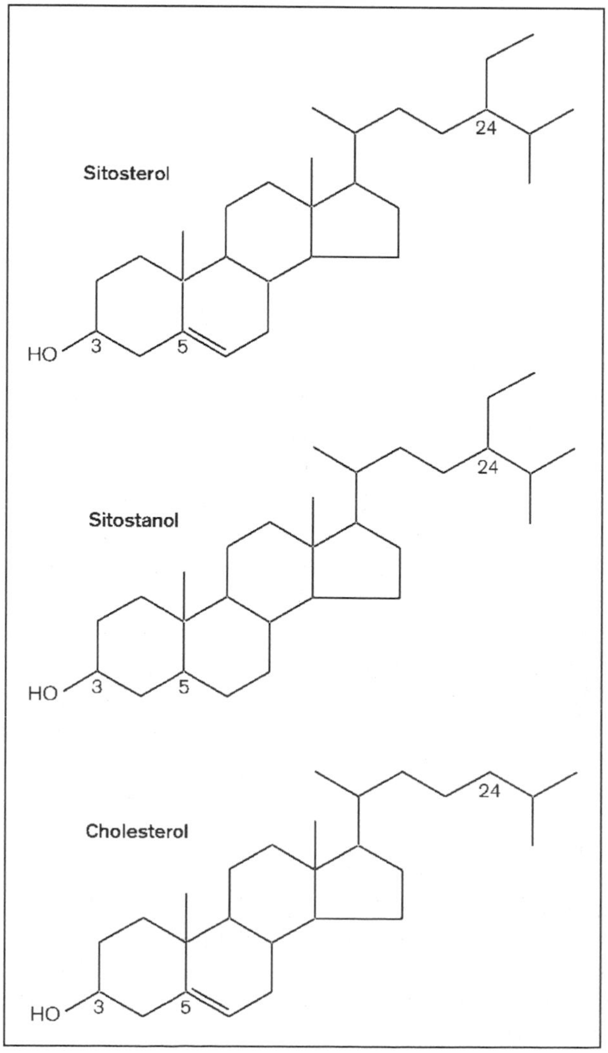

Figure 5. Common plant sterols. (Used with permission from Ostlund 2004.[14])

## Digestion

### *Triacylglycerol*

**Mouth, Esophagus, and Stomach.** Fat digestion begins at the point of entry, the oral cavity where salivation and mastication occur (Figure 6). Lingual lipase, released from the von Ebner (serous) glands of the tongue, along with saliva, can cause the release of small amounts of fatty acids from triacylglycerol.[16,17] The activity of lingual lipase is limited by the hydrophobic nature of dietary fat, the majority of which is triacylglycerol. The initial hydrolysis of triacylglycerol is augmented by chewing, which disperses the food, thus increasing the surface area on which the lipase can work. Lingual lipase cleaves the sn-3 position of the triacylglycerol molecule, with higher efficiency towards shorter-chain fatty acids. For this reason, the impact is thought to be greater in infants due to their high intake of milk fat, which contains a high proportion of short-chain fatty acids. When active, lingual lipase activity continues as food travels through the esophagus and into the stomach. In the stomach, gastric lipase is released from the gastric mucosa.[18-20] This enzyme cleaves triacylglycerol at the sn-3 position. Fat ingestion increases the expression of both lingual and gastric lipases. It has been estimated that 10% to 30% of fat hydrolysis occurs prior to the masticated bolus of food entering the small intestine. The pre-digestion of dietary fat may contribute to the efficiency of its intestinal digestion by the formation of hydrolysis products that increase the solubilization of triacylglycerol, the binding of colipase, and the free fatty acid concentration that stimulates the release of cholecystokinin.[18] The increased pH of the intestine on entry of the food bolus decreases the activity of the lingual and gastric lipases.

**Intestine.** The majority of triacylglycerol digestion and absorption occurs in the small intestine.[18] This process is co-dependent on pancreatic lipase and liver-derived bile salts. Bile is secreted from the gall bladder or directly from the liver in response to the presence of fat in the duodenum. Bile is composed of bile salts, phospholipids, and cholesterol. The major function of bile is to emulsify the chyme, or intestinal contents, thereby further increasing the surface area of the hydrophilic mass. This process maximizes the rate of fat digestion and is critical to the normal fat absorption process.

Bile salts have a steroid nucleus and an aliphatic side chain conjugated in an amide bond with taurine or glycine.[21,22] Bile acids are synthesized from cholesterol in the liver. The rate-limiting step in this process is catalyzed by 7α-hydroxylase.[23,24] The hydroxyl and ionized sulfonate or carboxylate groups of the conjugate

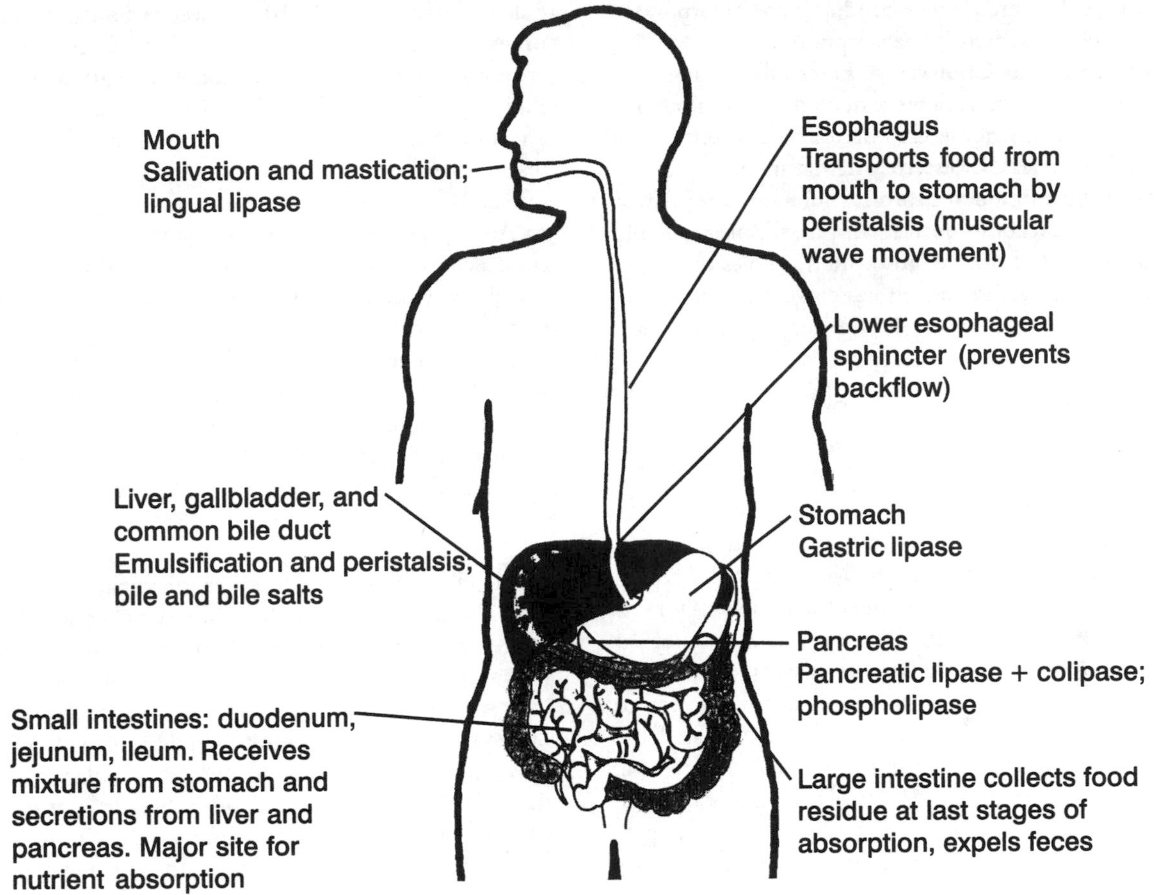


Figure 6. Diagram of absorption.

make bile salts water soluble. The primary bile salts are cholate and chenodeoxycholate (trihydroxy and dihydroxy bile salts, respectively), which are synthesized directly from cholesterol. The secondary bile salts, deoxycholate and lithocholate, are synthesized from primary bile salts (cholate and chenodeoxycholate, respectively) via bacterial action in the intestine. Secondary bile salts can be further modified by hepatocytes or bacteria. The products are sulfated esters of lithocholate and ursodeoxycholate.

The entry of fat into the duodenum, in addition to stimulating the contraction of the gall bladder, also causes the secretion of cholecystokinin and, as a result, the release of pancreatic lipase and colipase. The amount of fat habitually entering the duodenum is thought to regulate the gene expression of pancreatic lipase. In the intestine, pancreatic lipase is responsible for the majority of the triacylglycerol hydrolysis.[22,25] In addition to hydrolyzing the fatty acids in the sn-3 position (as do lingual and gastric lipases), pancreatic lipase also hydrolyzes the sn-1 position. The sn-2 (middle) position of glycerol is resistant to hydrolysis by lipases. Interestingly, pancreatic lipase is inhibited by bile salts via displacement from the lipid droplet. However, colipase, a protein also synthesized by the pancreas, binds pancreatic lipase and facilitates the enzyme's adhesion to the lipid droplets.[22,25,26]

The hydrolytic products of triacylglycerol (2-monoacylglycerol and free fatty acids), along with bile salts, phospholipids, and other fat-soluble substances present, form micelles in the small intestine. Cholesterol, normally secreted in bile, is also incorporated into the micellar particle.[27] Micelles only form when the critical micellar concentration of bile (about 2 mM) is reached. Colipase has an affinity for bile salts, phospholipids, and cholesterol. This property allows the protein to shuttle between the hydrolytic products of triacylglycerol—monoacylglycerol and free fatty acids—and micelles. The presence of monoacylglycerol increases the capacity of the micelle for free fatty acids and cholesterol. Deficits in the availability of an adequate amount of pancreatic lipase or bile acids can result in steatorrhea (the presence of undigested fat in the stool). Neither pancreatic lipase nor colipase is involved in the digestion of cholesteryl ester or phospholipids.

**Phospholipids.** The majority of the phospholipids in the small intestine are derived from bile, with a much smaller component coming from diet. The enzyme mediating phospholipid digestion is phospholipase $A_2$, a pancreatic enzyme secreted in the bile.[28] Phospholipase $A_2$ hydrolyzes the ester bond at the sn-2 position of the phospholipid, resulting in the production of free fatty acid and lysophosphoglyceride. Similar to the hydrolytic products of triacylglycerol, these products are incorporated into micelles for subsequent absorption.

**Cholesterol and Cholesteryl Esters.** Both bile, and to a lesser and more variable extent diet and sloughed intestinal cells, contribute cholesterol to the contents of the small intestine. Cholesterol originating from bile and intestinal cells is in the free form. Cholesterol originating from the diet occurs in both forms, free cholesterol and cholesteryl ester. Prior to absorption, cholesteryl ester must be hydrolyzed to free cholesterol and a fatty acid. This reaction is catalyzed by a bile-salt-dependent pancreatic enzyme, cholesteryl ester hydrolase.

# Absorption

## *Triacylglycerol*

Fat absorption occurs throughout the small intestine. Under normal conditions, the efficiency of fat absorption is approximately 95% in adults and 85% to 90% in infants (based on human milk fat). The high efficiency of fat absorption in adults is relatively consistent over a wide range of total fat intakes. Unsaturated fatty acids tend to be absorbed at a somewhat higher efficiency than saturated fatty acids, although from a practical perspective, these differences are small.[29] Fatty acids with 12 or more carbon atoms are absorbed into the lymphatic system as chylomicrons (see the section on intestinally derived particles). Fatty acids with 10 or fewer carbon atoms, sometimes referred to as short- or medium-chain fatty acids, are absorbed directly into the portal circulation. The positional distribution of the fatty acids on glycerol can also affect the efficiency of fatty acid absorption because of the resistance of the sn-2 position to hydrolysis by pancreatic lipase.[18,29]

Absorption of micellar components into intestinal mucosal cells is dependent on the penetration of micelles across the unstirred water layer that separates the intestinal contents from the brush border of the small intestine (Figure 7). The mechanism of absorption is passive diffusion. Under normal circumstances, micellar components exist in dynamic equilibrium with the surrounding environment and spontaneously exchange among micellar particles. This process is greatly facilitated by the peristaltic action of the small intestine, which continuously mixes the intestinal contents.

Micelles, in contrast to other intestinal contents such as lipid droplets, traverse the unstirred water layer because of their relatively small size (30 to 100 Δ) and hydrophilic nature (due to the presence of bile salts and phospholipids). As in the rest of the small intestine, the components of the micelle are in constant equilibrium with the surrounding environment. Since the intracellular concentration of the components and of the unstirred water layer are lower than that in the surrounding environment, the products of hydrolysis flow down the concentration gra-

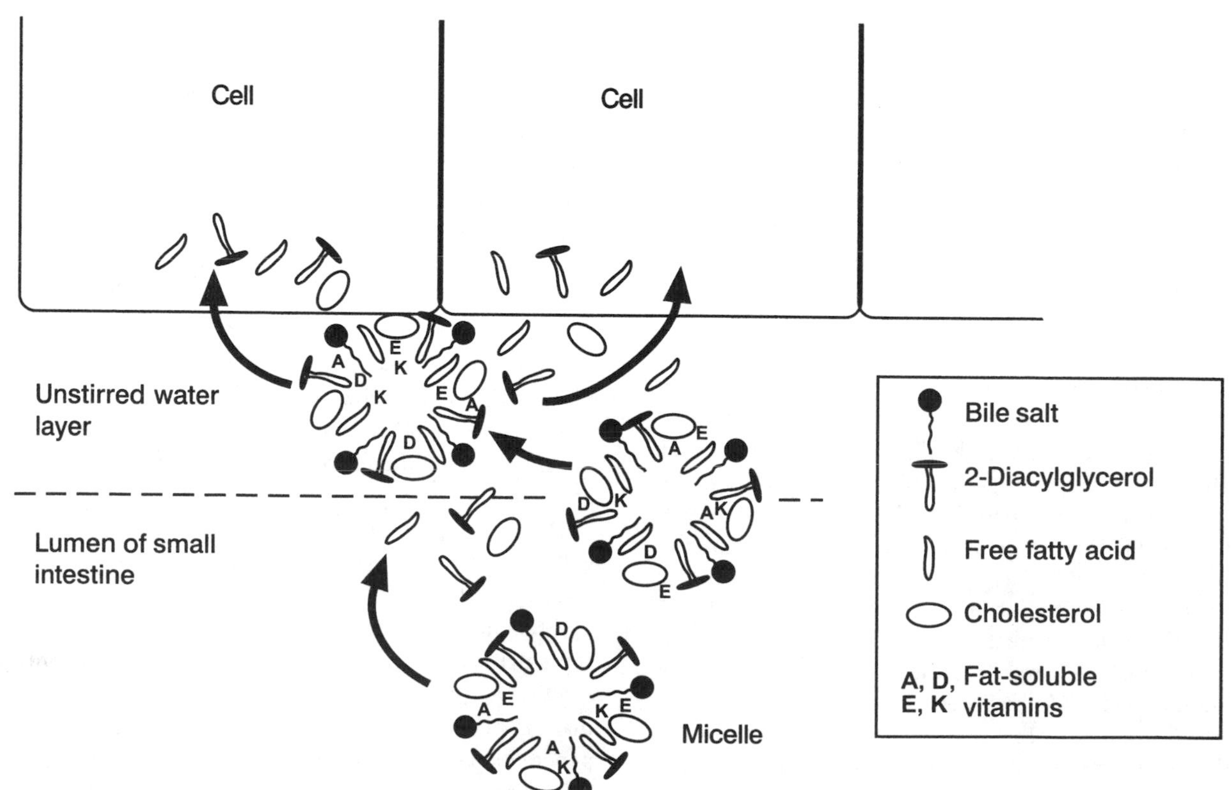


Figure 7. Lipid transport in blood. VLDL, very-low-density lipoprotein; IDl, intermediate-density lipoprotein; LDL, low-density lipoprotein; HDL, high-densityl liprotein; LCAT, lecithin cholesterol acyltransferase; ACAT, acyl coenzyme A cholesterol acytransferase.

dient, and thus into the cell. This net loss of micellar constituents results in a shift in the distribution of hydrolytic products from micelles in the intestinal lumen to micelles in the unstirred water layer, and from the unstirred water layer to intestinal cells. The small intestine contains a group of intracellular lipid-binding proteins of low molecular weight (e.g., retinol-binding proteins, sterol-carrier proteins, and cytosolic fatty acid-binding proteins). Three of these cytosolic fatty acid-binding proteins that may be important for fat absorption are liver-type fatty acid binding protein (L-FABP), intestinal fatty acid binding protein (I-FABP), and ileal lipid-binding protein.[30] These proteins are thought to facilitate the transmucosal transport of digestion products. Inter-individual variation in the metabolic response to diet has been partially attributed to polymorphism in the fatty acid-binding protein 2.[31,32]

Micellar bile salts are not absorbed with fat digestion products. There is a highly efficient system of re-absorbing bile salts in both the small intestine and colon, with re-secretion via bile in the duodenum for subsequent use. Bile salts are absorbed independently by both passive and active mechanisms. Passive absorption of unconjugated bile salts occurs along the entire length of the small intestine and colon. Active absorption occurs in the ileum and involves a brush border membrane receptor, cytosolic bile acid-binding protein, and basolateral anion-exchange proteins. Approximately 97% to 98% of bile acids are reabsorbed.[33] Interfering with the reabsorption of bile acids forces the liver to use cholesterol for synthesis. This cause/effect relationship has been exploited for the treatment of hypercholesterolemic patients with bile acid sequesterants, specifically designed to interfere with this process.

### *Phospholipids*

The products of phospholipid digestion, free fatty acid and lysophospholipids, are incorporated into intestinal micelles and are absorbed by a process similar to that described for the hydrolytic products of triacylglycerol.

### *Cholesterol and Cholesteryl Esters*

The efficiency of free and esterified cholesterol absorption is similar. It is not clear whether cholesteryl ester hydrolysis is rate limiting.[34,35] Free cholesterol and the free fatty acids resulting from the hydrolysis of cholesteryl esters are incorporated into intestinal micelles. A water-soluble lipid-exchange protein of low molecular weight, located on the luminal side of the brush border membrane, is involved in the transmembrane movement of cholesterol.[36]

Interestingly, the efficiency of cholesterol absorption is not regulated at the level of entry into the enterocyte; instead it is regulated by the balance between the incorporation of cholesterol into a newly synthesized chylomicron for secretion relative to the trafficking of cholesterol out of the enterocyte back into the small intestine.[37,38] This process is regulated by at least two proteins, ATP-binding cassette (ABC) G5 and G8 transporters: ABCG5 and ABCG8. Mutations in these proteins are characterized by the accumulation of cholesterol and other sterols in circulation and tissue. According to recent studies, a sterol-transporter protein, Niemann-Pick C1 like 1 (NPC1L1), also plays an important role in influx of cholesterol and plant sterols into the intestinal cell.[39,40] A mutation in this protein has been reported to be associated with non-response to ezetimibe, a cholesterol absorption-lowering agent.[41] As shown in Figure 8, trafficking of cholesterol and other sterols into the enterocyte, and their subsequent incorporation into chylomicrons, are regulated through the coordinated actions of influx and efflux transporter proteins.

### *Plant Sterols and Sterol Esters*

The efficiency of plant sterol absorption is relatively low: 0% to 10%, depending on the specific plant sterol. The poor efficiency of absorption is attributed to the activity of two genes (ABCG5 and ABCG8, which handle plant sterols as they do cholesterol, transporting them out of the enterocyte[38]), low solubility of the sterols in micelles, and the inability of the intestinal cell to re-esterify the sterols once absorbed.[42] Interestingly, despite the poor solubility of plant sterols in micelles, their presence interferes with the ability of cholesterol to be incorporated into micelles, thereby resulting in a lower efficiency of absorption of cholesterol.[43,44] As indicated earlier, the ability of plant sterols to displace cholesterol from micelles, resulting in a decreased absorption efficiency of cholesterol, is used in the treatment of hypercholesterolemia. The absence of ABCG5 and ABCG8 results in a rare genetic disorder called beta-sitosterolemia. This disorder is characterized by a 3-fold to 22-fold increase in plant sterol absorption, a 30-fold to 100-fold increase in plant sterol plasma levels, and a 13-fold to 100-fold increase in the plant sterol pool in the body.[38] Patients with beta-sitosterolemia are at markedly increased risk of premature cardiovascular disease.

## Transport and Metabolism

For the most part, due to the hydrophobic nature of fat, neither lipid itself nor the hydrolytic products thereof can be released directly into the aqueous milieu of the portal vein. The complex system for absorption and transport of lipid is in contrast to that of both protein and carbohydrate. Triacylglycerol and other lipid-soluble compounds are released into the circulation after being packaged within the enterocyte as lipoprotein particles called chylomicrons. These particles have a hydrophobic core and hydrophilic surface, and are similar in structure to lipoprotein particles synthesized and released by the liver, which are called very-low-density lipoproteins (VLDLs). The exception is short-chain fatty acids (≤10 carbons). These fatty acids tend to be absorbed directly

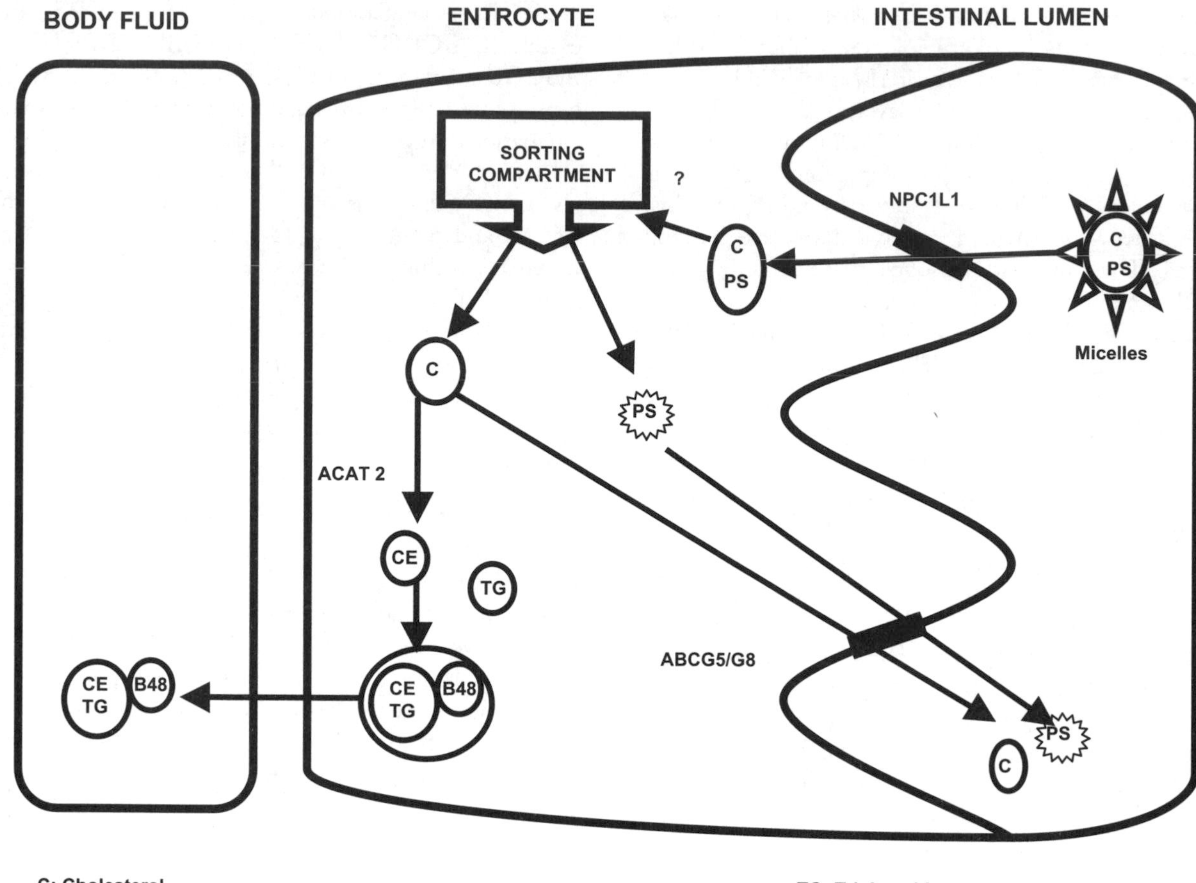


Figure 8. Cholesterol and plant sterol absorption at the enterocyte level.

into the portal circulation and, once in plasma, are bound to albumin. There is some evidence that the direct delivery of these short-chain fatty acids to the liver results in higher rates of oxidation than fatty acids endogenously present in the liver.

## *Intestinally Derived Particles*

Chylomicrons are intestinally derived lipoprotein particles formed and secreted after the ingestion of fat. Their main function is to provide a mechanism whereby dietary fat (triacylglycerol), cholesterol, and other fat-soluble compounds are carried from the site of absorption (intestine) to other parts of the body for subsequent uptake and potential metabolism or storage.[45,46]

The first step in the formation of chylomicron particles is the resynthesis of triacylglycerol and phospholipids from fatty acids, and glycerol, sn-2 monoacylglycerides or lysophospholipids, respectively.[47,48] This process occurs on the smooth endoplasmic reticulum. The fatty acid composition of the chylomicron triacylglycerol, but not the phospholipid composition, reflects for the most part, the fatty acid composition of the diet.[49] A large percentage of the cholesterol that enters the enterocyte is re-esterified, a reaction catalyzed by ACAT, prior to incorporation into the chylomicron particle.[11-13] The re-esterification processes are facilitated by fatty acid-binding protein.[50]

Chylomicron particles are the largest of all of the lipoprotein subclasses (Table 2).[51] The structure is similar to that of all the other lipoprotein particles that will be discussed. The core of the spherical particle is composed primarily of apolar components: triacylglycerol and cholesteryl ester. The surface of the particle is composed of the more polar constituents: phospholipid monolayer, apolipoproteins, and free cholesterol.[51] Fat-soluble vitamins are sequestered in the core of the chylomicron particle.

In humans, the distinguishing apolipoprotein of intestinally derived lipoproteins is apoB-48, whereas the distinguishing apolipoprotein of hepatically derived particles is apoB-100. apoB-48 is a large hydrophobic protein synthesized on the rough endoplasmic reticulum, which results from mRNA editing and is approximately 48% of the molecular weight of apoB-100. Additional apolipoproteins on the surface of chylomicron particles include apoA-I, apoA-IV, apoA-II, apoC, and apoE.[51] Recent work suggests that the release of apoA-IV is stimulated by lipid feeding and has a role in the regulation of upper gut function and satiety.[52] It has further been suggested

**Table 2.** Characteristics of Lipoproteins

| Lipoprotein | Density | Molecular Mass | Diameter | Lipid (%)* | | |
|---|---|---|---|---|---|---|
| | *g/dL* | *Daltons* | *nm* | Triacylglyerol | Cholesterol | Phospholipid |
| Chylomicron | 0.95 | $1400 \times 10^6$ | 75–1200 | 80–95 | 2–7 | 3–9 |
| VLDL | 0.95–1.006 | $10–80 \times 10^6$ | 30–80 | 55–80 | 5–15 | 10–20 |
| IDL | 1.006–1.019 | $5–10 \times 10^6$ | 25–35 | 20–50 | 20–40 | 15–25 |
| LDL | 1.019–1.063 | $2.3 \times 10^6$ | 18–25 | 5–15 | 40–50 | 20–25 |
| HDL | 1.063–1.21 | $1.7–3.6 \times 10^5$ | 5–12 | 5–10 | 15–25 | 20–30 |

* Percentage composition of lipids; apolipoproteins make up the rest.
HDL = high-density lipoprotein; IDL = intermediate-density lipoprotein; LDL = low-density lipoprotein; VLDL = very low-density lipoprotein.

that apoA-IV may be involved in the long-term regulation of food intake and that chronic ingestion of a high-fat diet blunts the intestinal apoA-IV response to lipid feeding, and therefore predisposes to obesity.[52]

Chylomicrons are assembled from apoB-48 and triacylglycerol accumulated in the smooth endoplasmic reticulum. Microsomal triacylglycerol transfer protein (MTP) is responsible for transporting and inserting the triacylglycerol into the nascent chylomicron core as the particle is then transferred into the lumen of the endoplasmic reticulum.[53] Some data suggest that small apoB-48-containing particles fuse with large, independently formed triacylglycerol apoB-48-free particles prior to secretion.[18,29] Carbohydrate is added to the nascent chylomicron particle just before release from the Golgi apparatus by exocytosis from the cell.

Chylomicrons are released from enterocytes into the lymph before being channeled from the thoracic duct to the subclavian vein. Once in circulation, the triacylglycerol component of chylomicron particles is hydrolyzed by lipoprotein lipase and apolipoproteins are transferred to other lipoprotein particles. Lipoprotein lipase is synthesized in adipose tissue, heart and skeletal muscle, and migrates to the capillaries where it functions.[54,55] apoC-II is a critical cofactor for the reaction whereas apoC-I and apoC-III inhibit the reaction.[55-57] The hydrolysis of triacylglycerol from chylomicrons in circulation accounts for the delivery of ingested fat from the gastrointestinal system to peripheral tissue for oxidation, metabolism and storage. This process also results in the production of lipids and apolipoproteins that form high-density lipoprotein (HDL).[55] Chylomicron particles depleted of the triacylglycerol component are termed chylomicron remnants and are taken up by the liver via either the LDL-receptor or LDL-receptor-like protein receptors.[58,59] The components of chylomicron particles are either used by the liver directly or are incorporated into newly synthesized hepatically derived lipoprotein particles.

## *Hepatically Derived Particles*

**Very-Low-Density, Intermediate-Density, and Low-Density Lipoproteins.** VLDL are hepatically derived particles that mediate the transport of fat from the liver to peripheral tissue.[60,61] The triacylglycerol in VLDL is synthesized from fatty acids derived from de novo lipogenesis, cytoplasmic triacylglycerol, lipoproteins taken up directly by the liver, and exogenous free fatty acids. The major apolipoprotein in VLDL is apoB-100.[60,61] apoB-100 is synthesized on the rough endoplasmic reticulum and transferred to the Golgi apparatus where, with the involvement of MTP, it is incorporated into the nascent VLDL particle. Inadequate triacylglycerol or the absence of MTP results in internal degradation of apoB-100.[62,63] This degradation is facilitated by the association of nascent apoB with a cytosolic chaperone protein called heat-shock protein-70.[64] In plasma, VLDL also contains apoE and apoC, which are either present at the time of secretion or acquired once in circulation.[60,61]

The lipid components of VLDL particles are similar to those of chylomicrons; however, the relative proportion of triacylglycerol is less (Table 2). This results in smaller, denser particles. Once in circulation, the initial stages of VLDL metabolism are similar to those of chylomicron metabolism. Lipoprotein lipase hydrolyzes the core triacylglycerol.[65,66] The resulting fatty acids are taken up by cells locally and are oxidized for energy, used for the synthesis of structural components (phospholipid) or bioactive compounds (leukotrienes, thromboxanes), or stored (triacylglycerol). Triacylglycerol-depleted particles, VLDL remnants, can either be taken up directly by receptor-mediated mechanisms in the liver or remain in circulation and be progressively depleted of triacylglycerol. The de-lipidation of VLDL results in a progressive shift in the composition of the lipoprotein particle from one defined as VLDL to an intermediate-density lipoprotein (IDL), and eventually an LDL.[65,66] This process is facilitated by not only lipoprotein lipase, but also by hepatic lipase.[65-67] This second lipase has the capacity to hydrolyze both triacylglycerol and phospholipids. The progressive depletion of triacylglycerol from the lipoprotein particle results in a marked increase in the relative proportion of cholesterol. As VLDL is depleted of triacylglycerol, apoC and apoE are transferred to other lipoproteins in circulation. The ultimate product is LDL, a cholesterol-rich particle containing only a single copy of apoB-100.

LDL can be taken up by an apolipoprotein-mediated or scavenger receptor.[68,69] There are a number of LDL receptors belonging to the sample gene family. These include the LDL receptor, LDL receptor-related protein (LRP), apoE receptor 2 protein, multiple epidermal growth factor-containing protein 7, VLDL receptor, LRP1B, megalin, LRP 5, and LRP 6. Whereas the LDL receptor mediates the uptake of apoB-100- or apoE-containing lipoproteins, the other members of the LDL receptor gene family recognize multiple ligands and appear to play diverse biological roles. Once LDL is taken up by the cell, it disassociates from the receptor and the receptor can be recycled. The LDL particle fuses with a lysosome and is subsequently degraded. This step is critical for whole-body cholesterol homoeostasis, because the cholesterol taken up from circulation and released from the lysosome has three distinct effects: it inhibits the activity of HMG CoA reductase, it down-regulates the synthesis of LDL receptors, and it increases ACAT activity. These actions have the effect of decreasing the rate of de novo cholesterol biosynthesis, the amount of LDL taken up by the cell, and the level of free cholesterol in the cytosol, respectively. Long-chain saturated fatty acids have been reported to further suppress LDL receptor activity.[70] Alternatively, LDL can be taken up by a scavenger receptor on macrophages in various tissues. This system predominates after LDL particles are modified or oxidized as they circulate in plasma.[68,69]

**High-Density Lipoprotein.** High-density lipoprotein (HDL) particles are derived from the liver, peripheral tissues, and the intestine. They participate in "reverse cholesterol transport" by shuttling cholesterol from the peripheral tissues to the liver for excretion, metabolism, or storage.[71,72] An integral part of this process is scavenger receptor (SR)-B1. This hepatic HDL receptor selectively takes up the cholesteryl ester component of HDL, thus promoting the ability of HDL to pick up additional cholesterol from peripheral tissue.[73,74]

HDL is a heterogeneous group of particles that differ both in apolipoprotein composition and size. All HDL particles contain apoA-I. However, other apolipoproteins associated with HDL can include apoA-II, apoA-IV, and apoC's. HDL particles reportedly protect other lipoproteins from oxidative modification. This activity appears to be related to the presence of apoA-I, paraoxonase, and platelet-activating factor acetylhydrolase.[75,76] Plasma HDL levels are inversely related to triglyceride and the risk of developing cardiovascular disease.[77,78]

Tangier disease is an autosomal recessive disorder characterized by the virtual absence of HDL cholesterol. HDL-mediated cholesterol efflux and intracellular lipid trafficking and turnover are abnormal in fibroblasts from Tangier patients. The genetic defect encoding for a member of the ABC transporter family has been identified in these individuals.[79,80] The ABC transporter is integral to the process of reverse cholesterol transport. Individuals with a mutation in the ABC transporter have very low levels of HDL cholesterol and develop premature atherosclerosis.

### *Lipoprotein Metabolism*

In addition to de-lipidation, lipoproteins are altered while in circulation.[81-84] This includes both exchange and modification of lipoprotein constituents. LCAT esterifies free cholesterol on the surface of HDL particles. ApoA-I serves as a cofactor and HDL-associated phosphotidylcholine as the source of fatty acid.[81,83] The formation of cholesteryl ester and its subsequent migration to the core of the HDL particle creates an environment receptive to the addition of more free cholesterol from peripheral tissue, and ensures that the cholesterol already on the HDL particle does not transfer back to peripheral tissue. Cholesterol ester transfer protein (CETP) facilitates the exchange of cholesteryl ester from HDL to VLDL or chylomicrons for triacylglycerol.[83,84] Phospholipid transfer protein activity results in HDL remodeling through the exchange of phospholipids.[82] These processes enhance reverse cholesterol transport.

## Modulation of Lipid Absorption in Disease Control

### *Obesity and Fat Absorption*

One of the many approaches being pursued in the treatment of obesity has been to interfere with fat digestion and absorption. The objective is to reduce the proportion of dietary fat energy that is absorbed either by substitution of natural food fat with materials that are not readily digested or by provision of agents that impair the process of digestion itself. One example is sucrose polyester, currently sold under the trade name Olestra. Sucrose polyesters contain several fatty acids esterified to the hydroxyl groups of sucrose.[85,86] This material possesses organoleptic properties similar to dietary fat and is heat stable, thereby facilitating its incorporation into a variety of foods. However, the sucrose polyester bonds are resistant to cleavage by digestive lipase enzymes, so the material passes through the gut unabsorbed. In so doing, sucrose polyesters provide neither dietary fatty acids nor energy.[85,86] As a direct consequence of the transit of unaltered sucrose polyester through the gastrointestinal system, other fat-soluble compounds may also be excreted. Those causing concern are one class of essential nutrients: the fat-soluble vitamins. In an attempt to remediate the situation, the US Food and Drug Administration (FDA) has approved the use of Olestra in savory snacks with the stipulation that foods must be fortified with adequate amounts of vitamins A, D, E, and K to prevent a drop in circulating levels of these nutrients.[87,88] Another potential consequence of the ingestion of sucrose polyester is gas, bloating, and diarrhea in a small proportion of the subjects consuming relatively large amounts of the material. Few other countries have approved the use of sucrose polyesters and consumer acceptance has been limited to date.

The most recent approach to altering fat absorption has targeted the activity of enzymes responsible for triacylglycerol digestion, gastric and pancreatic lipases. Orlistat is a chemically synthesized derivative of lipstatin and a product of the organism *Streptomyces toxytricini.* Orlistat directly inhibits lipase activity and results in the suppression of triacylglycerol digestion by around 30%, thus increasing fecal elimination of fat, and therefore overall energy. A recent systematic review concluded that Orlistat resulted in a 5% to 10% weight loss and improved total, LDL, and HDL cholesterol levels.[89] Adverse gastrointestinal events were common and were mild or moderate in intensity. Some studies reported non-significant declines in circulating vitamin A, D, and E, and beta-carotene concentrations.

### *Cardiovascular Disease Risk and Cholesterol Absorption*

The management of hypercholesterolemia is an essential component in the reduction of risk for cardiovascular disease. One dietary strategy aimed specifically at the process of cholesterol absorption has involved the addition of plant sterol or stanol esters to foods. As indicated previously, plant sterols are structurally related to cholesterol. Due to these structural similarities, they compete with and ultimately block the intestinal absorption of both dietary and biliary-originated cholesterol. These phytosterols are frequently esterified to fatty acids to increase their solubility in fat prior to incorporation into food products. Plant sterols are converted to stanols by hydrogenation. Both the esterified and free forms have also been shown to be effective in lowering cholesterol levels in hyperlipidemic individuals by about 5% to 15%.[14,90,91] This is attributed to an approximately 40% decrease in cholesterol absorption and only a 10% to 15% compensatory increase in de novo cholesterol biosynthesis. Maximum efficacy is reached at about 1.6 to 2 g/d of plant sterols. As with other agents that block fat absorption, supplementation with phytosterols is associated with a mild suppression of circulatory levels of fat-soluble vitamins.[92]

## Summary

Due to the hydrophobic nature of lipids, dietary fats are handled differently than protein or carbohydrates with respect to digestion and absorption. Dietary fats are broken down throughout the gastrointestinal system. A unique group of enzymes and cofactors allows this process to proceed in an efficient manner. Elegant systems operate to digest lipids, then ferry them from the gastrointestinal tract through the unstirred water layer into the enterocyte. Within the enterocyte, complex lipids are resynthesized and packaged into lipoprotein particles for release into the lymph system for subsequent metabolism by peripheral tissue. Once in the body, the apolar nature of lipids necessitates multiple complex transport systems that are unique relative to protein and carbohydrate. By the coordination of a number of plasma factors, cell surface receptors, and intracellular trafficking via plasma lipoproteins, dietary lipids are ultimately delivered to target tissues. Agents that replace dietary fat or block absorption may be useful in producing a negative energy balance consistent with risk reduction for obesity. Further work is needed to ascertain whether these approaches work over the very long term and what, if any, consequences are associated with prolonged usage. Similarly, agents that prevent the absorption of cholesterol are useful in the management of individuals with elevated LDL cholesterol levels.

## References

1. Wijendran V, Hayes KC. Dietary n-6 and n-3 fatty acid balance and cardiovascular health. Ann Rev Nutr. 2004;24:597–615.
2. Nakamura MT, Nara TY. Structure, function, and dietary regulation of delta6, delta5, and delta9 desaturases. Ann Rev Nutr. 2004;24:345–376.
3. Bretillon L, Chardigny JM, Gregoire S, Berdeaux O, Sebedio JL. Effects of conjugated linoleic acid isomers on the hepatic microsomal desaturation activities in vitro. Lipids. 1999;34:965–969.
4. Terpstra AH. Effect of conjugated linoleic acid on body composition and plasma lipids in humans: an overview of the literature. Am J Clin Nutr. 2004;79:352–361.
5. Larsen TM, Toubro S, Astrup A. Efficacy and safety of dietary supplements containing CLA for the treatment of obesity: evidence from animal and human studies. J Lipid Res. 2003;44:2234–2241.
6. Tada N, Shoji K, Takeshita M, et al. Effects of diacylglycerol ingestion on postprandial hyperlipidemia in diabetes. Clin Chim Acta. 2005;353:87–94.
7. Maki KC, Davidson MH, Tsushima R, et al. Consumption of diacylglycerol oil as part of a reduced-energy diet enhances loss of body weight and fat in comparison with consumption of a triacylglycerol control oil. Am J Clin Nutr. 2002;76:1230–1236.
8. Cocco L, Manzoli L, Barnabei O, Martelli A. Significance of subnuclear localization of key players of inositol lipid cycle. Adv Enzyme Regul. 2004;44:51–60.
9. Santamarina-Fojo S, Lambert G, Hoeg JM, Brewer HB, Jr. Lecithin-cholesterol acyltransferase: role in lipoprotein metabolism, reverse cholesterol transport and atherosclerosis. Curr Opin Lipidol. 2000;11:267–275.
10. Dobiasova M, Frohlich JJ. Advances in understand-

ing of the role of lecithin cholesterol acyltransferase (LCAT) in cholesterol transport. Clin Chim Acta. 1999;286:257–271.
11. Rudel LL, Lee RG, Cockman TL. Acyl coenzyme A: cholesterol acyltransferase types 1 and 2: structure and function in atherosclerosis. Curr Opin Lipidol. 2001;12:121–127.
12. Buhman KF, Accad M, Farese RV. Mammalian acyl-CoA:cholesterol acyltransferases. Biochim Biophys Acta. 2000;1529:142–154.
13. Chang TY, Chang CC, Cheng D. Acyl-coenzyme A:cholesterol acyltransferase. Ann Rev Biochem. 1997;66:613–638.
14. Ostlund RE Jr. Phytosterols and cholesterol metabolism. Curr Opin Lipidol. 2004;15:37–41.
15. Katan MB, Grundy SM, Jones P, et al. Efficacy and safety of plant stanols and sterols in the management of blood cholesterol levels. Mayo Clin Proc. 2003; 78:965–978.
16. Kawai T, Fushiki T. Importance of lipolysis in oral cavity for orosensory detection of fat. Am J Physiol Regul Integr Comp Physiol. 2003;285:R447–R454.
17. Lohse P, Chahrokh-Zadeh S, Seidel D. Human lysosomal acid lipase/cholesteryl ester hydrolase and human gastric lipase: site-directed mutagenesis of Cys227 and Cys236 results in substrate-dependent reduction of enzymatic activity. J Lipid Res. 1997; 38:1896–1905.
18. Mu H, Hoy CE. The digestion of dietary triacylglycerols. Prog Lipid Res. 2004;43:105–133.
19. Pafumi Y, Lairon D, de la Porte PL, et al. Mechanisms of inhibition of triacylglycerol hydrolysis by human gastric lipase. J Biol Chem. 2002;277: 28070–28079.
20. Canaan S, Riviere M, Verger R, Dupuis L. The cysteine residues of recombinant human gastric lipase. Biochem Biophys Res Commun. 1999;257:851–854.
21. Chiang JY. Regulation of bile acid synthesis: pathways, nuclear receptors, and mechanisms. J Hepatol. 2004;40:539–551.
22. Canaan S, Roussel A, Verger R, Cambillau C. Gastric lipase: crystal structure and activity. Biochim Biophy Acta. 1999;1441:197–204.
23. Davis RA, Miyake JH, Hui TY, Spann NJ. Regulation of cholesterol-7alpha-hydroxylase: BAREly missing a SHP. J Lipid Res. 2002;43:533–543.
24. Cohen JC. Contribution of cholesterol 7alpha-hydroxylase to the regulation of lipoprotein metabolism. Curr Opin Lipidol. 1999;10:303–307.
25. Lowe ME. The triglyceride lipases of the pancreas. J Lipid Res. 2002;43:2007–2016.
26. van Tilbeurgh H, Bezzine S, Cambillau C, Verger R, Carriere F. Colipase: structure and interaction with pancreatic lipase. Biochim Biophy Acta. 1999;1441: 173–184.
27. Nordskog BK, Phan CT, Nutting DF, Tso P. An examination of the factors affecting intestinal lymphatic transport of dietary lipids. Adv Drug Deliv Rev. 2001;50:21–44.
28. Chaminade B, Le Balle F, Fourcade O, et al. New developments in phospholipase A2. Lipids. 1999;34 (suppl):S49–S55.
29. Mu H, Hoy CE. Intestinal absorption of specific structured triacylglycerols. J Lipid Res. 2001;42: 792–798.
30. Agellon LB, Toth MJ, Thomson AB. Intracellular lipid binding proteins of the small intestine. Mol Cell Biochem. 2002;239:79–82.
31. Hanhoff T, Lucke C, Spener F. Insights into binding of fatty acids by fatty acid binding proteins. Mol Cell Biochem. 2002;239:45–54.
32. Weiss EP, Brown MD, Shuldiner AR, Hagberg JM. Fatty acid binding protein-2 gene variants and insulin resistance: gene and gene-environment interaction effects. Physiol Genomics. 2002;10:145–157.
33. Dawson PA, Rudel LL. Intestinal cholesterol absorption. Curr Opin Lipidol. 1999;10:315–320.
34. Lopez-Candales A, Grosjlos J, Sasser T, et al. Dietary induction of pancreatic cholesterol esterase: a regulatory cycle for the intestinal absorption of cholesterol. Biochem Cell Biol. 1996;74:257–264.
35. Shamir R, Johnson WJ, Zolfaghari R, Lee HS, Fisher EA. Role of bile salt-dependent cholesteryl ester hydrolase in the uptake of micellar cholesterol by intestinal cells. Biochemistry. 1995;34:6351–6358.
36. Lipka G, Schulthess G, Thurnhofer H, et al. Characterization of lipid exchange proteins isolated from small intestinal brush border membrane. J Biol Chem. 1995;270:5917–5925.
37. Wilund KR, Yu L, Xu F, Hobbs HH, Cohen JC. High-level expression of ABCG5 and ABCG8 attenuates diet-induced hypercholesterolemia and atherosclerosis in Ldlr-/- mice. J Lipid Res. 2004;45: 1429–1436.
38. Sehayek E. Genetic regulation of cholesterol absorption and plasma plant sterol levels: commonalities and differences. J Lipid Res. 2003;44:2030–2038.
39. Davis HR, Jr., Zhu LJ, Hoos LM, et al. Niemann-Pick C1 Like 1 (NPC1L1) is the intestinal phytosterol and cholesterol transporter and a key modulator of whole-body cholesterol homeostasis. J Biol Chem. 2004;279:33586–33592.
40. Altmann SW, Davis HR, Jr., Zhu LJ, et al. Niemann-Pick C1 Like 1 protein is critical for intestinal cholesterol absorption. Science. 2004;303: 1201–1204.
41. Wang J, Williams CM, Hegele RA. Compound heterozygosity for two non-synonymous polymorphisms in NPC1L1 in a non-responder to ezetimibe. Clin Genet. 2004;67:175–177.
42. Field FJ, Mathur SN. beta-sitosterol: esterification by intestinal acylcoenzyme A: cholesterol acyltransf-

erase (ACAT) and its effect on cholesterol esterification. J Lipid Res. 1983;24:409–417.
43. Sudhop T, Lutjohann D, Agna M, von Ameln C, Prange W, von Bergmann K. Comparison of the effects of sitostanol, sitostanol acetate, and sitostanol oleate on the inhibition of cholesterol absorption in normolipemic healthy male volunteers. A placebo controlled randomized cross-over study. Arzneimittelforschung. 2003;53:708–713.
44. Meijer GW, Bressers MA, de Groot WA, Rudrum M. Effect of structure and form on the ability of plant sterols to inhibit cholesterol absorption in hamsters. Lipids. 2003;38:713–721.
45. Redgrave TG. Chylomicron metabolism. Biochem Soc Trans. 2004;32:79–82.
46. Williams CM, Bateman PA, Jackson KG, Yaqoob P. Dietary fatty acids and chylomicron synthesis and secretion. Biochem Soc Trans. 2004;32:55–58.
47. White DA, Morris AJ, Burgess L, Hamburger J, Hamburger R. Facilitators and barriers to improving the quality of referrals for potential oral cancer. Br Dent J. 2004;197:537–540.
48. Gordon DA, Jamil H, Sharp D, et al. Secretion of apolipoprotein B-containing lipoproteins from HeLa cells is dependent on expression of the microsomal triglyceride transfer protein and is regulated by lipid availability. Proc Natl Acad Sci U S A. 1994;91: 7628–7632.
49. Hussain MM. A proposed model for the assembly of chylomicrons. Atherosclerosis. 2000;148:1–15.
50. Joyce C, Skinner K, Anderson RA, Rudel LL. Acyl-coenzyme A:cholesteryl acyltransferase 2. Curr Opin Lipidol. 1999;10:89–95.
51. Ginsberg HN. Lipoprotein metabolism and its relationship to atherosclerosis. Med Clin North Am. 1994;78:1–20.
52. Tso P, Liu M. Ingested fat and satiety. Physiol Behav. 2004;81:275–287.
53. White DA, Bennett AJ, Billett MA, Salter AM. The assembly of triacylglycerol-rich lipoproteins: an essential role for the microsomal triacylglycerol transfer protein. Br J Nutr. 1998;80:219–229.
54. Stein Y, Stein O. Lipoprotein lipase and atherosclerosis. Atherosclerosis. 2003;170:1–9.
55. Merkel M, Eckel RH, Goldberg IJ. Lipoprotein lipase: genetics, lipid uptake, and regulation. J Lipid Res. 2002;43:1997–2006.
56. Saito H, Lund-Katz S, Phillips MC. Contributions of domain structure and lipid interaction to the functionality of exchangeable human apolipoproteins. Prog Lipid Res. 2004;43:350–380.
57. Shachter NS. Apolipoproteins C-I and C-III as important modulators of lipoprotein metabolism. Curr Opin Lipidol. 2001;12:297–304.
58. Cooper AD. Hepatic uptake of chylomicron remnants. J Lipid Res 1997;38:2173–2192.
59. Havel RJ. Remnant lipoproteins as therapeutic targets. Curr Opin Lipidol. 2000;11:615–620.
60. Karpe F. Postprandial lipoprotein metabolism and atherosclerosis. J Intern Med. 1999;246:341–355.
61. Frost PH, Havel RJ. Rationale for use of non-high-density lipoprotein cholesterol rather than low-density lipoprotein cholesterol as a tool for lipoprotein cholesterol screening and assessment of risk and therapy. Am J Cardiol. 1998;81:26B–31B.
62. Shelness GS, Ingram MF, Huang XF, DeLozier JA. Apolipoprotein B in the rough endoplasmic reticulum: translation, translocation and the initiation of lipoprotein assembly. J Nutr. 1999;129:456S–462S.
63. Kendrick JS, Wilkinson J, Cartwright IJ, Lawrence S, Higgins JA. Regulation of the assembly and secretion of very low density lipoproteins by the liver. Biol Chem. 1998;379:1033–1040.
64. Ginsberg HN. Role of lipid synthesis, chaperone proteins and proteasomes in the assembly and secretion of apoprotein B-containing lipoproteins from cultured liver cells. Clin Exp Pharmacol Physiol. 1997;24:A29–A32.
65. Cilingiroglu M, Ballantyne C. Endothelial lipase and cholesterol metabolism. Curr Atheroscler Rep. 2004; 6:126–130.
66. Choi SY, Hirata K, Ishida T, Quertermous T, Cooper AD. Endothelial lipase: a new lipase on the block. J Lipid Res. 2002;43:1763–1769.
67. Zambon A, Bertocco S, Vitturi N, Polentarutti V, Vianello D, Crepaldi G. Relevance of hepatic lipase to the metabolism of triacylglycerol-rich lipoproteins. Biochem Soc Trans. 2003;31:1070–1074.
68. Boucher P, Gotthardt M. LRP and PDGF signaling: A pathway to atherosclerosis. Trends Cardiovasc Med. 2004;14:55–60.
69. Van Berkel TJ, Van Eck M, Herijgers N, Fluiter K, Nion S. Scavenger receptor classes A and B. Their roles in atherogenesis and the metabolism of modified LDL and HDL. Ann N Y Acad Sci. 2000;902: 113–126.
70. Knopp RH. Introduction: low-saturated fat, high-carbohydrate diets: effects on triglyceride and LDL synthesis, the LDL receptor, and cardiovascular disease risk. Proc Soc Exp Biol Med. 2000;225: 175–177.
71. Morgan J, Carey C, Lincoff A, Capuzzi D. High-density lipoprotein subfractions and risk of coronary artery disease. Curr Atheroscler Rep. 2004;6: 359–365.
72. Meagher EA. Addressing cardiovascular risk beyond low-density lipoprotein cholesterol: the high-density lipoprotein cholesterol story. Curr Cardiol Rep. 2004;6:457–463.
73. Marcil M, O'Connell B, Krimbou L, Genest J Jr. High-density lipoproteins: multifunctional vanguards of the cardiovascular system. Expert Rev Cardiovasc Ther. 2004;2:417–430.

74. Tall AR. An overview of reverse cholesterol transport. Eur Heart J. 1998;19 (suppl A):A31–A35.
75. Navab M, Ananthramaiah GM, Reddy ST, et al. The oxidation hypothesis of atherogenesis: the role of oxidized phospholipids and HDL. J Lipid Res. 2004;45:993–1007.
76. Ji Y, Wang N, Ramakrishnan R, et al. Hepatic scavenger receptor BI promotes rapid clearance of high density lipoprotein free cholesterol and its transport into bile. J Biol Chem. 1999;274:33398–33402.
77. Szapary PO, Rader DJ. The triglyceride-high-density lipoprotein axis: an important target of therapy? Am Heart J. 2004;148:211–221.
78. Taskinen MR. LDL-cholesterol, HDL-cholesterol or triglycerides—which is the culprit? Diabetes Res Clin Pract. 2003;61 (suppl 1):S19–S26.
79. Burris TP, Eacho PI, Cao G. Genetic disorders associated with ATP binding cassette cholesterol transporters. Mol Genet Metab. 2002;77:13–20.
80. Oram JF. ATP-binding cassette transporter A1 and cholesterol trafficking. Curr Opin Lipidol. 2002;13: 373–381.
81. Miller M, Rhyne J, Hamlette S, Birnbaum J, Rodriguez A. Genetics of HDL regulation in humans. Curr Opin Lipidol. 2003;14:273–279.
82. Huuskonen J, Olkkonen VM, Jauhiainen M, Ehnholm C. The impact of phospholipid transfer protein (PLTP) on HDL metabolism. Atherosclerosis. 2001; 155:269–281.
83. Tall AR, Jiang X, Luo Y, Silver D. 1999 George Lyman Duff memorial lecture: lipid transfer proteins, HDL metabolism, and atherogenesis. Arterioscler Thromb Vasc Biol. 2000;20:1185–1188.
84. Borggreve SE, De Vries R, Dullaart RP. Alterations in high-density lipoprotein metabolism and reverse cholesterol transport in insulin resistance and type 2 diabetes mellitus: role of lipolytic enzymes, lecithin: cholesterol acyltransferase and lipid transfer proteins. Eur J Clin Invest. 2003;33:1051–1069.
85. Stubbs RJ. The effect of ingesting olestra-based foods on feeding behavior and energy balance in humans. Crit Rev Food Sci Nutr. 2001;41:363–386.
86. Jandacek RJ, Kester JJ, Papa AJ, Wehmeier TJ, Lin PY. Olestra formulation and the gastrointestinal tract. Lipids. 1999;34:771–783.
87. Peters JC, Lawson KD, Middleton SJ, Triebwasser KC. Assessment of the nutritional effects of olestra, a nonabsorbed fat replacement: summary. J Nutr. 1997;127:1719S–1728S.
88. Koonsvitsky BP, Berry DA, Jones MB, et al. Olestra affects serum concentrations of alpha-tocopherol and carotenoids but not vitamin D or vitamin K status in free-living subjects. J Nutr. 1997;127:1636S–1645S.
89. Hutton B, Fergusson D. Changes in body weight and serum lipid profile in obese patients treated with orlistat in addition to a hypocaloric diet: a systematic review of randomized clinical trials. Am J Clin Nutr. 2004;80:1461–1468.
90. Miettinen TA, Gylling H. Plant stanol and sterol esters in prevention of cardiovascular diseases. Ann Med. 2004;36:126–134.
91. Law M. Plant sterol and stanol margarines and health. BMJ. 2000;320:861–864.
92. Richelle M, Enslen M, Hager C, et al. Both free and esterified plant sterols reduce cholesterol absorption and the bioavailability of beta-carotene and alpha-tocopherol in normocholesterolemic humans. Am J Clin Nutr. 2004;80:171–177.

# 10 Lipids: Cellular Metabolism

Peter J.H. Jones and Andrea A. Papamandjaris

The discovery of the importance of lipids in healthy nutrition has been a process spanning the 20th century. Before the 1920s, it was believed that fat did not play an essential dietary role if sufficient vitamins and minerals were in the diet. However, in 1927, Evans and Burr[1] demonstrated that animals fed semi-purified, fat-free diets had impaired growth and reproductive failure. This demonstration that fat was required for health led these authors to postulate that fat contained a new essential substance, which they called vitamin F. Subsequently, Burr and Burr[2] documented the nutritional essentiality of a specific essential component of fat, linoleic acid (C18:2n-6). In the absence of this nutrient, symptoms developed, including scaliness of the skin, water retention, impaired fertility, and growth retardation.[1-3] Thus, the concept of "essential" fatty acids was introduced to represent those dietary fatty acids required by mammals that are not synthesized in vivo.

Fatty acids are classified as essential based on the position of the first double bond from the methyl end of the acyl chain. Mammals do not possess enzymes able to synthesize double bonds at the n-6 and n-3 positions of the carbon chain of a fatty acid. Therefore, humans must obtain the essential fatty acids, linoleic acid and α-linolenic acid (C18:3n-3), and their chain-elongated derivatives, from dietary sources.

Identification of the dietary importance of essential fatty acids in humans followed discovery of their importance in animals. Beginning in 1958, studies in infants using skim milk-based, fat-free diets demonstrated a requirement for essential fatty acids in humans when the introduction of linoleic acid into the diet alleviated skin symptoms.[4] In human adults, the use of fat-free parenteral solutions containing only glucose, amino acids, and micronutrients resulted in clinical fatty acid deficiency, which was reversed by the inclusion of linoleic acid in the solution. In the 1970s, dietary deficiency of n-3 fatty acids was linked to abnormal electroretinographic recordings in animals.[5,6] A human n-3 fatty acid requirement was demonstrated in 1982, when deficiency symptoms, including neuropathy, were linked to a parenteral solution deficient in n-3 fatty acids in a young girl.[7] Symptoms were reversed with the addition of n-3 fatty acids to the solution.

Recent essential fatty acid research has focused on the importance of the dietary ratio of linoleic acid to α-linolenic acid, particularly as it is related to the development of disease.[8-10] Characterization of dietary needs of individual long-chain polyunsaturated fatty acids, arachidonic acid (ARA) (C20:4n-6), docosahexaenoic acid (DHA) (C22:6n-3), and eicosapentaenoic acid (EPA) (C20:5n-3), is also under investigation, notably in infant populations.[11-13] Additionally, the evolutionary importance of DHA in human brain development has been stressed.[14]

In addition to their important roles in membrane phospholipids and as energy sources, polyunsaturated fatty acids are required in the formation of metabolic regulators called eicosanoids. Eicosanoids, as a class of diverse components, function in cardiovascular, pulmonary, immune, secretory, and regulatory systems. The discovery of the unique properties of eicosanoids dates back to the 1930s, when the effect of seminal fluid on the relaxation of the uterus was documented. After further research, Von Euler[15] characterized the active lipid-soluble compound, naming it prostaglandin. In the 1960s, prostaglandin E1 and prostaglandin F1a were isolated from sheep prostate glands.[16,17] Characterization of other prostaglandins followed.[18] The biologically active compounds derived from 20-carbon unsaturated fatty acids were classified as eicosanoids in 1979.[18] The effects and mechanisms of eicosanoids in health and disease are the focus of active, ongoing research. These and additional aspects of essential fatty acid research are leading to a better understanding of their role in human nutrition and health.

## Dietary Sources of Lipids

Lipids are found in a variety of foods (Table 1; see also Table 1 in the Chapter "Lipids: Absorption and Transport" for fatty acid formulas). Butter is a source of short-chain fatty acids. Medium-chain fatty acids are found in coconut oil. Meat contains longer-chain saturates and monounsaturates, whereas vegetable oils are major dietary sources of essential fatty acids and other unsaturated fatty acids. The fatty acid profile of vegetable oils varies widely, and therefore different oils have different proportions of linoleic acid and α-linolenic acid. Safflower, sunflower, corn, and soybean oils are high in linoleic acid, yet, of these, only soybean oil is a significant source of α-linolenic acid. Flaxseed, linseed, and canola oils are also high in α-linolenic acid but relatively low in linoleic acid. Olive and peanut oils have a higher content of monounsaturated oleic acid. Consequently, the consumption of specific vegetable oils as a sole dietary fat source can lead to a deficiency of essential fatty acids.

**Table 1.** Average Triacylglycerol Fatty Acid Composition of Various Foods and Oils

| | | | Average fatty acid composition (%) | | | | | | |
|---|---|---|---|---|---|---|---|---|---|
| | | | Saturated | | | Mono- and polyunsaturated | | | |
| **Food** | **Average fat (%)** | **Total[a]** | **16:0** | **18:0** | **18:1n–9** | **18:2n–6** | **18:3n–3** | **20:4n–6** | |
| Almond oil | 100 | 8 | 6 | 1 | 65 | 23 | Trace | — | |
| Avocado oil | 100 | 11 | 10 | 1 | 67 | 15 | — | — | |
| Beef tallow | 100 | 53 | 29 | 20 | 42 | 2 | Trace | — | |
| Cashew nut | 68 | 24 | 14 | 10 | 30 | 35 | Trace | — | |
| Chicken | 15 | 30 | 25 | 4 | 42 | 21 | — | — | |
| Coconut oil | 100 | 88* | 10 | 3 | 6 | 2 | — | — | |
| Corn oil | 100 | 13 | 11 | 2 | 25 | 55 | Trace | — | |
| Cottonseed oil | 100 | 30 | 25 | 3 | 18 | 51 | Trace | — | |
| Grapeseed oil | 100 | 11 | 7 | 4 | 20 | 68 | Trace | — | |
| Groundnut oil | 100 | 19† | 11 | 3 | 40–55† | 20–43† | — | — | |
| Hazelnut oil | 100 | 7 | 5 | 2 | 80 | 11 | Trace | — | |
| Hemp oil | 100 | 9 | 6 | 3 | 13 | 55 | 16‡ | — | |
| Herring (menhaden) | 16–25 | 30 | 19 | 4 | 13 | 1 | 1§ | — | |
| Mackerel‖ | 25 | 25 | 17 | 5 | 18 | 1 | — | — | |
| Milk (cow) | 3.5 | 65* | 25 | 11 | 26 | 1–3 | 2 | Trace | |
| Olive oil | 100 | 17 | 14 | 3 | 71 | 10 | Trace | — | |
| Palm kernel oil | 100 | 80* | 7 | 2 | 14 | 1 | — | — | |
| Palm oil | 100 | 52 | 45 | 5 | 38 | 10 | — | — | |
| Pork fat (lard) | 100 | 42 | 28 | 13 | 46 | 6–8 | 2 | 2 | |
| Rapeseed oil | 100 | 7 | 5 | 2 | 53 | 22 | 10¶ | — | |
| Safflower seed oil | 100 | 10 | 7 | 3 | 15# | 75# | Trace | — | |
| Sesame oil | 100 | 15 | 9 | 5 | 39 | 40 | 1 | — | |
| Soybean oil | 100 | 15 | 11 | 4 | 23 | 51 | 7 | — | |
| Sunflower seed oil | 100 | 12 | 6 | 4 | 24 | 60–70 | Trace | — | |
| Walnut | 63 | 10 | 7 | 2 | 15 | 60 | 10 | — | |
| Wheat germ oil | 100 | 18 | 17 | Trace | 17 | 55 | 6 | — | |

Note: The percentages given are approximations, because climate, species, fodder composition, etc., cause great variations. Trace, <1% detected. Dash, nondetectable amounts.*The balance of saturated fatty acids is formed by fatty acids with chain lengths <12 (butter 14%) and chain lengths of 12 and 14 (butter 16%, coconut and palm kernel 65–70%).†Circa 4% of C20:0 and C22:0; groundnuts from Argentina have relatively low C18:1 and high C18:2 concentrations.‡Also contains 18:3n–6.§Menhaden herring oil has 11% C20:5n–3 and 9% C22:6n–3, but Norwegian herring oil has 13% C20:1n–9, 21% C22:1n–11, 7% C20:5n–3, and 7% C22:6n–3. ‖Depending on fishing grounds, mackerel oil is similar to menhaden or to Norwegian/North Sea herring.¶Contrary to new rapeseed varieties like Canbra and LEAR, old varieties of rapeseed oil as well as mustard seed oil have 10% C20:1n–9 and 30–50% C22:1n–9.#Safflower seed oil with the reverse C18:1/18:2 composition is also available.

Long-chain polyenoic fatty acids, products of intracellular elongation and desaturation of essential fatty acids, are not present in vegetable oils but are found in some animal products. Particularly, high-fat fish and marine mammals contain larger amounts of long-chain n-3 fatty acids, EPA and DHA. The longer-chain n-6 fatty acids, such as arachidonic acid, are found in foods of animal origin, including organ meats. Smaller quantities of very-long-chain fatty acids and alcohols (more than 24 carbons) are found in plant-derived foods. Cholesterol is found only in products of animal origin, while phytosterols (or plant sterols) occur in plant oils.

Recently, focus has shifted to the development of functional foods that incorporate essential fatty acids and other lipids to offer added healthful benefits to consumers. Examples include bakery products made with flaxseed oil, eggs containing marine n-3 fatty acids, and spreads incorporating phytosterols, or their saturated derivatives, phytostanols. Additionally, foods that require oil during preparation are currently made with vegetable-based rather than animal-based oils, thereby decreasing the amount of saturated and or trans fats incorporated in the diet.

## Cellular Roles of Lipids

Lipid constituents are required for a diverse array of cellular processes, including structure, function, and energy-related roles. Polyenoic fatty acids provide the hydrophobic moiety of phospholipids, which are critical for membrane structure and serve as precursors for eicosanoids, which regulate cellular activity. Fatty acids also play a pivotal role in providing fuel for adenosine triphosphate (ATP) and reducing equivalents and in generating body heat. Fat contains more than twice the energy per gram as does carbohydrate or protein, which explains why humans preferentially store fat as the primary energy reservoir. Dietary lipids are also a source of lipid-soluble vitamins and sterols. Although not essential in the diet, cholesterol is needed as an integral component of membranes to increase their fluidity. Cholesterol is also converted to bile salts through hepatic hydroxylation and conjugation. Bile salts are required for normal digestion and absorption of dietary lipids. Additionally, cholesterol serves as a precursor for steroid-based hormone systems, including sex and adrenocorticoid hormones. Cholesterol, as 7-dehydrocholesterol, exists as the precursor of vitamin D, formed at the skin surface through the action of ultraviolet irradiation. Approximately 50 mg of cholesterol is converted to steroid hormones daily.

To ensure normal cellular function, an elaborate system regulates lipid biosynthesis, oxidation, and intracellular trafficking. This homeostatic regulatory system ensures that pathways of lipid anabolism and catabolism mesh with those of other macronutrients. Dominating this regulatory system is the ability of dietary lipid selection to modulate several key metabolic pathways. For example, the fatty acid composition of the diet alters the composition of membrane phospholipids, which in turn changes membrane functions. Similarly, the blend of dietary fatty acids substantially alters adipose tissue fatty acid profiles.[19] Dietary fatty acid selection also modulates cellular synthesis of regulatory eicosanoids, influencing a series of physiological responses. Similarly, alterations in cholesterol or phytosterol intake modulate cholesterol synthesis, absorption, and subsequent metabolism. Consequently, the metabolism of fatty acids, sterols, and their derivatives responds to manipulation in dietary lipid intakes in many important ways. To appreciate the link between dietary lipid consumption and disease risk modification, it is important to individually consider the fundamental processes of cellular lipid metabolism.

## Lipid Biosynthesis

### *Fatty Acid Synthesis*

Fatty acids are synthesized de novo from acetyl coenzyme A (CoA) in the extramitochondrial space by a group of enzymes classified as fatty acid synthetases. The synthesis of fatty acids is governed by the enzyme acetyl CoA carboxylase, which converts acetyl CoA to malonyl CoA. A series of malonyl CoA units are added to the growing fatty acid chain to culminate in the formation of palmitic acid (C16:0). From this point, more complex fatty acids can be formed through elongation and desaturation; however, humans do not possess the enzymes capable of inserting points of unsaturation at sites below the n-7 carbon, making the n-6 and the n-3 fatty acids essential (see the chapter "Lipids: Absorption and Transport" for a discussion of nomenclature). Desaturase enzymes are membrane bound and occur in the endoplasmic recticulum of several tissues. Desaturases are specific for the position of the double bond in the carbon chain and require electrons supplied by nicotinamide adenine dinucleotide (NADH) or nicotinamide adenine dinucleotide phosphate (NADPH), which are catalyzed by cytochrome b5.

Longer-chain fatty acids are synthesized from C16:0, C18:0, C18:2n-6, and C18:3n-3 by alternating desaturation and elongation. The synthesis of C20:4n-6 from C18:2n-6 and of C20:5n-3 from C18:3n-3 is achieved through D6 desaturation followed by elongation and D5 desaturation (Figure 1). The synthesis of C22:6n-3 from C20:5n-3 occurs through elongation, desaturation, and partial $\alpha$-oxidation.[20] It was recently demonstrated that fatty acid elongation need not commence with 18-carbon precursors. To meet n-6 fatty acid requirements, it is possible to use C16:2n-6, derived from plant materials, in place of linoleic acid, thereby effectively reducing the requirement for the latter fatty acid.[21] The extent to which this pathway contributes substantially to in vivo linoleic acid levels remains to be assessed.

| | n–7 fatty acids | n–9 fatty acids | n–6 EFA | n–3 EFA |
|---|---|---|---|---|
| | Palmitic 16:0 | Stearic 18:0 | | |
| Δ9 Desaturase ↓ | Palmitoleic 16:1n–7 | Oleic 18:1n–9 | Linoleic 18:2n–6 | α-Linolenic 18:3n–3 |
| Δ6 Desaturase ↓ | 16:2n–7 | 18:2n–9 | γ-Linolenic 18:3n–6 | 18:4n–3 |
| Elongase ↓ | 18:2n–7 | 20:2n–9 | Dihomo-γ-linolenic 20:3n–6 | 20:4n–3 |
| Δ5 Desaturase ↓ | 18:3n–7 | Eicosatrienoic 20:3n–9 | Arachidonic 20:4n–6 | Eicosapentaenoic 20:5n–5 |
| Elongase ↓ | 20:3n–7 | 22:3n–9 | Docosatetraenoic 22:4n–6 | 22:5n–3 |
| Desaturase/oxidation ↓ | | | 22:5n–6 | Docosahexaenoic 22:6n–3 |

Figure 1. Interconversions of nonessential and essential fatty acids. EFA, essential fatty acid.

The synthesis of longer-chain fatty acids has been shown to be regulated by the D6 desaturase enzyme, which in turn is influenced by hormones and dietary constituents. The D6 desaturase preferentially targets the most highly unsaturated fatty acid; therefore, the preferential desaturation order is C18:3n-3 > C18:2n-6 > C18:1n-9. As such, the competitive nature of the fatty acid desaturation and elongation among the three classes of fatty acids (Figure 1) has nutritional implications. The consumption of diets rich in n-6 fatty acids can result in suppression of the elongation and desaturation of C18:3n-3 to C20:5n-3 and C22:6n-3. An example of this situation is infant formulas, in which high ratios of C18:2n-6 to C18:3n-3 potentially depress the production of important n-3 polyenoic fatty acids required for the developing nervous system. Alternatively, changing prostaglandin profiles through elevated intakes of n-3 fatty acids such as EPA and DHA from fish and fish oils can decrease the clotting capacity of blood. Hormonal shifts may also perturb desaturase activity: insulin increases, but glucagon and epinephrine decrease, desaturase enzyme activity.[22]

Reversal of the elongation and desaturation process may also occur intracellularly. Very-long-chain and long-chain n-3 and n-6 fatty acids may undergo shortening and saturation through retroconversion to other, shorter fatty acids.[23] This process occurs in peroxisomes and is probably necessary for some, if not all, of the endogenous synthesis of DHA in animals.[20]

## *Cholesterol Biosynthesis*

Cholesterol is synthesized in almost all human tissues in a process that has more than 20 steps; indeed, the pathway is one of the longest of any lipid produced intracellularly. Humans likely once relied extensively on endogenously produced cholesterol for cellular requirements, as ancestral daily dietary intakes have been estimated at as low as 50 mg. However, today, most people consume diets in which the dietary intake of cholesterol and fat is increased such that cholesterogenesis is less relied on to serve cellular cholesterol needs. Unlike animals, humans appear to synthesize most cholesterol in extrahepatic tissues. The total body pool of cholesterol is estimated to be 75 g. Of the 1200 mg cholesterol turned over daily, 300 to 500 mg are absorbed from the diet and de novo synthesis accounts for 700 to 900 mg.[24] How synthesis is coordinated across tissues remains to be defined.

As with fatty acids, the process of cholesterol synthesis begins with acetyl CoA generated through the oxidative decarboxylation of pyruvate or the oxidation of fatty acids. In the initial phase of the pathway, acetyl CoA molecules combine to form mevalonic acid. The final enzyme of this initial phase, hydroxymethylglutaryl (HMG) CoA reductase, is considered to be rate limiting in the overall cascade of cholesterogenesis and has been studied widely in relation to pathway control. In fact, statin drugs, currently the most widespread pharmacological intervention to lower cholesterol levels, work through inhibition of HMG CoA reductase. The later phase of cholesterol biosynthesis involves steps of phosphorylation, isomerization, and conversion to geranyl-B and farnesyl-pyrophosphate, which in turn form squalene. From the squalene stage, loss of three methyl groups, side chain saturation, and bond rearrangement result in the formation of cholesterol.

Diet modulates cholesterol biosynthesis in several ways. Curiously, it is a common misconception that high levels of dietary cholesterol increase circulating levels of cholesterol; however, total and low-density lipoprotein (LDL) cholesterol levels as well as cholesterol biosynthesis are minimally affected by even sizable increases in dietary cholesterol concentration.[25,26] Conversely, qualitative dietary fat intake more substantially perturbs the rate of cholesterol biosynthesis and circulating lipid levels. In particular, dietary polyunsaturated fat intake enhances,[27] whereas trans fatty acid intake suppresses,[28] cholesterol biosynthesis. Increasing the number of meals consumed per day, while holding total caloric intake constant, has also been shown to reduce sterol biosynthesis rates.[27] Of the dietary factors capable of modifying cholesterol synthesis, energy restriction has the greatest effect. Humans who fast for 24 hours exhibit complete cessation of cholesterol biosynthesis.[27] How synthesis responds to more minor energy imbalances has not been examined; however, substantial suppression of human de novo cholesterogenesis has been demonstrated with even modest levels of energy restriction and weight loss.[29]

## *Fatty Acid Oxidation*

Fatty acid oxidation generates acetyl CoA and occurs through β-oxidation, predominantly in mitochondria. During this process, the fatty acyl chain undergoes cyclical degradation through four stages, including dehydrogenation (removal of hydrogen), hydration (addition of water), dehydrogenation, and cleavage. At points of unsaturation within the acyl chain, the initial dehydration step does not take place. The four-stage oxidation process is repeated until the fatty acid is completely degraded to acetyl CoA, as shown by the absence of intracellular or circulatory n-3 or n-6 chain-shortened fatty acids. Fatty acids containing 18 carbons or fewer enter the mitochondria as fatty acyl CoA through transport by carnitine. Short- and medium-chain fatty acids do not require the presence of the carnitine shuttle to enter the mitochondria for oxidation.

Beta-oxidation also occurs in peroxisomes through a similar, but not identical, process that is tailored to the oxidation of long-chain fatty acids with more than 18 carbons. Also, the initial desaturation reaction in peroxisomal β-oxidation occurs via a fatty acyl CoA oxidase, whereas an acyl CoA dehydrogenase is the first enzyme in the mitochondrial pathway. Last, peroxisomal β-oxidation is not tightly linked to the electron transfer chain. Thus, in peroxisomes, electrons produced during the initial stage of oxidation transfer directly to molecular oxygen. This oxygen generates hydrogen peroxide that is degraded to water by catalase. The energy produced in the second oxidation step is conserved in the form of the high-energy-level electrons of NADH.

Evidence is emerging that the rate of fatty acid oxidation is not identical across all chain lengths and degrees of unsaturation, but exhibits structural specificity. For decades, it has been suggested that short- and medium-chain saturated fatty acids undergo more rapid combustion for energy compared with long-chain fatty acids, probably because of the preferential transport of the former linked to albumin through the portal circulation and the lack of need for carnitine to enter the mitochondria.[30] In addition, the notion that more highly unsaturated long-chain fatty acids are preferentially oxidized has also received some support,[31] although this concept is paradoxical given the essentiality of these highly unsaturated polyunsaturated fatty acids. Intriguingly, carbon from oxidized linoleic and α-linolenic acid is extensively recycled into de novo synthesis of long-chain fatty acids and cholesterol. This pathway is particularly evident in the brain during early development,[32] but is quantitatively important even when intake of these parent polyunsaturates is severely deficient.[33]

In addition to the effect exerted by the type of fatty acid consumed, variations in the metabolic state also influence the rate of fat oxidation. Conditions such as fasting and exercise at moderate intensity result in increased lipolysis and oxidation.[34-36] With respect to substrates and hormones, raised glucose and insulin levels suppress fatty acid oxidation.[37]

## Eicosanoid Production and Regulation

Structurally, as oxygenated 20-carbon derivatives from the n-3 and n-6 family of fatty acids, eicosanoid members include prostaglandins, thromboxanes, leukotrienes, hydroxy acids, and lipoxins. The production of specific categories of eicosanoids is governed by fast-acting and rapidly inactivated enzyme systems. Whereas prostaglandins and thromboxanes are generated via cyclooxygenase enzymes, leukotrienes, hydroxy acids, and lipoxins are produced through the action of lipoxygenase (LO). Major pathways for eicosanoid synthesis are depicted in Figure 2. The process begins with the action of phospholipase A2 on cell membrane phospholipids, splitting off fatty acids from the sn-2 position of the molecule. All membrane phospholipid species serve as substrates in the

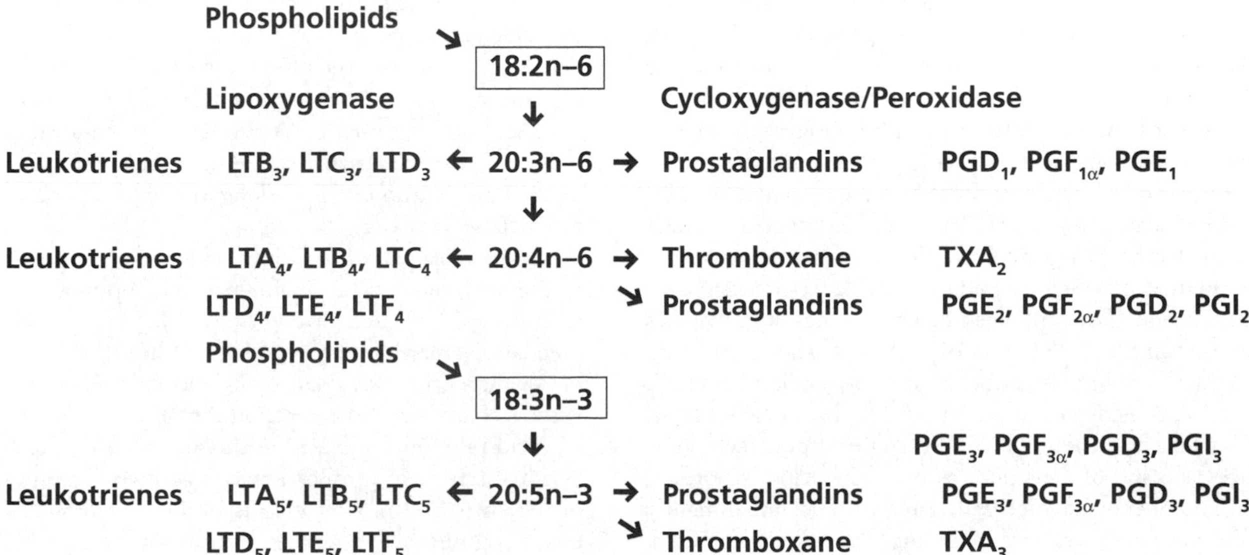


Figure 2. Synthesis of major eicosanoids from n-6 and n-3 fatty acids.

cleavage process; the resultant cleaved fatty acids serve directly as substrates for eicosanoid production via the cyclooxygenase and lipoxygenase enzyme cascades. With respect to the n-6 series, cleaved arachidonic acid is transformed to prostaglandins by prostaglandin H synthase-1 (PGHSB1) and prostaglandin H synthase-2 (PGHSB2). These enzymes catalyze the conversion of arachidonic acid to prostaglandin G2 (PGG2) via a cyclooxygenase reaction, and then the reduction of PGG2 to PGH2 via a peroxidase reaction. This latter intermediate then undergoes rapid conversion to other active forms of prostaglandins, thromboxanes, or prostacyclins. As an alternative pathway, arachidonic acid undergoes oxidation via a series of LO enzymes to form a series of active eicosanoids. The 5-LO pathway generates leukotrienes B4, C4, and D4 (LTB4, LTC4, and LTD4), which are believed to serve as mediators in the immune response. The 12-LO pathway generates 12-L-hydroxyeicosatetranoic acid (12-HETE) and 12-hydroperoxyeicosatetranoic acid (12-HPETE), which are also involved in the inflammatory response. The action of a third LO reaction pathway, 15-LO, results in the formation of 15-hydroeicosatetranoic acid (15-HETE), which possesses anti-inflammatory actions and may inhibit the activities of both 5-LO and 12-LO. Thus, several eicosanoid subtypes may be generated from arachidonic acid intracellularly.

Eicosanoids are also derived from the n-3 series of fatty acids cleaved from membrane phospholipids. Eicosanoids derived from n-3 fatty acids evoke less-active responses than do those of the corresponding n-6 eicosanoids. Thus, PGE3 formed from EPA possesses less inflammatory action than does PGE2 formed from arachidonic acid. Similarly, LTB5 derived from EPA is less active in the pro-inflammatory response than is LTB4, which is produced from arachidonic acid. On these bases, the two classes of eicosanoids compete, evoking opposing biological actions.

Dietary fatty acid composition has been shown to play an important role in eicosanoid-mediated function. The consumption of diets high in n-3-rich fats produces higher levels of n-3 fatty acids in phospholipids. These fatty acids, when cleaved from phospholipase, compete with arachidonic acid for incorporation into eicosanoids. The enhanced bleeding times observed in Inuit populations who consume higher levels of n-3 fatty acid containing fish reflect the shift from n-6 to n-3-based eicosanoid formation. PGI3, produced from EPA, has anti-aggregatory action. The prolonged bleeding times in individuals consuming high amounts of n-3 fatty acids containing marine-based foods are believed to be mediated through such anti-aggregatory action of n-3- based eicosanoids. Conversely, eicosanoid overproduction from arachidonic acid, a result of diets poor in n-3 fatty acids, may result in a number of disorders associated with the inflammatory and immune systems, including thrombosis, arthritis, lupus, and cancer (see section below). For instance, arthritic patients appear to benefit from increasing their intake of fish oil,[38] likely at least in part to the inhibition by n-3 fatty acids of the production of the pro-inflammatory eicosanoids LTB4 and PGE2. The demonstration that dietary fatty acid selection may modulate physiological function through eicosanoid generation underscores the importance of food selection in the prevention and treatment of disease.

# Dietary Requirements

Currently, dietary recommendations for omega-3 fatty acids are 1.6 g/d for men and 1.1 g/d for women, while omega-6 fatty acids recommendations are 17 g/d for men and 12 g/d for women.[39] These values were established based on the levels of fatty acids required to prevent or alleviate essential fatty acid deficiency. Deficiency symptoms were documented when patients were fed total parenteral nutrition solutions devoid of essential fatty acids in the 1960s. Skin irritations that developed during fat-free diets were alleviated when patients were fed solutions containing linoleic acid.[4] Recent evidence indicates that pure linoleate deficiency, in contrast to general unsaturated fatty acid deficiency categorized previously, can be reversed with as little as 2% of dietary energy fed as linoleic acid in the rat.[21] For α-linolenic acid, classification of deficiency symptoms has been difficult, since related deficiencies are more subtle than those found with linoleic acid. Also, pure deficiencies are hard to induce, because symptoms may remain absent in the presence of DHA.

Based on essential fatty acid metabolism, an indicator for essential fatty acid deficiency is the triene-to-tetraene ratio, which assesses the ratio of C20:3n-9 to C20:4n-6. The triene, C20:3n-9, is the product of the desaturation of C18:1n-9 to C20:3n-9 (Figure 2). Because of the affinity of the D6 desaturase for essential fatty acids more than 16 carbons in length, the triene concentrations increase only during essential fatty acid deficiency, when C16:0 and C18:1n-9 are the major substrates available. A triene-to-tetraene ratio above 0.4 indicates essential fatty acid deficiency. However, the ratio is not specific to deficiency of linoleic or α-linolenic acid. To assess for α-linolenic deficiency, the ratio of DPA to DHA can be a valuable index, because the absence of n-3 fatty acids results in the increased formation of n-6 elongation and desaturation products.

As the roles of essential fatty acids and their products in the achievement and maintenance of optimal health are further elucidated through research, dietary recommendations may be set on the basis of health promotion rather than on the avoidance of deficiency. An example is the recognition of the contribution of the ratio of linoleic acid to α-linolenic acid in the diet toward a healthy essential fatty acid profile. The competitive desaturation of n-3, n-6, and n-9 fatty acids by D6 desaturase is of major significance consistent with this rationale. If α-linolenic acid is lacking in the diet or if there is a large amount of linoleic acid present, EPA production will become elevated and little or no DHA will be produced. If both essential fatty acids are lacking, C20:3n-9 will accumulate. Inhibition of arachidonic acid and DHA production achieved through high levels of linoleic acid or essential fatty acid deficiency may be undesirable, based on the metabolic functions of these compounds and their roles in disease onset and progression (see below).

Beginning in the 1920s, the levels of linoleic acid in the Western diet have been increasing and the levels of α-linolenic acid decreasing.[8,40] Estimates of the current ratio of linoleic to α-linolenic acid in North America range from 9.8:1[41] to 20:1 to 30:1.[8] A ratio of 2:1 to 5:1 is currently recommended,[8,37,41,42] with the World Health Organization (WHO)-recommended level at 5: 1 to 10:1.[43] Achieving this recommended ratio would require a reversal in the trend of fatty acid consumption, with the inclusion of greater amounts of n-3 fatty acids from plant and marine oils in tandem with the consumption of lower amounts of n-6 fatty acids from seed oil in the diet. The consequences of the long-term consumption of a high ratio of n-6 to n-3 fatty acids are being studied and will provide further insight into healthy dietary essential fatty acid levels. At present, arachidonic acid and DHA are not considered essential to a healthy adult diet, unless the capacity for desaturation and elongation of essential fatty acids is compromised.

Dietary essential fatty acid requirements in infants are being widely investigated, because there might be a need to provide not only essential fatty acids, but arachidonic acid and DHA as well. Preterm infants, depending on age at birth, may not receive an intrauterine supply of arachidonic acid and DHA[40] and, if formula fed, may not receive arachidonic acid and DHA, but only 18-carbon essential fatty acids. Recently, conventional infant formulas have been produced that contain added DHA and ARA. DHA and ARA are often added at levels concurrent with the WHO guidelines, which are based on international levels of DHA and ARA in breast milk.[44,45] Because both brain and retina have high levels of DHA, it has been hypothesized that DHA in breast milk may confer a developmental advantage to both term and preterm infants, as has been reported with breast feeding.[46,47] These findings have been somewhat supported by the results of clinical intervention studies, in which direct supplementation of formula with n-3 fatty acids resulted in improvements in development-associated parameters.[48-50] Without the inclusion of arachidonic acid and DHA, there may not be sufficient capacity to convert essential fatty acids into arachidonic acid and, more specifically, into DHA to meet requirements for brain and visual function.[51] Results in preterm infants have demonstrated evidence that DHA supplementation may affect visual acuity and development,[52-56] but not all studies show positive benefits.[57] A recent review of the clinical trials published to date in preterm infants has concluded that the long-term benefits of DHA and ARA formula supplementation have yet to be demonstrated.[58] For infants born at term, research has demonstrated that formula supplementation with DHA may[59-65] or may not[66,67] affect development, and that any effect may disappear over time.[68,69] No differences were reported in age appropriate tests of receptive and expressive language, IQ, visual or motor function, or visual acuity in infants at 39 months that had either been breast-fed or formula-fed with formula that either did or did not contain DHA and ARA.[50] Continued research in this area in both term and preterm infants using well-controlled studies with large sample sizes will address the long-term and short-term effects of DHA and arachidonic acid supplementation on visual and cognitive development.[11,40]

## Dietary Fatty Acids and Disease Risk

Scientists and the general public alike are interested in the importance of comparative fatty acid selection in relation to health and longevity. Consensus is beginning to emerge concerning the role of qualitative fat intake in the management of disease risk. For certain diseases common to Western civilization, the evidence for reducing risk by adopting certain fat intake profiles is compelling; for other diseases, the link remains speculative. This rapidly progressing field will undoubtedly see further development as research advances our knowledge. Quantitative fat intake is undergoing renewed scrutiny as scientists debate the percentage of daily energy from fat that is necessary for optimal health.

Current recommendations relating to quantitative fat intake call for a reduction in total fat and saturated fat intakes.[70-73] The basis for such recommendations comes from epidemiological evidence indicating that body weight is positively correlated with quantitative fat and not carbohydrate intake.[74] Additionally, research has shown that increasing the fat content of a diet promotes fat storage in adipose tissue rather than fat oxidation[75,76] (see the chapters "Obesity," "Changing Dietary Behavior," and "Hunger and Appetite.") However, not all evidence establishes a link between quantitative fat intake and obesity. Willett[77] demonstrated that a decrease in dietary fat as a percentage of energy has not resulted in a decrease in overweight and obesity. Indeed, there is insufficient evidence to link percentage energy from dietary fat with obesity.[78] It may be more effective to focus on qualitative fat consumption—notably, decreased saturated fat and increased unsaturated fat—combined with recommendations to restrict energy intakes.[79,80] Such an approach would acknowledge the overall importance of the metabolic actions of all fatty acids in the diet, which is an increasing area of focus in fatty acid research.[81] This approach would also recognize the link between percent fat and energy density, and the influence on total caloric intake.[82,83]

**Table 2.** Diseases Influenced by Qualitative Polyunsaturated Fatty Acid Intake in Humans

| |
|---|
| Coronary heart disease and stroke |
| Essential fatty acid deficiency during development |
| Autoimmune disorders, including lupus and nephropathy |
| Type 2 diabetes |
| Inflammatory bowel disease |
| Breast, colon, and prostate cancers |
| Rheumatoid arthritis |

Table 2 lists diseases linked to the relationship between polyunsaturated and other fatty acids in the diet. Of these disorders, coronary heart disease is the most strongly linked with qualitative fat intake. Although it has been well established that the consumption of n-9 and n-6 fatty acids favorably reduces circulating levels of total cholesterol and LDL cholesterol, n-3 fatty acids recently have been the focus of much attention.[10,80,84-86] The surprisingly low cardiovascular mortality rate in Native Alaskans consuming traditional diets high in EPA and DHA alerted researchers to the fact that in the presence of elevated total fat intakes, n-3 fatty acids are effective in reducing disease risk. The influence of fish oils on cardiovascular disease risk is multifactorial. Fish oils reduce very-low-density lipoprotein (VLDL) secretion, lower triacylglycerol transport, and may enhance VLDL clearance.[84] The net effect often is a reduction of circulating triacylglycerol levels. For LDL cholesterol, the data are clearer for n-9 and n-6 fatty acids, as the consumption of these fats results in unequivocal depression of circulating levels. However, for n-3 fatty acids, the data are more controversial; evidence indicates that LDL cholesterol may increase marginally in humans fed fish oil. Similarly, in vitro plasma lipid oxidizability is enhanced in animals fed fish oil. The consumption of diets high in n-6 fatty acids generally results in the suppression of HDL cholesterol levels, whereas n-9 fatty acid intake does not affect values. Studies of the effects on blood lipids of n-3-containing fish oils suggest that HDL cholesterol levels are maintained or elevated with fish oil consumption.

The action of n-3 fatty acids in reducing coronary heart disease risk is not related solely to effects on circulating lipids. Fish oil-derived fatty acids may also increase endothelium-dependent dilatation of arteries, which is thought to be beneficial in risk reduction for atherosclerosis. Moreover, polyenoic n-3 fatty acids are receiving considerable attention as potential anti-inflammatory agents.[87-89] In vitro studies comparing the action of various long-chain polyunsaturated fatty acids on endothelial tissue activation as assessed by surface enzyme immunoassay or flow cytometry found no effect. However, a progressive increase in the inhibition of cytokine-induced expression of adhesion molecules was observed with increasing degrees of fatty acid unsaturation from monounsaturated fatty acids to polyenoic n-3 fatty acids. Endothelial activation was most highly inhibited with n-3 versus n-6 or n-9 fatty acids.

In addition, the beneficial effects of dietary n-3 fatty acids on coronary heart disease risk are thought to be mediated via the prevention of arrhythmias, particularly ventricular tachycardia and fibrillation, as well as by favorable modulation of prostaglandin and leukotriene production to reduce thrombogenesis.[90,91] It can be surmised that dietary fat selection consistent with maximal reduction in cardiovascular disease risk would result in lower levels of saturated fats and higher intakes of EPA and DHA from fish oil. Based on current knowledge, this approach would be appropriate for both primary and secondary disease prevention.

A second critical health issue regarding the selection of dietary fatty acids is the need for adequate intakes of essential fatty acids during fetal development and shortly following birth. As noted above, polyenoic unsaturated fatty acids are important components of neural structure membrane phospholipids. Major phospholipid classes in brain and retina contain high levels of DHA. DHA is considered a conditionally essential nutrient for adequate growth in humans.[92] Prolonged absence of dietary n-6 or n-3 fatty acids results in depressed levels of phospholipid polyenoic fatty acids. Of particular interest is the definition of what constitutes adequate dietary n-3 fatty acid levels; neural tissue DHA levels fall to one-fifth the normal amount in animals deprived of n-3 fats.[93] In addition to structural changes, n-3 fatty acid deficiency also results in pronounced behavioral changes. In rhesus monkeys, perinatal n-3 deficiency resulted in functional changes in offspring including reduced vision, electroretinogram irregularities, polydipsia, and possibly cognition disturbances.[94] Although the behavioral changes in animals deprived of n-3 fatty acids may be due directly to impaired neural cell function, secondary neurotransmitter-related effects arise from n-3 fatty acid deficiency. In rats deficient in n-3 fatty acids, behavioral disturbances were shown to be associated with changes in dopaminergic neurotransmission in the nucleus accumbens region of the brain.[95]

By extension, a critical issue relating to human health is the quantity and composition of n-3 fatty acids in infant formulas. Probably because of reduced levels of polyenoic long-chain fatty acids in infant formulas compared with human breast milk, formula-fed infants have lower levels of DHA in the brain.[96] Although earlier formulas had notoriously imbalanced ratios of n-3 to n-6 fatty acids, the use of soybean oil has markedly improved this ratio in modern formulas. However, the n-3 fatty acids are provided largely as α-linolenic acid, which may not be fully converted to DHA by developing infants. Current debate focuses on whether infant formula would benefit from direct supplementation with highly polyunsaturated fatty acids of both the n-6 and the n-3 classes.[46-68] Manufacturing processes presently add specific antioxidants to reduce the possibility of oxidative damage, which allows the routine addition of long-chain polyunsaturated fatty acids. Results at this time remain equivocal, but continued study with reliable sources of DHA and ARA, such as single-cell oils and standardized developmental tests, should permit the establishment of consensus in the near future.

The relationship between dietary fat composition and inflammatory bowel disease is increasingly recognized.[97,98] Although it has been proposed that olive oil and oils containing n-6 fatty acids are potentially beneficial, most interest is centered on the use of dietary fish oil to improve remission rates of Crohn's disease and to suppress the symptoms and histological appearance of ulcerative colitis. Results from recent studies are not unequivocal; however, evidence suggests that the consumption of n-3 fatty acids, particularly as fish oil, improves the clinical management of inflammatory bowel disease.[99] The likely reason is that n-3 fatty acids suppress LTB4 and thromboxane A2, both of which are derived from arachidonic acid and are associated with mucosal inflammation.

The role of dietary fat composition in cancer risk remains controversial. It has been demonstrated that the effects of specific fatty acids on mammary carcinogenesis vary in both in vitro and in vivo animal models, with stimulatory effects observed for linoleic acid compared with saturated fatty acids.[100] Mechanistically, cyclooxygenase and lipoxygenase products derived from n-6 fatty acids may stimulate the growth factors and oncogenes that are responsible for the increased carcinogenesis. Alternatively, the inhibition of calcium mobilization, which is linked to cell signaling and cell proliferation, may be affected by the presence of higher cellular concentrations of EPA and DHA.[101] The link with n-6 fatty acid consumption and prostate cancer remains weak. Mounting evidence does, however, suggest a beneficial role of n-3 fatty acids compared with other fats in the suppression of breast and prostate cancers.[100,102-106]

Evidence linking the consumption of n-3 fatty acids with reduced severity of arthritic symptoms remains controversial despite reported improvements in the incidence of tender joints and joint stiffness in a meta-analysis of studies reporting n-3 fatty acid supplement use.[105] The effect probably involves altered eicosanoid metabolism and interleukin-1α levels. In general, patients are advised to consume 3 to 6 g/d of n-3 fatty acids to achieve benefits against arthritis, although further confirmation of this association is needed.

A model demonstrating the possible effects of different levels of essential fatty acids and long-chain polyunsaturated fatty acids on the disease states discussed above is illustrated in Figure 3.[8,40,106,107] The model demonstrates the interrelated manner in which various dietary lipid components interact to influence disease outcome, and highlights the heterogeneity of dietary lipid constituents. It also points out potential beneficial actions of increasing the ratio of n-3 to n-6 fatty acid intake; however, the possible risk of increasing peroxidative status with the elevation in degree of unsaturation of the fat consumed must also be considered.

Overall, research suggests that dietary lipid selection plays a central role in the prevention and development of several important chronic diseases.[108] An emerging conclusion is that the ratio of linoleic acid to α-linolenic acid may be of importance in the etiology of several of these

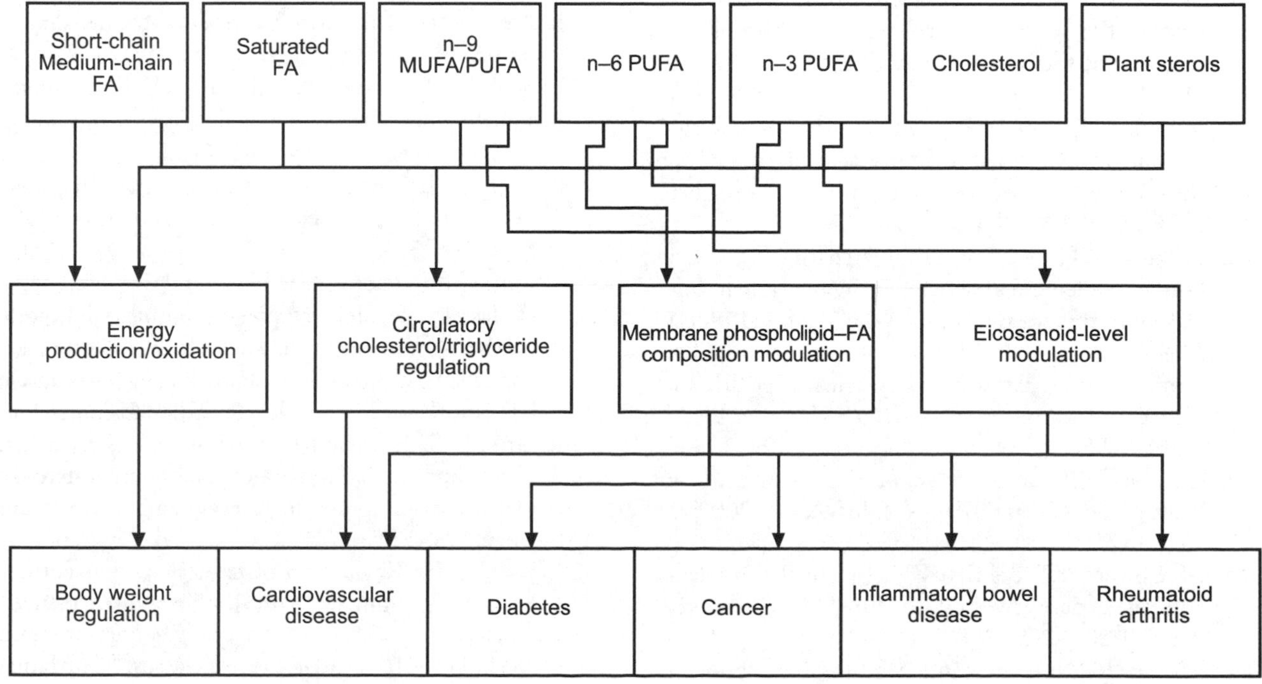


Figure 3. Interaction among dietary lipid components, metabolic systems, and disease/health outcomes.

conditions. Evidence suggests that a lower ratio may be protective. Given the present high ratio of 18:2n-6 to 18:3n-3 in the Western-style diet,[8] dietary recommendations to include greater amounts of n-3 fatty acids may be valuable in preventing disease.[8,40,42,109] However, safety issues related to increased n-3 fatty acid intakes also need to be fully explored, because it cannot be ruled out that peroxidative status increases along with the degree of unsaturation of dietary fat. Future well-controlled clinical trials are necessary to clearly elucidate the effects of qualitative fatty acid intake in relation to disease risk.

## Acknowledgment

We thank Stephanie Jew and Richard Bazinet for their assistance in preparing this chapter.

## References

1. Evans HM, Burr GO. New dietary deficiency with highly purified diets. Proc Soc Exp Biol Med.1927; 24:740–743.
2. Burr GO, Burr MM. A new deficiency disease produced by the rigid exclusion of fat from the diet. J Biol Chem. 1929;82:345–367.
3. Burr GO, Burr MM. On the nature and the role of fatty acids essential in nutrition. J Biol Chem. 1930;86:587–621.
4. Hansen AE, Haggard ME, Boelsche AN, et al. Essential fatty acids in infant nutrition. III. Clinical manifestations of linoleic acid deficiency. J Nutr. 1958;66:564–570.
5. Futterman S, Downer JL, Hendrickson A. Effect of essential fatty acid deficiency on the fatty acid composition, morphology, and electroretinograph response of the retina. Invest Opthalmol. 1971;10: 151–156.
6. Wheeler TG, Benolken RM, Anderson RE. Visual membranes: specificity of fatty acid precursors for the electrical response to illumination. Science. 1975;188:1312–1314.
7. Holman RT, Johnson SB, Hatch SF. A case of human linolenic acid deficiency involving neurological abnormalities. Am J Clin Nutr. 1982;35: 617–623.
8. Simopoulos A. Essential fatty acids in health and chronic disease. Am J Clin Nutr. 1999;70: 560S–569S.
9. Connor WE. Importance of n-3 fatty acids in health and disease. Am J Clin Nutr. 2000;71: 171S–175S.
10. McCowen KC, Bistrian BR. Essential fatty acids and their derivatives. Curr Opin Gastroenterol. 2005;21:207–215.
11. Morley R. Nutrition and cognitive development. Nutrition. 1998;14:752–754.
12. Uauy R, Hoffman DR. Essential fat requirements in preterm infants. Am J Clin Nutr. 2000;71: 245S–250S.
13. Gibson RA, Makrides M. n-3 Polyunsaturated fatty acid requirements of term infants. Am J Clin Nutr. 2000;71:251S–255S.
14. Cunnane SC, Crawford MA. Survival of the fattest: Fat babies were the key to evolution of the large human brain. Comp Biochem Physiol Part A. 2003; 136;17–36.
15. Von Euler US. Welcoming address. In: Bergstrom S, Samuelsson B, eds. *Prostaglandins: Proceedings of the Second Nobel Symposium*. New York: Interscience Publishers; 1967; 17–21.
16. Bergstrom S, Sjovall J. The isolation of prostaglandin F from sheep prostate glands. Acta Chem Scand. 1960;14:1693–1700.
17. Bergstrom S, Sjovall J. The isolation of prostaglandin E from sheep prostate glands. Acta Chem Scand. 1960;14:1701–1705.
18. Baker RR. The eicosanoids: a historical overview. Clin Biochem. 1990;23:455–458.
19. Field CJ, Angel A, Clandinin MT. Relationship of diet to the fatty acid composition of human adipose tissue structural and stored lipids. Am J Clin Nutr. 1985;42:1206–1220.
20. Voss A, Reinhart M, Sankarappa S, Sprecher H. The metabolism of 7,10,13,16,19-docosapentaenoic acid to 4,7,10,13,16,19-docosahexaenoic acid in rat liver is independent of a 4-desaturase. J Biol Chem. 1991;266:19995–20000.
21. Cunnane, SC. Enduring issues about essential fatty acids: Time for a new paradigm? Progr Lipid Res. 2003;48:544–568.
22. Brenner RR. Endocrine control of fatty acid desaturation. Biochem Soc Trans. 1990;18:773–775.
23. Schlenk H, Sand DM, Gellerman JL. Retroconversion of docosahexaenoic acid in the rat. Biochim Biophys Acta. 1969;187:201–207.
24. Dietschy JM. Regulation of cholesterol metabolism in man and other species. Klin Wochenschr. 1984; 62:338–345.
25. Jones PJH, Pappu AS, Hatcher L, et al. Dietary cholesterol feeding suppresses human cholesterol synthesis measured using deuterium incorporation and urinary mevalonic acid levels. Arterioscler Thromb Vasc Biol. 1996;16:1222–1228.
26. Grundy SM, Barrett-Connor E, Rudel LL, et al. Workshop on the impact of dietary cholesterol on plasma lipoproteins and atherogenesis. Arteriosclerosis. 1988;8:95–101.
27. Jones PJH. Regulation of cholesterol biosynthesis by diet in humans. Am J Clin Nutr. 1997;66: 438–446.
28. Matthan NR, Ausman LM, Lichtenstein AH, Jones PJH. Hydrogenated fat consumption affects

cholesterol synthesis in moderately hypercholesterolemic women. J Lipid Res. 2000;41:834–839.

29. Di Buono M, Hannah JS, Katzel LI, Jones PJ. Weight loss due to energy restriction suppresses cholesterol biosynthesis in overweight, mildly hypercholesterolemic men. J Nutr. 1999;129: 1545–1548.
30. Papamandjaris AA, MacDougall DE, Jones PJH. Medium chain fatty acid metabolism and energy expenditure: obesity treatment implications. Life Sci. 1998;14:1203–1215.
31. Leyton J, Drury PJ, Crawford MA. Differential oxidation of saturated and unsaturated fatty acids in vivo in the rat. Br J Nutr. 1987;57:383–393.
32. Cunnane SC, Ryan MA, Nadeau CR, Bazinet RP, Musa-Veloso K, McCloy, U. Why is lipid synthesis an integral target of β-oxidized and recycled carbon from polyunsaturates in neonates? Lipids. 2003;38: 477–484.
33. Cunnane SC, Belza K, Anderson MJ, Ryan MA. Substantial carbon recycling from linoleate into products of de novo lipogenesis occurs in rat liver even under conditions of extreme linoleate deficiency. J Lipid Res. 1998;39:2271–2276.
34. Wolfe RR. Metabolic interactions between glucose and fatty acids in human subjects. Am J Clin Nutr. 1998;67:519S–526S.
35. Phillips SM, Green HJ, Tarnopolsky MA, et al. Effects of training duration on substrate turnover and oxidation during exercise. J Appl Physiol. 1996; 81:2182–2191.
36. Achten J, Jeukendrup AE. Optimizing fat oxidation through exercise and diet. Nutrition. 2004;20: 716–727.
37. Jequier E. Response to and range of acceptable fat intake in adults. Eur J Clin Nutr. 1999;53:S84–S93.
38. Kremer JM. Effects of modulation of inflammatory and immune parameters in patients with rheumatic and inflammatory disease receiving dietary supplementation of n-3 and n-6 fatty acids. Lipids. 1996; 31:243S–247S.
39. Food and Nutrition Board, Institute of Medicine. Dietary Reference Intakes for Energy, Carbohydrate, Fiber, Fat, Fatty Acids, Cholesterol, Protein, and Amino Acids (Macronutrients). Washington, DC: National Academies Press; 2002. Available online at: http://www.nap.edu/books/0309085373/html.
40. Uauy R, Mena P, Valenzuela A. Essential fatty acids as determinants of lipid requirements in infants, children, and adults. Eur J Clin Nutr. 1999;53: S66–S77.
41. Kris-Etherton PM, Shaffer Taylor D, Yu-Poth S, et al. Polyunsaturated fatty acids in the food chain in the United States. Am J Clin Nutr. 2000;71: 179S–188S.
42. Holman RT. The slow discovery of the importance of 3 essential fatty acids in human health. J Nutr. 1998;128:427S–433S.
43. World Health Organization. Fats and oils in human nutrition: report of a joint expert consultation of the Food and Agriculture Organization of the United Nations and the World Health Organization. FAO Food and Nutrition Paper. Rome: FAO; 1995; 1–147.
44. FAO/WHO Joint Expert Consultation. Report of a joint expert consultation: FAO Food and Nutrition Paper No. 57. Rome: FAO; 1994; 49–55.
45. Jensen RG, Ferris AM, Lammi-Keefe CJ. Lipids in human milk. Annu Rev Nutr. 1992;12:417–441.
46. Lucas A, Morley R, Cole TJ, Gore SM. A randomised multicentre study of human milk versus formula and later development in preterm infants. Arch Dis Child. 1994;70:F141–F146.
47. Lucas A, Morley R, Cole TJ, et al. Breast milk and subsequent intelligence quotient in children born preterm. Lancet. 1992;339:261–264.
48. Neuringer M, Adamkin D, Auestad N, et al. Efficacy of dietary long-chain polyunsaturated fatty acids (LCP) for preterm (PT) infants [abstract]. FASEB J. 2000;14:LB179.
49. Birch EE, Hoffman DR, Uauy R, et al. Visual acuity and the essentiality of docosahexaenoic acid and arachidonic acid in the diet of term infants. Pediatr Res. 1998;44:201–209.
50. Uauy R, Hoffman DR, Mena P, et al. Term infant studies of DHA and ARA supplementation on neurodevelopment: results of randomized controlled trials. J Pediatr. 2003;143:S17–S25.
51. Cunnane, SC, Francescutti V, Brenna, JT, Crawford, MA. Breast-fed infants achieve a higher rate of brain and whole body docosahexaenoate accumulation than formula-fed infants not consuming dietary docosahexaenoate. Lipids. 2000;35:105–111.
52. Carlson SE, Werkman SH, Peeples JM, Wilson WM. Long-chain fatty acids and early visual and cognitive development of preterm infants. Eur J Clin Nutr. 1994;48:S27–S30.
53. Giovannini M, Riva E, Agostoni C. The role of dietary polyunsaturated fatty acids during the first 2 years of life. Early Hum Dev. 1998;53:S99–S107.
54. SanGiovanni JP, Parra-Cabrera S, Colditz GA, et al. Meta-analysis of dietary essential fatty acids and long-chain polyunsaturated fatty acids as they relate to visual resolution acuity in healthy preterm infants. Pediatrics. 2000;105:1292–1298.
55. Uauy R, Mena P, Rojas C. Essential fatty acids in early life: Structural and functional role. Proc Nutr Soc. 2000;59:3–15.
56. Lapillonne A, Picaud JC, Chirouze V, et al. The use of low-EPA fish oil for long-chain polyunsaturated fatty acid supplementation of preterm infants. Pediatr Res. 2000;48:835–841.
57. Simmer K, Patole S. Long chain polyunsaturated

fatty acid supplementation in preterm infants. Cochrane Database Syst Rev. 2004;1:CD000375.

58. van Wezel-Meijler G, van der Knaap MS, Huisman J, et al. Dietary supplementation of long-chain polyunsaturated fatty acids in preterm infants: effects on cerebral maturation. Acta Paediatr. 2002;91: 942–950.
59. Makrides M, Simmer K, Goggin M, Gibson RA. Erythrocyte docosahexaenoic acid correlates with the visual response of healthy, term infants. Pediatr Res. 1993;34:425–427.
60. Willatts P, Forsyth JS, DiMondugno JK, et al. The effects of long chain polyunsaturated fatty acids on infant habituation at 3 months and problem solving at 9 months. In: *PUFA in Infant Nutrition: Consensus and Controversies. Proceedings of American Oil Chemists Society*. Barcelona; 1996; 42A.
61. Hoffman DR, Birch EE, Castaneda YS, et al. Visual function in breast-fed term infants weaned to formula with or without long-chain polyunsaturates at 4 to 6 months: a randomized clinical trial. J Pediatr. 2003;142:669–677.
62. Larque E, Demmelmair H, Koletzko B. Perinatal supply and metabolism of long-chain polyunsaturated fatty acids: importance for the early development of the nervous system. Ann N Y Acad Sci. 2002;967:299–310.
63. Birch EE, Hoffman DR, Castaneda YS, et al A randomized controlled trial of long-chain polyunsaturated fatty acid supplementation of formula in term infants after weaning at 6 wk of age. Am J Clin Nutr. 2002;75:570–580.
64. Hoffman DR, Birch EE, Birch DG, et al. Impact of early dietary intake and blood lipid composition of long-chain polyunsaturated fatty acids on later visual development. J Pediatr Gastroenterol Nutr. 2000;31:540–553.
65. Birch EE, Garfield S, Hoffman DR, et al. A randomized controlled trial of early dietary supply of long-chain polyunsaturated fatty acids and mental development in term infants. Dev Med Child Neurol. 2000;42:174–181.
66. Innis SM, Nelson CM, Rioux FM, King DJ. Development of visual acuity in relation to plasma and erythrocyte w-6 and w-3 fatty acids in healthy term gestation infants. Am J Clin Nutr. 1994;60: 347–352.
67. Simmer K. Long chain polyunsaturated fatty acid supplementation in infants born at term. Cochrane Database Syst Rev. 2001;4:CD000376.
68. Agostoni C, Trojan S, Bellu R, et al. Neurodevelopment quotient of healthy long term infants at 4 months and feeding practice: the role of long-chain polyunsaturated fatty acids. Pediatr Res. 1995;38: 262–266.
69. Agostoni C, Trojan S, Bellu R, et al. Developmental quotient at 24 months and fatty acid composition of diet in early infancy: a follow up study. Arch Dis Child. 1997;76:421–424.
70. Summary of the second report of the National Cholesterol Education Program (NCEP) Expert Panel on Detection, Evaluation, and Treatment of High Blood Cholesterol in Adults. JAMA. 1993;269: 3015–3023.
71. Mann J. Complex carbohydrates: replacement energy for fat or useful in their own right? Am J Clin Nutr. 1987;45S:1202–1206.
72. Grundy SM, Denke MA. Dietary influences on serum lipids and lipoprotein. J Lipid Res. 1990;31: 1149–1172.
73. National Research Council. *Diet and Health: Implications for Reducing Chronic Disease Risk*. Washington DC: National Academies Press; 1989; 183.
74. Lissner L, Heitman B. Dietary fat and obesity: evidence from epidemiology. Eur J Clin Nutr. 1995; 49:79–90.
75. Schutz Y, Flatt JP, Jequier E. Failure of dietary fat intake to promote fat oxidation: a factor favoring the development of obesity. Am J Clin Nutr. 1989; 50:307–314.
76. Jequier E. Body weight regulation in humans: the importance of nutrient balance. News Physiol Sci. 1993;8:273–276.
77. Willett WC. Is dietary fat a major determinant of body fat? Am J Clin Nutr. 1998;67S:556S–562S.
78. Seidell JC. Dietary fat and obesity: an epidemiologic perspective. Am J Clin Nutr. 1998;67S:546S–550S.
79. Katan MB. High-oil compared with low-fat, high-carbohydrate diets in the prevention of ischemic heart disease. Am J Clin Nutr. 1997;66S: 974S–979S.
80. Lichtenstein AH. Dietary fat and cardiovascular disease risk: Quantity or quality? J Womens Health (Larchmt). 2003;12:109–114.
81. Grundy SM. Multifactorial causation of obesity: implications for prevention. Am J Clin Nutr. 1998; 67S:563S–572S.
82. Prentice AM, Jebb SA. Fast foods, energy density and obesity: a possible mechanistic link. Obes Rev. 2003;4:187–194.
83. French S, Robinson T. Fats and food intake. Curr Opin Clin Nutr Metab Care. 2003;6:629–634.
84. Nestel PJ. Fish oil and cardiovascular disease: lipids and arterial function. Am J Clin Nutr. 2000;71: 228S–2231S.
85. Zhao G, Etherton TD, Martin KR, et al. Dietary alpha-linolenic acid reduces inflammatory and lipid cardiovascular risk factors in hypercholesterolemic men and women. J Nutr. 2004;134:2991–2997.
86. Wolfram G. Dietary fatty acids and coronary heart disease. Eur J Med Res. 2003;8:321–324.
87. Flickinger BD, Huth PJ. Dietary fats and oils: technologies for improving cardiovascular health. Curr Atheroscler Rep. 2004;6:468–476.

88. Calder PC. n-3 Fatty acids and cardiovascular disease: evidence explained and mechanisms explored. Clin Sci (Lond). 2004;107:1–11.
89. Simopoulos AP. Omega-3 fatty acids in inflammation and autoimmune diseases. J Am Coll Nutr. 2002;21:495–505.
90. Renaud SC. Diet and stroke. J Nutr Health Aging. 2001;5:167–172.
91. Gerber MJ, Scali JD, Michaud A, et al. Profiles of a healthful diet and its relationship to biomarkers in a population sample from Mediterranean southern France. J Am Diet Assoc. 2000;100:1164–1171.
92. Uauy R, Hoffman DR, Peirano P, et al. Essential fatty acids in visual and brain development. Lipids. 2001;36:885–895.
93. Neuringer M, Connor WE, Lin DS, et al. Biochemical and functional effects of prenatal and postnatal omega-3 fatty acid deficiency on retina and brain in rhesus monkeys. Proc Natl Acad Sci U S A. 1986;83:40021–40025.
94. Reisbick S, Neuringer M, Connor WE. Effects of n-3 fatty acid deficiency in non-human primates. In: Bindels JG, Goedhardt AC, Visser HKA, eds. *Nutrica Symposium*. Lancaster, UK: Kluwer Academic Publishers; 1996; 157–172.
95. Zimmer L, Delion-Vancassel S, Durand G, et al. Modification of dopamine neurotransmission in the nucleus accumbens of rats deficient in n-3 polyunsaturated fatty acids. J Lipid Res. 2000;41:32–40.
96. Makrides M, Neumann MA, Byard RW, et al. Fatty acid composition of brain, retina, and erythrocytes in breast- and formula-fed infants. Am J Clin Nutr. 1994;60:189–194.
97. Mori TA, Beilin LJ. Omega-3 fatty acids and inflammation. Curr Atheroscler Rep. 2004;6: 461–467.
98. Shapiro H. Could n-3 polyunsaturated fatty acids reduce pathological pain by direct actions on the nervous system? Prostaglandins Leukot Essent Fatty Acids. 2003;68:219–224.
99. Belluzzi A, Boschi S, Brignola C, et al. Polyunsaturated fatty acids and inflammatory bowel disease. Am J Clin Nutr. 2000;71S:339S–342S.
100. Rose DP. Effects of dietary fatty acids on breast and prostate cancers: evidence from in vitro experiments and animal studies. Am J Clin Nutr. 1997;66S: 1513S–1522S.
101. Calviello G, Palozza P, Nicuolo FD, et al. n-3 PUFA dietary supplementation inhibits proliferation and store-operated calcium influx in thymoma cells growing in Balb/C mice. J Lipid Res. 2000; 41:182–188.
102. Rose DP, Connolly JM, Rayburn J, Coleman M. Influence of diets containing eicosapentaenoic or docosahexaenoic acid on growth and metastasis of breast cancer cells in nude mice. J Natl Canc Inst. 1995;87:587–592.
103. Dagnelie PC, Bell JD, William SCR, et al. Effect of fish oil in cancer cachexia and host liver metabolism in rats with prostate tumors. Lipids. 1994;29: 195–203.
104. de Deckere EA. Possible beneficial effect of fish and fish n-3 polyunsaturated fatty acids in breast and colorectal cancer. Eur J Cancer Prev. 1999;8: 213–221.
105. Kremer JM. n-3 Fatty acid supplements in rheumatoid arthritis. Am J Clin Nutr. 2000;71S: 349S–351S.
106. Simopoulos AP. Fatty acid composition of skeletal muscle membrane phospholipids, insulin resistance, and obesity. Nutrition Today. 1994;2:12–16.
107. Okuyama H, Kobayashi T, Watanabe S. Dietary fatty acids: the n-6/n-3 balance and chronic elderly diseases: excess linoleic acid and relative n-3 deficiency syndrome seen in Japan. Prog Lipid Res. 1997;35:409–457.
108. McCowen KC, Bistrian BR. Essential fatty acids and their derivatives. Curr Opin Gastroenterol. 2005;21:207–215.
109. Yam D, Eliraz A, Berry EM. Diet and disease-the Israeli paradox: possible dangers of a high omega-6 polyunsaturated fatty acid diet. Isr J Med Sci. 1996;32:1134–1143.

# 11 Alcohol: The Role in Health and Nutrition

Paolo M. Suter

## Introduction

Alcohol is a major component of the daily life in most Western countries. Presently, about 55% of US adults 18 years or older reported drinking at least once in the past month, 62.4% of these were men and 47.9% women.[1] Despite the wide acceptance of alcohol consumption in most societies, it remains an important cause and modulator of disease risk.[2] With approximately 85,000 deaths per year attributable to excessive drinking, alcohol consumption represents the third leading cause of death after tobacco and poor diet and physical inactivity.[3] Compared with other food items, alcohol has three characteristic features: depending on the absolute amount and frequency of consumption, it can be regarded as a nutrient, a toxin, or a psychoactive drug. Each consumer determines which aspect of alcohol will prevail for him or herself.

The energy content of alcohol, compared with other energy sources, is rather high (1 g alcohol = 7.1 kcal = 29.7 kJ), and thus alcohol represents an important source of energy for many alcohol consumers. Alcohol energy contributes depending on sex and age about 1.3% to 3.4% of total energy intake of the US diet,[4] but in heavy drinkers, it may contribute up to 50% of the daily energy intake. In view of the importance of alcoholic beverages as an important source of energy, alcohol has a high potential to displace other essential nutrients.

Because of its potential toxicity and the inability of the body to store alcohol, it has to be eliminated as quickly as possible from the body. This absolute priority in metabolism is a major cause of the metabolic effects of alcohol on nearly all nutrients, on most if not all organ systems, and, consequently, on disease risks (Figure 1).

In view of the large variability among alcohol drinkers in patterns of drinking, amounts ingested, ingestion of other nutrients, and metabolic characteristics, as well as lifestyle characteristics (such as exercise or smoking behavior), the heterogeneous effects of alcohol on nutritional status and disease risk are not surprising. These effects are further complicated by genetically determined differences in alcohol metabolism.[5] For the purposes of this discussion, one drink corresponds to 12 g of alcohol, the amount contained in approximately 270 mL of beer, 100 mL of wine (12% by volume), or 30 mL of liquor (40% by volume). A review of alcohol's effects on selected nutrients and on disease risk follows.

## Alcohol Metabolism

Alcohol is rapidly absorbed from the stomach and the jejunum and is distributed in the total water compartment of the body. Most of it is metabolized in the liver; however, a small amount may be metabolized in the stomach mucosa (i.e., during the first-pass metabolism).[6] The first-pass metabolism is higher in men then in women, declines with age, and is affected by different drugs such as aspirin, which decreases it. Alcohol can be metabolized via three different enzyme systems and, under usual conditions, depending on the dose and frequency of consumption, is metabolized by two major pathways: for light to moderate levels of intake, alcohol is metabolized in the alcohol dehydrogenase (ADH) pathway; for higher levels of intake, it is predominantly metabolized in the microsomal ethanol oxidizing system (MEOS).[7] The oxidation of alcohol in both the ADH and the MEOS pathway leads to the production of acetaldehyde, which is further metabolized to acetate by acetaldehyde dehydrogenase (ALDH). Acetate is shuttled to the peripheral tissues and used as a source of energy. The metabolism of alcohol induces a change in the redox potential in the liver. This change contributes to different metabolic and clinical consequences and to functional abnormalities such as

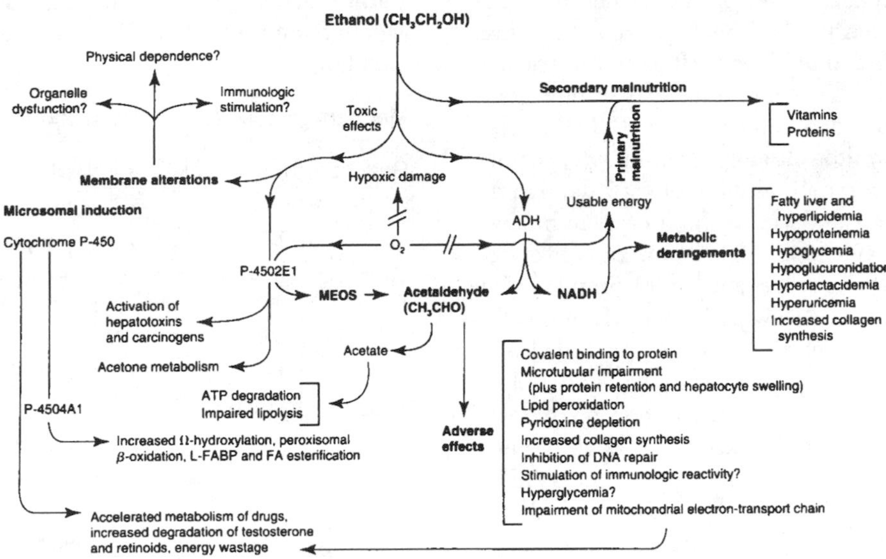


Figure 1. Metabolic and functional abnormalities due to alcohol consumption. (Used with permission from Lieber CS. Medical disorders of alcoholism. N Engl J Med 1995;333:1058–1065.)

suppression of the Krebs cycle, with an increased transformation of pyruvate to lactate, impaired gluconeogenesis and hypoglycemia, greater fatty acid synthesis, reduced urate excretion, and hyperuricemia.[8].

These alcohol-induced metabolic perturbations depend on the dose of alcohol and the duration of consumption, but most metabolic, endocrine, and functional systems of the body are affected (Figure 1). The metabolic consequences of alcohol may be mediated directly or indirectly. Direct alcohol toxicity leads to an alteration in cellular function resulting from alterations in membrane fluidity, in the intracellular redox potential, and acetaldehyde toxicity. Acetaldehyde elicits many different effects, such as increased free radical production and lipid peroxidation, inhibition of protein synthesis, and impaired of vitamin metabolism.[9]

The metabolism of alcohol shows a wide inter-individual variability that is modulated by different genotypes of the alcohol-metabolizing enzymes ADH and ALDH.[10] Depending on the ADH genotype, higher maximal alcohol and acetaldehyde concentrations and a slower alcohol elimination are found, a situation that may lead to increased direct and indirect alcohol toxicity and thus a different alcohol-related disease pattern. In many people of Asian origin, the activity of ALDH may be low and thus cause a typical facial flushing reaction and headaches after ingestion of even small amounts of alcohol.

Although the capacity to metabolize alcohol varies widely, a healthy person metabolizes alcohol on average at 5 to 7 g/h. There is no useful and safe strategy (except a high fructose intake leading to a reduced nicotinamide adenine dinucleotide reoxidation) known to increase the rate of alcohol degradation.

## The Nutritional Assessment of the Alcoholic Patient

Nutritional assessment of the alcoholic patient is a challenging task in either the clinical or the community setting. The clinical signs of alcohol-related malnutrition depend on the stage of alcoholism, the level of socioeconomic integration, social and familial networks, associated alcohol- and non-alcohol-related diseases (especially liver disease), and concomitant medication intake of the patient.[11] Socioeconomically integrated heavy drinkers, in the absence of any clinically manifested somatic diseases, rarely show signs of malnutrition.[12] With the progression of alcoholism, clinical signs from all organ systems and malnutrition may prevail. Different clinical signs of malnutrition may be found; for example, thin arms and legs due to muscle wasting,[13] edema (protein deficiency), glossitis (B-vitamin deficiency), and scaly, dry skin (zinc and essential fatty acid deficiency). Spider nevi and multiple hematomas due to easy bruising (vitamin C and K deficiency) may be found on the skin. The parotid glands are often enlarged due to chronic parotitis. The patients may present with new bone fractures and several old costal fractures, and advanced osteoporosis (especially in men), attributable in part to impaired vitamin D nutriture and metabolism.

Alcohol-associated endocrine pathologies may manifest themselves as gynecomastia, testicular atrophy, and loss of body hair. Neurological signs may be limited to peripheral neuropathy (B-vitamin deficiency), different central nervous system impairments (see section on thiamine), or the full clinical picture of stroke. An impaired dark adaptation due to zinc deficiency is fairly common. In general, the nutritional assessment of the alcoholic patient is not different from the assessment of other patients. The biochemical assessment includes measurement of the conventional alcohol markers (i.e., liver transaminase levels and red blood cell mean cell volume) in combination with biochemical markers of nutritional status. Carbohydrate-deficient transferrin (CDT), a specific marker to monitor chronic alcohol abuse, may be helpful. A chronic alcohol consumption (< 7 days) in the range of 50 to 70 g/d induces the hepatocyte to produce a transferring molecule that is deficient in carbohydrates. The CDT is a marker for sustained and harmful alcohol consumption and returns slowly (the half-life of CDT is approximately 14 d) to normal upon cessation of alcohol intake. CDT measurements may be especially useful for the follow-up of patients in detoxification programs.[14] The usefulness of alcohol markers such as the serum/plasma concentration of fatty acid ethyl esters (FAEE), ethyl glucuronide (EtG) in urine,[15] or urinary 5-hydroxytryptophol (5-HTOL)/5-hydroxyindole-3-acetic acid (5-HIAA) ratio[16] for the clinical setting are controversial and not yet established. Elevated levels of high-density lipoprotein (HDL) cholesterol, uric acid, and fasting triacylglycerol levels without other explanation may be signs of excessive alcohol intake.

The assessment of alcohol intake at either the population or individual level is very difficult, especially for drinking in the low to moderate range. Although heavy alcohol intake is detected sooner or later by typical clinical signs or laboratory test results, there is no reliable clinical sign of biochemical marker for the assessment of light to moderate alcohol intake. Intentional or unintentional underreporting and overreporting often lead to uncontrollable bias in epidemiological and clinical studies. The difficulty in assessing low to moderate levels of alcohol consumption represents probably one of the most important causes for inconsistent research findings.

## Alcohol and Nutrition

As a function of the amount of alcohol consumed, the duration of intake, and any associated diseases, drinking can impair the nutritional status of all nutrients. Alcohol-associated malnutrition includes both primary and secondary malnutrition. Because of the comparatively high energy content of alcohol, it displaces other energy sources and thus many essential nutrients in the diet, thereby lowering the intake of most nutrients (primary malnutrition). Gastrointestinal and metabolic complications of heavy alcohol intake (especially liver dysfunction) lead to so-called secondary malnutrition (Figure 1). Anorexia and vomiting from alcoholic gastritis further promote inadequate intakes of food. Malabsorption of nearly all nutrients can develop as a result of mucosal dysfunction, liver insufficiency, and pancreatic insufficiency.[17] Alcoholic liver dysfunction causes a reduced capacity to transport nutrients in the blood, a reduced storage capacity, and an insufficient activation of nutrients such as vitamins. In addition, alcohol increases the excretion of nutrients in the urine and bile. In alcoholic patients, several mechanisms for the development of malnutrition usually occur simultaneously (Table 1).[17]

**Table 1.** Alcohol and Nutritional Status: Possible Mechanisms of the Alcohol-Mediated Toxicity on Nutrition

| Mechanisms | Possible Causes |
|---|---|
| Reduced dietary intake | • Poverty |
| | • Displacement of normal food |
| | • Inappetence due to direct alcohol toxicity and secondary due to disease (e.g., alcoholic gastritis) |
| | • Anorexia due to medications |
| Impaired digestion | • Alcoholic gastritis |
| | • Impaired bile and pancreatic enzymes secretion |
| | • Direct mucosal damage and impairment of mucosal enzymes (e.g., folyl conjugase) |
| | • Altered gastrointestinal mobility |
| Malabsorption | • Direct mucosal damage |
| | • Indirect damage (e.g., due to folate deficiency) |
| | • Motility changes including accelerated small intestinal transit time and diarrhea |
| | • Pancreatic insufficiency |
| Impaired transport in the circulation | • Decreased synthesis of transport proteins due to liver damage |
| Impaired activation | • Liver damage |
| | • Inadequate supply of cofactors |
| Decreased storage | • Liver pathology |
| | • Alcoholic myopathy/sarcopenia |
| Increased losses | • Increased excretion in urine and bile |
| | • Increased urinary losses due to medications |
| | • Increased fecal losses |
| Increased requirements | • Due to the above factors |
| | • Increased metabolic rate |

## Effects of Alcohol on Energy Metabolism

In view of the increasing prevalence of obesity, the effects of alcohol on energy balance and metabolism are of great importance.[18] Because alcohol is mostly devoid of other nutrients and is not regulated (in contrast to other nutrients, there is no mechanism such as appetite regulation or hunger), alcohol's calories are unregulated, empty calories.[19,20] The importance of alcohol as a risk factor for weight gain and obesity is disputed.[18,21,22] For weight maintenance, the energy balance has to be equilibrated, and alcohol has been reported to affect all components of the energy balance negatively, favoring a positive energy balance.[23]

Because moderate drinkers generally add alcohol to their usual food intake, a positive energy balance with an increased risk for weight gain and obesity will result unless compensated for by other means. This risk is increased by the combination of a high-fat diet and even moderate alcohol intake because of the hyperphagic effect of alcohol.[24] Alcohol substitution (i.e., the usual food energy sources are substituted by alcohol) is the typical feature of the heavy drinker and will result in malnutrition and weight loss (Figure 2).

Depending on the amount and frequency of consumption, alcohol leads to an increase of energy expenditure. In young, moderate drinkers, the addition and the substitution of 25% of their energy requirements (corresponding to 96 ± 4 g alcohol) by alcohol leads to increasing energy expenditures of 7% ± 1% and 4% ± 1%, respectively.[25] These increases of energy expenditure correspond to a thermic effect of 20% to 25% of the energy content of the ingested alcohol. Other studies[18] reported a thermic effect of alcohol in healthy, moderate consumers in the range of 15% to 25%, which is rather high compared with other energy sources (e.g., the thermic effect of a mixed meal is approximately 12%).

Presently, it is not clear what fraction of the alcohol energy could be used for adenosine triphosphate (ATP) production. In their classical studies more than 100 years ago, Atwater and Benedict[26] suggested that alcohol energy seems to be equivalent to the energy of carbohydrates or fat. However, subsequent studies revealed that as a function of the pathway of the metabolic degradation of alcohol (i.e., ADH vs. MEOS), lower amounts of ATP are produced than theoretical calculations would suggest.[27] Nevertheless, epidemiological and experimental studies suggest that, despite some energy wastage, alcohol calories are largely a usable energy source in the moderate consumer.

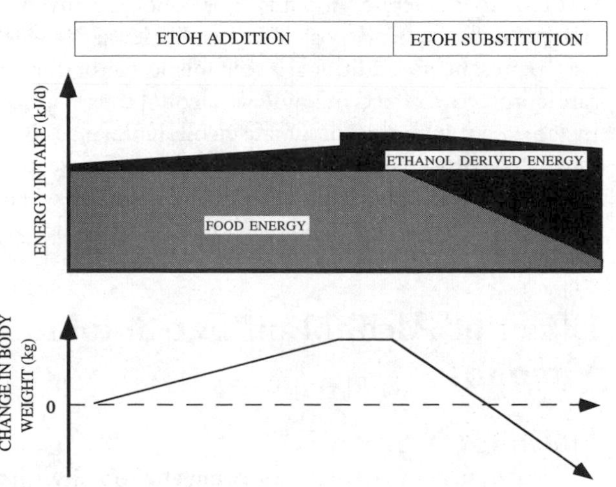

Figure 2. Effect of alcohol on energy intake and body weight.

Alcohol also affects the energy balance equation by its effects on substrate balance. Independently, whether alcohol is added to or substituted for usual food, lipid oxidation is suppressed approximately by a third,[25] producing a positive fat balance. The positive fat balance is not caused by a de novo lipogenesis from alcohol, but by acetate being used in the peripheral organs (mainly muscle) as a source of energy at the expense of a lower fat oxidation. Use off stable isotope mass spectrometry techniques has shown that most (98%) of the carbons of a moderate alcohol load (25 g) is transported as acetate to the peripheral tissues, and only a negligible amount of the ingested dose (<1%) is used for de novo lipogenesis.[28]

Despite these effects of alcohol on energy balance, some epidemiological and experimental studies were unable to identify moderate alcohol consumption as a risk factor for obesity.[21,29] This is not surprising in view of the difficulty in assessing alcohol intake and other lifestyle parameters that may compensate for some of the effects of alcohol. Because of the suppression of lipid oxidation and the resulting positive energy balance, even moderate amounts of alcohol have to be regarded as a risk factor for weight gain and obesity when not counterbalanced by other means. To counteract the effects of alcohol on fat oxidation, fat intake should be kept as low as possible, and whenever alcohol is consumed, fat intake has to be reduced in proportion to the amount of alcohol ingested to remain in substrate balance.

Alcohol enhances the abdominal deposition of fat, which is associated with several adverse health outcomes such as hypertension or dyslipidemia,[22,30] and represents a typical feature of the metabolic syndrome.[31] Again, the later relationship is complicated by recent epidemiologic findings reporting a lower prevalence of the typical features of the metabolic syndrome in mild to moderate alcohol consumers.[32,33]

## Effects of Alcohol on Lipid Metabolism

As a function of the amount consumed, the frequency of drinking, and presence of concomitant diseases (especially liver disease, overweight, and obesity), alcohol affects all lipoprotein fractions in the blood.[34] The development of a fatty liver, a characteristic early sign of alcoholic liver disease, is partially caused by the alcohol-induced suppression of lipid oxidation in the liver and by an increased influx of fat from the peripheral tissues.[25,35] These early changes are also associated with the typical signs of alcoholic hyperlipidemia, which include elevated serum triacylglycerol levels caused by an increased hepatic secretion of very-low-density-lipoproteins (VLDL) and alcohol-induced injury to peripheral removal of the VLDLs resulting from an impaired lipoprotein lipase. The rise in triacylglycerol levels is increased by the ingestion of a diet rich in fat. The effects of alcohol on triacylgylcerol levels are also seen during the postprandial phase; however, they can be partially counteracted by a concomitant reduction in fat intake and/or higher physical activity before or after the meal.[36]

The chronic moderate ingestion of alcohol leads to an increase in HDL cholesterol, which may be a major mechanism for the beneficial cardiovascular effects of alcohol.[37] The alcohol-associated increase in HDL cholesterol may have multiple causes, including an increased hepatic production and secretion of apoproteins, an increased peripheral production due to lipid exchange within the different lipoprotein fractions, and a decreased catabolism of the HDL particle caused by alcohol's effects on specific enzymes involved in lipid transfer or effects on postprandial lipemia.[38,39] The HDL-raising effects of alcohol are nonlinear, showing a threshold effect on HDL-cholesterol,[40] and depend on different factors such as gender, body mass index, smoking habits, and genotype (e.g., apolipoprotein E genotype).[41] One study[41] reported that only in women with the apolipoprotein E genotype *ε4/3* does alcohol consumption intensify the increase in LDL-cholesterol and the decrease in HDL-cholesterol associated with increasing BMI. In this context, it should be remembered that obesity represents one of the major causes of low HDL-cholesterol.

The effects of alcohol on low-density-lipoprotein (LDL) cholesterol are only minor and less consistent than the effects on the other lipoprotein fractions. In animal studies, alcohol led to a decrease in LDL clearance due to a decreased hepatic LDL-receptor expression.[42] Alcohol may unfavorably affect the size of the lipoprotein particles, especially LDL particles.[42] During the last few years, evidence has accumulated suggesting that lipoprotein subclass distributions according to particle size may be important modifiers of atherogenic risk. Individuals with a high concentration of small, dense LDL particles and their metabolic precursors, the large VLDL particles, have a higher cardiovascular risk than those with predominantly large LDL particles and small VLDL particles. The role of certain polyphenolic compounds of wine as modulators of LDL-oxidation rates in vivo is uncertain,[43] especially given the strong prooxidative effects of alcohol and the extremely variable bioavailability and bioefficacy of these compounds.[44] The atherogenic lipoprotein (a) is lowered by alcohol consumption. A minor fraction of ethanol is metabolized by the formation of fatty acid ethyl esters (FAEEs).[45] Because these FAEEs accumulate in different tissues, they may be of pathophysiologic relevance in the development of alcohol-related pathologies,[46] and they may represent useful markers of alcohol intake.[47]

## Alcohol and Carbohydrate Metabolism

The effects of alcohol on glucose handling are multiple as a function of the dosage, duration of alcohol intake, and overall nutritional status. In healthy, moderate drinkers with normal food intake, alcohol's effects on carbohydrate metabolism are hardly of any clinical relevance. By contrast, excessive alcohol consumption may be associated with the typical clinical entity of alcoholic pancreatitis,[48] which results in exocrine pancreatic insufficiency with maldigestion and malabsorption. Alcohol may also lead to life-threatening changes in glucose metabolism. The reduced forms of nicotinamide-adenine dinucleotide (NADH) and acetate produced during alcohol metabolism represent major modulators of glucose metabolism.

The increased production of reducing equivalents caused by the oxidation of alcohol leads to a decrease in gluconeogenesis.[49] This decrease may bring about clinically dangerous hypoglycemia, especially in the heavy drinker with an overall inadequate diet and poor intake of carbohydrates (and thus low glycogen stores).[50] This effect is being reinforced in people with diabetes by the ingestion of oral hypoglycaemic agents, insulin, or both.[51] The alcohol-induced reduction in gluconeogenesis also occurs in the fed state, but is usually compensated for by the glucose in the ingested food. The clinical features of hypoglycemia may share some of the signs of alcohol intoxication, and when it is misdiagnosed as simple alcohol intoxication, deleterious health consequences may result. In addition, alcohol produces changes in the secretory response of different counterregulatory hormones (such as epinephrine or growth hormone), thus resulting in an absence of the potential clinical warning signs of hypoglycemia.[50] Alcohol also inhibits the storage of glycogen, further increasing the predisposition to hypoglycemia when carbohydrate intake is insufficient.

Light to moderate amounts of alcohol are inversely related to fasting and post-load insulin levels,[52] which may represent an additional mechanistic factor for the cardioprotective effects of low-level alcohol consumption. In agreement with this, moderate alcohol intake has been associated with a reduction in coronary heart disease mortality in persons with older onset diabetes mellitus[53] and a lower risk for the development of the metabolic syndrome.[32,33]

## Effect of Alcohol on Fat-Soluble Vitamins

### *Vitamin A*

Alcohol may interfere with the metabolism of all fat-soluble vitamins. Retinol (vitamin A), also an alcohol, shares some metabolic pathways with ethanol and thus a high potential to be affected negatively by alcohol consumption. In light to moderate drinkers, vitamin A metabolism is not altered. Despite low intakes, frank vitamin A deficiency is rarely seen in alcoholics, probably because of the rather large hepatic stores of this vitamin. However, chronic alcohol consumption may lead to low levels of vitamin A in plasma, and when alcoholic liver disease is present, decreased hepatic vitamin A levels are found. These lower levels are a result of an increased degradation of the vitamin as a consequence of the induction of microsomal enzymes[54] and the alcohol-induced decreased synthesis of retinol-binding protein.[55] This condition may lead to the prescription of vitamin A supplements; however, higher levels of vitamin A intake (independent of alcohol intake) are associated with considerable hepatotoxicity,[54] and alcohol represents one of the most important modulators of vitamin A toxicity, especially in the presence of liver disease. In the setting of chronic alcohol consumption, an increased production of polar retinol metabolites seems to be a central mechanism of hepatocellular damage.[56]

Although the vitamin A precursor β-carotene is thought to bear no toxicity in humans, one epidemiological study reported an increased lung cancer rate in β-carotene-supplemented smokers, especially in those who were also drinking alcohol, an increase most likely due to alcohol-induced alterations in the β-carotene metabolism.[57] The negative effects of alcohol observed in the this study were seen at rather low dosage levels, starting at $\geq 12.9$ g/d. Although heavy drinkers ($\geq 200$ g/d) show lower β-carotene plasma concentrations than do control subjects, they show higher β-carotene serum levels than those drinking less.[58] These higher levels may be caused by an impaired utilization or excretion of β-carotene due to liver damage or a partial shift in the degradation of β-carotene from central cleavage to eccentric cleavage.[54] In view of the present evidence, it is not advisable to routinely prescribe either high-dose β-carotene or vitamin A supplements to heavy consumers of alcohol.

### *Vitamin E*

Levels of vitamin E are reduced in chronic alcohol consumers independent of cirrhosis as a result of reduced intake and higher requirements.[59] Vitamin E supplementation has been reported to reduce alcohol-induced lipid peroxidation; however, vitamin E supplementation did not affect laboratory or clinical outcomes.[60] If vitamin E supplements are given, an adequate vitamin K nutriture should be insured, given that a high dose of vitamin E may lead to impairment of the vitamin K cycle and an increased tendency to bleed.[61]

### *Vitamin K*

Data about the effect of alcohol on vitamin K nutriture is scarce. Acute and chronic alcohol consumption has been reported to lead to alterations in gamma-carboxylated molecules such as osteocalcin.[62] In the setting of alcoholic liver disease, vitamin K might have favorable effects on bone health.[63]

### *Vitamin D*

Heavier alcohol consumption may be associated with an increased fracture risk due to indirect and direct alcohol effects on bone metabolism and on vitamin D metabolism.[64] Heavier drinkers have a lower intake, absorption, and activation of vitamin D.[65] In addition, because of alcohol's effects on the target organs, tissue-specific vitamin D effects may be impaired.

## Effects of Alcohol on Water-Soluble Vitamins

The metabolism of all water-soluble vitamins may be affected by the ingestion of alcohol. Alcohol's effects on water-soluble vitamin metabolism are dose dependent, and in the range of light to moderate alcohol intake in healthy subjects eating a balanced diet, no adverse effects are expected. In heavy drinkers, a deficiency of several vitamins is usually present,[66] so the typical clinical signs of vitamin deficiency are not necessarily seen. In this section, alcohol's effects on a few selected water-soluble vitamins are summarized, but special attention is paid to thiamine and folic acid.

### *Thiamine*

Excessive alcohol intake represents the major cause of thiamine deficiency in the US population, and alcohol intake has been identified as the major predictor of thiamine status. Up to 80% of heavy drinkers have impaired thiamine nutriture independent of the presence of liver disease. Insufficient dietary intake is the major cause of thiamine deficiency in alcoholics; in addition, the small amounts of ingested thiamine are malabsorbed.[67] Low doses of thiamine are absorbed by a carrier-mediated active process or at high concentrations by passive diffusion. In the alcoholic, $B_1$ intake is generally low so that the vitamin is principally absorbed by the active process, which is, however, impaired by alcohol. Alcohol abstinence brings about an improvement of thiamine absorption.[68] Even in nonalcoholic subjects, active thiamine absorption is inhibited by an acute single dose of alcohol. Alcohol also induces a reduction in the activation of thiamine by phosphorylation and an increase in the dephosphorylation of phosphorylated thiamine. These effects are potentiated by the presence of liver disease. In addition, loss of the vitamin in urine may increase by alcohol intake. The thiamine storage capacity is reduced in the heavy drinker because of liver abnormalities and decreased muscle mass.[69] Because of the reduced storage capacity of vitamin $B_1$ in general and especially in heavy drinkers due to the aforementioned reasons, the vitamin has to be ingested regularly, on a more or less daily basis. Alcohol induces specific alterations of thiamine metabolism in the central nervous system, thereby producing the typical clinical symptoms of Wernicke-Korsakoff syndrome: encephalopathy, oculomotor dysfunction, and gait ataxia.[70] Wernicke-Korsakoff syndrome is probably the only medical emergency situation involving vitamin deficiencies: the neurological condition has to be treated immediately with parenteral thiamine.[71] The syndrome shows typical clinical features including altered consciousness, ataxia, eye muscle paralysis, and psychosis.

Although no prospective evidence supports the routine administration of several vitamins to alcoholic patients, present evidence suggest a high potential for benefit of B-vitamin supplementation. Research has shown that the neurotoxic effects of alcohol may be potentiated even in subclinical thiamine deficiency,[72] and, accordingly, if alcohol abuse cannot be controlled, the supplementation of thiamine and other B vitamins is indicated. Because of the interrelationship between thiamine and magnesium, an adequate supply of this mineral should be insured.[73] In the alcoholic patient (even when alcohol intake is reduced), thiamine deficiency may represent an important cause for heart failure, especially in combination with diuretics, which increase urinary thiamine losses.[74]

## *Riboflavin*

Riboflavin deficiency is common in the alcoholic patient and is due to low intakes and decreased bioavailability resulting from an alcohol-induced impairment of intraluminal hydrolysis of flavin adenin dinucleotide (FAD) in food sources.[75] In addition, alcohol inhibits the transformation and activation of the vitamin not only at the level of absorption but also at the level of the peripheral tissues.[76] Riboflavin is an essential cofactor in the conversion of vitamin $B_6$ and folate, and thus it represents an important modulator of the overall nutritional status of the B vitamins. Usually, riboflavin deficiency does not occur in isolation but in combination with a deficiency of other B-complex vitamins. Accordingly, the clinical entity is not typical. Because milk and milk products represent one of the major riboflavin sources, the low intake of this vitamin among heavy consumers of alcohol is not surprising.

## *Niacin*

Light to moderate alcohol consumption does not interfere with niacin nutriture. A deficiency in niacin (vitamin $B_3$) is often found in the setting of chronic excessive alcohol consumption, usually together with deficiencies of other B-complex vitamins[77] and other nutrients such as zinc. The prevalence of low niacin plasma levels in chronic alcohol consumers varies widely, probably due to fact that niacin can be obtained preformed from food and from synthesis in the liver from tryptophan. In chronic liver disease, the latter synthetic pathway is impaired.[78] In excessive alcohol consumers, a low intake, decreased synthesis from tryptophan, and an increased requirement might be of pathophysiological importance in the development of deficiency. The coenzyme forms of this vitamin (NAD and NADH) play an important role in alcohol metabolism.[79] In clinical practice, niacin deficiency symptoms (diarrhea, dermatitis, and dementia) might be confused with the Wernicke-Korsakoff syndrome.[80] Niacin supplementation might lead to an increase in liver transaminase levels, which could be misinterpreted as an alcohol-induced increase in transaminase levels. Further pharmacological doses of niacin in the form of a supplement may exacerbate gastric ulcer disease and gout, both conditions that are often found in chronic alcohol consumers. Due to the multinutrient deficiency in excessive alcohol consumers, polyvitamin preparations should be used for therapeutic purposes[81] and should include trace elements such as zinc.[82]

## *Vitamin $B_6$*

Depending on liver function, between 50% and 90% of alcoholics show low pyridoxal-5′-phosphate (PLP) serum levels. The PLP content in liver tissue is reduced independent of the presence of liver disease. As for most nutrients, the pathogenesis of the impaired vitamin $B_6$ nutriture is multifactorial. The formation of the active vitamin (PLP) in the liver is reduced or even completely blocked by the ingestion of alcohol.[83] Acetaldehyde increases the degradation of the vitamin by displacing the vitamin from binding sites and this, in turn, leads to an increased catabolism of the free vitamin and consecutively an increased urinary loss.[75] Because the vitamin has to be activated in a multi-step activation process at the level of the liver, supplementation of this vitamin does not necessarily lead to an improved vitamin $B_6$ nutriture in alcoholics if they continue to ingest alcohol. A recent population-based cohort study reported an inverse association between vitamin $B_6$ intake and the risk of colorectal cancer,[84] especially in women consuming $\geq$ 30 g of alcohol.

## *Folic Acid*

Folate deficiency is one of the most prevalent deficiencies in alcohol consumers. Up to 50% of heavy alcoholics show low concentrations of serum folate and or low red blood cell folate.[85] Beer consumers may show folate levels somewhat higher than these because of the folic acid content of this beverage. The clinical hallmark of folate deficiency is a megaloblastic anemia caused by damaged cell replication. It is found in all tissues, but especially in those with a high turnover rate, including the gastrointestinal mucosa.[86] The result is functional abnormalities and clinical symptoms such as diarrhea. Accordingly, folate deficiency leads to a malabsorption of other nutrients, such as other water-soluble vitamins, and also folic acid itself. The malabsorption is further exacerbated by an abnormal enterohepatic circulation. The metabolic transformation to different active folate metabolites is impaired as a consequence of altered liver function and toxic alcohol and acetaldehyde effects on different enzymes. In addition, alcohol increases the urinary losses of this vitamin.

The impairment of absorption at the level of the gut and the kidney may be due to alcohol's effects on specific folate transporters in these tissues.[87] Because of an alcohol-induced rise in free radical production, the degradation of the vitamin is increased and may cause a tissue-specific deficiency. The alcohol-induced local impairment of folate metabolism may play a role in colorectal carcinogenesis.[88] However, the alcohol-associated risk of colorectal carcinogenesis may vary in part according to the genetic polymorphisms of the 5,10-methylenetetrahydrofolate reductase (MTHFR) related to DNA methylation.[89] The same may also apply to the process of carcinogenesis in other tissues such as oropharyngeal tissue.[90] Several studies reported an inverse association between moderate alcohol intake and plasma homocysteine levels, whereas higher alcohol intake is consistently associated with increased plasma homocysteine levels, which is in part mediated by the alcohol-induced deficiency of folate, vitamin $B_6$ and also vitamin $B_{12}$.

## Effects of Alcohol on Mineral and Trace Element Metabolism

### *Magnesium*

Low serum and tissue levels of magnesium are a typical feature in heavy drinkers, and these alterations are more prevalent in the presence of liver disease.[91] The magnesium nutriture is impaired as a result of reduced intake, malabsorption, increased urinary losses, secondary hyperaldosteronism, and increased fecal losses due to diarrhea. A reduction of alcohol intake is associated with an increase of the magnesium content of red blood cells.[91] The decreased magnesium content of tissues may play a role in the development and progression of alcohol-associated pathologies. Magnesium content is especially decreased in heart tissue, a condition that may predispose to cardiac arrhythmias, a typical symptom in magnesium deficiency. Because of magnesium's effects in the maintenance of the membranes, a deficiency may exacerbate the development of organ damage, including liver damage. Magnesium plays a central role in over 300 biochemical reactions, one of them being thiamine phosphorlylation. In view of the low toxicity of magnesium, this mineral should be replaced in the medical treatment of heavy drinkers (e.g., supplementation with 200–300 mg elemental magnesium in chronic mild hypomagnesemia, where 1 mmol = 2mEq = 24 mg elemental magnesium).

### *Zinc*

Heavy alcohol consumption is associated with deceased serum zinc and lower hepatic zinc concentrations.[92] The lower zinc levels are correlated with the degree of liver damage, but low zinc levels in serum are also found in less-advanced liver disease, such as fatty liver disease.[92] The deficient zinc status results from low intakes, a reduced absorption, an increased urinary excretion, and an alteration of zinc distribution. Usually, zinc deficiency in the alcoholic is multifactorial, but a low dietary intake is found in most heavy consumers of alcohol. The zinc malabsorption is caused by direct and indirect alcohol effects, such as mucosal damage and altered synthesis of zinc ligands (such as metallothionein) owing to alcohol-induced impaired protein synthesis. The presence and the degree of exocrine pancreatic insufficiency represents an additional modulator of zinc status. Alcoholic liver disease, especially alcoholic hepatitis, has been identified as the major predictor for metabolic perturbations in zinc nutriture. The increased urinary excretion of zinc correlates with the degree of liver damage[93] and is caused by decreased peripheral tissue zinc uptake and decreased serum levels of albumin. In patients with liver cirrhosis, the increased urinary zinc excretion persists even after cessation of alcohol intake. The acute ingestion of alcohol among moderate drinkers causes increased urinary zinc excretion, a consequence that suggests direct effects of alcohol on zinc homeostasis at the level of the kidney.[93]

Malnutrition in combination with alcohol leads to a higher degree of zinc depletion. It has been suggested that alcohol-induced alterations in zinc metabolism may increase alcohol-associated carcinogenesis.[94] In view of the multiple effects of zinc, clinical signs of zinc deficiency—abnormalities of taste and smell, hypogonadism, infertility and an impaired dark adaptation—are often seen in alcoholics. An impaired dark adaptation is a characteristic symptom in alcohol consumers, one generally not caused by vitamin A deficiency but by zinc deficiency. Defective zinc nutriture may increase alcohol toxicity given that the rate-limiting enzyme in alcohol degradation, ADH, is a zinc metalloenzyme.

## Alcohol and Mortality

The effect of alcohol on morbidity and mortality is biphasic, and the relationship is J-shaped: low levels of ingestion are associated with a reduced morbidity and mortality risks, whereas abstinence and higher levels of ingestion are associated with a higher mortality risk due to different cancers, alcoholic liver disease, and cardiovacular diseases such as arrhythmias, alcoholic cardiomyopathy, hypertension, and stroke.[95,96] The reduced mortality risk at lower intakes is explained by a reduced risk of coronary artery disease[95,97,98] and gallstones.[99] The amount of alcohol ingestion at the nadir of mortality risk is not known and varies from study to study and from one individual to another. A study analyzing data from 20 international cohort studies found a substantial variation in the nadir (the level of consumption at which mortality is least).[100]

This meta-analysis estimated the nadir for US men to be 7.7 units of alcohol per week (95% confidence interval [CI] 6.4–9.1). In that study, 1 unit (1 drink) was considered to be 9 g alcohol for US men, 2.9 units per week (95% CI 2.0–4.0) for US women, and 12.9 units per week (95% CI 10.8–15.1) for UK men.[100]

The J-shaped relationship has been reported in different studies, one of them being the American Cancer Society investigation.[97] In that study in men and in women, a light alcohol intake was associated with a reduction in mortality risk because of a lower coronary artery disease risk. However, with increasing alcohol intake (even in the range of moderate intake), mortality risk rose, especially in women, whose risk of breast cancer also increased.[97] The hallmark of excessive alcohol intake is metabolic and structural alterations at the level of the liver, and liver cirrhosis is the leading cause of death in heavy drinkers.[97,101,102] Age-adjusted death rates of liver cirrhosis have been reported as 11.1 and 4.6 per 100,000 for US men and women, respectively. In addition, nearly one-third of all traffic crash fatalities in the United States are alcohol related.

## Alcohol and Cardiovascular Diseases

The protective effect of alcohol on coronary disease risk has been reported in men and women,[95,97,103,104] with a risk reduction in the range of 20% to 40%. A meta-analysis of 42 studies concluded that the ingestion of 30 g of alcohol per day would result in a 24.7% reduction in risk of coronary heart disease.[104] The intake levels related to the nadir of risk vary widely in different studies.[100] It is important to recognize that the protective effects are seen mainly in older people and those who do have one or more of the classical cardiovascular risk factors.[97,105-107] This finding suggests that alcohol may modulate the pathophysiological potential of some of the classic risk factors for coronary artery disease.

The mechanisms of the cardioprotective effects of alcohol (Table 2) are not completely elucidated, and about 50% of the potential protection seems to be mediated by the alcohol-induced increase in HDL-cholesterol levels.[105] Favorable effects on fibrinolysis, thromobogenesis, coronary blood flow, postprandial metabolism, prostaglandin and thromoboxane synthesis, arterial vasodilatation, other lipoprotein fractions than HDL-cholesterol, anti-inflammatory effects, antioxidative effects, ingestion of non-nutritive protective compounds, ischemic preconditioning, or behavioral aspects have also been suggested.[104,108,109]

The protective effects of alcohol are independent of the beverage type,[98] although studies reported a higher protection in red wine consumers[110] because of its content

**Table 2.** Summary and Classification of Possible Cardioprotective Mechanisms of Alcohol

| Lipid Effects | Blood Coagulation | Endocrine Effects |
|---|---|---|
| • Increase in HDL-cholesterol<br>• Decrease in composition, size, and concentration of LDL-cholesterol<br>• Decrease in Lipoprotein (a)<br>• LDL-receptor effects | • Modulation of coagulation factors<br>• Modulation of thrombogenesis<br>• Modulation of fibrinolysis | • Insulin metabolism<br>• Estrogen metabolism<br>• Steroid metabolism |
| **Psychological Effects** | **Non-Nutritive Compounds** | **Miscellaneous Effects** |
| • Control of type A behavior<br>• Anti-anxiety effects<br>• Stress control | • Polyphenolic compounds<br>• Phytoalexins (e.g., resveratrol) | • Vasoreactivity<br>• Ischemic preconditioning<br>• membrane fluidity<br>• Liver structure (liver sieve)<br>• Modulation of the metabolic syndrome |

HDL = high-density lipoprotein; LDL = low-density lipoprotein.

of polyphenols and flavonoids.[111] Red wine consumption may elicit a higher protection that is related to personality traits of the typical red wine consumer and the ingestion of red wine mainly together with a meal.[112]

If the cardioprotective effects or alcohol are really causal, then the central questions are "how much is enough?" and "how much is too much?" A systematic review (using data from England and Wales) reported that the level of alcohol intake with the lowest mortality ranges from 0 units a week in men and women under 35 years of age to three units a week in women over 65 years of age and 8 units a week in men over 65 years of age (in this article, 1 unit was defined as 9 g of alcohol).[107] Smoking is a major determinant of health, and the interaction between alcohol and smoking is of great importance. In a recent prospective cohort study of postmenopausal women,[113] alcohol ingestion among those who had never smoked was inversely associated with coronary heart disease mortality. Among current smokers, no association was found between alcohol ingestion and coronary heart disease mortality, but there was a positive association with cancer incidence among those consuming at least one drink daily. Based on data from White et al.[107] it can be concluded that the alcohol consumption levels with the greatest potential benefit are likely to be lower in the future due to a decline in coronary heart disease for reasons unrelated to alcohol intake. This also means that the cornerstone of coronary artery disease prevention remains in the control of the major classic cardiovascular risk factors (i.e., smoking, dyslipidemia, hypertension, and obesity). Despite the potentially favorable effects of alcohol on coronary artery disease risk, alcohol represents an important cause of hypertension,[114] hemorrhagic stroke,[115] alcoholic cardiomyopathy, heart insufficiency, and arrhythmias.[116]

The protective effects of alcohol on coronary artery disease risk in the French population has been termed "The French Paradox." The French do indeed show a more than one-third lower mortality rate for ischemic heart disease than the Americans or British; however, the all-cause mortality rate in France is not much different and the mortality rate for some of the typical alcohol-associated diseases, such as oropharyngeal cancer or liver cirrhosis, even higher is in France than in other countries.[117] Despite the many associations between alcohol and coronary artery disease mortality, recent data suggest that the protective effect of alcohol may be biased by "good habits" and not "just good wine,"[118] so that the drinker's habits become more important than the drink.[119] Several studies reported that moderate alcohol drinkers or wine drinkers do show a healthier diet and behavior compared with other drinkers or abstainers.[120-123] The cardioprotection may thus be mediated by synergistic effects of a low dose of alcohol in combination with health-prone behavior.

### *Alcohol and Hypertension*

The first description of the relationship between alcohol and blood pressure was published by Lian in 1915. Cross-sectional, prospective, and interventional studies have reported an increase in systolic and diastolic blood pressure with increasing alcohol intake.[124,125] Most studies reported a dose-response relationship between alcohol intake and blood pressure without a threshold level of alcohol intake, and cessation of alcohol intake in heavy consumers led to a reduction in blood pressure.[126] The decline in blood pressure upon cessation of excessive alcohol consumption shows a wide variability. Based on a recent meta-analysis with the exclusive reduction of alcohol intake a significant reduction of mean systolic (2.52 to 4.10 mmHg) and of mean diastolic (1.49 to 2.58 mmHg) blood pressure was achieved.[127] This decline in blood pressure would result in a 6% reduction of coronary heart disease risk and a 15% reduction in the risk of stroke of transient ischemic attacks.[127] Blood pressure effects are more pronounced in daily alcohol consumers. A recent study underlined the importance of the effect of the timing of blood pressure measurements after alcohol intake on the magnitude and direction of the blood pressure change,[128] and this may also be a reason for inconsistent effects of alcohol on blood pressure in epidemiological and some experimental studies. The pathophysiologic mechanisms for the pressor effects of alcohol are not known exactly, and multiple mechanisms involving direct and indirect effects of alcohol on autonomic regulation, neurohumoral effects, effects on peripheral resistance, calcium handling in the vascular smooth muscle cells, and altered stress perception have been suggested. Alterations in liver function may affect the metabolism of antihypertensive drugs.

### *Alcohol and Stroke*

Alcohol has been identified as an independent risk factor for hemorrhagic stroke.[126] The increased stroke risk is partly caused by the pressure effects of alcohol as well as effects on cerebrovascular vasculature.[115]

Because cardiovascular disease and ischemic stroke share some common pathophysiological features, alcohol may also have protective effects on ischemic stroke. In a study set in a multi-ethnic, urban society, moderate alcohol consumption (up to two drinks per day) had protective effects on ischemic stroke, with an odds ratio (OR) of 0.51, 95% CI 0.39–0.67).[129] However, excessive drinking, considered to be 7 or more drinks per day (OR 2.96, 95% CI 1.05–8.29) and binge drinking were associated with a 2- to 4-fold increased risk of ischemic stroke. A study by Jackson et al.[130] reported a possible inverse association between light to moderate alcohol intake and risks of total and cardiovascular mortality in men with a history of stroke. At present. it is controversial whether light to moderate alcohol intake increases the risk of atrial fibrillation,[131] an important risk factor for ischemic stroke. Recent data from the Health Professional Follow-up Study[132] reported that two drinks or fewer per day was not associated with an increased risk for ischemic stroke and that consuming red wine (not other beverages) was associated with a lower risk. Moderate alcohol consumption (especially wine consumption) is associated with a healthier lifestyle such as increased fruit and vegetable consumption,[120-123] and an increased fruit and vegetable intake is associated with a reduced risk of stroke.[133] Accordingly a study from western New York showed that wine drinkers had a higher education, higher household incomes, a lower prevalence of smoking, and a higher vitamin intake.[134]

Several recent studies reported that moderate alcohol consumption is associated with better cognitive functioning and a reduced risk of a cognitive decline with aging.[135] Once again, it is not completely clear whether the light alcohol drinking or the behavior of the drinker is the protective principle.

## Alcohol and Liver Disease

Alcoholic liver disease (steatosis, alcoholic hepatitis, and cirrhosis) represents the central feature of alcohol-related pathologies. There is a direct relationship between the per capita alcohol consumption (independent of the beverage type) and the death rate from liver cirrhosis. As with other alcohol-related pathologies, susceptibility to developing alcoholic cirrhosis varies from one individual to another as a function of the amount and duration of alcohol intake, gender, genetic predisposition, characteristics of alcohol metabolism, previous hepatitis B or C,[136,137] and potential nutritional factors.[138] The risk of developing alcoholic liver disease increases sharply with alcohol consumption over 40 g/d. For women, the threshold dose of alcohol is about half the threshold dosage of men. The mechanisms of alcoholic liver damage are multiple, and include direct toxic effects of alcohol, acetaldehyde-mediated toxicity, increased oxygen requirements, and free radical damage. In addition, immune-mediated phenomena such as a proinflammatory state seem to be of central importance.[139] In the development of alcoholic fatty liver, the altered redox potential (NADH/NAD+), impaired lipid oxidation, and increased lipogenesis seem to play a central role. The role of oxidative stress and injury in the pathogenesis of alcohol-induced hepatic injury is underlined by an inverse association between the serum alanin transaminase (ALT) and serum concentration of certain nutrients such as vitamin C, alpha- and beta-carotene, and lutein/zeaxanthin.

## Alcohol and Cancer

Alcohol consumption is related to an increased prevalence of oropharyngeal, esophageal, liver, and colorectal cancers.[2] The combination of smoking and drinking increases the risk of the oropharyngeal cancers. Alcohol per se has no direct carcinogenic properties, and the pathophysiologic bases of the alcohol-induced cancers are multiple and include effects of acetaldehyde or effects of alcohol on methyl-group metabolism.[140] Increased alcohol intake, in combination with a low micronutrient intake, increases cancer risk (e.g., colorectal cancer). A collaborative analysis of 53 studies in which the consumption was over 35 g/d of alcohol resulted in a significantly increased risk for breast cancer.[141] Whether small amounts of alcohol intake are associated with an increased risk of breast cancer in women is controversial.[97,142,143] In a pooled analysis of six prospective studies, the multivariate-adjusted relative risk for women whose total alcohol intakes were between 30 g/d and <60 g/d versus non-drinking women was 1.41 (95% CI, 1.18–1.69).[142] Alcohol has a high potential to modulate estrogen metabolism, leading to higher circulating estrogen levels,[144] so the potential detrimental effects of alcohol on estrogen-sensitive cancers is not surprising. Some of the controversy of the data can be explained by genetic factors and/or menopausal status or period of life with alcohol consumption. In view of the current evidence, light alcohol consumption seems to be safe for most women.

## Alcohol and Bone

The direct and indirect effects of alcohol on bone metabolism are multiple and depend on the amount and duration of alcohol intake. Acute and chronic effects of alcohol on bone have to be distinguished. In heavy drinkers, the calcium balance is negatively affected by low intakes and malabsorption of calcium due to direct mucosal damagee, an impaired vitamin D nutriture, and increased urinary calcium losses.[145] In heavy drinkers, different structural and functional changes in the bone can be found. Low to moderate amounts of alcohol have no adverse effects on bone mass in postmenopausal women[146] because of alcohol's effects on endogenous (and exogeneous) estrogens (see above). Despite some controversial data that have been reported about the effects of alcohol on bone metabolism, in the clinical setting any unexplained fracture or osteoporosis (especially in men) may point to alcohol-related problems.

## Fetal Alcohol Syndrome

Pregnancy is a period of life during which alcohol intake should be avoided completely. Nearly 40 years ago, it was first reported that heavy alcohol intake during pregnancy may be associated with fetal alcohol syndrome (FAS). FAS is characterized by typical physical and neurobehavioral features.[147] Children with FAS show a pre- and postnatal growth retardation, facial dysmorphy, and central nervous system dysfunctions that cause permanent cognitive impairment and learning disabilities. Present evidence suggests that even low to moderate amounts of alcohol at the critical time during the early phase of pregnancy may lead to FAS or a syndrome with only partial and/or minor phenotypic expression of the FAS (so-called alcohol-related birth defects). Despite the knowledge of the relationship between alcohol and the FAS, 1 in 8 women of childbearing age reportedly drink the amount known to cause FAS ( ≥7 drinks per week, or ≥5 on any one occasion). Alcohol intake during pregnancy, but also during the week of conception increases the risk of early pregnancy loss.

## Conclusion

As a function of the amount of alcohol consumed and individual factors (genetic factors and environmental factors, including lifestyle and nutritional factors), the health and nutritional effects of alcohol may be positive or negative. Often, both positive and negative effects occur. In view of the heterogeneity of responses for any given alcohol dose, the formulation of public health recommendations for safe consumption levels are becoming increasingly difficult. In today's world, the art of any patient counseling and public health counseling about alcohol consumption is not to forbid alcohol consumption, but to try to formulate safe consumption levels for those wishing to drink. In any case, alcohol should not be recommended for health reasons or for health maintenance.

Evidence suggests that the safe amount may vary considerably from one individual to another, even for those whose alcohol intake is in the light to moderate range. Identifying biochemical and genetic markers for risk assessment related to moderate alcohol consumption may help to formulate and implement specific individual recommendations. In addition, future research activities should focus on strategies to implement safe drinking practices in combination with an overall healthy lifestyle with respect to nutrition and physical activity. In such a setting, light to moderate alcohol consumption may add to the quality of life.

## References

1. Centers for Disease Control and Prevention, National Center for Chronic Disease Prevention and Health Promotion. *Measures of Alcohol Consumption and Alcohol-Related Health Effects from Excessive Consumption*. Available at: http://www.cdc.gov/alcohol/factsheets/general_information.htm. Accessed February 24, 2006.
2. Hamdy RC, Aukerman MM. Alcohol on trial: the evidence. South Med J. 2005;98:34–68.
3. Mokdad AH, Marks JS, Stroup DF, Gerberding JL. Actual causes of death in the United States, 2000. JAMA. 2004;291:1238–1245.
4. US Department of Agriculture, Food Surveys Research Group. *Results from USDA's 1994–96 Continuing Survey of Food Intakes by Individuals and 1994–96 Diet and Health Knowledge Survey Table Set 10*. Available at: http://199.133.10.189/SP2UserFiles/Place/12355000/pdf/Csfii3yr.pdf. Accessed February 24, 2006.
5. Higuchi S, Matsushita S, Masaki T, et al. Influence of genetic variations of ethanol-metabolizing enzymes on phenotypes of alcohol-related disorders. Ann N Y Acad Sci. 2004;1025:472–480.
6. Paton A. Alcohol in the body. BMJ. 2005;330: 85–87.
7. Lieber CS, DeCarli LM. Hepatic microsomal ethanol-oxidizing system: in vitro characteristics and adaptive properties in vivo. J Biol Chem. 1970; 245:2505–2512.
8. Watson RR, Preedy VR. *Nutrition and Alcohol: Linking Nutrient Interactions and Dietary Intake*. Boca Raton, FL: CRC Press; 2003.
9. Brooks PJ. DNA damage, DNA repair, and alcohol toxicity—a review. Alcohol Clin Exp Res. 1997;21: 1073–1082.
10. Li TK. Pharmacogenetics of responses to alcohol and genes that influence alcohol drinking. J Stud Alcohol. 2000;61:5–12.
11. Santolaria-Fernandez FJ, Gomez-Sirvent JL, Gonzalez-Reimers CE, et al. Nutritional assessment of drug addicts. Drug Alcohol Depend. 1995;38: 11–18.
12. Salaspuro M. Nutrient intake and nutritional status in alcoholics. Alcohol Alcohol. 1993;28:85–88.
13. Urbano-Marquez A, Fernandez-Sola J. Effects of alcohol on skeletal and cardiac muscle. Muscle Nerve. 2004;30:689–707.
14. Burke V, Puddey IB, Rakic V, et al. Carbohydrate-deficient transferrin as a marker of change in alcohol intake in men drinking 20–60 g of alcohol per day. Alcohol Clin Exp Res. 1998;22: 1973–1980.
15. Borucki K, Schreiner R, Dierkes J, et al. Detection of recent ethanol intake with new markers: comparison of fatty acid ethyl esters in serum and of ethyl glucuronide and the ratio of 5-hydroxytryptophol to 5-hydroxyindole acetic acid in urine. Alcohol Clin Exp Res. 2005;29:781–787.
16. Bisaga A, Laposata M, Xie S, Evans SM. Comparison of serum fatty acid ethyl esters and urinary 5-hydroxytryptophol as biochemical markers of recent ethanol consumption. Alcohol Alcohol. 2005; 40:214–218.
17. Seitz HK, Suter PM. Ethanol toxicity and the nutritional status. In: Kotsonis FN, Mackey M, Hjelle J, eds. *Nutritional Toxicology*. New York: Raven Press; 1994; 95–116.
18. Suter PM. Is alcohol consumption a risk factor for weight gain and obesity? Crit Rev Clin Lab Sci. 2005;42:197–227.
19. Westerterp-Plantenga MS, Verwegen CRT. The appetizing effect of an apéritif in overweight and normal-weight humans. Am J Clin Nutr. 1999;69: 205–212.
20. Yeomans MR. Effects of alcohol on food and energy intake in human subjects: evidence for passive and active over-consumption of energy. Br J Nutr. 2004;92 (suppl 1):S31–S34.
21. Liu S, Serdula MK, Williamson DF, et al. A prospective study of alcohol intake and change in body weight among US Adults. Am J Epidemiol. 1994; 140:912–920.
22. Sakurai Y, Umeda T, Shinchi K, et al. Relation of total and beverage-specific alcohol intake to body mass index and waist-to-hip ratio: A study of self-defense officials in Japan. Eur J Epidemiol. 1997; 13:893–898.
23. Suter PM. Is alcohol consumption a risk factor for weight gain and obesity? Crit Rev Clin Lab Sci. 2005;42:1–31.

24. Yeomans MR, Hails NJ, Nesic JS. Alcohol and the appetizer effect. Behav Pharmacol. 1999;10: 151–161.
25. Suter PM, Schutz Y, Jéquier E. The effect of ethanol on fat storage in healthy subjects. N Engl J Med. 1992;326:983–987.
26. Atwater WD, Benedict FG. An experimental inquiry regarding the nutritive value of alcohol. Mem Natl Acad Sci. 1902;8:235–272.
27. Lieber C. Perspectives: do alcohol calories count? Am J Clin Nutr. 1991;54:976–982.
28. Siler SQ, Neese RA, Hellerstein MK. De novo lipogenesis, lipid kinetics, and whole-body lipid balances in humans after acute alcohol consumption. Am J Clin Nutr. 1999;70:928–936.
29. Rohrer JE, Rohland BM, Denison A, Way A. Frequency of alcohol use and obesity in community medicine patients. BMC Fam Pract. 2005;6:17.
30. Suter PM, Maire R, Vetter W. Is an increased waist: hip ratio the cause of alcohol-induced hypertension. The AIR94 study. J Hypertens. 1995;13:1857–1862.
31. Eckel RH, Grundy SM, Zimmet PZ. The metabolic syndrome. Lancet. 2005;365:1415–1428.
32. Djousse L, Arnett DK, Eckfeldt JH, et al. Alcohol consumption and metabolic syndrome: does the type of beverage matter? Obes Res. 2004;12: 1375–1385.
33. Freiberg MS, Cabral HJ, Heeren TC, et al. Alcohol consumption and the prevalence of the metabolic syndrome in the US: a cross-sectional analysis of data from the Third National Health and Nutrition Examination Survey. Diabetes Care. 2004;27: 2954–2959.
34. Barona E, Lieber CS. Alcohol and lipids. In: Galanter M, ed. *Recent Developments in Alcoholism. Volume 14: Consequences of Alcoholism.* New York: Plenum Press; 1998; 97–134.
35. Eaton S, Record CO, Bartlett K. Multiple biochemical effects in the pathogenesis of alcoholic fatty liver. Eur J Clin Invest. 1997;27:719–722.
36. Suter PM, Gerritsen M, Häsler E, et al. Alcohol effects on postprandial lipemia with and without preprandial exercise. FASEB J (Part I) 1999;13: A208.
37. Manttari M, Tenkanen L, Alikoski T, Manninen V. Alcohol and coronary heart disease: the roles of HDL-cholesterol and smoking. J Intern Med. 1997;214:157–163.
38. Greenfield JR, Samaras K, Hayward CS, et al. Beneficial postprandial effect of a small amount of alcohol on diabetes and cardiovascular risk factors: modification by insulin resistance. J Clin Endocrinol Metab. 2005;90:661–672.
39. Liinamaa MJ, Kesaniemi YA, Savolainen MJ. Lipoprotein composition influences cholesteryl ester transfer in alcohol abusers. Ann Med. 1998;30: 316–322.
40. Johansen D, Andersen PK, Jensen MK, et al. Nonlinear relation between alcohol intake and high-density lipoprotein cholesterol level: results from the Copenhagen City Heart Study. Alcohol Clin Exp Res. 2003;27:1305–1309.
41. Lussier-Cacan S, Bolduc A, Xhignesse M, et al. Impact of alcohol intake on measures of lipid metabolism depends on context defined by gender, body mass index, cigarette smoking, and apolipoprotein E genotype. Arterioscler Thromb Vasc Biol. 2002;22:824–831.
42. Ayaori M, Ishikawa T, Yoshida H, et al. Beneficial effects of alcohol withdrawal on LDL particle size distribution and oxidative susceptibility in subjects with alcohol induced hypertriglyceridemia. Arterioscler Thromb Vasc Biol. 1997;17:2540–2547.
43. Fuhrman B, Lavy A, Aviram M. Consumption of red wine with meals reduces the susceptibility of human plasma and low-density-lipoprotein to lipid peroxidation. Am J Clin Nutr. 1995;61:549–554.
44. Manach C, Williamson G, Morand C, et al. Bioavailability and bioefficacy of polyphenols in humans. I. Review of 97 bioavailability studies. Am J Clin Nutr. 2005;81:230S–242S.
45. Lange LG. Nonoxidative ethanol metabolism: formation of fatty acid ethyl esters by cholesterol esterase. Proc Natl Acad Sci U S A. 1982;79:3954–3957.
46. Criddle DN, Raraty MG, Neoptolemos JP, et al. Ethanol toxicity in pancreatic acinar cells: Mediation by nonoxidative fatty acid metabolites. Proc Natl Acad Sci U S A. 2004;101:10738–10743.
47. Borucki K, Kunstmann S, Dierkes J, et al. In heavy drinkers fatty acid ethyl esters in the serum are increased for 44 hr after ethanol consumption. Alcohol Clin Exp Res. 2004;28:1102–1106.
48. Hanck C, Whitcomb DC. Alcoholic pancreatitis. Gastroenterol Clin North Am. 2004;33:751–765.
49. Siler SQ, Neese RA, Chrstiansen MP, Hellerstein MK. The inhibition of gluconeogenesis following alcohol in humans. Am J Physiol.1998;275: E897–E907.
50. Flanagan D, Wood P, Sherwin R, et al. Gin and tonic and reactive hypoglycemia: what is important - the gin, the tonic, or both? J Clin Endocrinol Metabol. 1998;796–800.
51. Pedersen-Bjergaard U, Reubsaet JL, Nielsen SL, et al. Psychoactive drugs, alcohol, and severe hypoglycemia in insulin-treated diabetes: analysis of 141 cases. Am J Med Sci. 2005;118:307–310.
52. Van-de-Wiel A. Alcohol and insulin sensitivity. Neth J Med. 1998;52:91–94.
53. Valmadrid CT, Klein R, Moss SE, et al. Alcohol intake and the risk of coronary heart disease mortality in persons with older-onset diabetes mellitus. JAMA. 1999;282:239–246.

54. Leo MA, Lieber CS. Alcohol, vitamin A, and beta-carotene: adverse interactions, including hepatotoxicity and carcinogenicity. Am J Clin Nutr. 1999;69: 1071–1085.
55. McClain CJ, Van-Thiel DH, Parker S, et al. Alteration in zinc, vitamin A and retinol-binding protein in chronic alcoholics: a possible mechanism for night blindness and hypogonadism. Alcohol Clin Exp Res. 1979;3:135–140.
56. Dan Z, Popov Y, Patsenker E, et al. Hepatotoxicity of alcohol-induced polar retinol metabolites involves apoptosis via loss of mitochondrial membrane potential. FASEB J. 2005;19:845–847.
57. Albanes D, Heinonen OP, Taylor PR, et al. a-Tocopherol and b-carotene supplements and lung cancer incidence in the Alpha-Tocopherol, Beta-Carotene Cancer Prevention Study: Effects of Base-line Characteristics and Study Compliance. J Natl Cancer Inst. 1996;88:1560–1570.
58. Ahmed S, Leo MA, Lieber CS. Interactions between alcohol and b-carotene in patients with alcoholic liver disease. Am J Clin Nutr. 1994;60: 430–436.
59. Bjørneboe GEA, Johnsen J, Bjørneboe A, et al. Diminished serum concentration of vitamin E and selenium in alcoholics. Ann Nutr Metabol. 1988;32: 56–61.
60. de-la-Maza MP, Petermann M, Bunout D, Hirsch S. Effects of long-term vitamin E supplementation in alcoholic cirrhotics. J Am Coll Nutr. 1995;14: 192–196.
61. Machlin L. Use and safety of elevated dosages of vitamin E in adults. Int J Vitam Nutr Res. 1989; 30(suppl):56–68.
62. Nyquist F, Ljunghall S, Berglund M, Oberant K. Biochemical markers of bone metabolism after short and long time ethanol withdrawal in alcoholics. Bone. 1996;19:51–54.
63. Shiomi S, Nishiguchi S, Kubo S, et al. Vitamin K2 (menatetrenone) for bone loss in patients with cirrhosis of the liver. Am J Gastroenterol. 2002;97: 978–981.
64. Nyquist F, Karlsson MK, Obrant KJ, Nilsson JA. Osteopenia in alcoholics after tibia shaft fractures. Alcohol Alcohol. 1997;32:599–604.
65. Laitinen K, Valimaki M, Lamberg-Allardt C, et al. Deranged vitamin D metabolism but normal bone mineral density in Finnish noncirrhotic male alcoholics. Alcohol Clin Exp Res. 1990;14:551–556.
66. Jamieson CP, Obeid OA, Powell-Tuck J. The thiamin, riboflavin and pyridoxine status of patients on emergency admission to hospital. Clin Nutr. 1999; 18:87–91.
67. Tomasulo PA, Kater RMH, Iber FL. Impairment of thiamine absorption in alcoholism. Am J Clin Nutr. 1968;21:1341–1344.
68. Holzbach E. Thiamine absorption in alcoholic delirum patients. J Stud Alcohol. 1996;57:581–584.
69. Preedy V, Reilly ME, Patel VB, et al. Protein metabolism in alcoholism: effects on specific tissues and the whole body. Nutrition. 1999;15:604–608.
70. Martin PR, Singleton CK, Hiller-Sturmhofel S. The role of thiamine deficiency in alcoholic brain disease. Alcohol Res Health. 2003;27:134–142.
71. Cook CC, Thomson AD. B-complex vitamins in the prophylaxis and treatment of Wernicke-Korsakoff syndrome. Br J Hosp Med. 1997;57:461–465.
72. Crowe SF, Kempton S. Both ethanol toxicity and thiamine deficiency are necessary to produce long-term memory deficits in the young chick. Pharmacol Biochem Behav. 1997;58:461–470.
73. McLean J, Manchip S. Wernicke's encephalopathy induced by magnesium depletion. Lancet. 1999; 353:1768.
74. Suter PM, Vetter W. Diuretics and vitamin B1: are diuretics a risk factor for thiamin malnutrition? Nutr Rev. 2000;58:319–323.
75. Pinto J, Huang YP, Rivlin RS. Mechanisms underlying the differential effects of ethanol on the bioavailability of riboflavin and flavin adenine dinucleotide. J Clin Invest. 1987;79:1343–1348.
76. Ono S, Takahashi H, Hirano H. Ethanol enhances the esterification of riboflavin in rat organ tissue. Int J Vitam Nutr Res. 1987;57:335.
77. Dastur DK, Santhadevi Q, Quadros EV. The B-vitamins in malnutrition with alcoholism. Br J Nutr. 1976;36:143–159.
78. Rossouw JE, Labadorios D, Davis M, Williams R. The degradation of tryptophan in severe liver disease. Int J Vit Nutr Res. 1978;48:281–289.
79. Hardman MJ, Page RA, Wiseman MS, Crow KE. Regulation of rates of ethanol metabolism and liver [NAD+]/[NADH] ratio. In: Palmer NT, ed. *Alcoholism. A Molecular Perspective*. New York: Plenum Press; 1991; 27–33.
80. Cook CCH, Hallwood PM, Thomson AD. B-Vitamin deficiency and neuropsychiatric syndromes in alcohol misuse. Alcohol Alcohol. 1998;33: 317–336.
81. Pitsavas S, Andreou C, Bascialla F, et al. Pellagra encephalopathy following B-complex vitamin treatment without niacin. Int J Psychiatry Med. 2004; 34:91–95.
82. Vannucchi H, Moreno FS. Interaction of niacin and zinc metabolism in patients with alcoholic pellagra. Am J Clin Nutr. 1989;50:364–369.
83. Mitchell D, Wagner C, Stone WJ, et al. Abnormal regulation of plasma pyridoxal-5′-phosphate in patients with liver disease. Gastroenterology. 1976;71: 1043–1049.
84. Larsson SC, Giovannucci E, Wolk A. Vitamin B6 intake, alcohol consumption, and colorectal cancer:

a longitudinal population-based cohort of women. Gastroenterology. 2005;128:1830–1837.

85. Gloria L, Cravo M, Camilo ME, et al. Nutritional deficiencies in chronic alcoholics: relation to dietary intake and alcohol consumption. Am J Gastroenterol. 1997;92:485–489.
86. Halsted CH. Alcohol and folate interactions: Clinical implications. In: Bailey LB, ed. *Folate in Health and Disease*. New York: Marcel Dekker; 1995; 313–327.
87. Ross DM, McMartin KE. Effect of ethanol on folate binding by isolated rat renal brush border membranes. Alcohol. 1996;13:449–454.
88. Kim YI. Role of folate in colon cancer development and progression. J. Nutr. 2003;133:3731S–3739S.
89. Le Marchand L, Wilkens LR, Kolonel LN, Henderson BE. The MTHFR C677T polymorphism and colorectal cancer: The Multiethnic Cohort Study. Cancer Epidemiol Biomarkers Prev. 2005; 14:1198–1203.
90. Capaccio P, Ottaviani F, Cuccarini V, et al. Association between methylenetetrahydrofolate reductase polymorphisms, alcohol intake and oropharyngolaryngeal carcinoma in northern Italy. Laryngol Otol. 2005;119:371–376.
91. Kisters K, Schodjaian K, Nguyen SQ, et al. Effect of alcohol on plasma and intracellular magnesium status in patients with steatosis or cirrhosis of the liver. Medical Science Research. 1997;25:805–806.
92. Bode JC, Hanisch P, Henning H, et al. Hepatic zinc content in patients with various stages of alcoholic liver disease and in patients with chronic active and chronic persistent hepatitis. Hepatology. 1988; 8:1605–1609.
93. Rodriguez-Moreno F, Gonzalez RE, Santolaria FF, et al. Zinc, copper, manganese, and iron in chronic alcoholic liver disease. Alcohol. 1997;14: 39–44.
94. Seitz HK, Pöschl G, Simanowski UA. Alcohol and cancer. In: Galanter M, ed. *Recent Advances in Alcoholism*. New York: Plenum Press; 1998; 67–134.
95. Hill JA. In vino veritas: alcohol and heart disease. Am J Med Sci. 2005;329:124–135.
96. Rehm J, Bondy S. Alcohol and all-cause mortality: an overview. In: Chadwick DJ, Goode JA, eds. *Alcohol and Cardiovascular Diseases*. Chichester: John Wiley & Sons; 1998; 68–85.
97. Thun MJ, Peto R, Lopez AD, et al. Alcohol consumption and mortality among middle aged and elderly U.S. adults. N Engl J Med. 1997;337: 1705–1714.
98. Rimm EB, Klatsky A, Grobbee D, Stampfer MJ. Review of moderate alcohol consumption and reduced risk of coronary heart disease: is the effect due to beer, wine, or spirits? Br Med J. 1996;312: 731–736.
99. Leitzmann MF, Giovannucci EL, Stampfer MJ, et al. Prospective study of alcohol consumption patterns in relation to symptomatic gallstone disease in men. Alcohol Clin Exp Res. 1999;23:835–841.
100. White IR. The level of alcohol consumption at which all-cause mortality is least. J Clin Epidemiol. 1999;52:967–975.
101. Rodés J, Salaspuro M, Sorensen TA. Alcohol and Liver Disease. In: Macdonald I, ed. *Health Issues Related to Alcohol Consumption*. Washington, DC: International Life Sciences Institute; 1999; 396–450.
102. Lieber CS. Hepatic and metabolic effects of ethanol: pathogenesis and prevention. Ann Med. 1994;26:325–330.
103. Gronbaek M. Epidemiologic evidence for the cardioprotective effects associated with consumption of alcoholic beverages. Pathophysiology. 2004;10: 83–92.
104. Rimm EB, Williams P, Fosher K, et al. Moderate alcohol intake and lower risk of coronary artery disease: meta-analysis of effects on lipids and haemostatic factors. BMJ. 1999;319:1523–1528.
105. Criqui MH. Do known cardiovascular risk factors mediate the effect of alcohol on cardiovascular disease? Novartis Found Symp. 1998;216:159–167.
106. Shaper A. Alcohol and mortaliy: A review of prospective studies. Br J Addiction. 1990;85:837–847.
107. White IR, Altmann DR, Nanchahal K. Alcohol consumption and mortality: modelling risks for men and women at different ages. BMJ. 2002;325:191.
108. Pagel PS, Kersten JR, Warltier DC. Mechanisms of myocardial protection produced by chronic ethanol consumption. Pathophysiology. 2004;10:121–129.
109. Mann LB, Folts JD. Effects of ethanol and other constituents of alcoholic beverages on coronary heart disease: a review. Pathophysiology. 2004;10: 105–112.
110. Renaud SC, Gueguen R, Siest G, Salamon R. Wine, beer, and mortality in middle-aged men from eastern France. Arch Intern Med. 1999;159: 1865–1870.
111. Ruf JC. Wine and polyphenols related to platelet aggregation and atherothrombosis. Drugs Exp Clin Res. 1999;25:125–131.
112. Trevisan M, Krogh V, Farinaro E. Alcohol consumption, drinking pattern and blood pressure: analysis of data from the Italian National Research Council Study. Int J Epidemiol. 1987;16:520–527.
113. Ebbert JO, Janney CA, Sellers TA, et al. The association of alcohol consumption with coronary heart disease mortality and cancer incidence varies by smoking history. J Gen Intern Med. 2005;20: 14–20.
114. Suter PM, Vetter W. The effect of alcohol on blood pressure. Nutr Clin Care. 2000;3:24–34.
115. Hillbom M, Numminen H. Alcohol and stroke:

Pathophysiologic mechanisms. Neuroepidemiology. 1998;17:281–287.
116. Lucas DL, Brown RA, Wassef M, Giles TD. Alcohol and the cardiovascular system: research challenges and opportunities. J Am Coll Cardiol. 2005; 45:1916–1924.
117. Zureik M, Ducimetière P. High Alcohol-related premature mortality in france: concordant estimates from a prospective cohort study and national mortality study. Alcohol Clin Exp Res. 1996;20: 428–433.
118. Rimm EB. Alcohol consumption and coronary heart disease: good habits may be more important than just good wine. Am J Epidemiol. 1996;143: 1094–1098.
119. Klatsky AL. Is it the drink or the drinker? Circumstantial evidence only raises a probability. Am J Clin Nutr. 1999;69:2–3.
120. Klatsky AL, Armstrong MA, Kipp H. Correlates of alcoholic beverage preference: traits of persons who choose wine, liquor or beer. Brit J Addiction. 1990;85:1279–1289.
121. Tjonneland A, Gronbæk M, Stripp C, Overvad K. Wine intake and diet in a random sample of 48763 Danish men and women. Am J Clin Nutr. 1999; 69:49–54.
122. Ruidavets J-B, Bataille V, Dallongeville J, et al. Alcohol intake and diet in France, the prominent role of lifestyle. Eur Heart J. 2004;25:1153–1162.
123. Rouillier P, Boutron-Ruault MC, Bertrais S, et al. Drinking patterns in French adult men—a cluster analysis of alcoholic beverages and relationship with lifestyle. Eur J Nutr. 2004;43:69–76.
124. Klatsky AL, Friedman GD, Siegelaub AB, Gérard MJ. Alcohol consumption and blood pressure: Kaiser-Permanente multiphasic health examination data. N Engl J Med. 1977;296:1194–1200.
125. Huntgeburth M, Ten-Freyhaus H, Rosenkranz S. Alcohol consumption and hypertension. Curr Hypertens Rep. 2005;7:180–185.
126. Grobbee DE, Rimm EB, Keil U, Renauld S. Alcohol and the cardiovascular system. In: Macdonald I, ed. *Health Issues related to Alcohol Consumption.* Washington, DC: International Life Sciences Institute; 1999.
127. Xin X, He J, Frontini MG, et al. Effects of alcohol reduction on blood pressure. Hypertension. 2001; 38:1112–1117.
128. McFadden CB, Brensinger CM, Berlin JA, Townsend RR. Systematic review of the effect of daily alcohol intake on blood pressure. Am J Hypertens. 2005;18:276–286.
129. Sacco RL, Elkind M, Boden-Albala B, et al. The protective effect of moderate alcohol consumption on ischemic stroke. JAMA. 1999;281:53–60.
130. Jackson VA, Sesso HD, Buring JE, Gaziano JM. Alcohol consumption and mortality in men with preexisting cerebrovascular disease. Arch Intern Med. 2003;163:1189–1193.
131. Frost L, Vestergaard P. Alcohol and risk of atrial fibrillation or flutter: a cohort study. Arch Intern Med. 2004;164:1993–1998.
132. Mukamal KJ, Ascherio A, Mittleman MA, et al. Alcohol and risk for ischemic stroke in men: the role of drinking patterns and usual beverage. Ann Intern Med. 2005;142:11–19.
133. Lock K, Pomerleau J, Causer L, et al. The global burden of disease attributable to low consumption of fruit and vegetables: implications for the global strategy on diet. Bull World Health Organ. 2005; 83:100–108.
134. McCann SE, Sempos C, Freudenheim JL, et al. Alcoholic beverage preference and characteristics of drinkers and nondrinkers in western New York (United States). Nutr Metab Cardiovasc Dis. 2003; 13:2–11.
135. Stampfer MJ, Kang JH, Chen J, et al. Effects of moderate alcohol consumption on cognitive function in women. N Engl J Med. 2005;352:245–253.
136. Lieber CS. New concepts of the pathogenesis of alcoholic liver disease lead to novel treatments. Curr Gastroenterol Rep. 2004;6:60–65.
137. Diehl AM. Recent Events in Alcoholic Liver Disease V. Effects of ethanol on liver regeneration. Am J Physiol Gastrointest Liver Physiol. 2005;288: G1–G6.
138. Halsted CH. Nutrition and alcoholic liver disease. Semin Liver Dis. 2004;24:289–304.
139. Mendez-Sanchez N, Almeda-Valdes P, Uribe M. Alcoholic liver disease. An update. Ann Hepatol. 2005;4:32–42.
140. Poschl G, Seitz HK. Alcohol and cancer. Alcohol Alcohol. 2004;39:155–165.
141. Hamajima N, Hirose K, Tajima K, et al.; Collaborative Group on Hormonal Factors in Breast Cancer. Alcohol, tobacco and breast cancer: collaborative reanalysis of individual data from 53 epidemiological studies, including 58,515 women with breast cancer and 95 067 women without the disease. Br J Cancer. 2002;87:1234–1245.
142. Smith-Warner SA, Spiegelman D, Yaun SS, et al. Alcohol and breast cancer in women: a pooled analysis of cohort studies. JAMA. 1998;279:535–540.
143. Byrne C, Webb PM, Jacobs TW, et al. Alcohol consumption and incidence of benign breast disease. Cancer Epidemiol Biomarkers Prev. 2002;11: 1369–1374.
144. Onland-Moret NC, Peeters PHM, van der Schouw YT, et al. Alcohol and endogenous sex steroid levels in postmenopausal women: a cross-sectional study. J Clin Endocrinol Metab. 2005;90:1414–1419.

145. Laitinen K, Valimaki M. Bone and the 'comforts of life'. Ann Med. 1993;25:413–425.
146. Feskanich D, Korrick SA, Greenspan SL, et al. Moderate alcohol consumption and bone density among postmenopausal women. J Womens Health. 1999;8:65–63.
147. Plant ML, Abel EL, Guerri C. Alcohol and Pregnancy. In: Macdonald I, ed. *Health Issues Related to Alcohol Consumption.* Washington, DC: International Life Sciences Institute; 1999; 182–213.
148. Lieber CS. Medical disorders of alcoholism. N Engl J Med. 1995;333:1058–1065.

# IV Fat-Soluble Vitamins and Related Nutrients

# 12 Vitamin A

Noel W. Solomons

## Introduction

The pioneering studies by E.V. McCollum and his co-workers recognized vitamin A as the first of the vitamins in 1913. A number of compounds of the carotenoid family (provitamin A compounds) can be oxidized to yield the retinoid forms of the vitamin, as first shown by Moore in 1929. Micronutrient deficiency disorders involving iron, iodine, vitamin A, and their combination, are today the most widespread public health nutrition problem worldwide: over a billion individuals are affected at any given time. The highest specific prevalence rates of hypovitaminosis A are seen in southern Asia and sub-Saharan Africa among pregnant women and young children.[1] Specifically, it has been estimated that approximately 127 million preschool children have vitamin A deficiency at any time, while 4.4 million have some stage of xerophthalmia.[2] In developing countries, more than 7.2 million pregnant women have a deficient, and another 13.5 million a marginal vitamin A status; annually, over 6 million women develop night blindness during pregnancy. Hypovitaminosis A can clearly be regarded as a public health nutrition scourge.[3] Moreover, vitamin A, along with other retinoids, has important health-related actions beyond its functions as a nutrient.

### *Nomenclature and Chemical Properties*

The term vitamin A refers to a subgroup of retinoids that possess the biological activity of all-*trans*-retinol. Retinol has a molecular weight of 286.5 Da. Retinoids typically have four isoprenoid units joined head-to-tail and, contain five conjugated carbon-carbon double-bonds. Figure 1 provides the molecular structures for selected retinoid and carotenoid compounds of interest to this chapter. The numbering system for the carbons of retinol is illustrated in Figure 1A.[4] Retinol can be reversibly oxidized to retinal (Figure 1B), which exhibits all of the biological activities of retinol, or further oxidized to retinoic acid (Figure 1C), which is insufficient for vision or animal reproduction.[5]. The form of vitamin A involved in the vision cycle is 11-*cis* etinal (Figure 1D), whereas the primary storage form is retinyl palmitate (Figure 1E).[6] Beyond their nutritional function, retinoids can be effective therapeutically for the treatment of skin disorders and some cancers.[7] Acitretin (Figure 1F) is one example of a less toxic, highly active, synthetic retinoid. The term "provitamin A" is given to several carotenoids, the archetype of which, β-carotene (Figure 1G), has a molecular weight of 536.9 Da and can be cleaved to yield active retinoids. An unsubstituted β-ionone ring is necessary for this function. Although more than 600 carotenoids have been isolated from natural sources, only about 50 possess vitamin A activity.

Retinoids and carotenoids are soluble to varying degrees in most organic solvents, but are insoluble in water. Both are susceptible to oxidation and isomerization when exposed to light, oxygen, reactive metals, and elevated temperatures. Under ideal conditions, both retinoids and carotenoids will remain stable for long periods in serum, tissue, or crystalline forms.[8,9]

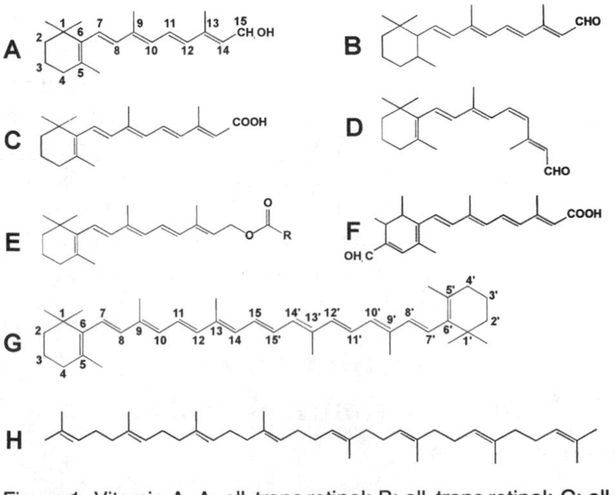

Figure 1. Vitamin A. A: all-*trans* retinol; B: all-*trans* retinal; C: all-*trans* retinoic acid; D: 11-*cis* retinal; E: retinyl esters, mainly retinyl palmitate; F: all-*trans* β-carotene; G: trimethyl methoxyphenol retinoic acid (etrin, acitretin); H; lycopene.

Vitamin A possesses several physical properties useful for its analysis. The series of conjugated double bonds in both classes of compounds produce characteristic ultraviolet or visible absorption spectra. The absorption maxima and molar extinction coefficients in ethanol are 325 nm (~ 52,480) for all-*trans*-retinol, 381 nm (~ 43,400) for all-*trans*-retinal, and 350 nm (~ 45,200) for all-*trans*-retinoic acid.[10] Retinol fluoresces at 470 nm when excited with UV light at 325 nm. Its ability to form a blue color with Lewis acids in anhydrous chloroform has been used as the basis of quantitation for decades. β-carotene, with nine conjugated double bonds, absorbs maximally in petroleum ether at 450 nm (~ 138,900). Lycopene, by contrast (Figure 1H), is an example of a carotene that lacks the properties to be provitamin A compound.

### *Analytical Methods*

The conjugated polyene structures of these compounds give them unique light absorption spectra and high molar absorptivities.[11] Historically, retinoids and carotenoids have been measured using their absorption or fluorescence properties. More recently, reversed-phase high-performance liquid chromatography, or HPLC, has become the method of choice for the analysis of retinoids and carotenoids in biological tissues.[11]

Reversed-phase HPLC (C18 column) followed by visible detection for carotenoids (approximately 450 nm) or UV detection for retinoids is the most common method of analysis.[12] In many cases, *cis-trans* isomers can be better separated using normal-phase HPLC (silica or alumina columns). During sample preparation and analysis, samples should be protected from heat, light, and oxidizing substances. Other techniques, such as gas chromatography (GC) and mass spectroscopy (coupled with GC and HPLC), immunoassays, supercritical fluid chromatography, and capillary electrophoresis, have proven useful in certain applications.[11]

Retinol is transported in serum associated with retinol-binding protein (RBP), whereas carotenoids are incorporated into lipoproteins. To analyze serum retinol, the RBP is denatured with alcohol or acetonitrile to release the retinol for organic-solvent extraction prior to analysis.

Vitamin A in tissues is stored as esters, predominantly retinyl palmitate. Although retinyl esters can be extracted directly into organic solvents, this step is usually preceded by the precipitation of cellular proteins and is followed by hydrolysis of the esters to release free retinol. Guidance for the analysis of provitamin A compounds in foods by both traditional open-column and advanced HPLC techniques have been published.[13-15]

## Intestinal Absorption of Preformed Vitamin A and Provitamin A

The first requirement for the ability of a nutrient to nourish is that it be absorbed into the body. The digestion of vitamin A-containing foods, the uptake of preformed vitamin A and provitamin A carotenoids across the intestinal membrane, and the handling within the enterocyte to allow transfer to the host for nutritional uses constitute the most fundamental underpinning for adequate vitamin A nutrition of the host.

### *Mechanisms of Absorption*

The starting point for accessing dietary nutrients is extracting them from foods. Dissociation and digestion, therefore, must be intact and efficient. The well-described constellation of actions by bile salts and pancreatic lipases within an appropriate pH milieu, in conjunction with forming mixed micellar formation within the lumen, is a prerequisite to freeing retinyl esters for intestinal uptake. Carotenes in the plant matrix of green leafy vegetables are compacted into the chloroplasts. In fruits, vegetables, and tubers of orange hue, they form part of chromoplasts, again in a highly structured organelle.[16] The dissociation of the matrix of solid foods through chewing and gastric action is a fundamental first step in making the dietary vitamin A components available to the host. Thereafter, the rest of digestive mission for rendering protein and carbohydrates to their essential elements is also important. In foods such as dairy items, and especially some fatty fruits, the carotenoids are dispersed and emulsified in an oily milieu within the foods, and the matrix factors represent less of a barrier to the uptake of the provitamin A.

The intracellular transport of vitamin A (see below) has now been revealed to be managed and mediated by a complement of cellular transport proteins not dissimilar from that in peripheral tissue cells. The particular routes of transport and roles and functions of transporters is illustrated diagrammatically in Figures 2 and 3 and described in the respective legends.[17] With respect to vitamin A compounds, luminal conditions and interactions influence the yield of vitamin A, as discussed in the following section. Once inside the intestinal cell, however, the provitamin A compound has the options of being passed intact into the lymphatic circulation, cleaved and converted into a retinoid, metabolized to an inactive species, or retained intact until the cell is desquamated.

The mechanisms of bioconversion of provitamin A to the active (retinoid) form of the vitamin have been reviewed.[18,19] The routine mechanism for conversion of β-carotene to retinaldehyde is via the 15,15′ monooxygenase enzyme in the intestine[20,21]; this leads to central cleavage, with the formation of up to two retinal molecules from each carotenoid moiety. The properties of 15,15′ monooxygenase (EC 1.13.11.21) have been established[22]; it is a cytosolic enzyme, with a slightly alkaline pH optimum, which utilizes molecular oxygen for cleavage. The enzyme has been cloned,[23] and it has been established that peroxisome proliferator-activated receptor-alpha is a transcriptional regulator in the expression of this monoxygenase.[24] This enzyme has recently been termed "carotene monoxygenase 1". Eccentric cleavage of β-carotene also occurs, with the conversion of β-carotene into β-apo-carotenals and eventually to retinoids. This is not

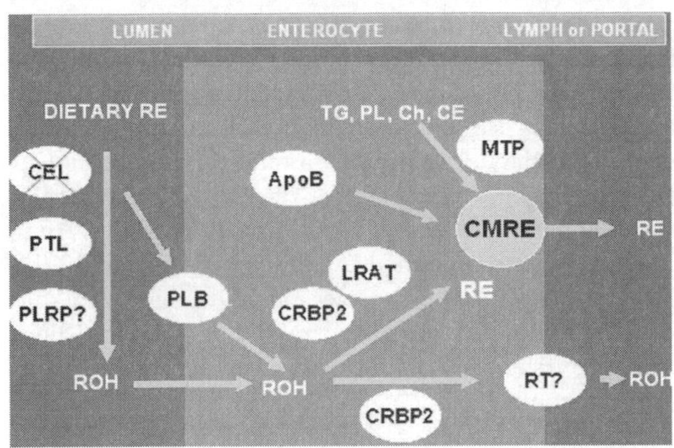


Figure 2. Overview of digestion and absorption of vitamin A. Dietary retinyl esters (REs) are hydrolyzed in the lumen by the pancreatic enzyme pancreatic triglyceride lipase (PTL) and intestinal brush border enzyme phospholipase B (PLB). Studies of the carboxylester lipase (CEL) knockout mouse suggest that CEL is not involved in dietary RE digestion. The possible roles of the pancreatic lipase-related proteins (PLRPs) 1 and 2 and other enzymes require further investigation. Unesterified retinol (ROH) is taken up by the enterocyte, perhaps facilitated by an as-yet-unidentified retinol transporter. Once in the cell, retinol is complexed with cellular RBP type 2 (CRBP2), and the complex serves as a substrate for reesterification of the retinol by the enzyme lecithin:retinol acyltransferase (LRAT). The REs are then incorporated into chylomicrons, intestinal lipoproteins containing other dietary lipids such as triglycerides (TGs), phospholipids (PLs), cholesterol (Ch), cholesteryl esters (CEs), and apolipoprotein B (ApoB). The incorporation of some of these lipids is dependent on the activity of microsomal triglyceride-transfer protein (MTP). Chylomicrons containing newly absorbed retinyl esters (CMREs) are then secreted into the lymph. Unesterified retinol is also absorbed into the portal circulation and its efflux from the basolateral cell membrane may also be facilitated by retinol transporter (RT) proteins. (Used with permission from Harrison 2005.[17])

exclusively related to spontaneous oxidation, and it has been found to be present in at least four mammalian species by enzymatic action (carotene monoxygenase 2). [25]

### *Considerations of Bioavailability and Bioconversion of Provitamin A*

A series of factors influence the yield of vitamin A one derives from provitamin A carotenoids, both those extrinsic to the body (i.e., diets that provide vitamin A) and those intrinsic to the host (i.e., the consequence of one's digestive and absorptive capacities). These factors can enhance or inhibit the uptake of vitamin A or provitamin A and the conversion of the latter into the active vitamin. This topic has been comprehensively reviewed.[26]

**Extrinsic Factors.** Our understanding of the dietary factors influencing the efficacy of conversion of provitamin A in foods has been aided by rapid advances in isotope tracer techniques and mathematical modeling.[27,28] It is known that the yield of vitamin A from carrots, for example, is generally low, and highly variable depending on the preparation: juiced, pureed, grated, or cooked.[29,30] When the provitamin A is in leaves or pulp of plants, the bioefficacy is well below 6:1 in relation to active vitamin A[31,32] in both marginal and replete subjects. Pectin also interferes with dietary carotene utilization.

Two drugs that achieve their therapeutic effects by producing fat malabsorption, orlistat and olestra, have been examined for their effects on vitamin A status. When these drugs were consumed by volunteers along with a daily vitamin A supplement, normal vitamin A status was maintained.[33,34] The consumption of plant sterols, commonly used to lower cholesterol, has been shown in two studies to interfere with beta-carotene uptake[35,36], but did not influence vitamin A status.[36] Indirect evidence suggests that dietary non-starch polysaccharides have no effect on the absorption of vitamin A.[37]

The amount of dietary fat accompanying vitamin A and provitamin A in meals is an enhancing factor. The presence of fat ensures the absorption of preformed vitamin A, but a minimum of 3 to 5 g is required to enhance the uptake of provitamin A for bioconversion.[38] Nagao[39] also suggests that lipids modulate the action of 15,15′ monoxygenase (CMO1). Carotenes dispersed and emulsified in fat or oil approach the biological efficacy of preformed vitamin A itself.[40]

**Intrinsic Factors.** The intrinsic factors for intestinal uptake begin with the nutritional demand of the organism for vitamin A, by which the intestine homeostatically regulates the conversion of provitamin A carotenoids to the vitamin A. That is, in the healthy individual, it depends upon the underlying adequacy of vitamin A status. Individuals who are replete have a low bioconversion drive,[41] and aging may reduce the efficiency of the conversion further.[42] The physical health of the alimentary tract is an additional factor in common for both preformed and provitamin A, insofar as fat maldigestion or injury or malfunction of the intestinal cells impairs the release of the constituents from the food and their transport out of the intestinal lumen.

## Metabolism of Preformed Vitamin A and Provitamin A

The appropriate fate of an absorbed nutrient is to become inserted into the sites of its essential physiological or structural roles or to be maintained in a storage reserve until needed.

### *Storage and Transport*

At any given time, the majority of the body's vitamin A, up to 90%, is in storage, with the remainder at peripheral sites in active functions.

**Cellular Uptake and Intracellular Metabolism.** As shown in the entero- and hepatocyte metabolic schemes in Figure 3,[43] the chemical actors are RBP from the circulation, cellular RBPs (CRBP I and CRBP II), cellular retinoic acid binding proteins (CRABP I and CRABP II), the retinaldehyde dehydrogenase type 2 (RALDH-2) and other enzymes, the retinoic acid receptors (RARs), and the retinoid X receptors (RXRs). The RARs are primed for activation by retinoic acid and its analogs, whereas the RXRs are receptors for the vitamin A metabolite 9-*cis* retinoic acid.[44-46] It has also recently been noted by Biesalski[47] that under certain circumstances and in selected tissues, such as buccal mucosa and vaginal epithe-

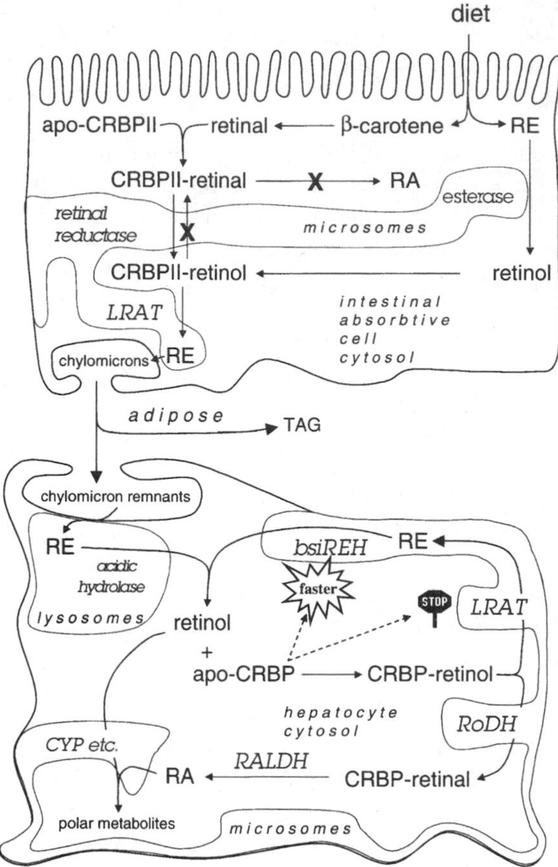


Figure 3. A model of retinol metabolism and retinoic acid (RA) biosynthesis that integrates cumulative data of interactions between cellular retinol-binding protein (CRBP) and CRBP(II) and enzymes that catalyze retinol metabolism. *Top panel*: Dietary carotenoids undergo central cleavage into retinal,which binds to CRBP(II). A microsomal retinal reductase recognizes retinal bound with CRBP(II) and converts it into retinol. Dietary retinyl esters (RE) undergo hydrolysis into retinol, which bind to (CRBP(II). Lecithin-retinol acyltransferase (LRAT) recognizes the complex CRBP(II)-retinol and synthesizes RE. CRBP(II) prevents oxidation of retinal and retinol, optimizing RE formation. Chylomicrons incorporate and deliver RE to the liver as chylomicron remnants formed after hydrolysis of triacylglycerol (TAG). *Bottom panel*: Chylomicron remnants deliver RE to the liver, where lysosomes engulf them and an acidic hydrolase releases retinol to bind with CRBP. The holo-CRBP formed serves as substrate for retinol esterification catalyzed by LRAT. A neutral bile salt-independent RE hydrolase (bsiREH) catalyzes RE mobilization. Apo-CRBP controls retinol metabolism by inhibiting LRAT and increasing the rate of hydrolysis via the bsiREH. Holo-CRBP also serves as substrate for retinal formation, catalyzed by retinol dehydrogenase (RoDH). Retinal dehydrogenase (RALDH) isozymes catalyze the irreversible and possibly rate-determining conversion of retinal into RA. Absence of CRBP potentially would allow numerous enzymes access to retinol, in addition to LRAT and RoDH, including perhaps medium-chain alcohol dehydrogenases, cytochromes P-450 (CY), oxidoreductases, etc. Reactive oxygen species, nucleophiles, and other intracellular reactive molecules also would have access to retinol in the absence of CRBP. The enhanced access of enzymes and reactive smaller molecular species would accelerate retinol metabolism and RE depletion. (Used with permission from Napoli 2000.[43])

lium, retinyl ester forms can be taken up directly by cells for nutritional purposes.

The transport of retinoids intracellularly is the purview of the cellular-binding proteins. Retinol first encounters the CRBP class of transport proteins to carry retinol to either esterifying or oxidizing enzymes.[46] We now recognize four relevant classes of alcohol dehydrogenases. After oxidation to the aldehyde, and then to an acid, the CRABP class assumes the relevance and a regulatory role as well.[43,48] These intracellular binding proteins show high specificity and affinity for specific retinoids, and seem to control retinoid metabolism both qualitatively and quantitatively. On the former side, they protect retinoids from nonspecific interactions, and on the quantitative side, they have been stated to "chaperone" access of metabolic enzymes to retinoids.[48]

**Hepatic Storage.** Immediately postprandially, vitamin A, packaged in chylomicra aggregates of enterocyte lipoprotein, move across the basement membrane of the enterocyte into the mesenteric lymphatic and via the thoracic duct into the systemic circulation. As noted, the storage organ for vitamin A is the liver. Newly absorbed retinyl esters are taken up by the liver (hepatocyte) cells,[43] as shown in Figure 3. Its uptake by the liver follows the normal metabolism and degradation of chylomicra to their remnants. In older persons, the clearance of the postprandial lipemia is half as fast as for younger persons, thus retarding the uptake of the retinyl esters into the liver.

From the hepatocyte, transport of vitamin A can be local or remote. Local storage involves its translocation to nearby, fat-storage stellate (Ito) cells. About half of the vitamin A in the liver of a vitamin-replete individual resides in hepatocytes, whereas the other half is in stellate cell deposits.

**Circulatory Transport.** The remote transport of vitamin A involves the tissue sites of its utilization in the body. Transport of vitamin A to peripheral tissues occurs primarily by way of a shuttle of recently absorbed vitamin from the liver to the periphery as part of the RPB-transthyretin (TTR) complex. Within the hepatocyte, retinol forms a complex with RPB, a 183-amino acid residue, 21,230-Da peptide; this in turn joins a binding site on TTR and is stored in the Golgi body until retinol for transport becomes available.[49] The stability of RBP's binding to retinol is enhanced by complexing with TTR, increasing the binding affinity of RBP for retinol.[50] This complexing into a 55-Da homotetramer prevents glomerular filtration of the smaller RPB.[51]

In states of vitamin A sufficiency, RBP synthesis and accumulation is modest; little if any newly absorbed vitamin moves out of the liver. In states of vitamin A deficiency, hepatic RBP levels are elevated, and a vitamin A-rich meal translates into a major release to feed deprived peripheral tissues. This is the biological basis for the relative dose response test.[52]

**Transplacental Transport.** The role of vitamin A in cell differentiation and rapid growth makes it indispensable for in utero embryogenesis and fetal development.

Nonetheless, there are major gaps in our understanding of maternal-fetal vitamin A transport. What appears to be most likely is that RBP-free retinol diffuses across the intravillous spaces to be captured by RBP of fetal amniochorionic membrane origin.[53] It has been suggested that fetal nutrition may derive from the 15 mL of amniotic fluid swallowed daily in utero, or even from the placenta as an extraintestinal site of bioconversion of β-carotene to the active vitamin.[54]

**Secretory Transport in Lactation.** The vitamin A supplied by lactation is adequate to supply all of the needs of the growing infant through the first 6 months of life.[55] The mechanism by which vitamin A is mobilized to the mammary glands for milk secretion either from hepatic stores or from recently absorbed vitamin has important practical importance to public health. Although two recent studies from south Asia[56,57] found a positive effect on maternal milk vitamin A concentrations after a single 200,000 IU (60 mg) postpartum dose of vitamin A, the overall literature is inconsistent and situational on the matter of its public health efficacy. Two recent publications of complementary studies in piglets[58] and rodents[59] showed the lack of a milk vitamin A response to a priming dose, as well as a rapid effect on milk of changes in dietary vitamin A. Derivative inferences from these animal models support the theory that recently absorbed retinyl esters, circulated postprandially on chylomicra and lipoprotein remnants, constitute the first line of maternal retinol supply to breast milk.[59]

Observations in Icelandic mothers suggesting that recommended intakes of vitamin A in lactation can be more easily met with maternal cod liver oil supplement than through diet alone[60] provide some confirmation of the continuous supply of vitamin A from diet as supporting the consequences of postprandial delivery of newly absorbed vitamin as a prime scenario for human lactation. By contrast, however, no relationship between the previous day's vitamin A intake and breast milk retinol content was found in Brazilian mothers.[61,62]

In a multinational collaborative study involving developed and transitional nations (Australia, Canada, China, Chile, Japan, Mexico, the Philippines, and the United Kingdom), milk retinol levels were generally adequate, but varied two-fold across countries.[63] Findings related to carotenoids as a source of infant vitamin A were more interesting. Overall, provitamin A species constituted 50% of total milk carotenoids. Total carotenoids were highest in Japanese milk samples and lowest in the Philippines, whereas beta-carotene content was highest in Chile and lowest in the Philippines.[63] In Brazilian mothers, the plasma-to-milk ratio for β-carotene was 17:1, with modest mutual association.[62] Observations comparing carotenoid patterns in colostrum and mature milk may provide some inferential insights into the distribution of provitamin A to human milk. In colostrum, the carotenoid pattern resembled that in LDL lipoproteins, whereas at 19 days (mature milk), it reflected that in HDL, suggesting that the transfer of carotenoids to milk involves different lipoproteins at different specific times of lactation.[64]

### *Excretion*

The primary excretion route for vitamin A and metabolites from the body is biliary. Based on rodent models,[65,66] vitamin A is excreted with a fixed concentration in bile, with net losses depending on biliary volume. With increased hepatic stores, output increases in a responsive manner.[66] The fractional loss of vitamin A in the urine is diminutive under usual circumstances. However, pathological situations such as toxemia,[67] acute renal failure,[68] multiple myeloma,[69] and febrile infections[70] increase urinary losses. An estimated 20% to 40% of a child's liver reserves can be lost in a severe diarrheal episode.[70]

## Physiology of Vitamin A: Functions and Actions

The late Prof. James A. Olson defined the "function" of a food constituent as "an essential role played by the nutrient in growth, development, and maturation"; by contrast, he defined "actions" as "demonstrable effects in various biologic systems that may or may not have general physiologic significance."[71]

### *Physiological Functions of Vitamin A*

Some form of retinoid is involved in functions of all cells of the body. Vision, intercellular communication, mucin production, embryogenesis, cell growth, and cell differentiation are prominent among the gamut of functions related to vitamin A; the latter involves vascular, hematopoietic, immunocyte, osteoblastic and osteoclastic, alveolar, and neuronal tissues.

**Retinol Isomer and Visual Pigments in the Visual Cycle.** The classical (archetypical) function for which vitamin A is known is in the visual cycle. Vitamin A is an active component of the visual pigments in the rods and cones of the retina. In dim-light (scotopic) vision with the dark-adapted eye, the cycle involves the regeneration of the rhodopsin pigment, with the insertion of 11-*cis*-retinol. Photons from low-intensity light energy produce the cleavage of the pigment-retinoid complex, liberating dissociated 11-*cis*-retinal and exciting neural transmission, as described by George Wald.[72] The regeneration of the retinol from the aldehyde form was the primary feature, and the molecular biology of this visual pathway has subsequently been elucidated. For high-resolution color (photopic) vision in daylight, the retinal cones of the retinal epithelium are involved in a similar, although less-well-understood, photon-activated excitation and transmission. The regeneration of 11-*cis*-retinal via all-trans-retinol to 11-*cis*-retinol has been shown to be distinct in the photopic vision cycle.[73]

**Retinoids and Intercellular Communication.** One of the macro-level functions for the integrity and function of tissues is the communication among adjacent cells. This can occur by various signaling mechanisms, the best understood of which is the connexin 36 mechanism at so-called "gap junctions" across the intercellular space.

All-*trans* retinal and retinoic acid have been shown to be a potent inhibitor of connexin-36 mediated gap junctional communication.[74] On the other hand, within the cell nucleus, retinoic acid induces adhesion proteins and membrane complexes necessary for cell-to-cell adhesion and communication in hepatocytes.[75]

**Mechanism of Action as a Nuclear Hormone.** The functions, metabolism, and nuclear receptors of natural retinoids have been reviewed.[76,77] The aforementioned wide variety of functions of vitamin A are derived from a complex retinoid signaling pathway system, in which various isometric forms of retinoic acid act as nuclear hormones.[78] These include all-*trans*-retinoic acid and 9-*cis*-retinoic acid as the principal players, with additional participation by 13-*cis*-retinoic acid.[79] A wide array of synthetic retinoid analogs can also participate in the signaling system in pharmacological situations.

The retinoids act as transcription factors, modulating and regulating either the activation or repression of messenger RNA formation in cell nuclei.[80] This is affected by their serving as binding ligands in nuclear receptor complexes. The basic elements of the genetic signaling system are the nuclear receptors. The receptors for retinoic acid (RAR) and its 9-*cis* isomer (RXR) each have three types (alpha, beta, and gamma). RARs can bind and respond to both retinoic acid and its isomer, whereas RXRs are specific for isomeric form (9-*cis* is retinoic acid). The receptors act through either dimerization to form homodimers (RAR-RAR, RXR-RXR) or heterodimers (RAR-RXR) with the various permutations of the Greek-letter subtypes. Cooperative binding to hormone response elements coordinates the regulation of target genes by RXR ligands.[81] The transcription regulation, moreover, can involve further heterodimer formation between the RXR receptor and either thyroid hormone receptor or the peroxisome proliferator activated receptor.[82,83] In addition, in some cell lines, interleukin-2[84,85] and other proinflammatory cytokines[86] can participate in the transcriptional signaling.

The best-known roles of the retinoid receptor system involve the regulation of the division and differentiation of cells. Signals involving the RXR are known to reduce cellular proliferation and enhance programmed cell death (apoptosis).[87] In terms of cellular differentiation, influencing the proteins involved in the cell cycle is pivotal to the action of intracellular retinoid regulatory roles via RAR.[85,88,89] An alternative mechanism for influencing genetic expression involves epigenetic regulation at the level of the chromatin conformation. Mammalian reflections of the uncoupling of histone acetylation in the HIV1 virus are postulated.[90] Interestingly, the alcohol form, retinol, has been shown to have potential epigenetic potential in modifying the chromatin conformation of a zinc-finger domain of the gene for serine/threonine kinase expression.[91]

Upregulated expression of mRNA for mucin proteins of the conjunctiva[92] and the respiratory tract[86] by retinoic acid is a classical example of signaling related to intracellular protein synthesis. The retinoid signaling system is central to embryogenesis such as of the brachial arches[93] and the alveolar membrane of the lungs.[94]

Retinoic acid, circulating in nanomolar concentrations in blood, accounts for the majority of the supply for the brain and liver, but is also locally produced in other tissues.[95] Beyond the serial oxidation of retinol is the intracorporeal bioconversion of carotenoids as a potential source of retinoids at the tissue and cellular level.[96]

### *Actions of Vitamin A*

Outside of the evolutionary functions of vitamin A for the metabolism in normal health, vitamin A exhibits a series of actions that are adjunctive to the correction of various pathological conditions.

**Antiproliferative Action.** The ability of vitamin A and its isomeric forms to promote terminal differentiation, inhibit proliferation, and promote apoptosis comes into play in neoplastic situations in which one tissue has undergone malignant transformation. High-dose retinoids have shown anti-neoplastic activity in vitro in a diverse array of cancer cell lines.[78,97,98]

**Improved Iron Uptake from Meals.** Iron is a vitally essential, but generally poorly bioavailable dietary trace element. There are a series of conflicting observations related to enhancement of the biological availability of iron. The amount of vitamin A,[99,100] including provitamin A forms,[101] improved absorption presumably by interdicting the interference of phytates. Swiss investigators examined iron absorption efficiency from iron-fortified maize porridge in vitamin A-deficient African children in the presence or absence of retinyl palmitate, and found no enhancement.[102] At this time, the final word on this potential dietary action of vitamin A is not yet established.

## Manifestations and Consequences of Vitamin A Deficiency and Variation in Vitamin A Nutriture

Deficiency of vitamin A is associated with clinical and functional manifestations. However, apparent variations of vitamin A status within the range that would be considered adequate also have some influence on human health and function.

### *Ocular Manifestations*

Xerophthalmia (literally, dryness of the eye) is the hallmark clinical feature of clinical vitamin A deficiency. It has been classified by stages according to specific ocular manifestations. Stage XN, the earliest stage, involves night blindness due to impaired dark adaptation. Stage X1A is conjunctival xerosis due to reduction in goblet cell mucus, followed by stage X1B, which is manifested by Bitot's spots, foamy excrescences on the temporal surface of the conjunctiva. Corneal xerosis constitutes the advancing stages, with X2 being simple drying of the cornea, with involvement of less than (X3A) or more than (X3B) one-third of the corneal surface with ulceration or corneal liquification, respectively. Past involvement leaves a corneal scar (XS), and a globe destroyed by advanced keratomalacia is xerophthalmic fundus.

### *Other Epithelial Dysfunction Syndromes*

Other epithelial tissues are affected by vitamin A deficiency. Thickening of the hair follicles (follicular hyperkeratosis) is a cutaneous manifestation of vitamin A deficiency. The reduction in mucin production in mucous membranes from the adenopharyngeal passages, bronchial and pulmonary tissue to the digestive tract, produces symptomatic distress and susceptibility to microbial invasion.

### *Excessive Mortality Rates*

It has been known since the 1980s, from the pioneering epidemiological observations of Sommer et al[103] in the Ache region of Indonesia, that marginal vitamin A status was associated with excessive mortality from childhood infections. This was confirmed first by a vitamin A intervention study in the same population[104] and then by meta-analyses across six sites.[105] Additional confirmatory intervention studies continue to emerge, including a 22% mortality reduction in newborn infants in southern India[106] and a 46% reduction in HIV-infected children in Uganda.[107]

In developed countries, sudden infant death syndrome (SIDS) may bear some relationship to differential vitamin A status. Observations from Sweden suggested a high association between SIDS and infants not being given vitamin A supplements during the first year of life.[108]

### *Excess Infectious Morbidity*

Although death from childhood infectious diseases are more common in low-income societies, and immune defense deficiencies result from marginal vitamin A deficiency, little evidence for reduced incidence of infectious episodes has been gleaned from community intervention trials. The odds ratio was 1.08 for the effect of prophylactic vitamin A supplementation on acute respiratory infections in a meta-analysis,[109] while a comparable analysis for efficacy also showed no efficacy.[110] Supplementation was effective to prevent cough among HIV-infected children in Uganda.[107] The prevention of diarrhea is another domain in which meta-analyses revealed no efficacy.[109] In the situation of HIV, however, reductions in the incidence of acute and chronic diarrhea[107] incidence have been noted. As tentative resolution of this apparent mortality-morbidity paradox, it is postulated that the specific intensity and lethality of infections is aggravated in the child with marginal vitamin A status.

### *Hematological Support*

A number of recent observational studies have documented an independent association of vitamin A status with hematological adequacy[111-113] beyond any direct action of meal vitamin A to enhance iron absorption. Historically, vitamin A interventions were shown to improved hemoglobin or hematocrits in a multiply deficient, anemic population. Semba and Bloem[114] propose several metabolic mechanisms whereby modulation of vitamin A exposure and status could influence red cell biology: stimulating progenitor cells, promoting resistance to infection, and mobilization of iron to the erythron. Basic research provides evidence for retinoids regulating hematopoiesis from the yolk sac stage in the embryo to the fetal liver production in utero to the bone marrow.[115]

Not only is the erythropoietic line of bone marrow proliferation related to vitamin A, but platelet production is also influenced by retinoid biology. Japanese oncologists observed increased thrombocytosis and thrombopoietin levels in patients treated with all-*trans*-retinoic acid for acute promyelocytic leukemia. Subsequent in vitro studies in bone marrow stromal cell culture, all-*trans*-retinoic acid triples thrombopoietin mRNA expression.[116]

### *Miscellaneous Considerations*

Endemic vitamin A deficiency and controlled observations of responses to vitamin A supplementations interventions have received so much interest in observational and intervention studies that commentary on consequences that do not appear to be part of the hypovitaminosis A context. Growth[117] and psychomotor function seem to relatively unaffected by vitamin A deficits and unimproved by restoration and maintenance of adequate nutriture. In the situation of HIV-infected preschoolers, however, maternal vitamin A supplementation improved postnatal growth of children in Tanzania,[118] and direct child supplementation improved growth in the same milieu.[119]

## Causes of Variation in Vitamin A Status and Epidemiology of Vitamin A Deficiency

Secondary vitamin A deficiency can arise in any situation or clinical condition or illness in which there is reduced absorption, increased excretion, enhanced destruction, impaired utilization, or exaggerated requirement for the nutrient.

### *Conditions Predisposing to Impaired Vitamin A Status*

A standard list of predisposing causes of vitamin A deficiency has been recognized for decades. These include a myriad of situations of low-intake bioconvertibility of dietary vitamin A, poor intestinal absorption, impaired utilization of the vitamin, and increased destruction or wastage. Recent concerns focus on impairment in vitamin A nutriture in novel conditions or emergent or re-emergent diseases. These include: bariatric surgical procedures for weight loss,[120,121] pancreaticoduodenostomy ablation surgery for malignancies,[122] peritoneal dialysis,[123] hematopoietic stem cell transplant,[124] acute respiratory syndromes,[125] pulmonary tuberculosis,[126] cigarette smoking,[127] HIV/AIDS,[128,129] and asthma.[130]

### *Population Epidemiology of Hypovitaminosis A*

The current estimates of hypovitaminosis A on a worldwide basis suggest that it is the second most common micronutrient deficiency. Singh and West[131] estimate that 23% of children between the ages of 5 to 15 years in southeast Asian nations have deficient vitamin A status. In a nationally representative sample of Mexico,[132] low retinol levels were found in a quarter of the sample, with highest rates in indigenous communities in the southern part of the country. Diverse, contemporary surveys have identified a prevalence of impaired vitamin A status in Inuit and First Nation newborns,[133] Israeli Bedouin toddlers,[134] black toddlers in the western cape of South Africa,[135] nomadic herder women in Chad,[136] and pregnant urban women in Nigeria.[137] Risk factors found variously across sites of hypovitaminosis A endemicity were male gender,[138] the youth of children,[132,138] low body-mass index (BMI),[132] stunting,[138] familial xerophthalmia history,[138] history of maternal diarrhea,[138] the nutritional quality of pastoralists' milk,[136] and warm seasons.[138]

# Nutrient Requirements and Recommended Intakes for Dietary Vitamin A

## *Quantitative Expression of Dietary Vitamin A Activity*

Units of expression of vitamin A in foods and pharmaceutical preparations have a tortuous history and present confusion. Historically, we have international units (IU) from early food science literature, retinol equivalents (RE), adopted by a Food and Agriculture Organization of the United Nations/World Health Organization (FAO/WHO) panel in 1967,[139] and retinol activity equivalents (RAE), proposed by the US Institute of Medicine for the 2001 *Dietary Reference Intakes* (DRI).[140] Certain measures can be taken to promote harmonization and reduce inconsistencies.

The IU expression can be found in food composition tables, and is still widely used in medicinal contexts. The conversion relationship is 1 IU = 3.3 RE (1 RE = 0.3 IU), which is valid only for preformed vitamin A. Interconversions involving the IU and provitamin A are universally invalid, and quantification of dietary vitamin A in mixed diets will grossly overestimate relative vitamin activity. The RE is related to vitamin A compounds in gravimetric units in the following manner:

1 RE = 1 μg of retinol

1 RE = 6 μg of all-*trans* beta-carotene

1 RE = 12 μg of other provitamin A carotenes

The "other" provitamin A carotenes include the stereoisomers of beta-carotene, as well as compounds such as alpha-carotene and beta-cryptoxanthin, etc.

The aforementioned considerations regarding the superior bioconversion of isolated carotenes in an oily matrix and inferior conversion for carotenes in the plant matrices of fruits, vegetables and herbs, reviewed in the section on bioavailability and bioconversion, guided the creation of the RAE. The definitions provided in the DRI[140] for RAEs were:

1 RAE = 1 μg of retinol

1 RAE = 2 μg of all-*trans* beta-carotene as supplement

1 RAE = 12 μg of all-*trans* beta-carotene in food matrix

1 RAE = 24 μg of other provitamin A carotenes in food matrix

Where preformed vitamin A in foods or supplements are concerned, RE and RAE are completely interchangeable. Moreover, it must be clarified that, implicitly, 4 μg of other provitamin A carotenoids alone or in oil could also be equivalent to 1 RAE. What still may be unresolved within the RAE convention is an appropriate value for carotenes that are free of plant matrices but in a relatively modest fatty milieu. This would apply to provitamin A in milk and most cheeses, as well as in eggs.

## *Estimated Human Requirements and Recommended Dietary Intakes*

For planning and evaluation, it is important to have estimates of the daily requirements of vitamin A. At the time of publication of the 8th edition of this textbook, the DRIs for the United States and Canada had just been released.[140] The WHO and the Food and Nutrition Organization released a set of vitamin and mineral requirements with worldwide applicability in 2004.[141] The former are based, when possible, around estimated average requirements (EAR) for relevant age groups, sexes, and physiological status. This allows for probabilistic estimates for the prevalence of individuals at risk in a population. The United Nations (UN) agencies also provide a mean requirement value, but this represents daily intakes adequate to prevent the appearance of deficiency-related syndromes."[141] The intake level of reference to assure a greater than 90% probability of covering one's own requirement of vitamin A, however, is the recommended nutrient intake (RNI)[141] in the UN system and the recommended dietary allowance (RDA)(Table 1).[140]

The discrepancy between the units of dietary vitamin A activity, RAE for the DRI[140] and RE for the UN system,[141] complicates the discussion of recommended intakes of vitamin A for an international forum. Nevertheless, there is a certain degree of correspondence in the estimates for protective intakes, RNI, and RDA for vitamin A between the two options in Table 1. The recommended intakes of the UN System agencies are slightly lower for infancy, higher for childhood, and lower again for adolescence and adulthood. The major discrepancy between the two panels of recommendations relates to the disproportion in estimated requirements for lactation.

# Food Sources and Dietary Intakes of Vitamin A

The richest animal sources of vitamin A in the human diet are fish liver oils, liver, other organ meats, cream,

**Table 1.** Recommendations for Daily Intake of Vitamin A from the US Institute of Medicine and the World Health Organization

| | United Nations System (WHO/FAO) | | United States and Canada Dietary Reference Intakes | |
|---|---|---|---|---|
| | **Mean Requirement** | **Recommended Nutrient Intake** | **Estimated Average Requirement** | **Recommended Dietary Allowance** |
| **Population** | *RE/d* | | *RAE/d* | |
| 0–6 mo | 180 | 375 | – | 400 AI |
| 7–12 mo | 190 | 400 | – | 500 AI |
| 0–1 y | 200 | 400 | – | – |
| 1–3 y | 200 | 450 | 210 | 300 |
| 4–6 y | 200 | 450 | – | – |
| 4–8 y | – | – | 275 | 400 |
| 7–9 y | 250 | 500 | – | – |
| 9–13 y | – | – | 445, 420 | 600 |
| 10–18 y | 330–400 | 600 | – | – |
| 14–18 y males | – | – | 630 | 900 |
| 14–18 y females | – | – | 485 | 700 |
| Adult males | 300 | 600 | 625 | 900 |
| Adult females | 270 | 500 | 500 | 750 |
| Pregnant females | 370 | 800 | 550 | 770 |
| Lactating females | 450 | 850 | 900 | 1300 |

RE = Retinol equivalents; RAE = retinol activity equivalents.

butter, and fortified milks. Certain tropical fatty fruits are the richest sources of plant origin.

## *Estimates of Average Dietary Intake and Adequacy of Selected Population Samples*

Combined with the prevalent distortion in the quantifying dietary vitamin A values inherited from a confused evolution of units of expression, data on average or median intakes are somewhat scarce and selective and data on average vitamin A intakes in truly representative populations samples across the world are scant. Within these constraints, an appreciation of the diversity of findings in the literature on central tendencies for dietary vitamin A intake in adults and children in affluent and low-income settings is shown in Table 2.[142-151] An important caveat in reviewing the extant literature on individual and population vitamin A intakes is the almost universal expression in REs. This generally has overestimated the consumption of vitamin A, more so to the extent it is based on plant sources, as would occur in vegetarians or residents of developing countries. Similarly, the relative contribution of plant sources are historically overvalued in the RE system.

Preformed vitamin A levels were above the EAR in adult women of all ethnic groups in small towns of the contemporary rural south of the United States[152] and generally among Mexican-American women.[143] From studies in selected European adult samples, over 10% of the Spanish population was shown to be consuming less than two-thirds of the referent standard for vitamin A intake[153]; among Portuguese elderly, 78% of men and 73% of women had intakes below the lowest European recommended dietary intake levels.[154]

Studies among juvenile populations in Germany[155] and the northern provinces of the United Kingdom[156] found generally adequate intakes of dietary vitamin A. In Spain, younger children's intakes were generally adequate, but a substantial number of adolescents had vitamin A intakes below two-thirds of the reference level.[150] South Asia has traditionally been an endemic area of hypovitaminosis A. In rural India, intakes of vitamin A were described as "woefully inadequate."[151] The situation was better in the metro Manila area of the Philippines.[157]

## *Dietary Sources of Vitamin A*

Dietary sources from two representative national survey samples, for the United States and the Netherlands, are available. Sixty-seven percent of cumulative intake of vitamin A in the US diet, as calculated in RE, comprised in descending order: carrots, milk, organ meats, ready-to-eat cereals, cheese, margarine, tomatoes, and eggs.[158] Carrots constitute 27% of all estimated intake. Comparable data for the Netherlands, also in RE but organized by food groups, found 91% of all vitamin A consumed

**Table 2.** Mean or Median Daily Vitamin A Intakes of Selected Populations in the Contemporary Literature

| Population | Estimated Intake | Reference |
|---|---|---|
| Adults | | |
| US, both sexes, 20–39 y, preformed vitamin A | 1484 RE | Ervin et al., 2004[142] |
| US, both sexes, 20–39 y, provitamin A | 450 RE | Ervin et al., 2004[142] |
| Mexican-American women, US born (food only) | 1035 RAE | Harley et al., 2005[143] |
| Mexican-American women, US born (plus supplement) | 2156RAE | Harley et al., 2005[143] |
| Mexican-American women, Mexican born (food only) | 1361 RAE | Harley et al., 2005[143] |
| Mexican-American women, Mexican born (plus supplement) | 2442 RAE | Harley et al., 2005[143] |
| Dutch (males) | 1100 RE | Goldbohm et al., 1998[144] |
| Dutch (females) | 900 RE | Goldbohm et al., 1998[144] |
| British (males) | 660 RE* | Henderson et al., 2003[145] |
| British (females) | 549 RE* | Henderson et al., 2003[145] |
| Italian (males) | 1013 μg* | Riccioni et al., 2004[146] |
| Bangladeshi (males) | 537 μg | Hels et al., 2003[147] |
| Bangladeshi (females) | 471 μg | Hels et al., 2003[147] |
| Children and Adolescents | | |
| German, 4–7 y (mixed gender) | 588 μg | Sichert-Hellert et al., 2001[148] |
| German, 7–10 y (mixed gender) | 697 μg | Sichert-Hellert et al., 2001[148] |
| German, 10–13 y (males) | 745 μg | Sichert-Hellert et al., 2001[148] |
| German 10–13 y (females) | 739 μg | Sichert-Hellert et al., 2001[148] |
| German 13–15 y (males) | 883 μg | Sichert-Hellert et al., 2001[148] |
| German 13–15 y (females) | 876 μg | Sichert-Hellert et al., 2001[148] |
| Northern UK 1–6 y (mixed gender) | 578 μg | Watt et al., 2001[149] |
| Spanish 6–14 y (males) | 502 μg | Serra-Majem et al., 2001[150] |
| Spanish 6–14 y (females) | 434 μg | Serra-Majem et al., 2001[150] |
| Indian 10–12 y (males) | 131 μg* | Venkaiah et al., 2002[151] |
| Indian 10–12 y (females) | 111 μg* | Venkaiah et al., 2002[151] |
| Indian 11–15 y (males) | 137 μg* | Venkaiah et al., 2002[151] |
| Indian 11–15 y (females) | 132 μg* | Venkaiah et al., 2002[151] |
| Indian 16–18 y (males) | 184 μg* | Venkaiah et al., 2002[151] |
| Indian 16–18 y (females) | 145 μg* | Venkaiah et al., 2002[151] |

* Median vitamin A intakes for the survey population.
RAE, retinol activity equivalents; RE, retinol equivalents.

came from meats (35%), fats and oils (24%), vegetables (16%), and dairy foods (16%).[144]

Among Inuits of Canada, the livers of seals, caribou, and fish provide half of the vitamin A and market foods the other half.[159] It has been estimated that fortified dairy products can contribute 39% of the RDA in three standard portions in Spain.[160] In central Java, where 83% of pregnant women consumed under 700 RE in the first trimester of pregnancy, plant sources contributed 64% to 79% of total vitamin A.[161] Dietary supplements make an important contribution to vitamin A intake. Through interval nationally representative surveys in the United States from 1987 to 1992 to 2000, the use of dietary supplements has increased steadily from 23.2% to 23.7% to 33.9%.[162] Supplement use by adults in Ireland was credited with reducing the number of adults consuming vitamin A below average requirement from 20% to 5%.[163]

With respect to juvenile populations, German children and adolescents received from 50% to 65% of reference intake needs of vitamin A from non-fortified foods in their diets, and an additional 10% to 20% from fortified foods.[148] This cohort had shown a 5% to 15% increase in the amount of the vitamin obtained from fortified beverages during the previous 15-year period.[155] On the island of Guam in the South Pacific, fruit drinks, milk, and fortified cereals contributed most of the vitamin A in Guamanian children; the median vitamin A intake was 76% of the age-appropriate RDA.[164] For the children living on the mainland of the United States, however, concern has been expressed that excessive sweetened drink consumption is associated with displacement of milk from children's diets, higher daily energy intake, and greater weight gain.[165]

Human milk can be a relatively important source of vitamin A, even beyond the first year of life. According to a study in Kenya, breast milk supplies more vitamin A than the complementary foods that replace it, making it an "irreplaceable source of fat and vitamin A."[166] The role of supplements as the source of vitamin A for juvenile populations is now beginning to emerge, even in the first two years of life. Among a cohort followed from infants to toddlers in the US state of Iowa, 32% were consuming vitamin A-containing supplements 40% to 60% of days by the age of 24 months.[167]

### *Factors Affecting Vitamin A Consumption*

A number of cultural, behavioral, and physical factors influence vitamin A intake in various populations of adults. In a study among pregnant women in the United States, Mexican-born women consumed more vitamin A than Mexican-American women during pregnancy.[143] Edentulous US white elderly consumed less vitamin A and carotene than peers with adequate dentition, although no gradient was seen in African-American contemporaries. No differences in vitamin A intake were found in greater Chicago residents with tobacco use status as smokers, ex-smokers, or never smokers.[168]

In an analysis of US Department of Agriculture (USDA) survey data, estimated vitamin A intakes were highest in those who derived the greatest portion of energy from carbohydrates.[169] Meals containing traditional native foods provide more vitamin A than non-traditional commodities among indigenous populations of the arctic of Canada.[170]

In children, adequacy of vitamin A intakes decreases with age.[150,171] Moreover, a gender gap emerges and widens over time, with boy's relative intakes better maintained than girls'.[171,172] Ethnicity plays a role among US children, with the Continuing Survey of Food Intakes showing that being black or being a female child of any race conferred the highest risk of consuming less than two-thirds of the RDA for vitamin A.[173]

A predictor of a preschool child's not meeting the RNI in the northern regions of the United Kingdom was being the son or daughter of a manual laborer.[149] In the metro Manila area, schoolchildren of higher socioeconomic status consumed more vitamin A than those of low socioeconomic status.[157] In British youth, low intake was inverse to dairy food consumption.[156] Consuming a more "Mediterranean" diet did not influence the relative adequacy of vitamin A intake.[174]

## Diagnostic Assessment of Vitamin A Nutriture

Approaches to the assessment of human vitamin A status are outlined in Table 3. The endeavor has numerous caveats, the most important of which is being clear that most of the diagnostic tests provide an assessment of the risk of hypovitaminosis A's being a public health problem for the population. An individual with an abnormal test is not necessarily deficient him- or herself. Only tests such as hepatic biopsies or deuterium dilution tests and, to a lesser degree, functional tests of dark adaptation provide a clinical diagnosis of vitamin A deficiency for the individual. Important advances and insights into the utility and application of diagnostic tests are ongoing.

**Table 3.** Clinical Assessment of Vitamin A Status and Estimation of Population Risk of Vitamin A Deficiency

**Dietary Intake Assessment**

Biological Fluid Markers
- Circulating retinol
- Retinol binding protein (RBP)
- RBP/transthyretin (TTR) ratio
- Breast milk retinol

Isotope Dilution Tests
- Deuterated retinol dilution test (DRD)

Tissue Biopsy Markers
- Invasive
  - Hepatic biopsy assay
- Non-invasive
  - Buccal cell vitamin A

Functional Tests
- Invasive
  - Relative dose response (RDR)
  - Modified RDR
  - 30-day RDR
- Mildly invasive
  - Conjunctival impression cytology
- Non-Invasive
  - Dark adaptation tests
  - Self-reported night blindness

The gold standard for individual assessment with some discomfort from blood drawing and major expense is deuterated retinol dilution, a stable-isotopic approach receiving increasing use in the field.[175-178] Dietary intake does not assess status, but rather gauges one of the risk factors. Rapid screening procedures are available at the field level.[179,180] Circulating retinol is the most commonly used approach, and RBP is a reasonable surrogate measure.[181] It only reflects systemic status at the extremes of deficiency and excess, while the presence of inflammatory conditions or infections distorts the assessment by depressing circulating concentrations of retinol.[182,184] Establishing the ratio of RBP to its TTR counterpart to account for the distortion of inflammation has proven to be disappointing for improving validity of diagnosis.[185]

Within the domain of more elaborate procedures that nevertheless have blood sampling or other discomforts associated, the RDR and MRDR continue to gain use in population studies.[186,187] The unique, 30-day dose response test, which measures the increment in retinol levels one month after a high-dose supplementation, has found favor in Brazil.[188] Conjunctival impression cytology finds occasional application[180] for screening for hypovitaminosis A.

Breast milk collection is totally non-invasive and, in relation to a standard of over 150 μmol/L,[188] systemic inflammation does not seem to distort the validity of assessment.[191] Buccal mucosa is a non-invasive biopsy tissue being explored.[192] On the technological front, recent years have seen continuing development of screening approaches for impaired dark adaptation in the field.[193,194] The opportunity to do sampling during in vitro fertilization has even opened a window on vitamin A status of ovarian tissue.[127,195]

# Vitamin A Interventions in Preventive Medicine and Public Health

A series of interventions are applied as public health measures to protect the vulnerable groups in the population from hypovitaminosis A. The four domains for population action are: general health, food selection, food and crop fortification, and periodic prophylactic supplementation.

## *General Health Interventions*

A healthy host is better able to absorb, retain, and utilize vitamin A. Sanitation and hygienic measures that reduce diarrhea and control intestinal parasites optimizes the intestine's capacity to take up the vitamin from the diet. Inflammation and febrile episodes provoke urinary wastage of the vitamin. Routine immunizations and control of systemic parasites can act to limit catabolic losses of micronutrients including vitamin A.

## *Food Choice Approaches*

Dietary diversification is the most fundamental and sustainable form to prevent hypovitaminosis A. It is based on increasing the selection and consumption of foods rich in dietary vitamin A activity to bring the habitual intake into the range of recommended intakes. Culture, cuisine and economic limitations, however, often interfere with achieving target intakes in low-income societies. Strategies appropriate to the intrinsic possibilities of the settings must be devised.

Given their content of preformed vitamin A, accessible animal sources of vitamin A have more specific potency. In Bangladesh, the consumption of small indigenous fish is widespread and promotes adequacy of intake[196,197]; different local species, however, have a wide range of vitamin A content. In Kenya, the addition of milk or meat to the school snack (a vegetable stew) improved overall vitamin A intake.[198]

Plant sources of vitamin A are more problematic as strategies for ensuring adequacy given the bioconversion issues of plant matrices. Nevertheless, home-gardening interventions in South Africa[199,200] and Thailand[201] were shown to support better vitamin A status. Varieties of bananas, extraordinarily rich in provitamin A carotenes, are cultivated throughout the Micronesian islands of the Pacific and have been recommended as a complement for that region.[202] To enhance the bioefficacy of mango's provitamin A, its consumption with fat has been advanced in the Gambia.[203]

Nature has supplied a number of oil-bearing fruits with high contents of vitamin A, which are exempt from the usual plant-matrix constrictions. Gac fruit (*Momordica cochinchinensis*)[204] from Vietnam and aguage or buriti fruit (*Maurita vinifera* Mart) from the Amazon valley[205] are the two tropical fatty fruits with the highest specific concentrations of provitamin A. Derivatives of the palm fruit (*Elaeis* spp.), such as red palm oil, are in third place, containing in excess of 50 mg of mixed provitamin A per 100 g of oil.[206] Intervention trials in India[207,208] and Burkina Faso[209] demonstrate the efficacy of cooking with red palm oil to improve vitamin A status. Tailored shortenings[210] or dishes of local cuisine[211] prepared with red palm oil represent the most highly developed approaches to dietary fortification with derivatives of oil-bearing fruits.

## *Food Fortification with Vitamin A and Provitamin A*

The addition of vitamin A to foods began in the 1930s with the enrichment of margarine so that it supported vitamin nutrition in a manner similar to natural butter. Homogenized milk, with its lower butterfat content, is also enriched with vitamin A, as is skim and low-fat milk and their powdered forms. Beginning in the 1970s, the idea of fortifying foods that were never natural sources of vitamin A emerged into public health thinking.[212,213]

Two food items, sugar and cooking oil, are currently the leading vehicles in the context of public health fortification of staple foods. Sugar is fortified with retinyl palmitate in four of the five republics of Central America, as well as in Zambia. A survey showed that 89% of Ugandan households consumed sugar during any given week, making this sweetener a feasible vehicle in that African country as well.[214] A pilot fortification of coconut oil in the Philippines made it the leading single source of the vitamin, providing one-third of dietary vitamin A and improved retinol status in the population[215]. Salt may soon become a third staple food vehicle because a triple-fortification strategy involving microencapsulation, which adds vitamin A to table salt without displacing iodine and iron, has been developed.[216] Rice may be a poor vehicle, as nutritional indicators were little affected by 6 weeks of supplementation to night-blind, vitamin A-deficient women in Nepal.[217]

Vitamin A fortification can also be targeted to a specific segment of the population, as shown in a low-cost complementary food for infants and toddlers that was pilot tested in South Africa.[218] Outside of public health programs, industrial fortification of commercial foods, especially breakfast cereals and fruit-flavored drinks, is adding more vitamin A to diets in both developing and developed countries.

## *Biofortification of the Food Supply*

Biofortification is an example of a food-based approach to improving vitamin A status in which food sources are modified to include greater than usual contents of dietary vitamin A. It has generally been applied to foods of vegetal origin, in which the provitamin A content is enhanced by genetic means, either cross-breeding hybridization or genetic modification.[219,220] An example of a biofortified food created through hybridization is the carotene-rich carrot,[221] which can have up to five times the provitamin A content of a conventional carrot. Similar successful efforts have been made to enhance the carotene of cauliflower, which is normally white. Both of these biofortified foods are part of the vegetable food group, which constitutes a variable contribution to the individual diet.

The major thrust of biofortification with provitamin A carotenes is aimed at the grains and tubers that constitute the major staple foods of populations. Where yams are a staple, hybridized varieties with augmented carotene content are being promoted. Cassava (yucca, manioc, tapioca), a normally beige-colored root crop, is widely used in Africa and South America. Both hybridization and biotechnological approaches are being explored to make a red variety as a source of dietary vitamin A.

The centerpiece of biofortified foods so far has been "golden rice," a genetically modified form of rice created by inserting the genetic apparatus of marigolds and daffodils.[222,223] It has been hailed as a major genetic-engineering achievement on the staple cereal grain for a plurality of the world's population. To date, however, neither the efficacy nor the effectiveness of golden rice for improving vitamin A nutriture has been tested.

The issue of acceptability to the consumer for produce with a deeper reddish hue is a challenge to the success of biofortification. At least in the case of carrots, provitamin A-enriched cultivars are appealing.[221] For vegetables, grains, tubers, or roots that are not conventionally pigmented, even greater barriers to acceptance may arise.

## *Vitamin A Supplementation Interventions*

Since the pioneering field trial by Sommer,[104] a myriad of vitamin A supplementation trials for prophylaxis against adverse health outcomes have been conducted. With their ongoing evaluation and meta-analyses, the recommendations for target populations and schedules of public health vitamin A supplementation continue in flux. The Annecy Accords[224] of the International Vitamin A Consultative Group (IVACG) was a guide around the time of the publication of the 8th edition of this textbook. These have been recently supplanted and superceded by the vitamin A-specific considerations of the Innocenti Micronutrient Research Report #1,[225] convened under the auspices of WHO, UNICEF, and IVACG in August 2005. The latter is the source of the guidance for the routine prophylactic vitamin A supplementation programs outlined in Table 4.

**Current Prophylactic Vitamin A Supplementation Recommendations.** The Innocenti process reviewed the literature and reports from ongoing research in the field to classify the strength of the evidence for or against supplementation programs, and found that there was strong supporting evidence to recommend prophylactic supplementation in certain circumstances. These included a delivery every 6 months of age-appropriate doses of supplements to children from 6 months to 5 years of age, living in deprived and unsanitary settings, and the delivery of

**Table 4.** Summary of Recommendations for Therapeutic and Prophylactic High-Dose Supplementation with Vitamin A using Conventional Age-Appropriate Dosages

Therapeutic Supplements

- Xerophthalmia: Single dosing on diagnosis; repeat dosing within 24 h, repeat dosing at least 2 weeks later*
- Measles: Single dosing on diagnosis; repeat dosing within 24 h
- Severe protein-energy malnutrition: Single dosing on admission, followed by low-dose maintenance supplements on a daily basis†

Prophylactic Supplements

- Six-monthly dosing from age 6 to 60 months of life
- One-time dosing within 48 h of birth in neonates of HIV-positive mothers

Age-Appropriate Supplement Doses

- <6 mo = 50,000 IU (15,150 RAE)
- 6–12 mo = 100,000 IU (30,300 RAE)
- >12 mo to adulthood = 200,000 IU (60,600 RAE)

RAE, retinol activity equivalents.

* For women of reproductive age, night blindness and Birot's spots can be treated with regimens of 10,000 (3030 RAE) daily or 25,000 (7575 RAE) weekly. With higher stages of corneal xerophthalmia, the dosage schedule for other adults would apply.

† This is to be followed by RDA-level daily doses of vitamin A, as from a multivitamin mix, for the duration of nutritional recover. One caveat is to withhold the high-dose supplement if the patient has received routine prophylaxis within the last month. Moreover, in children with HIV, who are constantly being readmitted, only repeat a high-dose supplement if there has been a 4-month hiatus since the previous dosing.

an age-appropriate supplement dosage to infants of HIV-positive mothers within 2 days of birth. Mentioned with major evidence, but not to be categorically recommended, is preconceptional or antenatal supplementation, possibly with low-dosage and high frequency, modeled on an experience in Nepal.

Concurrently, the panel mobilized categorical evidence that some formats for supplementation were not effective, and even injurious to recipients compared with not receiving the vitamin. These situations include giving supplements to infants in the 2-week to 4-month interval. Gestational daily supplementation with or without postpartum high-dose supplementation to reduce maternal-to-child-transmission is not effective, and in some circumstances could actually increase vertical transmission. The once-popular advice to give either 200,000 or 400,000 IU (60,600 or 121,200 RAE) within 42 days of birth to enhance breast milk vitamin A has been revealed to have limited efficacy for lactation support. These situations are no longer listed as indications.

**Programmatic Challenges to the Delivery of Vitamin A Supplements.** The worldwide effort to maintain dosing every 6 months with age-appropriate, high-dose vitamin A has recently run into obstacles. An apparent inadvertent overdosing of the vitamin in the Assam State of India[226] led to prohibition of campaign-style distribution programs. With the near conquest of polio and the winding down of the annual vaccination as part of the Expanded Program on Immunization, an important opportunity to give one of the periodic doses of vitamin A supplements to young children on National Immunization Days is disappearing.[227,228] Self-standing activities have problems of independent financing and coverage. It has also been shown that the poorer (and theoretically more vulnerable) the target family, the less likely a child is to have access to the vitamin A distribution system in Indonesia[229] and the Philippines.[230]

# Vitamin A in Clinical Medicine and Therapeutics

## *Uses for Vitamin A and Provitamin A*

Vitamin A supplements of both high and lower doses have been studied, and therapeutic supplementation is potentially indicated in a number of conditions and explicitly recommended in others (Table 4).

**Xerophthalmia.** Because of the danger of rapid deterioration of the physical integrity of the ocular tissues, xerophthalmia is a medical emergency, meriting high-dose and repeated therapeutic intervention with preformed vitamin A doses (Table 4).

**Measles.** When this viral exanthem occurs in the present era of vaccination, it is generally in more economically and nutritionally deprived populations. Complications from measles are more common in vitamin A-deficient populations.[231] Intervention trials in Africa showed improved survival from complicated measles when high-dose supplementation was given early in hospitalization. Systematic reviews show evidence for reduced mortality in complicated measles with vitamin A supplementation. As such (Table 4), two age-appropriate dosages on successive days are recommended for children with measles. This practice has equally been validated by the American Academy of Pediatrics.

**Clinical Protein-Energy Malnutrition.** The severe, endemic protein-energy malnutrition had been in decline in recent decades, resulting in a loss of the clinical acumen to manage sporadic cases. Recent famines, natural disasters, civil conflicts, and refugee situations, however, have produced a recrudescence in clinical protein-energy malnutrition. It has long been appreciated that multiple micronutrient deficiencies, including that of vitamin A, are common in these patients. The WHO initiative to improve care for protein-energy malnutrition[223] includes a provision to administer high-dose vitamin A (Table 4).

**Acute Diarrhea.** Clinical trials with vitamin A supplementation during episodes of acute diarrhea have shown mixed and selective results, generally with no greater efficacy for reducing disease severity than placebo.[234-236]

**Malaria.** Vitamin A administration has had a positive effect on malaria by reducing the severity of attacks. Shankar et al[237] demonstrated reduced morbidity from this parasitosis in an area of hyperendemicity of *Plasmodium falciparium* malaria in Papua, New Guinea with periodic high-dose vitamin A supplementation. Serghides and Kain[238] speculate that the mechanism could lie in enhancing protozoal clearance by phagocytic cells and in suppressing the tumor necrosis factor-alpha response. It also decreases C-reactive protein.[239]

Vitamin A supplementation ameliorated the adverse effect on growth of malaria-infected children in Tanzania.[119] Contrary to what was postulated, high-dose vitamin A suppressed erythropoeitin production in anemic, malaria-infected Zanzibari preschool children.[239]

**Tuberculosis.** A double-blind, placebo-controlled study of vitamin A and zinc supplementation in persons with tuberculosis was conducted in central Java in Indonesia.[240] A daily regimen of 5000 IU (1515 RAE) and 15 mg zinc in patients with tuberculosis under treatment produced earlier sputum clearance and radiographic resolution. The authors recommended this micronutrient combination as an adjunctive therapy for tuberculosis.

**Vaginal Herpes Virus Shedding.** An vitamin A intervention trial was conducted in HIV-seropositive Kenyan women who were also infected with genital herpes simplex virus.[241] Supplementation with 10,000 IU (3030 RAE) for 6 weeks had no effect on the rate of shedding of herpes simplex virus, and would therefore not contribute to reduced transmission.

**Radiation Proctopathy.** Preliminary encouraging results for reducing rectal symptoms 6 months after pelvic radiotherapy were obtained in a randomized clinical trial using 10,000 IU (3030 RAE) of retinyl palmitate for 90 days in oncology patients.[242]

**Retinitis Pigmentosa.** Vitamin A cycles from RPE to photoreceptors of the neural retina and conversion of all-*trans* retinol to 11-*cis*-retinal. Gene mutations in these pathways explain a series of retinal dystrophies.[234] The daily administration of 15,000 IU (4545 RAE) of retinyl palmitate slows the progression of the ocular defect in patients with retinitis pigmentosa.

**Prematurity-Associated Complications.** Because hepatic vitamin A stores are laid down in late gestation, babies born before term are notably deficient in vitamin A.[244] Moreover, lung prematurity or bronchopulmonary dysplasia, a common affliction of the small preterm infant, is more frequent the lower the circulating retinol concentration.[245] A major multicenter collaborative randomized clinical trial of thrice weekly doses of 5000 IU (1515 RAE) of intramuscular retinyl palmitate over the first 4 weeks of life in extremely low-birth-weight infants (under 1000 g), was conducted in US neonatal intensive care units in the 1990s[246]; it demonstrated a slight, but significant, 11% reduction in the combined outcomes of death or chronic lung disease at 36 weeks. In a subsequent study, neither doubling the doses nor combining the cumulative dosage into a single weekly dosing showed any difference in bronchopulmonary dysplasia, outcomes, or retinol status compared with the standard regimen[247]; most patients in all three treatment groups still had low retinol status. In somewhat larger, preterm children consuming either formula or breast milk through 3 months of postnatal life remained vitamin A deficient despite supplementation of both regimens with 3000 IU (909 RAE) of additional vitamin A.[248]

In another small trial in very-low-birth-weight preterm babies, administration of three doses of the standard intramuscular vitamin A regimen to preterm infants in the 500 to 1500 μg range provided no improvement to the 50% spontaneous closure of patent ductus arteriosus conditions.[249] In long-term follow-up of the initial cohort initially treated with IM vitamin A in the neonatal ICUs,[246] there were no differences in neurodevelopmental impairment or death at 18 to 22 months of postnatal life.[250]

### *Uses for Retinoid Derivative Compounds*

Retinoic acid and various isomers and synthetic analogues are being used in pharmacological dosages for an increasing number of therapeutic purposes.

**Severe Acne Vulgaris.** Both topical and systematic administration of retinoids has been successfully applied to the treatment of severe cases of acne vulgaris. Retinoids act to lyse the microcomedo before they develop into full-blown comedones.[251] Both all-*trans*-retinoic acid (tretinoin) and 13-*cis*-retinoic acid (isotretinoin) have successful track records in acne therapy.

**Malignancies.** Retinoids have also found application in therapy of both solid tumors and hematological malignancies. It was first observed that long-term remissions of chronic myelogenous leukemia could be induced by systemic application of all-*trans*-retinoic acid, and later its efficacy in chronic promyelocytic leukemia was also shown. In both dyscrasias, the retinoid induces terminal differentiation of the myeloid cells.[115] It is also effective in the treatment of Wilms tumors.[252] On the other side of the spectrum, in one randomized trial, low-dose application of all-*trans*-retinoic acid directly to the cervical cap of papilloma-virus positive women with low-grade cervical neoplasia failed to produce significant cytological regression.[253]

**Adjunctive Therapy in Hepatitis C Treatment.** Insight into a potential advance in adjunctive, interferon-1 therapy for hepatitic C virus comes from in vitro studies with 9-*cis*-retinoic acid on hepatic cells. The retinoid increases expression of the IFN1 receptors, enhancing the antiviral effect of the drug.[254]

## Adverse and Toxic Consequences of Exposures to Vitamin A and Retinoids

By virtue of their chemical nature and persistence in the body, excessive exposure to retinoids has recognized adverse consequences, and even toxic effects. In conjunction with the considerations of for nutritional adequacy, at least two organizations have offered systematic advice regarding tolerable upper intake levels (ULs) for habitual daily dietary intakes of preformed vitamin A: 1) the Food and Nutrition Board of the US Institute of Medicine[140] and 2) a panel of the European Union on Food.[255] The respective estimates of tolerable levels are shown in Table 5. They are largely homologous, concluding that habitual intake of 3000 μg of preformed vitamin A is the UL.

### *Systemic Toxicity of Vitamin A*

A hepatic concentration of over 300 mg/g of vitamin A is considered excessive, and could be associated with clinical toxicity manifestations. In fulminant overdoses of vitamin A, signs include severe skin rash, headache, and coma due to pseudotumor cerebri, resulting in rapid demise. In more chronic, but massive overdoses, hepatic fibrosis and ascites and skin lesions share the syndrome with central nervous system disturbances. Recently recognized toxic manifestations include bone marrow suppression in an infant with hypervitaminosis A[256] and hypercalcemia in an adult consuming commercial enteral formula for a prolonged period.[257]

In an interesting observation at the interface of pharmacology and toxicology, Myhre et al[258] reported that oil-based vitamin A or liver have one-tenth the toxic potential as water-miscible, emulsified, and solid forms of retinol supplements. In recent years, two prospective studies in healthy adult volunteers have compared daily consumption of oil-based retinyl ester supplements at dosages of 25,000 IU (7575 RAE), 50,000 IU (15,152 RAE), and 75,000 IU (23,727 RAE) for periods of 12

**Table 5.** Summary of Estimated Tolerance Limits for Average Daily Consumption of Preformed Vitamin A Supplementation with Vitamin A

| Population Group | Scientific Committee EU Commission (micrograms*) |
|---|---|
| 1–3 y | 800 |
| 4–6 y | 1100 |
| 7–10 y | 1500 |
| 11–14 y | 2000 |
| 15–17 y | 2600 |
| Adults | 3000 |
| Older adults | No finding |
| | **Dietary Reference Intakes (micrograms*)** |
| 0–1 y | 600 |
| 1–3 y | 600 |
| 4–8 y | 900 |
| 9–13 y | 1700 |
| 14–18 y | 2800 |
| Adults | 3000 |
| Pregnant women | 3000 |
| Lactating women | 3000 |

* Assumes micrograms of preformed vitamin A.

months[259] and 16 months.[260] The highest chronic dose represents 7.5 times the UL. No evidence of toxicity or adverse consequences were detected over the respective intervals.

With a public health perspective, Allen and Haskell[261] have examined the supplementation regimens current in 2002, and conclude that, on a single-dose or periodic basis, the schedules for high-dose supplements were safe for infants, children, and postpartum women. Although some exceeded the daily UL on a prorated basis, none would surpass the no-observed-adverse-effect level.

### *Systemic Toxicity of Retinoic Acid and Isomers*

Since the advent of high-dose treatment with systemic retinoic acid for leukemia and other malignant conditions, a condition known as "retinoic acid syndrome" has been recognized. It is characterized by weight gain, episodes of hypotension, acute renal failure, unexplained fever, and respiratory distress associated with interstitial pulmonary infiltrates and pleural and pericardial effusions seen on chest X-rays.[262] High doses of retinoid analogs can increase intracranial pressure as well.[263]

### *Teratogenesis*

Congenital birth defects can be induced by vitamin A deficiency and excess. The UL of vitamin A[140] is based on increased risk of teratogenesis, which is estimated to begin with habitual intakes of preformed vitamin A in excess of 10,000 IU (3030 RAE). The damage occurs in the embryogenic phase within days of conception. The manifestations of excess vitamin A include spectrum of malformations including ocular, pulmonary, cardiovascular, and urogenital defects.[80] These same birth defects can arise when systemic doses of the retinoid analogs are administered in dermatological practice to treat acne.[264] Provisional evidence suggests, however, that the topical use of these analogs in early pregnancy presents minimal to no risk of teratogenesis.[265]

### *Adverse Consequences*

Interest has arisen regarding adverse consequences of vitamin A on bone mineralization, cardiovascular risk, and repletion of iodine-deficient populations.

**Bone Demineralization and Osteoporotic Fracture Risk.** One of the areas of most recent toxicological concern is that of an adverse effect of vitamin A on bone mineralization and structural integrity. Adverse effects on skeletal tissue had long been associated with excessive vitamin A exposure. Spontaneous bone fractures are a common manifestation of vitamin A overfeeding in animals. From this mechanistic standpoint, vitamin A stimulates bone resorption and inhibits bone formation.[266] That this is a complex and long-range problem in adults is shown by the recent demonstration of no influence of 6 weeks of oral supplementation with 25,000 IU (7576 RAE) of retinyl palmitate on circulating biomarkers of bone turnover in a randomized trial of healthy adult men.[267]

The recent public health concern dates to the 1999 publication of observations on Swedish women by Mehlus et al,[268] who observed an inverse association between estimated preformed vitamin A intake and bone mineral density in a cross-sectional analysis for habitual daily vitamin A intakes above 1500 μg equivalents. A variety of subsequent investigations have examined the question with a mixture of evidence both confirming and refuting the premise of adverse effects of vitamin A excess on bone health. On the one hand, studies in Scandinavian men,[269] North American women,[270-272] and mixed-gender retirees in California[273] have provided evidence for accelerated bone demineralization or increased risk of osteoporotic fractures associated variously with baseline circulating retinol concentrations, total intake of preformed vitamin A, or with use of supplements containing the vitamin. In a study among North American nurses, a daily intake of over 2000 μg equivalents of preformed vitamin A defined the group at highest risk.[271] On the other hand, reports concerning postmenopausal Danish[274] and British[275] women and adult American women[276] found no associations between the same marker variables for comparable adverse outcomes for bone health.

The public health importance of this constellation of

observations has yet to be defined. Because of varying population vitamin A intakes across populations[277] or associations linked to circulating biomarkers,[269,270] agreement on threshold intake levels of preformed vitamin A conferring risk to bone health seems remote. A prudent interim conclusion comes from Crandall,[278] however: "It is not yet possible to set a specific level of retinol intake above which bone health is compromised. Pending further investigation, Vit A supplements should not be used with the express goal of improving bone health."

**Enhanced Cardiovascular Risk.** Another area of recent discovery, in which upward variations of dietary vitamin A exposure within the usual range may be to blame, comes from observational studies regarding cardiovascular disease as the outcome.[279,280] Higher vitamin A intake and higher serum levels were an independent risk factor for cardiovascular disease in Saudi adults.[279] In a cohort of US adults, higher baseline concentrations of retinol were associated with an increased risk, but in men only.[280]

# Thyroid Stimulation in Severely Iodine-Deficiency Populations

In field intervention studies in Morocco using iodization of salt in a goitrous population, Zimmermann et al[281] observed that children in the placebo group suffered increased volume of their goiters and biochemical signs of hypothyroidism (elevated thyroglobulin concentration) compared with those receiving a vitamin A supplement. They speculated that this effect could be due to decreased vitamin A-mediated suppression of the pituitary TSH-beta gene. Their recommendation was to introduce salt iodization in severely multiply deficient populations only after, or concurrent with, correction of vitamin A deficiency.

# Future Directions

Vitamin A and retinoid research need to advance on both the basic science and applied public health fronts. Cellular and molecular research will extend our insights into the actions of retinoids. Exhaustive exploration of the prophylactic and therapeutic utility of retinoids for malignant diseases, advancing the promise from in vitro cell culture studies to clinical trials in patients, is a high priority at the interface of basic science and clinical medicine.

With the ability to insert retinyl palmitate into commercial food processing and public health programs, safety issues are emerging as a prominent health concern. Further application of isolated provitamin A or carotenoids in oil bases could provide a high bioefficacy as safer alternatives to preformed vitamin A for periodic supplementation and food fortification. The promise of biofortification must be unlocked as potentially another approach to exploiting the contribution of provitamin A forms to support vitamin A nutrition.

Multiple micronutrient interventions are replacing single-nutrient concerns in program and policy. Advocacy to ensure that the vitamin A agenda is preserved as interventions become more integrated is needed, while ongoing inquiries into the efficacy and safety of vitamin A in the context of combined administration of micronutrients must be supported.

# References


1. Ramakrishnan U. Prevalence of micronutrient malnutrition worldwide. Nutr Rev. 2002;60:S46–52.
2. West KP Jr. Extent of vitamin A deficiency among preschool children and women of reproductive age. J Nutr. 2002;132(9 Suppl):2857S–2866S.
3. Underwood BA. Vitamin A deficiency disorders: international efforts to control a preventable "pox". J Nutr. 2004;134:231S–236S.
4. American Institute of Nutrition. Nomenclature policy: generic descriptions and trivial names for vitamins and related compounds. J Nutr. 1990;120: 12–9.
5. Frolik CA. Metabolism of retinoids. In: Sporn MB, Roberts AB, Goodman DS, eds. *The Retinoids, Vol. 2*. Orlando: Academic Press; 1984:177–208.
6. Blomhoff R, Green MH, Berg T, Norum FR. Transport and storage of vitamin A. Science. 1994; 250:399–404.
7. Dawson MJ, Okamura WH, eds. *Chemistry and Biology of Synthetic Retinoids*. Boca Raton, FL: CRC Press; 1990.
8. Comstock GW, Alberg AJ, Helzlsouer KJ. Reported effects of long-term freezer storage on concentrations of retinol, β-carotene, and α-tocopherol in serum or plasma summarized. Clin Chem. 1993; 39:1075–1078.
9. Klaui H, Bauernfeind JC. Carotenoids as food colorants. In: JC Bauernfeind, ed. *Carotenoids as Colorants and Vitamin A Precursors*. San Diego: Academic Press; 1981:47–317.
10. Kofler M, Rubin SH. Physiochemical assay of vitamin A and related compounds. Vitam Horm. 1960; 18:315–339.
11. Furr HC. Analysis of retinoids and carotenoids: problems resolved and unsolved. J Nutr. 2004;134: 281S–285S.
12. De Leenheer AP, Nelis HJ, Lambert WE. Chromatography of fat-soluble vitamins in clinical chemistry. J Chromatogr Biomed Applic. 1988;429: 3–58.
13. Rodriguez-Amaya DB. A Guide to Carotenoid Analysis in Foods. ILSI Press: Washington, DC; 1999.
14. Rodriguez-Amaya DB. Latin American food sources of carotenoids. Arch Latinoamer Nutr. 2000;49(Suppl 1):74S–84S.
15. Kimura M, Rodriguez-Amaya DB. Sources of error in the quantitative analysis of food carotenoids

by HPLC. Arch Latinoamer Nutr. 2000;49(Suppl 1):74S–84S.
16. West CE, Eilander A, van Lieshout M. Consequences of revised estimates of carotenoid bioefficacy for dietary control of vitamin A deficiency in developing countries. J Nutr. 2002;132((9 Suppl): 2920S–2926S.
17. Harrison EH. Mechanisms of digestion and absorption of dietary vitamin A. Annu Rev Nutr. 2005;25:87–103.
18. Ong DE. Absorption of vitamin A. In: Blomhoff R, ed. *Vitamin A in Health and Disease*. New York: Marcel Dekker; 1994:37–72.
19. Krinsky NI, Wang X-D, Tang G, Russell RM. Mechanism of carotenoid cleavage to retinoids. Ann NY Acad Sci. 1993;681:167–176.
20. Castenmiller JJ, West CE. Bioavailability and bioconversion of carotenoids. Annu Rev Nutr. 1998; 18:19–38.
21. Goodman DS, Huang HS. Biosynthesis of vitamin A with rat intestinal enzymes. Science. 1965;149: 879–880.
22. Olson JA, Hayaishi O. The enzymatic cleavage of β-carotene into vitamin A by soluble enzymes of rat liver and intestine. Proc Natl Acad Sci USA. 1965;54:1364–1370.
23. Lindqvist A, Andersson S. Biochemical properties of purified recombinant human beta-carotene 15,15′-monooxygenase. J Biol Chem. 2002;277: 23942–8.
24. Boulanger A, McLemore P, Copeland NG, et al. Identification of beta-carotene 15,15′-monooxygenase as a peroxisome proliferator-activated receptor target gene. FASEB J. 2003;17:1304–6.
25. Olson JA. Formation and function of vitamin A. In: Porter JW, Spurgeon SL, eds. *Biosynthesis of Isoprenoid Compounds, Vol 2*. New York: John Wiley & Sons; 1983:371–412.
26. Yeum KJ, Russell RM. Carotenoid bioavailability and bioconversion. Annu Rev Nutr. 2002;22: 483–504.
27. Furr HC, Green MH, Haskell M, et al. Stable isotope dilution techniques for assessing vitamin A status and bioefficacy of provitamin A carotenoids in humans. Public Health Nutr. 2005;8:596–607.
28. van Lieshout M, West CE, van Breemen RB. Isotopic tracer techniques for studying the bioavailability and bioefficacy of dietary carotenoids, particularly beta-carotene, in humans: a review. Am J Clin Nutr. 2003;77:12–28.
29. Thurmann PA, Steffen J, Zwernemann C, et al. Plasma concentration response to drinks containing beta-carotene as carrot juice or formulated as a water dispersible powder. Eur J Nutr. 2002;41:228–235.
30. Edwards AJ, Nguyen CH, You CS, Swanson JE, Emenhiser C, Parker RS. Alpha- and beta-carotene from a commercial puree are more bioavailable to humans than from boiled-mashed carrots, as determined using an extrinsic stable isotope reference method. J Nutr. 2002;132:159–167.
31. Haskell MJ, Jamil KM, Hassan F, et al. Daily consumption of Indian spinach (*Basella alba*) or sweet potatoes has a positive effect on total-body vitamin A stores in Bangladeshi men. Am J Clin Nutr. 2004; 80:705–714.
32. Tang G, Qin J, Dolnikowski GG, Russell RM, Grusak MA. Spinach or carrots can supply significant amounts of vitamin A as assessed by feeding with intrinsically deuterated vegetables. Am J Clin Nutr. 2005;82:821–828.
33. Tulley RT, Vaidyanathan J, Wilson JB, et al. Daily intake of multivitamins during long-term intake of olestra in men prevents declines in serum vitamins A and E but not carotenoids. J Nutr. 2005;135: 1456–1461.
34. McDuffie JR, Calis KA, Booth SL, Uwaifo GI, Yanovski JA. Effects of orlistat on fat-soluble vitamins in obese adolescents. Pharmacotherapy. 2002; 22:814–822.
35. Richelle M, Enslen M, Hager C, et al. Both free and esterified plant sterols reduce cholesterol absorption and the bioavailability of beta-carotene and alpha-tocopherol in normocholesterolemic humans. Am J Clin Nutr. 2004;80:171–177.
36. Ntanios FY, Homma Y, Ushiro S. A spread enriched with plant sterol-esters lowers blood cholesterol and lipoproteins without affecting vitamins A and E in normal and hypercholesterolemic Japanese men and women. J Nutr. 2002;132:3650–3655.
37. Greenwood DC, Cade JE, White K, Burley VJ, Schorah CJ. The impact of high non-starch polysaccharide intake on serum micronutrient concentrations in a cohort of women. Public Health Nutr. 2004;7:543–548.
38. Ribaya-Mercado JD. Influence of dietary fat on beta-carotene absorption and bioconversion into vitamin A. Nutr Rev. 2002;60:104–110.
39. Nagao A. Oxidative conversion of carotenoids to retinoids and other products. J Nutr. 2004;134: 237S–240S.
40. West CE, Eilander A, van Lieshout M. Consequences of revised estimates of carotenoid bioefficacy for dietary control of vitamin A deficiency in developing countries. J Nutr. 2002;132(9 Suppl): 2920S–2926S.
41. Hickenbottom SJ, Follett JR, Lin Y, et al. Variability in conversion of beta-carotene to vitamin A in men as measured by using a double-tracer study design. Am J Clin Ntur. 2002;75:900–907.
42. Wang Z, Yin S, Zhao X, Russell RM, Tang G. beta-Carotene-vitamin A equivalence in Chinese adults assessed by an isotope dilution technique. Br J Nutr. 2004;91:121–131.
43. Napoli JL. A gene knockout corroborates the integ-

rap function of cellular retinol-binding protein in retinoid metabolism. Nutr Rev. 200;58:230–235.
44. Glass CK, Rosenfeld MG, Rose DW, et al. Mechanisms of transcriptional activation by retinoic acid receptors. Biochem Soc Trans. 1997;25:602–605.
45. Rowe A. Retinoid X receptors. Biochem Cell Biol. 1997;29:275–278.
46. Troen G, Eskild W, Fromm SH, et al. Vitamin A-sensitive tissues in transgenic mice expressing high levels of human cellular retinol-binding protein type I are not altered phenotypically. J Nutr. 1999;129:1621–1627.
47. Biesalski HK, Nohr D. New aspects in vitamin a metabolism: the role of retinyl esters as systemic and local sources for retinol in mucous epithelia. J Nutr. 2004;134(12 Suppl):3453S–3457S.
48. Napoli JL. Interactions of retinoid binding proteins and enzymes in retinoid metabolism. Biochim Biophys Acta. 1999;1440:139–162.
49. Gaetani S, Bellovino D, Apreda M, Devirgiliis C. Hepatic synthesis, maturation and complex formation between retinol-binding protein and transthyretin. Clin Chem Lab Med. 2002;40:1211–1220.
50. Zanotti G, Berni R. Plasma retinol-binding protein: structure and interactions with retinol, retinoids, and transthyretin. Vitam Horm. 2004;69: 271–295.
51. Raghu P, Sivakumar B. Interactions amongst plasma retinol-binding protein, transthyretin and their ligands: implications in vitamin A homeostasis and transthyretin amyloidosis. Biochim Biophys Acta. 2004;1703:1–9.
52. Loerch JD, Underwood BA, Lewis KC. Response of plasma levels of vitamin A to a dose of vitamin A as an indicator of hepatic vitamin A reserves in rats. J Nutr. 1979;109:778–788.
53. Artacho CA, Piantedosi R, Blaner WS. Placental transfer of vitamin A. Sight & Life Newsletter. 1993;(3):23–28.
54. Dimenstein R, Trugo NMF, Donangelo CM, Trugo LC, Anastacio AS. Effect of subadequate maternal vitamin A status on placental transfer of retinol and β-carotene to the human fetus. Biol Neonate. 1996;69:230–234.
55. Dewey KG, Cohen RJ, Brown KH. Exclusive breast-feeding for 6 months, with iron supplementation, maintains adequate micronutrient status among term, low-birthweight, breast-fed infants in Honduras. J Nutr. 2004;134:1091–1098.
56. Bahl R, Bhandari N, Wahed MA, Kumar GT, Bhan MK; WHO/CHD Immunization-Linked Vitamin A Group. Vitamin A supplementation of women postpartum and of their infants at immunization alters breast milk retinol and infant vitamin A status. J Nutr. 2002;132:3243–3248.
57. Basu S, Sengupta B, Paladhi PK. Single megadose vitamin A supplementation of Indian mothers and morbidity in breastfed young infants. Postgrad Med J. 2003;79:397–402.
58. Valentine AR, Tanumihardjo SA. One-time vitamin A supplementation of lactating sows enhances hepatic retinol in their offspring independent of dose size. Am J Clin Nutr. 2005;81:427–33.
59. Akohoue SA, Green JB, Green MH. Dietary vitamin A has both chronic and acute effects on vitamin A indices in lactating rats and their offspring. J Nutr. 2006;136:128–32.
60. Olafsdottir AS, Wagner KH, Thorsdottir I, Elmadfa I. Fat-soluble vitamins in the maternal diet, influence of cod liver oil supplementation and impact of the maternal diet on human milk composition. Ann Nutr Metab. 2001;45:265–272.
61. Menses F, Torres AC, Trugo NMF. Influence of recent dietary intake on plasma and human milk levels of carotenoids and retinol in Brazilian nursing women. Adv Exp Med Biol. 2004;554:351–354.
62. Menses F, Trugo NMF. Retinol, β-carotene, and lutein + zeaxanthin in the milk of Brazilian nursing women: associations with plasma concentrations and influences of maternal characteristics. Nutr Res. 2005;25:443–451.
63. Canfield LM, Clandinin MT, Davies DP, et al. Multinational study of major breast milk carotenoids of healthy mothers. Eur J Nutr. 2003;42: 133–141.
64. Schweigert FJ, Bathe K, Chen F, Buscher U, Dudenhausen JW. Effect of the stage of lactation in humans on carotenoid levels in milk, blood plasma and plasma lipoprotein fractions. Eur J Nutr. 2004;43: 39–44.
65. Hicks VA, Gunning DB, Olson JA. Metabolism, plasma transport and biliary excretion of radioactive vitamin A and its metabolites as a function of liver rreserves of vitamin A in the rat. J Nutr. 1984;114: 1327–1333.
66. Skare KL, DeLuca HF. Biliary metabolites of all-*trans*-retinoic acid in the rat. Arch Biochem Biophys. 1983;224:13–18.
67. Raila J, Wirth K, Chen F, Buscher U, Dudenhausen JW, Schweigert FJ. Excretion of vitamin A in urine of women during normal pregnancy and pregnancy complications. Ann Nutr Metab. 2004;48: 357–364.
68. Gavrilov V, Weksler N, Ahmed A, Gorodischer R. Urinary excretion of vitamin A in critically ill patients complicated with acute renal failure. Ren Fail. 2004;26:589–590
69. Gavrilov V, Yermiahu T, Gorodischer R. Urinary excretion of retinol in patients with multiple myeloma: a preliminary study. Am J Hematol. 2003; 74:202–204.
70. Mitra AK, Wahed MA, Chowdhury AK, Stephensen CB. Urinary retinol excretion in children with acute watery diarrhoea. J Health Popul Nutr. 2002; 20:12–17.

71. Olson JA. Carotenoids. In: Shils ME, Olson JA, Ross AC, Shike M, eds. *Modern Nutrition in Health and Disease*. 9th Edition. Philadelphia: WB Saunders; 1998:525–541.
72. Wald G. Molecular basis of visual excitation. Science. 1968;162:230–239.
73. Wolf G. The visual cycle of the cone photoreceptors of the retina. Nutr Rev. 2004;62:283–286.
74. Pulukuri S, Sitaramayya A. Retinaldehyde, a potent inhibitor of gap junctional intercellular communication. Cell Commun Adhes. 2004;11:25–33.
75. Ara C, Devirgiliis LC, Massimi M. Influence of retinoic acid on adhesion complexes in human hepatoma cells: a clue to its antiproliferative effects. Cell Commun Adhes. 2004;11:13–23.
76. Bohnsack BL, Hirschi KK. Nutrient regulation of cell cycle progression. Annu Rev Nutr. 2004;24: 433–453.
77. Marill J, Idres N, Capron CC, Nguyen E, Chabot GG. Retinoic acid metabolism and mechanism of action: a review. Curr Drug Metab. 2003;4:1–10.
78. Evans T. Regulation of hematopoiesis by retinoid signaling. Exp Hematol. 2005;33:1055–1561.
79. Chu PW, Cheung WM, Kwong YL. Differential effects of 9-*cis*, 13-*cis* and all-*trans* retinoic acids on the neuronal differentiation of human neuroblastoma cells. Neuroreport. 2003;14:1935–1939.
80. Lefebvre P, Martin PJ, Flajollet S, Dedieu S, Billaut X, Lefebvre B. Transcriptional activities of retinoic acid receptors. Vitam Horm. 2005;70:199–264. Review.
81. DiRenzo J, Soderstrom M, Kurokawa R, et al. Peroxisome proliferator-activated receptors and retinoic acid receptors differentially control the interactions of retinoid X receptor heterodimers with ligands, coactivators, and corepressors. Mol Cell Biol. 1997;17:2166–2176.
82. Li D, Li T, Wang F, Tian H, Samuels HH. Functional evidence for retinoid X receptor (RXR) as a nonsilent partner in the thyroid hormone receptor/RXR heterodimer. Mol Cell Biol. 2002;22:5782–5792.
83. Wolf G. The regulation of the thyroid-stimulating hormone of the anterior pituitary gland by thyroid hormone and by 9-*cis*-retinoic acid. Nutr Rev. 2002; 60:374–377.
84. Blomhoff HK. Vitamin A regulates proliferation and apoptosis of human T- and B-cells. Biochem Soc Trans. 2004;32:982–984.
85. Ertesvag A, Engedal N, Naderi S, Blomhoff HK. Retinoic acid stimulates the cell cycle machinery in normal T cells: involvement of retinoic acid receptor-mediated IL-2 secretion. J Immunol. 2002;169: 5555–5563.
86. Beum PV, Basma H, Bastola DR, Cheng PW. Mucin biosynthesis: upregulation of core 2 beta 1,6 N-acetylglucosaminyltransferase by retinoic acid and Th2 cytokines in a human airway epithelial cell line. Am J Physiol Lung Cell Mol Physiol. 2005; 288:L116–124.
87. Crowe DL, Chandraratna RA. A Retinoid X Receptor (RXR)-selective retinoid reveals that RXR-alpha is potentially a therapeutic target in breast cancer cell lines, and that it potentiates antiproliferative and apoptotic responses to peroxisome proliferator-activated receptor ligand. Breast Cancer Res. 2004;6:R546–555.
88. Chen Q, Ross AC. Retinoic acid regulates cell cycle progression and cell differentiation in human monocytic THP-1 cells. Exp Cell Res. 2004;297: 68–81.
89. Amanatullah DF, Zafonte BT, Pestell RG. The cell cycle in steroid hormone regulated proliferation and differentiation. Minerva Endocrinol. 2002;27: 7–20.
90. Kiefer HL, Hanley TM, Marcello JE, Karthik AG, Viglianti GA. Retinoic acid inhibition of chromatin remodeling at the human immunodeficiency virus type 1 promoter. Uncoupling of histone acetylation and chromatin remodeling. J Biol Chem. 2004;279: 43604–43613.
91. Hoyos B, Jiang S, Hammerling U. Location and functional significance of retinol-binding sites on the serine/threonine kinase, c-Raf. J Biol Chem. 2005;280:6872–6878.
92. Hori Y, Spurr-Michaud S, Russo CL, Argueso P, Gipson IK. Differential regulation of membrane-associated mucins in the human ocular surface epithelium. Invest Ophthalmol Vis Sci. 2004;45: 114–122.
93. Mark M, Ghyselinck NB, Chambon P. Retinoic acid signalling in the development of branchial arches. Curr Opin Genet Dev. 2004;14:591–598.
94. Maden M, Hind M. Retinoic acid in alveolar development, maintenance and regeneration. Philos Trans R Soc Lond B Biol Sci. 2004;359:799–808.
95. Ross AC. On the sources of retinoic acid in the lung: understanding the local conversion of retinol to retinoic acid. Am J Physiol Lung Cell Mol Physiol. 2004;286:L247-L248.
96. Tang G, Qin J, Dolnikowski GG, Russell RM. Short-term (intestinal) and long-term (postintestinal) conversion of beta-carotene to retinol in adults as assessed by a stable-isotope reference method. Am J Clin Nutr. 2003;78:259–266.
97. Abu J, Batuwangala M, Herbert K, Symonds P. Retinoic acid and retinoid receptors: potential chemopreventive and therapeutic role in cervical cancer. Lancet Oncol. 2005;6:712–720.
98. Dawson MI, Zhang XK. Discovery and design of retinoic acid receptor and retinoid X receptor class- and subtype-selective synthetic analogs of all-*trans*-retinoic acid and 9-*cis*-retinoic acid. Curr Med Chem. 2002;9:623–637.
99. García-Casal MN, Layrisse M, Solano L, et al. A

new property of vitamin A and β-carotene on human non-heme iron absorption in rice, wheat and corn. J Nutr. 1998;128:646–650.

100. Layrisse M, García-Casal MN, Solano l, et al. The role of vitamin A on the inhibitors of nonheme iron absorption: Preliminary results. J Nutr Biochem. 1997;8:61–67.
101. Layrisse M, García-Casal MN, Solano L, et al. Vitamin A reduces the inhibition of iron absorption by phytates and polyphenols. Food Nutr Bull. 1998; 19:3–5.
102. Davidsson L, Adou P, Zeder C, Walczyk T, Hurrell R. The effect of retinyl palmitate added to iron-fortified maize porridge on erythrocyte incorporation of iron in African children with vitamin A deficiency. Br J Nutr. 2003;90:337–343.
103. Sommer A, Tarwojto I, Hussaini G, Susanto D. Increased mortality in children with mild vitamin A deficiency. Lancet. 1983;2:585–588.
104. Sommer A, Tarwotjo I, Djunaedi E, et al. The impact of vitamin A supplementation on childhood mortality. A randomised controlled community trial. Lancet. 1986;1:1169–1173.
105. Beaton GH, Martorell R, Aronson KJ, et al. Effectiveness of vitamin A supplementation in the control of young child morbidity and mortality in developing countries. ACC/SCN State-of-the-art Series Nutrition Policy Discussion Paper no. 13. Geneva, SubCommittee on Nutrition; 1993.
106. Rahmathullah L, Tielsch JM, Thulasiraj RD, et al. Impact of supplementing newborn infants with vitamin A on early infant mortality: community based randomised trial in southern India. BMJ. 2003;327: 254.
107. Semba RD, Ndugwa C, Perry RT, et al. Effect of periodic vitamin A supplementation on mortality and morbidity of human immunodeficiency virus-infected children in Uganda: A controlled clinical trial. Nutrition. 2005;21:25–31.
108. Alm B, Wennergren G, Norvenius SG, et al; Nordic Epidemiological SIDS Study. Vitamin A and sudden infant death syndrome in Scandinavia 1992–1995. Acta Paediatr. 2003;92:162–164.
109. Grotto I, Mimouni M, Gdalevich M, Mimouni D. Vitamin A supplementation and childhood morbidity from diarrhea and respiratory infections: a meta-analysis. J Pediatr. 2003;142:297–304.
110. Brown N, Roberts C. Vitamin A for acute respiratory infection in developing countries: a meta-analysis. Acta Paediatr. 2004;93:437–442.
111. Gamble MV, Palafox NA, Dancheck B, Ricks MO, Briand K, Semba RD. Relationship of vitamin A deficiency, iron deficiency, and inflammation to anemia among preschool children in the Republic of the Marshall Islands. Eur J Clin Nutr. 2004;58: 1396–1401.
112. Osorio MM, Lira PI, Ashworth A. Factors associated with Hb concentration in children aged 6–59 months in the State of Pernambuco, Brazil. Br J Nutr. 2004;91:307–315.
113. Kafwembe EM. Iron and vitamin A status of breastfeeding mothers in Zambia. East Afr Med J. 2001;78:454–457.
114. Semba RD, Bloem MW. The anemia of vitamin A deficiency: epidemiology and pathogenesis. Eur J Clin Nutr. 2002;56:271–281.
115. Oren T, Sher JA, Evans T. Hematopoiesis and retinoids: development and disease. Leuk Lymphoma. 2003;44:1881–1891.
116. Kinjo K, Miyakawa Y, Uchida H, Kitajima S, Ikeda Y, Kizaki M. All-*trans* retinoic acid directly up-regulates thrombopoietin transcription in human bone marrow stromal cells. Exp Hematol. 2004;32: 45–51.
117. Sarni RS, Kochi C, Ramalho RA, et al. Impact of vitamin A megadose supplementation on the anthropometry of children and adolescents with non-hormonal statural deficit: a double-blind and randomized clinical study. Int J Vitam Nutr Res. 2003; 73:303–311.
118. Villamor E, Saathoff E, Bosch RJ, et al. Vitamin supplementation of HIV-infected women improves postnatal child growth. Am J Clin Nutr. 2005;81: 880–888.
119. Villamor E, Mbise R, Spiegelman D, et al. Vitamin A supplements ameliorate the adverse effect of HIV-1, malaria, and diarrheal infections on child growth. Pediatrics. 2002;109:E6.
120. Mason ME, Jalagani H, Vinik AI. Metabolic complications of bariatric surgery: diagnosis and management issues. Gastroenterol Clin North Am. 2005;34:25–33.
121. Slater GH, Ren CJ, Siegel N, et al. Serum fat-soluble vitamin deficiency and abnormal calcium metabolism after malabsorptive bariatric surgery. J Gastrointest Surg. 2004;8:48–55.
122. Armstrong T, Walters E, Varshney S, Johnson CD. Deficiencies of micronutrients, altered bowel function, and quality of life during late follow-up after pancreaticoduodenectomy for malignancy. Pancreatology. 2002;2:528–534.
123. Aguilera A, Bajo MA, del Peso G, et al. True deficiency of antioxidant vitamins E and A in dialysis patients. Relationship with clinical patterns of atherosclerosis. Adv Perit Dial. 2002;18:206–211.
124. High KP, Legault C, Sinclair JA, Cruz J, Hill K, Hurd DD. Low plasma concentrations of retinol and alpha-tocopherol in hematopoietic stem cell transplant recipients: the effect of mucositis and the risk of infection. Am J Clin Nutr. 2002;76: 1358–1366.
125. Schmidt R, Luboeinski T, Markart P, et al. Alveolar antioxidant status in patients with acute respiratory distress syndrome. Eur Respir J. 2004;24:994–999.

126. van Lettow M, Harries AD, Kumwenda JJ, et al. Micronutrient malnutrition and wasting in adults with pulmonary tuberculosis with and without HIV co-infection in Malawi. BMC Infect Dis. 2004;4: 61.
127. Tiboni GM, Bucciarelli T, Giampietro F, Sulpizio M, Di Ilio C. Influence of cigarette smoking on vitamin E, vitamin A, beta-carotene and lycopene concentrations in human pre-ovulatory follicular fluid. Int J Immunopathol Pharmacol. 2004;17: 389–393.
128. Vorster HH, Kruger A, Margetts BM, et al. The nutritional status of asymptomatic HIV-infected Africans: directions for dietary intervention? Public Health Nutr. 2004;7:1055–1064.
129. Visser ME, Maartens G, Kossew G, Hussey GD. Plasma vitamin A and zinc levels in HIV-infected adults in Cape Town, South Africa. Br J Nutr. 2003; 89:475–482.
130. Arora P, Kumar V, Batra S. Vitamin A status in children with asthma. Pediatr Allergy Immunol. 2002;13:223–226.
131. Singh V, West KP Jr. Vitamin A deficiency and xerophthalmia among school-aged children in Southeastern Asia. Eur J Clin Nutr. 2004;58: 1342–1349.
132. Villalpando S, Montalvo-Velarde I, Zambrano N, et al. Vitamins A, and C and folate status in Mexican children under 12 years and women 12–49 years: a probabilistic national survey. Salud Publica Mex. 2003;45 Suppl 4:S508–S519.
133. Dallaire F, Dewailly E, Shademani R, et al. Vitamin A concentration in umbilical cord blood of infants from three separate regions of the province of Quebec (Canada). Can J Public Health. 2003;94: 386–390.
134. Coles CL, Levy A, Gorodischer R, et al. Subclinical vitamin A deficiency in Israeli-Bedouin toddlers. Eur J Clin Nutr. 2004;58:796–802.
135. Oelofse A, Van Raaij JM, Benade AJ, Dhansay MA, Tolboom JJ, Hautvast JG. Disadvantaged black and coloured infants in two urban communities in the Western Cape, South Africa differ in micronutrient status. Public Health Nutr. 2002;5: 289–294.
136. Zinsstag J, Schelling E, Daoud S, et al. Serum retinol of Chadian nomadic pastoralist women in relation to their livestocks' milk retinol and beta-carotene content. Int J Vitam Nutr Res. 2002;72: 221–228.
137. Ajose OA, Adelekan DA, Ajewole EO. Vitamin A status of pregnant Nigerian women: relationship to dietary habits and morbidity. Nutr Health. 2004; 17:325–333.
138. Semba RD, de Pee S, Panagides D, Poly O, Bloem MW. Risk factors for xerophthalmia among mothers and their children and for mother-child pairs with xerophthalmia in Cambodia. Arch Ophthalmol. 2004;122:517–523.
139. Food and Agricultural Organization/World Health Organization. *Requirement of Vitamin A, Thiamine, Riboflavin and Niacin*. Rome: FAO Food and Nutrition Series B; 1967.
140. Institute of Medicine, Food and Nutrition Board. *Dietary Reference Intakes for Vitamin A, Vitamin K, Arsenic, Boron, Chromium, Copper, Iodine, Iron, Manganese, Molybdenum, Nickel, Silicon, Vanadium and Zinc*. Washington, DC: National Academy Press; 2001.
141. World Health Organization/Food and Agricultural Organization. *Vitamin and Mineral Requirements in Human Nutrition*. Geneva, WHO; 2004.
142. Ervin RB, Wright JD, Wang CY, Kennedy-Stephenson J. Dietary intake of selected vitamins for the United States population: 1999–2000. Adv Data. 2004;(339):1–4.
143. Harley K, Eskenazi B, Block G. The association of time in the US and diet during pregnancy in low-income women of Mexican descent. Paediatr Perinat Epidemiol. 2005;19:125–134.
144. Goldbohm RA, Brants HA, Hulshof KF, van den Brandt PA. The contribution of various foods to intake of vitamin A and carotenes in the Netherlands. Int J Vitamin Nutr Res.
145. Henderson L, Irving K, Bates C, Prentics A, Perks J. Vitamin and mineral intake and urinary analytes. In: *The National Diet & Nutrition Survey Adults Aged 19 to 64 Years., Vol. 3*. London: Office for National Statistics, Food Standards Agency; 2003.
146. Riccioni G, Menna V, Di Ilio C, D'Orazio N. Food-intake and nutrients pattern in Italian adult male subjects. Clin Ter. 2004;155:283–286.
147. Hels O, Hassan N, Tetens I, Haraksingh Thilsted S. Food consumption, energy and nutrient intake and nutritional status in rural Bangladesh: changes from 1981–1982 to 1995–96. Eur J Clin Nutr. 2003;57:586–594.
148. Sichert-Hellert W, Kersting M, Manz F. Changes in time-trends of nutrient intake from fortified and non-fortified food in German children and adolescents—15 year results of the DONALD study. Dortmund Nutritional and Anthropometric Longitudinally Designed Study. Eur J Nutr. 2001;40: 49–55.
149. Watt RG, Dykes J, Sheiham A. Socio-economic determinants of selected dietary indicators in British pre-school children. Public Health Nutr. 2001;4: 1229–1233.
150. Serra-Majem L, Ribas L, Ngo J, et al. Risk of inadequate intakes of vitamins A, B1, B6, C, E, folate, iron and calcium in the Spanish population aged 4 to 18. Int J Vitam Nutr Res. 2001;71:325–331.
151. Venkaiah K, Damayanti K, Nayak MU, Vijayaraghavan K. Diet and nutritional status of rural ado-

lescents in India. Eur J Clin Nutr. 2002;56: 1119–1125.

152. Lewis SM, Mayhugh MA, Freni SC, et al. Assessment of antioxidant nutrient intake of a population of southern US African-American and Caucasian women of various ages when compared to dietary reference intakes. J Nutr Health Aging. 2003;7: 121–128.

153. Aranceta J, Serra-Majem L, Perez-Rodrigo C, et al. Vitamins in Spanish food patterns: the eVe Study. Public Health Nutr. 2001;4:1317–1323.

154. Martins I, Dantas A, Guiomar S, Amorim Cruz JA. Vitamin and mineral intakes in elderly. J Nutr Health Aging. 2002;6:63–65.

155. Sichert-Hellert W, Kersting M; Dortmund Nutritional and Anthropometric Longitudinally Designed Study. Significance of fortified beverages in the long-term diet of German children and adolescents: 15-year results of the DONALD Study. Int J Vitam Nutr Res. 2001;71:356–363.

156. Thane CW, Bates CJ, Prentice A. Zinc and vitamin A intake and status in a national sample of British young people aged 4–18 y. Eur J Clin Nutr. 2004; 58:363–375.

157. Florentino RF, Villavieja GM, Lana RD. Dietary and physical activity patterns of 8- to 10-year-old urban schoolchildren in Manila, Philippines. Food Nutr Bull. 2002;23:267–273.

158. Cotton PA, Subar AF, Friday JE, Cook A. Dietary sources of nutrients among US adults, 1994 to 1996. J Am Diet Assoc. 2004;104:921–930.

159. Egeland GM, Berti P, Soueida R, Arbour LT, Receveur O, Kuhnlein HV. Age differences in vitamin A intake among Canadian Inuit. Can J Public Health. 2004;95:465–469.

160. Herrero C, Granado F, Blanco I, Olmedilla B. Vitamin A and E content in dairy products: their contribution to the recommended dietary allowances (RDA) for elderly people. J Nutr Health Aging. 2002;6:57–59.

161. Persson V, Hartini TN, Greiner T, Hakimi M, Stenlund H, Winkvist A. Vitamin A intake is low among pregnant women in central Java, Indonesia. Int J Vitam Nutr Res. 2002;72:124–132.

162. Millen AE, Dodd KW, Subar AF. Use of vitamin, mineral, nonvitamin, and nonmineral supplements in the United States: The 1987, 1992, and 2000 National Health Interview Survey results. J Am Diet Assoc. 2004;104:942–950.

163. Kiely M, Flynn A, Harrington KE, et al. The efficacy and safety of nutritional supplement use in a representative sample of adults in the North/South Ireland Food Consumption Survey. Public Health Nutr. 2001;4:1089–1097.

164. Pobocik RS, Richer JJ. Estimated intake and food sources of vitamin A, folate, vitamin C, vitamin E, calcium, iron, and zinc for Guamanian children aged 9 to 12. Pac Health Dialog. 2002;9:193–202.

165. Mrdjenovic G, Levitsky DA. Nutritional and energetic consequences of sweetened drink consumption in 6- to 13-year-old children. J Pediatr. 2003;142: 604–610.

166. Onyango AW, Receveur O, Esrey SA. The contribution of breast milk to toddler diets in western Kenya. Bull World Health Organ. 2002;80: 292–299.

167. Eichenberger Gilmore JM, Hong L, Broffitt B, Levy SM. Longitudinal patterns of vitamin and mineral supplement use in young white children. J Am Diet Assoc. 2005;105:763–772.

168. Dyer AR, Elliott P, Stamler J, Chan Q, Ueshima H, Zhou BF; INTERMAP Research Group. Dietary intake in male and female smokers, ex-smokers, and never smokers: the INTERMAP study. J Hum Hypertens. 2003;17:641–654.

169. Bowman SA, Spence JT. A comparison of low-carbohydrate vs. high-carbohydrate diets: energy restriction, nutrient quality and correlation to body mass index. J Am Coll Nutr. 2002;21:268–274.

170. Kuhnlein HV, Receveur O, Soueida R, Egeland GM. Arctic indigenous peoples experience the nutrition transition with changing dietary patterns and obesity. J Nutr. 2004;134:1447–1453.

171. Lytle LA, Himes JH, Feldman H, et al. Nutrient intake over time in a multi-ethnic sample of youth. Public Health Nutr. 2002;5:319–328.

172. Lytle LA, Himes JH, Feldman Het. Nutrient intake over time in a multi-ethnic sample of youth. Public Health Nutr. 2002;5:319–328.

173. Ganji V, Hampl JS, Betts NM. Race-, gender- and age-specific differences in dietary micronutrient intakes of US children. Int J Food Sci Nutr. 2003;54: 485–490.

174. Serra-Majem L, Ribas L, Garcia A, Perez-Rodrigo C, Aranceta J. Nutrient adequacy and Mediterranean Diet in Spanish school children and adolescents. Eur J Clin Nutr. 2003;57(Suppl 1):S35–S39.

175. Tang G, Qin J, Hao LY, Yin SA, Russell RM. Use of a short-term isotope-dilution method for determining the vitamin A status of children. Am J Clin Nutr. 2002;76:413–418.

176. Ribaya-Mercado JD, Solomons NW, Medrano Y, et al. Use of the deuterated-retinol-dilution technique to monitor the vitamin A status of Nicaraguan schoolchildren 1 y after initiation of the Nicaraguan national program of sugar fortification with vitamin A. Am J Clin Nutr. 2004;80:1291–1298.

177. Ribaya-Mercado JD, Solon FS, Dallal GE, et al. Quantitative assessment of total body stores of vitamin A in adults with the use of a 3-d deuterated-retinol-dilution procedure. Am J Clin Nutr. 2003; 77:694–699.

178. Ribaya-Mercado JD, Solon FS, Fermin LS, et al. Dietary vitamin A intakes of Filipino elders with

adequate or low liver vitamin A concentrations as assessed by the deuterated-retinol-dilution method: implications for dietary requirements. Am J Clin Nutr. 2004;79:633–641.

179. Omidvar N, Ghazi-Tabatabie M, Harrison GG, Eghtesadi S, Mahboob SA, Pourbakht M. Development and validation of a short food-frequency questionnaire for screening women of childbearing age for vitamin A status in northwestern Iran. Food Nutr Bull. 2002;23:73–82.
180. Rose D, Meershoek S, Ismael C, McEwan M. Evaluation of a rapid field tool for assessing household diet quality in Mozambique. Food Nutr Bull. 2002;23:181–189.
181. de Pee S, Dary O. Biochemical indicators of vitamin A deficiency: serum retinol and serum retinol binding protein. J Nutr. 2002;132(9 Suppl):2895S–2901S.
182. Baeten JM, Richardson BA, Bankson DD, et al. Use of serum retinol-binding protein for prediction of vitamin A deficiency: effects of HIV-1 infection, protein malnutrition, and the acute phase response. Am J Clin Nutr. 2004;79:218–225.
183. Thurnham DI, McCabe GP, Northrop-Clewes CA, Nestel P. Effects of subclinical infection on plasma retinol concentrations and assessment of prevalence of vitamin A deficiency: meta-analysis. Lancet. 2003;362:2052–2058.
184. Wieringa FT, Dijkhuizen MA, West CE, Northrop-Clewes CA, Muhilal. Estimation of the effect of the acute phase response on indicators of micronutrient status in Indonesian infants. J Nutr. 2002; 132:3061–3061.
185. Donnen P, Dramaix M, Brasseur D, Bitwe R, Bisimwa G, Hennart P. The molar ratio of serum retinol-binding protein (RBP) to transthyretin (TTR) is not useful to assess vitamin A status during infection in hospitalised children. Eur J Clin Nutr. 2001; 55:1043–1047.
186. Verhoef H, West CE. Validity of the relative-dose-response test and the modified-relative-dose-response test as indicators of vitamin A stores in liver. Am J Clin Nutr. 2005;81:835–839.
187. Stephensen CB, Franchi LM, Hernandez H, et al. Assessment of vitamin A status with the relative-dose-response test in Peruvian children recovering from pneumonia. Am J Clin Nutr. 2002;76: 1351–1357.
188. Ferraz IS, Daneluzzi JC, Vannucchi H, et al. Detection of vitamin A deficiency in Brazilian preschool children using the serum 30-day dose-response test. Eur J Clin Nutr. 2004;58:1372–1377.
189. Courtright P, Fine D, Broadhead RL, Misoya L, Vagh M. Abnormal vitamin A cytology and mortality in infants aged 9 months and less with measles. Ann Trop Paediatr. 2002;22:239–243.
190. Ahmed L, Nazrul Islam S, Khan MN, Huque S, Ahsan M. Antioxidant micronutrient profile (vitamin E, C, A, copper, zinc, iron) of colostrum: association with maternal characteristics. J Trop Pediatr. 2004;50:357–358.
191. Dancheck B, Nussenblatt V, Ricks MO, et al. Breast milk retinol concentrations are not associated with systemic inflammation among breast-feeding women in Malawi. J Nutr. 2005;135:223–226.
192. Sobeck U, Fischer A, Biesalski HK. Determination of vitamin A palmitate in buccal mucosal cells: a pilot study. Eur J Med Res. 2002;7:287–289.
193. Wondmikun Y. Dark adaptation pattern of pregnant women as an indicator of functional disturbance at acceptable serum vitamin A levels. Eur J Clin Nutr. 2002;56:462–466.
194. Taren DL, Duncan B, Shrestha K, et al. The night vision threshold test is a better predictor of low serum vitamin A concentration than self-reported night blindness in pregnant urban Nepalese women. J Nutr. 2004;134:2573–2578.
195. Schweigert FJ, Steinhagen B, Raila J, Siemann A, Peet D, Buscher U. Concentrations of carotenoids, retinol and alpha-tocopherol in plasma and follicular fluid of women undergoing IVF. Hum Reprod. 2003;18:1259–1264.
196. Roos N, Islam MM, Thilsted SH. Small indigenous fish species in Bangladesh: contribution to vitamin A, calcium and iron intakes. J Nutr. 2003;133(11 Suppl 2):4021S–4026S.
197. Roos N, Leth T, Jakobsen J, Thilsted SH. High vitamin A content in some small indigenous fish species in Bangladesh: perspectives for food-based strategies to reduce vitamin A deficiency. Int J Food Sci Nutr. 2002;53:425–437.
198. Murphy SP, Gewa C, Liang LJ, Grillenberger M, Bwibo NO, Neumann CG. School snacks containing animal source foods improve dietary quality for children in rural Kenya. J Nutr. 2003;133(11 Suppl 2):3950S–3956S.
199. Faber M, Venter SL, Benade AJ. Increased vitamin A intake in children aged 2–5 years through targeted home-gardens in a rural South African community. Public Health Nutr. 2002;5:11–16.
200. Faber M, Phungula MA, Venter SL, Dhansay MA, Benade AJ. Home gardens focusing on the production of yellow and dark green leafy vegetables increase the serum retinol concentrations of 2–5-y-old children in South Africa. Am J Clin Nutr. 2002; 76:1048–1054.
201. Schipani S, van der Haar F, Sinawat S, Maleevong K. Dietary intake and nutritional status of young children in families practicing mixed home gardening in northeast Thailand. Food Nutr Bull. 2002; 23:175–180.
202. Englberger L, Darnton-Hill I, Coyne T, Fitzgerald MH, Marks GC. Carotenoid-rich bananas: a po-

tential food source for alleviating vitamin A deficiency. Food Nutr Bull. 2003;24:303–318.

203. Drammeh BS, Marquis GS, Funkhouser E, Bates C, Eto I, Stephensen CB. A randomized, 4-month mango and fat supplementation trial improved vitamin A status among young Gambian children. J Nutr. 2002;132:3693–3699.

204. Vuong LT, King JC. A method of preserving and testing the acceptibilolity of gac fruit oil, a good source of β-carotene and essential fatty acids. Food Nutr Bull. 2003;24:224–230.

205. Mariath JGR, Lima MCC, Santos LMP. Vitamin A activity of buriti (*Maurita vinifera* Mart) and its effectiveness in the treatment and prevention of xerophthalmia. Am J Clin Nutr. 1989;49:849–853.

206. Nagendran B, Unnithan UR, Choo YM, Sundram K. Characteristics of red palm oil, a carotene- and vitamin E-rich refined oil for food uses. Food Nutr Bull. 2000;21:189–194.

207. Radhika MS, Bhaskaram P, Balakrishna N, Ramalakshmi BA. Red palm oil supplementation: a feasible diet-based approach to improve the vitamin A status of pregnant women and their infants. Food Nutr Bull. 2003;24:208–217.

208. Sivan YS, Alwin Jayakumar Y, Arumughan C, et al. Impact of vitamin A supplementation through different dosages of red palm oil and retinol palmitate on preschool children. J Trop Pediatr. 2002;48: 24–28.

209. Zagre NM, Delpeuch F, Traissac P, Delisle H. Red palm oil as a source of vitamin A for mothers and children: impact of a pilot project in Burkina Faso. Public Health Nutr. 2003;6:733–742.

210. Benade AJ. A place for palm fruit oil to eliminate vitamin A deficiency. Asia Pac J Clin Nutr. 2003; 12:369–372.

211. Solomons NW, Orozco M. Alleviation of vitamin A deficiency with palm fruit and its products. Asia Pac J Clin Nutr. 2003;12:373–384.

212. Mora JO. Proposed vitamin A fortification levels. *J Nutr.* 2003;133:2990S–2993S.

213. Dary O, Mora JO; International Vitamin A Consultative Group. Food fortification to reduce vitamin A deficiency: International Vitamin A Consultative Group recommendations. J Nutr. 2002; 132(9 Suppl):2927S–2933S.

214. Kawuma M. Sugar as a potential vehicle for vitamin A fortification: experience from Kamuli district in Uganda. Afr Health Sci. 2002;2:11–15.

215. Candelaria LV, Magsadia CR, Velasco RE, Pedro MR, Barba CV, Tanchoco CC. The effect of vitamin A-fortified coconut cooking oil on the serum retinol concentration of Filipino children 4–7 years old. Asia Pac J Clin Nutr. 2005;14:43–53.

216. Zimmermann MB, Wegmueller R, Zeder C, et al. Triple fortification of salt with microcapsules of iodine, iron, and vitamin A. Am J Clin Nutr. 2004; 80:1283–1290.

217. Haskell MJ, Pandey P, Graham JM, Peerson JM, Shrestha RK, Brown KH. Recovery from impaired dark adaptation in nightblind pregnant Nepali women who receive small daily doses of vitamin A as amaranth leaves, carrots, goat liver, vitamin A-fortified rice, or retinyl palmitate. Am J Clin Nutr. 2005;81:461–471.

218. Oelofse A, Van Raaij JM, Benade AJ, Dhansay MA, Tolboom JJ, Hautvast JG. The effect of a micronutrient-fortified complementary food on micronutrient status, growth and development of 6- to 12-month-old disadvantaged urban South African infants. Int J Food Sci Nutr. 2003;54:399–407.

219. Genc Y, Humphries JM, Lyons GH, Graham RD. Exploiting genotypic variation in plant nutrient accumulation to alleviate micronutrient deficiency in populations. J Trace Elem Med Biol. 2005;8: 319–324.

220. Welch RM, Graham RD. Breeding for micronutrients in staple food crops from a human nutrition perspective. J Exp Bot. 2004;55:353–364.

221. Surles RL, Weng N, Simon PW, Tanumihardjo SA. Carotenoid profiles and consumer sensory evaluation of specialty carrots (*Daucus carota* L.) of various colors. J Agric Food Chem. 2004;52: 3417–3421.

222. Beyer P, Al-Babili S, Ye X, et al. Golden Rice: introducing the beta-carotene biosynthesis pathway into rice endosperm by genetic engineering to defeat vitamin A deficiency. J Nutr. 2002;132:506S–510S.

223. Potrykus I. Nutritionally enhanced rice to combat malnutrition disorders of the poor. Nutr Rev. 2003; 61:S101–S104.

224. Sommer A, Davidson FR; Annecy Accords. Assessment and control of vitamin A deficiency: the Annecy Accords. J Nutr. 2002;132(9 Suppl):2845S–2850S.

225. Sommer A (rapporteur). Innocenti micronutrient report #1. Sight & Life Newsletter. 2005(3):13–18.

226. Kapil U. Deaths in Assam during vitamin A pulse distribution: the needle of suspicion is on the new measuring cup. Indian Pediatr. 2002;39:114–115.

227. Aguayo VM, Baker SK, Crespin X, Hamani H, MamadoulTaibou A. Maintaining high vitamin A supplementation coverage in children: lessons from Niger. Food Nutr Bull. 2005;26:26–31.

228. Victora CG, Fenn B, Bryce J, Kirkwood BR. Co-coverage of preventive interventions and implications for child-survival strategies: evidence from national surveys. Lancet. 2005;366:1460–1466.

229. Pangaribuan R, Scherbaum V, Erhardt JG, Sastroamidjojo S, Biesalski HK. Socioeconomic and familial characteristics influence caretakers' adherence to the periodic vitamin A capsule supplementation program in Central Java, Indonesia. J Trop Pediatr. 2004;50:143–148.

230. Choi Y, Bishai D, Hill K. Socioeconomic differentials in supplementation of vitamin A: evidence from the Philippines. J Health Popul Nutr. 2005 Jun;23:156–164.
231. Perry RT, Halsey NA. The clinical significance of measles: a review. J Infect Dis. 2004;189 Suppl 1: S4–S16.
232. D'Souza RM, D'Souza R. Vitamin A for treating measles in children. Cochrane Database Syst Rev. 2002;(1):CD001479.
233. Ashworth A, Chopra M, McCoy D, et al. WHO guidelines for management of severe malnutrition in rural South African hospitals: effect on case fatality and the influence of operational factors. Lancet. 2004;363:1110–1115.
234. Bhandari N, Bahl R, Sazawal S, Bhan MK. Breastfeeding status alters the effect of vitamin A treatment during acute diarrhea in children. J Nutr. 1997;127:59–63.
235. Biswas R, Biswas AB, Manna B, Bhattacharya SK, Dey R, Sarkar S. Effect of vitamin A supplementation on diarrhoea and acute respiratory tract infection in children. A double blind placebo controlled trial in a Calcutta slum community. Eur J Epidemiol. 1994;10:57–61.
236. Andreozzi VL, Bailey TC, Nobre FF, et al. Random-Effects Models in Investigating the Effect of Vitamin A in Childhood Diarrhea. Ann Epidemiol. 2005 [Epub ahead of print]
237. Shankar AH, Genton B, Semba RD, e tal. Effect of vitamin A supplementation on morbidity due to Plasmodium falciparum in young children in Papua New Guinea: a randomised trial. Lancet. 1999;354: 203–209.
238. Serghides L, Kain KC. Mechanism of protection induced by vitamin A in falciparum malaria. Lancet. 2002;359:1404–1406.
239. Cusick SE, Tielsch JM, Ramsan M, et al. Short-term effects of vitamin A and antimalarial treatment on erythropoiesis in severely anemic Zanzibari preschool children. Am J Clin Nutr. 2005;82:406–412.
240. Karyadi E, West CE, Schultink W, et al. A double-blind, placebo-controlled study of vitamin A and zinc supplementation in persons with tuberculosis in Indonesia: effects on clinical response and nutritional status. Am J Clin Nutr. 2002;75:720–727.
241. Baeten JM, McClelland RS, Corey L, et al. Vitamin A supplementation and genital shedding of herpes simplex virus among HIV-1-infected women: a randomized clinical trial. J Infect Dis. 2004 Apr; 189:1466–1471.
242. Ehrenpreis ED, Jani A, Levitsky J, Ahn J, Hong J. A prospective, randomized, double-blind, placebo-controlled trial of retinol palmitate (vitamin A) for symptomatic chronic radiation proctopathy. Dis Colon Rectum. 2005;48:1–8.
243. Thompson DA, Gal A. Vitamin A metabolism in the retinal pigment epithelium: genes, mutations, and diseases. Prog Retin Eye Res. 2003;22: 683–703.
244. Mactier H, Weaver LT. Vitamin A and preterm infants: what we know, what we don't know, and what we need to know. Arch Dis Child Fetal Neonatal Ed. 2005;90:F103–F108.
245. Spears K, Cheney C, Zerzan J. Low plasma retinol concentrations increase the risk of developing bronchopulmonary dysplasia and long-term respiratory disability in very-low-birth-weight infants. Am J Clin Nutr. 2004;80:1589–1594.
246. Tyson JE, Wright LL, Oh W, et al. Vitamin A supplementation for extremely-low-birth-weight infants. National Institute of Child Health and Human Development Neonatal Research Network. N Engl J Med. 1999;340:1962–1968.
247. Ambalavanan N, Wu TJ, Tyson JE, Kennedy KA, Roane C, Carlo WA. A comparison of three vitamin A dosing regimens in extremely-low-birth-weight infants. J Pediatr. 2003;142:656–661.
248. Delvin EE, Salle BL, Claris O, et al. Oral vitamin A, E and D supplementation of pre-term newborns either breast-fed or formula-fed: a 3-month longitudinal study. J Pediatr Gastroenterol Nutr. 2005; 40:43–47.
249. Ravishankar C, Nafday S, Green RS, et al. A trial of vitamin A therapy to facilitate ductal closure in premature infants. J Pediatr. 2003;143:644–648.
250. Ambalavanan N, Tyson JE, Kennedy KA, et al; National Institute of Child Health and Human Development Neonatal Research Network. Vitamin A supplementation for extremely low birth weight infants: outcome at 18 to 22 months. Pediatrics. 2005; 115:e249–e254.
251. Chivot M. Retinoid therapy for acne. A comparative review. Am J Clin Dermatol. 2005;6:13–19.
252. Johanning GL, Piyathilake CJ. Retinoids and epigenetic silencing in cancer. Nutr Rev. 2003;61: 284–289.
253. Ruffin MT, Bailey JM, Normolle DP, et al. Low-dose topical delivery of all-trans retinoic acid for cervical intraepithelial neoplasia II and III. Cancer Epidemiol Biomarkers Prev. 2004;13:2148–2152.
254. Hamamoto S, Fukuda R, Ishimura N, et al. 9-cis retinoic acid enhances the antiviral effect of interferon on hepatitis C virus replication through increased expression of type I interferon receptor. J Lab Clin Med. 2003;141:58–66.
255. EU Commission, Scientific Committee on Food, Task-Force on Upper Levels for Vitamins and Minerals. Draft opinion of the Scientific Committee on Food on the Tolerable Upper Intake Level of preformed vitamin A (retinol and retinyl esters). Brussels; September 2002.
256. Perrotta S, Nobili B, Rossi F, et al. Infant hypervitaminosis A causes severe anemia and thrombocyto-

penia: evidence of a retinol-dependent bone marrow cell growth inhibition. Blood. 2002;99:2017–2022.

257. Bhalla K, Ennis DM, Ennis ED. Hypercalcemia caused by iatrogenic hypervitaminosis A. J Am Diet Assoc. 2005;105:119–121.
258. Myhre AM, Carlsen MH, Bohn SK, Wold HL, Laake P, Blomhoff R. Water-miscible, emulsified, and solid forms of retinol supplements are more toxic than oil-based preparations. Am J Clin Nutr. 2003;78:1152–1159.
259. Alberts D, Ranger-Moore J, Einspahr J, et al. Safety and efficacy of dose-intensive oral vitamin A in subjects with sun-damaged skin. Clin Cancer Res. 2004;10:1875–1880.
260. Sedjo RL, Ranger-Moore J, Foote J, et al. Circulating endogenous retinoic acid concentrations among participants enrolled in a randomized placebo-controlled clinical trial of retinyl palmitate. Cancer Epidemiol Biomarkers Prev. 2004;13:1687–1692.
261. Allen LH, Haskell M. Estimating the potential for vitamin A toxicity in women and young children. J Nutr. 2002;132(9 Suppl):2907S–2919S.
262. Larson RS, Tallman MS. Retinoic acid syndrome: manifestations, pathogenesis, and treatment. Best Pract Res Clin Haematol. 2003;16:453–461.
263. Friedman DI. Medication-induced intracranial hypertension in dermatology. Am J Clin Dermatol. 2005;6:29–37.
264. Miller RK, Hendrickx AG, Mills JL, Hummler H, Wiegand UW. Periconceptional vitamin A use: how much is teratogenic? Reprod Toxicol. 1998;8: 75–88.
265. Loureiro KD, Kao KK, Jones KL, et al. Minor malformations characteristic of the retinoic acid embryopathy and other birth outcomes in children of women exposed to topical tretinoin during early pregnancy. Am J Med Genet. 2005;136:117–121.
266. Genaro Pde S, Martini LA. Vitamin A supplementation and risk of skeletal fracture. Nutr Rev. 2004; 62:65–67.
267. Kawahara TN, Krueger DC, Engelke JA, Harke JM, Binkley NC. Short-term vitamin A supplementation does not affect bone turnover in men. J Nutr. 2002;132:1169–1172.
268. Melhus H, Michaelsson K, Kindmark A, et al. Excessive dietary intake of vitamin A is associated with reduced bone mineral density and increased risk for hip fracture. Ann Intern Med. 1999;131:392.
269. Michaelsson K, Lithell H, Vessby B, Melhus H. Serum retinol levels and the risk of fracture. N Engl J Med. 2003;348:287–294.
270. Opotowsky AR, Bilezikian JP; NHANES I follow-up study. Serum vitamin A concentration and the risk of hip fracture among women 50 to 74 years old in the United States: a prospective analysis of the NHANES I follow-up study. Am J Med. 2004; 117:169–174.
271. Feskanich D, Singh V, Willett WC, Colditz GA. Vitamin A intake and hip fractures among postmenopausal women. JAMA. 2002;287:47–54.
272. Lim LS, Harnack LJ, Lazovich D, Folsom AR. Vitamin A intake and the risk of hip fracture in postmenopausal women: the Iowa Women's Health Study. Osteoporos Int. 2004;15:552–559.
273. Promislow JH, Goodman-Gruen D, Slymen DJ, Barrett-Connor E. Retinol intake and bone mineral density in the elderly: the Rancho Bernardo Study. J Bone Miner Res. 2002;17:1349–1358.
274. Rejnmark L, Vestergaard P, Charles P, et al. No effect of vitamin A intake on bone mineral density and fracture risk in perimenopausal women. Osteoporos Int. 2004;15:872–880.
275. Barker ME, McCloskey E, Saha S, et al. Serum retinoids and beta-carotene as predictors of hip and other fractures in elderly women. J Bone Miner Res. 2005;20:913–920.
276. Wolf RL, Cauley JA, Pettinger M, et al. Lack of a relation between vitamin and mineral antioxidants and bone mineral density: results from the Women's Health Initiative. Am J Clin Nutr. 2005;82: 581–588.
277. Barker ME, Blumsohn A. Is vitamin A consumption a risk factor for osteoporotic fracture? Proc Nutr Soc. 2003;62:845–850.
278. Crandall C. Vitamin A intake and osteoporosis: a clinical review. J Womens Health (Larchmt). 2004; 13:939–953.
279. Alissa EM, Bahjri SM, Al-Ama N, Ahmed WH, Starkey B, Ferns GA. Dietary vitamin A may be a cardiovascular risk factor in a Saudi population. Asia Pac J Clin Nutr. 2005;14:137–144.
280. Sesso HD, Buring JE, Norkus EP, Gaziano JM. Plasma lycopene, other carotenoids, and retinol and the risk of cardiovascular disease in men. Am J Clin Nutr. 2005;81:990–997.
281. Zimmermann MB, Wegmuller R, Zeder C, Chaouki N, Torresani T. The effects of vitamin A deficiency and vitamin A supplementation on thyroid function in goitrous children. J Clin Endocrinol Metab. 2004;89:5441–5447.

# 13 Carotenoids

Brian L. Lindshield and John W. Erdman, Jr

## Introduction

Carotenoids are nonpolar, 40-carbon poly-isoprenoid compounds found throughout nature.[1] Of the approximately 600 known carotenoids, only 40 are typically ingested by humans and, of these, only 20 are commonly found in human tissues.[2] The six main carotenoids found in the diet, blood, and tissues are: β-carotene, α-carotene, β-cryptoxanthin, lutein, zeaxanthin, and lycopene. The latter carotenoid, lycopene, is the predominant carotenoid found in the diet and blood in the United States[3] (Table 1 and Figure 1). Carotenoids are classified in two ways: the first is based on whether the carotenoid is capable of being converted to vitamin A (provitamin A activity); the second on structural differences and polarity. Oxygenated carotenoids are known as xanthophylls, while hydrocarbon carotenoids are carotenes.

Carotenoid structures contain multiple conjugated double bonds that have the ability to efficiently scavenge free radicals (and thus serve as antioxidants) and to absorb light in the visible region. This absorption causes them to reflect their respective colors. Differences in the number of double bonds results in carotenoids ranging from colorless (due to an insufficient number of conjugated double bonds) to bright red[1] (Figure 1 and Table 1). This unsaturated structure also causes carotenoids to be labile to oxygen, light, and heat.

In plants, carotenoids are part of the light-harvesting complex that captures light for photosynthesis. Carotenoids are also found in bacteria, yeasts, molds, bird feathers, and crustaceans; however, mammals do not synthesize carotenoids and must obtain them from their diet. The carotenoids astaxanthin, lutein, and zeaxanthin are commonly used as animal feed supplements. Astaxanthin is responsible for the pink color of salmon, while lutein and zeaxanthin are used in poultry to increase the yellow pigmentation of egg yolks (Table 1 and Figure 1).

In this chapter, the factors that influence carotenoid bioavailability (how much carotenoid is actually absorbed) and bioconversion (how much carotenoid is converted to vitamin A) will be initially addressed, followed by a discussion of the enzymatic conversion of provitamin A carotenoids. The transport and accumulation of carotenoids, factors affecting circulating serum levels, deficiency, and toxicity will next be reviewed. The potential effects of carotenoids on the following health conditions will also be examined: lung cancer, prostate cancer, cardiovascular disease, macular degeneration and cataract formation, skin protection, coloration, and photosensitivity. Finally, future directions of carotenoid research will be discussed.

## Bioavailability and Bioconversion

A number of factors influence the absorption of carotenoids and the concomitant conversion of provitamin A carotenoids to vitamin A. To help remember these factors, the mnemonic "SLAMENGHI" (for "Species, Linkage, Amount, Matrix, Effectors, Nutrient status, Genetic factors, Host-related factors, and Interactions") was coined by Clive West and his colleagues.[6] The description under each factor first describes its effect on the absorption of carotenoids (bioavailability), followed by the role each factor plays in the conversion of provitamin A carotenoids to vitamin A (bioconversion).

### *Species*

**Bioavailability.** Among the types of carotenoids, xanthophylls are generally more readily absorbed than are carotenes. This is believed to be because the more hydrophilic nature of xanthophylls that allows them to be incorporated into the outer portion of lipid micelles in the gastrointestinal tract.[7] Carotenoids are normally found in nature in the all-*trans* form; however, they are easily isomerized to form *cis* isomers following exposure to heat and/or light. The relative absorption of *cis* isomers apparently differs between carotenoids. For example, absorption is decreased for β-carotene *cis* isomers, while uptake

**Table 1.** Color, Xanthophyll/Carotene Classification, Retinol Conversion Factors, US Mean Serum and Intake, and Good Food Sources of Selected Carotenoids

| | | | | | US Mean Serum Levels* | | US Mean Intake from Foods* | | |
|---|---|---|---|---|---|---|---|---|---|
| | | | | | M | F | M | F | |
| **Carotenoid** | **Color** | **Xanthophyll or Carotene** | **RE** | **RAE** | *μg/dL* | | *mg/d* | | **Good Food Sources**[3] |
| Lycopene | Red | Carotene | – | – | 26.4 | 23.9 | 11.27 | 6.71 | Tomatoes, watermelon, guava, pink grapefruit |
| β-Carotene | Yellow-orange | Carotene | 6 | 12 | 14.6 | 18.4 | 2.22 | 1.87 | Carrots, sweet potatoes, pumpkin, spinach, apricots |
| α-Carotene | Light yellow | Carotene | 12 | 24 | 3.8 | 4.4 | 0.44 | 0.36 | Carrots, pumpkin |
| β-Cryptoxanthin | Orange | Xanthophyll | 12 | 24 | 8.6 | 8.1 | 0.13 | 0.10 | Sweet red peppers, tangerines, papaya, persimmons |
| Lutein | Yellow | Xanthophyll | – | – | 20.1† | 18.2† | 2.11† | 1.86† | Kale, spinach, corn, collard greens, broccoli, eggs |
| Zeaxanthin | Yellow | Xanthophyll | – | – | | | | | |
| Canthaxanthin | Red-orange | Xanthophyll | – | – | – | – | – | – | Not consumed in significant quantities |
| Astaxanthin | Red | Xanthophyll | – | – | – | – | – | – | Not consumed in significant quantities |

F, female; M, male; RAE, retinol activity equivalent; RE, retinol equivalent.
* US mean serum levels and food intakes were calculated using the values for the 19–30 and 30–51 age groups.[4,5]
† Serum levels, intake, and food sources are presented together as the sum of lutein and zeaxanthin.

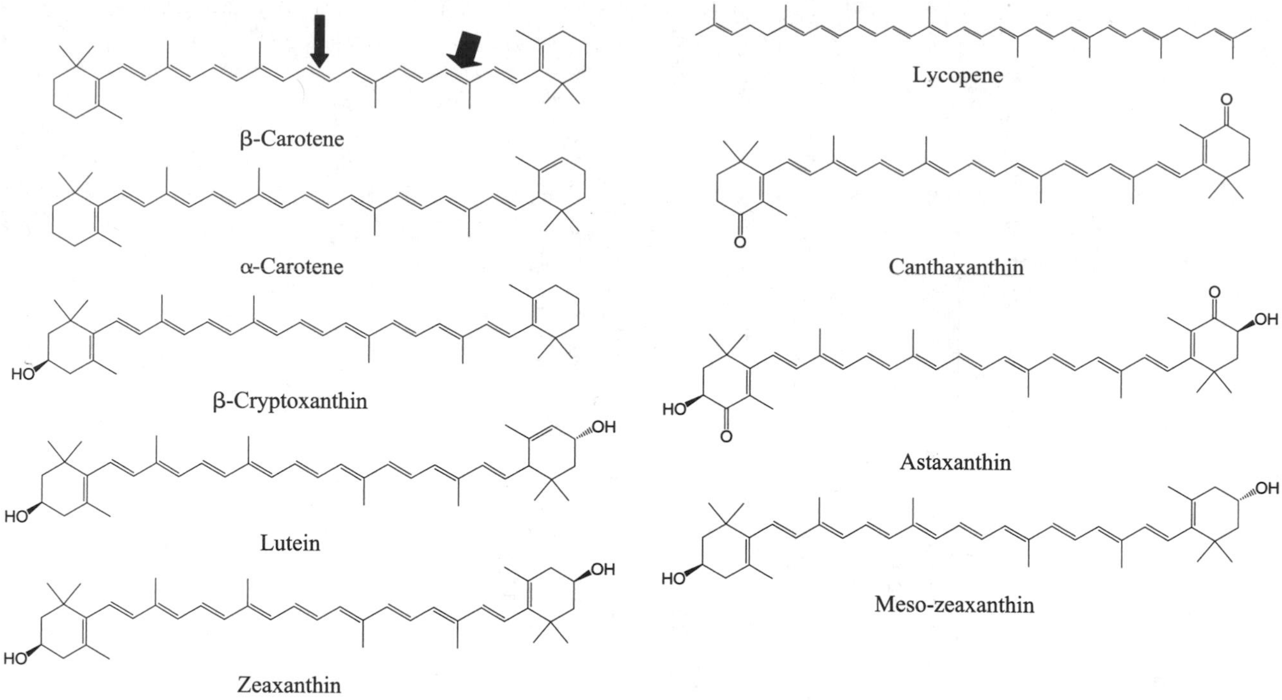

Figure 1. All-*trans* structures of common carotenoids. Narrow arrow on β-carotene indicates 15,15′ Carotenoid monooxygenase (CMO) I central cleavage; wide arrow on β-carotene indicates 9′,10′ CMO II eccentric cleavage site.

is increased for lycopene *cis* isomers compared with their respective all-*trans* forms.[6]

**Bioconversion.** The structure of carotenoids dictates the number of retinal molecules that can be formed from central cleavage. Among the provitamin A carotenoids, all-*trans*-β-carotene is the most efficient at producing vitamin A. This is because all-trans-β-carotene is the only carotenoid that can be cleaved to form two retinal molecules. However, *cis* isomerization decreases the conversion to retinal such that β-carotene *cis* isomers are defined as having half the vitamin A activity of all-*trans*-β-carotene.[8]

## Molecular Linkage

**Bioavailability.** In many fruits and vegetables, the hydroxyl groups of xanthophylls are esterified to fatty acids, increasing their stability but possibly hindering their absorption. Before esterified xanthophylls can be absorbed, the fatty acids must be cleaved to form free xanthophylls in the gastrointestinal tract. Xanthophyll ester hydrolysis appears to be an efficient process. For example, the absorption of lutein and β-cryptoxanthin esters is similar to the free carotenoid forms, while the uptake of zeaxanthin esters may actually be greater than that of free forms of this carotenoid.[9-11]

**Bioconversion.** Most provitamin A carotenoids are not esterified, but the hydroxyl, non-retinal-forming end of β-cryptoxanthin is found esterified in fruits and vegetables. However, most esters are cleaved prior to absorption, so they are unlikely to have an effect on the conversion to vitamin A.[12]

## Amount of Carotenoid Consumed

**Bioavailability.** The quantity of carotenoids consumed also plays a role in their uptake. As with many nutrients, absorption decreases with increasing dietary levels of carotenoids.[6]

**Bioconversion.** Similar to absorption, a large flux of carotenoids also decreases the efficiency of vitamin A conversion. It is important to note that vitamin A toxicity has not been reported, even with supplementation of extremely high levels (180 mg/d) of β-carotene.[5]

## Matrix

**Bioavailability.** What context, or matrix, that carotenoids are provided in appears to be the greatest factor affecting their bioavailability. For example, orange fruits such as papaya, mango, squash, and pumpkin yield twice as much vitamin A activity and four-fold higher serum β-carotene levels than do green leafy vegetables and carrots.[13] The difference between these fruits and vegetables is that in these fruits the carotenoids are found dissolved in oil droplets, whereas in vegetables they are sequestered as crystals, bound in chloroplasts, or associated with macromolecules such as fiber or protein. It is difficult for crystalline or bound carotenoids to become solubilized in micelles in the gastrointestinal tract, thus hindering their absorption. Mild heating and food processing increase the bioavailability of carotenoids by disrupting plant cell walls, binding proteins, and organelles, thus freeing carotenoids for uptake. In addition, because there is no matrix inhibiting their release, carotenoids provided in oil (e.g., red palm oil), or commercially available water-soluble beadlets, have superior bioavailability compared with fruits or vegetables.[13]

**Bioconversion.** There is no evidence that food matrix influences the conversion of carotenoids to vitamin A.

### *Effectors of Absorption*

**Bioavailability.** There are many effectors of carotenoid absorption. Fat intake increases carotenoid uptake by facilitating the formation of mixed micelles, which are important for lipid-soluble carotenoids to cross the unstirred water layer for uptake by the enterocyte. A modest amount of fat consumed in the same meal as carotenoids (e.g., salad dressing on salad) will enhance carotenoid absorption. Fiber, olestra, plant sterol, and stanol esters are dietary compounds that decrease the absorption of cholesterol and lipids. Thus, it is not surprising that these compounds also decrease uptake of carotenoids.[7] When provided at high levels, the consumption of one carotenoid can decrease the absorption of another. This most likely occurs because carotenoids share similar uptake and transport pathways.[7] In contrast, co-supplementation of other antioxidants actually may increase the bioavailability of carotenoids. Antioxidants such as vitamins C and E may increase the stability of the carotenoids in the gastrointestinal tract and thereby facilitate their absorption.[14]

**Bioconversion.** Some of the effectors of absorption may also have a similar effect on the conversion of carotenoids to vitamin A. For example, it appears that fat facilitates, while dietary fiber hinders, the conversion of provitamin A carotenoids to vitamin A.[8]

### *Nutrient Status of Host*

**Bioavailability.** Higher vitamin A status is believed to decrease the uptake of carotenoids.[6]

**Bioconversion.** The nutrient status of the host is important in the conversion of provitamin A carotenoids. Low vitamin A status increases the conversion to vitamin A to help meet the body's needs. In addition, protein deficiency decreases the level of the carotenoid central cleavage enzyme in rats.[8,12] Furthermore, because the central cleavage enzyme requires ferrous iron as a cofactor, iron status also is likely important to its activity.[15]

### *Genetic Factors*

**Bioavailability and Bioconversion.** As demonstrated in numerous clinical trials, there is large variability across the population in the relative absorption of carotenoids. The term "carotenoid non-responder" has been used to describe subjects who do not show an increase in plasma β-carotene following supplementation. It was previously believed that this phenotype was extremely inefficient in absorbing carotenoids. However, it may be that these subjects are actually more efficient converters of β-carotene to vitamin A, thereby giving the impression that they were not absorbing carotenoids. There are also individuals who poorly convert β-carotene to vitamin A, which is believed to be due to a polymorphism in the central cleavage enzyme. However, this polymorphism has not yet been extensively characterized.[12]

### *Host-Related Factors*

**Bioavailability.** Common conditions associated with aging that alter gastrointestinal function (e.g., atrophic gastritis) also alter carotenoid absorption. This condition of insufficient gastric acid secretion leads to decreased stomach acidity, which consequently decreases carotenoid uptake by disturbing the formation and absorption of mixed micelles.[7] Parasitic infections, which are prevalent in vitamin A-deficient populations, can also have a dramatic negative effect on carotenoid absorption.[12]

**Bioconversion.** Similar to food matrix, the identified host-related factors seem to mostly affect the absorption of carotenoids.

### *Mathematical Interactions*

**Bioavailability and Bioconversion.** Mathematical interactions between combinations of the above factors involved in carotenoid absorption and conversion have not been established.[6,12]

## Carotenoid Retinol Equivalents and Retinol Activity Equivalents

In 1989, the Food and Nutrition Board of the National Academies of Science established the conversion value of 2 μg of purified all-*trans*-β-carotene from supplements to be one retinol equivalent (RE = 1 μg all-*trans* retinol). Because of decreased bioavailability, 3 μg of dietary all-*trans*-β-carotene from food was thought to be equivalent to 1 μg of purified all-*trans*-β-carotene in oil. Thus, 6 μg of dietary all-*trans*-β-carotene was equivalent to 1 RE. Other dietary provitamin A carotenoids (mainly α-carotene and β-cryptoxanthin) were considered to have half the vitamin A activity of dietary all-*trans*-β-carotene and were set at 12 μg = 1 RE (Table 1). However, in 2001 the Food and Nutrition Board revised these conversion values based on human trials revealing the bioavailability of all-*trans*-β-carotene from foods was half of what was originally believed. To help alleviate the confusion in making the changes, a new term was coined: "retinol activity equivalent" (RAE = 1 μg all-*trans*-retinol). The RAE ratios of conversion for purified all-*trans*-β-carotene in oil, dietary all-*trans*-β-carotene, and other dietary provitamin A carotenoids were set at 2:1, 12:1, and 24:1, respectively[4] (Table 1).

## Carotenoid-Modifying Enzymes

The small intestine and selected other tissues contain high levels of the two main carotenoid-cleavage enzymes, carotenoid monooxygenase (CMO) I and II. Both of these enzymes are capable of cleaving provitamin A carotenoids to form different retinoids. CMO I primarily catalyzes the central cleavage of the 15,15′ β-carotene bond to form two retinal molecules (Figure 1). CMO II is reported to catalyze the eccentric cleavage of the 9′,10′ β-carotene bond, which subsequently can be shortened to one retinoic acid molecule by a mechanism similar to β-oxidation of fatty acids (Figure 1). Apparently, non-provitamin A carotenoids are not efficiently cleaved by CMO I; in contrast, CMO II appears to cleave both provitamin A and non-provitamin A carotenoids. For instance, purified CMO II has a high affinity for lycopene.[15] At this time, little is known about the in vivo function, catalytic mechanism (is it a monooxygenase-like CMO I?), or significance of CMO II or another potential carotenoid-modifying enzyme, RPE65. RPE65 was actually the first in the family to be cloned. This enzyme was named RPE65 because it was found in high levels in the retinol pigment epithelium of the eye and its molecular mass is 65 kD. Interestingly, inherited mutations in this gene lead to blindness in humans.[15]

Table 2 shows the relative tissue levels of CMO I in mice and humans and CMO II expression in mice. The expression varies between tissues, and the two different CMO isoforms are not always expressed in the same tissue. The significance of this differential tissue expression is under investigation.

# Transport and Accumulation

In the lumen of the small intestine, carotenoids are first incorporated into mixed micelles, which facilitate their absorption through an unresolved mechanism(s). Absorption may occur passively, or there may be carotenoid-binding proteins or transporters that facilitate their uptake.[21] In vitro evidence for the involvement of transporters has been found using a cholesterol transport inhibitor, which decreases the uptake of carotenoids.[22] Following absorption, carotenoids are incorporated into chylomicrons and, to a smaller extent, very-low-density lipoproteins (VLDL) of intestinal origin.[21] After incorporation, these lipoproteins are released into the lymph before entering general circulation. Carotenoids may be partially taken up by peripheral tissues before chylomicron remnants are taken up by the liver.[1,23] In the liver, carotenoids are repackaged into VLDL and secreted back into the blood.

Carotenoids are not equally distributed among lipoproteins; the hydrophobic carotenes are found predominately in low-density lipoproteins (LDL), while the more hydrophilic xanthophylls tend to be found in higher amounts in high-density lipoproteins (HDL).[21] The up-

**Table 2.** Relative Tissue Carotenoid Monooxygenase (CMO) Expression in Mice (CMO I and II mRNA Levels) and Humans (CMO I mRNA and Protein Levels)

| | Mouse mRNA | | Human CMO I | |
|---|---|---|---|---|
| **Tissue** | **CMO I[16,17]** | **CMO II[16]** | **mRNA[18,19]** | **Protein[20]** |
| Colon | – | – | + | + + + |
| Liver | + + | + + + | + + | + + + |
| Lung | – | + | – | NM |
| Prostate | NM | NM | + + | + |
| Retina pigment epithelium | NM | NM | + + + | NM |
| Skin | NM | NM | NM | + + + |
| Adrenal | NM | NM | NM | + + |
| Brain | – | + + | NM | NM |
| Endometrium | NM | NM | NM | + + + |
| Heart | – | + | – | NM |
| Kidney | + + + | + + + | + + + | + + |
| Ovary | NM | NM | + + | + |
| Pancreas | + | NM | NM | + + + |
| Retina | + | NM | – | NM |
| Skeletal muscle | NM | NM | + | + |
| Small intestine | + + + | + + + | + + + | + + + |
| Spleen | – | + | – | NM |
| Stomach | – | – | + | + + + |
| Testis | + + | + + | + + | + + |
| Thymus | + | NM | NM | NM |

–, Not detected; +, low; + +, medium; + + +, high; NM, not measured.

**Table 3.** Carotenoid Concentrations in Selected Human Tissues[21,24]

| Tissue | Lycopene | β-Carotene | α-Carotene | β-Cryptoxanthin | Lutein | Zeaxanthin |
|---|---|---|---|---|---|---|
| | | | *ng/g tissue* | | | |
| Colon | 534 | 256 | 128 | 35 | 452 | 32 |
| Liver | 352 | 470 | 67 | 363 | 1701 | 591 |
| Lung | 300 | 226 | 47 | 121 | 212 | 90 |
| Prostate | 374 | 163 | 50 | – | 128 | 35 |
| Skin | 69 | 26 | 8 | – | 26 | 6 |
| Retina pigment epithelium* | 8.64 | 10.80 | 2.97 | – | 18.27 | 4.85 |

* Concentrations in approximately 0.2 g of pooled retina pigment epithelium/choroid (n = 20).

take of carotenoids also varies between tissues. Table 3 gives the concentrations of the six major carotenoids in selected human tissues. Quantitatively, carotenoids are the highest in the liver and adipose; however, carotenoid concentrations are the highest in the liver, adrenal, and reproductive tissues (such as the prostate). The reason for this differential accumulation is not known, but it has been hypothesized that this differential uptake is a result of either high levels of LDL receptors in these tissues or specific carotenoid-binding proteins that have not yet been identified.[1]

## Factors Affecting Circulating Levels

A number of factors also affect the levels of circulating carotenoids. One major factor is the body composition of the subject. A number of studies have reported an inverse association between body-mass index (BMI) and plasma carotenoid concentrations. Further study of this association suggests that carotenoid plasma concentrations are inversely related not only to fat mass, but also to lean body mass. This indicates that non-fat tissues such as muscle may also serve as a reservoir for carotenoids.[21] Accordingly, people with anorexia nervosa have very high levels of plasma carotenoids, most likely due to high levels of mobilization in this catabolic condition.[25]

In general, circulating carotenoid levels are correlated with serum triglyceride and cholesterol levels. There are reported increases in serum levels as people age, which could be related to the upward shift in the serum lipid profile of older adults. In females, the concentrations of different carotenoids peak at different points of the menstrual cycle. The reason or significance is not known, but in men there also appears to be an inverse relationship between androgens and lycopene.[32] Smoking is associated with lower carotenoid levels, presumably due to an increase in oxidative stress, and alcohol intake has been shown to be inversely related to β-carotene levels. However, both smoking and alcohol intake are also associated with reduced dietary intakes of carotenoids. It is not clear whether differences in diet primarily account for these decreased serum carotenoid levels or if metabolism is altered.[5]

## Toxicity and Deficiency

Unlike vitamin A, there is no known toxicity or deficiencies for carotenoids. Low levels of carotenoids may increase people's risk for developing certain chronic conditions, but no deficiencies in the classical sense have been described. High intakes of β-carotene and lycopene can lead to carotenodermia and lycopenodermia, respectively. Carotenodermia is a condition that results in a yellowing of the skin due to accumulation of high levels of β-carotene. This disorder has been reported in subjects consuming large amounts of foods such as carrots or supplementing with 30 mg/d or more of β-carotene for long periods of time. Carotenodermia does not result in discoloring of the ocular sclera as occurs in jaundice, thus allowing carotenodermia to be distinguished from this malady. Similarly, lycopenodermia results from high intakes of tomatoes or lycopene and causes the skin to become orange.[5] Both of these conditions reverse days or weeks after reducing carotenoid intake. Two examples of adverse effects of high-dose carotenoid supplementation that are discussed below are β-carotene and lung cancer risk in smokers and canthaxanthin-induced retinopathy in the eye.

## Health and Disease States Related to Carotenoids

### *β-Carotene and Lung Cancer*

Lung cancer is the leading fatal cancer in both men and women in the United States, with the main risk factor being smoking.[26] In the early 1990s, there was strong evidence indicating an inverse association between the consumption of β-carotene-rich fruits and vegetables and lung cancer risk. Thus, two large, randomized, placebo-controlled trials were undertaken to examine the effectiveness of β-carotene supplementation on lung cancer occurrence in high-risk populations. The Alpha-Tocopherol Beta-Carotene Cancer Prevention Trial (ATBC) examined lung cancer risk in Finnish male smokers receiving daily placebo, 50 mg of dl α-tocopheryl acetate, 20 mg of β-carotene, or both antioxidants. In the Beta-Carotene and Retinol Efficacy Trial (CARET), American male and female smokers or asbestos-exposed workers received 30 mg of β-carotene and 25,000 IU of retinyl palmitate or placebo. The research community was shocked when ATBC and CARET results found significant 18% and 28% increases in lung cancer risk, respectively, among those receiving β-carotene supplements.[27]

These findings were not in agreement with reports from the Physicians' Health Study (39% former and 11% current male smokers) or the Women's Health Study (13% current smokers), which did not find adverse effects of 50 mg of β-carotene provided every other day to these lower-risk populations. One striking difference between these studies was that plasma β-carotene levels increased 18- and 14-fold for the ATBC and CARET trial subjects, respectively, compared with a four-fold increase in the Physicians' Health Study and the Women's Health Study participants.[28] Interestingly, 6 years after β-carotene supplementation ceased, the increased risk of lung cancer disappeared among ATBC and CARET subjects who received β-carotene supplements.[27]

The lack of coherence between epidemiological observations and the findings of the clinical trials has been clarified by studies with ferrets. Ferrets are an appropriate animal model for these studies because they metabolize and accumulate β-carotene in a manner similar to humans. Ferrets were fed β-carotene at levels equivalent to a human ingesting 6 mg/d (a normal dietary level) or 30 mg/d (to mimic supplement levels). High β-carotene intake with or without smoke exposure led to the generation of precancerous lung lesions, along with decreased lung retinoic acid, and retinoic acid receptor-β (RAR-β) levels. RAR-β is believed to be a tumor suppressor gene. High β-carotene intake was also associated with an upregulation of lung cytochrome P450 enzymes 1A1 and 1A2, which catabolize retinoic acid, possibly explaining some of the alterations observed. Low β-carotene intake, on the other hand, did not result in precancerous lesions, decreased retinoic acid, or RAR-β levels in ferret lungs. In fact, low β-carotene intake was mildly protective against the adverse effects of smoke on these parameters.[28] High levels of β-carotene intake are also likely to lead to the formation of β-carotene oxidation products, which have been found to increase the binding of benzo[-a]pyrene (the primary carcinogen in tobacco) metabolites to DNA, potentially leading to mutations.[28]

Overall, the clinical trials and animal studies suggest that β-carotene at levels from a diet rich in fruits and vegetables, is potentially protective against lung cancer, whereas pharmacologic levels increase the risk of lung cancer among smokers. The adverse effects associated with high levels of β-carotene intake do not appear to occur with all carotenoids. When smoke-exposed ferrets were fed lycopene at levels equivalent to a human consuming 15 or 60 mg/d (the amount of lycopene in approximately 5 and 20 medium-sized tomatoes, respectively), high lycopene intake prevented smoke-induced lung squamous metaplasia and cell proliferation more effectively than the lower intake level[28] (Figure 2).

## *Lycopene and Prostate Cancer*

The prostate is the most frequent site of cancer in males in the United States, estimated to account for approximately one-third of all diagnosed cases in 2005. Despite the high number of cases, familial predisposition is estimated to account for only 5% to 10% of prostate cancer occurrence.[26] Therefore, environmental factors such as diet have a significant impact on the development of this condition. In 1995, the Health Professional Follow-up Study,[29] a prospective male cohort in the United States, found that lycopene intake, as well as the consumption of raw tomatoes, tomato sauce, and pizza, were all significantly associated with a decreased risk of prostate cancer. Furthermore, after following this cohort for a total of 12 years, the significant inverse relationship between prostate cancer and intakes of both tomato sauce and lycopene remained.[29] A meta-analysis of published epidemiological studies reported that the highest levels of serum lycopene, lycopene intake, and cooked tomato consumption were all associated with a significant decrease in the risk of prostate cancer.[30]

Small clinical trials (N = 13–27) of men diagnosed with prostate cancer who elected to have their prostate removed found that tomato sauce consumption or lycopene supplementation was associated with improved outcomes. These outcomes include decreased DNA damage, less tumor invasiveness, and lower PSA (prostate specific antigen) levels, a common biochemical marker that increases in men with prostate cancer.[31] Thus, the evidence is encouraging for lycopene and tomato consumption being efficacious for men with prostate cancer. However, larger randomized studies are required before public health recommendations can be made.

Why the association between lycopene and prostate cancer? For reasons that are still not understood, lycopene preferentially accumulates in the prostate. In this tissue, the androgens testosterone and dihydrotestosterone play an important role in stimulating proliferation and the development of prostate cancer. There appears to be an interaction between androgens and lycopene levels, such that castration of male rats leads to a two-fold increase in hepatic lycopene, an effect that is normalized by testosterone replacement.[32]

In addition to possibly counteracting the mitogenic effects of androgens, lycopene and tomato intake have also been associated with decreased prostate and serum levels of insulin-like growth factor-I (IGF-I), which is associated with increased prostate cancer risk.[33] Further-

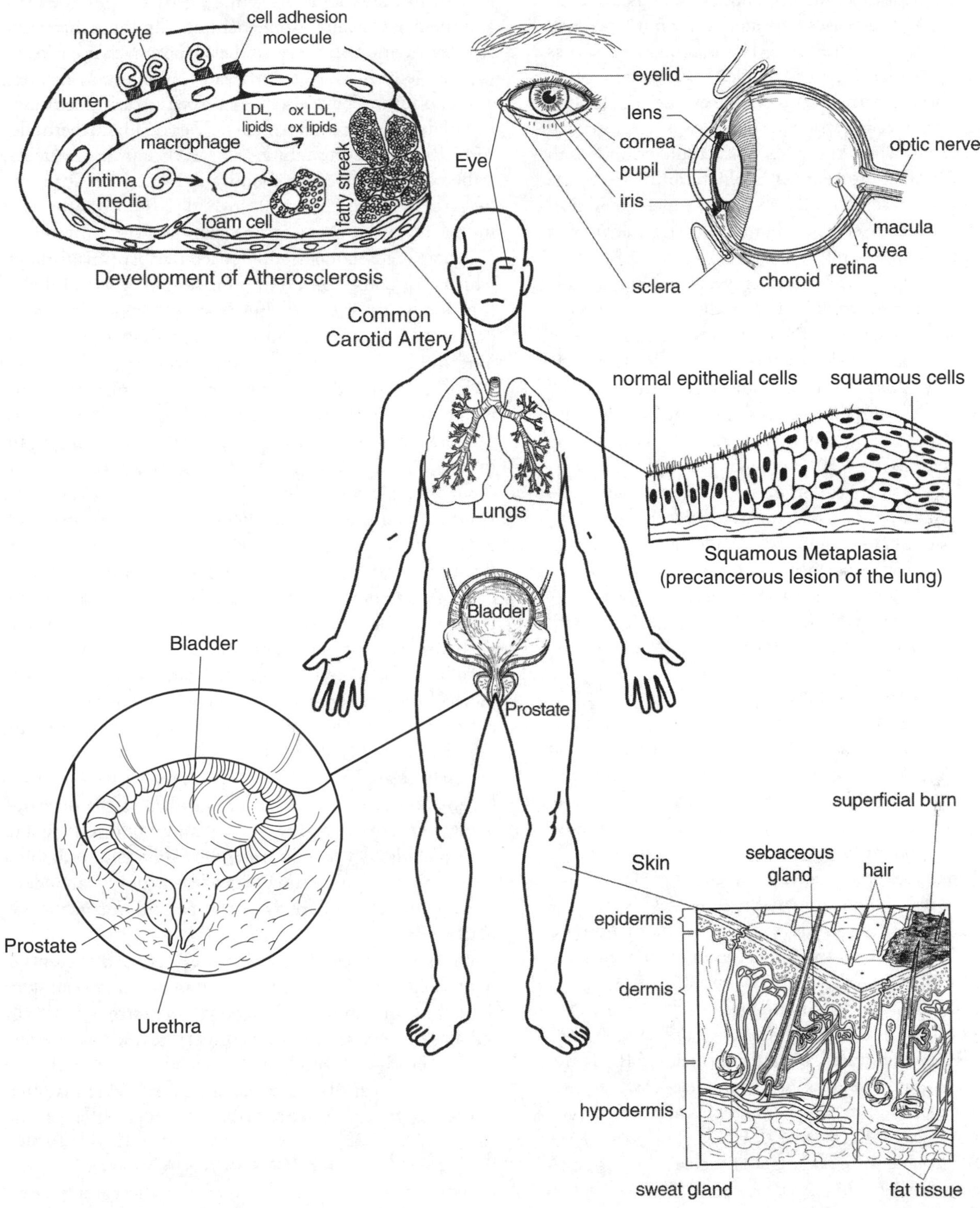


Figure 2. Health and disease states related to carotenoids. ox, oxidized.

more, lycopene is a potent antioxidant, inhibits cell cycle progression, and increases gap-junction communication. These gap junctions are formed by a protein known as connexin 43, which, when assembled together with other proteins, forms a small channel between cells. Through these channels, cells sense the presence of cells next to them, a phenomenon known as contact inhibition, which is believed to help prevent cell proliferation.[33] Lycopene appears to increase connexin 43 levels, which could lead to increased cell-to-cell communication and a lower risk of uncontrolled cell growth.

A common question is whether lycopene is responsible for the inverse association between tomato consumption and prostate cancer, or if there are other compounds in tomatoes that may also have anti-cancer action. In a study of chemically-induced prostate cancer, rats fed a 10% tomato powder diet experienced a significant 21% decrease in prostate cancer mortality, compared with a non-significant 9% decrease in diets supplemented with only lycopene.[34] This result suggests that there are other compounds in tomatoes (e.g., other carotenoids, polyphenols, vitamin E, and other compounds) in addition to lycopene, which may also be responsible for the anticancer action of tomatoes. In fact, animal and cell culture studies suggest that lycopene acts additively or synergistically with vitamin E and a number of other dietary compounds.[33]

## *Cardiovascular Disease*

Epidemiological studies have supported the relationship between carotenoid-rich foods and a decreased risk of developing cardiovascular disease. There have not been many clinical trials directly looking at the ability of β-carotene supplementation to prevent cardiovascular disease, but a number of randomized clinical trials primarily focused on cancer prevention have been conducted. While not a primary outcome, a meta-analysis of 131,551 subjects in six of these trials receiving the pharmacologic dose of 15 to 50 mg of β-carotene alone or in combination with other antioxidants found that supplementation was associated with a significant 10% increased risk of cardiovascular death.[35] This increased risk was driven by ATBC and CARET cardiovascular death rates; in CARET, the increased risk was found to be in females. However, like the lung cancer results, 6 years after β-carotene supplementation ceased, ATBC and CARET subjects who received β-carotene were no longer at increased risk of cardiovascular death.[27,36]

While β-carotene supplementation was not protective, other carotenoids have been associated with positive cardiovascular outcomes. Adipose and plasma lycopene levels have been found to be inversely related to coronary events in the European Study on Antioxidants, Myocardial Infarction, and Breast Cancer (EURAMIC) and the Women's Health Study, respectively. Furthermore, an inverse association was also found between intima-media thickness of the common carotid artery, an early marker of atherosclerosis, and serum and plasma lycopene levels in men in the Kuopio Ischemic Heart Disease (KIHD) and the Antioxidant Supplementation in the Atherosclerosis Prevention (ASAP) studies, respectively.[37] Like lycopene, serum levels of other carotenoids, such as lutein and zeaxanthin, have also been associated with decreased risk of developing cardiovascular disease. The Atherosclerosis Risk in Communities (ARIC) and Los Angeles Atherosclerosis studies found inverse associations between serum lutein, zeaxanthin, and β-cryptoxanthin and intima-media thickness of the common carotid artery.[38]

There are a number of potential mechanisms through which carotenoid consumption may maintain endothelial function and prevent atherosclerosis. Acting as antioxidants, lycopene and lutein have been shown to decrease lipid and LDL oxidation.[37,38] The oxidation of lipids and LDL increases their uptake by macrophages. After macrophages accumulate high levels of these lipids, they become what are known as foam cells, which aggregate to form the fibrous plaque that leads to the development of fatty streaks and ultimately atherosclerosis (Figure 2). Another step in the development of atherosclerosis that is potentially counteracted by carotenoids is the recruitment of monocytes to the intima by cell-adhesion molecules. After entering the intima, monocytes differentiate into macrophages and start to perform the functions described above. Lycopene and lutein serum concentrations have been found to be inversely related to cell-adhesion molecule expression, thereby potentially reducing the recruitment monocytes into the intima.[39] Furthermore, serum levels of carotenoids have also been found to be inversely related to the C-reactive protein, an acute inflammatory protein that has been linked to the development of atherosclerosis.[37,40-41] Inflammation is known to reduce serum levels of carotenoids, but it is unknown whether increasing serum levels of carotenoids can reduce inflammation and markers of this condition (such as C-reactive protein).

In addition to cardiovascular disease, serum concentrations of carotenoids have also been tied to a lower risk of developing other vascular diseases such as stroke.[38,41-42] It remains to be seen whether serum carotenoids specifically reduce the risk of developing vascular disease or if they are markers of fruit and vegetable intake, which is often associated with a decreased risk of vascular diseases.

## *Macular Degeneration and Cataract Formation*

In the United States and the rest of the Western world, age-related macular degeneration (AMD) is the leading cause of blindness, and is estimated to occur in greater than 20% of Americans over the age of 70.[43] AMD is characterized by the formation of druzen, an insoluble lipophilic material that can lead to the separation of photoreceptor cells from their nutrient and oxygen source. Photoreceptor cell death follows, leading to permanent vision loss.[44]

The retina, which is located at the back of the human

eye, contains a depression known as the fovea, on which light is focused after entering the lens (Figure 2). This region contains a high concentration of color-sensitive cones that affords humans our clearest, most distinct vision.[44,45] The fovea is in the center of the macula or macula lutea, which is Latin for "yellow spot." This yellow color is the result of large amounts of lutein and zeaxanthin in this area, which collectively is referred to as the macular pigment. The levels of carotenoids in the retina are almost 10,000-fold greater than levels typically found in the blood, indicating that there is preferential carotenoid accumulation in this region.[42] Lutein and zeaxanthin concentrations vary throughout the retina. In the central fovea, where zeaxanthin and its isomer meso-zeaxanthin are the predominate carotenoids, there is a low lutein-to-zeaxanthin ratio. However, this ratio rises with increasing distance from the fovea, such that lutein becomes the predominant carotenoid in the peripheral regions of the retina.[44,46]

Meso-zeaxanthin is not normally consumed; it is formed from lutein through what is believed to be a double-bond shift in the central fovea (Figure 1).[47] How this occurs is unknown, but a glutathione s-transferase Pi isoform has been isolated from the retina and characterized as a zeaxanthin-binding protein. This is the first known specific, vertebrate carotenoid-binding protein. It is found in high levels in the macula, near the fovea, and at lower levels elsewhere in the retina, which is consistent with the levels of carotenoids found in these regions. Glutathione s-transferases previously have been shown to catalyze reactions similar to the double-bond shift from lutein to meso-zeaxanthin, so it is possible that this protein may also be enzymatically involved in this transformation.[48]

The connection between lutein and zeaxanthin and AMD is that AMD has been found to be associated with lower levels of macular pigment.[44] Some, but not all, epidemiologic studies have found both intake and serum lutein and zeaxanthin levels to be associated with a reduced risk of developing AMD. Autopsied retinas with the highest levels of lutein and zeaxanthin were found to be at decreased risk of having AMD compared with retinas with the lowest levels of these carotenoids.[43] Furthermore, monkeys raised on a carotenoid-free diet lack macular pigment and form druzen, mimicking the early stages of AMD.[44] Feeding and supplementation studies have found that macular pigment levels can be increased by intake of lutein and zeaxanthin.[45] This leads researchers to be hopeful that consumption of these carotenoids might be able to prevent the development of AMD.

Lutein and zeaxanthin are thought to help prevent AMD by absorbing blue light and acting as antioxidants.[43] Because light is being focused on the fovea, it is important that the macular pigment prevents 40% to 90% of blue light from reaching the underlying structures of the eye. Blue light exposure leads the formation of the toxic lipofusion chromophore N-retinyl N-retinylidene ethanolamine (A2E) and reactive oxygen species, which can lead to photoreceptor cell apoptosis.[45] As evidence that this phenomenon occurs, zeaxanthin supplementation has been shown to prevent light-induced photoreceptor damage in Japanese quail.[44]

In addition to their effects on AMD, lutein and zeaxanthin intake have also been associated with a decreased risk of cataract incidence or surgery.[49] Cataracts are believed to be caused by photo-induced oxidation and precipitation of lens proteins. Surgery to correct this condition is the largest single-item cost in the Medicare budget.[49,50] Lutein and zeaxanthin are the only detectable carotenoids present in the lens, albeit at much lower levels than in the retina. It is believed that lutein and zeaxanthin lower the risk of cataract formation by preventing the oxidation of proteins, which ultimately leads to the development of this condition.[43,44]

### *Skin Protection, Coloration, and Photosensitivity*

In plants, carotenoids play an important role in protecting against excess sunlight and quenching of free radicals.[51] It is plausible that carotenoids might be capable of serving a similar role in protecting skin from excess sunlight. Excess sunlight can lead to ultraviolet (UV)-induced erythema, a reddening of the skin more commonly referred to as sunburn. Sunscreen is effective in helping to prevent sunburn, but most sun exposure occurs during times when sunscreen is not employed.[52] Therefore, antioxidants such as carotenoids may be beneficial in preventing UV-induced erythema during everyday exposure and may afford additional protection when used in combination with sunscreen.

High-dose β-carotene supplementation (24–180 mg/d) for greater than 10 weeks appears to be effective in increasing the minimum erythema exposure or decreasing erythema. A mixture of 8 mg each of lycopene, lutein, and β-carotene appears to be equally effective in decreasing UV-induced erythema as 24 mg of β-carotene. In addition to carotenoid supplementation, lycopene-rich tomato paste consumption has also been found to be effective in ameliorating erythema.[51] However, it should be noted that carotenoid intake provides modest UV protection and is not a replacement for sunscreen. Sunburn and excess sun exposure are also associated with an increased risk of skin cancer. However, two clinical trials with high-dose β-carotene failed to find that supplementation reduced the development of skin cancer.[53] The red-orange carotenoid canthaxanthin, which is approved for use as a food color by the Food and Drug Administration (FDA), is marketed at high-doses as a natural tanning pill. However, long-term supplementation needed to sustain the skin's tan color may lead to the development of canthaxanthin-induced retinopathy, a condition in which canthaxanthin crystals form in the retina. Luckily this condition is reversible: the crystals disappear several months after supplementation ceases.[53]

High doses of β-carotene are approved by the FDA for the management of erythropoietin protopoerphyria, a rare genetic disease caused by a defect in ferrochelatase. This defect leads to the accumulation of protophoryin in blood and tissues, which causes burning and possible ulceration of the skin when exposed to sunlight.[53] High-dose supplementation of 60 to 300 mg/d (dependent on age) of β-carotene has been found to help most patients tolerate at least three times more sun without symptoms. Approximately 1 to 2 months of supplementation are normally needed before the patient can expect to see benefits.[53] Despite the high doses administered, few cases of toxicity have been reported. Canthaxanthin has also been used along with β-carotene to manage erythropoietic protopoerphyria in Europe, but it is not approved in the United States for this use, and could potentially lead to canthaxanthin-induced retinopathy.[53]

## Summary

Of the more than 600 carotenoids found in nature, the six main carotenoids found in the diet, serum, and tissues are β-carotene, α-carotene, β-cryptoxanthin, lutein, zeaxanthin, and lycopene. Carotenoids are categorized in two ways: the first way is as provitamin A (β-carotene, α-carotene, β-cryptoxanthin) if they can be converted into retinal or retinoic acid through CMO I central cleavage or CMO II eccentric cleavage; the second way is when they are structurally divided into the hydrocarbon carotenes and the oxygenated xanthophylls (Table 1 and Figure 1). The mnemonic SLAMENGHI is helpful in remembering the factors affecting the bioavailability and bioconversion of carotenoids. Carotenoids preferentially accumulate in the liver, adrenal, and reproductive tissues, but the reason for differential accumulation of carotenoids in these and other tissues is not known (Table 2). A number of factors affect the circulating levels of carotenoids, such as body mass, hormones, smoking, and alcohol intake. There are no known carotenoid toxicities from foods, and extremely high intakes of β-carotene do not lead to vitamin A toxicity. Unlike essential micronutrients, there are no known deficiency signs of low carotenoid intake.

Pharmacologic levels of β-carotene may increase the risk for lung cancer and cardiovascular disease, especially in smokers, while dietary levels may be protective against these conditions. Lycopene may decrease atherogenesis, leading to decreased risk of cardiovascular disease (Figure 2). In addition, the intake of tomato products and serum levels of lycopene appear to be inversely related to prostate cancer risk, but there are other compounds in tomatoes that likely play a role in preventing this disease. Lutein and zeaxanthin, in addition to potentially preventing cardiovascular disease, make up the macular pigment, which appears to play a role in preventing the development of AMD. The glutathione s-transferase Pi isoform, a zeaxanthin-binding protein, appears to play an important role in concentrating meso-zeaxanthin. This isomer is found at high levels in the central fovea, but is not normally consumed in the diet. Finally, carotenoids in the skin may provide moderate protection from the harmful effects of UV light from the sun.

## Future Directions

The chemical characterization of carotenoids in foods and the vitamin A activity of carotenoids have received considerable research attention. In contrast, the study of the beneficial health aspects of these compounds is in its infancy. Many gaps in knowledge exist and are delineated below.

To date, β-carotene has been the primary carotenoid studied, but far less is known about other carotenoids commonly found in human diets and tissues. Tomatoes, in addition to lycopene, contain small amounts of β-carotene, and appreciable levels of the carotenoids phytoene, phytofluene, and ζ-carotene.[33] The latter three carotenoids may also play a role in human health. For example, consumption of tomato-based products protects against erythema better than lycopene supplementation alone. One potential explanation for this increased protection is that the maximum absorption of phytoene and phytofluene falls within the UV-visible light range.[54] This means they may be effective at absorbing UV light, thus preventing it from damaging the skin. Other lesser-studied carotenoids may also possess unique characteristics that could benefit human health. Studies examining the effect of lesser-known carotenoids and combinations of carotenoids are sorely needed.

The metabolic role and control of carotenoid cleavage enzymes is another area that needs elucidation. Following the cloning of RPE65, CMO I, and CMO II, more is being learned about these enzymes. Nevertheless, there may be other enzymes involved in carotenoid metabolism that have yet to be identified. Likewise, it is important to identify carotenoid cleavage products, because they may have biological functions. The identity and role of these metabolites are still not well understood.

Reasons for the varying carotenoid concentrations in different tissues are not clear, with the exception of the accumulation of zeaxanthin in the eye. The identification of the glutathione-s-transferase Pi isoform, which binds zeaxanthin, helps to explain the extremely high levels of this carotenoid in the macular pigment of the eye. However, this was only one of four potential carotenoid-binding proteins isolated from the macula. The other three proteins have not been identified and characterized.[48] Similarly, it is uncertain why lycopene preferentially accumulates in the prostate compared with its precursor carotenoids, phytoene, phytofluene, and ζ-carotene, all of which are remarkably similar in structure.[55] Factors that regulate either carotenoid storage in tissues or degradation of these compounds still need to be determined. Identifying factors that influence the levels of carotenoids in tissues is likely to help us begin to understand the role of individual carotenoids in tissues and, potentially, roles in health and disease prevention.

The genetic modification of plants to increase their carotenoid level is also an active area in research. "Golden Rice," which is genetically engineered to accumulate β-carotene, was produced to help combat vitamin A deficiency in developing countries. However, the levels of β-carotene in the rice were believed to be too low to realistically ameliorate this condition. In response to this concern, a corn-derived enzyme was inserted that increased the production of β-carotene 20-fold in "Golden Rice 2." This new β-carotene concentration is closer to a range that may prevent vitamin A deficiency. Nonetheless, it should be noted that the bioavailability of β-carotene from this rice has not been reported. Thus, it is unknown whether this product will provide enough β-carotene to be efficacious in improving vitamin A status, or if further increases in β-carotene concentrations will be needed because of poor bioavailability.[56,57] Overall, there are intriguing relationships between carotenoids and disease. Elucidating the mechanisms through which these relationships occur will be a major focus as carotenoid research moves toward understanding the role of these compounds in human health.

## References


1. Deming DM, Boileau TW, Heintz KH, et al. Carotenoids: linking chemistry, absorption, and metabolism to potential roles in human health and disease. In: Cadenas E, Packer L, eds. *Handbook of Antioxidants*. 2nd ed. New York: Marcel Dekker; 2001; 189–221.
2. Young AJ, Phillip DM, Lowe, GM. Carotenoid antioxidant activity. In: Krinsky NI, Mayne ST, Sies H, eds. *Carotenoids in Health and Disease*. New York: Marcel Dekker; 2004; 105-126.
3. Holden, JM, Eldridge AL, Beecher GR, Buzzard M. Carotenoid content of food: an update of the database. J Food Comp Anal. 1999;12:169–196.
4. Institute of Medicine. *Dietary Reference Intakes for Vitamin A, Vitamin K, Arsenic, Boron, Chromium, Copper, Iodine, Iron, Manganese, Molybdenum, Nickel, Silicon, Vanadium, and Zinc*. Washington, DC: National Academies Press; 2001. Available online at: http://www.nap.edu/books/0309072794/html/. Accessed August 2, 2005.
5. Institute of Medicine. *Dietary Reference Intakes for Vitamin C, Vitamin E, Selenium, and Carotenoids*. Washington, DC: National Academies Press; 2000. Available online at: http://www.nap.edu/openbook/0309069351/html/index.html. Accessed August 2, 2005.
6. Castenmiller JJ, West CE. Bioavailability and bioconversion of carotenoids. Annu Rev Nutr. 1998;18: 19–38.
7. Yeum KJ, Russell RM. Carotenoid bioavailability and bioconversion. Annu Rev Nutr. 2002;22: 483–504.
8. Tang G, Russell RM. Bioequivalence of provitamin A carotenoids. In: Krinsky NI, Mayne ST, Sies H, eds. *Carotenoids in Health and Disease*. New York: Marcel Dekker; 2004; 279–294.
9. Chung HY, Rasmussen HM, Johnson EJ. Lutein bioavailability is higher from lutein-enriched eggs than from supplements and spinach in men. J Nutr. 2004;134:1887–1893.
10. Breithaupt DE, Weller P, Wolters M, Hahn A. Plasma response to a single dose of dietary beta-cryptoxanthin esters from papaya (*Carica papaya* L.) or non-esterified beta-cryptoxanthin in adult human subjects: a comparative study. Br J Nutr. 2003;90: 795–801.
11. Breithaupt DE, Weller P, Wolters M, Hahn A. Comparison of plasma responses in human subjects after the ingestion of 3R,3R′-zeaxanthin dipalmitate from wolfberry (*Lycium barbarum*) and non-esterified 3R,3R′-zeaxanthin using chiral high-performance liquid chromatography. Br J Nutr. 2004;91:707–713.
12. Barua AB. Bioconversion of provitamin A carotenoids. In: Krinsky NI, Mayne ST, Sies H, eds. *Carotenoids in Health and Disease*. New York: Marcel Dekker; 2004; 295–312.
13. Boileau AM, Erdman JW Jr. Impact of food processing on content and bioavailability of carotenoids. In: Krinsky NI, Mayne ST, Sies H, eds. *Carotenoids in Health and Disease*. New York: Marcel Dekker; 2004; 209–228.
14. Tanumihardjo SA, Li J, Dosti MP. Lutein absorption is facilitated with cosupplementation of ascorbic acid in young adults. J Am Diet Assoc. 2005;105: 114–118.
15. Von Lintig J, Hessel S, Isken A, et al. Towards a better understanding of carotenoid metabolism in animals. Biochim Biophys Acta. 2005;1740:122–131.
16. Kiefer C, Hessel S, Lampert JM, et al. Identification and characterization of a mammalian enzyme catalyzing the asymmetric oxidative cleavage of provitamin A. J Biol Chem. 2001;276:14110–14116.
17. Wyss A. Carotene oxygenases: a new family of double bond cleavage enzymes. J Nutr. 2004;134: 246S–2450S.
18. Lindqvist A, Andersson S. Biochemical properties of purified recombinant human beta-carotene 15, 15′-monooxygenase. J Biol Chem. 2002;277: 23942–23948.
19. Yan W, Jang GF, Haeseleer F, et al. Cloning and characterization of a human beta,beta-carotene-15,15′-dioxygenase that is highly expressed in the retinal pigment epithelium. Genomics. 2001;72: 193–202.
20. Lindqvist A, Andersson S. Cell type-specific expression of beta-carotene 15,15′-mono-oxygenase in

human tissues. J Histochem Cytochem. 2004;52: 491–499.

21. Furr HC, Clark RM. Transport, uptake, and target tissue storage of carotenoids. In: Krinsky NI, Mayne ST, Sies H, eds. *Carotenoids in Health and Disease*. New York: Marcel Dekker; 2004; 229–278.
22. During A, Dawson HD, Harrison EH. Carotenoid transport is decreased and expression of the lipid transporters SR-BI, NPC1L1, and ABCA1 is down-regulated in Caco-2 cells treated with ezetimibe. J Nutr. 2005;135:2305–312.
23. Zaripheh S, Erdman JW Jr. The biodistribution of a single oral dose of [$^{14}$C]-lycopene in rats prefed either a control or lycopene-enriched diet. J Nutr. 2005;135:2212–2218.
24. Khachik F, Carvalho L, Bernstein PS, Muir GJ, Zhao DY, Katz NB. Chemistry, distribution, and metabolism of tomato carotenoids and their impact on human health. Exp Biol Med (Maywood). 2002; 227:845–851.
25. Curran-Celentano J, Erdman JW Jr. A case study of carotenemia in anorexia nervosa may support the interrelationship of vitamin A and thyroid hormone. Nutr Res. 1993;13:379–386.
26. American Cancer Society. *Cancer Facts and Figures 2005*. Atlanta: American Cancer Society; 2005. Available online at: http://www.cancer.org/downloads/STT/CAFF2005f4PWSecured.pdf. Accessed August 2, 2005.
27. Goodman GE, Thornquist MD, Balmes J, et al. The Beta-Carotene and Retinol Efficacy Trial: incidence of lung cancer and cardiovascular disease mortality during 6-year follow-up after stopping beta-carotene and retinol supplements. J Natl Cancer Inst. 2004; 96:1743–1750.
28. Wang XD. Carotenoid oxidative/degradative products and their biological activities. In: Krinsky NI, Mayne ST, Sies H, eds. *Carotenoids in Health and Disease*. New York: Marcel Dekker; 2004; 313–335.
29. Giovannucci E, Rimm EB, Liu Y, Stampfer MJ, Willett WC. A prospective study of tomato products, lycopene, and prostate cancer risk. J Natl Cancer Inst. 2002;94:391–398.
30. Etminan M, Takkouche B, Caamano-Isorna F. The role of tomato products and lycopene in the prevention of prostate cancer: a meta-analysis of observational studies. Cancer Epidemiol Biomarkers Prev. 2004;13:340–345.
31. Obermüller-Jevic UC, Packer L. Lycopene and prostate cancer. In: Packer L, Obermüller-Jevic UC, Kraemer K, Sies H, eds. *Carotenoids and Retinoids: Molecular Aspects and Health Issues*. Champaign, IL: AOCS Press; 2004; 295–302.
32. Boileau TW, Clinton SK, Zaripheh S, Monaco MH, Donovan SM, Erdman JW Jr. Testosterone and food restriction modulate hepatic lycopene isomer concentrations in male F344 rats. J Nutr. 2001;131: 1746–1752.
33. Campbell JK, Canene-Adams K, Lindshield BL, Boileau TW, Clinton SK, Erdman JW Jr. Tomato phytochemicals and prostate cancer risk. J Nutr. 2004;134(suppl 12):3486S–3492S.
34. Boileau TW, Liao Z, Kim S, Lemeshow S, Erdman JW Jr, Clinton SK. Prostate carcinogenesis in N-methyl-N-nitrosourea (NMU)-testosterone-treated rats fed tomato powder, lycopene, or energy-restricted diets. J Natl Cancer Inst. 2003;95: 1578–1586.
35. Vivekananthan DP, Penn MS, Sapp SK, Hsu A, Topol EJ. Use of antioxidant vitamins for the prevention of cardiovascular disease: meta-analysis of randomised trials. Lancet. 2003;361:2017–2023.
36. Tornwall ME, Virtamo J, Korhonen PA, et al. Effect of alpha-tocopherol and beta-carotene supplementation on coronary heart disease during the 6-year post-trial follow-up in the ATBC study. Eur Heart J. 2004;25:1171–1178.
37. Petr L, Erdman, JW Jr. Lycopene and risk of cardiovascular disease. In: Packer L, Obermüller-Jevic UC, Kraemer K, Sies H, eds. *Carotenoids and Retinoids: Molecular Aspects and Health Issues*. Champaign, IL: AOCS Press; 2004; 204–217.
38. Ribaya-Mercado JD, Blumberg JB. Lutein and zeaxanthin and their potential roles in disease prevention. J Am Coll Nutr. 2004;23(suppl 6):567S–587S.
39. van Herpen-Broekmans WM, Klopping-Ketelaars IA, Bots ML, et al. Serum carotenoids and vitamins in relation to markers of endothelial function and inflammation. Eur J Epidemiol. 2004;19:915–921.
40. Ford ES, Liu S, Mannino DM, Giles WH, Smith SJ. C-reactive protein concentration and concentrations of blood vitamins, carotenoids, and selenium among United States adults. Eur J Clin Nutr. 2003; 57:1157–1163.
41. Sesso HD, Gaziano JM. Heart and vascular diseases. In: Krinsky NI, Mayne ST, Sies H, eds. *Carotenoids in Health and Disease*. New York: Marcel Dekker; 2004; 473–490.
42. Hak AE, Ma J, Powell CB, et al. Prospective study of plasma carotenoids and tocopherols in relation to risk of ischemic stroke. Stroke. 2004;35:1584–1588.
43. Bone RA, Landrum LT. Macular carotenoids in eye health. In: Packer L, Obermüller-Jevic UC, Kraemer K, Sies H, eds. *Carotenoids and Retinoids: Molecular Aspects and Health Issues*. Champaign, IL: AOCS Press; 2004; 115–129.
44. Landrum JT, Bone RA. Mechanistic evidence for eye disease and carotenoids. In: Krinsky NI, Mayne ST, Sies H, eds. *Carotenoids in Health and Disease*. New York: Marcel Dekker; 2004; 445–472.
45. Krinsky NI, Landrum JT, Bone RA. Biologic mechanisms of the protective role of lutein and zeaxanthin in the eye. Annu Rev Nutr. 2003;23:171–201.

46. Semba RD, Dagnelie G. Are lutein and zeaxanthin conditionally essential nutrients for eye health? Med Hypotheses. 2003;61:465–472.
47. Johnson EJ, Neuringer M, Russell RM, Schalch W, Snodderly DM. Nutritional manipulation of primate retinas, III: Effects of lutein or zeaxanthin supplementation on adipose tissue and retina of xanthophyll-free monkeys. Invest Ophthalmol Vis Sci. 2005;46:692–702.
48. Bhosale P, Larson AJ, Frederick JM, Southwick K, Thulin CD, Bernstein PS. Identification and characterization of a Pi isoform of glutathione S-transferase (GSTP1) as a zeaxanthin-binding protein in the macula of the human eye. J Biol Chem. 2004;279: 49447–49454.
49. Mares JA. Carotenoids and eye disease: epidemiological evidence. In: Krinsky NI, Mayne ST, Sies H, eds. Carotenoids in Health and Disease. New York: Marcel Dekker; 2004; 427–444.
50. Alves-Rodrigues A, Shao A. The science behind lutein. Toxicol Lett. 2004;150:57–83.
51. Sies H, Stahl W. Carotenoids and UV protection. Photochem Photobiol Sci. 2004;3:749–752.
52. Sies H, Stahl W. Nutritional protection against skin damage from sunlight. Annu Rev Nutr. 2004;24: 173–200.
53. Mathews-Roth, MM. Therapeutic uses of carotenoids in skin photosensitivity diseases. In: Krinsky NI, Mayne ST, Sies H, eds. *Carotenoids in Health and Disease.* New York: Marcel Dekker; 2004; 519–529.
54. Aust O, Stahl W, Sies H, Tronnier H, Heinrich U. Supplementation with tomato-based products increases lycopene, phytofluene, and phytoene levels in human serum and protects against UV-light-induced erythema. Int J Vitam Nutr Res 2005; 75:54–60.
55. Campbell JK, Zaripheh S, Lila MA, Erdman JW Jr. Relative bioavailability of phytoene and phytofluene in male Fisher 344 rats. FASEB J. 2005;19:A472.
56. Grusak MA. Golden rice gets a boost from maize. Nat Biotechnol. 2005;23:429–430.
57. Paine JA, Shipton CA, Chaggar S, et al. Improving the nutritional value of Golden Rice through increased pro-vitamin A content. Nat Biotechnol. 2005;23:482–487.

# 14 Vitamin D

Anthony W. Norman and Helen H. Henry

## Background

### *Introduction*

Vitamin D is essential for life in higher animals. Classically, it has been shown to be one of the most important biological regulators of calcium homeostasis. It has been established that these important biological effects are only achieved as a consequence of the metabolism of vitamin D into a family of daughter metabolites, including the two key kidney-produced metabolites, $1\alpha,25(OH)_2$-vitamin $D_3$ [$1\alpha,25(OH)_2D_3$] and $24R,25(OH)_2$-vitamin $D_3$ [$24R,25(OH)_2D_3$] (Figure 2). $1\alpha,25(OH)_2D_3$ is considered to be a steroid hormone and there is evidence that $24R,25(OH)_2D_3$ may be as well.[1]

Since the 1980s, it has become increasingly apparent that $1\alpha,25(OH)_2D_3$ also plays an important role in differentiation and proliferation of a wide variety of cells and tissues not primarily related to mineral metabolism, including cells of the hematopoietic system, keratinocytes, and cells secreting parathyroid hormone and insulin. In addition, many types of cancer cells, including breast and prostate cancer cells, are targets of $1,25(OH)_2D_3$ action.[2] The purpose of this chapter is to provide a succinct overview of our current understanding of the important nutritional substance vitamin D and the mechanisms by which its biologically active metabolite, the steroid hormone $1\alpha,25(OH)_2D_3$, mediates biological responses. There have been more thorough reviews published that provide differing perspectives and more detail.[1,3-6]

### *Historical Review*

The first scientific description of rickets, which is the hallmark of a vitamin D deficiency, was provided in the 17th century by both Dr. Daniel Whistler in 1645 and Professor Francis Glisson in 1650.[7] The major breakthrough in understanding the causative factors of rickets was the development of nutrition as an experimental science and the appreciation of the existence of vitamins. Although through a historical accident, vitamin D was originally classified as a vitamin, it is now widely accepted that its biologically active form is a steroid hormone. In 1919–1920, Sir Edward Mellan raised dogs exclusively indoors (in the absence of sunlight or ultraviolet light) and fed them a diet that allowed him to unequivocally establish that rickets was caused by a deficiency of a trace component in the diet. In 1921 he wrote, "The action of fats in rickets is due to a vitamin or accessory food factor which they contain, probably identical with the fat-soluble vitamin." Furthermore, he established that cod-liver oil was an excellent anti-rachitic agent, leading to the classification of this anti-rachitic factor as a vitamin.[7]

The chemical structures of the D vitamins were determined in the 1930s in the laboratory of Professor A. Windaus at the University of Gottingen. Vitamin $D_2$, produced by ultraviolet irradiation of ergosterol (obtained from plants or yeast), was chemically characterized in 1932.[7] Vitamin $D_3$, the form produced in the skin of vertebrate animals, was not chemically characterized until 1936, when it was shown to result from the ultraviolet irradiation of 7-dehydrocholesterol.[7] Virtually simultaneously, the elusive anti-rachitic component of cod-liver oil was shown to be identical to the newly characterized vitamin $D_3$.[7] These results clearly established that the anti-rachitic substance vitamin D was chemically a steroid, more specifically a seco-steroid (see below).

The modern era of vitamin D began in the interval of 1965–1970 with the discovery[8] and chemical characterization of $1\alpha,25(OH)_2D_3$[9-11] and its nuclear receptor, the $VDR_{nuc}$.[12]

## Chemistry of Vitamin D

The structures of vitamin $D_3$ (cholecalciferol) and its provitamins 7-dehydrocholesterol, are presented in Figure 1. "Vitamin D" is a generic term and indicates a molecule of the general structure shown for rings A, B, C, and

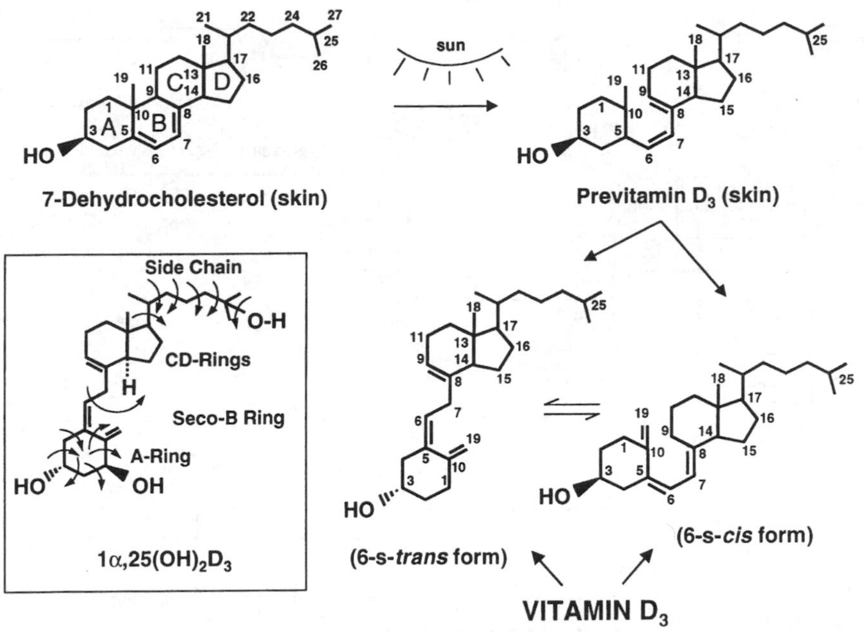

Figure 1. Chemistry and irradiation pathway for production of vitamin $D_3$. The provitamin, which is characterized by the presence in the B ring of a Δ5, Δ7 conjugated double bond system, is converted to a seco-B previtamin steroid, where the 9,10 carbon-carbon bond has been broken. Then the previtamin D, in a process independent of ultraviolet light, thermally isomerizes to the "vitamin" form, which is characterized by a Δ6,7, Δ8,9, Δ10,19 conjugated triple bond system. The extreme conformational flexibility potential of all vitamin D metabolites is illustrated in the inset box for the principal metabolite, 1α,25$(OH)_2D_3$. Each of the arrows indicates carbon-carbon single bonds present (in the side chain, the seco-B ring and the A ring) that have complete 360° rotational freedom. This results for the various vitamin D molecules in the generation in solution and in biological systems of a multitude of different shapes.[2] The main portion of the figure also illustrates the two principal conformations of the molecule that results as a consequence of rotation about the 6,7 carbon single bond of the seco-B ring. These are the 6-*s-cis* conformer (the steroid-like shape) and the 6-s-*trans* conformer (the extended shape) are illustrated.

D, with differing side chain structures. The A, B, C, and D ring structure is derived from the cyclopentanoperhydrophenanthrene ring structure for steroids. Technically, vitamin D is classified as a seco-steroid, in which one of the rings has been broken. In vitamin D, the 9,10 carbon-carbon bond of ring B is broken, as indicated by the inclusion of "9,10-seco" in the official nomenclature. A discussion of the conformational shapes attainable by vitamin D is given in the legend to Fig. 1.

Vitamin D (synonym calciferol) is named according to the revised rules of the International Union of Pure and Applied Chemists (IUPAC).[13] Because it is derived from a steroid, vitamin D retains its numbering from the parent compound cholesterol (Figure 1). Asymmetric centers are designated using the R,S notation;[14] the configuration of the double bonds are indicated as E (*trans*), and Z (*cis*). Thus, the official name of vitamin $D_3$ is 9,10-seco(5Z,7E)-5,7,10(19)cholestatriene-3β-ol. Vitamin $D_2$, which differs from vitamin $D_3$ by the presence of a 22-ene and 24-methyl group in the side chain, is 9,10-seco(5Z,7E)-5,7,10(19),22-ergostatetraene-3β-ol. From 1940 until about 1960, vitamin $D_2$ was used to supply vitamin D,[7] but in the United States today, vitamin $D_3$ is the form of calciferol that is used for food supplementation.

Vitamin $D_3$ can be produced photochemically from the provitamin D, 7-dehydrocholesterol, which is present in the epidermis or skin of most higher animals by the action of sunlight in most geographical locations or of artificial ultraviolet light. The conjugated double-bond system in ring B (Figure 1) allows the absorption of light quanta at certain wavelengths in the UV range, initiating a complex series of transformations of the provitamin (partially summarized in Figure 1) that ultimately result in vitamin $D_3$. Thus, it is important to appreciate that vitamin $D_3$ can be endogenously produced, and that as long as the animal (or human) has access on a regular basis to adequate sunlight, there may be no need for a dietary requirement for this vitamin.

# Physiology and Biochemistry of Vitamin D

## *Vitamin D Endocrine System*

Vitamin $D_3$ itself is not known to have any intrinsic biological activity, but must be metabolized, first to 25(OH)$D_3$ in the liver and then to 1α,25$(OH)_2D_3$ and/or 24R,25$(OH)_2D_3$ by the kidney. Altogether, some 37 vitamin $D_3$ metabolites have been isolated and chemically characterized.[15]

The elements of the vitamin D endocrine system[2,16] include the following (Figure 2): 1) the photoconversion of 7-dehydrocholesterol to vitamin $D_3$ in the skin or di-

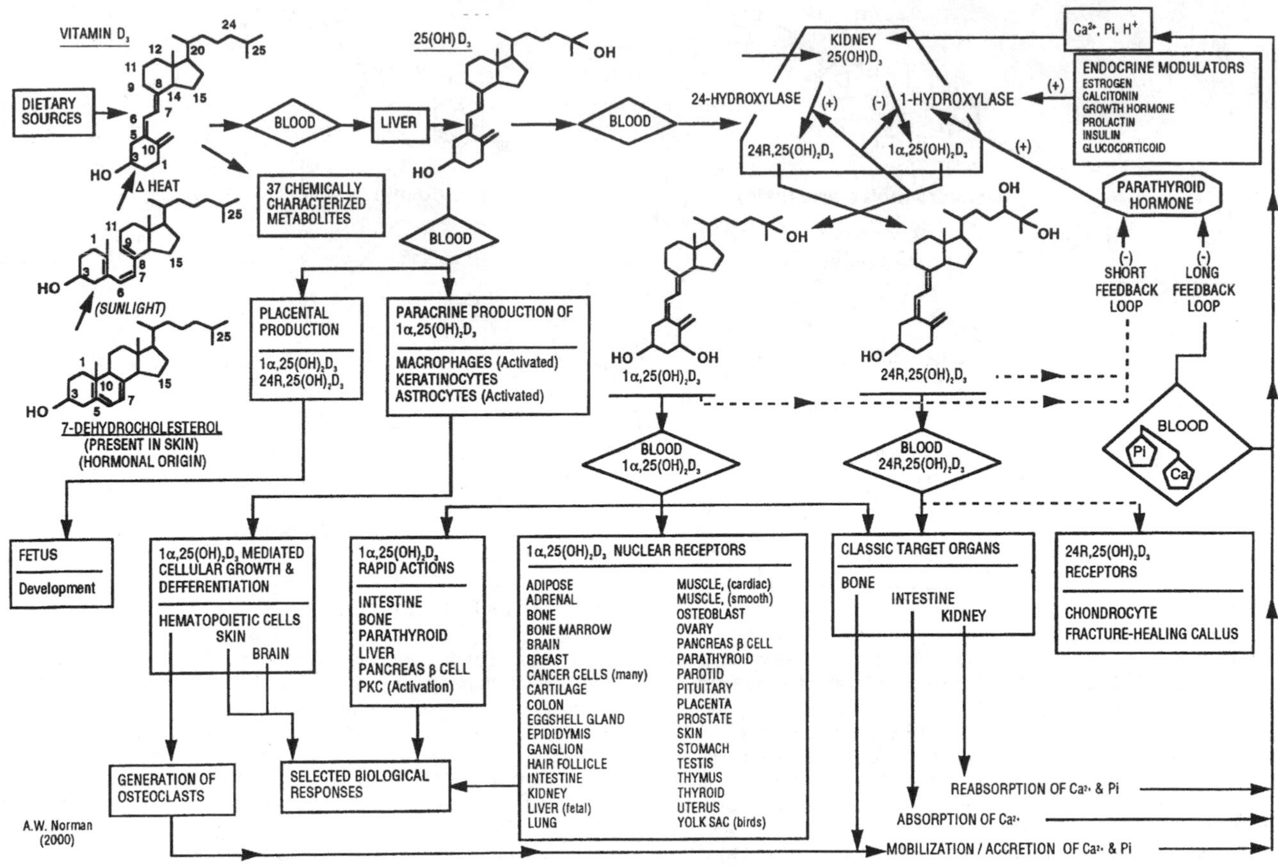


Figure 2. Summary of the vitamin D endocrine system. In this system, the biologically inactive vitamin $D_3$ is activated first in the liver, and then converted by the endocrine gland, the kidney, to the hormones $1\alpha,25(OH)_2D_3$ and $24R,25(OH)_2D_3$. Pi = inorganic phosphate. There is currently much research being conducted to understand structure-function relationships in the vitamin D endocrine system and their relation to the development of new drugs. (From Norman and Silva, 2001.[95] Used with kind permission of Springer Science and Business Media.)

etary intake of vitamin $D_3$; 2) metabolism of vitamin $D_3$ by the liver to $25(OH)D_3$, the major form of vitamin D circulating in the blood compartment; 3) conversion of $25(OH)D_3$ by the kidney (functioning as an endocrine gland) to produce the two principal dihydroxylated metabolites, $1\alpha,25(OH)_2D_3$ and $24R,25(OH)_2D_3$; 4) systemic transport of the dihydroxylated metabolites $24R,25(OH)_2D_3$ and $1\alpha,25(OH)_2D_3$ to distal target organs; and 5) binding of the dihydroxylated metabolites, particularly $1,25(OH)_2D_3$, to either a nuclear receptor or membrane receptor at the target organs, followed by the subsequent generation of the appropriate biological responses (Figure 3). An additional key component in the operation of the vitamin D endocrine system is the plasma vitamin D-binding protein, which carries vitamin $D_3$ and all of its metabolites to their sites of metabolism and various target organs.[17]

The three enzymes responsible for the conversion of vitamin $D_3$ into its two key daughter metabolites include the hepatic vitamin $D_3$-25-hydroxylase[1] and the two kidney enzymes, the $25(OH)D_3$-1α-hydroxylase(4) and the $25(OH)D_3$-24R-hydroxylase.[1] All three enzymes have been demonstrated to be cytochrome P450 mixed-function oxidases.[18] Both renal enzymes are localized in mitochondria of the proximal tubules of the kidney. The genes for all three cytochrome P450 molecules have been cloned,[1] and the specific sites of mutations of the $25(OH)D_3$-1α-hydroxylase that result in vitamin D-resistant rickets, type I (VDRR-I), have been identified.[19]

The most important point of regulation of the vitamin D endocrine system occurs through the stringent control of the activity of the renal $25(OH)D_3$-1α-hydroxylase. In this way, the production of the hormone $1\alpha,25(OH)_2D_3$ can be modulated according to the calcium and other endocrine needs of the organism. The chief regulatory factors are $1\alpha,25(OH)_2D_3$ itself, which down-regulates its own production, parathyroid hormone, which stimulates the renal production of $1,25(OH)_2D_3$, and the serum concentrations of calcium and phosphate.[15,18] Probably the most important determinant of the 1α-hydroxylase is the vitamin D status of the animal.[15] When the circulating concentration of $1\alpha,25(OH)_2D_3$ is low, the production of $1\alpha,25(OH)_2D_3$ by the kidney is high; when the circulating concentrations of $1\alpha,25(OH)_2D_3$ is high, the output of $1\alpha,25(OH)_2D_3$ by the kidney is sharply reduced.[4]

**Mechanism of Action of $1\alpha,25(OH)_2D_3$.** The steroid

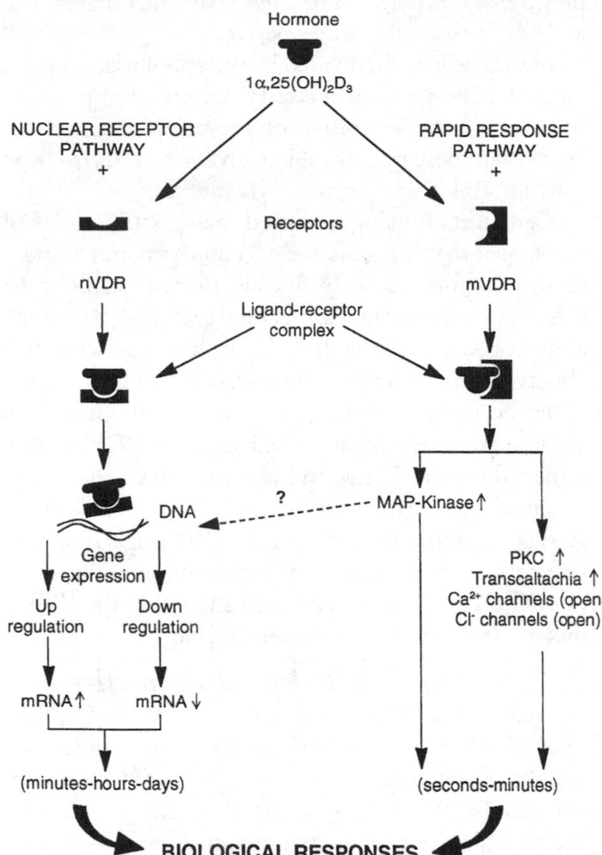


Figure 3. Model to describe how $1\alpha,25(OH)_2D_3$ and its analogs generate biological responses. A, Biological responses to $1\alpha,25(OH)_2D_3$ are believed to occur as a consequence of different shapes of the conformationally flexible $1\alpha,25(OH)_2D_3$ interacting with two separate receptors linked to different signal transduction pathways(20;36). Thus, 6-s-*trans* shaped analogs are preferred by the vitamin D-resistant (VDR) nucleus, while 6-s-*cis* shaped analogs are preferred by the VDR membrane. In the genomic pathway, occupancy of the nuclear receptor for $1\alpha,25(OH)_2D_3(VDR_{nuc})$ by a ligand of the correct shape (the hat icon) leads to up- or down-regulation of genes subject to hormone regulation. In the rapid response pathway, occupancy of a putative membrane receptor ($VDR_{mem}$), by a different (6-s-*cis*) shape (the half-hat icon) of $1\alpha,25(OH)_2D_3$, can produce a variety of rapid responses depending upon the cell type. These can include activation of protein kinase C (PKC), opening of voltage-gated $Ca^{2+}$ or $Cl^-$ channels, or activation of mitogen-activated protein (MAP)-kinase, which are linked to the generation of biological response(s).

hormone 1α,25(OH)2D3, as well as many other steroid hormones (e.g., estradiol, progesterone, testosterone, cortisol, and aldosterone) generate biological responses both by regulation of gene transcription (the classic genomic responses) and via the rapid activation of a variety of signal transduction pathways at or near the plasma membrane (referred to as either rapid or non-genotropic responses)[20] (21).

**Genomic Responses of $1\alpha,25(OH)_2D_3$.** The genomic responses to $1\alpha,25(OH)_2D_3$ result from its stereo-specific interaction with its nuclear receptor, $VDR_{nuc}$ (Figure 4). $VDR_{nuc}$ is a protein of 50-kD that binds $1\alpha,25(OH)_2D_3$ with high affinity ($K_d$ approximately 0.5 nM). $VDR_{nuc}$ does not bind the parent vitamin D; $25(OH)D_3$ and $1\alpha(OH)D_3$ only bind 0.1–0.3% as well as $1\alpha,25(OH)_2D_3$. The primary amino acid sequence of the $VDR_{nuc}$, as is true for all nuclear receptors for steroid hormones, consists of five functional domains involved in nuclear localization, DNA binding (the C domain), heterodimerization, ligand binding (the E domain), and transcriptional activation.[5] A detailed discussion of the $VDR_{nuc}$ and its participation in the regulation of gene transcription is available.[22]

Nuclear receptor-mediated regulation of gene transcription is dependent upon the structural relationship between the unoccupied receptor, which is transcription-

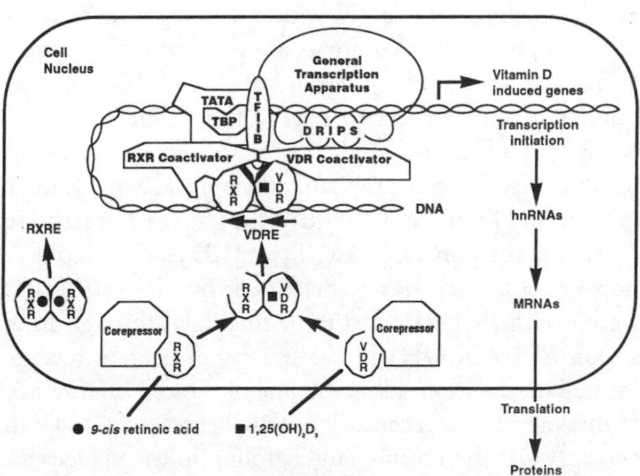


Figure 4. Model of $1\alpha,25(OH)_2D_3$ and $VDR_{nuc}$ activation of transcription. The vitamin D-resistant (VDR) form, after binding its cognate ligand $1\alpha,25(OH)_2D_3$, forms a heterodimer with retinoid-X receptor (RXR). This heterodimer complex then interacts with the appropriate vitamin D response element (VDRE) on the promoter of genes (in specific target cells) that are destined to be up- or down-regulated. The heterodimer-DNA complex then recruits necessary co-activator proteins, TATA, TBP, TFIIB, and other proteins, to generate a competent transcriptional complex capable of modulating mRNA production. A detailed discussion is given in Whitfield et. al., 2005.[22]

ally inactive, and its cognate ligand. Formation of the ligand-receptor complex results in conformational changes in the receptor protein, which allow it to interact with the transcriptional machinery. A detailed understanding of the complementarity of the ligand shape with that of the interior surface of the nuclear VDR receptor ligand-binding domain is the key to understanding not only the structural basis of receptor action and its formation of heterodimers and interactions with co-activators (Figure), but also to designing new drug forms of the various hormones, including 1α,25$(OH)_2D_3$.

The receptors for all steroid hormones (estrogen, progesterone, testosterone, cortisol, and aldosterone), and the nuclear receptors for 1α,25$(OH)_2D_3$, retinoic acid, and thyroid hormone are members of the same super gene family;[23] accordingly, there is substantial conservation of their amino acid sequences, particularly in the DNA-binding domains. Although there is considerably less conservation of amino acid sequence in the ligand-binding domains of the nuclear receptors, X-ray crystallographic studies of many of these ligand-binding domains shows the same overall secondary and tertiary structures.[24] These structures, including that of the $VDR_{nuc}$, consist of 12 α-helices arranged to create a three-layer "sandwich" that completely encompasses the ligand 1α,25 $(OH)_2D_3$ in a hydrophobic core.

Mice in which the gene for the $VDR_{nuc}$ has been deleted or rendered nonfunctional (VDR-KO) by targeted disruption of the DNA encoding the first or second zinc finger of the DNA-binding domain[25] display the phenotype of vitamin D-dependent rickets type II (VDDR-II). Except for the alopecia that appears at about 7 weeks, most of the features of this phenotype can be "rescued" by feeding the mice a diet high in calcium and lactose. Additionally, in spite of the widespread tissue distribution of the $VDR_{nuc}$, these animals are phenotypically normal at birth. These results suggest that there is biological redundancy with respect to many of the functions of the VDR. Interestingly, VDR KO mice have an impaired insulin secretory capacity[26] that may presage involvement of vitamin D nutritional status with glucose homeostasis.

**Rapid Responses of 1α,25$(OH)_2D_3$.** The "rapid" or non-genomic responses mediated by 1α,25$(OH)_2D_3$ were originally postulated to be mediated through interaction of 1α,25$(OH)_2D_3$ with a novel protein receptor located on the external membrane of the cell (Figure 3A); [27] this membrane receptor has now been shown to be the classic VDR (heretofore largely found in the nucleus and cytosol) associated with caveolae present in the plasma membrane of a variety of cells.[28] Using VDR knockout (KO) and wild-type mice, the rapid modulation of osteoblast ion channel responses by 1α,25$(OH)_2D_3$ was found to require the presence of a functional vitamin D nuclear/caveolae receptor.[29]

Rapid responses stimulated by 1α,25$(OH)_2D_3$ or 6-s-*cis* locked analogs of 1α,25$(OH)_2D_3$ (see below) acting through the $VDR_{mem}$ include the following: rapid stimulation by 1α,25$(OH)_2D_3$ of intestinal $Ca^{2+}$ absorption(transcaltachia);[30] opening of voltage-gated $Ca^{2+}$ and $Cl^-$[31] channels; store-operated $Ca^{2+}$ influx in skeletal muscle cells as modulated by phospholipase C, protein kinase C, and tyrosine kinases;[32] activation of protein kinase C;[33,34] and inhibition of activation of apoptosis in osteoblasts mediated by rapid activation of Src, phosphatidyl inositol 3′-kinase and JNK kinases.[35]

Careful study using structural analogs of 1,25$(OH)_2D_3$ has shown that the genomic and non-genomic responses to this conformationally flexible steroid hormone have different requirements for ligand structure.[21,36,37] For example, a key consideration is the position of rotation about the 6,7 single carbon-carbon bond, which can either be in the 6-s-*cis* or 6-s-*trans* orientation (Figure 1). The preferred shape of the ligand for $VDR_{nuc}$, determined from the X-ray crystal structure of the receptor occupied with ligand, is a 6-s-*trans* shaped bowl with the A-ring 30° above the plane of the C/D rings. In contrast, structure-function studies of rapid non-genomic actions of 1,25$(OH)_2D_3$ and its analogs show that the $VDR_{mem}$ prefers its ligand to have a 6-s-*cis* shape.[56]

### *24R,25$(OH)_2D_3$: Biological Properties*

**Background.** Compared with 1α,25$(OH)_2D_3$, the biological actions of 24R,25$(OH)_2D_3$ have been less studied. One key question that has attracted attention is whether 1α,25$(OH)_2D_3$ acting alone can generate all of the biological responses that are attributed to the parent vitamin $D_3$ or if, for some responses, a second vitamin $D_3$ metabolite may be required. Evidence has been presented to support the view that the combined presence of 1α,25$(OH)_2D_3$ and 24R,25$(OH)_2D_3$ are required to generate the complete spectrum of biological responses attributable to the parent vitamin $D_3$.[38] The key experiments demonstrated that when hens were raised from hatching to sexual maturity with only 1α,25$(OH)_2D_3$ as their sole source of vitamin D, fertile eggs appeared to develop normally but failed to hatch. However when the hens received a combination of 1α,25$(OH)_2D_3$ and 24R,25$(OH)_2$ $D_3$, hatchability was equivalent to that of hens given vitamin $D_3$.[39,40]

**24R,25$(OH)_2D_3$ and Bone.** Evidence for a biological role for 24R,25$(OH)_2D_3$ in the fracture-healing process has also been obtained using a chicken model system.[41,42] Preliminary evidence has been presented for the existence of a non-nuclear membrane receptor in the fracture-healing callus, which is specific for 24R,25$(OH)_2D_3$.[41,43] The work of Boyan and Schwartz[46] has focused directly on cartilage tissue and cells, and shows evidence for a unique membrane receptor for 24R,25$(OH)_2D_3$[44,45] that is linked to the initiation of rapid responses.

## Nutritional Aspects of Vitamin D

### *Recommended Dietary Allowance (RDA)*

The World Health Organization has defined the international unit (IU) of vitamin $D_3$ as "the vitamin D activity of 0.025 μg of the international standard preparation of crystalline vitamin $D_3$.[7]" Thus, 1.0 IU of vitamin $D_3$ is 0.025 μg, which is equivalent to 65.0 pmol. With the discovery of the metabolism of vitamin $D_3$ to other active seco-steroids, particularly $1\alpha,25(OH)_2D_3$, it was recommended that 1.0 IU of $1\alpha,25(OH)_2D_3$ be set equivalent in molar terms to that of the parent vitamin, $D_3$. Thus, 1.0 IU of $1\alpha,25(OH)_2D_3$ has been operationally defined to be equivalent to 65 pmol.

In addition to the fact that vitamin $D_3$ can be and is produced endogenously by sunlight exposure, it is also retained for relatively long periods of time in vertebrate tissues. For both of these reasons, it is difficult to determine with precision the minimum daily requirements for this seco-steroid and, in fact, the vitamin D requirement for healthy adults has never been precisely defined.

Since vitamin $D_3$ is produced in the skin after exposure to sunlight, the human does not have a requirement for vitamin D when sufficient sunlight is available. It has been estimated that exposure of just the face, hands, and wrists for 20 minutes 3 times per week to ambient sunlight at the latitude of Boston (42° N) will provide the equivalent of the daily dietary dose (200 IU) of vitamin $D_3$ for 1 week.[47] However man's tendency to wear clothes, to live in cities where tall buildings block adequate sunlight from reaching the ground, to live indoors, to use synthetic sunscreens that block ultraviolet rays, and to live in geographical regions of the world that do not receive adequate sunlight, all contribute to the inability of the skin to biosynthesize sufficient amounts of vitamin $D_3$.[48] Thus, vitamin D does become an important nutritional factor in the absence of adequate sunlight. The requirement for vitamin D is also known to be dependent on the age, sex, degree of exposure to the sun, season, and the amount of pigmentation in the skin.[49]

The current "adequate intake" (AI) allowance of vitamin D recommended in 1998 by the US Food and Nutrition Board of the Institute of Medicine is 200 IU/d (5 μg/d) for infants, children, and adult males and females (including during pregnancy and lactation) up to age 51. For males and females ages 51 to 70, the adequate indicated level is set at 400 IU/d (10 μg/d). For those over 70 years of age, the level is 600 IU (15 μg/d). Further, the currently stipulated tolerated upper intake level of vitamin $D_3$ is set at 2000 IU/d.[50]

It is known that a substantial proportion of the US population is exposed to suboptimal levels of sunlight; this is particularly true during the winter months.[51,52] Under these conditions, vitamin D becomes a true vitamin, which means that it must be supplied in the diet on a regular basis. Recent work suggests that winter-time vitamin D insufficiency is common in young Canadian women, and that the levels of vitamin D in food does not prevent this deficiency.[53] This has led Vieth and others[54,55] to ask whether the optimal requirement of vitamin D should be much higher than what is officially recommended. Further, a recent report documents the widespread deficiency of vitamin D in all regions of China, particularly in children.[56]

## *Food Sources*

Animal products constitute the bulk source of vitamin D that occurs naturally in unfortified foods. Saltwater fish such as herring, salmon, and sardines, and fish liver oils are good sources of vitamin $D_3$. Small quantities of vitamin $D_3$ are also derived from eggs, veal, beef, butter, and vegetable oils, whereas plants, fruits, and nuts are extremely poor sources of vitamin D. In the United States, fortification of foods such as milk (both fresh and evaporated), margarine and butter, cereals, and chocolate mixes help in meeting the RDA recommendations.[57] Because only fluid milk is fortified with vitamin D, other dairy products (e.g., cheese and yogurt) do not provide the vitamin.

## *Vitamin D Deficiency and Rickets*

The classic deficiency state resulting from a dietary absence of vitamin D or lack of ultraviolet (sunlight) exposure is the bone disease called rickets in children or osteomalacia in adults. The clinical features of rickets and osteomalacia depend upon the age of onset. The classical skeletal disorder of rickets includes deformity of the bones, especially in the knees, wrists, and ankles, as well as associated changes in the costochondral joint functions, sometimes called the rachitic rosary. If rickets develops in the first 6 months, infants may suffer from convulsions or develop tetany due to a low blood calcium level (usually $< 7$ mg/100 mL), but may have only minor skeletal changes. After 6 months, bone pain as well as tetany is likely to be present. Since osteomalacia occurs after growth and development of the skeleton are complete (i.e., the adult stage of life), its main symptoms are muscular weakness and bone pain, with little bone deformity.[14]

A characteristic feature of osteomalacia and rickets is the failure of the organic matrix of bone (osteoid) to calcify, leading to excessive uncalcified osteoid. In addition, there is often a high serum level of alkaline phosphatase, a fact that is often used to assist in the clinical diagnosis of osteomalacia. Low serum levels of $25(OH)D_3$ are also suggestive of rickets or osteomalacia. When the serum $25(OH)D_3$ level is below 5 ng/mL of serum, the individual is classified as being vitamin D deficient.[58-60] When the serum $25(OH)D_3$ level is below 10 ng/mL, the individual is "at risk" for the development of vitamin D deficiency.

The nutritional availability of vitamin D is particularly important in the newborn, the young child, and the elderly. Deprivation of sunlight through seasonal variation (winter),[49,61] skin pigmentation in Africans[62,63] or African Americans,[64] or clothing habits such as those of Muslims,[60,65] can all lead to the onset of clinical rickets or osteomalacia, characterized by low serum $25(OH)D_3$ levels. In the latter case, the clothing may cover the nursing infant as well, rendering the infant at risk for rickets if the mother is vitamin D deficient.

At the present time, it is not feasible to determine the circulating levels of vitamin D directly as a routine clinical chemistry assay. However, because of the rapid metabolism of both vitamin $D_3$ and vitamin $D_2$ to their cognate 25(OH)D's, Heaney[66] has proposed that nutritional vitamin D status can be inferred from the determination of circulating levels of 25(OH)$D_3$. One application is the demonstration in elderly subjects that optimal intestinal calcium absorption is only achieved when 25(OH)$D_3$ is present at 80 nmol/L of plasma.[66] This suggests, then, that that the daily intake of vitamin $D_3$ should be as high as 2200 IU to achieve the desired 25(OH)$D_3$ plasma concentration of 80 nmol/L.

This approach has also been applied to postmenopausal women and the elderly of both sexes.[67-70] The principal concern is that the presence of a chronic vitamin D deficiency in the elderly can lead to a deterioration in the quality of bone, thereby increasing the risk for traumatic fractures, which in the extreme can be life-threatening.[71,72] It has been reported that age-related changes in the 25(OH)$D_3$ versus parathyroid hormone relationship are why older adults require more vitamin D than that recommended by the official guidelines.[54,73]

When vitamin D deficiency is encountered in the clinical setting (e.g., in older or sick individuals and newborn infants), the physician naturally will want to provide replacement or supplemental vitamin D; this could be either be in the form of vitamin $D_3$ or vitamin $D_2$. It has been taught for the last 7 decades that in humans, vitamin $D_3$ and vitamin $D_2$ (Figure 1) are equally biologically efficacious. However, with the realization that the serum 25(OH)$D_3$ clinical assay provides the best assessment of vitamin D status,[74] it is appropriate to determine whether vitamin $D_2$ is as effective in elevating serum 25(OH)D levels in humans as is vitamin $D_3$. Earlier data suggesting that vitamin $D_3$ is substantially more effective than vitamin $D_2$[75] has been recently confirmed by Heaney et al.,[76] who found in a study in 20 healthy human volunteers that vitamin $D_2$ potency was less than one-third that of vitamin $D_3$, as judged by their relative ability to elevate serum 25(OH)D levels. Regrettably, for patients with poor vitamin D status, there are currently no high-dose vitamin $D_3$ formulations approved by the US Food and Drug Administration for clinical use; there are also no formulations of 25(OH)$D_3$ approved in the United States.

# Excess and Toxicity of Vitamin D

## *Dietary Vitamin D*

Vitamin D intoxication can result in nausea, vomiting, and poor appetite that can lead to weight loss and heart arrhythmias; serum calcium levels can become as elevated as 12 to 14 mg/dL,[7] and in the extreme can lead to soft tissue calcification in the heart and kidney.[77] Excessive amounts of vitamin D are not normally available from the usual dietary sources, so reports of vitamin D intoxication are rare. However, there is always the possibility that vitamin D intoxication may occur in individuals who are taking excessive amounts of supplemental vitamins. One report describes vitamin D intoxication occurring from drinking milk that had been fortified with inappropriately high levels of vitamin $D_3$.[78] A more recent report describes severe vitamin D intoxication of one family resulting from contamination of a household table sugar supply with extraordinary levels of vitamin D.[79] Symptoms of vitamin D intoxication include hypercalcemia, hypercalciuria, anorexia, nausea, vomiting, thirst, polyuria, muscular weakness, joint pains, diffuse demineralization of bones, and general disorientation. If allowed to go unchecked, death will eventually occur. The extent of toxicity has been shown in some instances to be related to the level of dietary intake of calcium.[80,81]

The Food and Nutrition Board of the National Institutes of Medicine have set the tolerable upper intake levels at 1000 IU/d for infants and 2000 IU/d for all other age groups.[74] The biological basis for intoxication resulting from the inappropriate intake of the parent vitamin $D_3$ is believed to be the unrestrained metabolism by the liver of the vitamin $D_3$ to 25(OH)$D_3$.

Vitamin D intoxication is thought to occur as a result of high plasma levels of 25(OH)D rather than high plasma $1\alpha$,25$(OH)_2D_3$ levels.[82,83] Patients suffering from hypervitaminosis D have been shown to exhibit a 15-fold increase in plasma 25(OH)D concentration compared with normal individuals; however, their $1\alpha$,25$(OH)_2D$ levels are not substantially altered.[84] It has also been shown that large concentrations of 25(OH)$D_3$ can mimic the actions of $1\alpha$,25$(OH)_2D_3$ at the level of the $VDR_{nuc}$,[84] which can lead to a massive stimulation of intestinal $Ca^{2+}$ absorption and bone $Ca^{2+}$ resorption, and ultimately the occurrence of soft tissue calcification and kidney stones.[77] The use of pamidronate, a bisphosphonate inhibitor of bone resorption, has been proposed to reduce the hypercalcemia secondary to acute vitamin D intoxication.[85]

## *Drug Forms of $1\alpha$,25$(OH)_2D_3$*

Table 1 lists the drug forms of $1\alpha$,25$(OH)_2D_3$ that are currently available for the treatment of several disease states, including hypoparathyroidism, vitamin D-resistant rickets, renal osteodystrophy (calcitriol[86,87] and paricalcitol[88]), osteoporosis (calcitriol[89,90]) and psoriasis (calcipotriene[91]). The potential for vitamin D intoxication, hypercalcemia and soft tissue calcification, is much higher when an individual has access to drug formulations of $1\alpha$,25$(OH)_2D_3$, since these medications bypass the stringent physiological control point of the vitamin D

**Table 1.** Drug Forms of Vitamin D Metabolites

| Compound Name | Generic Name | Commercial Name | Pharmaceutical Company | Effective Daily Dose* | Approved Use |
|---|---|---|---|---|---|
| 1α,25(OH)$_2$D$_3$ | Calcitriol | Rocaltrol | HoffmannLa Roche | 0.5–1.0 μg | RO, HP, O† |
| 1α,25(OH)$_2$D$_3$ | Calcitriol | Calcijex | Abbott | 0.5 μg (IV) | HC |
| 1α,25(OH)$_2$-19-nor-D$_2$ | Paricalcitol | Zemplar | Abbott | 2.8–7 μg (EOD) | SHP |
| 1α,24(OH)$_2$D$_3$ | Tacalcitol | Bonalfa | Teijin Ltd. (Japan) | 40–80 μg (topical) | PP |
| 1α,24S(OH)$_2$-22-ene-24-cyclopropyl-D$_3$ | Calcipotriene | Dovenex | Leo-Denmark | 40–80 μg (topical) | PP |
| 1α,24S(OH)$_2$-22-ene-24-cyclopropyl-D$_3$ | Calcipotriene | Dovenex | Westwood-Squibb | 40–80 μg (topical) | PP |
| 1α-OH-D$_3$ | Alfacalcidol | One-Alfa | Leo-Denmark | 1–2 μg | RO, HP, O, VDRR |
| 1α-OH-D$_3$ | Alfacalcidol | Alpha-D$_3$ | Teva-Israel | 0.25–1.0 μg | RO, O, HC, HP |
| – 1α-OH-D$_3$ | Alfacalcidol | OneAlfa | Teijin Ltd.-Japan | 0.25–1.0 μg | RO, O |
| 1α-OH-D$_3$ | Alfacalcidol | OneAlfa | Chugai- Japan | 0.25–1.0 μg | RO, O |
| 1α-OH-D$_2$ | Doxercalciferol | Hectorol | Bone Care | 10 μg four times/ week (15–30 mg/week) | SHP |
| 25(OH)D$_3$ | Calcifediol | Calderol | Organon-USA | 50–500 μg | RO |
| 25(OH)D$_3$ | Calcifediol | Dedrogyl | Roussel-UCLAF-France | 50–500 μg | RO |
| 10,19-dihydrotachysterol$_3$ | Dihydrotachysterol$_3$ | Hytakerol | Winthrop | 200–1000 μg | RO |
| 1α,25(OH)$_2$-22-oxa-D$_3$ | Maxacalcitol | Oxarol | Chugai-Japan | 5–10 μg three times/week (IV) | SHP |
| 1α,25(OH)$_2$-26,27-F$_6$-D$_3$ | Falecalcitriol | Fulstan Tablets | Sumitom D Pharmaceuticals-Japan | 0.15–0.35 μg | HC, SHP, RO,O |
| 1α,25(OH)$_2$-26,27-F$_6$-D$_3$ | Falecalcitriol | Hornel Tablets | Taisho Pharmaceuticals-Japan | 0.15–0.35 μg | HC, SHP, RO,O |

HC = hypocalcemia (frequently present in patients with renal osteodystrophy who are subjected to hemodialysis); HP = hypoparathyroidism and associated hypocalcemia which may frequently be encountered in patients with hypoparathyroidism, pseudohypoparathyroidism or in circumstances of post-surgical hypoparathyroidism; PO = postmenopausal osteoporosis; PP = plaque psoriasis; RO = renal osteodystrophy; SHP = secondary hyperparathyroidism associated with renal osteodystrophy; VDRR = vitamin D-resistant rickets.

* Oral dose unless otherwise indicated; eod = every other day.

† The use of Rocaltrol for postmenopausal osteoporosis is approved in Argentina, Australia, Austria, Czech Republic, Columbia, India, Ireland, Italy, Japan, Malaysia, Mexico, New Zealand, Peru, Philippines, South Korea, South Africa, Switzerland, Turkey, and the United Kingdom.

endocrine system, namely the 25(OH)D$_3$-1-hydroxylase of the kidney.

# Disease States in Man Related to Vitamin D

Figure 5 describes human disease states related to vitamin D and the vitamin D endocrine system. Conceptually, human clinical disorders related to vitamin D can be considered as those arising because of: 1) altered availability of vitamin D; 2) altered conversion of vitamin D$_3$ to 25(OH)D$_3$; 3) altered conversion of 25(OH)D$_3$ to 1α,25(OH)$_2$D$_3$ and/or 24R,25(OH)$_2$D$_3$; 4) variations in end organ responsiveness to 1α,25(OH)$_2$D$_3$ or possibly 24R,25(OH)$_2$D$_3$; and 5) other conditions with an uncertain relationship to vitamin D. Thus, the clinician/nutri-

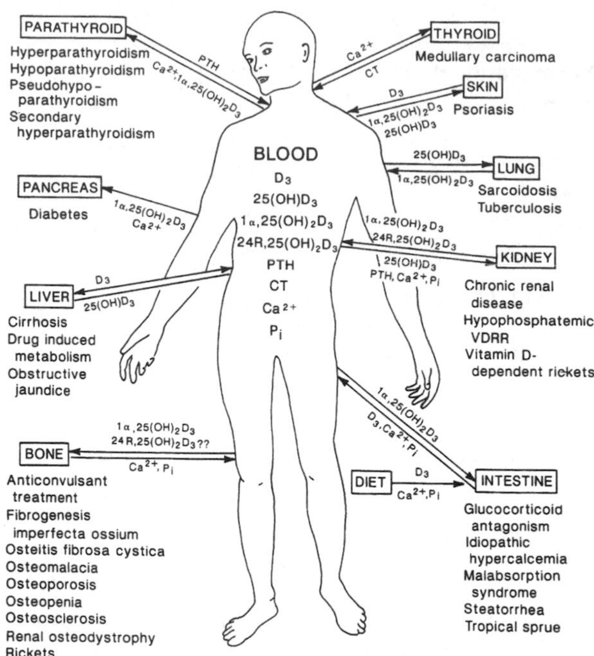


Figure 5. Human disease states related to the vitamin D endocrine system. Under the boxed headings (e.g., parathyroid, liver, bone, etc) are listed disease states occurring in man that have been shown or are believed to have some functional linkage between some aspect of the vitamin D endocrine system and that particular organ. The information associated with the arrows indicate the direction of flow of calcium, phosphate, or the calcium-regulating hormones vitamin $D_3$, $25(OH)D_3$, $1\alpha,25(OH)_2D_3$, $24R,25(OH)_2D_3$, parathyroid hormone (PTH), or calcitonin (CT). A presentation on each of these diseases states is given in Feldman, 2005.[1] VDRR, vitamin D-resistant rickets; Pi, inorganic phosphate.

tionist/biochemist is faced with the diagnostic problem of identifying parameters of hypersensitivity, antagonism, or resistance (including genetic aberrations) to vitamin D or one of the other of its metabolites, in addition to identifying perturbations of metabolism that result in problems in production and/or delivery of the hormonally active form, $1\alpha,25(OH)_2D_3$. A detailed consideration of this topic is beyond the scope of this presentation; more details are available elsewhere.[1,16]

# Vitamin D and Cancer

The relationship of vitamin D nutrition to cancer treatment and cancer chemoprevention was the topic of a recent meeting at the US National Institutes of Health (NIH), and the proceedings have recently been published.[92] One focus of the meeting was the pharmacological use of analogs of $1\alpha,25(OH)_2D_3$ to treat a variety of cancers, such as prostate cancer, colorectal cancer, leukemia, and breast cancer. It is becoming clear that drug surrogates for $1\alpha,25(OH)_2D_3$ may act at the site of the cancer to effect either an antiproliferative response or a cell differentiation response.

However, a nutritionally related vitamin D/cancer interface is possible because of the surprising number of extra-renal sites of the important $25(OH)D_3$-$1\alpha$-hydroxylase, the enzyme that produces the product steroid hormone.[93,94] Extra renal $1\alpha$-hydroxylase is present in breast, prostate, and colon cells and activated macrophages, and has been shown to produce small amounts of $1\alpha,25(OH)_2D_3$, which acts in a paracrine to cause beneficial anticancer effects. This then provides support for the concept of cancer chemoprevention. By administering high doses of vitamin D or $25(OH)D_3$ (the latter compound is the substrate for the $1\alpha$-hydroxylase), it is possible to enzymatically generate the steroid hormone that can operate locally to prevent both the early and later stages of transformation of normal into cancerous cells.

# Summary

Current evidence supports the concept that the classical biological actions of the nutritionally important fat-soluble vitamin D in mediating calcium homeostasis are supported by a complex vitamin D endocrine system that coordinates the metabolism of vitamin $D_3$ into $1\alpha,25(OH)_2D_3$ and $24R,25(OH)_2D_3$. It is now clear that the vitamin D endocrine system embraces many more target tissues than simply the intestine, bone, and kidney. Notable additions to this list include the pancreas, pituitary, breast tissue, placenta, hematopoietic cells, and skin and cancer cells of various origins (Figure 2). Key advances in understanding the mode of action of the $1\alpha,25(OH)_2D_3$ have been made by a thorough study of the vitamin D-resistant classical nuclear receptor as well as the emerging studies describing the presence of the classical vitamin D-resistant in the plasma membrane. Integral to these observations are efforts to define the signal transduction systems that are subservient to the nuclear and membrane receptors for $1\alpha,25(OH)_2D_3$ and to obtain a thorough study of the tissue distribution and subcellular localization of the gene products induced by this steroid hormone. There are clinical applications for $1\alpha,25(OH)_2D_3$ or related analogs for treatment of the bone diseases of renal osteodystrophy and osteoporosis, psoriasis, and hypoparathyroidism; other clinical targets for $1\alpha,25(OH)_2D_3$ currently under investigation include its use in leukemia, breast, prostate, and colon cancer, and as an immunosuppressive agent. An emerging human nutritional issue is the question of whether the RDA for vitamin $D_3$ should be adjusted upwards.

# References

1. Feldman D, Pike JW, Glorieux FH, eds. *Vitamin D.* San Diego: Elsevier; 2005; 1892 pp.
2. Bouillon R, Okamura WH, Norman AW. Structure-function relationships in the vitamin endocrine system. Endocr Rev. 1995;16:200–257.
3. Demay MB. Mouse models of vitamin D receptor

ablation. In: Feldman D, Pike JW, Glorieux FH, eds. *Vitamin D.* San Diego: Elsevier; 2005; 341–349.

4. Henry HL. The 25-Hydroxyvitamin D 1-α-hydroxylase. In: Feldman D, Pike JW, Glorieux FH, eds. *Vitamin D.* San Diego: Elsevier; 2005; 69–83.
5. Pike JW, Shevde NK. The vitamin D receptor. In: Feldman D, Pike JW, Glorieux FH, eds. *Vitamin D.* San Diego: Elsevier; 2005; 167–191.
6. Okamura WH, Zhu G-D. Chemistry and design: structural biology of vitamin D action. In: Feldman D, Pike JW, Glorieux FH, eds. *Vitamin D.* San Diego: Elsevier; 2005; 939–971.
7. Norman AW. *Vitamin D: The Calcium Homeostatic Steroid Hormone.* New York: Academic Press; 1979; 490 pp.
8. Haussler MR, Myrtle JF, Norman AW. The association of a metabolite of vitamin $D_3$ with intestinal mucosa chromatin, in vivo. J Biol Chem. 1968;243: 4055–4064.
9. Norman AW, Myrtle JF, Midgett RJ, et al. 1,25-Dihydroxycholecalciferol: identification of the proposed active form of vitamin $D_3$ in the intestine. Science. 1971;173:51–54.
10. Lawson DEM, Fraser DR, Kodicek E, et al. Identification of 1,25-dihydroxycholecalciferol, a new kidney hormone controlling calcium metabolism. Nature. 1971;230:228–230.
11. Holick MF, Schnoes HK, DeLuca HF. Identification of 1,25-dihydroxycholecalciferol, a form of vitamin $D_3$ metabolically active in the intestine. Proc Natl Acad Sci U S A. 1971;68:803–804.
12. Haussler MR, Norman AW. Chromosomal receptor for a vitamin D metabolite. Proc Natl Acad Sci U S A. 1969;62:155–162.
13. Commission on the Nomenclature of Biological Chemistry. Definitive rules for the nomenclature of amino acids, steroids, vitamins and carotenoids. J Am Chem Soc. 1960;82:5575–5586.
14. Norman AW, Litwack G. *Hormones.* Boca Raton, FL: Academic Press; 1987; 806 pp.
15. Norman AW, Henry HL. Vitamin D: Metabolism and mechanism of action. In: Favus MJ, ed. *Primer on the Metabolic Bone Diseases and Disorders of Mineral Metabolism.* New York: Raven Press; 1993; 63–70.
16. Reichel H, Koeffler HP, Norman AW. The role of the vitamin D endocrine system in health and disease. N Engl J Med. 1989;320:980–991.
17. Laing, CJ and Cooke, NE. Vitamin D binding protein. In: Feldman D, Pike JW, Glorieux FH, eds. *Vitamin D.* San Diego: Elsevier; 2005; 117–134.
18. Henry, HL. Vitamin D. In: Goodman HM, ed. *Handbook of Physiology. Section 7: The Endocrine System.* New York: Oxford; 2000; 699–718.
19. Kitanaka S, Takeyama K, Murayama A, et al. Inactivating mutations in the 25-hydroxyvitamin $D_3$ 1α-hydroxylase gene in patients with pseudovitamin D-deficiency rickets. N Engl J Med. 1998;338: 653–661.
20. Norman AW, Mizwicki MT, Norman DPG. Steroid hormone rapid actions, membrane receptors and a conformational ensemble model. Nature Reviews Drug Discovery. 2004;3:27–41.
21. Mizwicki MT, Keidel D, Bula CM, et al. Identification of an alternative ligand-binding pocket in the nuclear vitamin D receptor and its functional importance in 1α,25$(OH)_2$-vitamin $D_3$ signaling. Proc Natl Acad Sci U S A. 2004;101:12876–12881.
22. Whitfield, GK, Jurutka PW, Haussler CA, et al. Nuclear vitamin D receptor: Structure-function, molecular control of gene transcription and novel bioactions. In: Feldman D, Pike JW, Glorieux FH, eds. *Vitamin D.* San Diego: Elsevier; 2005; 219–328.
23. Mangelsdorf DJ, Thummel C, Beato M, et al. The nuclear receptor superfamily: The second decade. Cell. 1995;83:835–839.
24. Weatherman RV, Fletterick RJ, Scanlon TS. Nuclear receptor ligands and ligand-binding domains. Annu Rev Biochem. 1999;68:559–582.
25. Bula CM, Huhtakangas J, Olivera C, Bishop JE, Norman AW, Henry HL. Presence of a truncated form of the vitamin D receptor (VDR) in a strain of VDR-knockout mice. Endocrinology. 2005;146: 5581–5586.
26. Zeitz U, Weber K, Soegiarto DW, et al. Impaired insulin secretory capacity in mice lacking a functional vitamin D receptor. FASEB J. 2003;17:509–511.
27. Nemere I, Dormanen MC, Hammond MW, et al. Identification of a specific binding protein for 1α,25-dihydroxyvitamin $D_3$ in basal-lateral membranes of chick intestinal epithelium and relationship to transcaltachia. J Biol Chem. 1994;269:23750–23756.
28. Huhtakangas JA, Olivera CJ, Bishop JE, et al. The vitamin D receptor is present in caveolae-enriched plasma membranes and binds 1α,25$(OH)_2$-vitamin $D_3$ in vivo and in vitro. Mol Endocrinol. 2004;18: 2660–2671.
29. Zanello LP, Norman AW. Rapid modulation of osteoblast ion channel responses by 1α,25$(OH)_2$-vitamin $D_3$ requires the presence of a functional vitamin D nuclear receptor. Proc Natl Acad Sci U S A. 2004; 101:1589–1594.
30. Norman AW, Okamura WH, Farach-Carson MC, et al. Structure-function studies of 1,25-dihydroxyvitamin $D_3$ and the vitamin D endocrine system. 1,25-dihydroxy-pentadeuterio-previtamin $D_3$ (as a 6-s-*cis* analog) stimulates nongenomic but not genomic biological responses. J Biol Chem. 1993;268:13811–13819.
31. Zanello LP, Norman AW. Stimulation by 1α,25$(OH)_2$-vitamin $D_3$ of whole cell chloride currents in osteoblastic ROS 17/2.8 cells: A structure-function study. J Biol Chem. 1997;272:22617–22622.

32. Vazquez G, De Boland AR, Boland RL. 1α,25-Dihydroxy-vitamin-$D_3$-induced store-operated Ca2+ influx in skeletal muscle cells: modulation by phospholipase C, protein kinase C, and tyrosine kinases. J Biol Chem. 1998;273:33954–33960.
33. Schwartz Z, Ehland H, Sylvia VL, et al. 1α,25-Dihydroxyvitamin $D_3$ and 24R,25-dihydroxyvitamin $D_3$ modulate growth plate chondrocyte physiology via protein kinase C- dependent phosphorylation of extracellular signal-regulated kinase 1/2 mitogen-activated protein kinase. Endocrinology. 2002;143:2775–2786.
34. Schwartz Z, Sylvia VL, Larsson D, et al. 1α,25(OH)2$D_3$ regulates chondrocyte matrix vesicle protein kinase D (PKC) directly via G protein-dependent mechanisms and indirectly via incorporation of PKC during matrix vexicle biogenesis. J Biol Chem. 2002;277:11828–11837.
35. Vertino AM, Bula CM, Chen J-R, et al. Nongenotropic, anti-apoptotic signaling of 1α,25$(OH)_2$-vitamin $D_3$ and analogs through the ligand binding domain of the vitamin D receptor in osteoblasts and osteocytes. Mediation by Src, phosphatidylinositol 3-, and JNK kinases. J Biol Chem. 2005;280:14130–14137.
36. Norman AW, Henry HL, Bishop JE, et al. Different shapes of the steroid hormone 1α,25$(OH)_2$-vitamin $D_3$ act as agonists for two different receptors in the vitamin D endocrine system to mediate tenomic and rapid responses. Steroids. 2001;66:147–158.
37. Norman AW. 1α,25$(OH)_2$-vitamin $D_3$ mediated rapid and genomic responses are dependent upon critical structure-function relationships for both the ligand and receptor(s). In: Feldman D, Pike JW, Glorieux FH, eds. *Vitamin D*. San Diego: Elsevier; 2005; 381–407.
38. Norman AW, Henry HL, Malluche HH. 24R,25-dihydroxyvitamin $D_3$ and 1α,25-dihydroxyvitamin $D_3$ are both indispensable for calcium and phosphorus homeostasis. Life Sci. 1980;27:229–237.
39. Henry HL, Norman AW. Vitamin D: Two dihydroxylated metabolites are required for normal chicken egg hatchability. Science. 1978;201:835–837.
40. Norman AW, Leathers VL, Bishop JE. Studies on the mode of action of calciferol. XLVIII. Normal egg hatchability requires the simultaneous administration to the hen of 1α,25-dihydroxyvitamin $D_3$ and 24R,25-dihydroxyvitamin $D_3$. J Nutr. 1983;113:2505–2515.
41. Kato A, Seo E-G, Einhorn TA, et al. Studies on 24R,25-dihydroxyvitamin $D_3$: Evidence for a non-nuclear membrane receptor in the chick tibial fracture-healing callus. Bone. 1998;23:141–146.
42. Seo E-G, Einhorn TA, Norman AW. 24R,25-dihydroxyvitamin $D_3$: An essential vitamin $D_3$ metabolite for both normal bone integrity and healing of tibial fracture in chicks. Endocrinology. 1997;138:3864–3872.
43. Seo E-G, Kato A, Norman AW. Evidence for a 24R,25(OH)2-vitamin $D_3$ receptor/binding protein in a membrane fraction isolated from a chick tibial fracture-healing callus. Biochem Biophys Res Commun. 1996;225:203–208.
44. Pedrozo HA, Schwartz Z, Rimes S, et al. Physiological importance of the 1,25(OH)2$D_3$ membrane receptor and evidence for a membrane receptor specific for 24,25(OH)2$D_3$. J Bone Miner Res. 1999;14:856–867.
45. Boyan BD, Bonewald LF, Sylvia VL, et al. Evidence for distinct membrane receptors for 1α,25-(OH)2$D_3$ and 24R,25-(OH)2$D_3$ in osteoblasts. Steroids. 2002;67:235–246.
46. Boyan BD, Jennings EG, Wang L, Schwartz Z. Mechanisms regulating differential activation of membrane-mediated signaling by 1α,25(OH)(2) D(3) and 24R,25(OH)(2)D(3). J Steroid Biochem Mol Biol. 2004;89–90:309–315.
47. Adams JS, Clemens TL, Parrish JA, Holick MF. Vitamin-D synthesis and metabolism after ultraviolet irradiation of normal and vitamin-D-deficient subjects. N Engl J Med. 1982;306:722–725.
48. Holick MF. Environmental factors that influence the cutaneous production of vitamin D. Am J Clin Nutr. 1995;(61 suppl):638S–645S.
49. Harris SS, Dawson-Hughes B. Seasonal changes in plasma 25-hydroxyvitamin D concentrations of young American black and white women. Am J Clin Nutr. 1998;67:1232–1236.
50. Food and Nutrition Board, Institute of Medicine. Dietary Reference Intakes: A Risk Assessment Model for Establishing Upper Intake Levels for Nutrients. Washington, DC: National Academies Press; 1998. Available online at: http://www.nap.edu/openbook/0309063485/html/. Accessed February 27, 2006.
51. Webb AR, Holick MF. The role of sunlight in the cutaneous production of vitamin $D_3$. Ann Rev Nutr. 1988;8:375–399.
52. Webb AR, Pilbeam C, Hanafin N, Holick MF. An evaluation of the relative contributions of exposure to sunlight and of diet to the circulating concentrations of 25-hydroxyvitamin D in an elderly nursing home population in Boston. Am J Clin Nutr. 1990;51:1075–1081.
53. Vieth R, Cole DE, Hawker GA, et al. Wintertime vitamin D insufficiency is common in young Canadian women, and their vitamin D intake does not prevent it. Eur J Clin Nutr. 2001;55:1091–1097.
54. Vieth R. Why the optimal requirement for Vitamin $D_3$ is probably much higher than what is officially recommended for adults. J Steroid Biochem Mol Biol. 2004;89–90:575–579.
55. Whiting SJ, Calvo MS. Dietary recommendations

for vitamin D: a critical need for functional end points to establish an estimated average requirement. J Nutr. 2005;135:304–309.
56. Fraser DR. Vitamin D-deficiency in Asia. J Steroid Biochem Mol Biol. 2004;89–90:491–495.
57. Collins ED, Norman AW. Vitamin D. In: Machlin LJ, ed. *Handbook of Vitamins*. New York: Marcel Dekker; 1990; 59–98.
58. Seino Y, Ishii T, Shimotsuji T, et al. Plasma active vitamin D concentration in low birthweight infants with rickets and its response to vitamin D treatment. Arch Dis Child. 1981;56:628–632.
59. Dawson-Hughes B, Harris SS, Dallal GE. Plasma calcidiol, season, and serum parathyroid hormone concentrations in healthy elderly men and women. Am J Clin Nutr. 1997;65:67–71.
60. Mawer EB, Stanbury SW, Robinson MJ, et al. Vitamin D nutrition and vitamin D metabolism in the premature human neonate. Clin Endo. 1986;25: 641–649.
61. Salamone LM, Dallal GE, Zantos D, et al. Contributions of vitamin D intake and seasonal sunlight exposure to plasma 25-hydroxyvitamin D concentration in elderly women. Am J Clin Nutr. 1994;59: 80–86.
62. Thacher TD, Fischer PR, Pettifor JM, et al. A comparison of calcium, vitamin D, or both for nutritional rickets in Nigerian children. N Engl J Med. 1999; 341:563–568.
63. Oginni LM, Worsfold M, Oyelami OA, et al. Etiology of rickets in Nigerian children. J Pediat. 1996; 128:692–694.
64. Kreiter SR, Schwartz RP, Kirkman HN Jr, et al. Nutritional rickets in African American breast-fed infants. J Pediatr. 2000;137:153–157.
65. Preece MA, Ford JA, McIntosh WB, et al. Vitamin-D deficiency amoung Asian immigrants to Britain. Lancet. 1973;7809:907–910.
66. Heaney RP. The Vitamin D requirement in health and disease. J Steroid Biochem Mol Biol. 2005;97: 13–19.
67. Wishart JM, Horowitz M, Need AG, et al. Relations between calcium intake, calcitriol, polymorphisms of the vitamin D receptor gene, and calcium absorption in premenopausal women. Am J Clin Nutr. 1997;65: 798–802.
68. Utiger RD. The need for more vitamin D. N Engl J Med. 1998;338:828–829.
69. Harris SS, Dawson-Hughes B. Plasma vitamin D and 25OHD responses of young and old men to supplementation with vitamin $D_3$. J Am Coll Nutr. 2002;21:357–362.
70. Lips P. Which circulating level of 25-hydroxyvitamin D is appropriate? J Steroid Biochem Mol Biol. 2004; 89–90:611–614.
71. Heaney RP. Age considerations in nutrient needs for bone health: older adults. J Am Coll Nutr. 1996;15: 575–578.
72. Chapuy MC, Arlot ME, Delmas PD, Meunier PJ. Effect of calcium and cholecalciferol treatment for three years on hip fractures in elderly women. Brit Med J. 1994;308:1081–1082.
73. Vieth R, Ladak Y, Walfish PG. Age-related changes in the 25-hydroxyvitamin D versus parathyroid hormone relationship suggest a different reason why older adults require more vitamin D. J Clin Endocrinol Metab. 2003;88:185–191.
74. Food and Nutrition Board, Institute of Medicine. Dietary Reference Intakes for Calcium, Phosphorus, Magnesium, Vitamin D, and Fluoride. Washington, DC: National Academies Press; 1997. Available online at: http://www.nap.edu/books/0309063507/html. Accessed February 27, 2006.
75. Trang H, Cole DE, Rubin LA, et al. Evidence that vitamin $D_3$ increases serum 25-hydroxyvitain D more efficiently that does vitamin $D_3$. Am J Clin Nutr. 1998;68:854–858.
76. Armas LAG, Hollis BW, Heaney RP. Vitamin $D_2$ is much less effective than vitamin $D_3$ in humans. J Clin Endocrinol Metab 2004;89:5387–5391.
77. Hartenbower DL, Stanley TM, Coburn JW, Norman AW. Serum and renal histologic changes in the rat following administration of toxic amounts of 1,25-dihydroxyvitamin $D_3$. In: Norman AW, Schaefer K, von Herrath D, et al, eds. *Vitamin D: Biochemical, Chemical and Clinical Aspects Related to Calcium Metabolism*. Berlin: Walter de Gruyter; 1977; 587–589.
78. Jacobus CH, Holick MF, Shao Q, et al. Hypervitaminosis D associated with drinking milk. N Engl J Med. 1992;326:1173–1177.
79. Vieth R, Pinto TR, Reen BS, Wong MM. Vitamin D poisoning by table sugar. Lancet. 2002;359:672.
80. Beckman MJ, Johnson JA, Goff JP, et al. The role of dietary calcium in the physiology of vitamin D toxicity: Excess dietary vitamin $D_3$ blunts parathyroid hormone induction of kidney 1-hydroxylase. Arch Biochem Biophys. 1995;319:535–539.
81. Rubin MR, Thys-Jacobs S, Chan FKW, Koberle LMC, Bilezikian JP. Hypercalcemia due to vitamin D toxicity. In: Feldman D, Pike JW, Glorieux FH, eds. *Vitamin D*. San Diego: Elsevier; 2005; 1355–1377.
82. Hughes MR, Baylink DJ, Jones PG, Haussler MR. Radioligand receptor assay for 25-hydroxyvitamin $D_2/D_3$ and 1$\alpha$,25-dihydroxyvitamin $D_2/D_3$. J Clin Invest. 1976;58:61–70.
83. Kistler A, Galli B, Horst RL, et al. Effects of vitamin D derivatives on soft tissue calcification in neonatal and calcium mobilization in adult rats. Arch Toxicol. 1989;63:394–400.
84. Brumbaugh PF, Haussler MR. 1$\alpha$,25-Dihydroxyvi-

tamin $D_3$ receptor: Competitive binding of vitamin D analogs. Life Sci. 1973;13:1737–1746.

85. Lee DC, Lee GY. The use of pamidronate for hypercalcemia secondary to acute vitamin D intoxication. J Toxicol Clin Toxicol. 1998;36:719–721.
86. Brickman AS, Sherrard DJ, Jowsey J, et al. 1,25-Dihydroxy-cholecalciferol: Effect on skeletal lesions and plasma parathyroid hormone levels in uremic osteodystrophy. Ann Intern Med. 1974;134:883–888.
87. Henderson RG, Ledingham JGG, Oliver DO, et al. The effects of 1,25-dihydroxycholecalciferol on calcium absorption, muscle weakness and bone disease in chronic renal failure. Lancet. 1974;7854:379–384.
88. Martin KJ, González EA, Gellens M, et al. 19-Nor-1-α-25-dihydroxyvitamin $D_2$ (paricalcitol) safely and effectively reduces the levels of intact parathyroid hormone in patients on hemodialysis. J Am Soc Nephrol. 1998;9:1427–1432.
89. Gallagher JC. Metabolic effects of synthetic calcitriol (Rocaltrol) in the treatment of postmenopausal osteoporosis. Metabolism. 1990;39(suppl 1):27–29.
90. Tilyard MW, Spears GFS, Thomson J, Dovey S. Treatment of postmenopausal osteoporosis with calcitriol or calcium. N Engl J Med. 1992;326: 357–362.
91. Van de Kerkhof PC. An update on vitamin $D_3$ analogues in the treatment of psoriasis. Skin Pharmacol. 1998;11:2–10.
92. Bouillon R, Moody T, Sporn M, et al. NIH deltanoids meeting on vitamin D and cancer. Conclusion and strategic options. J Steroid Biochem Mol Biol. 2005;97:3–5.
93. Townsend K, Banwell CM, Guy M, et al. Autocrine metabolism of vitamin D in normal and malignant breast tissue. Clin Cancer Res. 2005;11:3579–3586.
94. Hewison M, Kantorovich V, Liker HR, et al. Vitamin D-mediated hypercalcemia in lymphoma: evidence for hormone production by tumor-adjacent macrophages. J Bone Miner Res. 2003;18:579–582.
95. Norman AW, Silva FR. Structure function studies: Identification of vitamin D analogs for the ligand-binding domains of important proteins in the vitamin D-endocrine system. Rev Endocr Metab Disord. 2001;2:229–238.

# 15 Vitamin E

Maret G. Traber

## Introduction

Unlike most vitamins, which function as cofactors or have specific metabolic functions, vitamin E is unique in human nutrition because its major, if not sole, function is as an antioxidant. Consequently, vitamin E deficiency symptoms in target tissues are dependent not only upon vitamin E concentrations, but also on the degree of oxidative stress. This chapter will describe vitamin E structures and antioxidant properties; its distribution in food; its role in lipoprotein transport, delivery to tissues, and metabolism; and its safety and role in chronic disease prevention.

## Definitions, Structures, and Antioxidant Activity

Vitamin E is the collective name for molecules that exhibit the antioxidant activity of α-tocopherol. Vitamin E was discovered in 1922 when it was found to be required by pregnant rats to prevent the resorption of fetuses.[1] At least eight different molecules (tocopherols and tocotrienols) have α-tocopherol antioxidant activity.[2] These forms vary in the number of methyl groups on the chromanol ring: trimethyl (α-), dimethyl (β- or γ-), and monomethyl (δ-). The tocopherols have a chromanol ring with a phytyl tail, while the tocotrienols have an unsaturated tail (Figure 1).

## Vitamin E Form Required By Humans: α-Tocopherol

The naturally occurring form of α-tocopherol is *RRR*-α-tocopherol.[2] This nomenclature means that the chiral carbons are in the *R*-conformation at positions 2, 4′, and 8′. Unlike most other vitamins, chemically synthesized α-tocopherol is not identical to the naturally occurring form. Synthetic α-tocopherol is called *all-rac*-α tocopherol (*all racemic* or *dl*) and contains an equal mixture of eight different stereoisomers (*RRR*, *RSR*, *RRS*, *RSS*, *SRR*, *SSR*, *SRS*, *SSS*), all of which have equal antioxidant, but differing biologic activities.

The 2 position of α-tocopherol (the junction of the ring and tail) is critical for α-tocopherol biologic activity. Only 2*R*-α-tocopherol forms meet human vitamin E requirements.[2] *SRR*-α-tocopherol is prototypic of the 2S-forms and has been used to study synthetic vitamin E kinetics.

Vitamin E supplements often contain esters of α-tocopherol such as α-tocopheryl acetate, succinate, or nicotinate. The ester form prevents the oxidation of vitamin E and prolongs its shelf life. Following oral administration, these esters are readily hydrolyzed and α-tocopherol (unesterified form) is absorbed.[3]

## Antioxidant Activity

Vitamin E, a potent peroxyl radical scavenger, is a chain-breaking antioxidant that prevents the propagation of free radicals in membranes and in plasma lipoproteins. When peroxyl radicals (ROO•) are formed, they react 1000 times faster with vitamin E (Vit E-OH) than with PUFA (RH).[4] The hydroxyl group of tocopherol reacts with the peroxyl radical to form the corresponding hydroperoxide and the tocopheroxyl radical (Vit E-O•):

In the presence of vitamin E:

$$\text{ROO}\bullet + \text{Vit E-OH} \rightarrow \text{ROOH} + \text{Vit E-O}\bullet$$

In the absence of vitamin E:

$$\text{ROO}\bullet + \text{RH} \rightarrow \text{ROOH} + \text{R}\bullet$$
$$\text{R}\bullet + O_2 \rightarrow \text{ROO}\bullet$$

The tocopheroxyl radical (Vit E-O•) reacts with vitamin C (or other hydrogen donors, AH), thereby oxidizing the latter and returning vitamin E to its reduced state:

$$\text{Vit E-O}\bullet + \text{AH} \rightarrow \text{Vit E-OH} + \text{A}\bullet$$

This phenomenon has led to the idea of "vitamin E recycling," in which the antioxidant function of oxidized vitamin E is continuously restored by other antioxidants.

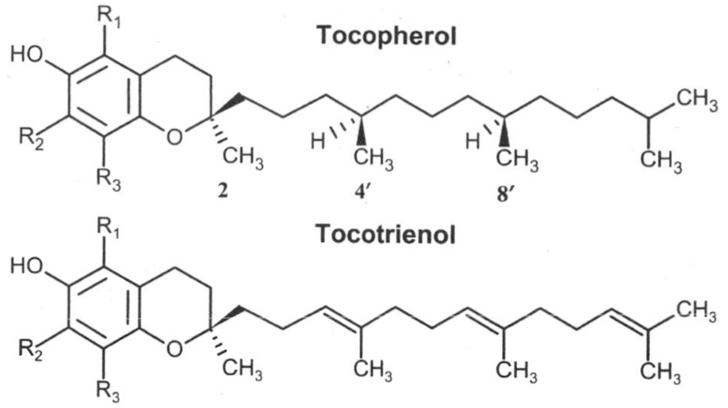

Tocopherol

Tocotrienol

| Compound | $R_1$ | $R_2$ | $R_3$ |
|---|---|---|---|
| α-tocopherol | $CH_3$ | $CH_3$ | $CH_3$ |
| β-tocopherol | $CH_3$ | H | $CH_3$ |
| γ-tocopherol | H | $CH_3$ | $CH_3$ |
| δ-tocopherol | H | H | $CH_3$ |
| α-tocotrienol | $CH_3$ | $CH_3$ | $CH_3$ |
| β-tocotrienol | $CH_3$ | H | $CH_3$ |
| γ-tocotrienol | H | $CH_3$ | $CH_3$ |
| δ-tocotrienol | H | H | $CH_3$ |

Figure 1. Tocopherols and tocotrienols. Compounds with vitamin E antioxidant activity have a chromanol head with a hydroxyl group and varying numbers of methyl groups, as indicated. Tocopherols have 3 chiral centers in the phytyl tail at positions 2, 4′, and 8′.

The "antioxidant network" depends upon the supply of aqueous antioxidants and the metabolic activity of cells. This interaction of vitamins E and C has been demonstrated in humans under oxidative stress. Specifically, cigarette smokers with the lowest plasma ascorbic acid concentrations had the fastest vitamin E disappearance rates.[5]

Further information concerning the reactions of tocopherols and tocotrienols in vivo and in vitro can be found in the extensive review by Kamal-Eldin and Appelqvist.[6] Since the tocopheroxyl radical can be reduced back to tocopherol by ascorbate or other reducing agents, oxidized tocopherols are usually not found in vivo. Liebler et al.[7] suggest that biologically relevant oxidation products formed from α-tocopherol include 4a,5-epoxy- and 7,8-epoxy-8a(hydroperoxy)tocopherones and their respective hydrolysis products, 2,3-epoxy-tocopherol quinone and 5,6-epoxy-α-tocopherol quinone. However, these products are formed during in vitro oxidation; their importance in vivo is unknown.[8]

## Content of Foods

γ-Tocopherol is the most abundant tocopherol found in the US diet.[9] However, α-tocopherol, not γ-tocopherol, and specifically only the 2*R*-forms of α-tocopherol, were defined by the Food and Nutrition Board of the US Institute of Medicine to meet human vitamin E requirements.[2] This change from the 1989 RDA makes vitamin E one of the most difficult nutrients to obtain from the diet. Only 8% of men and 2% of women in the United States had dietary vitamin E intakes[10] that met the 2000 Estimated Average Requirement (EAR, 12 mg α-tocopherol/d).[2] Moreover, most individuals obtain dietary vitamin E from high-energy, high-fat foods that are not particularly α-tocopherol rich.[10] Some examples of vitamin E food sources are shown in Table 1.

**Table 1.** 2*R*-α-Tocopherol Contents of Foods

| | Serving Size | mg/serving |
|---|---|---|
| Cereals ready-to-eat, fortified | 1 cup | 13.50 |
| Sunflower seeds, dry roasted | 1/4 cup | 8.35 |
| Almonds | 1 oz (24 nuts) | 7.33 |
| Spinach, cooked | 1 cup | 6.73 |
| Oil, sunflower | 1 tbsp | 5.59 |
| Tomato sauce | 1 cup | 5.10 |
| Oil, safflower | 1 tbsp | 4.64 |
| Hazelnuts | 1 oz | 4.26 |
| Carrot juice | 1 cup | 2.74 |
| Beet greens, cooked | 1 cup | 2.61 |
| Potato chips | 1 oz | 2.58 |
| Potato, french fried | 1 large | 2.57 |
| Sweet potato, canned | 1 cup | 2.55 |
| Broccoli, chopped, cooked | 1 cup | 2.43 |
| Oil, canola | 1 tbsp | 2.39 |
| Peppers, sweet, red, raw | 1 cup | 2.35 |
| Oil, olive | 1 tbsp | 1.94 |
| Oil, soybean | 1 tbsp | 1.65 |

USDA National Nutrient Database for Standard Reference. Available online at http://www.nal.usda.gov/fnic/foodcomp/search.

The richest dietary sources of vitamin E are edible vegetable oils.[9] Most oils contain varying amounts of the tocopherols; few oils contain tocotrienols. α-Tocopherol is especially high in wheat germ oil, safflower oil, and sunflower oil. Soybean and corn oils contain predominantly γ-tocopherol, as well as some tocotrienols. Cottonseed oil contains both α- and γ-tocopherols in equal proportion. Palm oil contains large amounts of α- and γ-tocotrienols and some α-tocopherol. Nuts, especially almonds, are also good sources of vitamin E, while fruits and vegetables—good sources of antioxidants such as vitamin C, flavonoids and carotenoids—are not good sources of vitamin E. Indeed, the major food source of vitamin E is dessert.[11]

## Dietary Reference Intakes

### *Recommended Dietary Allowance for α-Tocopherol*

In 2000, the Food and Nutrition Board published "Dietary Reference Intakes for Vitamin C, Vitamin E, Selenium, and Carotenoids."[2] The Recommended Dietary Allowances (RDAs) represent the daily α-tocopherol

**Table 2.** Criteria and Dietary Reference Intake Values for Vitamin E by Life Stage Group

| Life Stage Group | Criterion | EAR* | RDA† | AI‡ | UL§ |
|---|---|---|---|---|---|
| Premature infants | | | | | 21 |
| 0–6 months | Average vitamin E intake from human milk | | | 4 | |
| 7–12 months | Extrapolation from 0–6 months AI | | | 5 | |
| 1–3 years | Extrapolation from adult EAR | 5 | 6 | | 200 |
| 4–8 years | Extrapolation from adult EAR | 6 | 7 | | 300 |
| 9–13 years | Extrapolation from adult EAR | 9 | 11 | | 600 |
| 14–18 years | Extrapolation from adult EAR | 12 | 15 | | 800 |
| >18 years | Intakes sufficient to prevent hydrogen peroxide-induced erythrocyte hemolysis in vitro | 12 | 15 | | 1000 |
| Pregnancy | | | | | |
| ≤ 18 years | Adolescent EAR | 12 | 15 | | 800 |
| 19–50 years | Adult EAR | 12 | 15 | | 1000 |
| Lactation | | | | | |
| ≤ 18 years | Adolescent EAR plus average amount of vitamin E secreted in human milk | 16 | 19 | | 800 |
| 19–50 years | Adolescent EAR plus average amount of vitamin E secreted in human milk | 16 | 19 | | 1000 |

* EAR = Estimated Average Requirement: The intake that meets the estimated nutrient needs of half the individuals in a group.
† RDA = Recommended Dietary Allowance: The intake that meets the nutrient needs of almost all (97–98%) of individuals in a group.
‡ AI = Adequate Intake: The observed average or experimentally determined intake by a defined population or subgroup that appears to sustain a defined nutritional status. For healthy infants receiving human milk, the AI is the mean intake.
§ UL = Tolerable Upper Intake Level: The highest level of daily nutrient intake that is likely to pose no risk of adverse health effects in almost all individuals.
Data from Food and Nutrition Board, Institute of Medicine, 2000.[2]

intakes required to ensure adequate nutrition in 95% to 97.5% of the population, and are an overestimation of the level needed for most people in any given age or gender group (Table 2).[2]

The vitamin E requirement is based on the observation that only supplements containing α-tocopherol have been shown to reverse vitamin E deficiency symptoms in humans. The α-tocopherol amounts were based primarily on the amounts necessary to correct abnormal erythrocyte hemolysis in subjects who had consumed experimental vitamin E-deficient diets for 5 to 7 years.[2] Serum concentrations (in response to known supplemental vitamin E intakes) that prevented in vitro peroxide-induced erythrocyte hemolysis were used to determine EARs. Supplements containing either *RRR*- or *all-rac*-α-tocopherol were used to reverse vitamin E abnormal erythrocyte hemolysis, and therefore correction factors were developed to convert international units to milligrams of 2*R*-α-tocopherol.

The factors to convert international units to milligrams are 0.45 times the IU for *all-rac*- and 0.67 times the IU for *RRR*-α-tocopherol.[2] For example, if a vitamin E supplement is labeled 400 IU *dl*-α-tocopheryl acetate, then 400 times 0.45 equals 180 mg 2*R*-α-tocopherol, but if it is labeled 400 IU *d*-α-tocopheryl acetate, then 400 times 0.67 equals 268 mg 2*R*-α-tocopherol. These conversions are used only to estimate intakes relative to the RDA; different conversion factors are used to assess intakes relative to the upper limit (UL).

## Safety and Upper Limits

The recommendation by the Food and Nutrition Board is that the UL for any supplements containing α-tocopherol is 1000 mg for adults.[2] Reports of adverse effects of vitamin E supplements in humans are sufficiently rare that data from multiyear studies in rats fed high dietary vitamin E levels were used to set the ULs.[2] No UL was set for infants, as food was recommended as the only vitamin E source for them. However, a UL of 21 mg/d was suggested for premature infants with birth weights of 1.5 kg, based on the adult UL. The ULs are also shown in Table 2.

The UL was set only for vitamin E supplements and not for food, because it is almost impossible to consume enough α-tocopherol-containing foods to achieve a daily

1000 mg intake for prolonged periods of time. The UL was defined for both 2*R*- and 2*S*-α-tocopherols, because all of the stereoisomeric forms in *all-rac*-α-tocopherol are absorbed and delivered to the liver. The appropriate conversion factors are different from those above for *all-rac*-α-tocopherol. The factors to convert international units to milligrams are 0.9 times the IU for *all-rac*- and 0.67 times the IU for *RRR*-α-tocopherol. The UL amounts given in IU are 1100 IU for *all-rac*- and 1500 IU for *RRR*-α-tocopherol. The UL for *RRR*-α-tocopherol is apparently higher, because each capsule of *RRR*-α-tocopherol contains fewer milligrams of α-tocopherol than does one containing *all-rac*-α-tocopherol.

A review of the literature on vitamin E safety has been published recently,[12] and confirms the findings from the Food and Nutrition Board. However, reports from three clinical trials have suggested adverse vitamin E effects in humans under special circumstances. One study was a 3-year, double-blind trial of antioxidants (vitamins E and C, β-carotene, and selenium) in 160 subjects on simvastatin-niacin therapy.[13] In subjects taking antioxidants, there was less benefit of the drugs in raising high-density lipoprotein (HDL) cholesterol than was expected, and there was an increase in clinical end points (arteriographic evidence of coronary stenosis, or the occurrence of a first cardiovascular event, including death, myocardial infarction, stroke, or revascularization).[13] The Women's Angiographic Vitamin and Estrogen (WAVE) Trial, was a randomized, double-blind trial of 423 postmenopausal women with at least one coronary stenosis at baseline coronary angiography. In the postmenopausal women on hormone replacement therapy, all-cause mortality was increased in women assigned to antioxidant vitamins compared with placebo (HR, 2.8; 95% CI, 1.1–7.2; $P = .047$).[14] The "HopeToo" trial suggested that patients at high risk for coronary heart disease taking vitamin E were at increased risk of left-ventricular dysfunction.[15] Interestingly, none of these trials had the same adverse effect of vitamin E. Moreover, a meta-analysis evaluating the relationship of vitamin E supplements with all-cause mortality could not define a mechanism for adverse vitamin E effects.[16] Traber[17] proposed that the adverse effects seen in clinical trials in patients consuming a variety of pharmaceutical agents were a result of vitamin E-mediated alterations in xenobiotic metabolism. This hypothesis is based on the increase in vitamin E metabolism in response to supplements and the potential for alterations in xenobiotic metabolism and disposition, as discussed below.

High vitamin E intakes are associated with an increased tendency to bleed.[2] It is not known if increased bleeding is a result of decreased platelet aggregation caused by an inhibition of protein kinase C by α-tocopherol, some other platelet-related mechanism, or decreased clotting due to a vitamin K and E interactions causing abnormal blood clotting.[2] Patients on anticoagulant therapy should be monitored when taking vitamin E supplements to insure adequate vitamin K intakes.[18]

# Biological Activities of the Tocopherols

### *Intestinal Absorption*

All vitamin E forms are absorbed, along with fats, into intestinal cells and incorporated in chylomicrons for secretion into lymph.[19] The major steps from micellar uptake to enterocyte trafficking and incorporation into chylomicrons are largely unknown. Fat malabsorption syndromes (e.g., cholestatic liver disease) and genetic abnormalities in either lipoprotein synthesis (e.g., abetalipoproteinemia) or the α-tocopherol transfer protein (α-TTP) (e.g., ataxia with vitamin E deficiency, or AVED) result in vitamin E malabsorption or abnormally low plasma α-tocopherol transport, respectively.[19]

Vitamin E absorption from supplements is poor when the supplement is consumed without fat, as was observed when vitamin E pills were consumed without food.[20] Moreover, vitamin E bioavailability is highly influenced by prandial status.[21] However, the amount of dietary fat needed for optimal vitamin E absorption is unknown.

### *Lipoprotein Transport*

Unlike other fat-soluble vitamins that have specific plasma transport proteins, vitamin E is transported nonspecifically in all of the plasma lipoproteins. Once chylomicron remnants containing dietary vitamin E reach the liver, only one form of vitamin E, α-tocopherol, is preferentially secreted by the liver into the plasma in very-low-density lipoproteins (VLDL).[19] Once in the circulation, VLDL are delipidated to form low-density lipoproteins (LDL). During this process, vitamin E is transferred to HDLs, which can transfer vitamin E to all of the circulating lipoproteins.[19] Thus, the liver, not the intestine, discriminates between tocopherols. All lipoproteins transport vitamin E, and all mechanisms for delivery of lipids from lipoproteins to tissues (e.g., receptors) deliver vitamin E along with the lipoprotein contents. This phenomenon was demonstrated in a porcine blood-brain barrier model in which both the SR-B1 receptor and lipoprotein lipase were demonstrated to deliver α-tocopherol to cells.[22]

# α-Tocopherol-Transfer Protein

The liver preferentially secretes α-tocopherol into plasma under the control of the hepatic α-TTP, as shown in patients with genetic α-TTP defects[23,24] and in α-TTP-knockout mice (*Ttpa*$^{-/-}$).[25]

Liver α-TTP has been isolated and its cDNA sequences reported.[26] α-TTP has been crystallized and the α-tocopherol-binding pocket identified.[27,28] Interestingly, the pocket causes α-tocopherol to fold such that the 2 position is critical for the fit into the pocket.

## Plasma Vitamin E kinetics

A kinetic model of vitamin E transport in plasma has been described.[29] In normal subjects, the fractional disappearance rates of *RRR*-α-tocopherol (0.4 ± 0.1 pools/d) were significantly ($P < 0.01$) slower than for *SRR*-α-tocopherol (1.2 ± 0.6 pools/d). The apparent half-life of *RRR*-α-tocopherol was about 48 h, while *SRR*-α-tocopherol had a half-life of approximately 13 h.[29]

Vitamin E kinetics of α- and γ-tocopherols have also been studied.[30] Plasma γ-tocopherol exponential disappearance rates (1.39 ± 0.44 pools/d) were triple those of α-tocopherol (0.33 ± 0.11; $P < 0.001$). The γ-tocopherol half-lives were 13 ± 4 h, compared with 57 ± 19 h for α-tocopherol. Thus, *RRR*-α-tocopherol remains in the plasma about 4 times longer than does *SRR*-α-tocopherol or γ-tocopherol (Figure 2). The similarity in the disappearance rates for γ-tocopherol and *SRR*-α-tocopherol strongly support the idea that forms of vitamin E that are not actively re-secreted by α-TTP into the plasma are excreted or metabolized.

## Biliary Excretion

Vitamin E does not accumulate in the liver to "toxic" levels, suggesting that excretion and metabolism are important in preventing adverse vitamin E effects. However, the regulation of hepatic vitamin E concentrations has not been extensively studied. α-Tocopherol is excreted into bile via multi-drug resistance gene 2 (MDR2, ABC B4, or p-glycoprotein),[31] an ATP-binding cassette transporter that also facilitates biliary phospholipid excretion.

The ATP-binding cassette transporter (ABCAI) mediates the α-tocopherol efflux from cells to HDL, similarly to "cholesterol reverse transport."[32] HDL has been shown to deliver α-tocopherol to the liver via scavenger receptor-BI (SR-BI).[33] In SR-BI-null compared with wild-type mice, plasma α-tocopherol concentrations increased, biliary α-tocopherol decreased, but liver α-tocopherol was unchanged; therefore, it appears that SR-BI-mediated hepatic α-tocopherol uptake is coupled to its biliary excretion.[34] Importantly, SR-BI protein is increased in vitamin E-deficient rats, suggesting that the liver can increase SR-BI to increase hepatic α-tocopherol delivery.[35] Under normal conditions, α-tocopherol transport via HDL to the liver would allow uptake of α-tocopherol into a liver pool destined for excretion in bile or perhaps metabolism.

## Vitamin E Metabolism

The first vitamin E metabolites described were urinary "Simon metabolites," which are oxidized, tail-shortened vitamin E metabolites.[8] Unoxidized vitamin E metabolites, alpha-carboxyethyl hydroxychroman (α-CEHC) and γ-CEHC, are derived from α- and γ-tocopherol (as well as α- and γ-tocotrienols), respectively, and have been detected in urine, bile, and plasma,[8] as well as liver homogenates.[36] Modern techniques to prevent in vitro oxidation have shown that Simon metabolites largely occur during in vitro sample handling.[8]

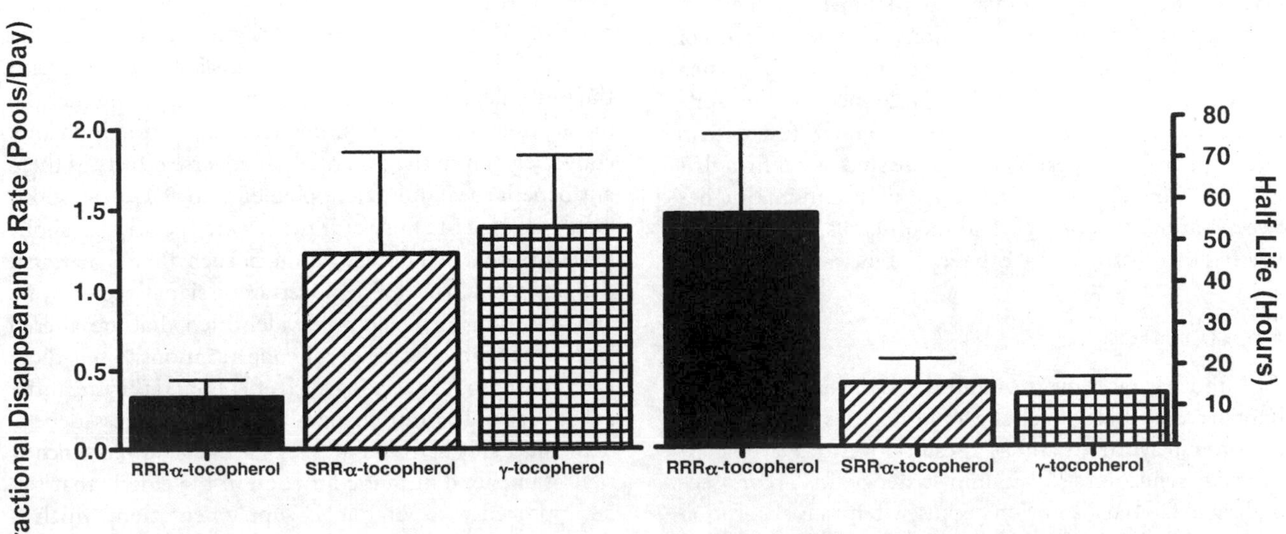


Figure 2. Plasma *RRR*- and *SRR*-α-tocopherol, and γ-tocopherol disappearance rates and half-lives. Vitamin E kinetics of *RRR*- and *SRR*-α-tocopherols[29] and γ-tocopherol[30] have been studied. The fractional disappearance rates of *RRR*-α-tocopherol (0.4 ± 0.1 pools/d) were significantly ($P < 0.01$) slower than for *SRR*-α-tocopherol (1.2 ± 0.6).[29] Plasma γ-tocopherol exponential disappearance rates (1.39 ± 0.44 pools/d) were triple those of α-tocopherol (0.33 ± 0.11, $P < 0.001$).[30] The apparent half-life of *RRR*-α-tocopherol was about 48 h, while *SRR*-α-tocopherol had a half-life of approximately 13 h.[29] The γ-tocopherol half-lives were 13 ± 4 h compared with 57 ± 19 h for α-tocopherol.[30]

Vitamin E metabolism is mediated by cytochrome P450s (CYPs), in that the tocopherols or tocotrienols are initially ω-oxidized by CYPs and then, following β-oxidation, are conjugated with sulfate or glucuronide and excreted in urine or bile.[8]

Hepatocytes produce γ-CEHC when incubated with γ-tocopherol. Initially, CYP3A appeared to be involved in γ-CEHC production because CYP3A stimulators and inhibitors appropriately altered vitamin E metabolism.[37,38] Subsequently, CYP4F2 was demonstrated to be involved in the ω-oxidation of α- and γ-tocopherols.[39] In mice with widely ranging liver α- (from 0.7 to 16 nmol/g) and γ-tocopherol (0 to 13 nmol/g) concentrations, hepatic α-CEHC was undetectable, but γ-CEHC concentrations (0.1 to 0.8 nmol/g) were correlated with both α- and γ-tocopherol concentrations ($P < 0.004$).[40] However, when Cyp4f and Cyp3a protein concentrations were measured, there were no variations in Cyp4f protein expression, but Cyp3a protein was correlated ($P < 0.0001$) with liver α- but not γ-tocopherol concentrations. Apparently, α-tocopherol increases Cyp3a protein expression, γ-CEHC formation, and the excretion of both γ-tocopherol and γ-CEHC.[40] This important relationship between α-tocopherol and Cyp3a mRNA expression has also been observed elsewhere.[41]

The regulatory mechanisms of CEHC production have not been extensively studied. CEHC production from γ-tocopherol is much greater than that from α-tocopherol,[37] and studies in isolated hepatocytes or liver cell lines have not provided answers to the mystery of why α- and γ-tocopherols, despite their very similar structures and antioxidant activities, are metabolized differently by the liver. When equimolar amounts of labeled tocopherols (about 50 mg each $d_6$-α- and $d_2$-γ-tocopheryl acetates) were administered to normal subjects,[30] plasma $d_6$-α-CEHC concentrations were below levels of detection for all subjects at all time points. Rates of plasma γ-CEHC and γ-tocopherol disappearance were not different from each other and were much faster than α-tocopherol disappearance.[30] These studies confirm that vitamin E metabolism is important in discriminating between various tocopherols and tocotrienols, and thus is a key regulator of vitamin E bioavailability.

# Deficiency

Although rare, overt vitamin E deficiency occurs in humans as a result of genetic abnormalities in α-TTP or lipoprotein synthesis and as a result of various fat malabsorption syndromes.[19] Vitamin E deficiency occurs secondary to fat malabsorption because vitamin E absorption requires biliary and pancreatic secretions.[19]

The large-caliber, myelinated axons in peripheral sensory nerves are the predominant target tissue in vitamin E deficiency in humans. A progressive peripheral neuropathy is observed, with a dying back of the large-caliber axons in the sensory neurons.[42] In deficient humans, axonal degeneration rather than demyelination is the primary sensory nerve abnormality. Thus, the axons degenerate first, then demyelination occurs.

Genetic defects in α-TTP are associated with a characteristic syndrome, AVED.[19] The ataxia observed in these patients has also been mimicked in α-TTP-null mice.[43] Gene analysis using high-density nucleotide arrays have shown repressed expression of retinoic acid-related orphan receptor alpha (ROR-α) in the cortex of α-TTP-null mice.[44] ROR-α absence causes ataxia in mice[45]; thus, some α-tocopherol actions may be mediated by ROR-α.

AVED patients have extraordinarily low plasma vitamin E concentrations (as low as 1/100 of normal), but if they are given vitamin E supplements, plasma concentrations reach normal levels within hours.[46] A dose of 800 to 1200 mg/d is usually sufficient to prevent further deterioration of neurologic function and, in some cases, improvements have been noted.[42,47] Postmortem analysis of an AVED patient demonstrated that vitamin E supplementation did allow brain vitamin E accumulation and prevention of Purkinje cell loss.[48] If supplementation is halted, plasma vitamin E concentrations decrease within days to deficient levels. The biochemical defect in AVED patients, shown using deuterated tocopherols, demonstrated that hepatic α-TTP is required to maintain plasma *RRR*-α-tocopherol concentrations[23,24] via secretion in VLDL. The molecular mechanism by which α-TTP facilitates α-tocopherol export from the liver remains under investigation.

# Chronic Disease Prevention and Public Health Implications

Given that vitamin E deficiency is very rare and that vitamin E intakes by most Americans are much less than their estimated requirements, questions arise whether the dietary α-tocopherol recommendations are too high and, conversely, given the potential for adverse effects, is there any benefit to vitamin E supplementation? The questions would be easier to answer if there were specific metabolic pathways that required vitamin E such that a marginal deficiency could be defined. Certainly, signaling pathways and specific genes have been identified that are altered by low or high α-tocopherol concentrations,[49] but there is no consensus concerning such effects, and they are difficult to separate from changes in oxidative stress-dependent mechanisms. One area of particular importance is that of impaired immune function in the elderly that can be improved with vitamin E supplementation, which is discussed further in the chapter in this volume on vitamin E.[50] Again, it is not clear if this result in the elderly a situation in which long-term suboptimal intakes of vitamin E allow increased oxidative stress to alter T-cell function. Similarly, aged patients with eye disease (macular degeneration) benefited from the daily use of a dietary supplement that included vitamin E.[51] Eyes are an extension of the nervous system, and vitamin E is particularly necessary for the maintenance of normal nerve function. It is therefore quite provocative that vitamin E supplements were associated with a decreased risk of amyotrophic lateral sclerosis,[52] and that supplements have been reported to delay the progression of Alzheimer's disease.[53]

Oxidative stress increases plasma vitamin E disappearance caused by endurance exercise[54] and in cigarette smokers.[5] Vitamin E supplementation decreases F2-isoprostanes, a measure of lipid peroxidation in exercisers[55] and in hypercholesterolemics.[56] Moreover, supplementation with both vitamin E and C slows atherosclerosis progression,[57] which is not surprising given that this is an oxidative stress disorder[58] and that low vitamin C status allows faster vitamin E disappearance.[5]

## Summary

Taken together, these findings suggest that long-term suboptimal vitamin E intakes will indeed allow the accumulation of oxidative damage. It is generally agreed that chronic diseases are associated with increased oxidative damage.[2] What remains an open question is whether vitamin E supplements in excess of daily requirements will decrease the risk of chronic disease. Although many vitamin E supplementation studies carried out in patients with various kinds of chronic diseases have failed to show benefit, these studies have largely attempted to reverse existing disease. The question of whether increased oxidative stress as a result of suboptimal vitamin E intake increases the risk of chronic disease has not yet been answered.

## Acknowledgments

This work was supported by a National Institutes of Health grant (NIH DK59576).

## References

1. Evans HM, Bishop KS. On the existence of a hitherto unrecognized dietary factor essential for reproduction. Science. 1922;56:650–651.
2. Food and Nutrition Board, Institute of Medicine. Dietary Reference Intakes for Vitamin C, Vitamin E, Selenium, and Carotenoids. Washington, DC: National Academies Press; 2000. Available online at: http://www.nap.edu/openbook/0309069351/html/index.html. Accessed March 1, 2006.
3. Cheeseman KH, Holley AE, Kelly FJ, et al. Biokinetics in humans of RRR-alpha-tocopherol: the free phenol, acetate ester, and succinate ester forms of vitamin E. Free Radic Biol Med. 1995;19:591–598.
4. Buettner GR. The pecking order of free radicals and antioxidants: lipid peroxidation, alpha-tocopherol, and ascorbate. Arch Biochem Biophys. 1993;300: 535–543.
5. Bruno RS, Ramakrishnan R, Montine TJ, et al. α-Tocopherol disappearance is faster in cigarette smokers and is inversely related to their ascorbic acid status. Am J Clin Nutr. 2005;81:95–103.
6. Kamal-Eldin A, Appelqvist LA. The chemistry and antioxidant properties of tocopherols and tocotrienols. Lipids. 1996;31:671–701.
7. Liebler DC, Burr JA, Philips L, Ham AJ. Gas chromatography-mass spectrometry analysis of vitamin E and its oxidation products. Anal Biochem. 1996;236: 27–34.
8. Brigelius-Flohé R, Traber MG. Vitamin E: function and metabolism. FASEB J. 1999;13:1145–1155.
9. Eitenmiller R, Lee J. *Vitamin E: Food Chemistry, Composition, and Analysis*. New York: Marcel Dekker; 2004.
10. Maras JE, Bermudez OI, Qiao N, et al. Intake of alpha-tocopherol is limited among US adults. J Am Diet Assoc. 2004;104:567–575.
11. Ma J, Hampl JS, Betts NM. Antioxidant intakes and smoking status: data from the continuing survey of food intakes by individuals 1994–1996. Am J Clin Nutr. 2000;71:774–780.
12. Hathcock JN, Azzi A, Blumberg J, et al. Vitamins E and C are safe across a broad range of intakes. Am J Clin Nutr. 2005;81:736–745.
13. Brown BG, Zhao XQ, Chait A, et al. Simvastatin and niacin, antioxidant vitamins, or the combination for the prevention of coronary disease. N Engl J Med. 2001;345:1583–1592.
14. Waters DD, Alderman EL, Hsia J, et al. Effects of hormone replacement therapy and antioxidant vitamin supplements on coronary atherosclerosis in postmenopausal women: a randomized controlled trial. JAMA. 2002;288:2432–2440.
15. Lonn E, Bosch J, Yusuf S, et al. Effects of long-term vitamin E supplementation on cardiovascular events and cancer: a randomized controlled trial. JAMA. 2005;293:1338–1347.
16. Miller ER 3rd, Paston-Barriuso R, Dalal D, et al. Meta-analysis: high-dosage vitamin E supplementation may increase all-cause mortality. Ann Intern Med. 2005;142:37–46.
17. Traber MG. Vitamin E, nuclear receptors and xenobiotic metabolism. Arch Biochem Biophys. 2004; 423:6–11.
18. Corrigan JJ Jr, Ulfers LL. Effect of vitamin E on prothrombin levels in warfarin-induced vitamin K deficiency. Am J Clin Nutr. 1981;34:1701–1705.
19. Traber MG. Vitamin E. In: Shils ME, Olson JA, Shike M, Ross AC, eds. *Modern Nutrition in Health and Disease*. Baltimore: Williams & Wilkins; 1999; 347–362.
20. Leonard SW, Good CK, Gugger ET, Traber MG. Vitamin E bioavailability from fortified breakfast cereal is greater than that from encapsulated supplements. Am J Clin Nutr. 2004;79:86–92.

21. Iuliano L, Micheletta F, Maranghi M, et al. Bioavailability of vitamin E as function of food intake in healthy subjects: effects on plasma peroxide-scavenging activity and cholesterol-oxidation products. Arterioscler Thromb Vasc Biol. 2001;21:E34–E37.
22. Goti D, Balazs Z, Panzenboeck U, et al. Effects of lipoprotein lipase on uptake and transcytosis of low density lipoprotein (LDL) and LDL-associated alpha-tocopherol in a porcine in vitro blood-brain barrier model. J Biol Chem. 2002;277:28537–28544.
23. Traber MG, Sokol RJ, Burton GW, et al. Impaired ability of patients with familial isolated vitamin E deficiency to incorporate alpha-tocopherol into lipoproteins secreted by the liver. J Clin Invest. 1990;85: 397–407.
24. Traber MG, Sokol RJ, Kohlschütter A, et al. Impaired discrimination between stereoisomers of α-tocopherol in patients with familial isolated vitamin E deficiency. J. Lipid Res. 1993;34:201–210.
25. Terasawa Y, Ladha Z, Leonard SW, et al. Increased atherosclerosis in hyperlipidemic mice deficient in alpha-tocopherol transfer protein and vitamin E. Proc Natl Acad Sci. U S A. 2000;97:13830–13834.
26. Arita M, Sato Y, Miyata A, et al. Human alpha-tocopherol transfer protein: cDNA cloning, expression and chromosomal localization. Biochem J. 1995; 306:437–443.
27. Meier R, Tomizaki T, Schulze-Briese C, et al. The molecular basis of vitamin E retention: structure of human alpha-tocopherol transfer protein. J Mol Biol. 2003;331:725–734.
28. Min KC, Kovall RA, Hendrickson WA. Crystal structure of human α-tocopherol transfer protein bound to its ligand: Implications for ataxia with vitamin E deficiency. Proc Natl Acad Sci U S A. 2003; 100:14713–14718.
29. Traber MG, Ramakrishnan R, Kayden HJ. Human plasma vitamin E kinetics demonstrate rapid recycling of plasma RRR-α-tocopherol. Proc Natl Acad Sci U S A. 1994;91:10005–10008.
30. Leonard SW, Paterson E, Atkinson JK, et al. Studies in humans using deuterium-labeled α- and γ-tocopherol demonstrate faster plasma g-tocopherol disappearance and greater g-metabolite production. Free Radic Biol Med. 2005;38:857–866.
31. Mustacich DJ, Shields J, Horton RA, et al. Biliary secretion of alpha-tocopherol and the role of the mdr2 P-glycoprotein in rats and mice. Arch Biochem Biophys. 1998;350:183–192.
32. Oram JF, Vaughan AM, Stocker R. ATP-binding cassette transporter A1 mediates cellular secretion of alpha-tocopherol. J Biol Chem. 2001;276:39898–39902.
33. Mardones P, Quinones V, Amigo L, et al. Hepatic cholesterol and bile acid metabolism and intestinal cholesterol absorption in scavenger receptor class B type I-deficient mice. J Lipid Res. 2001;42:170–180.
34. Mardones P, Strobel P, Miranda S, et al. Alpha-tocopherol metabolism is abnormal in scavenger receptor class B type I (SR-BI)-deficient mice. J Nutr. 2002;132:443–449.
35. Witt W, Kolleck I, Fechner H, et al. Regulation by vitamin E of the scavenger receptor BI in rat liver and HepG2 cells. J Lipid Res. 2000;41:2009–2016.
36. Leonard SW, Gumpricht E, Devereaux MW, et al. Quantitation of rat liver vitamin E metabolites by LC-MS during high-dose vitamin E administration. J Lipid Res. 2005;46:1068–1075.
37. Birringer M, Pfluger P, Kluth D, et al. Identities and differences in the metabolism of tocotrienols and tocopherols in HepG2 cells. J Nutr. 2002;132: 3113–3118.
38. Parker RS, Sontag TJ, Swanson JE. Cytochrome P4503A-dependent metabolism of tocopherols and inhibition by sesamin. Biochem Biophys Res Commun. 2000;277:531–534.
39. Sontag TJ, Parker RS. Cytochrome P450 omega-hydroxylase pathway of tocopherol catabolism: Novel mechanism of regulation of vitamin E status. J Biol Chem. 2002;277:25290–25296.
40. Traber MG, Siddens LK, Leonard SW, et al. α-Tocopherol modulates Cyp3a expression, increases γ-CEHC production and limits tissue γ-tocopherol accumulation in mice fed high γ-tocopherol diets. Free Radic Biol Med. 2005;38:773–785.
41. Kluth D, Landes N, Pfluger P, et al. Modulation of Cyp3a11 mRNA expression by alpha-tocopherol but not gamma-tocotrienol in mice. Free Radic Biol Med. 2005;38:507–514.
42. Sokol RJ. Vitamin E deficiency and neurological disorders. In: Packer L, Fuchs J, eds. *Vitamin E in Health and Disease*. New York: Marcel Dekker; 1993; 815–849.
43. Yokota T, Igarashi K, Uchihara T, et al. Delayed-onset ataxia in mice lacking alpha-tocopherol transfer protein: model for neuronal degeneration caused by chronic oxidative stress. Proc Natl Acad Sci U S A. 2001;98:15185–15190.
44. Gohil K, Godzdanker R, O'Roark E, et al. Alpha-tocopherol transfer protein deficiency in mice causes multi-organ deregulation of gene networks and behavioral deficits with age. Ann N Y Acad Sci. 2004; 1031:109–126.
45. Steinmayr M, Andre E, Conquet F, et al. *Staggerer* phenotype in retinoid-related orphan receptor alpha-deficient mice. Proc Natl Acad Sci U S A. 1998;95: 3960–3965.
46. Sokol RJ, Kayden HJ, Bettis DB, et al. Isolated vitamin E deficiency in the absence of fat malabsorption—familial and sporadic cases: characterization and investigation of causes. J Lab Clin Med. 1988; 111:548–559.
47. Gabsi S, Gouider-Khouja N, Belal S, et al. Effect of vitamin E supplementation in patients with ataxia

with vitamin E deficiency. Eur J Neurol. 2001;8: 477–481.
48. Yokota T, Uchihara T, Kumagai J, et al. Postmortem study of ataxia with retinitis pigmentosa by mutation of the alpha-tocopherol transfer protein gene. J Neurol Neurosurg Psychiatry. 2000;68:521–525.
49. Azzi A, Gysin R, Kempna P, et al. Regulation of gene expression by alpha-tocopherol. Biol Chem. 2004;385:585–591.
50. Meydani SN, Leka LS, Fine BC, et al. Vitamin E and respiratory tract infections in elderly nursing home residents: a randomized controlled trial. JAMA. 2004;292:828–836.
51. Age-Related Eye Disease Study Research Group. A randomized, placebo-controlled, clinical trial of high-dose supplementation with vitamins C and E, beta carotene, and zinc for age-related macular degeneration and vision loss: AREDS report no. 8. Arch Ophthalmol. 2001;119:1417–1436.
52. Ascherio A, Weisskopf MG, O'Reilly E J, et al. Vitamin E intake and risk of amyotrophic lateral sclerosis. Ann Neurol. 2005;57:104–110.
53. Sano M, Ernesto C, Thomas RG, et al. A controlled trial of selegiline, alpha-tocopherol, or both as treatment for Alzheimer's disease. The Alzheimer's Disease Cooperative Study. N Engl J Med. 1997;336: 1216–1222.
54. Mastaloudis A, Leonard SW, Traber MG. Oxidative stress in athletes during extreme endurance exercise. Free Radic Biol Med. 2001:911–922.
55. Mastaloudis A, Morrow JD, Hopkins DW, et al. Antioxidant supplementation prevents exercise-induced lipid peroxidation, but not inflammation, in ultramarathon runners. Free Radic Biol Med. 2004; 36:1329–1341.
56. Davi G, Alessandrini P, Mezzetti A, et al. In vivo formation of 8-Epi-prostaglandin F2 alpha is increased in hypercholesterolemia. Arterioscler Thromb Vasc Biol. 1997;17:3230–3235.
57. Salonen RM, Nyyssonen K, Kaikkonen J, et al. Six-year effect of combined vitamin C and E supplementation on atherosclerotic progression: the Antioxidant Supplementation in Atherosclerosis Prevention (ASAP) Study. Circulation. 2003;107:947–953.
58. Diaz MN, Frei B, Vita JA, Keaney JFJ. Antioxidants and atherosclerotic heart disease. N Engl J Med. 1997;337:408–416.

# 16 Vitamin K

Guylaine Ferland

## Introduction

The history of vitamin K dates back to 1929, when, as part of his work on sterol metabolism, Henrik Dam observed that chicks fed fat-free diets developed subcutaneous hemorrhages and anemia. Further work by Dam determined that the antihemorrhagic substance was fat soluble and occurred in extracts of liver and various plant tissues. In 1935, Dam named this new substance vitamin K. By 1939, the two naturally occurring forms of the vitamin, vitamin K1 and vitamin K2, had been isolated from alfalfa and putrefied fish meal, respectively.[1]

In 1941, the first vitamin K antagonist was discovered when Campbell and Link identified a new substance in spoiled sweet clover hay that had been reported to cause hemorrhagic disease in cattle in the United States and western Canada in the 1920s. This substance, 3,3′-methyl-bis-(4-hydroxycoumarin), later became known as dicoumarol. In the period after the discovery of dicoumarol, several derivatives of coumarin were synthesized for use as clinical agents in anticoagulant therapy. One of these, warfarin, or 3-(α-acetonyl-benzyl)-4-hydroxycoumarin, has been used successfully as a clinical agent since 1941. Access to vitamin K antagonists eventually helped to specify the role of vitamin K in blood coagulation and proved to be invaluable in vitamin K research in general.[1]

Although the bleeding condition reported by Dam was originally associated with decreased prothrombin (factor II) activity, it was later established that three other coagulation proteins (factors VII, IX, and X) were also depressed in vitamin K deficiency states. For many years, this participation in blood coagulation was assumed to be the sole physiological role for vitamin K. However, the discovery in the early 1970s of γ-carboxyglutamic acid (Gla), a new amino acid common to all vitamin K proteins, later led to the discovery of additional vitamin K-dependent proteins (VKDPs) not involved in hemostasis, and greatly contributed to our present understanding of the action of vitamin K at the molecular level. To this day, the participation of vitamin K in Gla synthesis remains the only well-defined function of this vitamin.[2]

## Chemistry and Nomenclature

Compounds with vitamin K activity have a common 2-methyl-1,4-naphtoquinone ring, but differ in the structure at the 3-position. Vitamin K occurs naturally in two forms (Figure 1). Phylloquinone, or vitamin K1 (2-methyl-3-phytyl-1,4-naphtoquinone), is synthesized in plants and represents the main source of dietary vitamin K in Western countries.[3] The menaquinone, or vitamin K2 (2-methyl-1,4-naphtoquinones), are produced by bacteria and form a family of compounds with unsaturated isoprenyl side chains of various length at the 3 position. The predominant forms of the menaquinone series contain 6 to 10 isoprenoid units, but menaquinones containing up to 13 units have been isolated.[4] One of the menaquinones, MK-4, is not a common product of bacte-

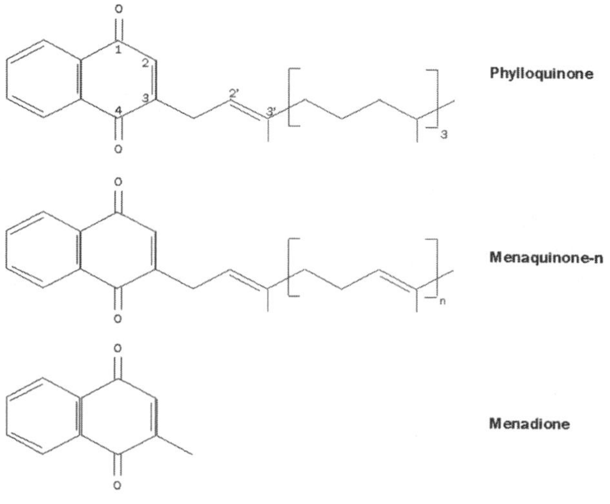

Phylloquinone

Menaquinone-n

Menadione

Figure 1. Chemical structures of phylloquinone, the menaquinones, and menadione.

rial synthesis, but can be produced from phylloquinone.[5] Animal studies have demonstrated that the conversion of phylloquinone to MK-4 is tissue specific and occurs independently of intestinal bacteria. The parent structure of all K vitamins, 2-methyl-1,4 naphtoquinone, also called menadione or vitamin K3 (Figure 1), does not occur in nature, but can be alkylated to MK-4 in avian and mammalian tissues. This synthetic form has been used as a source of vitamin K in a wide range of animal feeds.[1]

Current methods to assess vitamin K in plasma, biological tissues, and foods are based on high-performance liquid chromatography (HPLC). Vitamin K is first extracted from matrices with organic solvents, and then by solid-phase chromatography, before being selectively isolated by HPLC. Quantitation is now usually achieved using fluorescence detection, and procedures enabling simultaneous determination of phylloquinone and the menaquinones have been developed and used reliably.[5] A simple procedure for the determination of phylloquionone in small volumes of plasma or serum (0.1–0.25 mL) was described in 2004.[6] Methods based on gas chromatography and mass spectrometry have also been described, but are not routinely used.

## Absorption, Transport, Storage, and Turnover

### *Absorption*

Vitamin K is absorbed from the proximal intestine into the lymphatic system by a process that requires the presence of bile and pancreatic juices.[7] Consequently, conditions interfering with these functions or associated with fat malabsorption will impair vitamin K absorption.[8] In healthy adults, the absorption of phylloquinone has been estimated to be approximately 80% when administered in its free form, but decreases significantly when it is absorbed from foods.[7] Using the area under an absorption curve, the absorption of phylloquinone from spinach was found to be 4% to 17% that of phylloquinone from a suspension or a tablet.[9,10] Phylloquinone absorption from vegetables can be improved when consumed with fat,[9] but absorption efficiency remains lower than when phylloquinone is consumed in an oil form.[11] Data for the menaquinones are more limited, but in a study comparing the absorption efficiency of equivalent intakes of phylloquinone from cooked spinach and MK-7 from the Japanese food natto, absorption of that particular menaquinone was found to be significantly higher than that for phylloquinone.[12]

### *Transport*

Absorbed phylloquinone is incorporated into chylomicrons and transported to the liver, where it is cleared from chylomicron remnants through an apolipoprotein E (ApoE) receptor. Unlike other fat-soluble vitamins, vitamin K has no known carrier protein. In the circulation, phylloquinone is principally carried in triacylglycerol-rich lipoproteins (>50%), with each of the LDL and HDL fractions accounting for about 15% of the circulating vitamer.[13,14] This likely explains the strong positive correlation observed between circulating phylloquinone and triacylglycerols in some studies.[15] Data on the lipoprotein distribution of ingested menaquinones is limited but suggest different distributions for the short- and long-chain menaquinones.[13] Finally, recent in vitro studies indicate that, as in liver, internalization of phylloquinone in bone (osteoblasts) is mediated at least in part by the ApoE contained in the lipoprotein fractions.[16]

Compared with the other fat-soluble vitamins, phylloquinone circulates in blood in very small concentrations, and a normal range of 0.25 to 2.7 nmol/L was established by Sadowski et al.[15] Fasting plasma phylloquinone has been linked to the genetic polymorphism of ApoE, however, results have been inconsistent, differing in healthy subjects and certain groups of patients.[17] Circulating phylloquinone has also been linked to the lipid component of the diet. In a recent study, fasting phylloquinone was significantly reduced following ingestion of a polyunsaturated fatty acid-rich corn oil diet compared with diets enriched with a mixture of olive and safflower oils.[18] Finally, menaquinones are also present in plasma, notably MK-7 and MK-8; however, unlike phylloquinone, normal ranges for these are not yet available.[4]

### *Storage*

As the site of synthesis of the coagulation proteins, liver is usually considered to be the main storage organ, consisting of around 90% menaquinones (with MK-10 and MK-11 being particularly abundant) and 10% phylloquinone.[4] However, phylloquinone and the menaquinones are also present in extra hepatic tissues. In postmortem specimens, phylloquinone concentrations in heart and pancreas were found to be comparable to that in liver, while those in lung, kidney, and brain were much lower. Menaquinone-4, a K vitamer assumed to be a by-product of phylloquinone, is also widely distributed and present in tissues in variable amounts. In brain and kidney, for example, MK-4 concentrations largely exceed those of phylloquinone, whereas in the pancreas, MK-4 and phylloquinone are present in comparable amounts.[19] Vitamin K is also present in bone. When investigated from the femoral neck of patients undergoing hip replacement, phylloquinone, MK-6, MK-7, and MK-8 were present in both cortical and trabecular compartment in amounts as high as those observed in liver.[20] Animal research also points to a wide distribution of the different K vitamers in extra-hepatic tissues.[5]

### *Turnover*

Older studies using pharmacological dosage protocols showed phylloquinone to be rapidly metabolized, with about 20% being excreted in the urine and 40% to 50% excreted in the feces via the bile. When consumed in physiological amounts, postprandial plasma phylloquinone concentrations peak after about 6 hours, returning to baseline by 24 hours.[14] This is in contrast to the long-chain menaquinones, which remain in the circulation much longer when ingested in similar quantities (up 72 hours in the case of MK-7[12]). Evidence for the slower turnover of the long-chain menaquinones is also available from animal studies.[4] Urinary vitamin K metabolites consist mainly of glucuronide conjugates of derivatives in which the phytyl side chain has been oxidized. Biliary metabolites have not been clearly identified. A method for measuring two major urinary metabolites of phylloquinone, 5C- and 7C-aglycone, by HPLC with electrochemical detection in the redox mode, has been described previously.[21] Compared with the other fat-soluble vitamins, the total body pool of vitamin K is very small, and hepatic reserves are rapidly depleted when dietary vitamin K is restricted. Using radiolabeled vitamin, the total body pool for phylloquinone has been estimated to be approximately 1.5 days.[22]

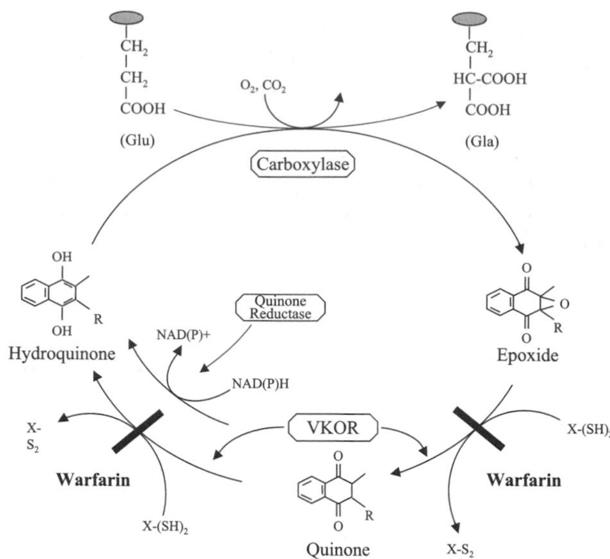


Figure 2. The vitamin K cycle. X-(SH)2 and X-S2 denote reduced and oxidized dithiols, respectively. The dithiol-dependent oxidoreductase is inhibited by coumarin-type drugs such as warfarin, while the NAD(P)H-dependent reductase is not.

# Biochemical and Physiological Functions

## *Vitamin K-Dependent Carboxylation*

Over 40 years after its discovery, it was shown that vitamin K acts as a cofactor in the posttranslational synthesis of Gla from glutamic acid (Glu) residues contained in precursor proteins. γ-Carboxyglutamic acid is common to all VKDPs, and increases the affinity of these proteins for calcium.[23] As illustrated in Figure 2, the γ-carboxylation of glutamate residues is catalyzed by a microsomal enzyme called vitamin K-dependent carboxylase, which is located at the luminal surface of the endoplasmic reticulum in a reaction that requires the reduced form of vitamin K, hydroquinone, as well as carbon dioxide and oxygen. It is currently believed that the vitamin K hydroquinone and oxygen react to form a strong base capable of abstracting a proton from the γ-carbon of the Glu residue to form a carbanion intermediate, which then undergoes carboxylation to yield Gla.[24] The carboxylase therefore uses the energy of vitamin K hydroquinone oxygenation to convert Glu to Gla in VKDPs. Carboxylation of the Glu residues is accomplished by a processive mechanism and is facilitated by a carboxylase recognition signal propeptide that tethers the Glu to the enzyme.[25]

Once formed, vitamin K 2,3-epoxide is recycled to its quinone and hydroquinone forms in successive reactions catalyzed by a vitamin K oxidoreductase, the activity of which is dependent on dithiol cofactors and is inhibited by 4-hydroxycoumarin derivatives such as warfarin. The blocking action of coumarin-type drugs toward this enzyme forms the basis of their pharmacological action as anticoagulants. However, at least in the liver, reduction of the vitamin K quinone to hydroquinone is also possible by a NAD(P)H-dependent quinone reductase that is insensitive to coumarin drugs, but cannot reduce vitamin K epoxide to the quinone form. This enzyme operates at high tissue concentrations of vitamin K and can therefore support carboxylation of the hepatic VKDPs in the presence of coumarins.[2] Collectively, these reactions make up the vitamin K cycle (Figure 2).

In the absence of vitamin K or in the presence of vitamin K antagonists, carboxylation of precursor proteins is incomplete and proteins are secreted in plasma in various undercarboxylated forms. These proteins, referred to as PIVKAs (protein induced by vitamin K absence or antagonism), lack biological activity and have been used to assess vitamin K nutritional status. Specific antibodies for the undercarboxylated forms of prothrombin, osteocalcin and matrix Gla protein (MGP), have been developed and their presence in blood and tissues is usually interpreted as reflecting a suboptimal vitamin K status (see below).

# Vitamin K-Dependent Proteins

Although γ-carboxyglutamic acid residues have been detected in both vertebrate and invertebrate species, only proteins of mammalian origins will be discussed here.

## *Blood Coagulation Proteins*

There are seven VKDPs involved in blood coagulation: prothrombin (factor II), factors VII, IX, and X, protein C, protein S, and protein Z. All of the vitamin K-dependent coagulation proteins (46,000 to 72,000 Da) are synthesized in the liver and contain between 10 and 13 Gla residues. The Gla residues enable $Ca^{2+}$-mediated binding of the proteins to the negatively charged phospholipid surfaces provided by blood platelets and endothelial cells at the site of injury. With the exception of proteins S and Z, Gla-containing blood proteins are zymogen forms of serine proteases and have considerable structural homology. Prothrombin and factors VII, IX, and X represent the classical vitamin K-dependent plasma clotting factors and participate in the cascade resulting in the formation of a fibrin clot. A key element in the formation of fibrin is the generation of thrombin from prothrombin by activated factor X. Vitamin K-dependent factors VII and IX activate factor X by the extrinsic and intrinsic pathways, respectively. In contrast, proteins C, S, and Z are inhibitors of the procoagulant system. Protein C exerts its inhibitory activity by inactivating factors Va and VIIIa, and enhances fibrinolysis with protein S as a cofactor, while protein Z serves as a cofactor for the inhibition of factor Xa by protein Z-dependent protease inhibitor.[2]

In addition to their hemostatic action at the cell surface, many of the coagulation proteins are now known to also possess cell signaling activity and influence a wide range of cellular events. Therefore, through its interaction with protease-activated receptors (PARs), thrombin has been shown to promote platelet aggregation and to be involved in such phenomena as tumor growth and metastasis, angiogenesis, atherosclerosis and inflammation, survival of glial cells, neurons and myoblasts, and chemotaxis of neutrophils and monocytes.[26] When complexed to tissue factor, factors VII and Xa activate PAR-1 and PAR-2 receptors and participate in pro-inflammatory cell signaling.[27] In contrast, protein C and its activated form have been shown to possess anti-inflammatory and anti-apoptotic properties through mechanisms that appear to involve interactions with the endothelial protein C receptor and PAR-1 in the membrane. For example, activated protein C has been found to be neuroprotective in different models of ischemia and in cultured cortical neurons, and both protein C and activated protein C have been shown to inhibit adhesion of neutrophils to endothelial cell surface, as well as their trans-migration.[28]

In contrast to the other vitamin K-dependent blood factors, which are principally associated with the liver, protein S is synthesized by different cell types (e.g., megakaryocytes, vascular smooth muscle cells, and osteoblasts), and has been found in many extra-hepatic tissues, including brain, testes, spleen, endothelium, and bone. Recently, it was found that protein S is involved in apoptotic processes, promoting phagocytosis when in its free form, but counteracting apoptotic processes when bound to the complement regulator C4b-binding protein.[28] Like protein C, protein S has been shown to confer neuronal protection in ischemic and hypoxic injury in a mouse model. Protein S has also been shown to possess mitogenic activity toward vascular smooth muscle cells and, as discussed below, has been linked to bone metabolism.[2] Finally, protein S was found to stimulate photoreceptor outer segment phagocytosis by cultured retinal pigment epithelial cells from rats, suggesting a role for this protein in vision.[29]

### *Bone Proteins*

There are three Gla proteins in bone: osteocalcin, MGP, and protein S. Osteocalcin, also known as bone Gla protein, is synthesized in osteoblasts and odontoblasts, and accounts for 15% to 20% of the non-collagenous bone protein in most vertebrate species. Osteocalcin has a molecular weight of about 5700 Da and three Gla residues, which allow binding to hydroxyapatite crystals in bone. Synthesis of osteocalcin by osteoblasts is notably stimulated by the active metabolite of vitamin D, 1,25(OH)2D3. About 20% of the newly synthesized protein is released in the circulation and is used as a measure of bone formation. In states of dietary restriction or following treatment with vitamin K antagonists, partially carboxylated osteocalcin appears in the circulation. Despite the interest osteocalcin has raised since its discovery, its physiological function remains elusive. The protein is expressed relatively late in the developmental stage and appears in bone with the onset of mineralization. Early studies showed osteocalcin to be involved in the differentiation and recruitment of osteoclast progenitor cells, suggesting a participation in bone resorption. Reports have since shown that rats rendered osteocalcin deficient following treatment with warfarin exhibit excessive bone mineralization and premature closure of the growth plate, and that mice lacking the osteocalcin gene exhibit a phenotype characterized by increased bone mass. Collectively, these data suggest a role for osteocalcin as a negative regulator of bone formation.[23,30]

The second vitamin K-dependent bone protein to be discovered, MGP, contains five Gla residues and has a molecular weight of about 9600. In contrast to osteocalcin, which is exclusively associated with mineralized tissues, MGP is expressed in many soft tissues and cell types (including vascular smooth muscle cells), although the protein itself only accumulates in calcified tissues. The physiological function of MGP as an inhibitor of calcification was established when mice lacking the gene coding for MGP showed calcification of their arteries that led to hemorrhagic death due to vessel rupture within 2 months. A similar phenotype, calcification of the arteries and of the aortic valves, was subsequently observed, although to a lesser degree of severity, in MGP-depleted rats treated with warfarin. Furthermore, because MGP in these animals was largely of the uncarboxylated form as a result of the warfarin treatment, this study also confirmed that the protein's action as a calcification inhibitor is dependent on the presence of the Gla residues.[23,31]

A role for protein S in bone metabolism was suggested back in 1990, when children with inherited protein S deficiency were found to suffer from osteopenia and presented with reduced BMD. Since this report, evidence has been obtained that protein S is synthesized and secreted by various human osteosarcoma cell lines and by human osteoblast-like cells.[23] Despite these findings, the exact role of protein S in bone remains undetermined at this point.

### *Other VKDPs*

Discovered in 1993, Gas6, named after it was found to be the product of the growth-arrest-specific gene 6, is a high-molecular weight protein (75,000 Da) that contains 11 to 12 Gla residues. It has a structure similar to that of protein S (44% amino acid homology) and is expressed in numerous tissues, including those in the nervous system.[23] Gas6 is a ligand for a family of receptor tyrosine kinases that include Axl (also referred to as Ark/Ufo/Tyro7), SKY (also referred to as Rse/Tyro3/Etk-2/Dtk/Brt), and Mer (also referred to as Tyro12/Eyk/Nyk), a property that is dependent on Gla residues. Since its discovery, Gas6 has been involved in a wide range of cellular processes that include cell proliferation, phagocytosis, protection against apoptosis, cell adhesion, and chemotaxis. Physiologically, Gas6 has been involved in the nervous system and vision, in platelet metabolism and the vascular system, in bone metabolism, and in the renal system. It has also been linked to pathologies such as neoplasia and angiogenesis, thrombotic events, glomerular kidney disease, and cancer.[2,23,29,32-34] Clearly, the actions of Gas6 are diverse and wide-ranging, and already appear to be of great importance to general cell physiology.

Among the other VKDPs that have been identified are those of the TMG (for transmembrane Gla) family, which comprises four proteins: PRPG1, PRPG2, TMG3, and TMGP4. In contrast to the previously discussed VKDPs, these are not secreted but, rather, are single-pass integral membrane proteins. Like Gas6, however, the TGMs have a wide tissue distribution. Their functions in vivo are presently unclear, but their chemical conformations suggest that they could be involved in cell transduction and have broad physiological activities.[2] A summary of the VKDPs and their functions is presented in Table 1.

## Vitamin K in Bone Health

Support for a role for vitamin K in human bone health was first suggested when osteoporotic patients with reduced bone mineral density (BMD) or having suffered a fracture were reported to have lower concentrations of circulating phylloquinone and menaquinones compared

**Table 1.** Summary of the Vitamin K-Dependent Proteins and Their Functions

| Protein category | Physiological functions | |
|---|---|---|
| Blood coagulation | Hemostasis | Cell Signaling-Related Actions |
| Prothrombin | Procoagulant | *Thrombin* |
| Factor VII | Procoagulant | Platelet aggregation, |
| Factor IX | Procoagulant | Tumor growth and metastasis |
| Factor X | Procoagulant | Angiogenesis |
| Protein C | Anticoagulant | Cell survival or apoptosis (glial cells, neurons, myoblasts) |
| Protein S | Anticoagulant | |
| Protein Z | Anticoagulant | Chemotaxis (neutrophils, monocytes) |
| | | *FVII-FIX-tissue factor complex* |
| | | Pro-inflammatory action |
| | | *Protein C* |
| | | Anti-inflammatory action |
| | | Anti-apoptotic action |
| | | Neuronal protection (in ischemic stroke) |
| | | *Protein S* |
| | | Apoptotic processes (pro- and anti-) |
| | | Mitogenesis (VSMC) |
| | | Neuronal protection (during ischemia) |
| | | Retinal integrity |
| Bone | | |
| Osteocalcin | Negative regulator of bone formation | |
| Matrix Gla protein | Inhibitor of calcification* | |
| Protein S | Undetermined | |
| Others | | |
| Gas6 | Cell adhesion, cell proliferation, phagocytosis protection against apoptosis, chemotaxis | |
| TMGs | Undetermined | |

TMG = transmembrane Gla; VSMC = vascular smooth muscle cells

*This role as calcification inhibitor applies to soft tissues as well as bone.

with healthy subjects. Epidemiological studies then showed partially carboxylated osteocalcin to be a predictor of BMD and hip fracture risk, these associations having been observed in both institutionalized and free-living elderly women.[31] In a study involving approximately 1600 men and women participating in the Framingham Heart Study, poor vitamin K status, as assessed by plasma phylloquinone and circulating partially carboxylated osteocalcin, was associated with low BMD in men (femoral neck) and in women (spine) not using estrogen replacements. No associations were observed in either premenopausal women or postmenopausal women undergoing estrogen therapy.[30] In another recent study of healthy young girls (3–16 years of age) consuming a typical US diet, better vitamin K status (i.e., higher plasma phylloquinone and lower levels of partially carboxylated osteocalcin) was associated with decreased bone turnover. However, indicators of vitamin K status were not consistently associated with current bone mineral content (BMC) or gain in BMC over 4 years.[35]

Associations between vitamin K and bone health have also been investigated from the point of view of dietary intake. In the Nurses' Health Study, which included women 38 to 63 years of age, phylloquinone intakes of over 109 μg/d were associated with a lower risk of hip fracture during a 10-year follow-up period. Similarly, in a report of about 900 men and women (mean age: 75.2 years) participating in the Framingham Heart Study, individuals in the highest quartile of phylloquinone intake (median: 254 μg/d) had a significantly lower adjusted relative risk of hip fracture than those in the lowest quartile (median: 56 μg /d). However, there were no associations between phylloquinone intake and BMD in either men or women.[30] Dietary and biochemical measures of phylloquinone have also been investigated with respect to bone quality as assessed by quantitative ultrasound of the heel, and, in general, associations have not been conclusive.[36]

Although these findings are of interest, one caveat with dietary associations is that they make it difficult to discern the specific role of vitamin K from those of other nutrients in the diet. For example, diets rich in vitamin K also tend to be rich in fruits and vegetables, which in themselves could be beneficial to bone health. Similarly, the clinical significance of partially carboxylated osteocalcin remains to be established. A dose-response study revealed that daily intake of about 1000 μg phylloquinone was required to achieve maximal γ-carboxylation of circulating osteocalcin, an amount nearly 10 times higher than current recommendations.[30] Although it is reasonable to think that full carboxylation is required for osteocalcin to optimally exert its action in bone, data supporting this hypothesis are not yet available. At this time, results from only one intervention study are available. When administered for 3 years, a dietary supplement containing a mineral mix (Ca, Zn, and Mg), vitamin D, and 1 mg of phylloquinone significantly reduced bone loss at the femoral neck in postmenopausal women 50 to 60 years of age compared with a placebo or a supplement containing the mineral mix and vitamin D only. In contrast, no effect of phylloquinone was observed in lumbar BMD.[30]

In Japan, MK-4 has been used as an anti-osteoporotic agent in pharmacological doses (45 mg/d) since 1995, with positive effects on BMD and fracture incidence. However, there is some indication that the anti-resorptive effect of pharmacological MK-4 is through a modulation of cellular differentiation by its geranylgeranyl side chain, an action that is independent of its usual role in the γ-carboxylation of proteins.[30] In vivo, high doses of MK-4 have been shown to reduce ovariectomy-induced bone loss in rats, although not all studies have observed such effects. In other studies, MK-4 has been observed to stimulate the synthesis of osteoblastic markers and the deposition of bone and to decrease bone resorption by inhibiting the formation of osteoclasts and their bone-resorptive activity. More specifically, high doses of MK-4 have been shown to stimulate apoptosis of osteoclasts while inhibiting apoptosis of osteoblasts.[37] Finally, because individuals on warfarin therapy are by definition in a state of chronic vitamin K deficiency, bone status in this category of patients has been investigated. In a meta-analysis, these patients have not been deemed to be at risk of bone disorders,[30] a conclusion that was confirmed in a stringently controlled study.[38]

## Vitamin K and Cardiovascular Health

In addition to the MGP-related animal work described earlier, indications that vitamin K could be involved in the mineralization process in humans came when it was reported that infants born to mothers who had received warfarin during the first trimester of pregnancy developed abnormal calcification that included nasal hypoplasia, stippled epiphyses, and irregular growth of the facial and long bones.[23] Although initially attributed to the teratogenic effect of warfarin, these bone defects have since been shown to result from maternal vitamin K deficiency during pregnancy and/or congenital deficiency of the vitamin K epoxide reductase in the infants (inhibiting recycling of the vitamin). More recently, individuals suffering from Keutel syndrome, an autosomal recessive disorder characterized by abnormal cartilage calcification, midfacial hypoplasia, and peripheral pulmonary stenosis, have been shown to possess mutations of the MGP gene that result in nonfunctional MGP. However, in contrast to the MGP knockout mouse model (described above), these individuals do not exhibit gross vascular calcification or aortic rupture.[31]

Initial immunohistochemical studies comparing normal and atherosclerotic human tissues showed MGP to be constitutively expressed in the vessel wall during calcification. The development of an assay for MGP in serum then led to reports of increased and decreased serum MGP levels in association with atherosclerosis. However, interpretation of such correlations is complicated by polymorphisms of the MGP gene, which have been shown to influence MGP serum levels and/or be associated with increased risks of myocardial infarction and vascular calcification.[2] Furthermore, because MGP is expressed by numerous tissues, all of which can contribute to circulating MGP, the clinical value of serum MGP as an indicator of arterial calcification is unclear at this point. Novel conformation specific antibodies against MGP have been developed and used for immunohistochemical analyses of healthy and sclerotic human tissues. Compared with arteries from healthy subjects, those from individuals suffering from atherosclerosis or Mönckeberg's sclerosis were associated with the presence of undercarboxylated MGP, suggesting a link between suboptimal vitamin K status and vascular health.[39]

Insight into this association was gained in a series of reports comparing the vitamin K intakes of healthy individuals and those of subjects who later developed coronary heart disease (CHD). In the Nurses' Health Study (N = 72,874; age = 38–65 years), women in the highest four quintile categories of phylloquinone intake had a 23% to 33% lower age-adjusted risk of CHD than women in the lowest quintile. However, when intakes were further adjusted for dietary variables known to be related to CHD (e.g., saturated fats, trans fatty acids, and folate), this association was attenuated, suggesting that dietary patterns associated with phylloquinone intake, rather than intake of the nutrient itself, may have accounted for the weak association with CHD. In this study, rates of total or ischemic strokes were also investigated and were not found to be associated with phylloquinone intake.[40] A non-significant association between phylloquinone intake and premature coronary calcification was also observed in a group of 807 healthy adults 39 to 45 years of age.[41]

Dietary vitamin K intakes, both phylloquinone and menaquinones, were also investigated with respect to incident CHD, all-cause mortality, and aortic atherosclerosis in the Rotterdam Study, a population-based study of 4807 men and women over the age of 55 years with no history of myocardial infarction at the start of the study. While no stastistically significant associations were observed between phylloquinone intakes and any of these conditions, the relative risk of incident CHD was significantly reduced in subjects in the middle and upper tertile of menaquinone intakes compared with those in the lower tertile. Intake of menaquinone was also inversely related to all-cause mortality and severe aortic calcification. In this study, intake of menaquinone comprised 10% of the total vitamin K intake, and the menaquinones were mainly derived from dairy products, notably cheese.[42] In animal studies, MK-4 but not phylloquinone, has been shown to accumulate in the aorta and to inhibit warfarin-induced arterial calcification.[43] In the only intervention study currently available, supplementation with 1 mg of phylloquinone plus vitamin D and a mineral cocktail for 3 years maintained the elastic properties of the common carotid artery in a group of postmenopausal women, while these deteriorated in the placebo group. In contrast, the supplement had no effect on the vessel wall's intima media thickness.[44] The effect of chronic vitamin K deficiency on arterial calcification was also investigated in patients receiving (n = 10) or not receiving (n = 35) preoperative oral anticoagulant treatment. In this preliminary study, duration of the anticoagulant treatment varied between 16 and 35 months (mean 25 months) and target international normalized ratio were between 2 and 3. Calcification in patients receiving preoperative oral anticoagulant therapy were found to be 2-fold larger than in untreated group (37% vs. 16%).[45]

# Vitamin K and Brain Function

The notion that vitamin K could be involved in the nervous system was first suggested following reports that the administration of warfarin to growing animals led to significant reductions in brain sphingolipids, a class of lipids found in high concentrations in cell membranes of the nervous system. These changes in sphingolipids were subsequently linked to alterations of their synthetic enzymes, all of which could be reversed by subsequent administration of either phylloquinone or MK-4.[32] Following that report, MK-4, which represents over 98% of total vitamin K in rat brain, was found to be present in significantly higher concentrations in myelinated (pons medulla and midbrain) than in non-myelinated regions of the brain.[46] Vitamin K, mainly in the form of MK-4, has also been shown to be protective of the retina during aging.[47] Furthermore, there is now evidence to suggest that both phylloquinone and MK-4 possess nerve-growth factor potentiating activity and have survival-promoting effects on different neuronal cells. Finally, it was demonstrated that MK-4 and, to a lesser extent, phylloquinone prevent oxidative injury as defined by free radical accumulation and cell death, in primary cultures of oligodendrocyte precursors and immature fetal cortical neurons.[32] Whether these findings are dependent on the action of the VKDPs remain to be established, but both Gas6 and protein S have been linked to the nervous system. In addition to the findings presented in the previous sections, Gas6 and, to a lesser extent, protein S, have been shown to be widely expressed in the rat central nervous system. Furthermore, Gas6 has been shown to possess neurotrophic activity towards hippocampal neurons and to prevent apoptosis and/or promote the growth and survival of cells such as oligodendrocytes, gonadotropin-releasing hormone neurons, and Schwann cells.[2,32]

# Vitamin K Deficiency

Clinically significant vitamin K deficiency is associated with an increase in prothrombin time and, in severe cases, bleeding. However, overt vitamin K deficiency is uncommon in adults and has mainly been associated with gastrointestinal disorders associated with fat malabsorption (e.g., bile duct obstruction, inflammatory bowel disease, chronic pancreatitis, and cystic fibrosis) and liver disease.[8] Hospitalized patients with low food intake or poor nutritional status may also be at increased risk of vitamin K deficiency, especially if treated with antibiotics or other drugs interfering with vitamin K metabolism. Although bleeding episodes in antibiotic-treated patients have often been attributed to an acquired vitamin K deficiency resulting from a suppression of menaquinone-synthesizing organisms in the gut, data to substantiate this hypothesis are lacking. Furthermore, interpretation of these reports have generally been complicated by the possibility of general malnutrition in the patients under investigation.[48]

Newborn infants, on the other hand, are a clinical population with a well-established risk for vitamin K deficiency. Factors contributing to the condition are poor placental transfer, low concentrations of plasma clotting factors due to hepatic immaturity, and low vitamin K content of breast milk. Individually or in concert, these factors increase the risk of bleeding in infants in the first weeks of life, a condition known as hemorrhagic disease of the newborn.[48] Because hemorrhagic disease of the newborn can be effectively prevented by administration of vitamin K, the American Academy of Pediatrics recommends that phylloquinone be given to all newborns as a single, intramuscular dose of 0.5 to 1 mg within 6 hours of birth.[49] Although some authors have questioned the appropriateness of this recommendation for premature infants, specific recommendations for preterm infants are not yet available. Reports in the early 1990s of an increased risk of leukemia and other forms of cancer in children who had received vitamin K intramuscularly at birth were not corroborated in subsequent studies, confirming the innocuous nature of this prophylactic measure.

High doses of vitamin E have been shown to interfere with vitamin K and precipitate deficiency states, especially in subjects with low vitamin K status. In one study, 12 weeks of supplementation with 1000 IU RRR-alpha-tocopherol/d increased PIVKA-prothrombin (PIVKA-II) levels in adults not receiving oral anticoagulant therapy. In contrast, neither plasma phylloquinone nor partially carboxylated osteocalcin were significantly affected by the supplementation regimen.[50] Although the clinical significance of the PIVKA-II changes observed in this study warrants further investigation, the results do show that high-dose vitamin E supplementation has the potential to interfere with vitamin K status.

Patients treated with coumarin drugs undergo a particular drug-nutrient interaction because warfarin blocks the vitamin K cycle by inhibiting vitamin K epoxide reductase activity. In light of this tight coupling, any alteration in vitamin K intake will influence warfarin efficacy, as has been reported on numerous occasions. In one review, it was concluded that very large amounts of vitamin K from a single meal that includes vegetables (e.g., 400 g of vegetables providing 700–1500 μg of phylloquinone) can measurably affect coagulation as measured by the International Normalized Ratio (INR), but occasional typical servings (<100 g) would probably have little lasting impact on INR. The Institute of Medicine recommends that once the dose of warfarin has been established, individuals can avoid any complications resulting from variations in vitamin K intake by continuing to follow their normal dietary patterns.[48]

## Vitamin K Requirements

The Food and Nutrition Board of the National Academy of Sciences updated the recommendations for vitamin K in 2001.[48] The Adequate Intake (AI) for vitamin K is 120 μg/d for men and 90 μg/d for women. The AI for children during the first 6 months of life is 2 μg/d and from 7 to 12 months is 2.5 μg/d. AIs for children are 30 μg/d for ages 1 to 3 years, 55 μg/d for ages 4 to 8 years, 60 μg/d for ages 9 to 13 years, and 75 μg/d for ages 14 to 18 years. The recommendations for pregnancy and lactation are the same as for nonpregnant females of similar age (90 μg/d). No Tolerable Upper Intake Level for vitamin K has been established.

## Sources of Vitamin K

The application of HPLC analysis to vitamin K and the development of relatively straightforward assay procedures have enabled analysis of a large number of foods in the last decade, in both the United States and in Europe. Vitamin K is found in a limited number of foods, with the green leafy vegetables contributing 40% to 50% of total intake, followed by certain oils. Mixed dishes were reported to contribute 15% of total intake by virtue of the oils added to the foods. Vegetables such as Swiss chard, spinach, and kale contain in excess of 300 μg phylloquinone/100 g, while broccoli, brussels sprouts, and cabbage contain between 100 and 200 μg phylloquinone/100 g.[3] The phylloquinone contents of oils is variable, with soybean and canola oils being the richest sources (100 and 200 μg/100 g, respectively), followed by olive oil (50–100 μg/100 g). Oils derived from corn and sunflower seeds are not good sources of phylloquinone (<10 μg/100 g). Hydrogenation of plant oils to form solid shortenings results in some conversion of phylloquinone to 2′,3′-dihydrophylloquinone. This form of the vitamin is most prevalent in margarines and prepared foods, and has been reported to contribute 15% to 30% of total phylloquinone intakes in the United States. The bioavailability and the relative biological activity of dihydrophylloquinone were shown to be lower than those of phylloquinone.[52] The menaquinones are not widely distributed in commonly consumed foods, but can be found in meats and some cheeses. Natto, a traditional Japanese dish made of fermented soybeans, is an excellent source of MK-7.[12]

The availability of reliable data on the vitamin K content of foods has now made it possible to obtain reasonable estimates of the dietary phylloquinone intake of the

North American, European, and Asian populations. The results of a number of studies on phylloquinone intake have been summarized by Booth and Suttie.[3] These data are somewhat variable, but indicate a mean phylloquinone intake of about 150 μg/d for older (>55 years) and 80 μg/d for younger men and women. Reported phylloquinone intakes in the United Kingdom[53] and Ireland[54] are comparable to these, albeit slightly lower, while those in the Netherlands[3] and in China[53] are higher. Intake and sources of phylloquinone from British children have also been published.[55]

## Vitamin K Toxicity

No toxicity for the natural form vitamins K1 and K2 has been documented, even when large amounts are administered.[48] However, synthetic menadione has been shown to produce hemolytic anemia, hyperbilirubinemia, and kernicterus when administered in amounts of more than 5 mg/d to infants. Consequently, menadione is no longer used as a therapeutic agent.

## Future Directions

Significant ground has been covered since the discovery of vitamin K. From a nutrient assumed to be strictly involved in blood coagulation, this vitamin has become a nutrient of many physiological systems. The family of the VKDPs now comprises proteins involved in such fundamental cellular events as signaling, proliferation, survival, and death, as well as proteins that specifically participate in skeletal, cardiovascular, and nervous systems. Still, many aspects of vitamin K metabolism remain to be specified. For example, with respect to the role of vitamin K in bone health, it has to be clarified whether the vitamin acts synergistically with other nutrients involved in bone metabolism or independently of them. Similarly, because the beneficial effects of MK-4 in bone have all been observed following pharmacological rather than physiological treatments of the vitamer, the nutritional pertinence of these results remains to be established.

As for the role of vitamin K in cardiovascular health, although animal studies have provided strong evidence that MGP acts as an inhibitor of calcification, intervention studies using the different K vitamers are needed before we know whether vitamin K nutriture can significantly influence cardiovascular risks. Furthermore, research to that end will require taking into consideration the actions of all of the VKDPs. As pointed out in a previous report,[45] a vitamin K nutritional status that is beneficial to hemostasis (warfarin treatment) could end up being detrimental to the vasculature, promoting calcification through suboptimal MGP carboxylation. Finally, much remains to be established about the role of vitamin K in brain function and whether dietary vitamin K can significantly influence cognition at different stages of life. In light of this research agenda, the vitamin K field will continue to be an exciting one in the years to come.

## References

1. Suttie JW. Vitamin K. In: Diplock AT, ed. *The Fat-Soluble Vitamins*. Lancaster: Technomic Publishing; 1985; 225–311.
2. Berkner KL, Runge KW. The physiology of vitamin K nutriture and vitamin K-dependent protein function in atherosclerosis. J Thromb Haemost. 2004;2: 2118–2132.
3. Booth SL, Suttie JW. Dietary intake and adequacy of vitamin K. J Nutr. 1998;128:785–788.
4. Suttie JW. The importance of menaquinones in human nutrition. Ann Rev Nutr. 1995;15:399–417.
5. Thijssen HHW, Drittij-Reijnders MJ. Vitamin K distribution in rat tissues: dietary phylloquinone is a source of tissue menaquinone-4. Br J Nutr. 1994;72: 415–425.
6. Wang LY, Bates CJ, Yan L, et al. Determination of phylloquinone (vitamin K1) in plasma and serum by HPLC with fluorescence detection. Clin Chim Acta. 2004;347:199–207.
7. Shearer MJ, McBurney A, Barkhan P. Studies on the absorption and metabolism of phylloquinone (vitamin K1) in man. Vitam Horm. 1974;32:513–542.
8. Savage D, Lindenbaum J. Clinical and experimental human vitamin K deficiency. In: Lindenbaum J, ed. *Nutrition in Hematology*. New York: Churchill Livingstone; 1983; 271–320.
9. Gijsbers BLMG, Jie KS, Vermeer C. Effect of food composition on vitamin K absorption in human volunteers. Br J Nutr. 1996;76:223–229.
10. Garber AK, Binkley NC, Krueger DC, Suttie JW. Comparison of phylloquinone bioavailability from food sources or a supplement in human subjects. J Nutr. 1999;129:1201–1203.
11. Booth SL, Lichtenstein AH, Dallal GE. Phylloquinone absorption from phylloquinone-fortified oil is greater than from a vegetable in younger and older men and women. J Nutr. 2002;132:2609–2612.
12. Schurgers LJ, Vermeer C. Determination of phylloquinone and menaquinones in food. Effect of food matrix on circulating vitamin K concentrations. Haemostasis. 2000;30:298–307.
13. Schurgers LJ, Vermeer C. Differential lipoprotein transport pathways of K-vitamins in healthy subjects. Biochim Biophys Acta. 2002;1570:27–32.
14. Erkkilä AT, Lichtenstein AH, Dolnikowski GG, et al. Plasma transport of vitamin K in men using deuterium-labeled collard greens. Metabolism. 2004;53: 215–221.
15. Sadowski JA, Hood SJ, Dallal GE, Garry PJ. Phylloquinone in plasma from elderly and young adults: Factors influencing its concentration. Am J Clin Nutr. 1989;50:100–108.

16. Newman P, Bonello F, Wierzbicki AS, et al. The uptake of lipoprotein-borne phylloquinone (vitamin K1) by osteoblasts and osteoblast-like cells: role of heparan sulfate proteoglycans and apolipoprotein E. J Bone Miner Res. 2002;17:426–433.
17. Yan L, Zhou B, Nigdikar S, et al. Effect of apolipoprotein E genotype on vitamin K status in healthy older adults from China and the UK. Br J Nutr. 2005; 94:956–961.
18. Schurgers LJ, Shearer MJ, Soute BA, et al. Novel effects of diets enriched with corn oil or with an olive oil/sunflower oil mixture on vitamin K metabolism and vitamin K-dependent proteins in young men. J Lipid Res. 2002;43:878–884.
19. Thijssen HHW, Drittij-Reijnders MJ. Vitamin K status in human tissues: Tissue-specific accumulation of phylloquinone and menaquinone-4. Br J Nutr. 1996;75:121–127.
20. Hodges SJ, Bejui J, Leclercq M, Delmas PD. Detection and measurement of vitamins K1 and K2 in human cortical and trabecular bone. J Bone Miner Res. 1993;8:1005–1008.
21. Harrington DJ, Soper R, Edwards C, et al. Determination of the urinary aglycone metabolites of vitamin K by HPLC with redox-mode electrochemical detection. J Lipid Res. 2005;46:1053–1060.
22. Olson RE, Chao J, Graham D, et al. Total body phylloquinone and its turnover in human subjects at two levels of vitamin K intake. Br J Nutr. 2002 ;87: 543–553.
23. Ferland G. The vitamin K-dependent proteins: An update. Nutr Rev. 1998;56:223–230.
24. Dowd P, Hershline R, Ham SW, Naganathan S. Vitamin K and energy transduction: a base strength amplification mechanism. Science. 1995;269:1684–1691.
25. Berkner KL. The vitamin K-dependent carboxylase. Annu Rev Nutr. 2005;25:127–149.
26. Di Cera E. Thrombin interactions. Chest. 2003; 124(suppl 3):11S–17S.
27. Riewald M, Ruf W. Orchestration of coagulation protease signaling by tissue factor. Trends Cardiovasc Med. 2002;12:149–154.
28. Dahlback B, Villoutreix BO. Regulation of blood coagulation by the protein C anticoagulant pathway: novel insights into structure-function relationships and molecular recognition. Arterioscler Thromb Vasc Biol. 2005;25:1311–1320.
29. Hall MO, Obin MS, Heeb MJ, et al. Both protein S and Gas6 stimulate outer segment phagocytosis by cultured rat retinal pigment epithelial cells. Exp Eye Res. 2005;81:581–591.
30. Booth SL, Charette AM. Vitamin K, oral antigoagulants, and bone health. In: Holick MF, Dawson-Hughes B, eds. *Nutrition and Bone Health*. Totowa, NJ: Humana Press; 2004; 475–478.
31. Shearer MJ. Role of vitamin K and Gla proteins in the pathophysiology of osteoporosis and vascular calcification. Curr Opin Clin Nutr Metab Care. 2000; 3:433–438.
32. Denisova NA, Booth SL.Vitamin K and sphingolipid metabolism: evidence to date. Nutr Rev. 2005; 63:111–121.
33. Yanagita M. The role of the vitamin K-dependent growth factor Gas6 in glomerular pathophysiology. Curr Opin Nephrol Hypertens. 2004;13:465–470.
34. Holland SJ, Powell MJ, Franci C, et al. Multiple roles for the receptor tyrosine kinase axl in tumor formation. Cancer Res. 2005;65:9294–9303.
35. Kalkwarf HJ, Khoury JC, Bean J, Elliot JG. Vitamin K, bone turnover, and bone mass in girls. Am J Clin Nutr. 2004;80:1075–1080.
36. McLean RR, Booth SL, Kiel DP, Broe KE, Gagnon DR, et al. Association of dietary and biochemical measures of vitamin K with quantitative ultrasound of the heel in men and women. Osteoporos Int. 2006 Jan 6:1–8 [Epub ahead of print].
37. Iwamoto J, Takeda T, Sato Y. Effects of vitamin K2 on osteoporosis. Curr Pharm Des. 2004;10:2557–2576.
38. Pilon D, Castilloux AM, Dorais M, LeLorier J. Oral anticoagulants and the risk of osteoporotic fractures among elderly. Pharmacoepidemiol Drug Saf. 2004; 13:289–294.
39. Schurgers LJ, Teunissen KJ, Knapen MH, et al. Novel conformation-specific antibodies against matrix gamma-carboxyglutamic acid (Gla) protein: undercarboxylated matrix Gla protein as marker for vascular calcification. Arterioscler Thromb Vasc Biol. 2005;25:1629–1633.
40. Erkkila AT, Booth SL, Hu FB, Jacques PF, et al. Phylloquinone intake as a marker for coronary heart disease risk but not stroke in women. Eur J Clin Nutr. 2005;59:196–204.
41. Villines TC, Hatzigeorgiou C, Feuerstein IM, et al. Vitamin K1 intake and coronary calcification. Coron Artery Dis. 2005;16:199–203.
42. Geleijnse JM, Vermeer C, Grobbee DE, et al. Dietary intake of menaquinone is associated with a reduced risk of coronary heart disease: the Rotterdam Study. J Nutr. 2004;134:3100–3105.
43. Spronk HM, Soute BA, Schurgers LJ, et al. Tissue-specific utilization of menaquinone-4 results in the prevention of arterial calcification in warfarin-treated rats. J Vasc Res. 2003;40:531–537.
44. Braam LA, Hoeks AP, Brouns F, et al. Beneficial effects of vitamins D and K on the elastic properties of the vessel wall in postmenopausal women: a follow-up study. Thromb Haemost. 2004;91:373–380.
45. Schurgers LJ, Aebert H, Vermeer C, et al. Oral anticoagulant treatment: friend or foe in cardiovascular disease? Blood. 2004;104:3231–3232.
46. Carrié I, Portoukalian J, Vicaretti R, et al. Menaquinone-4 concentration is correlated with sphingolipid

concentrations in rat brain. J Nutr. 2004;134: 167–172.

47. Carrié I, Ferland G, Obin, MS. Effects of long-term vitamin K (phylloquinone) intake on retina aging. J Nutr Neurosci. 2003;6:351–359.
48. Food and Nutrition Board, Institute of Medicine. Dietary Reference Intakes for Vitamin A, Vitamin K, Arsenic, Boron, Chromium, Copper, Iodine, Iron, Manganese, Molybdenum, Nickel, Silicon, Vanadium, and Zinc. Washington, DC: National Academies Press; 2001. Available online at: http://www.nap.edu/books/0309072794/html/. Accessed March 17, 2006.
49. American Academy of Pediatrics Committee on Fetus and Newborn. Controversies concerning vitamin K and the newborn. American Academy of Pediatrics Committee on Fetus and Newborn. Pediatrics. 2003;112(1 part 1):191–192.
50. Booth SL, Golly I, Sacheck JM, et al. Effect of vitamin E supplementation on vitamin K status in adults with normal coagulation status. Am J Clin Nutr. 2004;80:143–148.
51. Johnson MA. Influence of vitamin K on anticoagulant therapy depends on vitamin K status and the source and chemical forms of vitamin K. Nutr Rev. 2005;63:91–97.
52. Booth SL, Lichtenstein AH, O'Brien-Morse M, et al. Effects of a hydrogenated form of vitamin K on bone formation and resorption. Am J Clin Nutr. 2001;74:783–790.
53. Yan L, Zhou B, Greenberg D, Wang L, et al. Vitamin K status of older individuals in northern China is superior to that of older individuals in the UK. Br J Nutr. 2004;92:939–945.
54. Duggan P, Cashman KD, Flynn A, Bolton-Smith C, Kiely M. Phylloquinone (vitamin K1) intakes and food sources in 18–64-year-old Irish adults. Br J Nutr. 2004;92:151–158.
55. Prynne CJ, Thane CW, Prentice A, Wadsworth ME. Intake and sources of phylloquinone (vitamin K(1)) in 4-year-old British children: comparison between 1950 and the 1990s. Public Health Nutr. 2005; 8:171–180.

# V Water-Soluble Vitamins and Related Nutrients

# 17 Vitamin C

Carol S. Johnston

Long before vitamin C was utilized as a cofactor for enzymes in mammalian systems, it was a crucial constituent of land plants, scavenging hydrogen peroxide in chloroplasts to permit efficient photosynthesis. Plant mutants deficient in vitamin C are hypersensitive to ozone, sulfur dioxide, and ultraviolet B irradiation, and the genetic engineering of plants to enhance the ascorbate biosynthesis pathway has been considered as a way of increasing the plant's resistance to oxidative stress. Recent data demonstrating that ascorbic acid concentrations modulate plant gene expression indicate a role for the vitamin in plant development, with high concentrations promoting growth and buffering against the high oxidative load that accompanies rapid metabolism and low concentrations favoring dormancy.[1]

In the animal kingdom, invertebrates and fish cannot manufacture vitamin C; the transition of vertebrates from water to land was accompanied by an ability to manufacture vitamin C. Amphibians first appeared 345 to 395 millions of years ago during the Devonian period, about 100 million years after the appearance of the early terrestrial plants. The extremely stressful conditions associated with terrestrial life, including high oxygen tension, desiccation by dry air, and hot sun, may have necessitated selection pressure for species capable of vitamin C synthesis.[2] Reptiles, birds, and most mammals retained the capacity for vitamin C synthesis over the course of evolution. However, guinea pigs and the highly evolved mammalian species (flying mammals, monkeys, apes, and man) lost the ability to synthesize vitamin C due to the absence of L-gulonolactone oxidase, the terminal enzyme of the synthetic pathway from glucuronic acid. However, these vitamin C-dependent animals possessed a marked increase in both copper and zinc superoxide dismutases compared with the vitamin C-synthesizing amphibians, reptiles, and mammals, thereby maintaining a strong defense system against oxygen toxicity.[3]

Chatterjee[2] calculated that the rate of vitamin C synthesis in small mammals ranged from 150 mg/kg body weight/d in rats to nearly 275 mg/kg body weight/d in rabbits and mice. In these species, the body pool of vitamin C ranged from 30 to 100 mg/kg and blood vitamin C concentrations varied from 0.5 to 1.0 mg/dL (28–57 μmol/L).[4] In contrast, vitamin C-dependent humans consume only about 1 mg of vitamin C/kg body weight/d and maintain a body pool of vitamin C near 20 mg/kg and a plasma vitamin C concentration near 0.5 to 0.7 mg/dL (28–40 μmol/L).[5] Therefore, it would appear that humans, although incapable of manufacturing vitamin C, are adept at conserving the vitamin. Early tracer studies demonstrated that the calculated half-life for vitamin C in humans was several orders of magnitude above that calculated for both rats and guinea pigs.

The ability of humans to effectively retain vitamin C may be explained in part by differences in vitamin C catabolism. In guinea pigs and rats, as well as in primates, there is considerable conversion of ascorbic acid to carbon dioxide. Over 65% of an injected dose was excreted as carbon dioxide within 10 days in guinea pigs, with 40% of the dose catabolized to carbon dioxide within the first 24 hours.[7] In humans, this respiratory pathway is seemingly absent, since less than 5% of an injected dose appeared as carbon dioxide after a 10-day period.[6] The principal route of excretion of vitamin C and its metabolites in humans is through the urine, mainly as oxalate and unmetabolized ascorbic acid. In 10 days, about 40% of an injected dose of ascorbic acid is excreted in the urine in humans[6] compared with only 10% in guinea pigs. These metabolic differences among vitamin C-dependent species imply that interspecies comparisons must be carefully considered.

## Chemistry and Metabolism

Vitamin C is a redox system comprising L-ascorbic acid, the free radical monodehydro-L-ascorbic acid (AFR), and oxidized ascorbate or dehydro-L-ascorbic

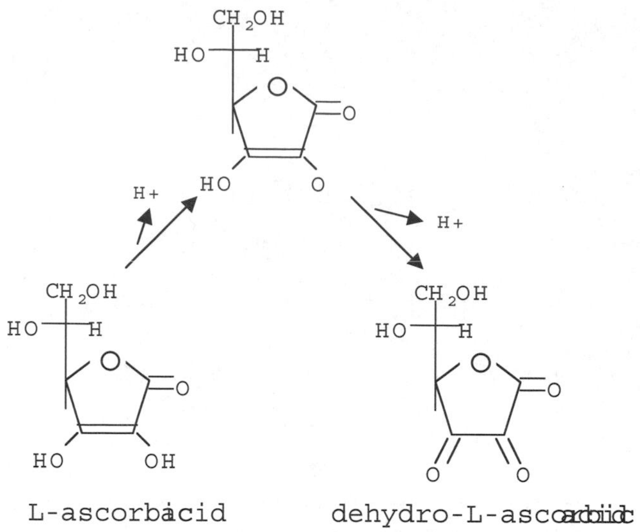

L-ascorbic acid dehydro-L-ascorbic acid

Figure 1. The catabolism of ascorbic acid.

acid (DHA) (Figure 1). The ascorbate radical/ascorbate thermodynamic couple, the one-electron reduction potential, is below that of most physiological redox systems. Hence, vitamin C acts as an antioxidant with many systems, including the α-tocopherol free radical, the glutathione radical, peroxyl radicals, the hydroxyl free radical, the superoxide radical, and the urate free radical. This strong reducing agent was first isolated from the adrenal glands of cows in 1928 and termed "hexuronic acid" by the Hungarian scientist Albert Szent-Györgyi. By 1932, the antiscorbutic property of hexuronic acid was established independently by Szent-Györgyi and by Professor C.G. King of the University of Pittsburgh, and the compound was renamed "ascorbic acid." Chemist Norman Haworth, at Birmingham, England, working in collaboration with Szent-Györgyi, elucidated the structure of ascorbic acid in 1933. Both men received a Nobel Prize in 1937 for their work leading to the discovery and structure of vitamin C.

Ascorbic acid is a six carbon, water-soluble (33 g/100 $cm^3$ at 20°C) γ-lactone (MW 176.14). Its acidic nature results from the ionization of the enolic OH on C-3 ($pK_a$ 4.25), and the molecule exists as a monovalent anion at physiological pH. In most animal species, ascorbic acid is synthesized from glucose units in the hexuronic acid pathway of the liver or kidney. In humans, a genetic lesion inhibits the synthesis of L-glulonolactone oxidase, the terminal enzyme for ascorbic acid synthesis, and diet is the sole source of the vitamin. Ascorbic acid is transported into cells via high-affinity, low-capacity, sodium-dependent transporters: SVCT1 expression is largely confined to epithelial cells (intestine, kidney, and liver), and SVCT2 is ubiquitously expressed in various tissues, including brain, eye, placenta, osteoblast cells, and endothelial tissues.[8] The requirement for ascorbic acid is evidenced in SVCT2-knockout mice (*S1c23a2*$^{-/-}$), which display respiratory distress and fatal brain hemorrhaging within minutes of birth.

As a sensitive single electron donor, ascorbic acid is readily oxidized to AFR in blood and tissues, and this radical is rapidly recycled to ascorbic acid via NADPH-dependent reduction by thioredoxin reductase or NADH-dependent reduction by microsomal or mitochondrial AFR reductases. Therefore, a free radical chain reaction involving other substrates is avoided. At sites of marked oxidant stress, the dismutation of two molecules of AFR to DHA and ascorbic acid will likely occur. DHA undergoes irreversible hydrolysis with a half-life of less than 1 minute, but the rapid uptake of DHA via glucose transporters by many cell types, followed by the immediate two-electron reduction of DHA to ascorbic acid by several mechanisms (glutathione-dependent systems or NADPH-dependent systems mediated by thioredoxin reductase or by 3α-hydroxysteroid dehydrogenase), suggests an efficient system for the recycling and salvaging of vitamin C.[9] This "bystander effect" would ensure increased intracellular antioxidant defense capacity at sites of extracellular oxidative stress.

In individuals with pathologies that could interfere with the DHA uptake and recycling process, such as diabetes and glucose transporter protein syndrome, vitamin C status may be compromised. Smoking may also alter these processes, thereby impacting vitamin C status. If not recycled to ascorbate, DHA is irreversibly delactonized to 2,3-diketogulonic acid, and its further degradation to oxalic acid likely represents the major catabolic pathway of ascorbic acid in non-supplementing individuals. In subjects observed for a 10-day period following injection of L-ascorbic acid-1-14C, over 40% of the administered dose appeared in urine, and nearly one-half of the excreted dose was oxalic acid. About 20% of the dose was excreted as unmetabolized ascorbic acid and 2,3-diketogulonic acid, and DHA represented 20% and less than 2% of the excreted metabolites, respectively.[6] Other possible catabolic products of ascorbic acid include L-threonic acid, L-xylonic acid, L-lyxonic acid, and L-xylose (Figure 2).

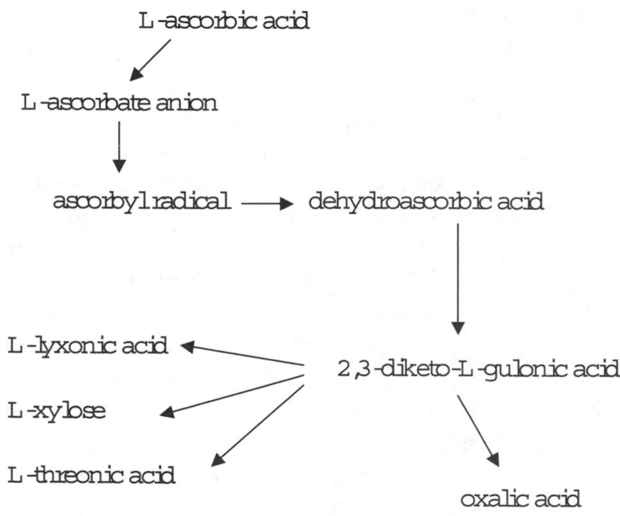


Figure 2. The vitamin C redox system.

As dosage levels increase, the amount of unmetabolized ascorbic acid excreted in urine increases substantially. In steady-state subjects receiving 100 mg of vitamin C daily, approximately 25% of the injected dose was excreted in urine within 24 hours.[10] At a 200 mg dosage, urinary excretion of ascorbic acid rose to over 50% of the injected dose. At 500 and 1000 mg dosages, 100% of the injected dose was excreted unmetabolized in urine within 24 hours. Urinary oxalic acid levels did not vary at vitamin C dosages ranging from 30 to 200 mg daily.[10] At higher dosage levels of 400 and 1000 mg of vitamin C daily, urinary oxalic acid rose 15% and 35%, respectively, reaching urinary concentrations in the range of 35 to 40 mg/d. In a separate study, pharmacologic dosages of vitamin C (5000 to 10,000 mg/d) raised urinary oxalic acid 20% to 40%, equating to concentrations from 32 to 37 mg/d.[11] Thus, at high intakes of ascorbic acid (>1000 mg/d), only about 1% of the dose is converted to oxalic acid and the remainder appears to be excreted unmetabolized in urine. In healthy, non-supplementing adults, oxalate excretion averages about 25 mg/d, and normal oxalate excretion is considered to be less than 40 mg/d.

## Analytical Measures

Liquid chromatography-electrochemical detection methods are generally employed to measure total ascorbic acid (the sum of ascorbic acid and DHA) in plasma samples.[12] For these methods, total ascorbic acid is effectively preserved in frozen (−70°C) lyophilized plasma samples containing dithiothreitol for at least 6 years, and in frozen (−70°C) serum containing 50 g/L metaphosphoric acid for 2 years. The inter-laboratory reproducibility for total ascorbic acid using similar chromatographic methods is large (coefficient of variation = 15%–25%), impacting comparisons between epidemiological or clinical investigations. Electrochemical detection cannot be used for the direct measurement of DHA, so most chromatographic methods measure DHA indirectly by subtraction after its pre- or post-column reduction to ascorbic acid using dithiothreitol or tris[2-carboxyethyl]phosphine hydrochloride.

Spectrophotometric procedures, the dinitrophenylhydrazine and dichlorophenolindophenol methods, are also used for ascorbic acid analyses of biological samples. The dinitrophenylhydrazine method utilizes copper to oxidize ascorbic acid to DHA, and these products react with 2,4-dinitrophenylhydrazine to form the chromophore with an absorption band at 520 nm. To differentiate DHA from ascorbic acid, copper is omitted from the reagent mixture, permitting the measurement of DHA specifically, and ascorbic acid is determined by calculation.[13] Although some investigations suggest that these spectrophotometric procedures have similar sensitivity and specificity as the chromatographic procedures,[13] others do not.[14] A simple and rapid enzymatic procedure using ascorbate oxidase and o-phenylenediamine has recently been described for the routine analysis of total ascorbic acid in a clinical setting.[15] This procedure can be automated and correlated well ($r^2 > 0.95$) with standard chromatographic analyses.

## Biochemical Functions

As a cofactor for mixed function oxidases, ascorbic acid participates in the synthesis of various macromolecules including collagen, carnitine, and norephinephrine. In many of these reactions, ascorbic acid promotes enzyme activity by maintaining metal ions in the reduced form. Other reductants (e.g., glutathione, cysteine, tetrahydrofolate, dithiothreitol, and 2-mercaptoethanol) can replace vitamin C in these reactions in vitro, but vitamin C is the most effective. Moreover, depletion/repletion studies in animals and man clearly demonstrate the physiological relevance of vitamin C in these pathways. In collagen and carnitine syntheses, α-ketoglutarate-dependent dioxygenases incorporate one atom of oxygen into succinate and one into the oxidized product of the substrate in the presence of ferrous iron. Three dioxygenases are required for the synthesis of the connective tissue protein collagen: prolyl 4-hydroxylase, prolyl 3-hydroxylase, and lysyl-hydroxylase. The hydroxylation of proline and lysine residues in nascent collagen polypeptide chains is a post-translational event that permits the intermolecular cross-linking required for the formation of the triple helical structure characteristic of collagen. In the absence of ascorbic acid, peptidyl hydroxylation does not occur, and the folding of pro-collagen molecules is prevented, resulting in intracellular accumulation of non-helical trimers. Many of the symptoms of the vitamin C deficiency disease scurvy can be attributed to weakened collagenous structures, including bruising, muscle weakness, gum deterioration, and poor wound healing.

In vivo investigations in vitamin C-deficient guinea pigs, controlling for effects of inanition, clearly demonstrated the essential role of vitamin C in collagen synthesis required for bone, skin, and tendon formation.[16] Furthermore, symptoms similar to scurvy are noted in patients with Ehlers-Danlos syndrome type VI, a condition characterized by reduced lysyl hydroxylase activity, a result of mutations in the DNA encoding this enzyme. Vitamin C supplementation in these patients (5 g/d for 3 weeks) improved wound healing and muscle strength and increased urinary excretion of hydroxylysine and hydroxyproline. In vitro investigations with fibroblasts extracted from these patients demonstrated that ascorbic acid stimulated collagen production 60% to 100%.[17] Thus, under conditions of low lysyl hydroxylase activity, vitamin C administration enhanced enzyme activity, peptidyl hydroxylation, and collagen production, providing evidence of its utilization in this pathway.

Two enzymes involved in the carnitine biosynthetic pathway are dependent on ascorbic acid for optimal activity: 6-N-trimethyl-L-lysine hydroxylase (in the conversion of 6-N-trimethyl-L-lysine to γ-trimethylaminobutyraldehyde) and γ-butyrobetaine hydroxylase (in the conversion of γ-butyrobetaine to carnitine). Carnitine is necessary for the transport of long-chain fatty acids into the mitochondrial matrix for oxidation, and the reverse flow of acetylcarnitine from the intra- to the extra-mitochondrial space promotes substrate oxidation and increases the availability of mitochondrial free coenzyme A. About 98% of total body carnitine is in muscle, and skeletal and heart muscle carnitine concentrations are reduced by 50% in vitamin C-deficient guinea pigs compared with pair-fed controls.[18] In cultured guinea pig hepatocytes, supplemental ascorbic acid resulted in enhanced carnitine synthesis and the stimulation of beta-oxidation.[19] Hughes et al.[20] first postulated that reduced muscle carnitine was responsible for the marked fatigue and lassitude characteristic of vitamin C depletion and early scurvy. Work efficiency during exercise, a measure of vigor, increased significantly in vitamin C-depleted subjects repleted with vitamin C (500 mg/d),[21] but it is not clear whether this change in performance was related to improved carnitine status.

Ascorbic acid is also considered the predominant reductant for two copper-dependent enzymes: dopamine β-hydroxylase (used in the synthesis of norepinephrine from dopamine[22]) and peptidylglycine α-amidating monooxygenase (used in the amidation, and therefore activation, of various hormones and neurotransmitters[23]). A role for ascorbic acid in these reactions may explain the high concentrations of ascorbic acid in the adrenal and pituitary glands: 30–40 mg/100 g versus 10–15 mg/100 g in most other tissues including liver, spleen, brain, and pancreas. Given the influence of norepinephrine on the vascular system, and the many autocrine and paracrine roles for α-amidated peptides, the involvement of ascorbic acid in these processes suggests an important yet unexplored role of this nutrient in neuroendocrine biology. Recent investigations utilizing cDNA microarray analysis showed that ascorbic acid treatment induced upregulation of numerous genes, including pro-collagen type 1 alpha 2, apolipoprotein E, transferrin, tyrosine hydroxylase, and interferon alpha-inducible protein,[24] suggesting novel molecular mechanisms of ascorbic acid.

# Physiological Functions

## *Immune Function*

As an effective scavenger of reactive oxygen species, ascorbic acid minimizes the oxidative stress associated with the respiratory burst of activated phagocytic leukocytes, thereby functioning to control the inflammation and tissue damage associated with immune responses.[25] Ascorbic acid also directly inhibited NF-κB activation in vitro[26] and selectively influenced inflammatory cytokine production in monocytes,[27] suggesting an antioxidant-independent effect of vitamin C in controlling inflammatory responses. Some evidence indicates that vitamin C may have antiviral activities. In vitro, ascorbic acid reduced virus activity by degrading phage/viral nucleic acids and by inhibiting viral replication. Topical application of ascorbic acid in patients with Herpes simplex virus infections decreased the duration of the lesions and viral shedding.[28] Several reports show an anti-*Helicobacter pylori* effect of ascorbic acid in vitro, and serum ascorbic acid was inversely related to seroprevalence of both *H. pylori* and the pathogenic cagA-positive strain of *H. pylori* in a large, population-based US sample.[29]

Vitamin C supplementation may also reduce the severity of cold symptoms. Based on standardized clinical assessment, elderly patients hospitalized with acute respiratory infections who received 200 mg of vitamin C daily fared better than patients receiving placebo.[30] Hyperresponsiveness to histamine is responsible for many of the symptoms associated with respiratory tract infections, allergic disorders, bronchial asthma, and colitis ulcerosa. Vitamin C destroys histamine spontaneously. In vivo, vitamin C supplementation (2000 mg/d for 2 weeks) reduced blood histamine concentrations 30% to 40% in adult subjects.[31] Oral dosages of vitamin C significantly reduced bronchial responsiveness to inhaled histamine in patients with allergy.[32] Also, supplementation with 250 mg of vitamin C/d for 6 weeks significantly reduced (by 50%) monocyte ICAM-1 mRNA expression in healthy male subjects,[33] which is an important observation because the expression of this adhesion molecule by inflammatory/endothelial cell types is associated with the airway hyperresponsiveness that is characteristic of the common cold, allergic asthma, and seasonal allergic rhinitis.

Supplemental vitamin C enhances neutrophil chemotaxis in healthy subjects. In patients with Chediak-Higashi syndrome, chronic granulomatous disease, or recurrent furunculosis, all conditions characterized by neutrophil dysfunction, vitamin C supplementation improves neutrophil motility and reduces infection rates. Some evidence indicates that vitamin C administration may augment natural killer cell activity, which is important for immunosurveillance against tumor cells in the early stages of tumor development.

## *Atherosclerosis*

Vascular health represents a balance between endothelial-derived vasodilative substances (e.g., nitric oxide) and the constrictor substances that promote endothelial dysfunction, smooth muscle proliferation, and the formation of plaque. The major atherosclerotic risk factors—hypercholesterolemia, hypertension, smoking, diabetes, and family history of premature coronary artery disease—are associated with reduced nitric oxide formation and endothelial dysfunction. Ascorbic acid stimulates endothelial nitric oxide synthesis in vitro by stabilizing, via chemical reduction, intracellular concentrations of the essential cofactor, tetrahydrobiopterin.[34] Intra-arterial infusion of ascorbic acid (approximately 25 mg/min) improved nitric oxide-mediated endothelium vasodilation in some investigations[35] but not others.[36] In a double-blind, placebo-controlled trial, both short (a single 2000 mg dose) and long-term (500 mg/d for 30 days) vitamin C supplementation of patients with clinically documented coronary artery disease improved endothelial vasomotor function by 40% to 50%[35]; however, combined antioxidant therapy (800 IU/d vitamin E and 1000 mg/d vitamin C for 6 months) did not improve brachial artery endothelial function in patients with coronary artery disease.[36] Epidemiological investigations suggest only a modest benefit of supplemental vitamin C for reducing cardiovascular disease mortality in low-risk populations. In a 5-year prospective study of 1605 randomly selected men ages 42 to 60, those with vitamin C deficiency at baseline (plasma vitamin C $< 0.2$ mg/dL) were at significantly increased risk of myocardial infarction after controlling for potentially confounding variables (RR = 2.5; 95% CI: 1.3,5.2).[37]

Vitamin C may also protect the vasculature against LDL-induced cytotoxicity. In vitro, pretreatment of arterial smooth muscle cells with vitamin C inhibited the muscle cell fragmentation and reactivity induced by oxidized LDL.[38] For patients receiving cardiac catheterization treatment, a low plasma vitamin C concentration predicted the presence of an unstable coronary syndrome, as indicated by athersclerotic lesion activity.[39] Vitamin C-induced improvements in endothelium vasodilation may also contribute to the reported hypotensive effects of vitamin C supplementation.

### *Cancer*

Damage to biomolecules by reactive free radicals is considered a major contributing factor in cancer, and as a particularly effective antioxidant in physiological systems, vitamin C has been promoted as an anti-cancer agent. Vitamin C supplementation was associated with modest reductions in mortality from stomach cancer and colorectal cancers in large study cohorts drawn from the Cancer Prevention Study II after a 16-year follow-up. A short-term prospective intervention trial, however, did not demonstrate a beneficial effect of vitamin C (120 mg/d for 5 years) on the incidence of esophageal, stomach, or colon cancers.[40] However, the progression of *H. pylori* infection to gastric dysplasia or gastric cancer was reduced by 80% in individuals with adequate serum vitamin C status ($>0.55$ mg/dL) compared with those who had below-adequate status.[41]

Many investigations have attempted to link vitamin C supplementation with reduced DNA oxidative damage in vivo, but the results are inconsistent and inconclusive. Epidemiological studies consistently indicate that cancer risks are inversely related to high intakes of fruits and/or vegetables, implying that vitamin C in isolation may function differently from the mixtures of antioxidants and phytochemicals found naturally in fruits and vegetables.

### *Other Physiological Effects*

As a major water-soluble antioxidant, ascorbic acid detoxifies reactive radicals in plasma and in the cytoplasm and mitochondria of cells. As discussed above for atherosclerosis and cancer, the data indicate only a neutral-to-modest role of vitamin C in attenuating the progression of diseases associated with oxidative stress. In the many disease states adversely affected by oxidative stress and reactive radicals, including cataract, macular degeneration, Alzheimer's disease, and rheumatoid arthritis, the total antioxidant capacity of tissues may be the protective factor, not a single antioxidant. Vitamin C enhanced vitamin E activity in human erythrocytes by regenerating α-tocopherol from its oxidized derivative,[42] and dietary vitamin C was associated with increased plasma vitamin E concentrations in vivo. Vitamin C supplementation also increased cellular glutathione concentrations by 18% in healthy adults.[43] Thus, vitamin C may help to maximize total tissue antioxidant capacity, the characteristic likely to be most physiologically relevant.

Vitamin C is required for collagen synthesis and may impact bone matrix formation. In postmenopausal women there was no evidence that dietary vitamin C (daily dietary intake of approximately 115 mg) was associated with bone mineral density. However, in several investigations, older women who used vitamin C supplements for 10 years or more (averaging 400–700 mg vitamin C daily) had a higher bone mineral density than non-supplement users of the same age.[44]

Iron absorption from test meals is enhanced 2- to 3-fold in the presence of 25 to 70 mg of vitamin C, presumably due to the ascorbate-induced reduction of ferric iron to ferrous iron, which is less likely to form insoluble complexes with phytates. However, indices of iron status, including hemoglobin, serum ferritin, and percent transferrin saturation, are generally not improved in iron-deficient subjects consuming vitamin C-fortified diets.[45] In animal models, ascorbic acid deficiency reduces the activity of hepatic cholesterol 7 alpha-hydroxylase, affecting the catabolism of cholesterol to bile acids and the risk for gallbladder disease. In patients with cholesterol gallstones, vitamin C supplementation (2000 mg/d for 2 weeks) altered bile acid composition and significantly increased nucleation time.[46] Epidemiological investigations have indicated an independent association between serum ascorbic acid level and a significantly lower prevalence of clinical gallbladder disease and asymptomatic gallstones.

## Deficient and Marginal Status

Functional measures for vitamin C status are not currently available, so it is generally evaluated based on vitamin C concentrations in the plasma or leukocytes. Although these indices are closely related over a wide range of vitamin C intakes, leukocyte concentrations are considered to be the more sensitive indicator of vitamin C status. The measurement of leukocyte vitamin C is technically complex, and interpretation of data is complicated by the variable content in different leukocyte fractions and the lack of standardized reporting procedures. Therefore, the measurement of plasma vitamin C concentration is currently the most practiced and widely applied test for vitamin C status. Plasma concentrations less than 0.2 mg/dL (11 μmol/L) indicate vitamin C deficiency, and concentrations between 0.2 and 0.5 mg/dL (11 and 28 μmol/L) represent marginal vitamin C status, defined as moderate risk for developing vitamin C deficiency due to inadequate tissue stores. Intakes at the recommended level, 75 to 90 mg/d, are associated with plasma vitamin C concentrations near 0.8 mg/dL (45 μmol/L), and tissue saturation is achieved at intakes from 100 to 200 mg/d, corresponding to plasma concentrations near 1.0 mg/dL (about 60 μmol/L).[10]

Subcutaneous and intramuscular hemorrhages, leg edema, neuropathy, and cerebral hemorrhage characterize scurvy, the vitamin C deficiency disease, and these symptoms are generally attributed to weakened collagenous structures. If untreated, the condition is ultimately fatal. Throughout the course of civilization, scurvy has plagued whole populations without access to fresh fruits and vegetables. However, scurvy is also occasionally observed in developed nations, particularly among alcoholics, institutionalized elderly, men who live alone, and individuals who consume restrictive diets containing little or no fruits and vegetables. Patients complain of lassitude, weakness, and vague myalgias, and seek medical advice following the appearance of a skin rash or lower extremity edema.

Data from the Second National Health and Nutrition Examination Survey (NHANES II) conducted from 1976–1980 and generalizable to the non-institutionalized civilian population of the United States indicated that the prevalence of vitamin C deficiency (plasma vitamin C concentrations less than 0.2 mg/dL or 11 μmol/L) ranged from 0.1% in children 3 to 5 years of age to 3% in females 25 to 44 years of age and 7% in males 45 to 64 years of age.[47] The prevalence of marginal vitamin C status (plasma vitamin C concentrations greater than 0.2 mg/dL and less than 0.5 mg/dL or from 11–28 μmol/L) ranged from 17% in adult females to 24% in adult males.[47] NHANES III data collected from 1988 to 1994 indicated that 17% of adult males and 12% of adult females 25 to 44 years of age were vitamin C deficient, and that 20% to 23% of adults had marginal vitamin C status.[48]

**Table 1.** Dietary Reference Intakes (DRI) for Vitamin C for All Age and Gender Groups

| Group | EAR* | RDA† |
|---|---|---|
| | *mg* | |
| **Infants‡** | | |
| 0–6 months | 40 | — |
| 7–12 months | 50 | — |
| **Children** | | |
| 1–3 years | 13 | 15 |
| 4–8 years | 22 | 25 |
| **Boys** | | |
| 9–13 years | 39 | 45 |
| 14–17 years | 63 | 75 |
| **Girls** | | |
| 9–13 years | 39 | 45 |
| 14–17 years | 56 | 65 |
| **Men** | | |
| 19–30 years | 75 | 90 |
| 31–50 years | 75 | 90 |
| 51–70 years | 75 | 90 |
| >70 years | 75 | 90 |
| **Women** | | |
| 19–30 years | 60 | 75 |
| 31–50 years | 60 | 75 |
| 51–70 years | 60 | 75 |
| >70 years | 60 | 75 |
| **Pregnant women** | | |
| 14–18 years | 66 | 80 |
| 19–30 years | 70 | 85 |
| 31–50 years | 70 | 85 |
| **Lactating women** | | |
| 14–18 years | 96 | 115 |
| 19–30 years | 100 | 120 |
| 31–50 years | 100 | 120 |

* EAR, Estimated Average Requirement (the intake estimated to meet the requirement of half the healthy individuals in a group)
† RDA, Recommended Daily Allowance (the intake sufficient to meet the nutrient requirement of 97% to 98% of healthy individuals in a group)
‡ Values represent Adequate Intake (AI, observed or estimates of intake by group of health individuals that are assumed to be adequate)

# Dietary Requirements

Historically, the Recommended Dietary Allowance (RDA) for vitamin C was set at a level to prevent scorbutic symptoms for several weeks if vitamin C were omitted from the diet. In 2000, the Panel on Dietary Antioxidants and Related Compounds of the Food and Nutrition Board of the Institute of Medicine released the Dietary Reference Intakes (DRI) for vitamin C (Table 1).[49] For adult men, the Estimated Average Requirement (EAR) for vitamin C, the level of intake that is estimated to meet the requirements of half the healthy individuals in a life stage and gender group, was set at 75 mg/d to maintain near-maximal tissue concentrations of vitamin C and provide antioxidant protection. The estimated requirement for adult women, 60 mg/d, was extrapolated based on body weight differences from the EAR for men.

The RDAs were calculated as 120% of the EAR, and

are believed to cover the needs of 97% to 98% of individuals in a group (90 and 75 mg/d for adult men and women, respectively). Older age groups (>50 years) have decreased lean body mass compared with their younger counterparts; however, the DRIs for older men and women were not decreased from that for younger adults because oxidative stress, which causes higher vitamin C needs, increases with age. Smokers should consume an additional 35 mg of vitamin C daily, totaling 125 mg/d for adult men and 110 mg/d for adult women, due to increased oxidative stress. Although dietary recommendations for vitamin C were not increased for passive smokers or for those under excessive physical or emotional stress, these individuals were urged to ensure that they meet the RDA for vitamin C.

Higher vitamin C intakes were recommended for pregnant and lactating women to offset losses from maternal body pools (Table 1). RDAs for children ranged from 15 to 25 mg/d for younger children and from 45 to 75 mg/d for preadolescents and adolescents (Table 1). Since there were no functional criteria for vitamin C status in infants, the recommended intakes of vitamin C at this age level were based on Adequate Intakes (AI) reflecting the vitamin C ingestion of mainly breast-fed infants (Table 1).

## Toxicity

High doses of vitamin C (as high as 2 g/d) are well tolerated by healthy individuals, and epidemiological data indicate that individuals who regularly supplement their diets with vitamin C may be at lower risk for some cancers, lens opacities, gall and kidney stones, and cardiovascular disease mortality. Claims that high-dose vitamin C regimens may lead to rebound scurvy, red blood cell hemolysis, and vitamin $B_{12}$ deficiency do not withstand scientific scrutiny.

Because dietary vitamin C may enhance mealtime iron absorption, some have speculated that high-dose vitamin C regimens may aggravate conditions associated with increased iron absorption and storage, notably hemochromatosis. About 0.5% and 10% of the US population are homozygous and heterozygous, respectively, for the hemochromatosis *HFE* gene mutation. Ascorbic acid fortification of foods did increase non-heme iron absorption in homozygous patients compared with wild-type controls, but increased iron absorption was not observed in heterozygous patients.[50]

Vitamin C supplementation may also have adverse effects on thalassemia major, an iron-overload disease characterized by impaired globin chain synthesis, ineffective erythroporesis, and anemia. Cases are usually diagnosed in the first year of life, and blood transfusions are often required for survival. In the absence of chelation therapy, iron accumulation in parenchymal tissues is associated with progressive dysfunction of the heart, liver, and endocrine glands. Vitamin C deficiency is common among these patients and may contribute to disease symptoms. However, vitamin C repletion of patients may mobilize iron stores, creating iron-overloaded plasma and risk for increased oxidative stress. Vitamin C supplementation in these patients should be coordinated with chelation therapy.

Although in vitro investigations have indicated that the $Fe^{3+}$-catalized oxidation of ascorbic acid promotes free radical formation in culture medium, experiments conducted in serum showed no such effect, even under conditions of iron overload. In animal models, ascorbic acid supplementation did not increase the oxidative stress induced by dietary iron.[51] High-dose vitamin C regimens may increase urinary excretion of oxalic acid and uric acid, constituents of renal calculi, and thus may theoretically promote the formation of kidney stones. Recently, a modest association between supplemental vitamin C use and incident kidney stones was observed in the Health Professionals Follow-up Study[52], but only after controlling for potassium intake. Hence, calcium oxalate stone formers should be cautioned on the use of supplemental vitamin C.

Nausea, diarrhea, and abdominal cramping are observed in a small portion of subjects (10%–30%) consuming large doses of vitamin C (≥3 g/d). Based strictly on reports of gastrointestinal disturbances, a tolerable upper intake level for vitamin C was set at 2000 mg/d for adults.[49] The upper intake level represents a dosage level that is with high probability tolerated biologically and provides guidance to individuals using dietary supplements.

## Summary

Ascorbic acid is a potent reducing agent/antioxidant in animal species and land plants. Humans rely on vitamin C for the activity of enzymes involved in collagen, carnitine, and norepinephrine synthesis and for non-enzymatic roles that impact physiological parameters. The recommended daily intake for vitamin C is 90 mg/d for adult men and 75 mg/d for adult women, and the tolerable upper limit is 2000 mg/d. Supplemental vitamin C should not replace high intakes of fruits and vegetables, but may offer health benefits under certain circumstances for some individuals. Scurvy continues to be observed in malnourished populations worldwide. Low intakes of fresh fruits and vegetables, either by choice or due to scarcity, increases the risk for vitamin C deficiency, a concern for isolated populations such as the Canadian Inuit, refugees dependent on standard relief food, cancer patients and the critically ill, and the elderly. Other population groups at risk for suboptimal vitamin C status include smokers and diabetics. Research into the contribution of poor vitamin C status to morbidity and mortality in these populations is warranted. Furthermore, because it is inexpensive and relatively non-toxic, continued investigation of the potential benefits of pharmacologic intakes of vitamin C should be pursued as well.

# References


1. Pastori GM, Kiddle G, Antoniw J, et al. Leaf vitamin C contents modulate plant defense transcripts and regulate genes that control development through hormone signaling. Plant Cell. 2003;15:939–951.
2. Chatterjee IB. Evolution and the biosynthesis of ascorbic acid. Nature. 1973;182:1271–1272.
3. Nandi A, Mukhopadhyay CK, Ghosh MK, Chattopadhyay DJ, Chatterjee IB. Evolutionary significance of vitamin C biosynthesis in terrestrial vertebrates. Free Radic Biol Med. 1997;22:1047–1054.
4. Dash JA, Jenness R, Hume ID. Ascorbic acid turnover and excretion in two arboreal marsupials and in laboratory rabbits. Comp Biochem Physiol B. 1984; 77:391–397.
5. Bluck LJ, Izzard AP, Bates CJ. Measurement of ascorbic acid kinetics in man using stable isotopes and gas chromatography/mass spectrometry. J Mass Spectrom. 1996;31:741–748.
6. Hellman L, Burns JJ. Metabolism of L-ascorbic acid-1-C14 in man. J Biol Chem. 1958;230:923–930.
7. Burns JJ, Burch HB, King CG. The metabolism of 1-C14-L-ascorbic acid in guinea pigs. J Biol Chem 1951;191:501–514.
8. Takanaga H, Mackenzie B, Hediger MA. Sodium-dependent ascorbic acid transporter family SLC23. Pflugers Arch. 2004;447:677–682.
9. Nualart FJ, Rivas CI, Montecinos VP, et al. Recycling of vitamin C by a bystander effect. J Biol Chem. 2003;278:10128–10133.
10. Levine M, Conry-Cantilena C, Wang Y, et al. Vitamin C pharmacokinetics in healthy volunteers: evidence for a recommended dietary allowance. Proc Natl Acad Sci U S A. 1996;93:3704–3709.
11. Wandzilak TR, D'Andre SD, Davis PA, Williams HE. Effect of high dose vitamin C on urinary oxalate levels. J Urol. 1994;161:834–837.
12. Margolis SA, Vangel M, Duewer DL. Certification of standard reference material 970, ascorbic acid in serum, and analysis of associated interlaboratory bias in the measurement process. Clin Chem. 2003;49: 463–469.
13. Schaus EE, Kutnink MA, O'Conner DK, Omaye ST. A comparison of leukocyte ascorbate levels measured by the 2,4-dinitrophenylhydrazine method with high-performance liquid chromatography using electrochemical detection. Biochem Med Metab Biol. 1986;36:369–376.
14. Margolis SA, Duewer DL. Measurement of ascorbic acid in human plasma and serum: stability, intralaboratory repeatability, and interlaboratory reproducibility. Clin Chem. 1996;42(8 part 1):1257–1262.
15. Ihara H, Shino Y, Aoki Y, Hashizume N, Minegishi N. A simple and rapid method for the routine assay of total ascorbic acid in serum and plasma using ascorbate oxidase and o-phenylenediamine. J Nutr Sci Vitaminol (Tokyo). 2000;46:321–324.
16. Kipp DE, McElvain M, Kimmel DB, Akhter MP, Robinson RG, Lukert BP. Scurvy results in decreased collagen synthesis and bone density in the guinea pig animal model. Bone. 1996;18:281–288.
17. Pasquali M, Still MJ, Vales T, et al. Abnormal formation of collagen cross-links in skin fibroblasts cultured from patients with Ehlers-Danlos syndrome type VI. Proc Assoc Am Physicians. 1997;109: 33–41.
18. Nelson PJ, Pruitt RE, Henderson LL, Jenness R, Henderson LM. Effect of ascorbic acid deficiency on the in vivo synthesis of carnitine. Biochim Biophys Acta. 1981;672:123–127.
19. Hughes RE, Hurley RJ, Jones E. Dietary ascorbic acid and muscle carnitine (β-OH-γ-(trimethyl amino) butyric acid) in guinea pigs. Br J Nutr. 1980; 43:385–387.
20. Ha TY, Otsuka M, Arakawa N. Ascorbate indirectly stimulates fatty acid utilization in primary cultured guinea pig hepatocytes by enhancing carnitine synthesis. J Nutr. 1994;124:732–737.
21. Johnston CS, Swan PD, Corte C. Substrate utilization and work efficiency during submaximal exercise in vitamin C depleted-repleted adults. Int J Vitam Nutr Res. 1999;69:41–44.
22. Bornstein SR, Yoshida-Hiroi M, Sottriou S, et al. Impaired adrenal catecholamine system function in mice with deficiency of the ascorbic acid transporter (SVCT2). FASEB J. 2003;17:1928–1930.
23. Prigge ST, Mains RE, Eipper BA, Amzel LM. New insights into copper monooxygenases and peptide amidation: structure, mechanism and function. Cell Mol Life Sci. 2000;57:1236–1259.
24. Yu DH, Lee KH, Lee JY, et al. Changes of gene expression profiles during neuronal differentiation of central nervous system precursors treated with ascorbic acid. J Neurosci Res. 2004;78:29–37.
25. Chien CT, Chang WT, Chen HW, et al. Ascorbate supplement reduces oxidative stress in dyslipidemic patients undergoing apheresis. Arterioscler Thromb Vasc Biol. 2004;24:1111–1117.
26. Bowie AG, O'Neill LA. Vitamin C inhibits NF-κB activation by TNF via the activation of p38 mitogen-activated protein kinase. J Immunol. 2000;165: 7180–7188.
27. Härtel C, Strunk T, Bucsky P, Schultz C. Effects of vitamin C on intracytoplasmic cytokine production in human whole blood monocytes and lymphocytes. Cytokine. 2004;27:101–106.
28. Hamuy R, Berman B. Treatment of Herpes simplex virus infections with topical antiviral agents. Eur J Dermatol. 1998;8:310–319.
29. Simon JA, Hudes ES, Perez-Perez GI. Relation of serum ascorbic acid to Helicobacter pylori serology in US adults: the Third National Health and Nutrition Examination Survey. J Am Coll Nutr. 2003;22: 283–289.
30. Hunt C, Chakravorty NK, Annan G, Habibzadeh

N, Schorah CJ. The clinical effects of vitamin C supplementation in elderly hospitalized patients with acute respiratory infections. Int J Vitam Nutr Res. 1994;64:212–219.

31. Johnston CS, Retrum KR, Srilakshmi JC. Antihistamine effects and complications of supplemental vitamin C. J Am Diet Assoc. 1992;92:988–989.
32. Bucca C, Rolla G, Oliva A, Farina JC. Effect of vitamin C on histamine bronchial responsiveness of patients with allergic rhinitis. Ann Allergy. 1990;65:311–314.
33. Rayment SJ, Shaw J, Woollard KJ, Lunec J, Griffiths HR. Vitamin C supplementation in normal subjects reduces constitutive ICAM-1 expression. Biochem Biophys Res Comm. 2003;308:339–345.
34. Heller R, Unbehaun A, Schellenberg B, Mayer B, Werner-Felmayer G, Werner ER. L-Ascorbic acid potentates endothelial nitric oxide synthesis via a chemical stabilization of tetrahydrobiopterin. J Biol Chem. 2001;276:40–47.
35. Gokce N, Keaney JF, Frei B, et al. Long-term ascorbic acid administration reverses endothelial vasomotor dysfunction in patients with coronary artery disease. Circulation. 1999;99:3234–3240.
36. Kinlay S, Behrendt D, Fang JC, et al. Long-term effect of combined vitamins E and C on coronary and peripheral endothelial function. J Am Coll Cardiol. 2004;43:629–634.
37. Nyyssonen K, Parviainen MT, Salonen R, Tuomilehto J, Salonen JT. Vitamin C deficiency and risk of myocardial infarction: prospective population study of men from Eastern Finland. BMJ. 1997;314:634–638.
38. Siow RC, Richards JP, Pedley KC, Leake DS, Mann GE. Vitamin C protects human vascular smooth muscle cells against apoptosis induced by moderately oxidized LDL containing high levels of lipid hydroperoxides. Arterioscler Thromb Vasc Biol. 1999;19:2387–2394.
39. Vita JA, Keaney JF, Raby KE, et al. Low plasma ascorbic acid independently predicts the presence of an unstable coronary syndrome. J Am Coll Cardiol. 1998;31:980–986.
40. Blot WJ, Li JY, Taylor PR, et al. Nutrition intervention trials in Linxian, China: supplementation with specific vitamin/mineral combinations, cancer incidence, and disease-specific mortality in the general population. J Natl Cancer Inst. 1993;85:1483–1492.
41. You WC, Zhang L, Gail MH, et al. Gastric dysplasia and gastric cancer: Helicobacter pylori, serum vitamin C, and other risk factors. J Natl Cancer Int. 2000;92:1607–1612.
42. May JM, Qu ZC, Mendiratta S. Protection and recycling of alpha-tocopherol in human erythrocytes by intracellular ascorbic acid. Arch Biochem Biophys. 1998;349:281–189.
43. Lenton KJ, Sane AT, Therriault H, Cantin AM, Payette H, Wagner JR. Vitamin C augments lymphocyte glutathione in subjects with ascorbate deficiency. Am J Clin Nutr. 2003;77:189–195.
44. Morton DJ, Barrett-Connor EL, Schneider DL. Vitamin C supplement use and bone mineral density in postmenopausal women. J Bone Miner Res. 2001;16:135–140.
45. Garcia OP, Diaz M, Rosado JL, Allen LH. Ascorbic acid from lime juice does not improve the iron status of iron-deficient women in rural Mexico. Am J Clin Nutr. 2003;78:267–273.
46. Gustafsson U, Wang FH, Axelson M, Kallner A, Sahlin S, Einarsson K. The effect of vitamin C in high doses on plasma and biliary lipid composition in patients with cholesterol gallstones: prolongation of the nucleation time. Eur J Clin Invest. 1997;27:387–391.
47. Fulwood R, Johnson CL, Bryner JD, Gunter EW, McGrath CR: Hematological and nutritional biochemistry reference data for persons 6 months - 74 years of age: United States, 1976–1980. DHHS Publication No. (PHS) 83-1682. Hyattsville, MD: US Department of Health and Human Services, Public Health Service, National Center for Health Statistics; 1982.
48. Hampl JS, Taylor CA, Johnston CS. Vitamin C deficiency and depletion in the United States: the Third National Health and Nutrition Examination Survey, 1988 to 1994. Am J Public Health. 2004;94:870–875.
49. Food and Nutrition Board, Institute of Medicine. Dietary Reference Intakes for Vitamin C, Vitamin E, Selenium, and Carotenoids. Washington, DC: National Academies Press; 2000. Available online at: http://www.nap.edu/openbook/0309069351/html/index.html.
50. Hunt JR, Zeng H. Iron absorption by heterozygous carriers of the HFE C282Y mutation associated with hemochromatosis. Am J Clin Nutr. 2004;80:924–931.
51. Premkumar K, Bowlus CL. Ascorbic acid does not increase the oxidative stress induced by dietary iron in C3H mice. J Nutr. 2004;134:435–438.
52. Taylor EN, Stampfer MJ, Curhan GC. Dietary factors and the risk of incident kidney stones in men: New insights after 14 years of follow-up. J Am Soc Nephrol. 2004;15:3225–3232.

# 18 Thiamin

C.J. Bates

Beriberi, or "kakke," a disease of human populations commonly characterized by a polyneuritic paralysis that affects mainly the lower limbs, has been encountered historically much more often in Far Eastern, rice-growing countries than in the west. Beriberi has been described throughout recorded history, but became especially prevalent during the 19th century, when the introduction of steam-powered mills began to permit highly efficient "polishing," or removal of the aleurone layer, of the rice. This appeared to improve the quality and thus increase the acceptability of the product, but it is now known that the highest concentration of B vitamins in general, and of thiamin (vitamin $B_1$) in particular, occurs in the narrow aleurone layer of cells between the germ and the starchy endosperm. Therefore, most of the B vitamins in rice are removed and discarded by the polishing process.

Theories of toxic or infectious causes of beriberi were favored until the end of the 19th century. The first accepted demonstration that food and nutrition were implicated is generally attributed to Dr. K. Takaki, surgeon-general of the Japanese navy, who in 1885 improved the quality of the naval diet by introducing protein-rich foods, and thereby greatly reduced the prevalence of beriberi. A few years later, Christian Eijkman, a Dutch medical officer working in Java, discovered that a polyneuritic disease closely resembling human beriberi could be induced in chickens by feeding them polished rice. This discovery of an animal model of the disease permitted rapid progress, and Eijkman then found that the affected chickens could be cured, and the disease prevented, by feeding them rice bran, or "silverskin," polishings. A detailed description of Eijkman's contribution is available.[1] The curative factor was shown by Eijkman's successor, Gerrit Grijns, to be water-soluble. Further studies of the anti-neuritic factor, by Casimir Funk in London, led to the coining of the term "vitamine" in 1911.

The chemical structure of the anti-neuritic vitamin, which was first known as aneurin, and later as vitamin $B_1$, thiamine, or thiamin (Figure 1), was established by Williams in 1936.[2] The achievement of a chemical synthesis in the same year[3] was the first step toward large-scale manufacture of this vitamin.

Biochemical studies, mainly during the 1930s, helped to elucidate the intracellular metabolic role of thiamin in the form of its phosphorylated derivative co-carboxylase, later renamed as thiamin pyrophosphate or thiamin diphosphate (TDP), as an essential catalytic center present in several key enzymes involved mainly in carbohydrate metabolism. The role of co-carboxylase in the metabolism of pyruvate proved especially important as a link between the anaerobic and aerobic oxidation of carbohydrates.

## Chemistry of Thiamin, Thiamin Cofactors, and Thiamin Antagonists

Figure 1 shows that thiamin consists of two linked organic ring structures: a pyrimidine ring bearing an amino group and a sulfur-containing thiazole ring linked to the pyrimidine by a methylene bridge. The thiazole ring bears a primary alcohol side chain that becomes phosphorylated in vivo to give the thiamin phosphate esters that have cofactor activity. The most widely available commercially produced form of the free vitamin is thiamin chloride hydrochloride, in which the thiazole nitrogen is in the chloride form and the basic amino group is present as its hydrochloride. The dry, crystalline vitamin salt is very stable, and solutions in dilute (e.g., 0.1 N) mineral acids are also very stable, provided that they are protected from ultraviolet light. The usual procedure employed to extract thiamin from food and tissues for analysis is to autoclave them in 0.1 N hydrochloric acid, which ensures complete conversion of its phosphorylated forms to free thiamin. If this simple acid extraction process fails to ensure complete liberation, the use of diastase enzyme treatment before acid extraction may be necessary.[4]

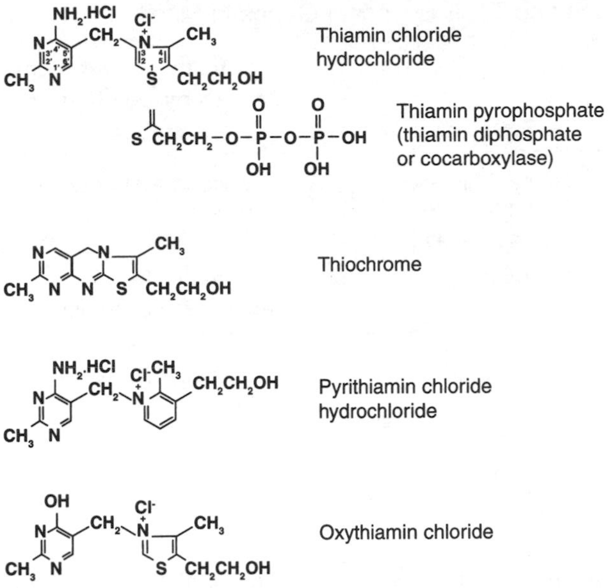

Thiamin chloride hydrochloride

Thiamin pyrophosphate (thiamin diphosphate or cocarboxylase)

Thiochrome

Pyrithiamin chloride hydrochloride

Oxythiamin chloride

Figure 1. Thiamin and its derivatives.

In alkaline solution, thiamin is much less stable, and is readily oxidized even at room temperature, firstly to the dimer thiamin disulfide and then with more vigorous oxidation (e.g., in alkaline potassium ferricyanide) to the biologically inactive, highly fluorescent, triple-ring structure known as thiochrome (Figure 1; see also the thiamin analysis section).

Thiamin is also readily inactivated by reaction with sulfite, which results in cleavage of the methylene bridge, even at room temperature. Certain enzymes that occur in fish, ferns, and some bacteria can destroy thiamin by their thiaminase activity. By this means, diets that contain large amounts of raw fish can cause thiamin deficiency in humans, and ferns and some other thiaminase-containing plants also produce deficiency, mostly in farm animals. There is a fascinating account of the hazard to humans who relied on a diet with a high thiaminase content coming from the nardoo fern (*Marsilea drummondii*) and from raw freshwater mussels during an ill-fated expedition by Burke and Wills through the center of Australia in the middle of the 19th century.[5]

Certain polyhydroxyphenols, such as caffeic acid, chlorogenic acid, and tannins, that occur in plants and plant foods can exhibit thiamin-inactivating properties by oxidizing the thiazole ring to the disulfide, which reduces absorption. Two compounds with very specific, competitive-type antithiamin activity that have been widely used in studies of thiamin deficiency in animal models are pyrithiamin and oxythiamin (Figure 1). Pyrithiamin, which accumulates in the brain, is a powerful inhibitor of the conversion of thiamin to TDP. It has proven very useful as a means of mimicking in animals the abnormalities characteristic of Wernicke's encephalopathy. Oxythiamin, by contrast, does not cross the blood-brain barrier and produces thiamin-deficiency symptoms only in peripheral tissues.

## Thiamin Analysis and Status Assessment

Several different approaches have been taken in the measurement of thiamin content of foods and tissues and the estimation of thiamin status in human individuals and populations.[4,6,7] In early studies, animal growth assays were used to quantitate thiamin potency, but these proved too slow and cumbersome. They were replaced by microbiological assays, which depend on the extent of growth of a thiamin-dependent organism such as *Lactobacillus fermentum* or *L. viridescens* in a growth medium in which the only source of thiamin is the test extract or calibration standard.[4] This approach is still used, especially for food analysis, and has the advantage of not requiring any preliminary separation or purification of the vitamin because the assay is highly specific for thiamin. However, this approach is not well suited to most modern analytical laboratories, in which chemical assay methods are usually preferred. The conversion of thiamin to fluorescent thiochrome (Figure 1) by oxidation in alkaline medium provides the basis for a highly sensitive assay. If combined with an efficient separation procedure, such as that afforded nowadays by high-performance liquid chromatography,[4,6,7] good sensitivity and specificity can usually be achieved.

Measurement of thiamin status in animals or humans has employed several different techniques, and there is little consensus about which technique is preferable. Thiamin excretion rates in urine have been widely used,[6,7,9] but ideally this requires a 24-hour sample, and thus depends on considerable subject cooperation. Also, it is not very sensitive at the borderline of deficiency. Several laboratories measure thiamin ester (or total thiamin) concentrations in serum, plasma, whole blood, or separated red cells. The preferred choice of assay depends on the precise question being asked.[8] Another approach depends on the sensitivity of red cell transketolase, a thiamin-dependent enzyme, to variations in tissue thiamin status and in medium-term intake. The ratio of transketolase activities in vitro with and without its TDP cofactor, varies with the thiamin supply and therefore tissue thiamin content. It is advisable to measure the basal activity (e.g., as a ratio to hemoglobin) as well as the response to TDP in vitro, which is known as the "activation coefficient." This method has been widely used for human population studies, and can be run as a rate assay on some programmable clinical chemistry analyzers. Unfortunately, there are no widely available quality control materials with defined values, nor are there external quality assurance schemes for any of the thiamin status assays.

**Table 1.** Thiamin and Reduced Folate Transporter Proteins and Their Encoding Genes in Man

| Transporter Protein | Gene | Chromosome Locus | Substrates | Abnormality or Pathology Caused by Deletion or Mutation |
|---|---|---|---|---|
| Reduced Folate Transporter (RFT) | SLC19A1 | 21q22.3 | Reduced folates and thiamin phosphates | Resistance to methotrexate (in mice) |
| Thiamin Transporter 1 (ThTr1) | SLC19A2 | 1q23.3 | Free thiamin | Thiamin-responsive megaloblastic anemia or Rogers syndrome |
| Thiamin Transporter 2 (ThTr2) | SLC19A3 | 2q37 | Free thiamin | Seizure susceptibility (in mice) |

# Mechanisms of Absorption and Bioavailability

Efficient utilization by the body of the low concentrations of thiamin liberated in the intestinal lumen during digestion of most unfortified foods and diets is achieved through a specific energy-dependent, saturable active transport process, with conversion in the gut wall to thiamin phosphate esters. This occurs in all animals that have been studied, including man,[9] and it is most active in the duodenum, especially the jejunum. In a study of thiamin uptake by human intestinal biopsies,[10] the active transport process was shown to exhibit Michaelis-Menten kinetics, with a $K_m$ of 4.4 μmol/L, and was competitively inhibited by the thiamin analogs pyrithiamin, oxythiamin, and amprolium. It was concluded, from a comparison of one deficient and several non-deficient human subjects, that the active transporter can be down-regulated when thiamin supplies are adequate. At higher concentrations of thiamin (e.g., above 5 μmol/L in the gut lumen), absorption by passive diffusion predominates. Because this process is less efficient than active transport, the proportion of the administered dose that is absorbed decreases sharply as its size increases.

During the past decade, considerable advances have been made in characterizing the specific thiamin transporter proteins, and the genes that encode them, in mammalian tissues.[11,12] Two microtubule-associated transporter proteins (Table 1) actively transport free thiamin by a hydrogen ion gradient-dependent process with which thiamin antagonists such as pyrithiamin strongly compete. One of these thiamin transporters, ThTr1, is mutated and nonfunctional in humans with the genetic disease called thiamin-responsive megaloblastic anemia (TRMA or Rogers syndrome). Its pathology includes megaloblastic anemia (probably resulting from impaired ribose metabolism in erythroblasts), sensorineural deafness, and diabetes (possibly due to impaired thiamin transport in the cochlea and pancreas, respectively). The anemia and diabetes respond to high oral doses of thiamin that bypass the impaired transporter. A mouse ThTr1-knockout model exhibits similar pathologies.

Less is known about the second thiamin transporter, ThTr2, which is encoded by the gene SLC19A3 (Table 1). A third, closely (structurally) related gene, SLC19A1, encodes RFT (reduced folate transporter), a protein that transports both reduced folates (e.g., 5-methyltetrahydrofolate) and the mono- and diphosphates of thiamin.

Active transport of thiamin occurs at the brush border surface of intestinal epithelial cells (maximally in the proximal ileum), in the renal tubular epithelium, in the placenta, and in many other cells and tissues, including fibroblasts and erythrocytes. Conversion to thiamin phosphates occurs abundantly within these cells, thus helping to retain the vitamin, but these are converted back to free thiamin before being transported across the basolateral surfaces of epithelia for delivery into the circulation. There is evidence of transport modulation by thiamin status variations, by the age of the animal, and possibly by factors such as the diabetic state, thyroid hormone levels, and calcium and calmodulin.

Although the bioavailability of thiamin in food has appeared to vary considerably,[9] this may have been an artifact of the assay procedures used, and in practice it is thought that most food sources of thiamin are readily available in healthy human subjects. The thiamin phosphate esters in tissues are readily converted to free thiamin in the gut.[13] Some drugs can impair thiamin availability, but the most common cause of impaired absorption is thought to be alcohol abuse.[9] Several lipophilic thiamin derivatives have been developed as a means of achieving a high percentage absorption of pharmacological doses. These have been used to treat people with impaired absorption and/or increased requirements, such as patients with Wernicke-Korsakoff syndrome (see below). The allithiamin compound benfotiamine, which contains an open thiazole ring that can be closed within the body, seems especially promising.[14]

If thiamin is infused as a large dose intravenously,[15] there is considerable intracellular accumulation of thiamin phosphates (e.g., in the red cells), as well as rapid renal excretion of the excess above requirements. A study of the half-life of thiamin at normal body loads using radioactively labeled thiamin probes[13] yielded an estimate of 9.5 to 18.5 days, and a large number of labeled breakdown products were detected in the urine. Compared with most other vitamins, tissue deficiency of thiamin occurs relatively quickly when a low intake is encountered. Because of this, thiamin deficiency is often one of the first deficiencies to appear when food quality has deteriorated rapidly, as may occur during famines or in refugee camps.

A specific thiamin-binding protein has been identified at a number of sites, including rat serum and liver and chicken eggs, that is hormonally controlled and essential for the carriage of thiamin between tissues. It forms an equimolar complex with another vitamin binding-protein, but the biological significance of this is not known.

## Biochemical Functions

The mammalian enzymes that require thiamin diphosphate as one of their cofactors are involved in carbohydrate, lipid, and amino acid metabolism.[16] The best known are pyruvate dehydrogenase, which provides a key link between the glycolytic pathway and the citric acid cycle; α-ketoglutarate dehydrogenase, which is part of the citric acid cycle; and tranketolase, which is involved in the pentose phosphate pathway. These enzymes are regulated in a complex manner. Each consists of a decarboxylase moiety that binds TDP at the active site, a lipoic acid-binding moiety, a flavoprotein (with dihydrolipoamide dehydrogenase activity), and one or more regulatory components that toggle the enzyme complex between the active (non-phosphorylated) form and the inactive (phosphorylated) form. Their activities are also controlled more directly by feedback interaction with the enzyme products. The phosphokinase that controls enzyme activity by phosphorylation is in turn controlled by changes in the ratio of adenosine triphosphate (ATP) to adenosine diphosphate (ADP) and by calcium ion concentrations. Because of these control mechanisms, and the excess capacity that they imply, it has proven difficult to trace a direct link between changes in the activity of the dehydrogenase enzymes in thiamin deficiency and the clinical (e.g., neurological) symptoms. A fourth thiamin-requiring enzyme is branched-chain ketoacid dehydrogenase, which plays a key role in the metabolism of branched-chain amino acids. A fifth, recently identified TDP-requiring enzyme is a peroxisomal enzyme that catalyzes the α-oxidation of 3-methyl branched chain fatty acids such as phytanic acid.

Thiamin deficiency results in the accumulation of lactate and pyruvate after a glucose load and exercise due to impairment of pyruvate dehydrogenase. However, despite the thiamin-requirement of α-ketoglutarate dehydrogenase, thiamin deficiency apparently does not usually affect substrate flux through the citric acid cycle, because an alternative or "shunt" pathway via γ-amino butyric acid can bypass it.[16]

There is some evidence of an additional function of thiamin as the triphosphate TTP in membrane function and nerve action potentials. This is poorly understood; however, the TTP in membranes tends to be conserved in thiamin deficiency. Thiamin is partly able to restore the nerve action potential of ultraviolet light-damaged isolated nerves. In Leigh's disease, encephalopathy is accompanied by a reduction in TTP synthesis, which can be treated with high-dose thiamin. TTP thus appears to have a function different from that of TDP, mainly in nerves and brain, where it may activate chloride ion transport, possibly by phosphorylation of a chloride ion channel.[16,17]

Recently, the detailed pathophysiology and biochemistry of thiamin deficiency-induced processes in the brain have been studied in human subjects, animal models, and cultured cells.[18-20] Neurodegeneration becomes apparent, initially as a reversible lesion and later irreversibly, in very specific areas of the brain, notably the submedial thalamic nucleus and parts of the cerebellum, especially the superior cerebellar vermis. Many of the biochemical changes that affect neurons and non-neuronal brain cells (e.g., astrocytes, glial cells, endothelial cells, and neutrophils) are chararacteristic of oxidative stress, and affect specific endothelial cell activation markers, including nitric oxide synthetase, hemoxygenase, and non-protein-bound iron. Microglial cells become activated, there are changes in the blood-brain barrier, and oxidation damage markers such as 4-hydroxynonenal, advanced glycation end products, and fragmentation damage to DNA have been observed in cultured neurons deprived of thiamin. Some of these changes are preventable by traditional antioxidants such as vitamin E or butylated hydroxyanisole. Mouse knockout models, with deletion of biochemical pathways that are activated by oxidant stress, may become partly protected from neuronal loss during thiamin deficiency.

Sufferers from Wernicke's encephalopathy (see below) are reported to have increased peroxidase activity in the neurons of their basal forebrain. Apoptosis of thiamin-deprived neuronal cells in culture has been linked to the decline of a specific regulatory protein kinase, Jnk1. It has been proposed that in the early stages of thiamin deficiency, biochemical changes in the (relatively robust) non-neuronal cells of the brain can be neuroprotective, but at the later stages of deficiency they are likely to exacerbate neuronal degeneration. Such mechanistic studies are potentially relevant, not only to the understanding of the sequelae of thiamin deficiency, but also of human diseases such as Wernicke-Korsakoff syndrome, Alzheimer's, and Parkinson's diseases, in which similar biochemical changes have been reported. Clearly, there are important aspects of the biochemical functions of thiamin that are only now being elucidated.

## Human Requirements, Dietary Reference Intakes, and Toxicity

Because thiamin is needed mainly for the metabolism of carbohydrate, fat, and alcohol, and because there is strong evidence that thiamin requirements increase as energy expenditure increases, its reference intake values are commonly expressed as ratios to food energy.

At intakes of thiamin below 0.16 mg/1000 kcal (0.038 mg/MJ), clinical symptoms of beriberi are likely to occur in the form of edema and heart failure (wet) and polyneuropathy (dry). In normal adult humans, as thiamin intake increases from 0.16 to 0.3 mg/1000 kcal (0.038–0.072 mg/MJ), the risk of beriberi symptoms becomes negligible and urinary excretion rates and red cell transketolase indices move into the normal range. For most subjects, this occurs at or below an intake of 0.23 mg/1000 kcal (0.055 mg/MJ).[21,22] In the United Kingdom,[21] the Lower Reference Nutrient Intake (LRNI) is set at 0.23 mg/1000 kcal (0.055 mg/MJ); the Estimated Average Requirement (EAR) at 0.3 mg/1000 kcal (0.072 mg/MJ); and the Reference Nutrient Intake (RNI), which is equivalent to the older Recommended Daily Intake (RDI), at 0.4 mg/1000 kcal (0.096 mg/MJ). Values for children younger than one year are slightly lower. Dietary Reference Intakes (DRI) for the United States[22] are 1.2 mg for adult males and 1.1 mg for adult females. For pregnant women in the United States the reference intake is 1.4 mg, and for lactating women it is 1.5 mg. Clearly, judgment must be used in setting these values, and caution is needed in their use and interpretation. Nevertheless, they can be very useful for the purpose of comparing populations and predicting risk in vulnerable groups.

Thiamin is remarkably non-toxic at high intakes, even in doses three orders of magnitude higher than the normal requirement, when given either orally or intravenously. If given orally, the majority is not absorbed and is therefore wasted. If given intravenously (e.g., at 100–500 mg/d), it can provide rapid relief from life-threatening deficiency conditions before the excess not required by the body is excreted in the urine. Concerns about allergic reactions are probably unfounded.[23]

## Food Sources of Thiamin

Particularly good sources of thiamin, which provide more than 0.3 mg per 1000 kcal (0.072 mg/MJ) of food energy, include wheat germ and yeast extract, pork and ham, organ meats from most animals, and some green vegetables, including peas, asparagus, and okra. Wholegrain foods are good sources, but white flour and bread made from it are poor sources unless there is mandatory fortification (as in the case in the United Kingdom, United States, and some other countries). Other types of meat, fish, and eggs, along with most vegetables, are moderate sources, whereas cow's milk and most fruits are rather poor sources. By far the poorest sources are polished rice (as noted earlier), refined sugars, and fats. An alkaline pH during cooking can result in increased losses; thus, more than 50% of thiamin in flour is lost during baking with bicarbonate baking powder (as in soda bread). The addition of sulfite to fruit, juices, and minced meat can result in major destruction of thiamin, and heat sterilization of milk causes a greater loss (30%–50%) than does pasteurization (10%–20%).

## Thiamin Deficiency in Human Populations at the End of the 20th Century

Whereas the older descriptions of beriberi focused mainly on the polyneuritic form of the disease, two separate clinical entities are now attributable to thiamin deficiency: an edematous form known as wet beriberi and a non-edematous neurological form known as dry beriberi. Affected individuals may exhibit either form or a mixture of both. The wet form is associated with heart failure, which may be rapidly fatal, while the dry form tends to be chronic but not usually life-threatening. A recent reanalysis of descriptions of the signs and symptoms of the pathology of thiamin deficiency[24] has suggested that a severe acute deficiency in animal models resembles human deficiency less well than a milder chronic deficiency does. Chronic marginal deficiency models may therefore be preferable for the study of human disease.

Recently, endemic thiamin deficiency has been reported in Indonesia,[25] the Seychelles,[26] the Amazonian Indians of South America,[27] and a refugee camp in Thailand,[28] and these are likely to be only a small proportion of the communities affected worldwide. In some countries, there have been several sporadic outbreaks in vulnerable groups. For example, in The Gambia in West Africa, which was closely monitored during the last half of the 20th century, there was an outbreak of edematous beriberi in adult male palm wine tappers in 1952; in 1967, there was a report of edema in urban policemen, which peaked during the rainy season every year for several years; in 1988, there was a severe outbreak in the rural village of Chilla, with 22 deaths of previously healthy adults[29]; and in 1990–1991, there was a report of 38 cases of beriberi (13 dry, 14 wet, and 11 mixed) from the main hospital in the capital, Banjul.[30] In all cases, the prevalence of the condition peaked during the rainy season, which is typically a time of food shortages, stress, and hard physical work, and the affected groups responded well to thiamin supplements alone.

Myeloneuropathies are relatively common in tropical developing countries[31]; some are endemic and others are epidemic in character. The etiology of these conditions is poorly understood but is likely to be multifactorial. A severe epidemic of optic and peripheral neuropathies occurred without warning in Cuba, starting in 1992 and peaking in 1993, with approximately 50,000 cases reported in a total population of 11 million. It began soon after a major economic upheaval associated with the breakup of the USSR, which caused a deterioration of living standards, including poor nutrition. In the early stages of the epidemic, the symptoms were mainly optic, with central or cecocentral scotoma, and were seen mainly in male tobacco and alcohol users. A few months later, there was a second peak, this time involving cases of painful sensory neuropathy that was sometimes associated with deafness.[32] Biochemical evidence of thiamin depletion was widespread, and in the clinically affected subjects there was a correlation between poor thiamin status and high alcohol consumption.[33] The incidence of new cases decreased rapidly during the later part of 1993 following the introduction of country-wide multivitamin supplementation. Other risk factors were also present in the affected population.[31,34]

Another report from Thailand[35] suggested that thiamin deficiency may increase the risk of cerebral complications of malaria. Although the amount of morbidity and mortality that is currently attributable, or partly attributable, to thiamin deficiency worldwide is difficult to estimate, it is likely to be a significant public health problem in many parts of the world. Sporadic outbreaks can clearly occur, without warning, in conditions of stress coupled with poor diet. Refugee camps, famines, and other emergencies are typical high-risk situations.

## Wernicke-Korsakoff Syndrome

Chronic alcohol abuse is frequently associated with a constellation of symptoms that can include Wernicke's encephalopathy, Korsakoff psychosis, or a combination of these, known as Wernicke-Korsakoff syndrome. Alcoholics often have a low intake of thiamin, impaired absorption, and possibly impaired utilization. Thiamin supplements frequently produce dramatic clinical improvement. At autopsy, there are pathological lesions in the middle and lower brain of Wernicke-Korsakoff syndrome victims, and it has been suggested that the accumulation of neurotoxic extracellular glutamate may be largely responsible.[36]

Australia has a relatively high prevalence of the disease, and the mandatory addition of thiamin to bread flour in 1991 was followed by some improvement.[37,38] Although alcohol consumption and thiamin fortification are significant factors, they do not appear to provide a complete explanation for the observed variation in prevalence among countries.[38] In the United Kingdom, concern has been expressed about under-diagnosis and poor clinical management,[23] and a wider use of parenteral thiamin supplements for treatment is recommended. Improved clinical criteria have been suggested, and the use of magnetic resonance imaging[39] for diagnosis is gaining favor.

Evidence of a possible genetic predisposition to Wernicke-Korsakoff syndrome in some individuals, based on subtle genetic changes in the properties of the thiamin-dependent enzyme transketolase, remains controversial.[16,18,40] There is evidence that low thiamin levels may have a deleterious effect on mRNA and apoenzyme protein synthesis for transketolase and pyruvate dehydrogenase without affecting those of α-ketoglutarate dehydrogenase to the same extent.[41] A study of thiamin deficiency using oxythiamin in rats suggested that the deficient state may dispose them to increased voluntary alcohol intake.[42]

Wernicke-Korsakoff syndrome has sometimes been observed in the absence of alcohol abuse. One example of increased risk is seen in gastrectomy patients long after surgery,[43] which may be a result of either poor diet or impaired thiamin absorption.

## Thiamin Needs of Older People: Possible Relation to Some Forms of Dementia

Because of reduced appetite, difficulty in eating, increased dependence on medication, and other risk factors, some older people are at high risk of poor micronutrient status. There is also evidence that thiamin compounds decrease in some parts of the human brain, such as the external globus pallidus, throughout life.[44] A review of the literature on thiamin intake and status of older people living in North America,[45] who were mostly poor or ill, and many of whom were living in institutions, had suboptimum status. However, conditions such as thiamin-responsive heart disease and Wernicke-Korsakoff syndrome were no more common in older than in younger people. The claim that iatrogenic effects of drugs can cause deficiency, for example, by an increased loss of thiamin associated with chronic diuretic use,[46] needs further investigation.

In a recent survey of older people living in the United Kingdom,[47,48] poor biochemical thiamin status, defined as erythrocyte transketolase activation coefficients above 1.25, was encountered in 9% of the free-living participants and in 14% of those living in institutions such as nursing homes. There was a highly significant ($P < 0.0001$) between-subject correlation between estimated thiamin intake and thiamin status as measured by the erythrocyte transketolase activation coefficient.

One question often raised in recent years is whether there is a relationship between poor thiamin status and risk of dementia, especially of Alzheimer's disease. If so, are thiamin (or multinutrient) supplements beneficial for people at high risk?[16,18] Low plasma thiamin concentrations have repeatedly been observed in patients with senile dementia of the Alzheimer's type, but were not found in patients with Parkinson's disease.[8,49] Patients with Alzheimer's disease appear to have decreased brain activity of some thiamin cofactor-dependent enzymes, and also have low levels of thiamin diphosphate and possibly of thiamin diphosphatase in their brains at autopsy. Some, but not all, thiamin supplementation studies found evidence of a mild beneficial effect in Alzheimer's sufferers.[16,18] A study in New Zealand[50] reported functional benefits of thiamin supplements given to older people with persistently low red cell thiamin diphosphate levels. There is a need for better biochemical and functional indices to help identify the particularly vulnerable and potentially responsive subgroups of the older population.

## Conclusion

We now know a great deal more about the body's need for thiamin than was known at the beginning of the 20th century, and widespread overt thiamin deficiency is now uncommon. Nevertheless, there remain some regions of the world and some subgroups of society that remain vulnerable and this should be investigated and monitored further. People living in tropical countries, especially when they suffer some catastrophic change in lifestyle and food quality such that "empty" calories and alcohol are heavily used, are clearly at risk. This often seems to include adult manual laborers, whose high energy expenditure is also likely to be a risk factor. Alcohol abuse, especially when it becomes chronic, is a major risk factor for Wernicke-Korsakoff Syndrome in some societies. This syndrome may be under-diagnosed, and may warrant more widespread thiamin fortification of staple foods. Some older people appear to be at risk of biochemical and functional deficiency, and some of these may benefit (e.g., with improved brain function) from supplementation, although this needs further study and confirmation. In public health terms, the benefits of reducing the risk levels in these high-risk groups are likely to be considerable.

## References


1. Carpenter KJ, Sutherland B. Eijkman's contribution to the discovery of the vitamins. J Nutr. 1995;125: 155–163.
2. Williams RR. Structure of vitamin B1. J Am Chem Soc. 1936;58:1063–1064.
3. Williams RR, Cline JK. Synthesis of vitamin B1. J Am Chem Soc. 1936;58:1504–1505.
4. Ball GFM. Thiamin (vitamin B1). In: Ball GFM, ed. *Bioavailability and Analysis of Vitamins in Foods*. London: Chapman and Hall; 1998: 267–292.
5. Earl JW, McCleary BV. Mystery of the poisoned expedition. Nature 1994;368:683–684.
6. Bates CJ. Vitamins: fat and water soluble: analysis of. In: Meyers RA, ed. *Encyclopaedia of Analytical Chemistry: Instrumentation and Applications*. Chichester, UK: John Wiley & Sons; 2000: 7390–7425.
7. Lynch PL, Young IS. Determination of thiamine by high-performance liquid chromatography. J Chromatogr A. 2000;881:267–284.
8. Gold M, Chen MF, Johnson K. Plasma and red blood cell thiamine deficiency in patients with dementia of the Alzheimer's type. Arch Neurol. 1995; 52:1081–1086.
9. Gregory JF 3rd. Bioavailability of thiamin. Eur J Clin Nutr. 1997;51(suppl 1):S34–S37.
10. Laforenza U, Patrini C, Alvisi C, Faelli A, Licandro A, Rindi G. Thiamine uptake in human biopsy specimens, including observations from a patient with acute thiamine deficiency. Am J Clin Nutr. 1997;66: 320–326.
11. Rindi G, Laforenza U. Thiamine intestinal transport and related issues: recent aspects. Proc Soc Exp Biol Med. 2000;224:246–255.
12. Ganapathy V, Smith SB, Prasad PD. SLC19: the folate/thiamine transporter family. Pflugers Arch. 2004;447:641–646.
13. Ariaey-Nejad MR, Balaghi M, Baker EM, Sauberlich HE. Thiamin metabolism in man. Am J Clin Nutr. 1970;23:764–778.
14. Loew D. Pharmacokinetics of thiamine derivatives especially of benfotiamine. Int J Clin Pharmacol Ther. 1996;34:47–50.
15. Zempleni J, Hagen M, Hadem U, Vogel S, Kübler W. Utilization of intravenously infused thiamin hydrochloride in healthy adult males. Nutrition Research. 1996;16:1479–1485.
16. Bender DA. Optimum nutrition: thiamin, biotin and pantothenate. Proc Nutr Soc. 1999;58:427–433.
17. Bettendorf L, Kolb HA, Schoffeniels E. Thiamine triphosphate activates an anion channel of large unit conductance in neuroblastoma cells. J Membr Biol. 1993;136:281–288.
18. Gibson GE, Zhang H. Interactions of oxidative stress with thiamine homeostasis promote neurodegeneration. Neurochem Int. 2002;40:493–504.
19. Martin PR, Singleton CK, Hiller-Sturmhofel S. The role of thiamine deficiency in alcoholic brain disease. Alcohol Res Health. 2003;27:134–142.
20. Ke ZJ, Gibson GE. Selective response of various brain cell types during neurodegeneration induced by mild impairment of oxidative metabolism. Neurochem Int. 2004;45:361–369.
21. Department of Health. *Report of the Panel on Dietary Reference Values of the Committee on Medical Aspects of Food Policy: Dietary Reference Values for Food Energy and Nutrients for the United Kingdom. Report on Health and Social Subjects 41*. London: Her Majesty's Stationery Office; 1995.
22. Institute of Medicine. Dietary Reference Intakes for Thiamin, Riboflavin, Niacin, Vitamin B6, Folate, Vitamin B12, Pantothenic Acid, Biotin, and Choline; 1998. Available online at: http://www.nap.edu/openbook/0309065542/html/. Accessed
23. Cook CC, Hallwood PM, Thomson AD. B vitamin deficiency and neuropsychiatric syndromes in alcohol misuse. Alcohol Alcohol. 1998;33:317–336.

24. Carpenter KJ. Acute versus marginal deficiencies of nutrients. Nutr Rev. 2002;60:277–280.
25. Djoenaidi W, Notermans SL, Verbeek AL. Subclinical beriberi polyneuropathy in the low income group: An investigation with special tools on possible patients with suspected complaints. Eur J Clin Nutr. 1996;50:549–555.
26. Bovet P, Larue D, Fayol V, Paccaud F. Blood thiamin status and determinants in the population of Seychelles (Indian Ocean). J Epidemiol Community Health. 1998;52:237–242.
27. San Sebastian M, Jativa R. Beriberi in a well-nourished Amazonian population. Acta Trop. 1998;70: 193–196.
28. McGready R, Simpson JA, Cho T et al. Postpartum thiamine deficiency in a Karen displaced population. Am J Clin Nutr. 2001,74:808–813.
29. Tang CM, Rolfe M, Wells JC, Cham K. Outbreak of beri-beri in The Gambia. Lancet. 1989;2:206–207.
30. Rolfe M, Walker RW, Samba KN, Cham K. Urban beri-beri in The Gambia, west Africa. Trans R Soc Trop Med Hyg. 1993;87:114–115.
31. Roman GC. An epidemic in Cuba of optic neuropathy, sensorineural deafness, peripheral sensory neuropathy and dorsolateral myeloneuropathy. J Neurol Sci. 1994;127:11–28.
32. Thomas PK, Plant GT, Baxter P, Bates C, Santiago Luis R. An epidemic of optic neuropathy and painful sensory neuropathy in Cuba: clinical aspects. J Neurol. 1995;242:629–638.
33. Macias-Matos C, Rodriguez-Ojea A, Chi N, Jimenez S, Zulueta D, Bates CJ. Biochemical evidence of thiamine depletion during the Cuban neuropathy epidemic, 1992–1993. Am J Clin Nutr. 1996;64: 347–353.
34. Bowman BA, Bern C, Philen RM. Nothing's simple about malnutrition: complexities raised by epidemic neuropathy in Cuba. Am J Clin Nutr. 1996;64: 383–384.
35. Krishna S, Taylor AM, Supanaranond W, et al. Thiamine deficiency and malaria in adults from southeast Asia. Lancet. 1999;353:546–549.
36. McEntee WJ. Wernicke's encephalopathy: an excitotoxicity hypothesis. Metab Brain Dis. 1977;12: 183–192.
37. Rolland S, Truswell AS. Wernicke-Korsakoff syndrome in Sydney hospitals after 6 years of thiamin enrichment of bread. Public Health Nutr. 1998;1: 117–122.
38. Harper C, Fornes P, Duyckaerts C, Lecomte D, Hauw JJ. An international perspective on the prevalence of the Wernicke-Korsakoff syndrome. Metab Brain Dis. 1995;10:17–24.
39. Pagnan L, Berlot G, Pozzi-Mucelli RS. Magnetic resonance imaging in a case of Wernicke's encephalopathy. Eur J Radiol. 1998;8:977–980.
40. Wang JJ, Martin PR, Singleton CK. A transketolase assembly defect in a Wernicke-Korsakoff syndrome patient. Alcohol Clin Exp Res. 1997;21:576–580.
41. Pekovich SR, Martin PR, Singleton CK. Thiamin deficiency decreases steady-state transketolase and pyruvate dehydrogenase but not α-ketoglutarate dehydrogenase mRNA levels in three human cell types. J Nutr. 1998;128:683–687.
42. Zimatkin SM, Zimatkina TI. Thiamine deficiency as predisposition to, and consequence of, increased alcohol consumption. Alcohol Alcohol. 1996;31: 421–427.
43. Shimomura T, Mori E, Hirono N, Imamura T, Yamashita H. Development of Wernicke-Korsakoff syndrome after long intervals following gastrectomy. Arch Neurol. 1998;55:1242–1245.
44. Bettendorff L, Mastrogiacomo F, Kish SJ, Grisar T. Thiamine, thiamine phosphates and their metabolizing enzymes in human brain. J Neurochem. 1996;66: 250–258.
45. Iber FL, Blass JP, Brin M, Leevy CM. Thiamin in the elderly–relation to alcoholism and to neurological degenerative disease. Am J Clin Nutr. 1982;6(suppl 50):1067–1082.
46. Suter PM, Vetter W. Diuretics and vitamin B1: Are diuretics a risk factor for thiamine malnutrition? Nutr Rev. 2000;58:319–323.
47. Finch S, Doyle W, Lowe C, et al. *National Diet and Nutrition Survey: People Aged 65 Years and Over. Vol. 1: Report of the Diet and Nutrition Survey*. London: Her Majesty's Stationery Office; 1998.
48. Bates CJ, Prentice A, Cole TJ, et al. Micronutrients: highlights and research challenges from the 1994–5 National Diet and Nutrition Survey of people aged 65 years and over. Br J Nutr. 1999;82:7–15.
49. Gold M, Hauser RA, Chen MF. Plasma thiamine deficiency associated with Alzheimer's disease but not Parkinson's disease. Met Brain Dis. 1998;13: 43–53.
50. Wilkinson TJ, Hanger HC, Elmslie J, George PM, Sainsbury R. The response to treatment of subclinical thiamine deficiency in the elderly. Am J Clin Nutr. 1997;66:925–928.

# 19 Riboflavin

Richard S. Rivlin

## Introduction

Like many of the B vitamins, riboflavin by itself has little metabolic activity. Rather, the physiological role of riboflavin resides largely in its being the precursor of riboflavin-5′-phosphate (flavin mononucleotide or FMN) and flavin adenine dinucleotide (FAD), two coenzymes that are required for a wide variety of enzymes in intermediary metabolism. In addition, riboflavin is the precursor of several other flavins that are covalently bound to tissue proteins. Nutritional factors, hormones, and drugs regulate the conversion of riboflavin into these active coenzyme derivatives. Disturbances in such regulation assume major significance in various diseases.

Advances in understanding the structure and function of the plethora of tissue flavins, their associated proteins, and their metabolic end products have been covered in detail by McCormick[1] in a previous edition of this volume. Other comprehensive reviews have emphasized medical aspects of riboflavin metabolism.[2-5] The chemical and nutritional aspects of riboflavin have been discussed elsewhere.[6-8] This chapter provides updated knowledge of riboflavin's role in physiology and medicine and newer proposed therapeutic roles.

## Chemistry

Riboflavin, as well as its coenzyme derivatives and all other tissue flavins, are isoalloxazines. The structure of riboflavin and its two major coenzyme derivatives are given in Figure 1. FMN is formed first from riboflavin by the addition of a phosphate group, which is catalyzed by the enzyme flavokinase. The second biosynthetic step consists of the combination of FMN with one molecule of adenosine triphosphate (ATP) to form flavin adenine dinucleotide (FAD), a step catalyzed by FAD synthetase, also called pyrophosphorylase. FAD can be converted further into forms covalently bound to tissue proteins.

Several important mammalian enzymes contain FAD modified at the 8-a position covalently bound to the tissue proteins. Included in this category are succinic and sarcosine dehydrogenase found in the inner mitochondrial membrane, monoamine oxidase in the outer mitochondrial membrane, and L-gulonolactone oxidase, present in liver microsomes of animals capable of making ascorbic acid. Human tissues do not contain L-gulonolactone as a functional holoenzyme. Results of measurements at intervals following the administration of radioactive riboflavin to intact animals suggest that the covalent linkage

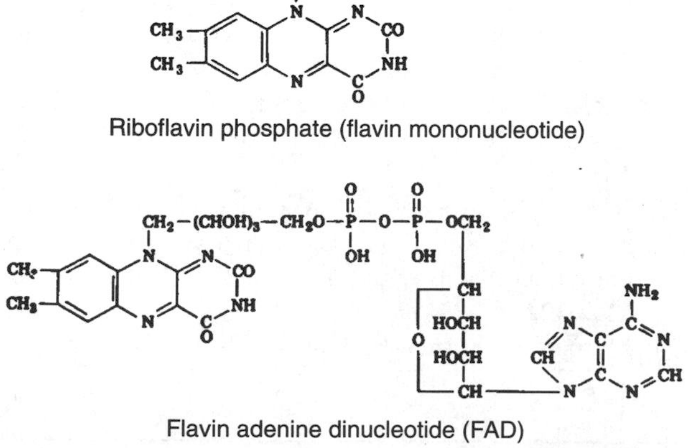

Riboflavin

Riboflavin phosphate (flavin mononucleotide)

Flavin adenine dinucleotide (FAD)

Figure 1. Structural formulas of riboflavin and the 2 coenzymes derived from riboflavin—riboflavin-5′-phosphate (flavin mononucleotide, FMN) and flavin adenine dinucleotide (FAD). FMN is formed from riboflavin by the addition in the 5′ position of a phosphate group derived from ATP. FAD is formed from FMN after combination with a molecule of ATP.

of flavins to tissue proteins occurs after the synthesis of FAD from riboflavin.[9,10]

Riboflavin is chemically defined as 7, 8-dimethyl-10-(1′-D-ribityl) isoalloxazine, and is a planar structure, yellow and highly fluorescent. There are many variations in structure in naturally occurring flavins. Riboflavin and its coenzymes are both alkali and acid sensitive, particularly in the presence of light. Riboflavin is photodegraded under alkaline conditions to yield lumiflavin (7, 8, 10-trimethylisoalloxazine), which is relatively inactive biologically. In acidic conditions, riboflavin is photodegraded to lumichrome (7, 8-dimethylalloxazine). Structure-function relationships of derivatives of riboflavin are discussed more fully in a previous edition of this volume.[1]

Riboflavin has only limited solubility in aqueous solutions, which is of practical importance because therapeutic solutions prepared for intravenous use can deliver only small amounts of the vitamin. FMN can be administered intravenously at higher concentrations. Most clinical studies with riboflavin have administered it orally.

## Absorption, Transport, Storage, and Turnover

Because dietary sources of riboflavin are largely in the form of coenzyme derivatives, these must be hydrolyzed before being absorbed. Absorption occurs predominantly in the upper gastrointestinal tract by specialized transport involving a phosphorylation-dephosphorylation mechanism rather than by passive diffusion.[11] This process is sodium dependent and involves an ATPase active transport system that can be saturated. Under normal conditions, the upper limit of intestinal absorption of riboflavin at any time has been estimated to be approximately 66.4 mmol (25 mg). Delaying the intestinal transit time of the food item consumed may result in an increase in the total amount of riboflavin absorbed from the intestine.[12] Dietary covalently bound flavins are largely but not entirely inaccessible as nutritional sources.

The uptake of riboflavin by human colonic epithelial cells,[13] as well as by human renal epithelial cells[14] and liver cells,[15] was described by Said et al. Intestinal uptake is increased in cellular riboflavin deficiency and decreased with high riboflavin status. Evidence was presented that a pathway mediated by calcium and calmodulin is involved. It was also suggested by this group that riboflavin is synthesized by intestinal bacteria and then absorbed by the colon, thereby making a contribution to overall riboflavin nutrition. The physiological role of this putative colonic absorption of riboflavin needs to be defined further.

Diets high in psyllium gum appear to decrease the rate of riboflavin absorption, whereas wheat bran has no detectable effect.[16] The time from oral administration to peak urinary excretion of riboflavin is prolonged by the antacids aluminum hydroxide and magnesium hydroxide. Total urinary excretion is unchanged by these drugs, however, and their major effect appears to be on rates of intestinal absorption rather than on urinary excretion.[17] Alcohol intake interferes with both the digestion of food flavins into riboflavin and the direct absorption of this vitamin.[18] This observation suggests that the initial rehabilitation of malnourished alcoholic patients would be accomplished more rapidly and efficiently with vitamin supplements containing riboflavin rather than with food sources of flavin derivatives.

There is some evidence that the amount of riboflavin absorbed by the intestine is increased by the presence of food.[11] This effect of food may be due to its decreasing the rates of gastric emptying and intestinal transit, thereby permitting more prolonged contact of dietary riboflavin with the absorptive surfaces of intestinal mucosal cells. In general, delaying the rate of gastric emptying tends to increase the overall intestinal absorption of riboflavin.[19] Bile salts also increase the absorption of both riboflavin and FMN. Several metals and drugs form chelates or complexes with riboflavin and FMN that may affect their bioavailability. Among the agents in this category are the metals copper, zinc, and iron; the drugs caffeine, theophylline, and saccharin; the vitamins nicotinamide and ascorbic acid; and tryptophan and urea.[20] The clinical significance of this binding under ordinary circumstances needs to be clarified.

In human blood, the transport of flavins involves loose binding to albumin and tight binding to a number of specific globulins. The major binding of riboflavin and its phosphorylated derivatives in serum is to several classes of immunoglobulins: IgA, IgG, and IgM.[21-24] Pregnancy induces the formation of proteins that bind flavins. It has been known for many years that a genetically controlled avian riboflavin carrier protein determines the amount of riboflavin in chicken eggs.[25] The absence of this protein in autosomal recessive hens results in massive riboflavinuria, because there is no mechanism for retaining and binding the vitamin in serum. Eggs become riboflavin deficient, and embryonic death occurs between 10 and 14 days of incubation.[26,27] The administration of antiserum to the chicken riboflavin carrier protein leads to termination of the pregnancy.[28]

A new dimension to concepts of protein binding of riboflavin in sera of mammals was provided by the demonstration that riboflavin-binding proteins can also be found in serum from pregnant cows, monkeys, and humans.[29-32] A comprehensive review of riboflavin-binding proteins covers the nature of the proteins in various species and provides evidence that in mammals, as in birds, these proteins are crucial for successful reproduction.[33] The pregnancy-specific binding proteins may help transport riboflavin to the fetus. Serum riboflavin-binding proteins also may influence placental transfer and fetal-maternal distribution of riboflavin. The maternal and fetal surfaces of the human placenta have different rates of riboflavin uptake.[34,35] Riboflavin-binding proteins also influence the activity of flavokinase, the first biosynthetic enzyme in the pathway of riboflavin to FAD.[36]

Concentrations of riboflavin-binding protein in serum were found to be markedly elevated with high specificity and high sensitivity in women with breast cancer.[37] The highest levels were found in women with estrogen-receptor-positive status, but a correlation with estrogen status in the women studied was not provided. Levels were generally higher in Black than in Caucasian women. It will be of interest to determine whether serum levels of riboflavin-binding protein have diagnostic significance or may be of value in following the course of patients with breast cancer and their response to treatment.

Flavins are excreted in the urine predominantly as riboflavin; FMN and FAD are not found in urine. McCormick and his group have been active in identifying many flavins and their derivatives in human urine. Aside from the 60% to 70% of urinary flavins contributed by riboflavin itself, other derivatives include 7-α-hydroxymethylriboflavin (10%–15%), 8-α-sulfonylriboflavin (5%–10%), 8-α-hydroxymethylriboflavin (4%–7%), riboflavinyl peptide ester (5%), and 10-hydroxyethylflavin (1%–3%). Lumiflavin and other derivatives have also been found. Ohkawa et al.[38] found that only 25% of dietary flavins were excreted as riboflavin and greater amounts as 7-α-hydroxyriboflavin. These findings were described more fully by McCormick in the previous edition of this volume[1] and studied further by his group.[39]

The ingestion of boric acid greatly increases the urinary excretion of riboflavin.[40] Boric acid forms a complex with riboflavin and other molecules having polyhydroxy groups, such as glucose and ascorbic acid. In rodents, riboflavin treatment greatly ameliorates the toxicity of administered boric acid.[41] This treatment should also be effective in humans suffering from accidental exposure to boric acid, although it may be difficult to provide adequate amounts of riboflavin because of its low solubility and limited absorption from the intestinal tract.

The urinary excretion of riboflavin in rats is greatly increased by chlorpromazine. Urinary levels of riboflavin are twice those of age- and sex-matched pair-fed control rats.[42] In addition, chlorpromazine accelerates the urinary excretion of riboflavin during dietary deficiency (Figure 2). Urinary concentrations of riboflavin are increased within 6 hours of treatment with this drug. These observations raise the possibility that nutritional deficiency may influence the action and toxicity of psychotropic drugs. This general concept requires further study and exploration.

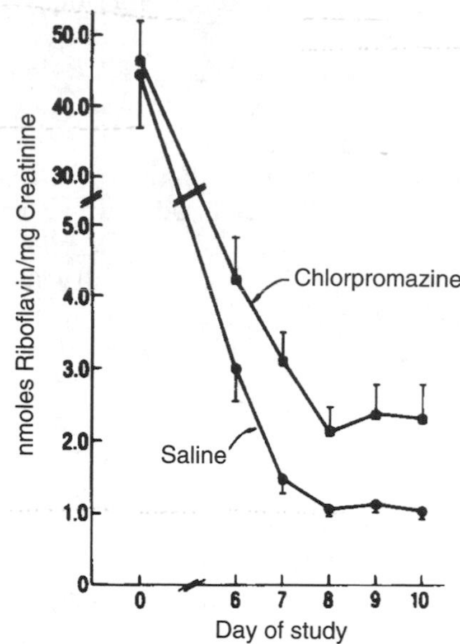


Figure 2. Urinary excretion of riboflavin in chlorpromazine-treated rats and in pair-fed, saline-treated controls during the development of riboflavin deficiency. (Data from Pelliccione et al., 1983.[42])

# Physiological (Biochemical) Function

The major function of riboflavin, as noted above, is to serve as the precursor of the coenzymes FMN and FAD and of covalently bound flavins. These coenzymes are widely distributed in metabolism. Riboflavin catalyzes numerous oxidation-reduction reactions. Because FAD is part of the respiratory chain, riboflavin is central to energy production. Other major functions of riboflavin include drug metabolism (in conjunction with the cytochrome P450 enzymes) and lipid metabolism. The redox functions of flavoenzymes include one-electron transfers. Two-electron transfers from substrate to flavin are also accomplished by flavoproteins.

Flavoproteins catalyze dehydrogenation reactions as well as hydroxylations, oxidative decarboxylations, deoxygenations, and reductions of oxygen to hydrogen peroxide. Thus, many different kinds of reactions are catalyzed by flavoproteins.[1]

Although FAD is the flavin coenzyme most widely utilized in intermediary metabolism, other enzymes utilize FMN. More recently, it has become recognized that some flavoenzymes contain both FMN and FAD as coenzymes. The first enzyme shown to be in this category of diflavin reductases is microsomal NADPH-cytochrome P450-reductase, which has FMN and FAD in equimolar ratios.[43] Other diflavin reductases include nitric oxide synthase, methionine synthase, and human novel reductase 1.[44–46]

It is not often recognized that riboflavin has powerful potential for antioxidant activity that is derived from its role as a precursor to FMN and FAD.[47] Among the FAD-requiring enzymes is glutathione reductase. The glutathione redox cycle provides a major protective role against lipid peroxides. Glutathione peroxidase, which breaks down lipid peroxides, requires reduced glutathione, which in turn is generated by glutathione reductase. Riboflavin deficiency is associated with increased lipid peroxidation, a process that can be inhibited by riboflavin.[48] Riboflavin was observed to ameliorate the cardiac damage to rabbit hearts caused by experimental ischemia and reperfusion, and to reduce damage to rat lungs from toxins and to rat brains from ischemia. This subject is covered more fully in a review that also discusses the antimalarial effects of riboflavin deficiency.[3]

## Deficiency at the Cellular Level

Because the coenzymes derived from riboflavin are distributed so widely in intermediary metabolism, the biochemical consequences of riboflavin deficiency may be extensive. Furthermore, flavin coenzymes are involved in the metabolism of four other vitamins: folic acid, pyridoxine, vitamin K, and niacin.[49] Thus, a profound deficiency of riboflavin has consequences for many enzyme systems in addition to those directly requiring flavin coenzymes.

In riboflavin deficiency, tissue concentrations of FMN and FAD decrease, as does the activity of the biosynthetic enzyme flavokinase, which converts riboflavin to FMN.[50] Concentrations of FMN are decreased proportionately more than those of FAD. The pattern of liver flavoprotein enzymes is greatly influenced by riboflavin deficiency. Some enzymes are more sensitive than others to a decrease in availability of their flavin coenzyme. The decrease in the activities of enzymes requiring FMN generally parallels the reduction of its tissue concentration, and activities of FAD-requiring enzymes variably follow the reduction of tissue FAD concentrations.[51]

Hepatic architecture is markedly disrupted in riboflavin deficiency. Mitochondria in riboflavin-deficient mice increase greatly in size and cristae increase in both number and size.[52] Hepatic concentrations of RNA and DNA are normal in early riboflavin deficiency, but are depressed in its later stages.[53]

Riboflavin deficiency has many other effects on intermediary metabolism, particularly on fat and protein metabolism. The conversion of vitamin $B_6$ to its coenzyme derivative may be impaired.[54] Decreased FMN-dependent pyridoxine-5′-phosphate oxidase activity has been described in most cases of deficiency of glucose-6-phosphate dehydrogenase.[55,56]

The increase in de novo synthesis of reduced glutathione from its amino acid precursors (Figure 3) likely represents an adaptation to riboflavin deficiency.

## Deficiency in Animals

Riboflavin deficiency has been studied in many animal species and has a number of detrimental effects, the foremost of which is failure to grow. Additional effects include loss of hair, disturbances in the skin, degenerative changes in the nervous system, and impaired reproduction. The conjunctivae become inflamed, the cornea is vascularized and eventually opaque, resulting in cataract formation.[57]

Changes in the skin consist of scaliness and incrustation of red-brown material. Alopecia may develop, lips become red and swollen, and filiform papillae on the

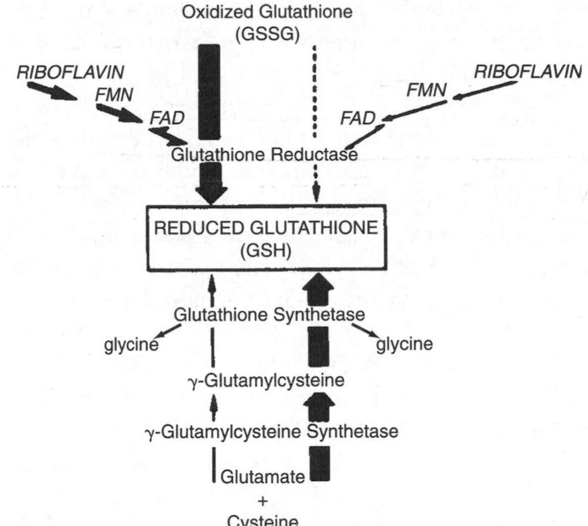


Figure 3. Regeneration of GSH under normal and riboflavin-deficient conditions. The diagram represents 2 major pathways for the formation of reduced glutathione in erythrocytes—reduction of GSSG via the glutathione reductase pathway and de novo biosynthesis via glutamylcysteine synthetase and glutathione synthetase. Bold arrows emphasize the predominant pathways, thin arrows represent pathways that are operating below maximal levels, and the dotted arrow indicates diminished enzymatic activity.

tongue deteriorate. A decrease in hemoglobin formation during late deficiency leads to anemia. Fatty degeneration of the liver occurs. Perhaps as a result of mitochondrial dysfunction, riboflavin-deficient rats require 15% to 20% more energy intake than do control animals to maintain the same body weight.

Thus, in all species studied to date, riboflavin deficiency causes profound structural and functional changes in an ordered sequence. Early changes are readily and completely reversible; later changes such as cataracts may not be.

## Deficiency in Humans

The clinical features of human riboflavin deficiency do not have the specificity that may characterize deficits of other vitamins such as ascorbic acid. Isolated deficiency of riboflavin is rarely encountered. Early symptoms may include weakness, fatigue, mouth pain and tenderness, eye burning and itching, and possibly personality changes. More advanced deficiency may give rise to cheilosis, angular stomatitis, dermatitis, corneal vascularization, anemia, and brain dysfunction. It is now recognized that the prevalence of cataract formation is decreased by a higher intake of riboflavin.[58] In patients with keratoconus, the administration of eye drops containing riboflavin delayed the progression of the disorder.[59] These findings suggest that riboflavin may have potential clinically in both the prevention and treatment of cataracts. Larger long-term clinical trials are needed to establish the efficacy and feasibility of this approach for the general population.

Based on the evidence accumulated to date, the syndrome of dietary riboflavin deficiency in humans has many similarities to that in animals. There is one notable exception, however: the spectrum of congenital malformations observed in rodents with maternal riboflavin deficiency has not been clearly identified in humans.[60]

Riboflavin deficiency may result not only from poor dietary intake of the vitamin but also from those diseases, drugs, and endocrine abnormalities that interfere specifically with vitamin utilization. The conversion of riboflavin into its active coenzyme derivatives is inhibited by thyroid and adrenal insufficiency; psychotropic drugs such as chlorpromazine, imipramine, and amitriptyline; the cancer chemotherapeutic drug doxorubicin; and antimalarial drugs such as quinacrine.[42,47-50] Alcohol causes riboflavin deficiency by interfering with both its digestion and intestinal absorption.[18] Structural similarities among riboflavin, imipramine, chlorpromazine, and amitriptyline are shown in Figure 4.

Clinical confirmation of these concepts is provided by the finding that riboflavin status is impaired in patients with hypothyroidism,[61] and can be corrected by treatment with thyroid hormones while maintaining a constant riboflavin intake. Further clinical confirmation of the findings in animals is provided by the observation that riboflavin metabolism is impaired in severe anorexia with low erythrocyte FAD concentrations in association with low serum triiodothyronine levels.[62]

The diagnosis of riboflavin deficiency in practice is based first on showing a reduction in the urinary excretion of riboflavin. This is a reliable test if the sample is properly collected in a dark bottle and a complete collection is made. The results may be misleading, however, if the subject has recently consumed a large amount of riboflavin. In that case, there will be an abrupt increase in urinary riboflavin excretion that does not accurately reflect overall body stores.

A useful functional test for clinical riboflavin deficiency is the activity coefficient (i.e., the ratio of activity of erythrocyte hemolysate glutathione reductase, an FAD-requiring enzyme, with and without the addition of FAD in vitro. When FAD is added in vitro to an erythrocyte hemolysate, the increase in enzyme activity observed is greater in hemolysates from riboflavin-deficient than from riboflavin-replete individuals, reflecting the lesser degree of saturation of the apoenzyme with its cofactor in the deficient group. Activity coefficients over 1.2 to 1.3 generally signify some degree of riboflavin deficiency, with higher activity coefficients indicative of greater deficiency.[45]

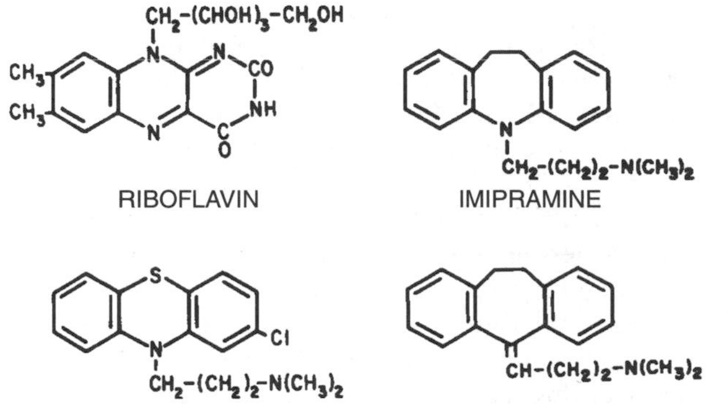

RIBOFLAVIN

IMIPRAMINE

CHLORPROMAZINE

AMITRIPTYLINE

Figure 4. Structural formulas showing the similarities of riboflavin, chlorpromazine, imipramine, and amitriptyline.

# Dietary Reference Intakes

The Dietary Reference Intakes (DRIs) for riboflavin and other B vitamins have been published and widely distributed[63] periodically. To meet the needs of adult males who are 19 to 50 years of age, 1.3 mg of riboflavin should be consumed daily; women 19 years of age and older should consume 1.1 mg daily. Amounts are increased to 1.4 mg/d throughout pregnancy and to 1.6 mg/d during lactation.

Measures of urinary riboflavin excretion and erythrocyte hemolysate glutathione reductase activity coefficients from a study of elderly patients in Guatemala suggested that the requirements of healthy individuals 60 years of age or older probably do not differ from those for individuals under 51 years of age.[64] Among elderly residents of a nursing home in the United States, increasing the riboflavin intake through a supplement from 1.7 to 3.4 mg/d doubled riboflavin excretion, strongly suggesting that the higher level of intake is above the requirement for the older age group.[65]

On the basis of studies of urinary riboflavin excretion after a test load, it was suggested that the requirement for riboflavin in Chinese people may be lower than the figures noted above.[66,67] More research is needed around the world to determine more completely the factors that determine riboflavin requirements in various populations.

Several nutritional and physiological factors also govern riboflavin requirements. Riboflavin excretion is accelerated when there is negative nitrogen balance.[68,69] Periods of major physical activity in young men and moderate exercise in young women have both been shown to reduce urinary riboflavin excretion.[69,70] Decreased urinary excretion of riboflavin with constant dietary intake may reflect enhanced tissue uptake. These results suggest an increased requirement for riboflavin during exercise, particularly because the study in women showed a small increase in the activity coefficient of erythrocyte glutathione reductase activity.

Further research is required to clarify the effects of exercise to determine whether it is physical activity per se that affects metabolism of riboflavin and not some consequence of exercise, such as increased metabolic rate or increased hormone release, and to determine what kinds of physical activity may be most clinically relevant. Tucker et al.[69] observed that sleep decreases riboflavin excretion, whereas heat stress and prolonged bed rest increase riboflavin excretion.

# Food and Other Sources

In the United States, the most significant dietary sources of riboflavin are meat and meat products, including poultry and fish, and milk and dairy products, such as eggs, yogurt, and cheese. In developing countries, plant sources contribute most of the dietary riboflavin intake. The dietary intake of riboflavin in developing countries such as China that rely predominantly on plant sources is much lower than that in the United States.[66,67] However, green vegetables such as broccoli, asparagus, and spinach are fairly good sources of riboflavin.

Natural grain products tend to be relatively low in riboflavin, but fortification and enrichment of grains and cereals has led to a great increase in riboflavin intake from these sources. Some fortified cereals contain 100% of the DRI for riboflavin. Multivitamin supplement use, which is a widespread practice among large segments of the US population, provides riboflavin at levels that may greatly exceed the DRIs. Any evaluation of an individual's or a group's diet must take into account sources of riboflavin obtained from fortified foods and dietary supplements.

The food sources of riboflavin are similar to those of other B vitamins. Therefore, it is not surprising that if an individual's diet has inadequate amounts of riboflavin, it will very likely be inadequate in other vitamins as well.

Several factors in food preparation and processing influence the amount of riboflavin that is actually consumed. Appreciable amounts may be lost with exposure to light, particularly during cooking and during storage of milk in clear bottles or glasses.[71] Fortunately, most milk is no longer sold in clear bottles. There is some uncertainty as to whether opaque plastic containers provide greater protection than cartons. It is highly likely that large amounts of riboflavin are lost during the sun-drying of fruits and vegetables, but the size of the loss is not known precisely. The practice of adding sodium bicarbonate (baking soda) to green vegetables to make them appear fresher accelerates the photodegradation of riboflavin.

## Excess and Toxicity

There is general agreement that dietary riboflavin intake at many times the RDA is without demonstrable toxicity.[64,72] Because riboflavin absorption is limited to about 66.4 mmol (25 mg) as a maximum at any time, as noted above, consuming megadoses of this vitamin would not be expected to increase the amount absorbed unless there were very unusual circumstances.

Furthermore, classical animal investigations showed an apparent upper limit to tissue storage of riboflavin and its derivatives that cannot be exceeded under ordinary conditions.[51] Thus, several protective mechanisms prevent tissue accumulation of excessive amounts of riboflavin. Because riboflavin also has very low solubility, even intravenous administration of the vitamin would not introduce large amounts into the body. FMN is more water soluble than riboflavin, but is ordinarily not available for routine clinical use.

Nevertheless, the photosensitizing properties of riboflavin raise the possibility of some potential risks. Phototherapy in vitro leads to the degradation of DNA and increases in lipid peroxidation. Both of these effects may have implications for carcinogenesis and mutagenesis. FMN increases the potassium loss observed in rat erythrocytes after irradiation.[73] Riboflavin forms an adduct with tryptophan and accelerates its photooxidation.[74] Further research is needed to explore completely the full implications of the photosensitivity of riboflavin and its flavin derivatives.

## Newer Therapeutic Applications of Riboflavin

Following up on the promising results of an open pilot study suggesting benefit of high-dose oral riboflavin (400 mg/d) in the treatment of migraine attacks,[75] Schoenen et al.[76] confirmed its efficacy in a randomized, controlled trial. The frequency of attacks of migraine and the number of days with migraine attacks were significantly reduced by riboflavin. This dose is known to exceed the intestinal absorptive capacity of humans, and suggests that much lower doses are likely to be effective. The hypothesis underlying the application of riboflavin in the treatment of migraine headaches is that it improves mitochondrial energy production in a condition in which mitochondrial dysfunction has been proposed as an underlying pathogenic mechanism.

A similar hypothesis of improving mitochondrial function underlies the application of riboflavin to treat lactic acidosis caused by nucleoside reverse transcriptase inhibitors in patients with AIDS.[77] Riboflavin deficiency is common in AIDS as a result of poor diet, anorexia, and, in some instances, diarrhea and malabsorption. An additional mechanism that may intensify the effects of poor dietary intake of riboflavin is treatment with amitriptyline, a drug commonly used in patients with AIDS, which in animal studies interferes with riboflavin conversion to FMN and FAD.[78] A dramatic reduction in urinary lactate excretion resulted from treatment with 50 mg riboflavin.

Genetic defects of the mitochondrial respiratory chain, such as infantile lactic acidosis, skeletal myopathy with or without cardiomyopathy, and Leigh's disease, respond to riboflavin administration. In one case report, a sustained remission in neuromuscular function was achieved by 25 mg of riboflavin given twice daily.[79] The authors proposed that all individuals with complex I deficiency be given a trial of riboflavin administration. Further research is needed before a formal recommendation can be made for riboflavin use in this disorder.

A practical therapeutic use of riboflavin has been described in enhancing the entry of protein molecules into cells. Low permeability of large protein molecules precludes significant entry, but conjugation of riboflavin with bovine serum albumin greatly facilitates protein entry into a variety of human cells in culture.[80] Whether riboflavin is as effective as other ligands, such as monoclonal antibodies or transferrin, is important to determine in future studies.

Evidence is accumulating that riboflavin joins $B_6$, $B_{12}$, and folic acid in regulating serum homocysteine concentrations. The flavin coenzyme FAD is utilized by methyltetrahydrofolate reductase, which converts N-5,10-methylenetetrahydrofolate into N-5-methyltetrahydrofolate.[81] Because of this requirement for FAD, the efficient utilization of dietary folic acid depends upon adequate dietary intake of riboflavin as well.[82]

This relationship assumed a new dimension with the identification of a genetic mutation that results in a heat-sensitive form of methylenetetrahydrofolate reductase.[63,64,83,84] This mutation is not rare, and is found in as many as 10% to 15% of the general population in North America and Europe.[65,85] Those individuals who are homozygous for the mutation are unusually sensitive to folic acid and riboflavin,[82,86] both of which serve to stabilize the enzyme variation. Because of their sensitivity to folic acid and riboflavin, individuals who are homozygous for this mutation have serum homocysteine levels that are closely governed by the levels of both folic acid and riboflavin.[82]

Further evidence of the significance of riboflavin is that its dietary intake from food, as well as that of folic acid, is inversely related to the serum concentration of homocysteine.[81] Other investigators have observed a lowering of serum homocysteine levels not only in individuals homozygous for this mutation but also in those with normal genotypes.[87]

## Future Directions

Future studies are needed to determine more accurately the interactions among drugs, hormones, and phytochemicals in relation to riboflavin metabolism. These relationships are particularly relevant with respect to the effects of psychotropic drugs on riboflavin metabolism. Riboflavin metabolism needs to be evaluated in relationship to that of other vitamins for several reasons. First, a clinical deficiency of riboflavin very rarely occurs by itself, being much more common under conditions of deficits of other B vitamins. Also, several vitamins utilize flavin cofactors in their own synthesis or degradation. The finding of greatly elevated serum concentrations of riboflavin in women with breast cancer may have diagnostic or therapeutic applications that need to be defined. Riboflavin as the dietary precursor to FAD, the coenzyme of glutathione reductase, has antioxidant potential that needs further evaluation. Thus, while much has been learned, there remain a number of aspects of riboflavin metabolism that deserve future exploration.

## Summary

Much knowledge has been gained on the structural and functional aspects of riboflavin and its coenzyme derivatives, as well as the spectrum of tissue flavins. The effects of riboflavin deficiency are widespread and extend beyond the depletion of flavin-requiring proteins. Deficiency results not only from dietary inadequacy but also from the effects of drugs, hormones, various diseases, and nutritional factors that regulate vitamin utilization. Recent advances have been made in understanding the pathogenesis of riboflavin deficiency and the factors that determine riboflavin requirements. Riboflavin in its role as a precursor to FAD is needed for functioning of glutathione reductase, and therefore has significant antioxidant activity. New therapeutic roles for riboflavin have been proposed in preventing attacks of migraine, treating lactic acidosis (particularly that associated with AIDS), treating genetic defects of the respiratory chain, and reducing elevated serum levels of homocysteine.

## References

1. McCormick DB. Riboflavin. In: Brown ML, ed. *Present Knowledge in Nutrition*. 6th ed. Washington, DC: ILSI Press; 1990; 146–154.
2. Powers HJ. Riboflavin (vitamin B2) and health. Am J Clin Nutr. 2003;77:1352–1360.
3. Rivlin RS, Dutta P. Vitamin B2 (riboflavin): relevance to malaria and antioxidant activity. Nutr Today. 1995;30:62–67.
4. Rivlin RS. Riboflavin (Vitamin B2) In: McCormick DB, Suttie JW, Zempleni J, Rucker RB, eds. *Handbook of Vitamins*. 4th ed. Boca Raton, CRC Press; 2006; In press.
5. Becker K, Schirmer M, Kansok S, Schirmer RH. Flavins and flavoenzymes in diagnosis and therapy. Methods Mol Biol. 1999;131:229–245.
6. McCormick DB. Riboflavin. In: Shils ME, Olson JA, Shike M, eds. *Modern Nutrition in Health and Disease*. 8th ed. Philadelphia: Lea and Febiger; 1994; 366–375.
7. Rivlin RS. Vitamin deficiency. In: Rakel RE, ed. *Conn's Current Therapy*. Philadelphia: W.B. Saunders; 1998; 579–587.
8. Rivlin RS, Pinto JT. Riboflavin (vitamin B2). In: Rucker R, Suttie JW, McCormick DM, Machlin LJ, eds. *Handbook of Vitamins*. 3rd ed. New York: Marcel Dekker; 2000; 255–273.
9. Yagi K, Nakagawa Y, Suzuki O, Ohishi N. Incorporation of riboflavin into covalently-bound flavins in rat liver. J Biochem. 1976;79:841–843.
10. Pinto J, Rivlin RS. Regulation of formation of covalently bound flavins in liver and cerebrum by thyroid hormones. Arch Biochim Biophys. 1979;194:313–320.
11. Jusko WJ, Levy G. Absorption, metabolism and excretion of riboflavin-5′ phosphate in man. J Pharm Sci. 1967;56:58–62.
12. Levy G, Mosovich LL, Allen JE, et al, Biliary excre-

tion of riboflavin in man. J Pharm Sci. 1972;61: 143–144.
13. Said HM, Ortiz A, Meyer MP, et al. Riboflavin uptake by human-derived colonic epithelial NCM460 cells. Am J Physiol. 2000;278:C270–C276.
14. Kumar CK, Yanagawa N, Ortiz A, et al. Mechanism and regulation of riboflavin uptake by human renal proximal epithelial cell line HK-2. Am J Physiol. 1998;274:F104–F110.
15. Said HM, Ortiz A, Ma TY, et al, Riboflavin uptake by the human-derived liver cells HepG2: mechanism and regulation. J Cell Physiol. 1998;176:588–594.
16. Roe DA, Kalkwarf H, Stevens J. Effect of fiber supplements on the apparent absorption of pharmacological doses of riboflavin. J Am Diet Assoc. 1998; 88:211–213.
17. Feldman S, Hedrick W. Antacid effects on the gastrointestinal absorption of riboflavin. J Pharm Sci. 1983;72:121–123.
18. Pinto JT, Huang YP, Rivlin RS. Mechanisms underlying the differential effects of ethanol upon the bioavailability of riboflavin and flavin adenine dinucleotide. J Clin Invest. 1987;79:1343–348.
19. Roe DA. Fiber and riboflavin absorption [letter]. J Am Diet Assoc. 1988;88:783.
20. Jusko WJ, Levy G. Absorption, protein binding and elimination of riboflavin. In: Rivlin RS, ed. *Riboflavin*. New York: Plenum Press; 1975; 99–152.
21. Merrill AH Jr, Froehlich JA, McCormick DB. Isolation and identification of alternative riboflavin-binding proteins from human plasma. Biochem Med. 1981;25:198–206.
22. Innis WSA, McCormick DB, Merrill AH Jr. Variations in riboflavin binding by human plasma: identification of immunoglobulins as the major proteins responsible. Biochem Med. 1985;34:151–165.
23. Innis WS, Nixon DW, Murray DR, et al. Immunoglobulins associated with elevated riboflavin binding by plasma from cancer patients. Proc Soc Exp Biol Med. 1986;181:237–241.
24. Merrill AH Jr, Innis-Whitehouse WSA, McCormick DB. Characterization of human riboflavin-binding immunoglobulins. In: Edmondson DE, McCormick DB, eds. *Flavins and Flavoproteins*. Berlin: De Gruyter; 1987; 445–448.
25. Clagett CO. Genetic control of the riboflavin carrier protein. Fed Proc. 1971;30:127–129.
26. Winter WP, Buss EG, Clagett CO, Boucher RV. The nature of the biochemical lesion in avian renal riboflavinuria. II. The inherited change of a riboflavin-binding protein from blood and eggs. Comp Biochem Physiol. 1967;22:897–906.
27. Clagett CO, Buss EG, Saylor EM, Girsh SJ. The nature of the biochemical lesion in avian renal riboflavinuria. 6. Hormone induction of the riboflavin-binding protein in roosters and young chicks. Poult Sci. 1970;49:1468–1472.
28. Natraj U, Kumar AR, Kadam P. Termination of pregnancy in mice with antiserum to chicken riboflavin-carrier protein. Biol Reprod. 1987;36:677–685.
29. Merrill AH Jr, Froehlich JA, McCormick DB. Purification of riboflavin-binding proteins from bovine plasma and discovery of a pregnancy-specific riboflavin-binding protein. J Biol Chem. 1979;254: 9362–9364.
30. Visweswariah SS, Adiga PR. Purification of a circulatory riboflavin carrier protein from pregnant bonnet monkey (M. radiata): comparison with chicken egg vitamin carrier. Biochim Biophys Acta. 1987;915: 141–148.
31. Murthy CVR, Adiga PR. Isolation and characterization of a riboflavin-carrier protein from human pregnancy serum. Biochem Int. 1982;5:289–296.
32. Visweswariah SS, Adiga PR. Isolation of riboflavin carrier proteins from pregnant human and umbilical cord serum; similarities with chicken egg riboflavin carrier protein. Biosci Rep. 1987;7:563–571.
33. White HB III, Merrill AH Jr. Riboflavin-binding proteins. Annu Rev Nutr. 1988;8:279–299.
34. Dancis J, Lehanka J, Levitz M. Transfer of riboflavin by the perfused human placenta. Pediatr Res. 1985; 19:1143–1146.
35. Dancis J, Lehanka J. Levitz M. Placental transport of riboflavin: differential rates of uptake at the maternal and fetal surfaces of the perfused human placenta. Am J Obstet Gynecol. 1988;158:204–210.
36. Slomczynska M, Sak Z. The effect of riboflavin binding protein (RBP) on flavokinase catalytic activity. Comp Biochem Physiol. 1987;37B:681–685.
37. Rao PN, Levine E, Myers MO, et al. Elevation of serum riboflavin carrier protein in breast cancer. Cancer Epidemiol Biomark Prev. 1999;8:985–900.
38. Ohkawa H, Ohishi N, Yagi K. New metabolites of riboflavin appear in human urine. J Biol Chem. 1983; 258:5623–5628.
39. Zempleni J, Galloway Jr, McCormick DB. Pharmacokinetics of orally and intravenously administered riboflavin in healthy humans. Am J Clin Nutr. 1996; 63:54–66.
40. Pinto JT, Huang YP, McConnell RJ, Rivlin RS. Increased urinary riboflavin excretion resulting from boric acid ingestion. J Lab Clin Med. 1978;92: 126–134.
41. Roe DA, McCormick DB, Lin RT. Effects of riboflavin on boric acid toxicity. J Pharm Sci. 1972;61: 1081–1085.
42. Pelliccione N, Pinto JT, Huang YP, Rivlin RS. Accelerated development of riboflavin deficiency by treatment with chlorpromazine. Biochem Pharmacol. 1983;32:2949–2953.
43. Paine MJ, Garner AP, Powell D, et al. Cloning and characterization of a novel human dual flavin reductase. J Biol Chem. 2000;275:1471–1478.

44. Finn RD, Basran J, Roitel O, et al. Determination of the redox potentials and electron transfer properties of the FAD- and FMN-binding domains of the human oxidoreductase NRI. Eur J Biochem. 2003; 270:1164–1175.
45. Bredt DS, Hwang PM, Glatt CE, et al. Cloned and expressed nitric oxide synthase structurally resembles cytochrome P-450 reductase. Nature. 1991;351: 714–718.
46. Dignam J, Strobel H. Preparation of homogeneous NADPH-cytochrome P-450 reductase from rat liver. Biochim Biophys Res Commun. 1975;63: 845–852.
47. Dutta P. Disturbances in glutathione metabolism and resistance to malaria: current understanding and new concepts. J Soc Pharm Chem. 1993;2:11–48.
48. Dutta P, Serafi J, Halpin D, et al. Acute ethanol exposure alters hepatic glutathione metabolism in riboflavin deficiency. Alcohol. 1995;12:43–47.
49. Rivlin RS. Disorders of vitamin metabolism: deficiencies, metabolic abnormalities and excesses. In: Wyngaarden JH, Smith LH Jr, Bennett JC, Plum F, eds. *Cecil Textbook of Medicine*. 19th ed. Philadelphia: WB Saunders; 1991; 1170–1183.
50. Rivlin RS, Menendez C, Langdon RG. Biochemical similarities between hypothyroidism and riboflavin deficiency. Endocrinology. 1968;83:461–469.
51. Burch HB, Lowry OH, Padilla AM, Combs AM. Effects of riboflavin deficiency and realimentation on flavin enzymes of tissues. J Biol Chem. 1956;223: 29–45.
52. Tandler B, Erlandson RA, Wynder EL. Riboflavin and mouse hepatic cell structure and function. I. Ultrastructural alterations in simple deficiency. Am J Pathol. 1968;52:69–95.
53. Chatterjee AK, Roy AK, Ghosh BB. Effect of riboflavin deficiency on nucleic acid metabolism of liver in the rat. Br J Nutr. 1969;23:657–663.
54. McCormick DB. Two interconnected B vitamins: riboflavin and pyridoxine. Physiol Rev. 1989;69: 1170–1198.
55. Powers HJ, Bates CV. A simple fluorometric assay for pyridoxamine phosphate oxidase in erythrocyte hemolysates: effects of riboflavin supplementation and of glucose 6-phosphate dehydrogenase deficiency. Hum Nutr Clin Nutr. 1985;39:107–115.
56. Anderson BB, Clements JE, Perry GM, et al. Glutathione reductase activity in G6PD deficiency. Eur J Haematol. 1987;38:12–20.
57. Goldsmith GA. Riboflavin deficiency. In: Rivlin R, ed. *Riboflavin*. New York: Plenum Press; 1975; 221–244.
58. Jacques PF, Taylor A, Moeller S, et al. Long-term nutrient intake and 5-year change in nuclear lens opacities. Arch Ophthalmol. 2005;123:517–526.
59. Sandner D, Sporl E, Kohlhaas M, Unger G, Pillunat LE, et al. Collagen crosslinking by combined riboflavin/ultraviolet-A(UVA) treatment can stop progression of keratoconus. Invest Ophthalmol Vis Sci. 2004;451E2887(abstract).
60. Warkany J. Riboflavin deficiency and congenital malformations. In: Rivlin R, ed. *Riboflavin*. New York: Plenum Press; 1975; 279–302.
61. Cimino JA, Jhangiani S, Schwartz E, et al. Riboflavin metabolism in the hypothyroid human adult. Proc Soc Exp Biol Med. 1987;184:151–153.
62. Capo-Chichi CD, Gueant JL, Lefebvre E, et al. Riboflavin and riboflavin-derived cofactors in adolescent girls with anorexia nervosa. Am J Clin Nutr. 1999;69:672–678.
63. Food and Nutrition Board, Institute of Medicine. Dietary Reference Intakes for Thiamin, Riboflavin, Niacin, Vitamin B6, Folate, Vitamin B12, Pantothenic Acid, Biotin, and Choline. Washington, DC: National Academies Press; 1998. Available online at: http://www.nap.edu/openbook/0309065542/html/. Accessed March 16, 2006.
64. Boisvert WA, Mendoza I, Castaneda C, et al. Riboflavin requirement of healthy elderly humans and its relationship to macronutrient composition of the diet. J Nutr. 1993;123:915–925.
65. Alexander M, Emanuel G, Golin T, et al. Relation of riboflavin nutriture in healthy elderly to intake of calcium and vitamin supplements: evidence against riboflavin supplementation. Am J Clin Nutr. 1984; 39:540–546.
66. Brun TA, Chen J, Campbell TC, et al, Urinary riboflavin excretion after a load test in rural China as a measure of possible riboflavin deficiency. Eur J Clin Nutr. 1990;44:195–206.
67. Campbell TC, Brun T, Junshi C, et al. Questioning riboflavin recommendations on the basis of a survey in China. Am J Clin Nutr. 1990;51:436–445.
68. Windmueller HG, Anderson AA, Mickelsen O. Elevated riboflavin levels in urine of fasting human subjects. Am J Clin Nutr. 1964;15:73–76.
69. Tucker RG, Mickelsen O, Keys A. The influence of sleep, work, diuresis, heat, acute starvation, thiamine intake and bed rest on human riboflavin excretion. J Nutr. 1960;72:251–261.
70. Belko AZ, Obarzanek E, Kalkwarf HJ, et al. Effects of exercise on riboflavin requirements of young women. Am J Clin Nutr. 1983;37:509–517.
71. Wanner RL. Effects of commercial processing of milk and milk products on their nutrient content. In: Harris RS, Loesecke HV, eds. *The Nutritional Evaluation of Food Processing*. New York: John Wiley; 1960; 173–196.
72. Rivlin RS. Effect of nutrient toxicities (excess) in animals and man: riboflavin. In: Rechcigl M, ed. *Handbook of Nutrition and Foods*. Cleveland: CRC Press; 1979; 25–27.

73. Ghazy FS, Kimura T, Muranishi S, Sezaki H. The photodynamic action of riboflavin on erythrocytes. Life Sci. 1977;21:1703–1708.
74. Salim-Hanna M, Edwards AM, Silva E. Obtention of a photo-induced adduct between a vitamin and an essential amino acid. Binding of riboflavin to tryptophan. Int J Vitam Nutr Res. 1987;57:155–159.
75. Schoenen J, Lenaerts M, Bastings E. High-dose riboflavin as a prophylactic treatment of migraine: results of an open pilot study. Cephalalgia. 1994;14: 328–329.
76. Schoenen J, Jacquy J, Lenaerts M. Effectiveness of high-dose riboflavin in migraine prophylaxis. A randomized controlled trial. Neurology. 1998;50:466–470.
77. Fouty B, Frerman F, Reves R. Riboflavin to treat nucleoside analogue-induced lactic acidosis. Lancet. 1998;352:291–292.
78. Pinto JT, Huang YP, Pelliccione N, et al. Cardiac sensitivity to the inhibitory effects of chlorpromazine, imipramine and amitriptyline upon formation of flavins. Biochem Pharmacol. 1982;31:3495–3499.
79. Ogle RF, Christodoulou J, Fagan E, et al. Mitochondrial myopathy with tRNA-Leu (UUR) mutation and complex I deficiency responsive to riboflavin. J Pediatr. 1997;130:138–145.
80. Holladay SR, Yang Z-F, Kennedy MD, et al. Riboflavin mediated delivery of a macromolecule into cultured human cells. Biochim Biophys Acta. 1999; 1426:195–204
81. Rozen, R. Methylenetetrahydrofolate reductase: A link between folate and riboflavin? Am J Clin Nutr. 2002;76:301–302.
82. Hustad, S. et. al. Riboflavin as a determinant of plasma total homocysteine: Effect modification by the methylenetetrahydrofolate reductase C677T polymorphism Clin Chem. 2000;46:1065–1071.
83. Frosst P, Blom HJ, Milos R, et al. A candidate genetic risk factor for vascular disease: a common mutation in methylenetetrahydrofolate reductase. Nature Genet. 1995;10:111–113.
84. Jacques PF, Kalmbach R, Bagley PJ, et al. The relationship between riboflavin and plasma total homocysteine in the Framingham offspring cohort is influenced by folate status and the C677T transition in the methylenetetrahydroreductase gene. J Nutr. 2002; 132:283–288.
85. McNulty, H, et al. Impaired functioning of thermolabile methylenetetrhydrofolate reductase is dependent on riboflavin status: implications for riboflavin requirements. Am J Clin Nutr. 2002;76:436–441.
86. Stern LL, et al, Combined marginal folate and riboflavin status affect homocysteine methylation in cultured immortalized lymphocytes from persons homozygous for the MTHFR C677T mutation. J Nutr. 2003;133:2716–2720.
87. Ganji G, Kafai MR. Frequent consumption of milk, yogurt, cold breakfast cereals, peppers and cruciferous vegetables and intakes of dietary folate and riboflavin but not vitamins B12 and B6 are inversely associated with serum total homocysteine concentrations in the US population. Am J Clin Nutr. 2004;80: 1500–1507.

# 20 Niacin

Robert A. Jacob

The term niacin is the generic descriptor for nicotinic acid (pyridine-3-carboxylic acid, sometimes known as vitamin $B_3$) and derivatives exhibiting qualitatively the biological activity of nicotinamide (nicotinic acid amide and niacinamide). Nicotinic acid was isolated as a pure chemical substance in 1867, but it was not until 1937 that it was demonstrated to be the "anti-black-tongue factor" in dogs and the anti-pellagra vitamin for humans.[1] Before 1937, it had been suggested that pellagra was due to a deficiency of tryptophan in corn, but the biosynthetic pathway for the formation of a niacin derivative from tryptophan was not established until after both nicotinamide and nicotinic acid were shown separately to be anti-pellagragenic.

## Chemistry and Analytical Methods

The structures of nicotinic acid and nicotinamide (niacinamide) are shown in Figure 1. Both compounds are stable, white, crystalline solids. Nicotinamide is more soluble in water, alcohol, and ether than is nicotinic acid. The acid or amide form can be determined using a chemical reaction with cyanogen bromide and organic bases, liquid chromatography, or microbiological methods employing a variety of bacteria requiring niacin for growth.[2,3] The active coenzyme forms of niacin, nicotinamide adenine dinucleotide (NAD) and NAD phosphate (NADP), can be determined by enzyme-cycling colorimetric, fluorimetric, or high-performance liquid chromatography (HPLC) or by spectrophotometric methods.[4,5,6]

Nicotinamide, nicotinic acid, and their metabolites can be measured in blood plasma and urine by HPLC and capillary electrophoresis techniques, as well as by traditional chemical methods.[2,7-9] The urinary metabolites of niacin, including the methylated derivatives $N^1$-methylnicotinamide (NMN) and $N^1$-methyl-2-pyridone-5-carboxamide (2-pyridone), can be determined by fluorescence or HPLC techniques. Ketones react with NMN in alkaline solution to form a fluorescent product. The relative biological activity of niacin-containing foods can be determined by measuring weight gain or hepatic pyridine nucleotides after feeding the test foods to niacin-deprived chicks or weanling rats.[10]

## Metabolism and Biochemistry

### *Absorption and Transport*

Nicotinic acid and nicotinamide are rapidly absorbed from the stomach and the intestine.[11-13] At physiological concentrations intestinal niacin absorption occurs as pH-dependent facilitated diffusion, but at higher concentrations passive diffusion predominates. Three to four grams of niacin given orally can be almost completely absorbed. Nicotinamide is the major form in the bloodstream and arises from enzymatic hydrolysis of NAD in the intestinal mucosa and liver. The intestinal mucosa is rich in niacin conversion enzymes such as NAD glycohydrolase. Nicotinamide is released from NAD in the liver and intestines by glycohydrolases and transported to tissues that synthesize their own NAD as needed. Tissues apparently take up both forms of the vitamin by simple diffusion, but evidence indicates a facilitated transport of niacin into erythrocytes.

### *Excretion*

Excess niacin is methylated in the liver to NMN, which is excreted in the urine along with the 2- and 4-pyridone oxidation products of NMN (Figure 2). The two major excretion products are NMN and 2-pyridone, but minor amounts of niacin or niacin oxide and hydroxyl forms are also excreted.[14] The pattern of niacin products excreted after niacin ingestion depends somewhat on the amount and form of niacin ingested and the niacin status of the individual.

### *Biosynthetic Pathways and Their Regulation*

Niacin is biosynthesized from quinolinate in all organisms that have been studied thus far. In mammals, quino-

Tryptophan | Nicotinic Acid | Nicotinamide | ADP-Ribose NAD⁺(NADP⁺)

NIACIN PRECURSOR | NIACIN FORMS | NIACIN COENZYME

Figure 1. Niacin-related structures.

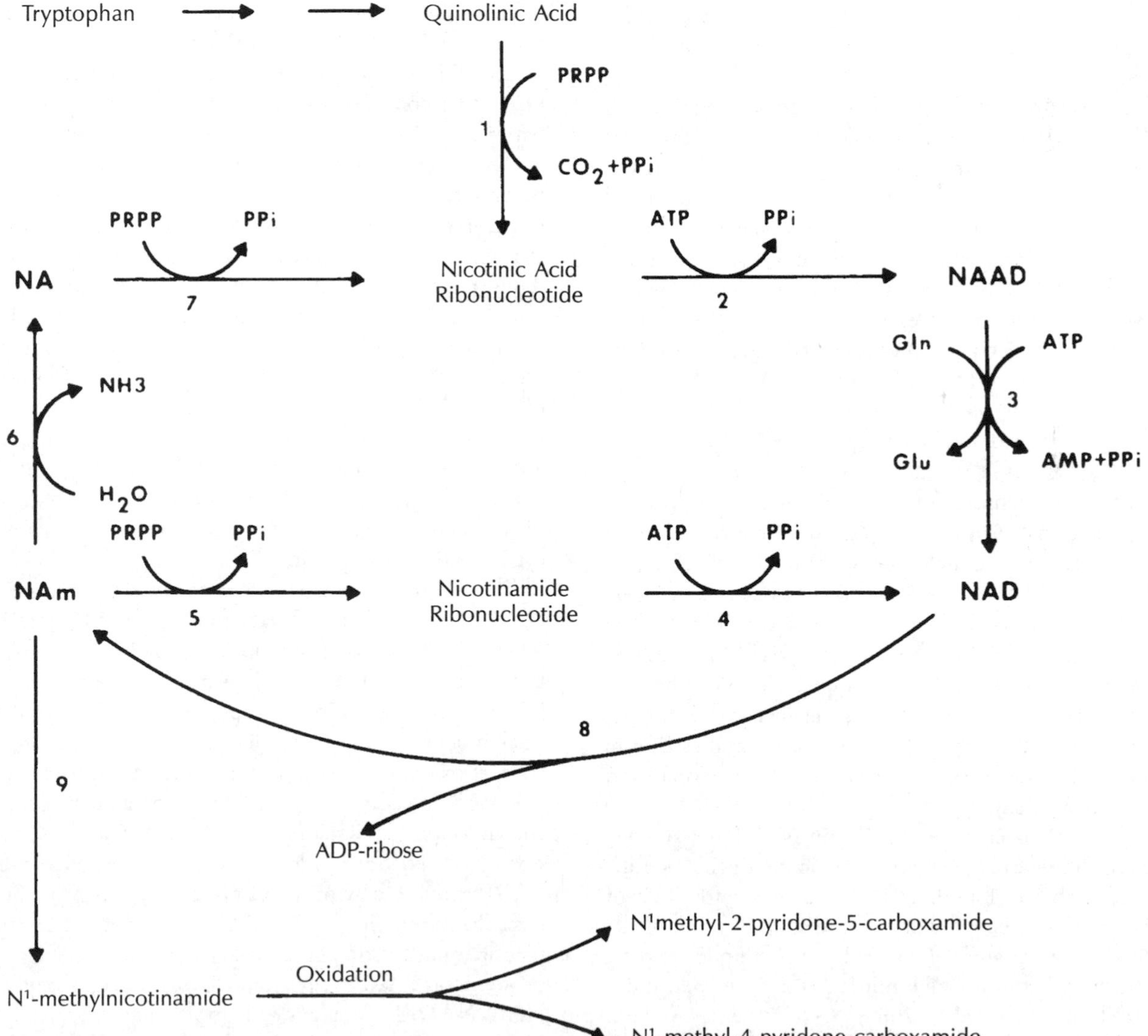


Figure 2. Pathways of niacin metabolism. NA, nicotinic acid; NAM, nicotinamide; NAAD, nicotinic acid adenine dinucleotide; PPPP, phosphoribosyl pyrophosphate. Enzymes: 1, quinolinate phosphoribosyltransferase; 2 & 4, adenyltransferases; 3, NAD synthetase; 5, nicotinamide phosphoribosyltransferase; 6 nicotinamide deamidase; 7, nicotinate phosphoribosyltransferase; 8, poly (ADP-ribose) synthetase or NAD glycohydrolase; 9, N¹-methyltransferase.

linic acid arising from dietary tryptophan through the kynurenine pathway is converted to nicotinic acid ribonucleotide (Figure 2).[15] This conversion is regulated by the enzyme quinolinate phosphoribosyltransferase. In humans, the biosynthesis of niacin from the essential amino acid tryptophan is an important route for meeting the body's niacin requirement. The efficiency of the conversion of dietary tryptophan to niacin is affected by a variety of nutritional and hormonal factors. Deficiencies of vitamin $B_6$, riboflavin, and iron slow the conversion because these micronutrients are essential cofactors for enzymes involved in the pathway. Conversion efficiency increases with restricted protein, tryptophan, energy, and niacin intakes because of changes in activities of pathway enzymes, including tryptophan oxygenase, quinolinate phosphoribosyltransferase, and picolinate carboxylase.[15,16] Regardless of dietary factors, large individual differences in the conversion efficiency of tryptophan to niacin have been reported.[17]

To estimate nutritional intake or niacin equivalents (NE) from tryptophan, an average conversion ratio of 60 mg tryptophan to 1 mg niacin was recommended by the Food and Nutrition Board of the Institute of Medicine.[18] This conversion value is based primarily on human studies measuring the conversion of tryptophan to niacin metabolites.[19] A threefold increase in tryptophan-to-niacin conversion efficiency in pregnant women and women taking oral contraceptives is presumably due to the stimulation by estrogen of tryptophan oxygenase, an enzyme in the pathway suggested to be rate limiting.[20]

An amino acid imbalance (particularly excessive dietary leucine) has been reported to antagonize the tryptophan-to-niacin conversion, probably by altering kynureninase activity.[21] Other studies showed that the addition of 5% leucine to the diet increased the activity of hepatic NADP glycohydrolase and thereby decreased NAD concentration. In isolated rat liver cells, 2-oxoisocaproate (the 2-oxo analog of leucine) decreases NAD biosynthesis from both tryptophan and nicotinic acid.[22] Whether excess dietary leucine compromises niacin status, however, remains open to question, because some studies in rats and humans showed no effects of excess leucine on niacin metabolism or status.[17,23-25]

The niacin coenzymes NAD and NADP are synthesized in all tissues of the body from nicotinic acid, nicotinamide, or both (Figure 2).[26] Tissue concentrations of NAD appear to be regulated by the concentration of extracellular nicotinamide, which in turn is under hepatic control and is hormonally influenced. In the liver, nicotinamide is converted to storage NAD (i.e., NAD not bound to enzymes) and to metabolites of niacin that are excreted. Tryptophan and nicotinic acid also contribute to storage NAD, and studies suggest that in rats the liver synthesizes NADP predominantly from tryptophan rather than from preformed niacin.[27] The nicotinamide formed in the degradation of NAD can be reconverted to NAD via nicotinamide ribonucleotide. Hepatocytes contain little nicotinamide deamidase, but nicotinamide can be deamidated in the intestinal tract by intestinal microflora.[28] Hydrolysis of hepatic NAD allows the release of nicotinamide for transport to tissues that lack the ability to synthesize the NADP coenzymes from tryptophan.

## *Biochemical Functions*

Niacin is essential in the form of the coenzymes NAD and NADP, in which the nicotinamide moiety acts as electron acceptor or hydrogen donor in many biological redox reactions. Thus, NAD functions as an electron carrier for intracellular respiration as well as a codehydrogenase with enzymes involved in the oxidation of fuel molecules such as glyceraldehyde 3-phosphate, lactate, alcohol, 3-hydroxybutyrate, pyruvate, and α-ketoglutarate dehydrogenases. NADP functions as a hydrogen donor in reductive biosyntheses such as fatty acid and steroid syntheses and, like NAD, it also functions as a co-dehydrogenase, for example, in the oxidation of glucose 6-phosphate to ribose 5-phosphate in the pentose phosphate pathway.

The niacin cofactor NAD is also required for important nonredox reactions. It is the substrate for three classes of enzymes that cleave the β-*N*-glycosylic bond of NAD to free nicotinamide and catalyze the transfer of adenosine diphosphate (ADP)-ribose. Two classes of enzymes catalyze ADP-ribose transfer to proteins: poly-ADP-ribose polymerases (PARP) and mono-ADP-ribosyltransferases.[29] A third class of enzymes promotes the formation of cyclic ADP-ribose, which mobilizes calcium from intracellular stores in many types of cells. Nicotinic acid adenine dinucleotide phosphate (NAADP), formed in vivo by the deamidation of NADP, also acts as a regulator of cellular calcium transport by a mechanism distinct from cyclic ADP-ribose action.[30]

The PARP nuclear enzymes catalyze the transfer of ADP-ribose units from NAD to acceptor proteins. The poly-ADP-ribosylated proteins function in DNA replication and repair, as well as in various cellular processes including differentiation and apoptosis.[29] In vitro and animal model studies show that DNA-damaging agents such as oxidant stressors and chemical carcinogens activate PARP, leading to altered NAD metabolism and the consumption of cellular NAD and energy via ATP depletion.[29,31,32] Nicotinamide, a product of NAD-dependent PARP activity, may provide anti-inflammatory action as a feedback inhibitor of the PARP-1 enzyme. However, nicotinamide exerts pharmacologic effects that are independent of PARP activity, including replenishment of NAD/NADPH pools and anti-inflammatory and antioxidant actions.[31] NAD is also required for the activity of silent information regulator (SIR or sirtuins) enzymes, protein deacetylases involved in transcriptional regulation, genome stability, neuronal protection, metabolism, and longevity.[33] NAD-dependent mono-ADP-ribosyltransferases function in cell signaling by modulating G-protein activity and in other less-well-known roles.[29]

Thus, the non-redox roles of niacin, as NAD and/or nicotinamide, can modulate or regulate DNA and genome fidelity, critical cellular processes, and inflammatory and immune responses. Some evidence suggests that niacin's roles in these pathways, and therefore niacin nutriture, may affect the progression of age-related degenerative diseases such as cancer, diabetes, and dementia.[29,32-34]

The metal-chelating ability of nicotinic acid may explain some of its biological interactions with essential trace metals. Nicotinic acid is part of a proposed glucose tolerance factor, an organo-chromium complex isolated from yeast that may potentiate the insulin response in some individuals.[35] Supplementing nicotinic acid into the diets of rats and mice enhanced zinc and iron use.[36]

### *Biochemical Assessment of Niacin Status*

Measurement of the urinary excretion of the two major methylated metabolites, NMN and 2-pyridone, has been used to determine niacin status. The Interdepartmental Committee on Nutrition for National Defense published criteria for interpreting urinary NMN excretion amounts in adults and pregnant women, and suggested 24-hour excretions for adults of under 5.8 μmol/d (0.8 mg/d) as representing deficient niacin status.[37] Use of random urine samples for the determination of niacin status is complicated by diurnal variations in metabolite excretion.[9,38] The use of creatinine corrections to allow for assay of random fasting urine samples rather than 24-hour collections can be difficult to interpret because of differences in creatinine excretion by age.

The ratio of urinary 2-pyridone to NMN has been suggested as a niacin deficiency marker independent of age and creatinine excretion.[37] A study of an outbreak of pellagra in Mozambican women showed that the ratio of 6-pyridone to NMN correlated well with the clinical symptoms, principally dermatitis.[39] However, studies in rats and humans found that the urinary pyridone-NMN ratio depended strongly on the level of protein intake and was a measure of protein adequacy rather than niacin status.[40] An experimental study of niacin deficiency in adult males found the ratio to be insensitive to a marginal niacin intake of 10 niacin equivalents (NE)/d and not totally reliable for evaluating an intake of 6 NE/d.[24]

Concentrations of niacin and niacin metabolites in plasma are normally quite low and generally have not been shown to be useful markers of niacin status. Results from an experimental study, however, indicated that 2-pyridone but not NMN in plasma could be a reliable marker of niacin deficiency, because 2-pyridone dropped below detection limits after a low niacin intake.[24] With an oral niacin load (20 mg nicotinamide/70 kg body weight), post-dose changes in the 2-pyridone metabolite reflected niacin status more so than changes in the NMN metabolite. These changes occurred in plasma as well as in urine.[24] Concentrations of 2-pyridone increase in plasma and decrease in urine with increasing age.[41]

Although Vivian et al.[42] reported a nearly 40% decrease in blood pyridine nucleotides in human subjects fed a niacin-deficient experimental diet, subsequent studies reported mixed results on the effects of pellagra or experimental niacin deficiency on concentrations of blood pyridine nucleotides. In the experimental study of niacin deficiency cited above,[24] erythrocyte NAD levels decreased by approximately 70%, whereas NADP levels remained unchanged when adult male subjects were fed low-niacin diets of either 6 or 10 NE/d. These results suggest that the erythrocyte NAD concentration may be a sensitive indicator of niacin depletion, and that a ratio of erythrocyte NAD to NADP of less than 1 may identify subjects at risk of developing niacin deficiency.[25] This is consistent with earlier findings of a similar decrease in NAD relative to NADP in fibroblasts grown in low-niacin culture medium.[43] The rationale for using the NAD-NADP ratio in whole blood or erythrocytes (termed niacin number) as an index of niacin status has been summarized previously.[44] The mean niacin number ([NAD/NADP] × 100) for healthy US adults is estimated as 175, with a range of 127 to 223 for 95% of the population. However, niacin status varies widely among different populations and is modulated by niacin supplementation.

## Requirement for Niacin

Experimental niacin depletion-repletion studies with healthy adults have indicated that urinary excretion of 7.3 μmol/d (1.0 mg/d) of the NMN metabolite reflects a niacin intake above that resulting in clinical symptoms of niacin deficiency (pellagra). Because no other functional measures of niacin status have been quantitatively related to niacin intake, the Recommended Dietary Allowance (RDA) for niacin was set based on estimation of the niacin intake equivalent to excretion of 1.0 mg/d of the NMN metabolite.[18] Accordingly, the RDA for males and females ages 14 years and above was set as 16 and 14 mg NE/d, respectively (1 mg NE = 1 mg niacin or 60 mg dietary tryptophan). These amounts allow for differences in energy use and size between men and women, differences in the bioavailability of niacin from various diets, and variations that occur in the amount of tryptophan converted to niacin.

Because of a lack of information about niacin requirements in children, the RDA for children was extrapolated from the RDA for adults, allowing for differences in body weight, metabolism, and growth needs. For children of both sexes ages 1 to 13 years, the RDA values range from 6 to 12 mg NE/d.[18] Because data are not sufficient for calculating a requirement for infants, an Adequate Intake (AI) was set based on the amounts consumed by healthy infants fed principally with human milk: 2 mg/d (0.3 mg/kg) of preformed niacin for infants ages 0 to 5 months and 4 mg NE/d (0.4 mg/kg) for infants 6 to 11 months of age. There is also no direct evidence defining niacin requirements during pregnancy and lactation. The RDA for pregnant women is 18 mg NE/d, the additional amount based on increased energy and growth needs. The RDA for lactating women is 17 mg NE/d, the additional amount based on the niacin content of milk and energy required for milk production.

## Food Sources

Niacin is widely distributed in plant and animal foods. Good sources are yeast, meats (including liver), cereals, legumes, and seeds. Milk, green leafy vegetables, fish, coffee, and tea also contain appreciable amounts of niacin. An estimated 20% of the total niacin intake of US adults is derived from enriched bread products and ready-to-eat cereals. The consumption of niacin supplements by approximately one-quarter of the US population adds substantially to total niacin intake by factors 0.5 to 6 times above dietary intakes. For healthy elderly in the Boston area, the median niacin intake from supplements was estimated as 20 and 30 mg/d for men and women, respectively.[18] Niacin is present in uncooked foods mainly as the pyridine nucleotides NAD and NADP, but some hydrolysis of these nucleotides to free forms may occur during food preparation.

Niacin in plants may be bound to macromolecules, making it unavailable to mammals.[12] In wheat, several forms of bound niacin contain various peptides, hexoses, and pentoses (sometimes referred to as niacinogen or niacytin). In corn, the bioavailability of bound niacin is increased by pretreatment with lime water, a procedure used in Central America and Mexico for preparing tortillas. Some newer varieties of corn contain more tryptophan and niacin than traditional varieties. Roasting green coffee beans removes the methyl group from trigonellin (1-methylnicotinic acid), resulting in an increase in nicotinic acid. Niacin is unique among the vitamins in that an amino acid, tryptophan, is a precursor that can contribute substantially to niacin nutriture by its conversion to a niacin derivative in mammalian liver tissue. Because most proteins contain about 1% tryptophan, it is theoretically possible to maintain adequate niacin status on a diet devoid of niacin but containing more than 100 g of protein.

## Deficiency States

The classic dietary niacin deficiency disease, pellagra, was observed in the mid-18th century in Spain, and was described more fully a few years later by physicians in northern Italy, who used the term pellagra ("raw skin") for the first time. The disease is associated with poorer social classes, whose chief dietary staple often consists of some type of cereal such as maize (corn) or sorghum. The connection between pellagra and eating maize was shown by Goldberger, who in 1920 conducted studies in the southeastern United States, where pellagra was endemic. The results indicated that pellagra was caused by the absence of a dietary factor in maize, a staple in the diet of the region's poor. In 1937, nicotinic acid was established as this factor by its demonstrated effectiveness in curing pellagra.[1]

In experimental studies with humans, clinical signs of pellagra develop 50 to 60 days after the initiation of a corn diet. Pellagra is characterized by the "three Ds": dermatitis, diarrhea, and dementia.[45] The most common signs of a niacin deficiency are changes in the skin, the mucosa of the mouth, tongue, stomach, and intestinal tract, and the nervous system. The skin lesions are most characteristic. A pigmented rash develops symmetrically in areas exposed to sunlight and is similar to sunburn, although in chronic cases a darker color may develop. Changes in the digestive tract are associated with vomiting, constipation, or diarrhea, and the tongue becomes bright red. Neurological symptoms include depression, apathy, headache, fatigue, and loss of memory. Pellagra was common in the United States and parts of Europe in the early 20th century, but fortification of cereal grain products and improved economies and diets have caused pellagra to virtually disappear from industrialized countries (except for its occurrence in some alcoholics). It still appears in poor sections of India, China, and Africa.

An analysis of diets described in historical studies of human pellagra indicated that many people consumed NEs in excess of the RDA, but a low intake of riboflavin was common. These results suggest that the etiology of the US pellagra epidemic of the early 1900s has not been completely explained.[46] Deficiencies of other micronutrients required in the tryptophan-to-niacin conversion pathways (e.g., riboflavin, pyridoxine, iron) may also be involved in the appearance of pellagra.

Pellagra-like syndromes have also been described in the absence of dietary niacin deficiency.[47] In most cases, the pellagra results from a problem with the use of tryptophan as a niacin precursor. Pellagra sometimes occurs with the carcinoid syndrome, in which tryptophan is preferentially hydrolyzed to 5-hydroxytryptophan and serotonin. Prolonged treatment with the drug isoniazid may also lead to niacin deficiency by competition of the drug with pyridoxal phosphate, a cofactor required in the tryptophan-to-niacin pathway.[48] Patients with Hartnup's disease, an autosomal recessive disorder, develop pellagra because of a defect in the absorption process for tryptophan and other monocarboxylic amino acids in the intestine and kidney.[49] Treatment of pellagra patients with oral nicotinamide or nicotinic acid (40–250 mg/d) resolves the skin and neurological abnormalities. Evidence of low plasma tryptophan and lymphocyte NAD in HIV-infected patients and the similarities between AIDS and pellagra symptoms have prompted the hypothesis that HIV infection induces systemic tryptophan-niacin depletion and therefore that therapeutic niacin may be beneficial.[50]

Niacin deficiency has been produced in dogs, pigs, monkeys, chickens, trout, and rats.[51] Pigs are particularly sensitive and exhibit a scaly dermatitis. There is generally poor growth and lack of appetite, as well as inflammation of mouth and tongue mucosa (black tongue disease in dogs). Skin lesions do not always occur (e.g., rats and young monkeys). Niacin deficiency states have also been produced in animals by administration of synthetic niacin antagonists such as acetylpyridine, 6-aminonicotinamide, and 2-amino, 1, 3, 4 thiazole.[52]

## Clinical, Pharmacologic Effects and Toxicity

Molecular and clinical evidence suggests that niacin, as nicotinamide or NAD, acts as a neuroprotectant and may reduce the risk of age-related cognitive decline and neurodegenerative diseases such as Alzheimer's.[34,53,54] However, research on the potential of niacin as a neuroprotectant has not always shown positive results, as treatment of mildly demented patients with 10 mg/d of NADH showed no evidence of cognitive improvement.[55]

Niacin given as nicotinic acid in doses of 1 to 4 g/d exerts a broad spectrum of effects that improve abnormal lipid profiles, including those of individuals with hyperlipidemia, the metabolic syndrome, and type 2 diabetes.[56] Niacin reduces plasma total and LDL cholesterol, triglycerides, lipoprotein, and is the most effective drug for increasing HDL cholesterol (nicotinamide does not have a similar effect).[57] Clinical trials of niacin, given alone or in combination with other lipid-lowering drugs, have shown significant improvements in cardiovascular disease risk factors, as well as reductions in atherosclerotic progression, adverse clinical events, and mortality.[57-60] Evidence suggests that niacin works in part by altering fat metabolism and improving HDL-mediated reverse cholesterol transport.[61,62] Nicotinic acid treatment also provides anti-atherothrombotic effects that improve endothelial function, reduce inflammation, increase plaque stability, and diminish thrombosis.[63]

Large oral doses of nicotinic acid produce flushing—a skin reddening, burning, tingling, and itching sensation that occurs with nicotinic acid but not with nicotinamide. The severity of this effect may be reduced by treatment with low doses of aspirin or ibuprofen, and often decreases with continued doses. Niacin applied topically produces a skin flush that is markedly reduced in schizophrenics and therefore may aid in early diagnosis of the disorder.[64] In addition to flushing, high-dose niacin treatment can also cause gastrointestinal problems, headache, and liver or muscle damage when used in combination with statin drugs, and may also aggravate hyperuricemia (gout).[65,66] Nicotinic acid as a drug is available in three formulations, which differ in their efficacy and safety: immediate release, sustained (long acting) release, and extended release. The extended-release form has shown advantages over the other forms in that it is effective, only needs to be taken once daily, and has fewer side effects.[56,65]

Whereas treatment of diabetics with immediate-release niacin is known to impair glucose control, the dyslipidemia of well-controlled type 2 diabetics responded favorably to treatment with low doses (1.0 or 1.5 g/d) of extended-release nicotinic acid without compromising glycemic control.[62] While the extended-release form shows a lower incidence of side effects, all patients treated with large doses of niacin should be monitored for possible toxic symptoms. Some evidence suggests that pharmacologic doses of nicotinamide may delay the loss of pancreatic beta cell function and the onset of type 1 diabetes,[67] but this action has not been well established by clinical trials.

Nicotinamide sensitizes tumors to radio- and chemotherapy, largely due to increased vasorelaxation and tumor oxygenation.[68] The pharmacokinetics of nicotinamide in healthy adults and cancer patients undergoing radiotherapy have been reported previously.[69,70] Plasma concentrations and clearance rates are dose dependent, with half-lives ranging from 1.5 to 9 hours for oral doses of 1 to 6 g, respectively. Peak concentrations ranged from 0.7 to 1.1 mmol/L after a 6 g dose. For doses of 3 to 10 g, the time to peak plasma concentration ranges from 0.5 to 3 hours. High plasma levels in patients were maintained longer with doses of 10 g than 6 g, but the larger doses were less well tolerated.[70] Comparison of immediate- and sustained-release nicotinamide in young adult men showed similar non-linear kinetics at higher doses, but the bioavailability of the immediate-release form was greater.[71] Toxic effects accompanying the use of nicotinamide with radiotherapy (nausea and vomiting, mucosal damage, and renal dysfunction) are considered manageable, with caution against use in patients with impaired renal function.[66,72]

The Tolerable Upper Intake Level (UL) of niacin, the highest level of daily nutrient intake likely to pose no risks of adverse health effects to almost all individuals in the general population, is 35 mg NE/d for adults and ranges from 10 to 30 mg/d for children and adolescents 1 to 18 years of age.[18] The UL is based on the transient flushing effect of nicotinic acid, but applies to intakes of nicotinamide also.

Injection of rats with 1 g/kg of nicotinamide causes phosphaturia due to increased NAD concentration in the renal cortex and altered renal phosphate transport.[73] Large doses of nicotinamide given to rats induce drug-metabolizing enzymes and produce increased lipid and decreased choline concentrations in the liver.[73,74] The oral lethal dose for the rat is 3.5 g/kg for nicotinamide and 4.5 to 5.2 g/kg for nicotinic acid. Nicotinamide fed at concentrations of 1% to 2% of the diet inhibits growth.[75]

## Summary and Future Directions

Niacin (as nicotinic acid or nicotinamide) is essential in the form of the coenzymes NAD and NADP, in which the nicotinamide moiety acts as electron acceptor or hydrogen donor in many biological redox reactions. Important non-redox roles of niacin involve NAD as substrate for three classes of nuclear enzymes that transfer ADP-ribose units to proteins and SIR enzymes involved in gene expression. The non-redox roles of niacin involve modulating or regulating DNA and genome fidelity, critical cellular processes, and inflammatory and immune responses, and therefore may affect the progression of age-related degenerative diseases including cancer, diabetes, and dementia.

Niacin is provided in the diet primarily as the pyridine nucleotides NAD and NADP, but both niacin and NAD are biosynthesized from dietary tryptophan. Therefore, the RDA (16 and 14 mg NE/d for males and females ages ≥ 14 years, respectively) is expressed in NE, where 1 mg NE equals 1 mg niacin or 60 mg tryptophan.

Pellagra, the classic niacin deficiency disease, is characterized by bilateral dermatitis and is often associated with a largely cereal diet containing little bioavailable niacin and lacking in tryptophan and other micronutrients needed for the biosynthesis of niacin from tryptophan. As a result of the fortification of cereal grain products and widespread supplement use, the disease is now rarely seen in industrialized countries, but still appears in some poor Asian, Chinese, and African populations. Clinical uses of niacin include therapy with nicotinic acid to improve the blood lipid profile and use of nicotinamide to sensitize tumors to radio- or chemotherapy. Large doses of nicotinic acid may produce flushing of the skin, gastrointestinal symptoms, and liver or muscle damage. The UL for niacin, based on flushing produced by nicotinic acid, is 35 mg NE/d for adults.

The best method for assessing niacin status currently is the determination of urinary metabolites, so research on blood and functional measures is needed. Information is also needed to determine the requirement for niacin based on the non-redox roles of NAD in fundamental genomic, molecular, and cellular processes involving protein ADP-ribosylation and SIR enzyme activity. Research is also needed to determine the value of various niacin formulations, especially extended-release forms and combinations with other drugs, for reducing the risk of degenerative and inflammatory disorders including heart disease, stroke, cancer, diabetes, arthritis, and neurodegenerative diseases.

## References

1. Spies TD, Cooper C, Blankenhorn MA. The use of nicotinic acid in the treatment of pellagra. JAMA. 1938;110:622–627.
2. Henderson LM. Niacin. Annu Rev Nutr. 1983;3: 289–307.
3. Baker H, Frank O, eds. *Clinical Vitaminology, Methods, and Interpretation*. New York: Interscience Publishers; 1968.
4. Uppal A, Ghosh N, Datta A, Gupta PK. Fluorimetric estimation of the concentration of NADH from human blood samples. Biotechnol Appl Biochem. 2005;41(part 1):43–47.
5. Stocchi V, Cucchiarini L, Canestrari F, Piacentini MP, Fornaini G. A very fast ion-pair reversed-phase HPLC method for the separation of the most significant nucleotides and their degradation products in human red blood cells. Anal Biochem. 1987;167: 181–190.
6. Wagner TC, Scott MD. Single extraction method for the spectrophotometric quantification of oxidized and reduced pyridine nucleotides in erythrocytes. Anal Biochem. 1994;222:417–426.
7. Iwaki M, Murakami E, Kakehi K. Chromatographic and capillary electrophoretic methods for the analysis of nicotinic acid and its metabolites. J Chromatogr B Biomed Sci Appl. 2000;747:229–240.
8. Pfuhl P, Karcher U, Haring N, et al. Simultaneous determination of niacin, niacinamide and nicotinuric acid in human plasma. J Pharm Biomed Anal. 2005; 36:1045–1052.
9. Creeke PI, Seal AJ. Quantitation of the niacin metabolites 1-methylnicotinamide and l-methyl-2-pyridone-5-carboxamide in random spot urine samples, by ion-pairing reverse-phase HPLC with UV detection, and the implications for the use of spot urine samples in the assessment of niacin status. J Chromatogr B Analyt Technol Biomed Life Sci. 2005; 817:247–253.
10. Behl R, Deodhar AD. Hepatic pyridine nucleotides content in rat–a better indicator for determining available niacin values of food. Indian J Exp Biol. 1999;37:32–36.
11. Bechgaard H, Jespersen S. GI absorption of niacin in humans. J Pharm Sci. 1977;66:871–872.
12. van den Berg H. Bioavailability of niacin. Eur J Clin Nutr 1997;51(suppl 1):S64–S65.
13. Nabokina SM, Kashyap ML, Said HM. Mechanism and regulation of human intestinal niacin uptake. Am J Physiol Cell Physiol. 2005;289:C97–C103.
14. Mrochek JE, Jolley RL, Young DS, Turner WJ. Metabolic response of humans to ingestion of nicotinic acid and nicotinamide. Clin Chem. 1976;22: 1821–1827.
15. Van Eys J. Niacin. In: Machlin LH, ed. *Handbook of Vitamins*. 2nd ed. New York: Marcel Dekker; 1991; 311–340.
16. Shibata K. Nutritional factors that regulate on the conversion of L-tryptophan to niacin. Adv Exp Med Biol. 1999;467:711–716.
17. Patterson JI, Brown RR, Linkswiler H, Harper AE. Excretion of tryptophan-niacin metabolites by young men: effects of tryptophan, leucine, and vitamin B6 intakes. Am J Clin Nutr. 1980;33:2157–2167.
18. Institute of Medicine. *Dietary Reference Intakes for Thiamin, Riboflavin, Niacin, Vitamin B6, Folate, Vitamin B12, Pantothenic Acid, Biotin, and Choline*;

1998. Available online at: http://www.nap.edu/openbook/0309065542/html/.

19. Horwitt MK, Harper AE, Henderson LM. Niacin-tryptophan relationships for evaluating niacin equivalents. Am J Clin Nutr. 1981;34:423–427.
20. Rose DP, Braidman IP. Excretion of tryptophan metabolites as affected by pregnancy, contraceptive steroids, and steroid hormones. Am J Clin Nutr. 1971; 24:673–683.
21. Pellagragenic effect of excess leucine. Nutr Rev. 1986;44:26–27.
22. Bender DA. Effects of a dietary excess of leucine and of the addition of leucine and 2-oxo-isocaproate on the metabolism of tryptophan and niacin in isolated rat liver cells. Br J Nutr. 1989;61:629–640.
23. Cook NE, Carpenter KJ. Leucine excess and niacin status in rats. J Nutr. 1987;117:519–526.
24. Jacob RA, Swendseid ME, McKee RW, Fu CS, Clemens RA. Biochemical markers for assessment of niacin status in young men: urinary and blood levels of niacin metabolites. J Nutr. 1989;119:591–598.
25. Fu CS, Swendseid ME, Jacob RA, McKee RW. Biochemical markers for assessment of niacin status in young men: levels of erythrocyte niacin coenzymes and plasma tryptophan. J Nutr. 1989;119:1949–1955.
26. Magni G, Amici A, Emanuelli M, et al. Enzymology of NAD+ homeostasis in man. Cell Mol Life Sci. 2004;61:19–34.
27. Bender DA, Olufunwa R. Utilization of tryptophan, nicotinamide and nicotinic acid as precursors for nicotinamide nucleotide synthesis in isolated rat liver cells. Br J Nutr. 1988;59:279–287.
28. Bernofsky C. Physiology aspects of pyridine nucleotide regulation in mammals. Mol Cell Biochem. 1980;33:135–143.
29. Kirkland JB. Niacin and carcinogenesis. Nutr Cancer. 2003;46:110–118.
30. Guse AH. Cyclic ADP-ribose (cADPR) and nicotinic acid adenine dinucleotide phosphate (NAADP): novel regulators of Ca2+-signaling and cell function. Curr Mol Med. 2002;2:273–282.
31. Szabo C. Nicotinamide: a jack of all trades (but master of none?). Intensive Care Med. 2003;29:863–866.
32. Virag L. Structure and function of poly(ADP-ribose) polymerase-1: role in oxidative stress-related pathologies. Curr Vasc Pharmacol. 2005;3:209–214.
33. Denu JM. Vitamin B3 and sirtuin function. Trends Biochem Sci. 2005;30:479–483.
34. Araki T, Sasaki Y, Milbrandt J. Increased nuclear NAD biosynthesis and SIRT1 activation prevent axonal degeneration. Science. 2004;305:1010–1013.
35. Mertz W. Effects and metabolism of glucose tolerance factor. Nutr Rev. 1975;33:129–135.
36. Agte VV, Paknikar KM, Chiplonkar SA. Effect of nicotinic acid on zinc and iron metabolism. Biometals. 1997;10:271–276.
37. Sauberlich HE, Dowdy RP, Skala JH. *Laboratory Tests for the Assessment of Nutritional Status.* Boca Raton, FL; CRC Press; 1974; 284–288.
38. Okamoto H, Ishikawa A, Yoshitake Y, et al. Diurnal variations in human urinary excretion of nicotinamide catabolites: effects of stress on the metabolism of nicotinamide. Am J Clin Nutr. 2003;77:406–410.
39. Dillon JC, Malfait P, Demaux G, Foldi-Hope C. The urinary metabolites of niacin during the course of pellagra [in French]. Ann Nutr Metab. 1992;36: 181–185.
40. Shibata K, Matsuo H. Effect of supplementing low protein diets with the limiting amino acids on the excretion of $N^1$-methylnicotinamide and its pyridones in the rat. J Nutr. 1989;119:896–901.
41. Slominska EM, Rutkowski P, Smolenski RT, Szutowicz A, Rutkowski B, Swierczynski J. The age-related increase in N-methyl-2-pyridone-5-carboxamide (NAD catabolite) in human plasma. Mol Cell Biochem. 2004;267:25–30.
42. Vivian VM, Chaloupka MM, Reynolds MS. Some aspects of tryptophan metabolism in human subjects. 1. Nitrogen balances, blood pyridine nucleotides, and urinary excretion of N-methylnicotinamide and N-methyl-2-pyridone-5-carboxamide on a low niacin diet. J Nutr. 1958;66:587–598.
43. Jacobson EL, Lange RA, Jacobson MK. Pyridine nucleotide synthesis in 3T3 cells. J Cell Physiol. 1979; 99:417–425.
44. Jacobson EL, Jacobson MK. Tissue NAD as a biochemical measure of niacin status in humans. Methods Enzymol. 1997;280:221–230.
45. Hegyi J, Schwartz RA, Hegyi V. Pellagra: dermatitis, dementia, and diarrhea. Int J Dermatol. 2004;43: 1–5.
46. Carpenter KJ, Lewin WJ. A reexamination of the composition of diets associated with pellagra. J Nutr. 1985;115:543–552.
47. McCormick DB. Niacin. In: Shils ME, Young VR, eds. *Modern Nutrition in Health and Disease.* 7th ed. Philadelphia: Lea and Febiger; 1988; 370–375.
48. Darvay A, Basarab T, McGregor JM, Russell-Jones R. Isoniazid induced pellagra despite pyridoxine supplementation. Clin Exp Dermatol. 1999;24:167–169.
49. Oakley A, Wallace J. Hartnup disease presenting in an adult. Clin Exp Dermatol. 1994; 19:407–408.
50. Murray MF. Tryptophan depletion and HIV infection: a metabolic link to pathogenesis. Lancet Infect Dis. 2003;3:644–652.
51. Sauberlich HE. Nutritional aspects of pyridine nucleotides. In: Dolphun D, Poulson R, Aramovic O, eds. *Pyridine Nucleotide Coenzymes.* New York: John Wiley & Sons; 1987; 608–609.
52. Weiner M, Van Eys J. Nicotinic acid antagonists. In: Weiner M, ed. *Nicotinic Acid: Nutrient-Cofactor-Drug.* New York: Marcel Dekker; 1983; 109–131.

53. Li F, Chong ZZ, Maiese K. Navigating novel mechanisms of cellular plasticity with the NAD+ precursor and nutrient nicotinamide. Front Biosci. 2004;9: 2500–2520.
54. Morris MC, Evans DA, Bienias JL, et al. Dietary niacin and the risk of incident Alzheimer's disease and of cognitive decline. J Neurol Neurosurg Psychiatry. 2004;75:1093–1099.
55. Rainer M, Kraxberger E, Haushofer M, Mucke HA, Jellinger KA. No evidence for cognitive improvement from oral nicotinamide adenine dinucleotide (NADH) in dementia. J Neural Transm. 2000; 107:1475–1481.
56. McKenney J. New perspectives on the use of niacin in the treatment of lipid disorders. Arch Intern Med. 2004;164:697–705.
57. Birjmohun RS, Hutten BA, Kastelein JJ, Stroes ES. Efficacy and safety of high-density lipoprotein cholesterol-increasing compounds A meta-analysis of randomized controlled trials. J Am Coll Cardiol. 2005;45:185–197.
58. Levy DR, Pearson TA. Combination niacin and statin therapy in primary and secondary prevention of cardiovascular disease. Clin Cardiol. 2005;28: 317–320.
59. Goldberg AC. A meta-analysis of randomized controlled studies on the effects of extended-release niacin in women. Am J Cardiol. 2004;94:121–124.
60. Canner PL, Furberg CD, Terrin ML, McGovern ME. Benefits of niacin by glycemic status in patients with healed myocardial infarction (from the Coronary Drug Project). Am J Cardiol. 2005;95:254–257.
61. Pike NB, Wise A. Identification of a nicotinic acid receptor: is this the molecular target for the oldest lipid-lowering drug? Curr Opin Investig Drugs. 2004;5:271–275.
62. Davidson MH. Niacin: a powerful adjunct to other lipid-lowering drugs in reducing plaque progression and acute coronary events. Curr Atheroscler Rep. 2003;5:418–422.
63. Rosenson RS. Antiatherothrombotic effects of nicotinic acid. Atherosclerosis. 2003;171:87–96.
64. Messamore E. Relationship between the niacin skin flush response and essential fatty acids in schizophrenia. Prostaglandins Leukot Essent Fatty Acids. 2003; 69:413–419.
65. Xydakis AM, Jones PH. Toxicity of antilipidemic agents: facts and fictions. Curr Atheroscler Rep. 2003;5:403–410.
66. Knip M, Douek IF, Moore WP, et al.; European Nicotinamide Diabetes Intervention Group. Safety of high-dose nicotinamide: a review. Diabetologia. 2000;43:1337–1345.
67. Greenbaum CJ, Kahn SE, Palmer JP. Nicotinamide's effects on glucose metabolism in subjects at risk for IDDM. Diabetes 1996;45:1631–1634.
68. Ruddock MW, Hirst DG. Nicotinamide relaxes vascular smooth muscle by inhibiting myosin light chain kinase-dependent signaling pathways: implications for anticancer efficacy. Oncol Res. 2004;14:483–489.
69. Stratford MR, Rojas A, Hall DW, et al. Pharmacokinetics of nicotinamide and its effect on blood pressure, pulse and body temperature in normal human volunteers. Radiother Oncol. 1992;25:37–42.
70. Dragovic J, Kim SH, Brown SL, Kim JH. Nicotinamide pharmacokinetics in patients. Radiother Oncol. 1995;36:225–228.
71. Petley A, Macklin B, Renwick AG, Wilkin TJ. The pharmacokinetics of nicotinamide in humans and rodents. Diabetes. 1995;44:152–155.
72. Kaanders JH, Pop LA, Marres HA, van der Maazen RW, van der Kogel AJ, van Daal WA. Radiotherapy with carbogen breathing and nicotinamide in head and neck cancer: feasibility and toxicity. Radiother Oncol. 1995;37:190–198.
73. Nomura K, Shin M, Sano K, Umezawa C, Shimada T. Effect of nicotinamide administration to rats on the liver microsomal drug metabolizing enzymes. Int J Vitam Nutr Res. 1983;53:36–43.
74. Kang-Lee YA, McKee RW, Wright SM, Swendseid ME, Jenden DJ, Jope RS. Metabolic effects of nicotinamide administration in rats. J Nutr. 1983;113: 215–221.
75. Friedrich W. *Vitamins*. New York: W. de Gruyter; 1988.

# 21 Vitamin $B_6$

Donald B. McCormick

Vitamin $B_6$ comprises a triad of closely related heterocycles that in free form are called pyridoxine, pyridoxal, and pyridoxamine.[1] The intertwined studies on B vitamins that led to the identity of the vitamin $B_6$ group have been documented in some detail.[2] Among those investigators especially active during the 1930s in distinguishing vitamin $B_6$ from other members of the water-soluble B complex was Gyorgy, who helped to clarify the role of vitamin $B_6$ in curing acrodynia in rats. Then, several groups of investigators succeeded in obtaining a crystalline vitamin $B_6$ from plant sources, which led in 1939 to the structural elucidation of pyridoxine and its synthesis by Harris and Folkers at Merck. When Snell and his associates recognized that at least another form of vitamin $B_6$ was responsible for the growth activities of some bacteria, proposed structures were synthesized by the Merck group to verify pyridoxal and pyridoxamine as the other natural forms of free vitamin $B_6$. The occurrence in the 1950s of epileptiform seizures and dermatitic lesions in infants receiving too little free vitamin $B_6$ in their formula brought new interest to the problem of vitamin B deficiency in humans. Investigations beginning with Gunsalus and colleagues that led to the recognition of pyridoxal 5′-phosphate (PLP) as the functional coenzyme were reviewed by Snell.[3] Periodic symposia continue to detail new findings on vitamin $B_6$ and PLP-dependent enzymes; the most recent was published in 2003.[4]

## Chemistry of Vitamin $B_6$

### *Structures*

The natural base forms of the three vitamin $B_6$ vitamers vary in the substituent at position 4 of 2-methyl-3-hydroxy-5-hydroxymethyl-pyridines. There is a hydroxymethyl function in pyridoxine, a formyl function in pyridoxal, and an aminomethyl function in pyridoxamine. With their natural 5′-phosphates (PNP, PLP, and PMP), esterification is at the hydroxymethyl substituent in position 5. This phosphate is an essential electrostatic group for protein interaction with coenzymic PLP. A relatively common form of vitamin $B_6$ stored in many plant foods is the 5′-O-(β-D-glucopyranosyl)pyridoxine. These compounds, present in ionic forms predominant at physiologic pH values, are illustrated in Figure 1.

### *Properties*

Salts of vitamin $B_6$, particularly the commercially available hydrochlorides, are quite water soluble. So too are the phosphate esters. The protonated pyridinium species that occur in neutral to acid ranges of pH absorb light near 290 nm, whereas anionic phenolate forms have absorption spectra that extend into the near ultraviolet and even visible region. Principal absorption maxima for vitamin $B_6$ vitamers and analogs have been collated,[5] as have their fluorescent properties.[6] Photodecomposition becomes significant in alkaline media, especially for the coenzyme PLP, in which oxidation of the aldehyde to the carboxylate occurs. It is notable that the 4-formyl function of pyridoxal reacts intramolecularly with its 5′-hydroxy group to form the relatively stable hemiacetal. The presence of the phosphate prevents this from occurring with PLP, which thereby retains the aldehyde function that can readily undergo Schiff base reactions with amino groups of substrates and proteins, including those using the coenzyme during enzymic operations.

### *Analyses*

The methods commonly used in determining vitamin $B_6$ content include biological, biochemical, and chemical techniques.[7] Microbiological, enzymatic, and high-performance liquid chromatographic techniques are available for extracts from foods and other materials.[8,9] Chemical differentiation of vitamin $B_6$ and analogs includes nuclear magnetic resonance spectroscopy and mass spectrometry.[10-13]

## Sources of Vitamin $B_6$

Vitamin $B_6$ in free and bound forms is widely distributed in foods, with good sources being meats, whole-

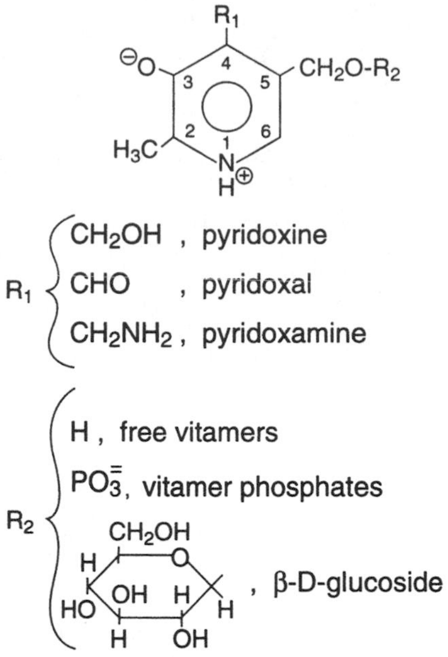

R1: $CH_2OH$, pyridoxine; CHO, pyridoxal; $CH_2NH_2$, pyridoxamine

R2: H, free vitamers; $PO_3^{=}$, vitamer phosphates; β-D-glucoside

Figure 1. Structures of vitamers of vitamin B-6, their phosphates, and the β-D-glucoside.

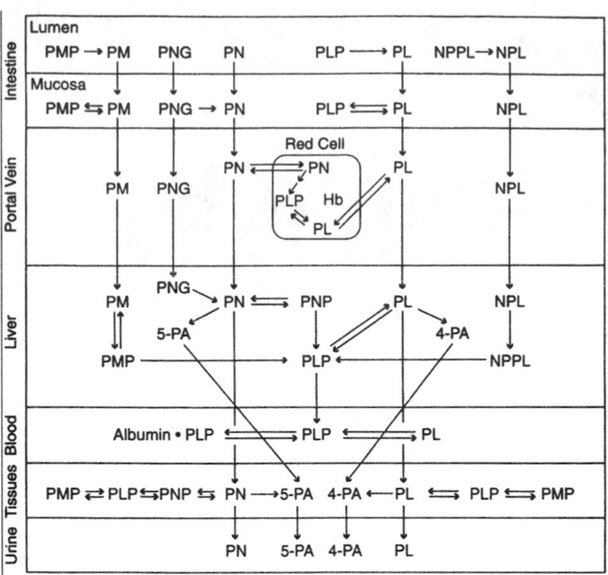


Figure 2. Disposition of ingested forms of vitamin B-6 with an indication of organ interplay. PL, pyridoxal; PM, pyridoxamine; PN, pyridoxine; PLP, PMP, PNP, their respective 5′-phosphates; PNG, pyridoxine β-D-glucoside; NPPL, ε-N-(5′-phospho-4′-pyridoxal)-L-lysine; NPL, ε-N-(4′- pyridoxal)-L-lysine; 4-PA, 5-PA, 4- and 5-pyridoxic acids. Hb, hemoglobin.

grain products, vegetables, and nuts.[2,14] Cooking and storage losses that may range from a few percent to nearly half the vitamin $B_6$ originally present are greater with animal products. Plant foods generally contain the more stable pyridoxine, its 5′-O-β-D-glucoside (PNG), and PNP; animal tissues have more pyridoxal and PLP, which are mainly bound to proteins via ε-amino groups of lysyl residues and sulfhydryl groups of cysteinyl residues. The bioavailability of vitamin $B_6$ in foods is not only affected by how much vitamin is released from such natural bound forms as the glucoside, but also by that from such forms as the ε-N-(4′-pyridoxyl)lysine, which results from canning under conditions whereby the PLP lysyl Schiff base is reduced followed by hydrolysis.[15] Compounds and factors involved in vitamin $B_6$ bioavailability were reviewed recently.[16] Because vitamin $B_6$ is available over the counter and in supplements, some individuals receive amounts well above requirement levels. Data from the Third National Health and Nutrition Examination Survey indicate 9 mg/d as the highest mean intake from food and supplements for any sex and life stage group. Highest intakes were in pregnant females.

# Vitamin $B_6$ Disposition In Vivo

The overall fate of most forms of vitamin $B_6$ consumed by mammals, particularly humans, is summarized in Figure 2, which is an update from that published earlier.[17]

## *Uptake*

During transit through the small intestine, the phosphorylated vitamers and PLP-protein adducts are dephosphorylated by membrane-bound alkaline phosphatase. Entry of the free vitamers occurs by passive diffusion and is facilitated by metabolic trapping as the 5′-phosphates reformed by adenosine triphosphate (ATP)-using pyridoxal kinase in the cytosol.[1,18] There is a decreased bioavailability of vitamin $B_6$ in foods with a high glucosylated pyridoxine content.[19] About 58% of PNG administered to humans is bioavailable as vitamin $B_6$.[20] Some PNG is absorbed intact, as reflected by urinary excretion,[14] and there is some inhibition of the use of co-ingested pyridoxine.[21] A cytosolic PNG hydrolase has been purified from porcine jejunal mucosa.[22] PNG is taken in by hepatocytes in a manner competitive with pyridoxine. The glucoside can then effect slow release of vitamin $B_6$.[23]

The less frequently encountered 4′-α- and 5′-α-D-glucosides of pyridoxine can also be taken up and metabolized by isolated rat liver cells.[24] The ε-N-(4′-pyridoxyl)-L-lysine remaining after hydrolytic cleavages of the phosphate and peptide bonds of PLP reductively bound to protein during thermal processing can also be absorbed in a manner competitive with vitamin $B_6$. Only after pyridoxal kinase-catalyzed rephosphorylation in somatic cells (e.g., liver and kidney) can the ε-N-(5′-phospho-4′-pyridoxyl)-L-lysine become oxidized to generate PLP and lysine plus hydrogen peroxide in a reaction catalyzed by the riboflavin 5′-phosphate-dependent pyridoxine (pyridoxamine) 5′-phosphate oxidase.[25-28] Overall efficiency of such conversion, at least as measured in rats, is such as to reduce the bioavailability of vitamin $B_6$.[29] Because ε-N-(4′-pyridoxyl)-L-lysine is a substrate for both kinase and oxidase responsible for converting natural forms of vitamin $B_6$ to the functional PLP, it competes with the use and uptake of the vitamin. This can accelerate deficiency in animals on diets deficient in vitamin $B_6$.[29,30]

## *Transport*

Under normal conditions, most of the vitamin $B_6$ in blood is present as PLP that is mainly Schiff base-linked to proteins, largely albumin in the plasma and hemoglobin in the erythrocytes. Although over 90% of vitamin $B_6$ in plasma typically is PLP (and the rest as lesser amounts of pyridoxal, pyridoxine, and derivatives[28]), the total is less than 0.1% of the total body vitamin $B_6$.[2] The plasma PLP concentration, usually over 50 nmol/L in adults, declines during pregnancy, partly attributable to a shift in distribution in favor of erythrocytes over plasma. Renal failure also causes a reduction in plasma PLP. Conditions in which plasma alkaline phosphatase is elevated, including pregnancy and metabolic bone disease, are associated with low plasma PLP and a corresponding increase in pyridoxal; conversely, with hypophosphatasia the plasma PLP is much higher than the normal level of around 62 nmol/L in humans.[2,31] Free vitamers of vitamin $B_6$ are readily taken into the blood cells and converted to PLP.[32]

## *Metabolism*

The ability of different organs to take in and convert vitamin $B_6$ to functional PLP is generalized, but the liver is the site of much of this conversion, which depends on sequential action of pyridoxal kinase and pyridoxine (pyridoxamine) 5′-phosphate oxidase.[1,2,31] The kinase has been characterized from both prokaryotic and eukaryotic sources.[33,34] The mammalian enzyme was found to operate with Zn·ATP, be stimulated by K+, and catalyze phosphorylation of all three natural vitamin $B_6$ vitamers,[33,35] whereas an additional pyridoxal-specific kinase[36] recently was found in organisms such as *Escherichia coli*, which biosynthesize vitamin $B_6$ in a pathway that produces PNP from condensation of 1-deoxy-D-xylulose with 4-phosphohydroxy-L-threonine.[37] This more specific kinase plays a salvage role in recovering pyridoxal released from PLP that is formed by oxidase conversion of PNP.

The kinase with broader specificity that functions in humans and most organisms has been known for some time to be inhibited by carbonyl reagents, including such drugs as cycloserine, dopamine, isoniazid, and thiamphenicol glycinate.[34,38] The recent discovery that the general pyridoxal kinase is also a benzodiazepine-binding protein[39] adds to its potential interest. The anti-anxiety action of benzodiazepines may be related to sequential events that enhance the inhibitory neuronal activity of γ-aminobutyrate. The oxidase that converts PNP and PMP to PLP was first purified from liver[26] and has been studied in such detail as to reveal the catalytically involved sequence found in both prokaryotic and eukaryotic organisms.[40] The riboflavin 5′-phosphate-dependent enzyme is affected by riboflavin status[41,42] and is subject to product inhibition by PLP.[43] Its major characteristics related to vitamin $B_6$ use in mammals and its interconnection to riboflavin have been reviewed in detail previously.[44,45] Interestingly, this oxidase is lacking in certain liver tumors and neural tumors,[46] and its expression is developmentally regulated.

Catabolism of vitamin $B_6$ is also most active in liver, although other tissues (e.g., kidney) contribute to such processes as aldehyde oxidase-catalyzed oxidation of pyridoxal to 4-pyridoxic acid, which is excreted in urine.[47] The 4-pyridoxic acid is a major excretory catabolite; about half the daily intake of vitamin $B_6$ by humans is lost in such a manner.[48] However, with higher intakes of pyridoxine, increasing amounts of the 5-pyridoxic acid are also excreted.[49,50] Assessments of body pools of vitamin $B_6$ reveal that of the approximately 1 mmol present, at least 80% is present in muscle, where most is the PLP bound in glycogen phosphorylase,[51-53] so the total vitamin $B_6$ in circulation is less than 1 mmol. The vitamin $B_6$ content of human milk varies with maternal intake of vitamin $B_6$ but is approximately 10 to 20 μg/L during the first days of lactation and thereafter increases to 100 to 250 μg/L.[1]

Defects in the metabolism or use of vitamin $B_6$ related to human diseases have been reviewed elsewhere.[54] Some more recent reports on particular genetic bases for deficiencies in PLP-dependent enzymes include pyridoxine-responsive convulsions resulting from inadequate γ-aminobutyrate synthesis in children,[55] homocystinuria due to cystathionine β-synthase deficiency,[56,57] and cystathionuria due to inadequate cystathionase. Other known defects include xanthurenic aciduria caused by inadequate kynureninase, ornithinemia (gyrate atrophy) caused by a defective ornithine aminotransferase, and primary oxalosis (type I), in which pyridoxine seems to increase the removal of glycolate to glycine.

# Functions of Vitamin $B_6$

## *Mechanisms*

By virtue of the ability of PLP to condense its 4-formyl substituent with an amine (usually the α-amino group of an amino acid) to form an azomethine (Schiff base) linkage, a conjugated double bond system extending from the α-carbon of the amine (amino acid) to the pyridinium nitrogen in PLP results in reduced electron density around the α-carbon.[1] This potentially weakens each of the bonds from the amine (amino acid) carbon to the adjoined functions (hydrogen, carboxyl, or side chain). An apoenzyme then locks in a particular configuration of the coenzyme-substrate compound such that maximal overlap of the bond to be broken will occur with the resonant, coplanar, electron-withdrawing system of the coenzyme complex. These steps of reversible condensation, dehydration, and replacement of groups on the

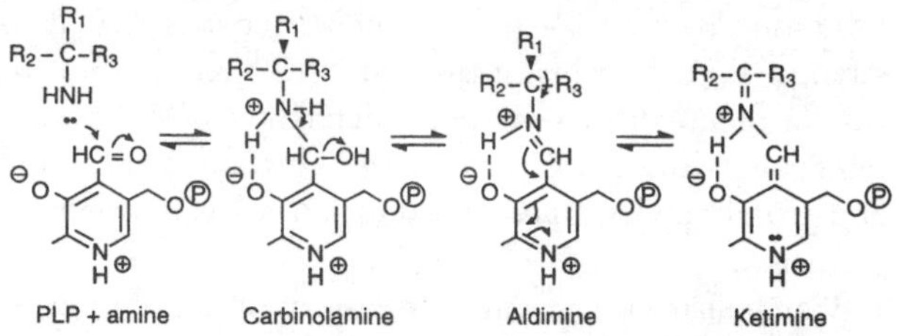

PLP + amine ⇌ Carbinolamine ⇌ Aldimine ⇌ Ketimine

Figure 3. Mechanism by which groups on a carbon bearing an amino function of a substrate can be made more labile by reaction with pyridoxal phosphate.

α-carbon are illustrated in Figure 3, and have been reviewed in encyclopedias[58,59] and symposia.[4] With crystallographic detail now available for a number of PLP-dependent enzymes, their structures, evolution, and detailed mechanisms have also been clarified.[60]

Aminotransferases (transaminases) effect rupture of the α-hydrogen bond of an amino acid with ultimate formation of an α-keto acid and PMP; this reversible reaction provides an interface between amino acid metabolism and ketogenic and glycogenic reactions (e.g., aspartate/oxaloacetate). Amino acid decarboxylases catalyze breakage of the α-carboxyl bond and lead to irreversible formation of amines, including several that are functional in nervous tissue (e.g., epinephrine, norepinephrine, serotonin, and γ-aminobutyrate). In some cases, decarboxylations are connected with new carbon-carbon bond formation. For example, the biosynthesis of heme depends on the early formation of δ-aminolevulinate from the synthase that catalyzed condensation of glycine and succinyl-coenzyme A followed by decarboxylation. The formation of 3-dehydrosphinganine, a precursor of sphingolipids, depends on condensation of L-serine with palmitoyl-coenzyme A that is catalyzed by a so-called transferase. There are many examples of enzymes, such as cysteine desulfhydrase and serine hydroxymethyltransferase, that effect the loss or transfer of amino acid side chains. There is also the special case of glycogen phosphorylase, wherein the PLP moiety functions as an ionic rather than as a condensation center to catalyze phosphorolysis of α-1, 4-linkages of glycogen. The mechanism has been envisioned as protonation of the glucosidic oxygen of the polysaccharide by inorganic phosphate in the initial stage, thus generating an oxycarbonium-phosphate ion pair. PLP interacts to stabilize this ion pair, thereby permitting covalent addition of phosphate to form glucose 1-phosphate.[61]

### *Systems*

As seen in the useful overview in a preceding volume in this series,[14] the roles of PLP are diverse and essential in numerous specialized cellular systems. A synopsis of such processes is given in Figure 4. Just as the formation of PLP from other 5′-phospho forms of vitamin $B_6$ requires riboflavin 5′-phosphate, PLP is required in the formation of such niacin equivalents as those derived from L-tryptophan.[1,2] The importance of PLP in several reac-

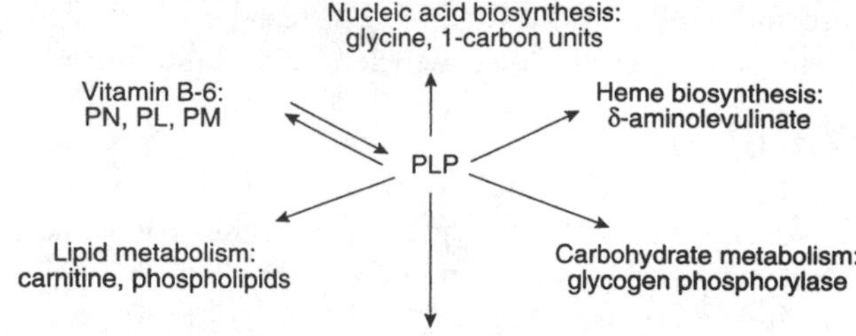


Figure 4. Cellular processes requiring participation of pyridoxal 5′-phosphate.

tions leading to neurotransmitters is illustrated by a report in which a deficit of vitamin $B_6$ in infant formula led to abnormal electroencephalograms (EEGs) and convulsions.[62] Adults fed diets low in vitamin $B_6$ can also develop abnormal EEGs.[63,64]

Participation of PLP in numerous other enzyme reactions of amino acid metabolism includes the requirements in sulfur amino acid turnover, which is sensitive to PLP level. As mentioned above, homocystinuria (and homocysteinemia) result from too little cystathionine synthase and potentially from poorly active methionine synthase, which is a vitamin $B_{12}$-dependent enzyme using methyl folate. The role of PLP in effecting one-carbon metabolism may be especially important in nucleic acid biosynthesis and immune system function.[14] PLP is also needed for gluconeogenesis by way of transaminases active on glucogenic amino acids and for lipid metabolism that involves several aspects of PLP function; for example, for production of carnitine needed to act as a vector for long-chain fatty acids for mitochondrial β-oxidation and of certain bases for phospholipid biosynthesis. Some evidence also exists for PLP modulation of steroid hormone action by its binding to receptors,[65] although the extent to which PLP mediates such effects in vivo is less clear.

# Assessment of Vitamin $B_6$ Status

### *Methods*

There are several indices that can be used for assessing the vitamin $B_6$ status of an individual. These have been reviewed over the past decade.[1,3,14,31,66-68] Vitamin $B_6$ status is most appropriately evaluated using a combination of indicators, including those considered direct (e.g., vitamer concentration in cells or fluids) and those that are indirect or functional (e.g., erythrocyte aminotransferase saturation by PLP or tryptophan metabolites).[69] Indicators used to estimate vitamin $B_6$ requirements are listed in Table 1. Plasma PLP may be the best single indicator, because it appears to reflect tissue stores.[70] Diets containing less than 0.05 mg of vitamin $B_6$ given to 11 young women for 11 to 28 days led to abnormal EEG patterns in two of the women and a plasma PLP of approximately 9 nmol/L.[64] Therefore, a level of approximately 10 nmol/L is considered suboptimal. A plasma PLP cutoff of 20

**Table 1.** Some Indicators for Assessing Vitamin $B_6$ Status

| Indicator | Assessment |
|---|---|
| Plasma PLP | Major vitamin B-6 form in tissue and reflects liver PLP; changes fairly slowly in response to vitamin intake |
| Urinary vitamin $B_6$ catabolite excretion | Excretion rate of vitamin and particularly 4-pyridoxate reflects intake; 5-pyridoxate appears with excess intake |
| Erythrocyte aminotransferases activity coefficients | Enzymes for aspartate and alanine reflect PLP levels; large variation in activity coefficients |
| Tryptophan catabolites | Urinary xanthurenate excretion, especially after a tryptophan load test |
| Other | Erythrocyte and whole-blood PLP, plasma homocysteine |

PLP, pyridoxal 5′-phosphate.

to 25 nmol/L has been proposed as an index of adequacy[68] on the basis of recent findings.[71] Plasma PLP levels have been reported to decrease with age.[14] The urinary 4-pyridoxic acid level changes promptly with changes in vitamin $B_6$ intake[70] and is therefore of questionable value in assessing status. However, a value of greater than 3 mmol/d has been suggested to reflect adequate intake.[66]

Erythrocyte aminotransferases for aspartate and alanine are commonly measured before and after addition of PLP to ascertain amounts of apoenzymes, the proportion of which increases with vitamin $B_6$ depletion. Values of 1.5 to 1.6 for the aspartate aminotransferase and approximately 1.2 for the alanine aminotransferase have been suggested as adequate.[66,72] Catabolites from tryptophan and methionine have also been used to assess vitamin $B_6$ status. A 24-hour urinary excretion of less than 65 mmol xanthurenate after a 2 g oral dose of tryptophan was suggested to indicate normal vitamin $B_6$ status.[66]

## *Deficiency*

Recognition of deficiency symptoms ultimately attributed to lack of vitamin $B_6$ was gained through the use of experimental animals (e.g., rat acrodynia) before the sequelae of events that occur in the human were determined. Investigations of the consequences of vitamin $B_6$ deficiency in humans have used diets deficient in the vitamin, diets containing an antagonist (usually 4′-deoxypyridoxine), or both.[1,2,31] A deficiency of vitamin $B_6$ alone is relatively uncommon; it is more common in association with deficits in other vitamins of the B complex.[72] However, both elderly adults and alcoholics may be at risk for deficiency of vitamin $B_6$ and other micronutrients.

Biochemical changes occur early and become more marked as vitamin $B_6$ deficiency progresses.[72] Plasma PLP and urinary output of vitamin $B_6$ and 4-pyridoxic acid decrease within 1 week of removal of the vitamin from the diet. There is increased xanthurenic acid in urine because liver kynureninase activity is decreased. Transaminases in serum and erythrocytes also decrease. EEG abnormalities appear within 3 weeks. Epileptiform convulsions, probably the result of insufficient activity of PLP-dependent L-glutamate decarboxylase, which is responsible for production of the inhibitory neurotransmitter γ-aminobutyrate, are a common finding in young subjects deficients in vitamin $B_6$. In addition, skin changes such as dermatitis with cheilosis and glossitis may occur. Hematological manifestations may include a decrease in circulating lymphocytes and possibly a normocytic, microcytic, or sideroblastic anemia.

The ongoing interest in the relationship of blood homocyst(e)ine levels to cardio- and cerebrovascular diseases has led to numerous studies examining the ameliorating effects of vitamin $B_6$ as well as folate and vitamin $B_{12}$, all with long-known biochemical functions as coenzymes necessary for sulfur amino acid metabolism. Some more recent reviews include consideration of homocyst(e)ine levels in neurologic disease[73] and cardiovascular disease.[74,75] It has also been reported that there is a decrease in the rate of coronary restenosis after lowering plasma homocysteine with a combination of pyriodoxine, folate, and vitamin $B_{12}$.[76]

Causes for deficiency vary. There have been infrequent reports of improperly constituted infant formulas (e.g., those singularly inadequate in vitamin $B_6$). There are instances in which chemotherapy or fortuitous ingestion of antagonists has led to hypovitaminosis $B_6$.[72] These include the tuberculostatic drug isoniazid, which can form hydrazones with pyridoxal and PLP. As with other carbonyl reagents, such compounds not only cause loss by displacement and urinary excretion, but the Schiff bases formed with pyridoxal inhibit pyridoxal kinase,[34,35] and the PLP Schiff bases may also inhibit some PLP-dependent enzymes. Several naturally occurring substituted hydrazines and hydroxylamines pose such risk.[77] Abnormalities in the function of vitamin $B_6$ occur in several genetic conditions. Pyridoxine-responsive genetic diseases include: infantile convulsions where the apoenzyme for glutamate decarboxylase has a poor affinity for the coenzyme; a type of chronic anemia in which the number but not the morphological abnormality of erythrocytes is improved by pyridoxine supplementation; xanthurenic aciduria, in which the affinity of the mutant kynureninase for PLP is decreased; primary cystathioninuria due to similarly defective cystathionase; and homocystinuria, in which there is less than the normal level of cystathionine synthase. Usually these inborn errors of metabolism respond to increased levels (5–50 mg/d) of administered vitamin $B_6$.[78]

### *Toxicity*

That neuropathy can result from high-dose pyridoxine has been documented in animals,[79] but the problem only became evident for humans when doses of >1 g/d were given for the treatment of premenstrual syndrome, asthma, and certain sensory neuropathies.[68,79] Both neurotoxicity and photosensitivity have been documented. Sensory neuropathy was selected as the critical end point on which to base a tolerable upper intake level of 100 mg/d for adults,[68] although supplements higher than this may be safe for most individuals.[14]

## Vitamin $B_6$ Requirements

Because there have been recent extensive considerations given to requirements and recommendations for vitamin $B_6$ intake by humans,[68,80] there is now reasonable confidence that numbers will not change much in the future. Recommendations, generally 20% higher than the estimated average requirements, are given in Table 2. Representative US surveys indicate mean daily intakes of approximately 2 mg/d for men and 1.5 mg/d for women. However, there are insufficient long-term studies with graded levels of vitamin $B_6$ to allow the cutoff values for clinical adequacy and inadequacy to be defined clearly. Also, as with most vitamins, there is a relative paucity of data for deducing more exact values for children after infancy and into adolescence.

**Table 2.** Recommendations for Vitamin $B_6$ for Humans

| Life Stage and Age | Amount (mg/d) |
|---|---|
| Infants | |
| 0–5 months | 0.1 |
| 6–11 months | 0.3 |
| Children | |
| 1–3 years | 0.5 |
| 4–6 years | 0.6 |
| 7–9 years | 1.0 |
| 10–18 years | |
| Females | 1.2 |
| Males | 1.3 |
| Adults | |
| Women | |
| ≤50 years | 1.3 |
| >50 years | 1.5 |
| Men | |
| ≤50 years | 1.3 |
| >50 years | 1.7 |
| Pregnancy | 1.9 |
| Lactation | 2.0 |

From Allgood and Cialowski,[65] copyright 1991, with permission from Elsevier.

## Summary

Vitamin $B_6$ is a group of compounds comprising three free forms, pyridoxine, pyridoxal, and pyridoxamine, and their 5′-phosphates. Foods contain mainly bound forms, especially PLP (animals), pyridoxine β-glucoside (plants), and some pyridoxyl peptides (processed foods), with varied bioavailability as vitamin $B_6$. Digestion and metabolism involve the release of most of the vitamin from glycosides and peptides with the formation of PLP to serve as coenzyme for over 100 characterized enzymatic reactions involved with the metabolism of glycogen, the biosynthesis of phospholipids, and numerous reactions with amino acids. Some vitamin is wasted as urinary 4-pyridoxate and, at higher intakes, 5′-pyridoxate. Requirements vary largely on the basis of metabolic size, pregnancy, lactation, and age. Large excesses are toxic. Future human nutrition research may be best aimed at better defining estimated average requirements for children, adolescents, pregnant and lactating women, and elderly adults.

## References

1. McCormick DB. Vitamin $B_6$. In: Bowman BB, Russell RM, eds. *Present Knowledge in Nutrition*. 8th ed. Washington, DC: ILSI Press; 2001; 207–213.
2. Combs GF Jr. *The Vitamins: Fundamental Aspects in Nutrition and Health*. 2nd ed. San Diego: Academic Press; 1998.
3. Snell EE. Pyridoxal phosphate: history and nomenclature. In: Dolphin D, Poulson R, Avramovic O, eds. *Pyridoxal Phosphate: Chemical, Biochemical and Medical Aspects*. part A, vol 1A. New York: Wiley; 1986; 1–12.
4. Proceedings of the 3rd International Symposium on Vitamin $B_6$, PQQ, Carbonyl Catalysis and Quinoproteins, Southampton, UK, 14–19 April 2002. Biochim Biophys Acta. 2003;1647:1–394.
5. Sober HA, ed. *Handbook of Biochemistry*. Cleveland: CRC Press; 1968; J222–J236.
6. Fasman GD, ed. *Handbook of Biochemistry and Molecular Biology*. Cleveland: CRC Press; 1976; 215.
7. Leklem JE, Reynolds RD, eds. *Methods in Vitamin B6 Nutrition, Analysis and Assessment*. New York: Plenum Press; 1980.
8. Polansky MM, Reynolds RD, Vandersclice JT. Vitamin B6. In: Augustine J, Klein BP, Becker DA, Venigopal PB, eds. *Methods of Vitamin Assay*. 4th ed. New York: Wiley; 1985; 417–443.
9. Gregory JF 3rd. Methods for determination of vita-

min $B_6$ in foods and other biological materials: a critical review. Journal of Food Composition and Analysis. 1988;1:105–123.

10. McCormick DB, Wright LD, eds. Vitamins and Coenzymes, Part A. San Diego: Academic Press; 1970. Methods in Enzymology Series, Vol. 18A.
11. McCormick DB, Wright LD. Vitamins and Coenzymes, Part D. San Diego: Academic Press; 1979. Methods in Enzymology Series, Vol. 62.
12. Chytil F, McCormick DB, eds. Vitamins and Coenzymes, Part G. San Diego: Academic Press; 1986. Methods in Enzymology Series, Vol. 122.
13. McCormick DB, Suttie JW, Wagner C, eds. Vitamins and Coenzymes, Part I. San Diego: Academic Press; 1997. Methods in Enzymology Series, Vol. 280.
14. Leklem JE. Vitamin B6. In: Ziegler EE, Files LJ, eds. *Present Knowledge in Nutrition*. 7th ed. Washington, DC: ILSI Press; 1996; 174–183.
15. Tsuge H, Maeno M, Hayakawa T, Suzuki Y. Comparative study of pyridoxine-alpha, beta-glucosides, and phosphopyridoxyl-lysine as a vitamin B6 nutrient. J Nutr Sci Vitaminol (Tokyo). 1996;42: 377–386.
16. Gregory JF 3rd. Bioavailability of vitamin B-6. Eur J Clin Nutr. 1997;51(suppl 1):S43–S48.
17. Merrill A, Burnham F. Vitamin B6. In: Brown M, ed. *Present Knowledge in Nutrition*. 6th ed. Washington, DC: ILSI Press; 1990; 155–162.
18. Henderson LM. Intestinal absorption of B6 vitamins. In Reynolds RD, Leklem JE, eds. *Vitamin B6: Its Role in Health and Disease*. New York: Liss; 1985; 22–23.
19. Kabir H, Leklem JE, Miller LT. Relationships of the glycosylated vitamin B6 content of foods on vitamin B6 bioavailability in humans. Nutr Rep Int. 1983;28:709–716.
20. Gregory JF 3rd, Trumbo PR, Bailey LB, Toth JP, Baumgartner TG, Cerda JJ. Bioavailability of pyridoxine-5-β-D-glucoside determined in humans by stable isotopic methods. J Nutr. 1991;121:177–186.
21. Nakano H, McMahon LG, Gregory JF 3rd. Pyridoxine-5′-β-glucoside exhibits incomplete bioavailability as a source of vitamin B6 and partially inhibits the utilization of co-ingested pyridoxine in humans. J Nutr. 1997;127:1508–1513.
22. McMahon LG, Nakano H, Levy MD, Gregory JF 3rd. Cytosolic pyridoxine-β-D-glucoside hydrolase from porcine jejunal mucosa. Purification properties, and comparison with broad specificity β-glucosidase. J Biol Chem. 1997;272:32025–32033.
23. Zhang Z, Gregory JF 3rd, McCormick DB. Pyridoxine-5′-β-D-glucoside competitively inhibits uptake of vitamin B6 into isolated rat liver cells. J Nutr. 1993;123:85–89.
24. Joseph T, Tsuge H, Suzuki Y, McCormick DB. Pyridoxine 4′-α- and 5′-α-D-glucosides are taken up and metabolized by isolated rat liver cells. J Nutr. 1996;126:2899–2903.
25. Kazarinoff MN, McCormick DB. N-(5′-Phospho-4′-pyridoxyl) amines as substrates for pyridoxine (pyridoxamine) 5′-phosphate oxidase. Biochem Biophys Res Commun. 1973;52:440–446.
26. Kazarinoff MN, McCormick DB. Rabbit liver pyridoxamine (pyridoxine) 5′-phosphate oxidase: purification and properties. J Biol Chem. 1975;250: 3436–3442.
27. Zhang Z, McCormick DB. Uptake of N-(4′-pyridoxyl) amines and release of amines by renal cells: a model for transporter-enhanced delivery of bioactive compounds. Proc Natl Acad Sci U S A. 1991;88: 10407–10410.
28. Zhang Z, McCormick DB. Uptake and metabolism of N-(4′-pyridoxyl) amines by isolated rat liver cells. Arch Biochem Biophys. 1992;294:394–397.
29. Gregory JF 3rd. Effects of ε-pyridoxyllysine bound to dietary protein on the vitamin B6 status of rats. J Nutr. 1980;110:995–1005.
30. Gregory JF 3rd. Effects of ε-pyridoxyl-lysine and related compounds on liver and brain pyridoxal kinase and liver pyridoxamine (pyridoxine) 5′-phosphate oxidase. J Biol Chem. 1980;255:2355–2359.
31. Bender DA. *Nutritional Biochemistry of the Vitamins*. Cambridge: Cambridge University Press; 1992; 223–268.
32. Ink SL, Henderson LM. Vitamin B6 metabolism. Annu Rev Nutr. 1984;4:455–470.
33. McCormick DB, Gregory ME, Snell EE. Pyridoxal phosphokinases. I. Assay, distribution, purification, and properties. J Biol Chem. 1961;236:2076–2084.
34. McCormick DB, Snell EE. Pyridoxal phosphokinases. II. Effects of inhibitors. J Biol Chem. 1961; 236:2085–2088.
35. McCormick DB, Snell EE. Pyridoxal kinase of human brain and its inhibition by hydrazine derivatives. Proc Natl Acad Sci U S A. 1959;45: 1371–1379.
36. Yang Y, Tsui HC, Man TK, Winkler ME. Identification and function of the pdxY gene, which encodes a novel pyridoxal kinase involved in the salvage pathway of pyridoxal 5′-phosphate biosynthesis in Escherichia coli K-12. J Bacteriol. 1998;180:1814–1821.
37. Winkler ME. Genetic and genomic approaches for delineating the pathway of pyridoxal 5′-phosphate coenzyme biosynthesis in *Escherichia coli*. In: Martinez-Carrion M, ed. 10th International Symposium on Vitamin B6 and Carbonyl Catalysis. 4th Meeting on PQQ and Quinoproteins. Basel: Birkhauser Verlag; 2000; 3–10.
38. Laine-Cessac P, Cailleux A, Allain P. Mechanisms of the inhibition of human erythrocyte pyridoxal kinase by drugs. Biochem Pharmacol. 1997;54: 863–870.
39. Hanna MC, Turner AJ, Kirkness EF. Human pyri-

doxal kinase: cDNA cloning, expression, and modulation by ligands of the benzodiazepine receptor. J Biol Chem. 1997;272:10756–10760.

40. McCormick DB, Chen H. Update on interconversions of vitamin B6 with its coenzyme. J Nutr. 1999; 129:325–327.
41. Rasmussen KM, Barsa PM, McCormick DB. Pyridoxamine (pyridoxine) 5′-phosphate oxidase activity in rat tissues during development of riboflavin or pyridoxine deficiency. Proc Soc Exp Biol Med. 1979; 161:527–530.
42. Rasmussen KM, Barsa PM, McCormick DB, Roe DA. Effect of strain, sex, and dietary riboflavin on pyridoxamine (pyridoxine) 5′-phosphate oxidase activity in rat tissues. J Nutr. 1980;110:1940–1946.
43. Merrill AH Jr, Horiike K, McCormick DB. Evidence for the regulation of pyridoxal 5′-phosphate formation in liver by pyridoxamine (pyridoxine) 5′-phosphate oxidase. Biochem Biophys Res Commun. 1978;83:984–990.
44. McCormick DB, Merrill AH Jr. Pyridoxamine (pyridoxine) 5′-phosphate oxidase. In: Tryfiates GP, ed. *Vitamin B6. Its Metabolism and Influence on the Processes of Growth*. Westport, CT: Food and Nutrition Press; 1980; 1–26.
45. McCormick DB. Two interconnected B vitamins: riboflavin and pyridoxine. Physiol Rev. 1989;69: 1170–1198.
46. Ngo EO, LePage GR, Thanassi JW, Meisler N, Nutter LM. Absence of pyridoxine-5′-phosphate oxidase (PNPO) activity in neoplastic cells: isolation, characterization, and expression of PNPO cDNA. Biochemistry. 1998;37:7741–7748.
47. Merrill AH Jr, Henderson JM, Wang E, McDonald BW, Millikan WJ. Metabolism of vitamin B-6 by human liver. J Nutr. 1984;114:1664–1674.
48. Wozenski JR, Leklem JE, Miller LT. The metabolism of small doses of vitamin B6 in men. J Nutr. 1980;110:275–285.
49. Mahuren JD, Coburn SP. Determination of 5-pyridoxic acid, 5-pyridoxic acid lactone, and other vitamin B6 compounds by cation-exchange high-performance liquid chromatography. Methods Enzymol. 1997;280:22–29.
50. Mahuren JD, Pauly TA, Coburn SP. Identification of 5-pyridoxic acid and 5-pyridoxic acid lactone as metabolites of vitamin $B_6$ in humans. J Nutr Biochem. 1991;2:449–453.
51. Coburn SP, Lewis DL, Fink WJ, Mahuren JD, Schal. Estimation of human vitamin B6 pools through muscle biopsies. Am J Clin Nutr. 1988;48: 291–294.
52. Coburn SP. Location and turnover of vitamin B6 pools and vitamin B6 requirements of humans. Ann N Y Acad Sci. 1990;585:75–85.
53. Krebs EG, Fischer EH. Phosphorylase and related enzymes of glycogen metabolism. In: Harris RS, Wol IG, Lovaine JA, eds. *Vitamins and Hormones*. vol 22. New York: Academic Press; 1964; 399–410.
54. Merrill AH Jr, Henderson JM. Diseases associated with defects in vitamin B6 metabolism or utilization. Annu Rev Nutr. 1987;7:137–156.
55. Pearl Pl, Gibson KM. Clinical aspects of the disorders of GABA metabolism in children. Curr Opin Neurol. 2004:17;107–113.
56. Yap S, Rushe H, Howard PM, Naughten ER. The intellectual abilities of early-treated individuals with pyridoxine-nonresponsive homocystinuria due to cystathionine beta-synthase deficiency. J Inherit Metab Dis. 2001;14:437–447.
57. Yap S, Boers GH, Wilcken B, et al. Vascular outcome in patients with homocystinuria due to cystathionine β-synthases deficiency treated chronically: a multicenter observational study. Arterioscler Thromb Vasc Biol. 2001;21:2080–2085.
58. McCormick DB. Coenzymes, biochemistry of. In: Meyers RA, ed. *Encyclopedia of Molecular Biology and Molecular Medicine*. Weinheim, Germany: VCH Publishers. 1996; 244–252.
59. McCormick DB. Coenzymes. In: *Encyclopedia of Human Biology*. vol 2. New York: Academic Press; 1997; 847–964.
60. Jansonius JN. Structure, evolution and action of vitamin B6-dependent enzymes. Curr Opin Struct Biol. 1998;8:759–769.
61. Palm D, Klein HW, Schinzel R, Buehner M, Helmreich EJ. The role of pyridoxal 5′-phosphate in glycogen phosphorylase catalysis. Biochemistry. 1990;29: 1099–1107.
62. Coursin DB. Convulsive seizures in infants with pyridoxine-deficient diet. JAMA. 1954;154:406–408.
63. Grabow JD, Linkswiler H. Electroencephalographic and nerve-conduction studies in experimental vitamin B6 deficiency in adults. Am J Clin Nutr. 1969; 22:1429–1434.
64. Kretsch MJ, Sauberlich HE, Newbrun E. Electroencephalographic changes and periodontal status during short-term vitamin B6 depletion of young, nonpregnant women. Am J Clin Nutr. 1991;53: 1266–1274.
65. Allgood VE, Cidlowski JA. Novel role for vitamin B6 in steroid-hormone action: a link between nutrition and the endocrine system. J Nutr Biochem. 1991;2:523–534.
66. Leklem J. Vitamin B6: a status report. J Nutr. 1990; 120(suppl 11):1503–1507.
67. Reynolds RD. Biochemical methods for status assessment. In: Raiten DJ, ed. *Vitamin B6 Metabolism in Pregnancy, Lactation and Infancy*. Boca Raton: CRC Press; 1995; 41–59.
68. Institute of Medicine. *Dietary Reference Intakes for Thiamin, Riboflavin, Niacin, Vitamin B6, Folate, Vitamin B12, Pantothenic Acid, Biotin, and Choline*;

1998. Available online at: http://www.nap.edu/openbook/0309065542/html/.
69. McCormick DB, Greene HL. Vitamins. In: Burtis CA, Ashwood ER, eds. *Tietz Textbook of Clinical Chemistry*. 3rd ed. Philadelphia: W.B. Saunders; 1994; 999–1028.
70. Liu A, Lumeng L, Aronoff GR, Li T-K. Relationship between body store of vitamin $B_6$ and plasma pyridoxal-P clearance: metabolic balance studies in humans. J Lab Clin Med. 1985;106:491–497.
71. Bailey AL, Wright AJ, Southon S. High performance liquid chromatography method for the determination of pyridoxal-5-phosphate in human plasma: how appropriate are cut-off values for vitamin B6 deficiency? Eur J Clin Nutr. 1999;53: 448–455.
72. Wilson JA. Disorders of vitamins: deficiency, excess, and errors of metabolism. In: Petersdorf RG, et al., eds. *Harrison's Principles of Internal Medicine*. 10th ed. New York: McGraw-Hill; 1983; 461–470.
73. Diaz-Arrastia R. Homocysteine and neurologic disease. Arch Neurol. 2000;57:1422–1427.
74. Spence JD. Patients with atherosclerotic vascular disease: how low should plasma homocyst(e)ine go? Am J Cardiovasc Drugs. 2001;1:85–89.
75. Graham IM, O'Callaghan P. Vitamins, homocysteine and cardiovascular risk. Cardiovasc Drugs Ther. 2002;16:383–389.
76. Schnyder G, Roffi M, Pin R, et al. Decreased rate of coronary restenosis after lowering of plasma homocysteine levels. N Engl J Med. 2001;345: 1593–1600.
77. Klosterman HJ. Vitamin B6 antagonists of natural origin. Methods Enzymol. 1979;62:483–495.
78. Rosenberg LE. Vitamin-responsive inherited diseases affecting the nervous system. Res Publ Assoc Nerv Ment Dis. 1974;53:263–272.
79. Schaumburg HH, Kaplan J, Windebank A, et al. Sensory neuropathy from pyridoxine abuse: a new megavitamin syndrome. N Engl J Med. 1983;309: 445–448.
80. Food and Agriculture Organization/World Health Organization. Human *Vitamin and Mineral Requirements: Report of a Joint FAO/WHO Expert Consultation Bangkok, Thailand*. Rome: FAO; 2002.

# 22 Folate

Lynn B. Bailey and Jesse F. Gregory III

Folate is a generic term for this water-soluble vitamin and includes naturally occurring food folate and folic acid in supplements and fortified foods. Folate coenzymes function in the acceptance and transfer of one carbon (1-C) moieties involved in the synthesis, interconversion, and modification of nucleotides, amino acids, and other cellular components. This chapter provides a review of current knowledge related to 1-C metabolism, a discussion of factors that may cause metabolic abnormalities (including inadequate folate intake), incomplete bioavailability, and folate-related genetic polymorphisms. Each of these factors is addressed by providing an overview of current knowledge regarding the interactions between the physiological, biochemical, and genetic aspects of folate metabolism coupled with an extrapolation to human health, including developmental abnormalities and chronic disease. In addition, this chapter addresses issues related to dietary folate intake recommendations based on current knowledge of food folate content and the effect of folate intake on status, as well as the potential public health consequences of these recommendations.

## Chemistry

Common structural features of the folate family include a pteridine bicyclic ring system, p-aminobenzoic acid, and one or more glutamic acid residues (Figure 1). Most naturally occurring folates have a side chain composed of five to eight glutamate residues joined in γ-peptide linkages. The term folic acid specifically refers to the fully oxidized monoglutamate form of the vitamin that is used in supplements and fortified foods and rarely occurs in nature. The folate molecule can vary in structure through reduction of the pteridine moiety to dihydrofolic acid and tetrahydrofolic acid (THF), elongation of the glutamate chain, and substitution of 1-C units at the N-5, N-10, or both positions.[1,2] The 1-C-substituted folates exist with methyl ($—CH_3$), formyl (—CH=O), formimino (—CH=NH), methylene ($—CH_2—$), or methenyl (—CH=) groups, mainly in polyglutamyl form of the THF molecule.

## Dietary Sources and Folic Acid Fortification

Naturally occurring dietary folate is concentrated in certain foods, including orange juice, dark green leafy vegetables, asparagus, strawberries, peanuts, and legumes such as black beans and kidney beans.[3] As of January 1, 1998, all cereal grain products in the United States labeled as "enriched" (e.g., bread, pasta, flour, breakfast cereal, and rice) and mixed food items containing these grains were required by the Food and Drug Administration (FDA) to be fortified with folic acid.[4] It is estimated that several thousand food items in the US food supply have been modified by fortification and now contain folic acid derived from enriched cereal grain ingredients.[5] In addition, folic acid is an ingredient in a large number of other food products, including meal replacements, infant formulas, and an increasing number of ready-to-eat breakfast cereals and snack foods. Outside of the United States, mandatory fortification also has been implemented in Canada,[6] Chile,[7] and some other Latin American countries.[8]

### *Effect of Folic Acid Fortification on Folate Intake and Status in the United States*

Significant increases in blood folate concentration in response to folic acid fortification in the United States have been documented in a number of studies.[9] Recently, the first nationally representative data for blood folate for the US population (≥3 years of age) after fortification was reported for individuals in the National Health and Nutrition Examination Survey (NHANES) IV (1999–2000) and compared with folate status during the prefortification survey from NHANES III (1988–1994).[10] From NHANES III to NHANES IV, the median serum folate concentration increased from 12.5 to

**Folic (Pteroyl-L-Glutamic) Acid**

**Polyglutamyl Tetrahydrofolates**

| Substituent (R) | Position |
|---|---|
| —$CH_3$ (methyl) | 5 |
| —CH=O (formyl) | 5 or 10 |
| —CH=NH (formimino) | 5 |
| —$CH_2$— (methylene) | 5 and 10 |
| —CH= (methenyl) | 5 and 10 |

Figure 1. Folic acid structures. Folic acid consists of a p-aminobenzoic acid molecule linked at one end to a pteridine ring, and at the other end to a molecule of glutamic acid. Food folates exist in various forms, containing from two to ten additional glutamate residues (**n**) joined to the first glutamate. The folate/folic acid structure can vary by reduction of the pteridine moiety to form dihydrofolic acid and tetrahydrofolic acid (THF), elongation of the glutamate chain, and substitution of 1-C units at the N5, N10, or both positions (**R**). Folate coenzymes are formed by the attachment of 1-C units including methyl (—$CH_3$), formyl (—CH═O), formimino (—CH═NH), methylene (—$CH_2$—), or methenyl (—CH═) groups to the polyglutamyl form of the THF molecule.

32.2 nmol/L and the median red blood cell folate concentration increased from 392 to 625 nmol/L. The significant upward shift in serum and red blood cell folate concentrations after fortification in the United States is illustrated in Figure 2.[10] The observed increase in blood folate post-fortification is greater than expected and, based on the analysis of a large number of fortified foods, has been attributed to overages by the food industry.[11] Two research groups using different approaches[54,55] have estimated that the increase in folic acid intake due to fortification is actually around 200 μg/d, which is about two times greater than the 100 μg/d originally predicted by FDA.[4]

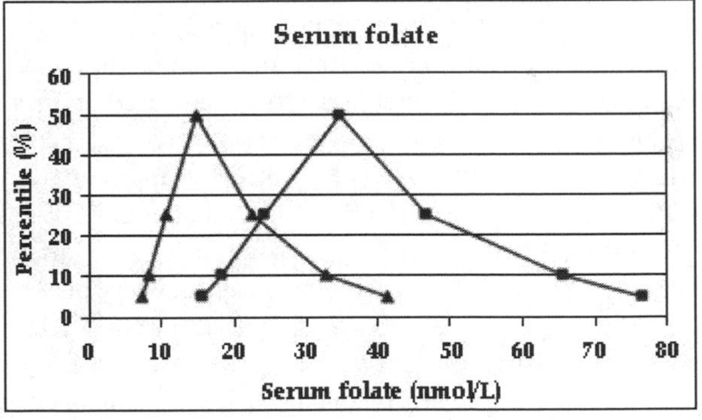


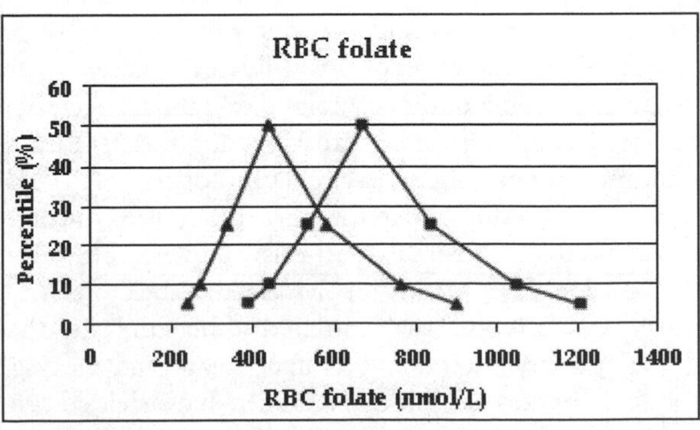


Figure 2. Frequency distribution of serum and red blood cell folate for persons 3 years of age and older from NHANES 1999–2000 (▲) compared with persons 4 years of age or older from NHANES III (■). (Adapted from Pfeiffer et al., 2005[10] with permission from *The American Journal of Clinical Nutrition.* © Am J Clin Nutr. American Society for Nutrition.)

# Physiology and Metabolism

When naturally occurring food folate is consumed, it must first be converted to the monoglutamate form by the enzyme folylpoly-γ-glutamate carboxypeptidase (EC 3.4.12.10), also referred to as pteroylpolyglutamate hydrolase or folate conjugase, located primarily in the jejunal brush border membrane.[12,13] The pH optimum for folylpoly-γ-glutamate carboxypeptidase is 6.5 to 7.0. Changes in luminal pH associated with chronic drug use or diseases that alter jejunal pH can impair folate absorption.[14] Following deconjugation to the monoglutamyl form, folates are transported across the membrane by a pH-dependent carrier-mediated mechanism.[15] A nonsaturable ion-mediated transport process predominates at high intraluminal concentrations of folate (>10 μmol/L).[16]

Prior to entry into the portal blood, folic acid undergoes reduction to THF and conversion to either methyl or formyl forms in mucosal cells.[17] The reduction process is readily saturated, such that significant amounts of folic acid are found in plasma and urine of humans ingesting 400 to 800 μg/d or more than 200 μg in a single dose.[18] The predominant form of folate in plasma is 5-methylTHF, which is primarily bound loosely to albumin, while a smaller percentage is bound with high affinity to folate-binding protein.[1] Folate transport into certain cells occurs by membrane-associated folate-binding proteins that act as folate receptors and thereby facilitate cellular uptake of folate.[19-22] In the proximal tubular cells of the kidney, the high-affinity folate-binding proteins appear to transport 5-methylTHF selectively.[22-24] The reduced folate carrier specifically targets reduced folates for uptake.[20,21]

Once within cells, 5-methylTHF is demethylated through the action of methionine synthase (MTR) (EC 1.16.1.8) and converted to a polyglutamyl form by folypolyglutamate synthetase (EC 6.3.2.17).[25] Since folate polyglutamates do not cross cell membranes due to the charge on the side chain and favorable binding to folate enzymes, polyglutamylation serves as a mechanism to help sequester folate inside the cell.[25] Prior to release from tissues into circulation, folate polyglutamates are reconverted to the monoglutamate form by γ-glutamyl hydrolase (EC 3.4.19.9).[1,26] Tissues are limited in their ability to store folate beyond that required for metabolic function. The total body content of folate in humans is estimated to be approximately 15 to 30 mg based on measurements of liver tissue concentration[27,28] and taking into account the estimated liver weight (approximately 1400 g) and the assumption that the liver contains 50% of total body folate.[29] Calculations based on in vivo kinetic studies yield similar estimates of body folate pools,[30,31] whereas another kinetic study suggested an almost four times greater amount of folate in humans.[32]

The fraction of plasma folate that is not associated with protein is freely filtered at the glomerulus, and most is reabsorbed in the proximal renal tubules.[33] Urinary excretion occurs mainly as the products of folate cleavage, and the urinary excretion of intact folates represents only a small percentage of dietary folate.[34,35] Biliary secretion of folate has been estimated to be as high as 100 μg/d, providing for enterohepatic circulation of folate.[33] Fecal folate losses are difficult to measure due to the contribution of colonic microbial synthesis of folate. However, based on data from a study involving radiolabeled folate,[36] fecal folate excretion was estimated to be similar to that of total urinary excretion of intact folate and cleavage products. Studies using isotopic tracers have yielded conflicting results regarding the actual magnitude of fecal excretion as a route of folate turnover.[30,32]

### *In vivo Kinetics*

Knowledge of in vivo kinetics aids in understanding the requirements of a nutrient and provides an insight into experimental designs involving interventions to alter nutritional status. Such is the case with folate, for which studies have been conducted using stable-isotopic and radioisotopic labeling methods.[37] Most kinetic studies of folate metabolism in humans have shown one or more fast-turnover pools with mean residence times of 0.5 to 2 days, and larger, very slow-turnover pools with mean residence times of 100 to 200 days at intakes of <400 μg/d.[30,36,38,39] Studies of folate kinetics during periods of controlled folate intake of 200, 300, and 400 μg/d have indicated mean residence times for whole-body folate of 212, 169, and 124 days, respectively, in nonpregnant women.[30] These findings indicate that approximately 0.5% to 1% of the whole-body folate pool is catabolized or excreted per day, and thus must be replaced by exogenous folate from the diet or supplements.

Another implication of these findings is that very long periods of nutritional intervention, as seen with supplementation or depletion regimens, are necessary for all body folate pools to attain fully their new steady-state levels. Particular priorities in future work include determining the effects of pregnancy and other conditions of altered physiology, effects of various disease states, and effects of genetic polymorphism of key enzymes of folate metabolism on whole-body folate kinetics.

## Bioavailability

The concept of folate bioavailability is most appropriately used in a broad sense to describe the overall efficiency of utilization, including physiological and biochemical processes involved in intestinal absorption, transport, metabolism, and excretion. Folate from naturally occurring food sources exhibits variable and often incomplete bioavailability. Many dietary variables, physiological conditions, and pharmaceuticals may affect the bioavailability of food folate. These include: 1) entrapment of naturally occurring folates in the cellular structure or insoluble matrix of certain foods; 2) instability of certain labile tetrahydrofolates during passage through the gastric environment; 3) inhibition of the intestinal deconjugation of polyglutamyl folates by certain food constituents; and 4) indirect impairment of folate deconjugation and absorption by alteration of jejunal pH. Because of variation among individuals in folate digestion, absorption, and metabolism, considerable variability in the bioavailability of food folate is a common finding, and substantial conflicts exist within published studies.[40-42] For example, a study reporting that folate in mixed fruits and vegetables is 60% to 90% bioavailable[43] appears to contradict another study reporting that such dietary folate sources did not improve folate status.[44] In addition to variation among individuals, the disparity among these observations also can be attributed to differences in protocols and analytical discrepancies.

Traditional estimates of folate bioavailability in naturally occurring foods have frequently been expressed relative to a folic acid standard consumed under fasting conditions. Folic acid is a frequent reference because of its stability and nearly complete absorption.[45,46] Recent data suggest that (6S)-5-methylTHF or (6S)-5-formylTHF may be preferable because they exhibit kinetics of absorption and distribution more consistent with food folates.[47] It is often assumed that the bioavailability of naturally occurring folate in a mixed diet is approximately 50% based on data provided by a study in humans,[48] in which blood folate response was compared between food folate and folic acid. However, it should be noted that these investigators actually concluded that the bioavailability of food folate was "no more than 50% that of folic acid."[48]

A series of studies conducted by Colman et al.[49] suggested that the bioavailability of folic acid added to South African cereal-based foods was comparable to that reported for naturally occurring food folate. Based on these data, a number of human metabolic studies were conducted in which the bioavailability of folic acid mixed with food exhibited limited bioavailability similar to that which occurs with naturally occurring food folate.[50] Shortly before the implementation of the 1998 cereal-grain enrichment program, contrasting results were obtained using stable-isotopic tracer studies. These findings indicated that folic acid incorporated into bread, pasta, and rice is highly available for absorption in humans.[51] When folic acid was consumed with a light breakfast meal, the absorption was reduced by approximately 15% relative to an equivalent dose of folic acid alone taken while fasting.[51] It was assumed that these data mean that folic acid consumed with food (as is the case with fortified foods) is approximately 85% bioavailable. Thus, the addition of folic acid to enriched foods is an effective means of delivering available folate to the population. This conclusion has been supported by further experimentation with human subjects[44,52] and by examination of population-based data following the implementation of the national enrichment of most cereal-based foods.[53] The very substantial rise in the folate status of the US population[53] can be attributed both to the high bioavailability of added folic acid and to the higher-than-anticipated level of this addition.[54,55]

The bioavailability of folic acid consumed in tablet form appears to be very high, as evidenced by the many studies documenting the efficacy of commercial folic acid preparations. However, an examination in 1997 of selected commercial prenatal multivitamin products in an in vitro dissolution protocol indicated that incomplete dissolution was common.[56] Because in vivo dissolution of a multivitamin supplement is necessary for absorption to occur, these observations indicate the need for further examination of folate bioavailability from nutritional supplements. The extent to which in vitro dissolution tests predict in vivo bioavailability is unclear. More detailed summaries of folate bioavailability and techniques for its assessment have been reported.[17,45,57]

# Biochemical Functions

## *Overview of Biochemical Functions*

Folate-requiring reactions, collectively referred to as 1-C metabolism, include those involved in phases of amino acid metabolism, purine and pyrimidine synthesis, and the formation of the primary methylating agent, S-adenosylmethionine (SAM). Figure 3 illustrates the central role of the folate acceptor molecule, a polyglutamyl form of THF, in the folate-dependent pathways with an emphasis on nucleotide synthesis and methylation reactions. THF is converted to 5,10-methyleneTHF in conjunction with the interconversion of serine and glycine by serine hydroxymethyltransferase (SHMT) (EC 2.1.2.1) (Figure 3, reaction 3). Pyrimidine synthesis is dependent on the availability of 5,10-methyleneTHF, a coenzyme required to donate the 1-C group in the production of thymidylate (dTMP) from deoxyuridylate (dUMP) by thymidylate synthase (EC 2.1.1.45) (Figure 3, reaction 1). This is the rate-limiting step during the cell cycle that enables DNA replication to proceed. The transfer includes the methylene group and one hydrogen from the coenzyme. The oxidized folate product is DHF, which is subsequently reduced to THF by dihydrofolate reductase (EC 1.5.1.3) (Figure 3, reaction 2).

An additional function of folate in nucleotide production involves the de novo synthesis of adenine and guanine, which requires 10-formylTHF, an enzyme produced from 5,10-methyleneTHF in reactions catalyzed by C1-THF synthetase (EC 6.3.4.3) (Figure 3, reaction 4) and from the coupling of formate to THF catalyzed by 10-formylTHF synthetase (Figure 4, reaction C3). 10-FormylTHF is used in two steps of purine synthesis that add 1-C units at positions C8 and C2 during synthesis of the purine ring (Figure 3, reactions 12 and 13). These reactions also regenerate folate to the THF form. 5, 10-methyleneTHF is a compound that can have several fates, one of which is reduction to 5-methylTHF in a reaction catalyzed by methylenetetrahydrofolate reductase (MTHFR) (EC 1.7.99.5) (Figure 3, reaction 5).

The production of 5-methylTHF by MTHFR is an important functional and regulatory component of the folate-dependent pathway for the production of methionine from homocysteine (Figure 3, reaction 6). The remethylation process in folate-dependent remethylation is catalyzed by MTR (EC 2.1.1.13), and requires cobalamin and 5-methylTHF. Homocysteine remethylation to produce methionine is the only known reaction involving 5-methylTHF. In the MTR reaction, a methyl group is sequentially transferred from 5-methylTHF to the cobalamin coenzyme and then to homocysteine, thus forming methionine and releasing THF, which is available for further participation in 1-C metabolism. The dependence of MTR on both folate and cobalamin provides a biochemical explanation of why a single deficiency of either vitamin leads to the same megaloblastic changes in the bone marrow and other tissues with rapidly dividing cells.

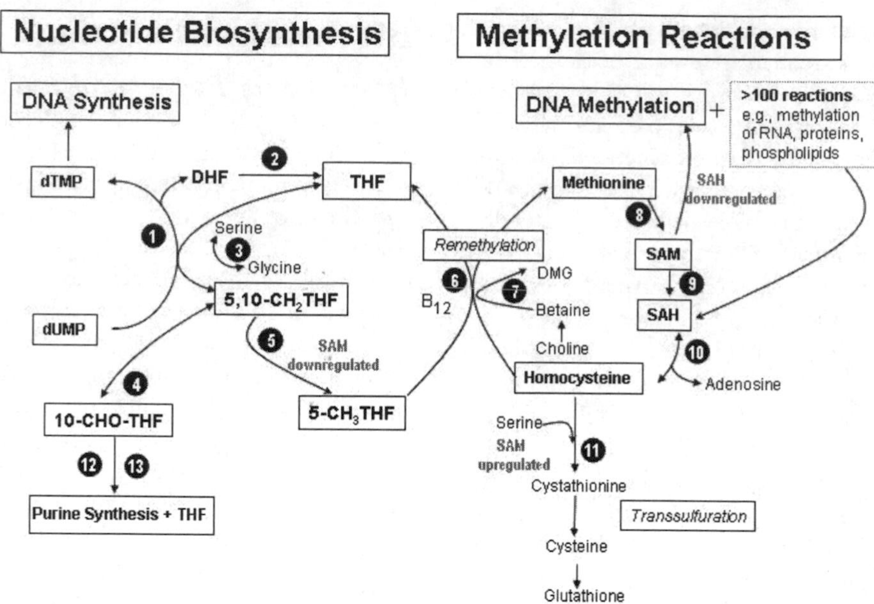


Figure 3. Major metabolic reactions and interconversions of folates (polyglutamates). DHF = dihydrofolate; DMG = dimethylglycine; SAM = S-adenosylmethionine; SAH = S-adenosylhomocysteine; THF = tetrahydrofolate. The enzymes and reactions are noted in Table 1.

**Table 1.** Major Metabolic Reactions for Folate (as shown in Figure 2)

| Reaction | Enzyme | EC Number |
|---|---|---|
| 1 | Thymidylate synthase | 2.1.1.45 |
| 2 | Dihydrofolate reductase | 1.5.1.3 |
| 3 | Serine hydroxymethyltransferase | 2.1.2.1 |
| 4 | 10-FormylTHF synthetase (trifunctional C1-THF enzyme) | 6.3.4.3 |
| 5 | 5,10-MethyleneTHF reductase | 1.1.99.5 |
| 6 | Methionine synthase | 2.1.1.3 |
| 7 | Betaine: homocysteine methyltransferase | 2.1.1.5 |
| 8 | S-adenosylmethionine synthase | 2.5.1.6 |
| 9 | Cellular methyltransferases | Various |
| 10 | S-adenosylhomocysteine hydrolase | 3.3.1.1 |
| 11 | Cystathionine β-synthase | 4.2.1.22 |
| 12 | Glycinamide ribonucleotide transformylase | 2.1.2.2 |
| 13 | Phosphoribosylamino-imidazole carboxamide transformylase | 2.1.2.3 |

In a cobalamin deficiency, folate is "trapped" in the 5-methylTHF form and THF is not regenerated for the formation of 5,10-methyleneTHF, which is required for dTMP and thus DNA synthesis.

Methionine, either from dietary protein or produced from homocysteine, can serve as a methyl group donor through conversion to SAM (Figure 3, reaction 8). Folate and SAM therefore are considered the primary 1-C carriers in biosynthetic pathways. SAM is the methyl donor in over 100 transmethylation reactions, including methylation of DNA, RNA, and membrane phospholipids. In these reactions, SAM donates the labile methyl group it accepted from folate. As a result of methyl group transfer, SAM is converted to S-adenosylhomocysteine (SAH) by a variety of methyltransferases present in all cells (Figure 3, reaction 9). SAH is hydrolyzed to homocysteine and adenosine by SAH hydrolase (EC 3.3.1.1) (Figure 3, reaction 10) via a reversible reaction in which the equilibrium actually favors SAH synthesis.[58] The utilization of adenosine by adenosine kinase and the remethylation of homocysteine provide the kinetic impetus that pulls this reaction in the direction of SAH hydrolysis.

Alternatively, homocysteine can be catabolized via the transsulfuration pathway leading ultimately to cysteine synthesis. Cystathionine β-synthase (CBS) (EC 4.2.1.22) (Figure 3, reaction 11) catalyzes the committing step in transsulfuration in which homocysteine and serine are coupled to form cystathionine in a pyridoxal phosphate-dependent reaction activated by SAM. The net result of CBS activation by SAM is the enhanced entry of homocysteine into the transsulfuration pathway under conditions of surplus methionine.

## *Subcellular Compartmentalization*

Research over the past decade has expanded our understanding of the compartmentalization of 1-C metabolism between cytosol and mitochondria and the specific roles of the folate-dependent enzymes in each of these subcellular compartments.[2]

## *Cytosolic Folate Metabolism*

Cytosolic folate metabolism involves a series of interconnected pathways (Figure 4). In each of these pathways, a specific form of the folate coenzyme donates a 1-C unit to the reaction, resulting in regeneration of THF, which is then free to accept other 1-C units from the folate pool and thus continue the cycle. Interconversion of 10-formylTHF, 5,10-methenylTHF, and 5,10-methyleneTHF is accomplished by the bifunctional cytosolic C1-THF synthase, which catalyzes the reversible oxidation/reduction and cyclohydrolase reactions in the cytosol (EC 1.5.1.5; EC 3.5.4.9) (Figure 4, reactions C1, C2, C3; M1, M2, M3). The sources of the various 1-C units donated to the folate pool include serine from the cytosolic SHMT (EC 2.1.2.1) reaction, which converts THF to 5,10-methyleneTHF (Figure 3, reaction 3 and Figure 4, reaction C5). Additional 1-C units are provided by formate entering from both mitochondrial and cytosolic sources as 10-formylTHF (Figure 4, reactions M5 and C5). Another source is the C-2 carbon of histidine, which enters the cytosolic pool via formiminoglutamic acid in the production of 5,10-methenylTHF.

An often unrecognized aspect of 1-C metabolism is the role of folates as regulatory molecules. Polyglutamyl forms of both 5-formylTHF and 5-methylTHF act as inhibitors of SHMT (Figure 4, reaction C5), whereas 5-methylTHF pentaglutamate is an inhibitor of glycine N-methyltransferase (Figure 4, reaction C4). In this manner, the generation of methyl groups for homocysteine remethylation tends to be maintained even during periods of reduced folate status, and the generation of new 1-C units is down-regulated during periods of their abundance.

## *Mitochondrial Folate Metabolism*

The interconversion of serine and glycine occurs both in cytosol and mitochondria (Figure 4, reactions C5 and M5). The mitochondrial form of SHMT (mSHMT) (EC 2.1.2.1) is a distinct protein from the cytosolic form.[59,60] The glycine cleavage system (Figure 4, reaction M13) is only found in the mitochondria and is not present in all tissues. The glycine cleavage system consists of four mitochondrial proteins whose activity results in pyridoxal phosphate-dependent catabolism of glycine to produce 5,10-methyleneTHF.

The final steps of choline catabolism occur in the mitochondria and are dependent on folate. The catabolism of choline begins in the liver, where it is converted to betaine. Betaine can be used in a pathway that parallels folate-dependent remethylation for the conversion of homocysteine to methionine via betaine-homocysteine methyltransferase (EC 2.1.1.5) (Figure 3, reaction 7). In

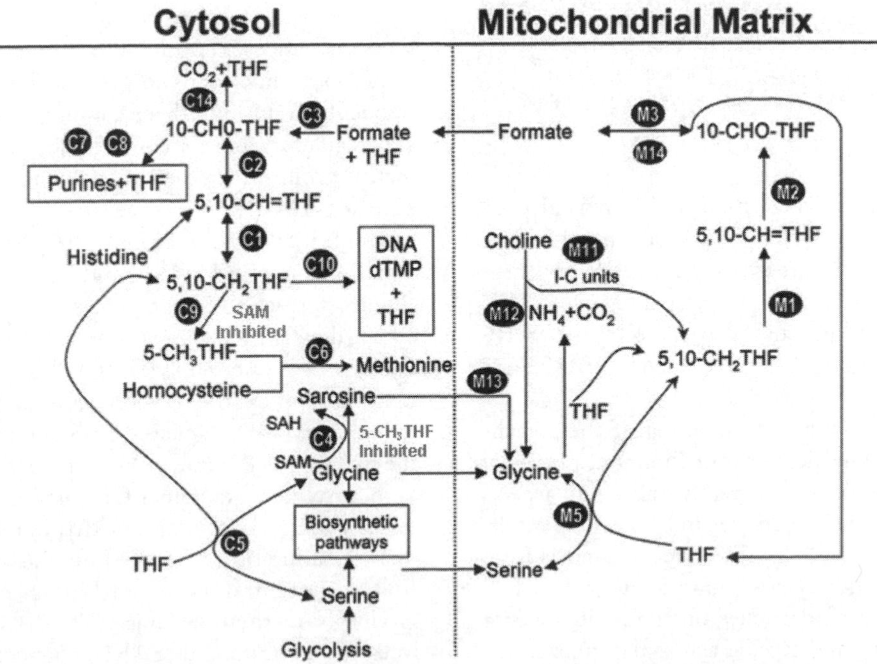


Figure 4. Unidirectional flow of 1-C units from serine, glycine, and choline through the mitochondrial folate pool to formate, which is transferred to the cytosol for conversion to 10-formylTHF. The dashed vertical line represents transport between the cytosol and the mitochondria. Cytosolic 10-formylTHF provides the pool of 1-C units that may be used directly for purine synthesis, reduced to 5,10-methyleneTHF for dTMP synthesis, or further reduced to 5-methylTHF for methionine synthesis. Each reaction shows the product plus tetrahydrofolic acid (THF), which is recycled to accept another formate from the mitochondria. The enzymes and reactions in this diagram are described in Table 2.

**Table 2.** Compartmentalization of Enzymes and Reactions (as shown in Figure 3)

| Reaction* | Enzyme | EC Number |
|---|---|---|
| C1:*M1* | 5,10-MethyleneTHF dehydrogenase | 1.5.1.5 |
| C2:*M2* | 5,10-MethenylTHF cyclohydrolase | 3.5.4.9 |
| C3:*M3* | 10-FormylTHF synthetase | 6.3.4.3 |
| C4 | Glycine N-methyltransferase | 2.1.1.20 |
| C5:*M5* | Serine hydroxymethyltransferase | 2.1.2.1 |
| C6 | Methionine synthase | 2.1.1.3 |
| C7 | Glycinamide ribonucleotide transformylase | 2.1.2.2 |
| C8 | Phosphoribosylamino-imidazole carboxamide transformylase | 2.1.2.3 |
| C9 | 5,10-MethyleneTHF reductase | 1.1.99.5 |
| C10 | Thymidylate synthase | 2.1.1.45 |
| M11 | Dimethylglycine dehydrogenase | 1.5.99.2 |
| M12 | Sarcosine dehydrogenase | 1.5.99.1 |
| M13 | Glycine cleavage system | 2.1.2.10 |
| C14:*M14* | 10-FormylTHF dehydrogenase | 1.5.1.6 |

* The letters C and M refer to the cytosolic and mitochondrial isozymes, respectively. Enzymes 1, 2, and 3 represent the three activities associated with the trifunctional C1-THF synthase. Italicized numbers refer to mitochondrial enzyme activities that have been identified but are yet to be purified and fully characterized.

the process, betaine is converted to dimethylglycine, which can then undergo two sequential mitochondrial oxidations catalyzed by dimethylglycine dehydrogenase (EC 1.5.99.2) and sarcosine dehydrogenase (EC 1.5.99.1) to form glycine and two molecules of 5,10-methyleneTHF (Figure 4, reactions M11, M12, and M13).

During the 1990s, our understanding of the coordinated roles of the cytosolic and mitochondrial phases of 1-C metabolism was expanded greatly,[2] although aspects still remain unclear. The current generally accepted model separates the synthesis of 1-C units in mitochondria from the biosynthetic reactions that require folate-linked 1-C units in cytosol. The model relies on the rapid transfer of 1-C units as serine and glycine across the inner mitochondrial membrane, and the unidirectional transfer of formate out of mitochondria and into the cytosol. In Cook's model,[2] serine provides the majority of the 1-C groups from which 5,10-methyleneTHF is formed through the action of mSHMT (Figure 4, reaction M5), with additional contributions from the choline catabolic pathway (Figure 4, reaction M11 and M12) and the glycine cleavage system (Figure 4, reaction M13). This mitochondrial 5,10-methyleneTHF is converted to 10-formylTHF by 10-formylTHF dehydrogenase (Figure 4, reaction M14), then to formate and THF by 10-formylTHF synthetase[61] (Figure 4, reaction M3). The formate is then delivered to the cytosol, where it is converted to 10-formylTHF for purine synthesis (Figure 4, reaction C3) or is reduced to 5,10-methyleneTHF for homocysteine remethylation (via 5-methylTHF) or dTMP synthesis (Figure 4, reaction C2). The 1-C unit in the form of 10-formylTHF may also be oxidized to $CO_2$, which removes excess 1-C groups (Figure 4, reaction C14). A more in-depth description of the enzymatic conversions involved in the sub-cellular compartmentalization of folate-dependent reactions has been published previously.[2]

## *Regulation of 1-C Metabolism*

The metabolism of serine, glycine, and methionine is integrally related to the regulation of 1-C metabolism (Figure 3). Serine provides the majority of the glycine requirement via the action of SHMT in a reaction in which the 1-C unit in the form of 5,10-methyleneTHF is then available for methionine, dTMP, or purine synthesis or may be oxidized to $CO_2$ via 10-formylTHF. The glycine cleavage system (Figure 4) cleaves glycine to produce $CO_2$, $NH_4^+$, and 5,10-methyleneTHF, which can be employed directly or oxidized to 10-formylTHF to recover 1-C units via glycine catabolism.

## *SAM Regulation*

Serine is believed to be the major source of 1-C units used in homocysteine remethylation.[62,63] The recycling of homocysteine tends to preserve methionine, which is frequently a limiting dietary amino acid (Figure 3). Several regulatory points control the synthesis of de novo methyl groups from the 1-C pool and the use of methionine as SAM.[64] In response to a surplus of SAM caused by ample intake of methionine, SAM binds to the regulatory domain of MTHFR and inhibits enzyme activity (Figure 3, reaction 5). Therefore, under conditions of adequate dietary methionine supply, SAM controls the production of 5-methylTHF by MTHFR, and therefore tends to suppress the recycling of homocysteine to methionine. SAM also regulates CBS (Figure 3, reaction 11), the first step in the transsulfuration pathway that converts homocysteine to cysteine. CBS is activated by SAM, so under conditions of ample SAM, homocysteine disposal by transsulfuration is favored over its remethylation.

The concentration of SAM in the liver is regulated by glycine N-methyltransferase (EC 2.1.1.20), which catalyzes the nonessential, SAM-dependent methylation of glycine to sarcosine and the consequent production of SAH (Figure 4 reaction C4).[65] Sarcosine is converted back to glycine by 5,10 methyleneTHF via sarcosine dehydrogenase (EC 1.5.99.1) (Figure 4, reaction M12) following transport into the mitochondria. These two reactions regulate the cytosolic SAM concentration while conserving the methyl group as a folate-linked 1-C unit. The end result is that SAM and SAH levels are maintained in a relatively constant ratio. The ratio of SAM to SAH is important because the rate of most methyltransferase reactions depends on the concentration of its substrate (SAM) as well as that of SAH, a product inhibitor; consequently, methyltransferase activities are regulated by the SAM/SAH ratio.

In the manner described above, reciprocal regulation of 1-C and methyl group metabolism is mediated largely by SAM and 5-methylTHF. When dietary methionine is low, less SAM is produced from dietary sources and this attenuates the inhibition of the MTHFR reaction, enabling an increase in production of 5-methylTHF required for remethylation of homocysteine. The production of 5-methylTHF promotes remethylation of homocysteine to generate a supply of methionine. 5-methylTHF inhibits glycine N-methyltransferase by binding tightly to the enzyme, with resulting inhibition of glycine methylation, which serves as another mechanism of methionine conservation.

### *SAH Regulation*

James et al.[58,66] have proposed that the regulatory importance of SAH in the maintenance of balanced 1-C metabolism may be underestimated. Cytosolic SAH concentrations have been shown to have tissue-specific regulatory functions and have been reported to up-regulate CBS activity, decrease betaine-homocysteine methyltransferase activity, and decrease MTHFR activity.[58]

The conversion of SAM to SAH is a one-way process subject to competitive inhibition by SAH, which has higher affinity for the active site of cellular methyltransferases.[58] The accumulation of SAH can lead to a decrease in the SAM/SAH ratio and inhibition of most cellular methyltransferases.[58] The accumulation of SAH and the associated inhibition of cellular methyltransferases will therefore occur under metabolic conditions that interfere with product removal of homocysteine or adenosine.[58]

## Genetic Polymorphisms

Normal folate metabolism is dependent on genes encoding the approximately 150 proteins directly or indirectly involved in folate metabolism and transport.[67] An alteration or mutation in the DNA sequence of any of these genes can yield a protein variant that can be either deleterious or benign. When a mutation is present in a population at a frequency of 1.0% or more of alleles, it is referred to as a polymorphism.[68] An increasingly large number of single-nucleotide polymorphisms have been linked to folate-related biochemical changes and, in some cases, clinical abnormalities, as discussed below.[67-69]

The most extensively studied of the folate-related polymorphisms is a C→T substitution at base pair 677 in the gene encoding the enzyme MTHFR, which catalyzes the reduction of 5,10-methyleneTHF to 5-methylTHF, the methyl donor for homocysteine remethylation to methionine.[68] Individuals who are homozygous for the 677C→T variant (i.e., the TT genotype) exhibit lower specific activity of MTHFR and reduced stability of the enzyme in vitro.[68] The MTHFR 677C →T polymorphism is prevalent in the overall population: approximately 12% are homozygous (TT genotype) and approximately 50% are heterozygous (CT genotype).[70]

The MTHFR 677C→T polymorphism has been associated with significantly increased plasma homocysteine concentrations, increased neural tube defect (NTD) risk, and chronic disease risk, especially when folate status is low.[68] The combined influence of the MTHFR polymorphism and inadequate dietary folate intake on folate status and homocysteine response was evaluated in women consuming low-folate diets (115–135 μg dietary folate equivalents [DFE]/d) followed by repletion with either 400 μg DFE/d[71,72] or 800 μg DFE/d.[72] Throughout folate depletion, women with the TT genotype had significantly lower serum folate and red blood cell folate concentrations than those with the CC genotype.[71,72] Folate status was low (serum folate <13.6 nmol/L) in more women with the TT (59%) compared with the CC genotype (15%) following consumption of the low-folate diet.[71] The influence of the MTHFR 677C→T polymorphism was also evident by differences in homocysteine response to folate depletion[71] and repletion with 400 μg DFE/d.[71,72] When repleted with a higher folate intake, 800 μg DFE/d, Guinotte et al.[72] found no differences in folate status between the TT and CC genotype groups, illustrating how dietary folate intake can significantly modify the metabolic response to the MTHFR 677C→T polymorphism.

The potential for the MTHFR 677C→T polymorphism to reduce global DNA methylation when coupled with poor folate status has been evaluated in population-based studies[73,74] and in one controlled feeding study conducted in the United States.[75] In an Italian population, significantly less DNA methylation was observed in subjects with the TT genotype compared with those with the CC genotype.[74] In contrast, differences in DNA methylation were not observed at baseline between genotypes in the US study,[75] which may be explained by the much higher folate status in the US study compared with the Italian study (serum folate concentration approximately 47.2 vs 11.6 nmol/L, respectively). In response to repletion with the Recommended Dietary Allowance (RDA) for folate (400 μg DFE/d) for 7 weeks following folate depletion (115 μg DFE/d), a significant increase in DNA methylation was observed in subjects with the TT genotype but not the CC genotype, which suggests a genotype difference in DNA methylation response to folate repletion.

The methionine synthase reductase (MTRR) enzyme is required for maintaining MTR in an active state by facilitating the reductive methylation of cobalamin.[76] Wilson et al.[77] identified a common variant of MTRR (66A→G) with a reported population frequency of about 30%. The coexistence of the MTRR 66A→G and MTHFR 677C→T polymorphisms has been reported to exacerbate the negative effect of the MTHFR variant on plasma homocysteine concentration.[76]

A polymorphism (1561C→T) in the glutamate carboxypeptidase II gene that encodes for the folylpoly-γ-glutamyl carboxypeptidase enzyme responsible for the deconjugation of polyglutamate folate in the small intestinal brush border was first reported by Devlin et al.[78] The presence of the T allele was not found to be associated with lower bioavailability of polyglutamyl folate[79] but, interestingly, has been reported to be associated with higher folate status.[79-81]

# Clinical Deficiency, Birth Defects, Chronic Disease

## *Severe Clinical Deficiency*

Clinically, chronic severe folate deficiency is associated with megaloblastic anemia characterized by large, abnormally nucleated erythrocytes that accumulate in the bone marrow.[82] There are also decreased numbers of white cells and platelets as a result of general impairment of cell division related to folate's role in nucleic acid synthesis.[82] Since the intestinal mucosa undergoes continuous regeneration, with replacement of epithelial cells every 3 days, its folate requirements are greater than other tissues.[82] Gastrointestinal symptoms frequently result from severe folate deficiency and are often associated with impaired absorption.[82]

Pregnant women are at increased risk of developing a folate deficiency due to the increased demands placed on the supply of folate for the synthesis of DNA and other 1-C transfer reactions.[83] In addition to megaloblastic anemia, inadequate folate intake and low serum folate concentrations have been associated with poor pregnancy outcomes, as reviewed previously.[83] There is evidence associating impaired folate status with increased risk of preterm delivery, low infant birth weight, and fetal growth retardation.[83] An elevation of maternal homocysteine concentrations has been associated both with increased habitual spontaneous abortion and pregnancy complications (e.g., abruptio placentae or placental infarction with fetal growth retardation and preeclampsia), which increase the risk of low birth weight and preterm delivery.[84,85] Folate deficiency and hyperhomocysteinemia, as well as the MTHFR 677C→T polymorphism, appear to be at least modest risk factors for placenta vascular disease, warranting continued investigation.[86]

## *Neural Tube Defects*

Embryological malformations of the central nervous system, commonly referred to as NTDs, result from a failure of fusion of neural folds in the developing embryo.[87] Folic acid taken periconceptionally significantly reduces the risk of NTDs, a conclusion based on definitive evidence from randomized, controlled intervention trials supported by observational studies.[87,88] The pathogenesis of NTDs is likely to be multifactorial, involving both genetic defects and environmental factors that may impair normal folate metabolic functions. Proposed mechanisms by which abnormalities in folate metabolism may increase the risk of NTD-affected pregnancies include elevations in homocysteine, decreased rates of DNA synthesis due to impaired dTMP synthesis, and elevations in the SAH/SAM ratio.[89] Evidence from human studies supporting the existing hypotheses indicates that impaired homocysteine remethylation or other affected SAM-dependent methylation reactions can impair embryonic development.[90] An increased risk for NTDs has been associated with moderate elevations in maternal homocysteine concentration.[67,68] Other proposed mechanisms by which elevations in homocysteine may increase NTD risk include the observation that elevated homocysteine may induce abnormal development of neural tube cells by acting as an antagonist of the N-methyl-D-aspartate glutamate receptor involved in neuronal development and migration.[91]

When the homocysteine concentration is elevated, the resulting increased SAH/SAM ratio can lead to abnormalities in DNA methylation that may affect expression of genes involved in neural tube formation.[92] Finally, impaired synthesis of dTMP has also been proposed to affect cell migration/proliferation during the period of rapid cell division associated with neural tube closure.[93] In addition to the proposed associations between NTD risk and folate-related metabolic abnormalities, data suggest that absorption of folate present as naturally occurring food folate and as folic acid in fortified foods or supplements may be somewhat impaired in women at risk of NTD-affected pregnancies.[94] A recent report found that serum from women with a pregnancy complicated by a NTD contains autoantibodies that bind to folate receptors and may block the cellular uptake of folate.[95] This finding warrants further study.

The fact that up to 70% of NTDs are considered "folic acid preventable"[89] has focused the search for NTD-genetic risk factors to major groups of genes that encode for folate-related enzymes, receptors, and binding proteins.[96] The association between specific polymorphisms in folate-related candidate genes and NTD risk has been evaluated in population-based studies for a series of genes including MTHFR, folate receptor alpha (FRα), reduced folate carrier (RFC), CBS, MTR, MTRR, methylenetetrahydrofolate dehydrogenase (MTHFD), and SHMT, to name just a few.[67] To date, very few polymorphisms appear to serve as significant NTD risk factors,[67,96,97] and the magnitude of the risk has been reported to be inversely associated with folate status.[97-99] The MTHFR 677C→T polymorphism is the first genetic risk factor reported to increase risk for NTD,[68] a conclusion supported by a large number of investigations,[70,100,101] although not all studies have found an association with NTDs.[67] A polymorphism affecting the trifunctional enzyme MTHFD1 was associated with an increased risk factor for NTDs in one study.[102] The MTHFD1 enzyme is critical for catalyzing the entry of mitochondrially derived formate into the cytoplasmic folate 1-C pool by catalyzing the conversion of tetrahydrofolate to 10-formylTHF (Figure 4).

Although many studies have focused on folate metabolic enzymes and NTD risk, studies with mouse models have highlighted the importance of folate-binding proteins and receptors on normal embryonic development.[103,104] The human folate receptor alpha (hFR-α) is a membrane-bound protein with high affinity for 5-methylTHF that is localized in high concentrations in the placenta and the developing neural tube.[67] Support for the folate receptor gene's involvement in risk for NTDs comes from studies with mouse models in which the homolog for hFR-α, folate binding protein-1, was inactivated, and the nullizygous mice exhibited NTDs and other folate-dependent congenital defects.[67,103,105] Mouse model studies in which embryo rescue from the lethal effects of homozygous deletion of the genes coding for hFR-α or RFC1 can be achieved with maternal folic acid rescue treatments conclusively demonstrate that fetal folate deficiency results in developmental anomalies including NTDs.[90,104]

The question of whether the dose of folic acid most frequently included in multivitamin supplements (400 μg) would significantly impact the occurrence of NTDs when given alone has been addressed in the largest intervention trial to date.[106] This very large-scale intervention trial was conducted in two regions of China, and included approximately 250,000 women followed prospectively beginning prior to the periconceptional period. When a daily supplement containing folic acid alone (400 μg) was taken more than 80% of the time, the reduction in risk was 85% in the northern region (high baseline frequency) and 40% in the southern region (low baseline frequency). The lower baseline frequency in the southern region was suggested to be associated with a higher dietary folate intake.[106]

Public health NTD policies include the 1992 US Public Health Service[107] and the 1998 Institute of Medicine (IOM) recommendation.[108] The IOM recommendation is not the same as the RDA, a common misconception, since the recommendation specifies that the supplemental form of the vitamin, folic acid (400 μg/d), be taken (or consumed as a fortified food) in addition to folate in a varied diet. In addition to the NTD-public health recommendations, the FDA mandated regulations requiring food manufacturers to fortify enriched products with folic acid.[4] Estimates of the effect of folic acid fortification on NTD prevalence are based on reports from the US, Canada, and Chile,[109-113] which indicate that fortification was associated with a significant reduction in NTDs, although the estimated reductions are quite variable (19%–50%) depending on the type of data evaluated.

## Congenital Heart Defects

One in 110 infants is born with heart defects, which account for more deaths than NTDs or any other congenital anomaly.[114-116] As previously reviewed,[117] the strongest evidence associating periconceptional folic acid use with a reduction in risk for congenital heart defects comes from a Hungarian randomized, controlled trial[118] and two population-based case-control studies in the United States.[119,120] These data provide evidence that multivitamins containing folic acid taken periconceptionally significantly reduce the risk of congenital heart defects.[118-120] In the Hungarian randomized, controlled intervention trial, the effectiveness of prenatal multivitamins containing 800 μg of folic acid to reduce the risk of NTDs was evaluated.[118] Further analysis of these and other data from Hungary[121,122] indicated that prenatal multivitamins were associated with an overall 50% reduction in risk for a broad range of heart defects. In the United States, a 24% reduction in the odds for congenital heart defects was associated with periconceptional use of multivitamins containing folic acid. This supports the conclusion from the Hungarian study that periconceptional use of multivitamins significantly reduces the occurrence of congenital heart defects.[119]

Data suggest that the specific types of heart defects primarily affected by folic acid-containing multivitamins are ventricular septal defects and some conotruncal defects (tetralogy of Fallot and D-transposition of the great arteries).[123] In both the Hungarian randomized, controlled intervention trial[118] and a US population-based case-control study,[119] the occurrence of conotruncal defects was reduced by about 50%. The conclusion that periconceptional multivitamins are associated with a reduction in the occurrence of conotruncal defects is also supported by data from a second population-based case-control study in the United States.[120] Other studies in the United States[124,125] did not detect a protective effect of periconceptional multivitamin use and heart defects; however, the majority of evidence supports the conclusion that periconceptional use of multivitamins containing folic acid is associated with a reduction in risk for congenital heart defects.

## Vascular Disease

A large body of epidemiological evidence indicates that elevated plasma homocysteine concentration is a significant risk factor for vascular disease. The conclusion from two recent meta-analyses[126,127] was that a 25% reduction in plasma homocysteine concentration is associated with an approximate 15% decrease in risk for ischemic heart disease (Figure 5)[126] and a 20% decrease in risk for stroke.[126,127]

Folic acid supplementation lowers blood homocyste-

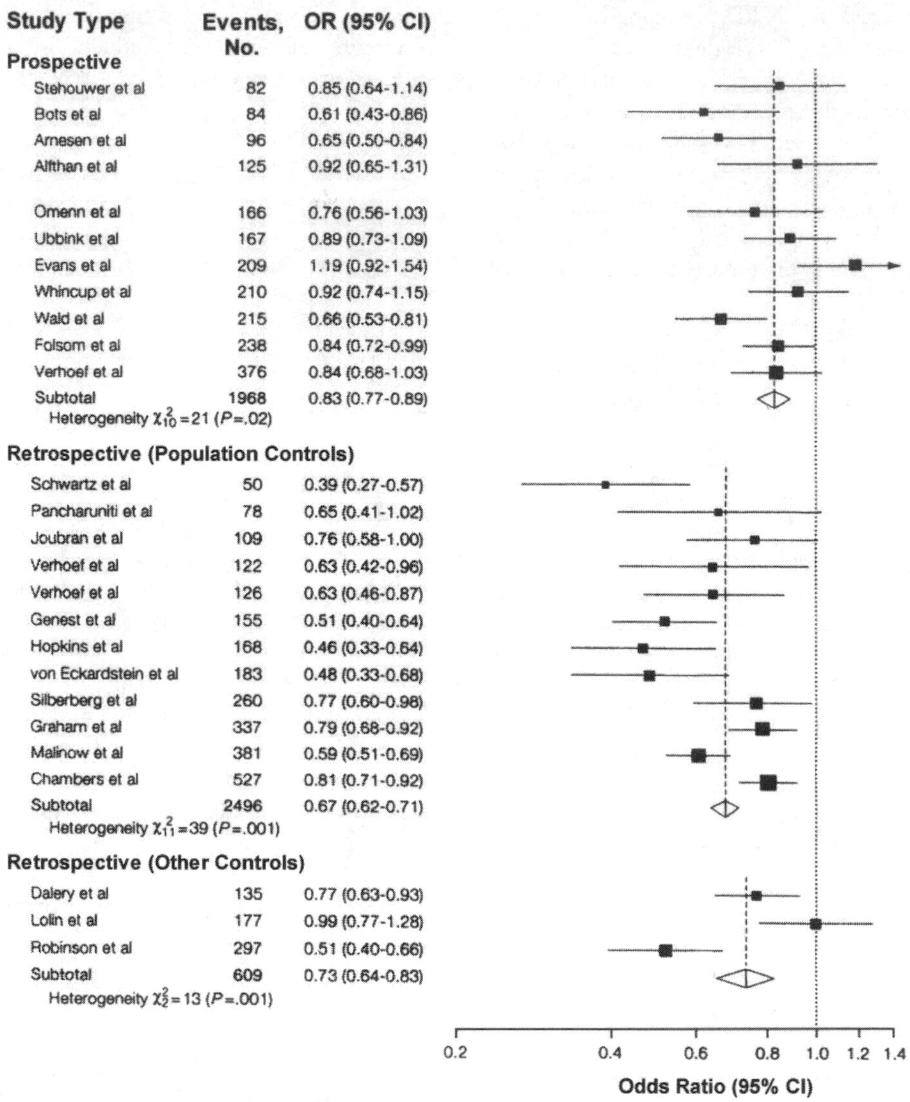


Figure 5. Odds ratios of ischemic heart disease for a 25% lower homocysteine level in individual studies cited in the referenced publication. Data were adjusted for study, sex, and age at enrollment and were corrected for regression dilution. The size of the square is inversely proportional to the variance of the log odds ratio (OR). The horizontal lines represent the 95% confidence intervals (CIs). The combined ORs in the subtotals for each study design and their 95% CI are indicated by diamonds. (Used with permission from JAMA 2002.[127] Copyright 2002 American Medical Association.)

ine concentration, with the greatest response observed in individuals with the highest pretreatment homocysteine concentration and the lowest pretreatment folate concentrations. Daily doses of at least 800 μg folic acid have been associated with a maximal reduction (23%) in plasma homocysteine concentrations, and doses of 200 and 400 μg folic acid were associated with 13% and 20% reductions, respectively, in studies in which the pretreatment homocysteine concentration was standardized to 12 μmol/L.[128]

In individuals with lower baseline homocysteine concentrations (comparable to that observed in countries with mandatory folic acid fortification), the maximum homocysteine lowering response to folic acid supplementation would be expected to be considerably less than that in individuals with higher baseline concentrations, such as those currently observed in European countries.[129] The potential for fortification to reduce plasma homocysteine concentrations of population groups consuming folic acid-fortified foods is of considerable interest because of its link to vascular disease risk.[130] Jacques et al.[53] reported that the prevalence of elevated homocysteine concentrations was reduced by about 50% in the Framingham population post-fortification compared with pre-fortification. A recent report of plasma homocysteine concentrations from a nationally representative sample in the United States (NHANES 1999–2000) indicates that approximately 80% of the entire US population currently have homocysteine concentrations ≤9 μmol/L and 5% (approximately 14% in the elderly) have elevated (≥13 μmol/L) concentrations.[10]

A major unresolved issue is whether supplemental folic acid will reduce the incidence of vascular disease, and this is the focus of ongoing randomized, controlled intervention trials in the United States, Canada, Europe, and Australia.[131] Since folic acid fortification has been shown to decrease baseline plasma homocysteine concentration significantly, trials conducted in the United States and Canada would not be expected to achieve the same reduction in homocysteine that would occur in populations not exposed to fortification. The loss of statistical power necessary to detect a significant effect of folic acid vitamin supplementation on vascular disease outcome is illustrated by the inconclusive results from the recent Vitamin Intervention for Stroke Prevention trial,[132] in which the reduction in homocysteine concentration was much smaller than predicted when the study was designed due to concomitant folic acid fortification of the food supply.

Ongoing randomized trials in countries that do not have mandatory folic acid fortification are likely to show a sustained homocysteine-lowering effect of folic acid that would increase the probability of detecting vascular benefits.[133] Among other factors that will interfere with the interpretation of the effect of folic acid on vascular disease risk in ongoing trials is the fact that, with few exceptions, the folic acid treatment is in combination with other nutrients (e.g., vitamins $B_6$ and $B_{12}$) that may also significantly affect homocysteine concentration. In addition, the multifactorial nature of vascular disease may further confound the results of these secondary intervention trials.

The 677C→T polymorphism in the MTHFR gene significantly influences vascular disease risk, according to a series of large meta-analyses providing evidence of a significant association between MTHFR genotype and vascular disease.[126,134,125] In the largest meta-analysis to date of studies examining the association between MTHFR and stroke (111 studies), Casas et al.[135] found that individuals with the TT genotype for the MTHFR 677C→T polymorphism who are homozygous (TT) for the MTHFR polymorphism have a significantly greater risk of stroke than individuals with the CC genotype. A key finding in this meta-analysis was that the magnitude of the increased risk associated with the TT genotype was the same as that associated with the higher homocysteine concentrations in TT versus CC genotype groups. In another large meta-analysis conducted by Wald et al.,[126] the risk for ischemic heart disease and deep vein thrombosis was significantly higher in individuals with the TT versus CC genotype for the MTHFR 677C→T polymorphism. Klerk et al.[134] conducted a meta-analysis involving 11,162 coronary heart disease cases and 12,758 controls from 40 studies, and found that individuals with the MTHFR 677 TT genotype had a 16% higher odds of coronary heart disease compared with individuals with the CC genotype.

Observed differences in homocysteine concentration and vascular disease risk associated with the TT genotype for the MTHFR polymorphism were attenuated in studies conducted in North America where folate intake was higher. The odds ratios of coronary heart disease within strata of the MTHFR 677C→T genotype and folate status for a subset of studies for which data on folate status was available are presented in Table 3. These data indicate that the TT genotype for the 677C→T polymorphism was only associated with increased coronary heart disease risk when folate status was low, which illustrates the modulating effect of folate status on vascular disease risk associated with the MTHFR 677C→T polymorphism.

## *Cancer*

Increased cancer risk has been associated with poor folate status in a number of different epidemiological studies, with the strongest support being for colorectal cancer and its precancerous lesion, adenoma.[9,129] For example, in the Nurses' Health Study[136] and the Health Professionals' Follow-Up Study,[137] the risk for colorectal adenoma and cancer was reduced by 30% to 40% in individuals with the highest folate intake (primarily supplement users) compared with those with the lowest folate intake.

The presence of the MTHFR 677C→T polymorphism has been associated with a significant reduction in cancer risk.[138-140] In the Physician's Health Study, for example, the risk for colorectal cancer was three-fold less in individuals homozygous for the MTHFR 677C→T polymorphism (TT genotype) with normal folate status

**Table 3.** Odds Ratios (ORs) of Coronary Heart Disease (CHD) by Strata of the MTHFR 677C→T Polymorphism and Folate Status*

| | MTHFR 677C→T Genotype | | |
|---|---|---|---|
| | **CC** | **CT** | **TT** |
| Cases, No. | 1543 | 1355 | 364 |
| Controls, No. | 2180 | 1847 | 445 |
| Risk of CHD, OR (95% confidence interval) | | | |
| High folate status | 1.00 | 0.91 (0.78–1.06) | 0.99 (0.77–1.29) |
| Low folate status | 1.24 (1.06–1.44) | 1.32 (1.13–1.54) | 1.44 (1.12–1.83) |

* Folate status was defined as below or above the median serum or plasma concentration per continent.
Used with permission from Klerk et al., 2002.[134] 

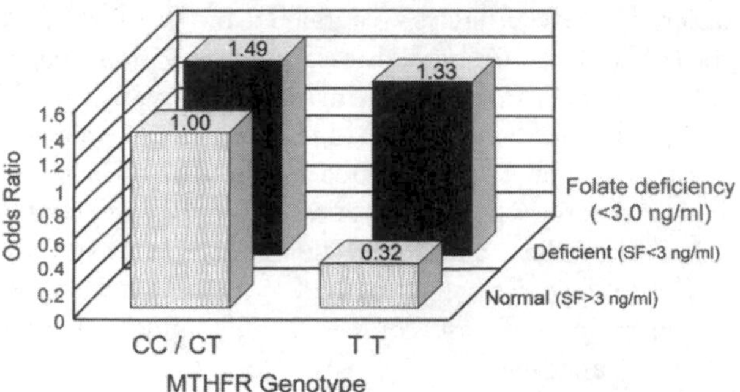


Figure 6. Combined effects of the methylenetetrahydrofolate reductase (MTHFR) TT genotype and folate status on colorectal cancer risk in the Physician's Health Study. Among men with normal folate status, there was a three-fold decrease in risk among individuals with the TT genotype compared with the homozygous CC and heterozygous genotypes combined (CC/CT). The protection associated with the MTHFR TT genotype was lost in men with deficient folate status. (Used with permission from Ma et al., 1997.[138])

than in the group with CC and CT genotypes combined.[138] In contrast, in individuals with deficient folate status, the protection attributed to the MTHFR 677C→T polymorphism was absent (Figure 6). The MTHFR enzyme reduces 5,10 methyleneTHF to 5-methylTHF, which is required for the production of methionine and SAM, the methyl donor for DNA. A reduction in MTHFR activity associated with the 677C→T polymorphism may lead to an increase in 5,10-methyleneTHF, which is required for DNA synthesis.[141] When folate status is low, the presence of the MTHFR 677C→T polymorphism (TT genotype) has been associated with elevations in homocysteine concentration and DNA hypomethylation.[142-145] A plausible explanation for the observed protective effect of the MTHFR 677C→T variant on cancer risk is that when folate status is adequate, the MTHFR 677C→T polymorphism leads to an increased availability of 5,10-methyleneTHF required for normal DNA synthesis and cell division.[146] Evidence of enhanced dTMP synthesis in the TT genotype has been observed.[141]

Chronic consumption of moderate amounts of alcohol (≥15 g/d, or approximately one drink of any kind daily) is a common lifestyle pattern that has been shown to significantly increase the risk for cancer.[147-149] Chronic alcohol exposure has been shown to impair folate absorption by inhibiting expression of the reduced folate carrier and decreasing the hepatic uptake and renal conservation of circulating folate,[150] thus providing a rationale for the observation that higher folate intake may significantly reduce the increased cancer risk associated with alcohol consumption. Evidence from two large epidemiological investigations suggests that the increased breast cancer risk associated with moderate alcohol consumption can be significantly reduced by increased folate intake (Figure 7).[147,148] When folate intake was increased to 600 μg/d or more, the higher breast cancer risk associated with moderate alcohol consumption was reduced by 45% compared with that observed in individuals with the lowest dietary intake who consumed moderate amounts of alcohol.[148] A dietary pattern that couples alcohol consumption with low folate and methionine intake (a "low-methyl diet") has been associated with a significant increase (7-fold) in colon cancer risk compared with a "high-methyl" diet.[149] Data from both the Health Professional Follow-Up Study and the Physician's Health Study indicate that individuals with the TT genotype for the MTHFR 677C→T variant are especially sensitive to the carcinogenic effects of alcohol.[138,151] These and other studies[149] support the conclusion that higher folate in-

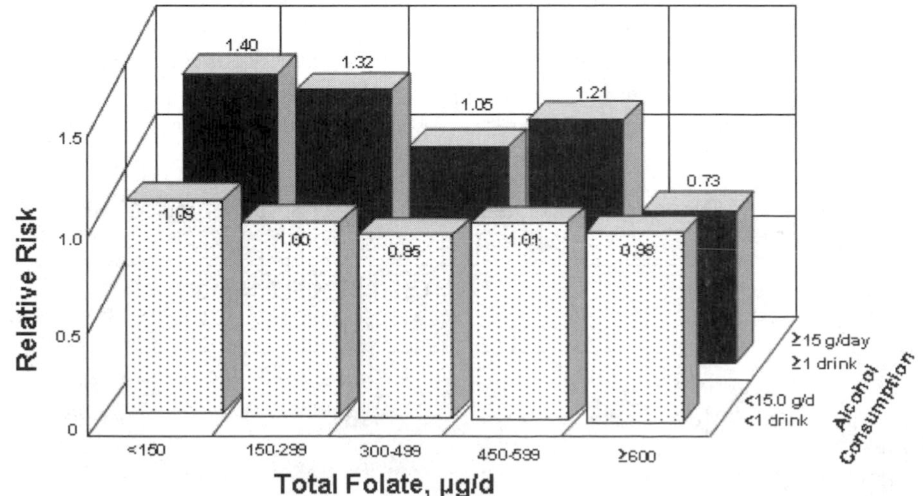


Figure 7. Effect of total folate intake and alcohol on the relative risk of breast cancer in the Nurses' Health Study. The two categories for alcohol consumption were 15 g/d or more, which is the approximate quantity of alcohol in one drink of any kind. In women who consumed 15 g/d or more, the breast cancer risk was significantly elevated, except in the highest folate intake group (≥ 600 μg/d), which included diet plus supplements. Folate intake was not associated with breast cancer risk for women who consumed less than 15 g/d of alcohol. (Used with permission from Zhang et al., 1999.[148] Copyright 1999 American Medical Association.)

takes may be associated with a significant reduction in cancer risk in individuals who consume alcohol on a regular basis.

The mechanisms by which folate inadequacy enhances and supplementation suppresses carcinogenesis have not been elucidated, but potential mechanisms include those that influence DNA stability or methylation.[146] In response to a folate deficiency, the synthesis of dTMP is impaired and the resulting nucleotide imbalance results in uracil misincorporation into DNA, which may lead to strand breaks associated with increased cancer risk. In folate-deficient humans, excessive DNA uracil content, as well as increased numbers of chromosomal breaks, have been observed and both defects were reversed by folate administration.[152] DNA methylation is a mechanism by which gene function is selectively activated or inactivated without changing the DNA sequence. Neoplastic cells simultaneously harbor widespread global hypomethylation involved with maintenance of gene stability and more specific regional areas of hypermethylation, which has been associated with the inactivation of tumor suppressor genes.[153] Changes in genomic methylation in human lymphocytic DNA in response to a low-folate diet have been demonstrated in three studies with healthy human volunteers,[75,153,154] and the observed hypomethylation effect was reversible in one study.[154]

Most of the epidemiological studies conducted in North America, in which an inverse association between folate status and cancer was observed, were conducted prior to fortification, and the risk reduction was associated with higher folate intake due to supplement use.[9] The increase in folate intake from the consumption of "enriched" cereal grain products is estimated to be about 200 μg, which is 50% of that provided by the majority of folic acid-containing multivitamins.[54,55] Whether this increased folate intake due to fortification will have an impact on the incidence of cancer may be difficult to ascertain; however, one study indicates that folic acid fortification is associated with a significant reduction in the incidence of pediatric neuroblastoma.[155]

## *Drug and Alcohol Impairment of Folate Metabolism*

A large number of drugs can affect the absorption and metabolism of folates, and the effects of certain pharmaceutical products can be considerable. Methotrexate (amethopterin) is one example. It has a molecular structure that differs from folic acid only slightly, having an amino group in place of the 4-hydroxyl group on the pteridine ring and a methyl group at the N-10 position. These modifications give methotrexate more affinity for dihydrofolate reductase, the target of the drug, than its natural folate substrate.[156] Other folate antagonists include aminopterin, trimethoprim, trimetrexate, and triamterene. These compounds can block the production of thymidine and inhibit de novo synthesis of purine nucleotides, and have played a key role in cancer treatment for half a century.[156]

Methotrexate also has been used frequently and successfully in the treatment of non-neoplastic diseases such as rheumatoid arthritis, psoriasis, asthma, and inflammatory bowel disease. Patients with rheumatoid arthritis are frequently reported to be folate deficient, and folate stores are decreased in patients with rheumatoid arthritis who take methotrexate.[157] Some of the side effects of methotrexate administration, such as gastrointestinal intolerance, mimic severe folate deficiency.[157] When patients also are given high-folate diets or supplemental folic acid, there is a significant reduction in toxic side effects with no reduction in drug efficacy.[157] A careful balance must be maintained between drug therapy and adjunct folic acid supplementation to ensure both drug efficacy and prevention of a severe folate deficiency. An increased risk of birth defects has been associated with doses of methotrexate as low as 10 mg weekly, and may be associated with the antifolate drug action.[158] The anti-neoplastic drug 5-fluorouracil has been used as a chemotherapeutic agent. Its efficacy is related to the inhibition of the dTMP synthase reaction in which 5-fluorouracil is incorporated into the nucleotide to produce 5-fluorodeoxyuridylate, an analog of dUMP.[156] The analog forms a covalent bond with the dTMP synthase enzyme to inhibit DNA synthesis and promote a subsequent buildup of dUMP/dUTP in the cell.[156] The impaired nucleotide synthesis leads to reduced cell proliferation, which is a treatment goal in neoplastic disease.

There are numerous reports of impaired folate status associated with chronic use of the anticonvulsants diphenylhydantoin or phenytoin (brand name Dilantin®) and phenobarbital. Some reports suggest that these drugs interfere with folate metabolism,[159] but the precise mechanism of the drug-nutrient interaction has not been elucidated. Salicylazosulfapyridine or sulfasalazine (brand name Aztilfidine®) is an anti-inflammatory drug commonly used for the treatment of ulcerative colitis. It is known to inhibit folate absorption and metabolism.[157] The biguanides (such as metformin) are used for glycemic control in diabetes and in certain types of cardiovascular disease, and their chronic use is associated with an increased risk for impaired folate status and hyperhomocystenemia.[160]

Based on a series of studies conducted in humans and in primate and pig models,[150] alcohol consumed chronically in large amounts has been shown to contribute to folate deficiency by interfering with folate absorption, decreasing hepatic folate uptake, and increasing urinary excretion. Chronic alcohol exposure was shown to lead to decreased activity of two proteins that regulate folate absorption, intestinal glucose carboxypeptidase II (GCPII) and RFC.[150] The combination of a folate-deficient diet and chronic alcohol consumption accentuates abnormal hepatic methionine metabolism and accelerates the development of alcoholic liver injury.[150]

## Dietary Reference Intakes

In establishing the 1998 Dietary Reference Intake (DRI) for folate, which replaced the RDA, the IOM shifted the focus of folate intake recommendations from quantities to prevent severe deficiency symptoms to intakes that promote optimum health.[108] The DRI for folate is a set of reference values that include the following: Estimated Average Requirement (EAR), RDA, Adequate Intake (AI), and Tolerable Upper Intake Level (UL) (Table 4).

The IOM considered differences in bioavailability between synthetic folic acid in fortified foods and naturally occurring dietary folate when expressing the DRIs as DFEs.[108] The conversion of dietary folate intake to DFEs is a method to convert all forms of dietary folate, including folic acid in fortified food, to an amount that is equivalent to naturally occurring food folate. DFEs are defined as the micrograms of naturally occurring food folate plus 1.7 times the micrograms of synthetic folate. The 1.7 multiplier for converting folic acid to DFEs was based on the assumption that added folic acid (consumed with a meal as a supplement or fortificant) is about 85% available[51] and food folate is about 50% available[48]; the ratio 85/50 yielded the multiplier of 1.7 in the DFE calculation. A recent long-term feeding study was designed to evaluate the validity of the bioavailability estimates that were the basis of the 1.7 multiplier used to calculate DFE.[161] In this study, the folate status response to multiple combinations of food folate and folic acid (micrograms of food folate or food folate plus micrograms of folic acid multiplied by 1.7) was compared and found not to differ among the treatment groups consuming either 400 or 800 μg DFE/d, thus supporting the 1.7 equivalency factor used to calculate DFEs.[161]

A UL for folic acid was estimated as 1000 μg/d,[108] but no UL was established for naturally occurring food folate. The UL for folic acid is based on historical case reports describing vitamin $B_{12}$-deficient patients whose anemia responded to folic acid alone. The reported hematological response to folic acid in these vitamin $B_{12}$-deficient patients was referred to as "masking" and is the sole basis of the UL for folic acid.[162] Unlike the case for other nutrients for which there is a UL, there are no substantiated toxic side effects and no dose response associated with high doses of folic acid.[108] Fortification of enriched cereal grains with folic acid has raised concerns that individuals who consume large quantities of fortified foods, particularly the elderly, may be at increased risk of masking (having vitamin $B_{12}$ deficiency without anemia). Mills et al.[163] found no evidence that masking of vitamin $B_{12}$ deficiency is increasing as a result of folic acid fortification.

**Table 4.** Folate Dietary Reference Intakes

| Population | Adequate Intake | Recommended Dietary Allowance μg of DFE*/d |
|---|---|---|
| Infants | | |
| 0–6 mo | 65 | |
| 6–11 mo | 80 | |
| Children and Adolescents | | |
| 1–3 yr | | 150 |
| 4–8 yr | | 200 |
| 9–13 yr | | 300 |
| 14–18 yr | | 400 |
| Adults (≥19 yr) | | 400 |
| Pregnant women (all ages) | | 600 |
| Lactating women (all ages) | | 500 |

* DFE = Dietary folate equivalents.

## Analytical Methods

Essentially all aspects of folate nutrition and folate research are predicated on reliable measurement of the vitamin in biological specimens and dietary components. The major approaches to the measurement of folate in biological specimens and foods or diet samples include microbiological growth procedures, protein-ligand binding methods, and chromatographic and mass spectrometric methods.[164,165] Microbiological assays using *Lactobacillus casei* provide measurement of total folate. Ligand-binding assays are commonly used in clinical settings because of their simplicity in well-standardized applications; however, non-uniform response among different folates tends to limit their application to foods or other samples containing multiple forms of the vitamin. High-performance liquid chromatography (HPLC) methods allow for the measurement of each form of folate if the samples are well purified; however, the preparation of reliable standards for all forms of folate constitutes a challenge. Several liquid chromatography-tandem mass spectrometry methods have been developed for the analysis of foods and clinical specimens.[166-169] Improvement and standardization of methods for measurement of folate analysis remains a research need of high priority.

The results of an international analysis of folate in serum and whole blood indicated that there are substantial differences in the response of methods commonly used in clinical folate analysis[170,171]; thus, reference ranges, calibration, and quality control protocols must be carefully established to avoid inaccurate results. A potentially important new variation of folate assays for nutritional status assessment is the measurement of whole blood folate on samples preserved as dried blood spots from "finger stick" samples on filter paper.[172] The Centers for Disease Control and Prevention and the National Institute of Standards and Technology recently have collaborated on the development and release of standard reference materials.

With respect to food analysis, several analytical approaches are capable of providing reliable data for the experienced analyst. However, a major research need remains the development of a fully optimized and validated method for the measurement of food folate. Traditional and contemporary analytical methods for the measurement of folate in foods have been reviewed previously.[141,164,165,173] Comparisons of folate HPLC methods for several reference food samples have generally yielded poor agreement among laboratories[174]; however, several methods exist that are very well suited to the HPLC measurement of food folate.[175-178]

The assessment of folate intake in most nutritional studies requires the use of food composition databases. Food folate composition data mainly have been obtained using microbiological assay procedures. The key elements of food folate methodology, whether by HPLC or microbiological assay, are the preparative stages that include extraction from sample matrix and enzymatic deconjugation of polyglutamyl folates if needed. Although unresolved issues concerning the conditions of the microbiological growth assay do exist,[164] many more problems can arise if the conditions of sample preparation (extraction, etc.) are not optimized. The apparent folate content of foods can be underestimated due to incomplete folate extraction and possibly incomplete deconjugation that may occur when using traditional conditions of sample preparation.[179,180] Insufficient enzymatic deconjugation results in underestimation of folate in either microbiological or HPLC assays.[176,180] Several studies have shown that treatment of food homogenates with amylase and/or protease enzymes (termed "trienzyme" methods) enhances the yield of measurable folate in folate assays, although this effect is highly variable.[173,176,181,182] Efforts have been made to standardize a microbiological assay method that incorporates preliminary protease and amylase treatments,[183] leading to the adoption of such a method for regulatory use. Comparisons with validated HPLC results are needed in a wide range of food types to confirm the specificity of trienzyme-based *L. casei* assay methods.

The details of analytical methods used to generate the major nutrient databases often have not been reported. In view of the limitations of traditional methods for food folate analysis, it is likely that many database values underestimate actual folate content. Many of the analyses used to generate common database values involved the use of extraction conditions that would yield incomplete extraction.[179] Improvements in food folate databases based on direct analysis with validated assay procedures are greatly needed, and efforts toward this goal are under way.

It is highly likely that many estimates of folate intake reported in population studies do not reflect actual folate intake, but the clinical relevance of any disparity is unclear. Estimates of intake derived from food frequency analysis are effectively predictive of folate nutritional status.[184] In a study of over 80,000 nurses, the relative risk of coronary heart disease was inversely related to estimated total folate intake from food alone or from food and supplements.[185] Thus, the food composition data, mainly from the USDA Nutrient Database, enabled reliable classification of subjects by quintile of folate intake, which indicated that intake was inversely related to relative risk of coronary heart disease. A similar relationship between measures of folate nutritional status and estimates of intake ranked by decile has also been observed in the Framingham Heart Study.[186,187] Thus, food composition data are clearly suitable for accurately classifying folate intakes, although quantitative estimates might be underestimated. The currently mandated addition of folic acid to many cereal-based foods[183] amplifies the need for improvements in food folate databases. While attempts have been made to calculate post-fortification folate content,[5] there is no alternative to direct analysis.

## Status Assessment

Folate status assessment in the research setting and in population surveys routinely includes blood folate concentrations and some indicators of metabolic function.[108] Since hematological findings such as macrocytic anemia occur late in the development of a folate deficiency, the emphasis in status assessment studies is on changes that precede clinical indicators.[108]

Serum folate concentrations are generally determined when folate status is assessed; however, changes may indicate a transient reduction in folate intake and may not represent body stores.[108] Serum folate is considered to be a sensitive indicator of recent dietary folate intake, and may require repeated measurements over time in the same individual to reflect long-term status.[108] The criterion for serum folate concentration routinely used to define inadequate folate status is less than 7 nmol/L (<3 ng/mL).[108]

In contrast to serum folate concentration, red blood cell folate concentration is considered an indicator of long-term status. Since folate is not taken up by the mature red blood cell in circulation, red blood cell folate concentration represents folate taken up in the developing reticulocyte early in the approximately 120-day erythrocyte lifespan. Based on associations with liver folate concentrations determined by biopsy,[108] red blood cell folate concentration is considered representative of tissue folate stores. A cutoff value of <305 nmol/L (<140 ng/mL) is the criterion commonly used to define inadequate folate status.[108]

In addition to blood folate concentrations, it is important to also evaluate folate status indices that may indicate changes in metabolic function. One such "functional" indicator is total plasma homocysteine concentration, which increases when there is a deficiency of 5-methylTHF necessary to convert homocysteine to methionine. The inverse association between blood folate concentrations and plasma total homocysteine concentration is well established.[108] Plasma homocysteine concentration is considered a sensitive functional indicator; however, it is not a highly specific indicator for folate status because it may be influenced by a number of other nutrient deficiencies, genetic abnormalities, and renal insufficiency.[108] Various cutoff values have been reported to define normal folate status and most frequently have ranged from 12 to 16 μmol/L.[108]

Human studies have shown that DNA methylation significantly decreases as a function of dietary folate depletion[75,144,154] and is dependent on an adequate supply of 5-methylTHF for the synthesis of SAM (Figure 3, reaction 8). DNA methylation has been determined on the basis of the ability of genomic DNA to incorporate [$^3$H]methyl groups from labeled SAM in an in vitro assay[188] or by direct analysis of hydrolyzed DNA for methylcytosine.[75,189] A sensitive new method for the rapid detection of abnormal methylation patterns in global DNA and within CpG islands has been reported.[190]

Studies have suggested that the estimation of uracil misincorporation into DNA may be used as a functional index of folate status.[152,154] Folate in the form of 5,10-methyleneTHF is required for the conversion of dUMP to dTMP by thymidylate synthase (Figure 2, reaction 1). When this reaction is impaired due to poor folate status, deoxuridylate may accumulate, leading to deoxynucleotide pool imbalances and an increase in the dUMP:dTTP ratio. As a result, uracil, which is normally only present in RNA, may be incorporated into DNA in place of thymine, setting off an excision-repair cycle that may cause DNA strand breaks and chromosome damage.[152]

## Summary and Public Health Implications

The potential for optimizing folate intake and metabolism to positively impact human health has provided the impetus for major collaborative research efforts in the area of folate nutrition. Our understanding of how 1-C moieties flow between folate-dependent pathways and subcellular compartments has increased dramatically within the past few years. A series of regulatory control mechanisms conserve 1-C compounds when folate is deficient; however, metabolic abnormalities and imbalances may result, including hyperhomocysteinemia and impaired nucleotide synthesis and methylation. The identification of common genetic polymorphisms of folate-related enzymes has led investigators to estimate their relationship to risk of disease and developmental defects. Future analysis of genes encoding the various enzymes and proteins involved in folate metabolism and transport, coupled with continued assessment of the interactions of polymorphism, nutrition, and disease prevalence, will greatly enhance our understanding of these issues.

The strength of the scientific evidence related to folic acid and NTDs resulted in the implementation of major public health policies worldwide coupled with folic acid fortification in select countries. Data suggest that consumption of foods fortified with folic acid and related improvements in folate status have been associated with a reduction in NTDs. The potential for folic acid supplements to reduce other types of birth defects and chronic disease risk has enormous implications for public health because of the large percentage of the population likely to be affected. The outcomes of intervention trials in countries in which mandatory fortification is not a confounding factor are likely to lead to more definitive conclusions regarding the efficacy of folic acid intervention to reduce the disease incidence. The collaborative nature of ongoing research efforts in the folate field is essential to link our rapidly expanding knowledge of the interrelationship between dietary folate intake, genetics, and metabolism with the maintenance of optimum health.

## References


1. Stokstad ELR. Historical perspective on key advances in the biochemistry and physiology of folates. In: Picciano MF, Stokstad ELR, Gregory JF, eds. *Folic Acid Metabolism in Health and Disease.* New York: Wiley-Liss; 1990; 1–15.
2. Cook RJ. Folate Metabolism. In: Carmel R, Jacobsen D, eds. *Homocysteine in Health and Disease.* New York: Cambridge University Press; 2001; 113–134.
3. Suitor CW, Bailey LB. Dietary folate equivalents: interpretation and application. J Am Diet Assoc. 2000;100:88–94.
4. Department of Health and Human Services, Food and Drug Administration. Food standards: amendment of standards of identity for enriched grain products to require addition of folic acid. Fed Regist. 1996;61:8781–8797.
5. Lewis CJ, Crane NT, Wilson DB, Yetley EA. Estimated folate intakes: data updated to reflect food fortification, increased bioavailability, and dietary supplement use. Am J Clin Nutr. 1999;70:198–207.
6. Health Canada. Regulations amending the food and drug regulations (1066). Canada Gazette, Part I. 1997;131:3702–3737.
7. Freire WB, Hertrampf E, Cortes F. Effect of folic acid fortification in Chile: preliminary results. Eur J Pediatr Surg. 2000;10(suppl 1):42–43.
8. Freire WB, Howson CP, Cordero JF. Recommended levels of folic acid and vitamin B12 fortification: a PAHO/MOD/CDC technical consultation. Nutr Rev. 2004;62(6 part 2):S1–S2.
9. Bailey LB. Folate, methyl-related nutrients, alco-

hol, and the MTHFR 677C→T polymorphism affect cancer risk: intake recommendations. J Nutr. 2003;133(11 suppl 1):3748S–3753S.

10. Pfeiffer CM, Caudill SP, Gunter EW, Osterloh J, Sampson EJ. Biochemical indicators of B vitamin status in the US population after folic acid fortification: results from the National Health and Nutrition Examination Survey 1999–2000. Am J Clin Nutr. 2005;82:442–450.
11. Rader JI, Weaver CM, Angyal G. Total folate in enriched cereal-grain products in the United States following fortification. Food Chem. 2000;70:275–289.
12. Halsted CH, Ling E, Luthi-Carter R, Villanueva JA, Gardner JM, Coyle JT. Folylpoly-gamma-glutamate carboxypeptidase from pig jejunum. Molecular characterization and relation to glutamate carboxypeptidase II. J Biol Chem. 1998;273: 20417–20424.
13. Halsted CH. Intestinal absorption of dietary folates. In: Picianno MF, Stokstad ELR, Gregory JF, eds. *Folic Acid Metabolism in Health and Disease.* New York: Wiley-Liss; 1990; 23–45.
14. Reisenauer AM, Krumdieck CL, Halsted CH. Folate conjugase: two separate activities in human jejunum. Science. 1977;198:196–197.
15. Zimmerman J, Gilula Z, Selhub J, Rosenberg IH. Kinetic analysis of the effect of luminal pH on transport of folic acid in the small intestine. Int J Vitam Nutr Res. 1989;59:151–156.
16. Mason JB. Intestinal transport of monoglutamyl folates in mammalian systems. In: Picianno MF, Stokstad ELR, Gregory JF, eds. *Folic Acid Metabolism in Health and Disease.* New York: Wiley-Liss; 1990; 47–64.
17. Gregory J. The bioavailability of folate. In: Bailey L, ed. *Folate in Health and Disease.* New York: Marcel Dekker; 1995; 195–235.
18. Kelly P, McPartlin J, Goggins M, Weir DG, Scott JM. Unmetabolized folic acid in serum: acute studies in subjects consuming fortified food and supplements. Am J Clin Nutr. 1997;65:1790–1795.
19. Henderson GB. Folate-binding proteins. Annu Rev Nutr 1990;10:319–335.
20. Antony AC. The biological chemistry of folate receptors. Blood. 1992;79:2807–2820.
21. Ratnman N and Freisheim JH. Proteins involved in the transport of folates and antifolates by normal and neoplastic cells. In: Picianno MF, Stokstad ELR, Gregory JF, eds. *Folic Acid Metabolism in Health and Disease.* New York: Wiley-Liss; 1990: 93–120.
22. Selhub J. Rosenberg IH. Folic acid. In: Ziegler EE, Fowler LJ, eds. *Present Knowledge in Nutrition.* 8th ed. Washington DC: ILSI Press; 1996:206–219.
23. Selhub J, Emmanouel D, Stavropoulos T, Arnold R. Renal folate absorption and the kidney folate binding protein. I. Urinary clearance studies. Am J Physiol. 1987;252(4 part 2):F750–F756.
24. Selhub J, Nakamura S, Carone FA. Renal folate absorption and the kidney folate binding protein. II. Microinfusion studies. Am J Physiol. 1987;252(4 part 1):F757–F760.
25. Shane B. Folylpolyglutamate synthesis and role in the regulation of one-carbon metabolism. Vitam Horm. 1989;45:263–335.
26. McGuire JJ, Coward JK. Pteropolyglutamates: biosynthesis, degradation, and function. In: Blakley RL, Benkovik SJ, eds. *Folates and Pterins.* New York: John Wiley & Sons; 1984; 135–190.
27. Hoppner K, Lampi B. Folate levels in human liver from autopsies in Canada. Am J Clin Nutr. 1980; 33:862–864.
28. Whitehead VM. Polygammaglutamyl metabolites of folic acid in human liver. Lancet. 1973;1: 743–745.
29. Herbert V, Zalusky R. Interrelations of vitamin B12 and folic acid metabolism: folic acid clearance studies. J Clin Invest. 1962;41:1263–1276.
30. Gregory JF 3rd, Williamson J, Liao JF, Bailey LB, Toth JP. Kinetic model of folate metabolism in nonpregnant women consuming [$^2H_2$]folic acid: isotopic labeling of urinary folate and the catabolite para-acetamidobenzoylglutamate indicates slow, intake-dependent turnover of folate pools. J Nutr. 1998;128:1896–1906.
31. Gregory JF 3rd, Caudill MA, Opalko FJ, Bailey LB. Kinetics of folate turnover in pregnant women (second trimester) and nonpregnant controls during folic acid supplementation: stable-isotopic labeling of plasma folate, urinary folate and folate catabolites shows subtle effects of pregnancy on turnover of folate pools. J Nutr. 2001;131:1928–1937.
32. Lin Y, Dueker SR, Follett JR, et al. Quantitation of in vivo human folate metabolism. Am J Clin Nutr. 2004;80:680–691.
33. Whitehead VM. Pharmacokinetics and physiological disposition of folate and its derivatives. In: Blakley RL, Whitehead VM, eds. *Folates and Pterins.* New York: John Wiley & Sons; 1986; 177–205.
34. Scott JM. Catabolism of folates. In: Blakley RL, Whitehead VM, eds. *Folates and Pterins.* New York: John Wiley & Sons; 1986; 307–327.
35. Caudill MA, Gregory JF, Hutson AD, Bailey LB. Folate catabolism in pregnant and nonpregnant women with controlled folate intakes. J Nutr. 1998; 128:204–208.
36. Krumdieck CL, Fukushima K, Fukushima T, Shiota T, Butterworth CE Jr. A long-term study of the excretion of folate and pterins in a human subject after ingestion of $^{14}C$ folic acid, with observations on the effect of diphenylhydantoin administration. Am J Clin Nutr. 1978;31:88–93.
37. Gregory JF 3rd, Quinlivan EP. In vivo kinetics of

folate metabolism. Annu Rev Nutr. 2002;22: 199–220.
38. Clifford AJ, Arjomand A, Dueker SR, Schneider PD, Buchholz BA, Vogel JS. The dynamics of folic acid metabolism in an adult given a small tracer dose of $^{14}$C-folic acid. Adv Exp Med Biol. 1998;445: 239–251.
39. Stites TE, Bailey LB, Scott KC, Toth JP, Fisher WP, Gregory JF 3rd. Kinetic modeling of folate metabolism through use of chronic administration of deuterium-labeled folic acid in men. Am J Clin Nutr. 1997;65:53–60.
40. Tamura T, Stokstad EL. The availability of food folate in man. Br J Haematol. 1973;25:513–532.
41. Babu S, Srikantia SG. Availability of folates from some foods. Am J Clin Nutr. 1976;29:376–379.
42. Prinz-Langenohl R, Bronstrup A, Thorand B, Hages M, Pietrzik K. Availability of food folate in humans. J Nutr. 1999;129:913–916.
43. Brouwer IA, van Dusseldorp M, West CE, et al. Dietary folate from vegetables and citrus fruit decreases plasma homocysteine concentrations in humans in a dietary controlled trial. J Nutr. 1999;129: 1135–1139.
44. Cuskelly GJ, McNulty H, Scott JM. Effect of increasing dietary folate on red-cell folate: implications for prevention of neural tube defects. Lancet. 1996;347:657–659.
45. Gregory JF 3rd. Bioavailability of folate. Eur J Clin Nutr. 1997;51(suppl 1):S54–S59.
46. Bhandari SD, Gregory JF 3rd. Folic acid, 5-methyl-tetrahydrofolate and 5-formyl-tetrahydrofolate exhibit equivalent intestinal absorption, metabolism and in vivo kinetics in rats. J Nutr. 1992;122: 1847–1854.
47. Wright AJ, Finglas PM, Dainty JR, et al. Differential kinetic behavior and distribution for pteroylglutamic acid and reduced folates: a revised hypothesis of the primary site of PteGlu metabolism in humans. J Nutr. 2005;135:619–623.
48. Sauberlich HE, Kretsch MJ, Skala JH, Johnson HL, Taylor PC. Folate requirement and metabolism in nonpregnant women. Am J Clin Nutr. 1987; 46:1016–1028.
49. Colman N. Addition of folic acid to staple foods as a selective nutrition intervention strategy. Nutr Rev. 1982;40:225–233.
50. O'Keefe CA, Bailey LB, Thomas EA, et al. Controlled dietary folate affects folate status in nonpregnant women. J Nutr. 1995;125:2717–2725.
51. Pfeiffer CM, Rogers LM, Bailey LB, Gregory JF 3rd. Absorption of folate from fortified cereal-grain products and of supplemental folate consumed with or without food determined by using a dual-label stable-isotope protocol. Am J Clin Nutr. 1997;66: 1388–1397.
52. Malinow MR, Duell PB, Hess DL, et al. Reduction of plasma homocyst(e)ine levels by breakfast cereal fortified with folic acid in patients with coronary heart disease. N Engl J Med. 1998;338:1009–1015.
53. Jacques PF, Selhub J, Bostom AG, Wilson PW, Rosenberg IH. The effect of folic acid fortification on plasma folate and total homocysteine concentrations. N Engl Med. 1999;340:1449–1454.
54. Quinlivan EP, Gregory JF 3rd. Effect of food fortification on folic acid intake in the United States. Am J Clin Nutr. 2003;77:221–225.
55. Choumenkovitch SF, Selhub J, Wilson PW, Rader JI, Rosenberg IH, Jacques PF. Folic acid intake from fortification in United States exceeds predictions. J Nutr. 2002;132:2792–2798.
56. Hoag SW, Ramachandruni H, Shangraw RF. Failure of prescription prenatal vitamin products to meet USP standards for folic acid dissolution. J Am Pharm Assoc (Wash). 1997;NS37:397–400.
57. Gregory JF, Quinlivan EP, Davis SR. Integrating the issues of folate bioavailability, intake and metabolism in the era of fortification. Trends Food Sci Technol. 2005;16:229–240.
58. Melnyk S, Pogribna M, Pogribny IP, Yi P, James SJ. Measurement of plasma and intracellular S-adenosylmethionine and S-adenosylhomocysteine utilizing coulometric electrochemical detection: alterations with plasma homocysteine and pyridoxal 5′-phosphate concentrations. Clin Chem. 2000;46: 265–272.
59. Narkewicz MR, Sauls SD, Tjoa SS, Teng C, Fennessey PV. Evidence for intracellular partitioning of serine and glycine metabolism in Chinese hamster ovary cells. Biochem J. 1996;313(part 3):991–996.
60. Stover PJ, Chen LH, Suh JR, Stover DM, Keyomarsi K, Shane B. Molecular cloning, characterization, and regulation of the human mitochondrial serine hydroxymethyltransferase gene. J Biol Chem. 1997;272:1842–1848.
61. Christensen KE, Patel H, Kuzmanov U, Mejia NR, MacKenzie RE. Disruption of the mthfd1 gene reveals a monofunctional 10-formyltetrahydrofolate synthetase in mammalian mitochondria. J Biol Chem. 2005;280:7597–7602.
62. Davis SR, Stacpoole PW, Williamson J, et al. Tracer-derived total and folate-dependent homocysteine remethylation and synthesis rates in humans indicate that serine is the main one-carbon donor. Am J Physiol Endocrinol Metab. 2004;286: E272–E279.
63. Schalinske KL, Steele RD. Quantitation of carbon flow through the hepatic folate-dependent one-carbon pool in rats. Arch Biochem Biophys. 1989;271: 49–55.
64. Finkelstein JD. The regulation of homocysteine metabolism. In: Graham I, ed. *Homocyteine Metabolism: From Basic Science to Clinical Medicine.* Boston: Kluwer Academic Publishers; 1997; 3–9.

65. Ogawa H, Gomi T, Takusagawa F, Fujioka M. Structure, function and physiological role of glycine N-methyltransferase. Int J Biochem Cell Biol. 1998;30:13–26.
66. Melnyk S, Pogribna M, Pogribny I, Hine RJ, James SJ. A new HPLC method for the simultaneous determination of oxidized and reduced plasma aminothiols using coulometric electrochemical detection. J Nutr Biochem. 1999;10:490–497.
67. Finnell RH, Gould A, Spiegelstein O. Pathobiology and genetics of neural tube defects. Epilepsia. 2003;44(suppl 3):14–23.
68. Rozen R. Polymorphisms of folate and cobalamin metabolism. In: Carmel R, Jacobsen D, eds. *Homocysteine in Health and Disease.* Cambridge UK: Cambridge University Press; 2001; 259–270.
69. Molloy AM. Folate and homocysteine interrelationships including genetics of the relevant enzymes. Curr Opin Lipidol. 2004;15:49–57.
70. Botto LD, Yang Q. 5,10-Methylenetetrahydrofolate reductase gene variants and congenital anomalies: a HuGE review. Am J Epidemiol. 2000;151: 862–877.
71. Shelnutt KP, Kauwell GP, Chapman CM, et al. Folate status response to controlled folate intake is affected by the methylenetetrahydrofolate reductase 677C→T polymorphism in young women. J Nutr. 2003;133:4107–4111.
72. Guinotte CL, Burns MG, Axume JA, et al. Methylenetetrahydrofolate reductase 677C→T variant modulates folate status response to controlled folate intakes in young women. J Nutr. 2003; 133: 1272–1280.
73. Stern LL, Mason JB, Selhub J, Choi SW. Genomic DNA hypomethylation, a characteristic of most cancers, is present in peripheral leukocytes of individuals who are homozygous for the C677T polymorphism in the methylenetetrahydrofolate reductase gene. Cancer Epidemiol Biomarkers Prev. 2000;9:849–853.
74. Friso S, Choi SW, Girelli D, et al. A common mutation in the 5,10-methylenetetrahydrofolate reductase gene affects genomic DNA methylation through an interaction with folate status. Proc Natl Acad Sci U S A. 2002;99:5606–5611.
75. Shelnutt KP, Kauwell GP, Gregory JF 3rd, et al. Methylenetetrahydrofolate reductase 677C→T polymorphism affects DNA methylation in response to controlled folate intake in young women. J Nutr Biochem. 2004;15:554–560.
76. Vaughn JD, Bailey LB, Shelnutt KP, et al. Methionine synthase reductase 66A→G polymorphism is associated with increased plasma homocysteine concentration when combined with the homozygous methylenetetrahydrofolate reductase 677C→T variant. J Nutr. 2004;134:2985–2990.
77. Wilson A, Platt R, Wu Q, et al. A common variant in methionine synthase reductase combined with low cobalamin (vitamin B12) increases risk for spina bifida. Mol Genet Metab. 1999;67:317–323.
78. Devlin AM, Ling EH, Peerson JM, et al. Glutamate carboxypeptidase II: a polymorphism associated with lower levels of serum folate and hyperhomocysteinemia. Hum Mol Genet. 2000;9: 2837–2844.
79. Melse-Boonstra A, Lievers KJ, Blom HJ, Verhoef P. Bioavailability of polyglutamyl folic acid relative to that of monoglutamyl folic acid in subjects with different genotypes of the glutamate carboxypeptidase II gene. Am J Clin Nutr. 2004;80:700–704.
80. Lievers KJ, Kluijtmans LA, Boers GH, et al. Influence of a glutamate carboxypeptidase II (GCPII) polymorphism (1561C→T) on plasma homocysteine, folate and vitamin B12 levels and its relationship to cardiovascular disease risk. Atherosclerosis. 2002;164:269–273.
81. Afman LA, Trijbels FJ, Blom HJ. The H475Y Polymorphism in the glutamate carboxypeptidase II gene increases plasma folate without affecting the risk for neural tube defects in humans. J Nutr. 2003; 133:75–77.
82. Lindenbaum J, Allen R. Clinical spectrum and diagnosis of folate deficiency. In: Bailey L, ed. *Folate in Health and Disease.* New York: Marcel Dekker; 1995; 43–73.
83. Scholl TO, Johnson WG. Folic acid: influence on the outcome of pregnancy. Am J Clin Nutr. 2000; 71(suppl 5):1295S–1303S.
84. Vollset SE, Refsum H, Irgens LM, et al. Plasma total homocysteine, pregnancy complications, and adverse pregnancy outcomes: the Hordaland Homocysteine study. Am J Clin Nutr. 2000;71: 962–968.
85. van der Molen EF, Arends GE, Nelen WL, et al. A common mutation in the 5,10-methylenetetrahydrofolate reductase gene as a new risk factor for placental vasculopathy. Am J Obstet Gynecol. 2000; 182:1258–1263.
86. Ray JG, Laskin CA. Folic acid and homocyst(e)ine metabolic defects and the risk of placental abruption, pre-eclampsia and spontaneous pregnancy loss: a systematic review. Placenta. 1999;20: 519–529.
87. Botto LD, Moore CA, Khoury MJ, Erickson JD. Neural-tube defects. N Engl J Med. 1999;341: 1509–1519.
88. Food and Nutrition Board, Institute of Medicine. *Evolution of Evidence for Selected Nutrient and Disease Relationships. Committee on Examination of the Evolving Science for Dietary Supplements.* Washington, DC: National Academies Press; 2002. Available online at: http://www.nap.edu/books/0309083087.html.
89. Scott JM. Evidence of folic acid and folate in the

prevention of neural tube defects. Bibl Nutr Dieta. 2001;55:192–195.

90. Stover PJ. Physiology of folate and vitamin B12 in health and disease. Nutr Rev. 2004;62(6 part 2): S3–S13.
91. Rosenquist TH, Schneider AM, Monogham DT. N-methyl-D-aspartate receptor agonists modulate homocysteine-induced developmental abnormalities. FASEB J. 1999;13:1523–1531.
92. Clarke S, Banfield K. S-adenosylmethionine-dependent methyltransferases. In: Carmel R, Jacobsen D, eds. *Homocysteine in Health and Disease.* Cambridge UK: Cambridge University Press; 2001; 63–78.
93. Fleming A, Copp AJ. Embryonic folate metabolism and mouse neural tube defects. Science. 1998;280: 2107–2109.
94. Boddie AM, Dedlow ER, Nackashi JA, et al. Folate absorption in women with a history of neural tube defect-affected pregnancy. Am J Clin Nutr. 2000; 72:154–158.
95. Rothenberg SP, da Costa MP, Sequeira JM, et al. Autoantibodies against folate receptors in women with a pregnancy complicated by a neural-tube defect. N Engl J Med. 2004;350:134–142.
96. Harris MJ. Why are the genes that cause risk of human neural tube defects so hard to find? Teratology. 2001;63:165–166.
97. Shaw GM, Lammer EJ, Zhu H, Baker MW, Neri E, Finnell RH. Maternal periconceptional vitamin use, genetic variation of infant reduced folate carrier (A80G), and risk of spina bifida. Am J Med Genet. 2002;108:1–6.
98. Christensen B, Arbour L, Tran P, et al. Genetic polymorphisms in methylenetetrahydrofolate reductase and methionine synthase, folate levels in red blood cells, and risk of neural tube defects. Am J Med Genet. 1999;84:151–157.
99. Molloy AM, Daly S, Mills JL, et al. Thermolabile variant of 5,10-methylenetetrahydrofolate reductase associated with low red-cell folates: implications for folate intake recommendations. Lancet. 1997;349: 1591–1593.
100. van der Put NM, Eskes TK, Blom HJ. Is the common 677C→T mutation in the methylenetetrahydrofolate reductase gene a risk factor for neural tube defects? A meta-analysis. QJM. 1997;90:111–115.
101. Shields DC, Kirke PN, Mills JL, et al. The "thermolabile" variant of methylenetetrahydrofolate reductase and neural tube defects: An evaluation of genetic risk and the relative importance of the genotypes of the embryo and the mother. Am J Hum Genet. 1999;64:1045–1055.
102. Brody LC, Conley M, Cox C, et al. A polymorphism, R653Q, in the trifunctional enzyme methylenetetrahydrofolate dehydrogenase/methenyltetrahydrofolate cyclohydrolase/formyltetrahydrofolate synthetase is a maternal genetic risk factor for neural tube defects: report of the Birth Defects Research Group. Am J Hum Genet. 2002;71:1207–1215.
103. Piedrahita JA, Oetama B, Bennett GD, et al. Mice lacking the folic acid-binding protein Folbp1 are defective in early embryonic development. Nat Genet. 1999;23:228–232.
104. Spiegelstein O, Eudy JD, Finnell RH. Identification of two putative novel folate receptor genes in humans and mouse. Gene. 2000;258:117–125.
105. Finnell RH, Spiegelstein O, Wlodarczyk B, et al. DNA methylation in Folbp1 knockout mice supplemented with folic acid during gestation. J Nutr. 2002;132(suppl 8):2457S–2461S.
106. Berry RJ, Li Z, Erickson JD, et al. Prevention of neural-tube defects with folic acid in China. China-U.S. Collaborative Project for Neural Tube Defect Prevention. N Engl J Med. 1999;341:1485–1490.
107. Centers for Disease Control and Prevention. Recommendations for the use of folic acid to reduce the number of cases of spina bifida and other neural tube defects. MMWR Recomm Rep. 1992;41(RR-14):1–7.
108. Food and Nutrition Board, Institute of Medicine. *Dietary Reference Intakes for Thiamin, Riboflavin, Niacin, Vitamin B6, Folate, Vitamin B12, Pantothenic Acid, Biotin, and Choline.* Washington, DC: National Academies Press; 1998. Available online at: http://www.nap.edu/openbook/0309065542/html/.
109. Honein MA, Paulozzi LJ, Mathews TJ, Erickson JD, Wong LY. Impact of folic acid fortification of the US food supply on the occurrence of neural tube defects. JAMA. 2001;285:2981–2986.
110. Williams LJ, Mai CT, Edmonds LD, et al. Prevalence of spina bifida and anencephaly during the transition to mandatory folic acid fortification in the United States. Teratology. 2002;66:33–39.
111. Gucciardi E, Pietrusiak MA, Reynolds DL, Rouleau J. Incidence of neural tube defects in Ontario, 1986–1999. CMAJ. 2002;167:237–240.
112. Persad VL, Van den Hof MC, Dube JM, Zimmer P. Incidence of open neural tube defects in Nova Scotia after folic acid fortification. CMAJ. 2002; 167:241–245.
113. Lopez-Camelo JS, Orioli IM, de Graca Dutra M, et al. Reduction of birth prevalence rates of neural tube defects after folic acid fortification in Chile. Am J Med Genet A. 2005;135:120–125.
114. Botto LD, Correa A, Erickson JD. Racial and temporal variations in the prevalence of heart defects. Pediatrics. 2001;107:E32.
115. Botto LD, Correa A. Decreasing the burden of congenital heart anomalies: an epidemiologic evaluation of risk factors and survival. Prog Pediatr Cardiol. 2003;18:111–121.
116. Botto LD, Olney RS, Erickson JD. Vitamin supple-

ments and the risk for congenital anomalies other than neural tube defects. Am J Med Genet C Semin Med Genet. 2004;125:12–21.

117. Bailey LB, Berry RJ. Folic acid supplementation and the occurrence of congenital heart defects, orofacial clefts, multiple births, and miscarriage. Am J Clin Nutr. 2005;81:1213S–1217S.

118. Czeizel AE, Dudas I. Prevention of the first occurrence of neural-tube defects by periconceptional vitamin supplementation. N Engl J Med. 1992;327: 1832–1835.

119. Botto LD, Mulinare J, Erickson JD. Occurrence of congenital heart defects in relation to maternal multivitamin use. Am J Epidemiol. 2000;151: 878–884.

120. Shaw GM, O'Malley CD, Wasserman CR, Tolarova MM, Lammer EJ. Maternal periconceptional use of multivitamins and reduced risk for conotruncal heart defects and limb deficiencies among offspring. Am J Med Genet. 1995;59:536–545.

121. Czeizel AE. Folic acid and prevention of birth defects. JAMA. 1996;275:1635–1636.

122. Czeizel AE. Periconceptional folic acid containing multivitamin supplementation. Eur J Obstet Gynecol Reprod Biol. 1998;78:151–161.

123. Botto LD, Mulinare J, Erickson JD. Do multivitamin or folic acid supplements reduce the risk for congenital heart defects? Evidence and gaps. Am J Med Genet A. 2003;121:95–101.

124. Scanlon KS, Ferencz C, Loffredo CA, et al. Preconceptional folate intake and malformations of the cardiac outflow tract. Baltimore-Washington Infant Study Group. Epidemiology. 1998;9:95–98.

125. Werler MM, Hayes C, Louik C, Shapiro S, Mitchell AA. Multivitamin supplementation and risk of birth defects. Am J Epidemiol. 1999;150:675–682.

126. Wald DS, Law M, Morris JK. Homocysteine and cardiovascular disease: evidence on causality from a meta-analysis. BMJ. 2002;325:1202–1206.

127. Homocysteine Studies Collaboration. Homocysteine and risk of ischemic heart disease and stroke: a meta-analysis. JAMA 2002;288:2015–2022.

128. Homocysteine Lowering Trialists' Collaboration. Dose-dependent effects of folic acid on blood homocysteine concentrations: a meta-analysis of the randomized trials. Am J Clin Nutr. 2005;82: 806–812.

129. Bailey LB, Rampersaud GC, Kauwell GP. Folic acid supplements and fortification affect the risk for neural tube defects, vascular disease and cancer: evolving science. J Nutr. 2003;133:1961S–1968S.

130. Selhub J. Homocysteine metabolism. Annu Rev Nutr. 1999;19:217–246.

131. Clarke S. Design of clinical trials to test the homocysteine hypothesis of vascular disease. In: Carmel R, Jacobsen D, eds. *Homocysteine in Health and Disease.* Cambridge UK: Cambridge University Press; 2001; 477–484.

132. Toole JF, Malinow MR, Chambless LE, et al. Lowering homocysteine in patients with ischemic stroke to prevent recurrent stroke, myocardial infarction, and death: the Vitamin Intervention for Stroke Prevention (VISP) randomized controlled trial. JAMA. 2004;291:565–575.

133. Hankey GJ, Eikelboom JW, Loh K, et al. Sustained homocysteine-lowering effect over time of folic acid-based multivitamin therapy in stroke patients despite increasing folate status in the population. Cerebrovasc Dis. 2005;19:110–116.

134. Klerk M, Verhoef P, Clarke R, et al.; MTHFR Studies Collaboration Group. MTHFR 677C→T polymorphism and risk of coronary heart disease: a meta-analysis. JAMA. 2002;288:2023–2031.

135. Casas JP, Bautista LE, Smeeth L, Sharma P, Hingorani AD. Homocysteine and stroke: evidence on a causal link from mendelian randomisation. Lancet. 2005;365:224–232.

136. Giovannucci E, Stampfer MJ, Colditz GA, et al. Multivitamin use, folate, and colon cancer in women in the Nurses' Health Study. Ann Intern Med. 1998;129:517–524.

137. Giovannucci E, Stampfer MJ, Colditz GA, et al. Folate, methionine, and alcohol intake and risk of colorectal adenoma. J Natl Cancer Inst. 1993;85: 875–884.

138. Ma J, Stampfer MJ, Giovannucci E, et al. Methylenetetrahydrofolate reductase polymorphism, dietary interactions, and risk of colorectal cancer. Cancer Res. 1997;57:1098–1102.

139. Giovannucci E. Epidemiologic studies of folate and colorectal neoplasia: a review. J Nutr. 2002; 132(suppl 8):2350S–2355S.

140. Robien K, Ulrich CM. 5,10-Methylenetetrahydrofolate reductase polymorphisms and leukemia risk: a HuGE minireview. Am J Epidemiol. 2003;157: 571–582.

141. Quinlivan EP, Davis SR, Shelnutt KP, et al. Methylenetetrahydrofolate reductase 677C→T polymorphism and folate status affect one-carbon incorporation into human DNA deoxynucleosides. J Nutr. 2005;135:389–396.

142. Jacques PF, Bostom AG, Williams RR, et al. Relation between folate status, a common mutation in methylenetetrahydrofolate reductase, and plasma homocysteine concentrations. Circulation. 1996;93: 7–9.

143. Kauwell GP, Wilsky CE, Cerda JJ, et al. Methylenetetrahydrofolate reductase mutation (677C→T) negatively influences plasma homocysteine response to marginal folate intake in elderly women. Metabolism. 2000;49:1440–1443.

144. Rampersaud GC, Kauwell GP, Hutson AD, Cerda JJ, Bailey LB. Genomic DNA methylation de-

creases in response to moderate folate depletion in elderly women. Am J Clin Nutr. 2000;72: 998–1003.

145. Friso S, Choi SW. Gene-nutrient interactions and DNA methylation. J Nutr. 2002;132(suppl 8): 2382S–2387S.

146. Kim YI. Folate and DNA methylation: a mechanistic link between folate deficiency and colorectal cancer? Cancer Epidemiol Biomarkers Prev. 2004;13: 511–519.

147. Rohan TE, Jain MG, Howe GR, Miller AB. Dietary folate consumption and breast cancer risk. J Natl Cancer Inst. 2000;92:266–269.

148. Zhang S, Hunter DJ, Hankinson SE, et al. A prospective study of folate intake and the risk of breast cancer. JAMA. 1999;281:1632–1637.

149. Giovannucci E, Rimm EB, Ascherio A, Stampfer MJ, Colditz GA, Willett WC. Alcohol, low-methionine-low-folate diets, and risk of colon cancer in men. J Natl Cancer Inst. 1995;87:265–273.

150. Halsted CH, Villanueva JA, Devlin AM, Chandler CJ. Metabolic interactions of alcohol and folate. J Nutr. 2002;132(suppl 8):2367S–2372S.

151. Chen J, Giovannucci EL, Hunter DJ. MTHFR polymorphism, methyl-replete diets and the risk of colorectal carcinoma and adenoma among U.S. men and women: an example of gene-environment interactions in colorectal tumorigenesis. J Nutr. 1999; 129(suppl 2S):560S–564S.

152. Blount BC, Mack MM, Wehr CM, et al. Folate deficiency causes uracil misincorporation into human DNA and chromosome breakage: implications for cancer and neuronal damage. Proc Natl Acad Sci U S A. 1997;94:3290–3295.

153. Davis CD, Uthus EO. DNA methylation, cancer susceptibility, and nutrient interactions. Exp Biol Med (Maywood). 2004;229:988–995.

154. Jacob RA, Gretz DM, Taylor PC, et al. Moderate folate depletion increases plasma homocysteine and decreases lymphocyte DNA methylation in postmenopausal women. J Nutr. 1998;128:1204–1212.

155. French AE, Grant R, Weitzman S, et al. Folic acid food fortification is associated with a decline in neuroblastoma. Clin Pharmacol Ther. 2003;74: 288–294.

156. Priest DG, Bunni MA. Folates and folate antagonists in cancer chemotherapy. In: Bailey L, ed. *Folate in Health and Disease.* New York: Marcel Dekker; 1995; 379–404.

157. Morgan S, Baggot J. Folate antagonists in nonneoplastic disease: proposed mechanism of efficacy and toxicity. In: Bailey L, ed. *Folate in Health and Disease.* New York: Marcel Dekker; 1995; 435–462.

158. Lloyd ME, Carr M, McElhatton P, Hall GM, Hughes RA. The effects of methotrexate on pregnancy, fertility and lactation. QJM. 1999;92: 551–563.

159. Young SN, Ghadirian AM. Folic acid and psychopathology. Prog Neuropsychopharmacol Biol Psychiatry. 1989;13:841–863.

160. Carlsen SM, Folling I, Grill V, Bjerve KS, Schneede J, Refsum H. Metformin increases total serum homocysteine levels in non-diabetic male patients with coronary heart disease. Scand J Clin Lab Invest. 1997;57:521–527.

161. Yang TL, Hung J, Caudill MA, et al. A long-term controlled folate feeding study in young women supports the validity of the 1.7 multiplier in the dietary folate equivalency equation. J Nutr. 2005; 135:1139–1145.

162. Savage DG, Lindenbaum J. Folate-cobalamin interactions. In: Bailey L, ed. *Folate in Health and Disease.* New York: Marcel Dekker; 1995; 237–285.

163. Mills JL, Von Kohorn I, Conley MR, et al. Low vitamin B-12 concentrations in patients without anemia: the effect of folic acid fortification of grain. Am J Clin Nutr. 2003;77:1474–1477.

164. Gregory JF 3rd. Chemical and nutritional aspects of folate research: analytical procedures, methods of folate synthesis, stability, and bioavailability of dietary folates. Adv Food Nutr Res. 1989;33:1–101.

165. Quinlivan EP, Hanson AD, Gregory JF. The analysis of folate and its metabolic precursors in biological samples. Anal Biochem. 2006;348:163–184.

166. Pawlosky RJ, Flanagan VP. A quantitative stable-isotope LC-MS method for the determination of folic acid in fortified foods. J Agric Food Chem. 2001;49:1282–1286.

167. Pawlosky RJ, Flanagan VP, Pfeiffer CM. Determination of 5-methyltetrahydrofolic acid in human serum by stable-isotope dilution high-performance liquid chromatography-mass spectrometry. Anal Biochem. 2001;298:299–305.

168. Pfeiffer CM, Fazili Z, McCoy L, Zhang M, Gunter EW. Determination of folate vitamers in human serum by stable-isotope-dilution tandem mass spectrometry and comparison with radioassay and microbiologic assay. Clin Chem. 2004;50:423–432.

169. Freisleben A, Schieberle P, Rychlik M. Specific and sensitive quantification of folate vitamers in foods by stable isotope dilution assays using high-performance liquid chromatography-tandem mass spectrometry. Anal Bioanal Chem. 2003;376:149–156.

170. Gunter EW, Bowman BA, Caudill SP, Adams MJ, Sampson EJ. Results of an international round robin for serum and whole-blood folate. Clin Chem. 1996;42:1689–1694.

171. van den Berg H, Finglas PM, Bates C. FLAIR intercomparisons on serum and red cell folate. Int J Vitam Nutr Res. 1994;64:288–293.

172. O'Broin SD, Gunter EW. Screening of folate status with use of dried blood spots on filter paper. Am J Clin Nutr. 1999;70:359–367.

173. Tamura T. Determination of food folate. J Nutr Biochem. 1998;9:285–293.
174. Finglas PM, Wigertz K, Vahteristo L, Witthoft CM, Southon S, de Froidmont-Gortz I. Standardisation of HPLC techniques for the determination of naturally-occurring folates in food. Food Chem. 1999;64:245–255.
175. Konings EJ. A validated liquid chromatographic method for determining folates in vegetables, milk powder, liver, and flour. J AOAC Int. 1999;82: 119–127.
176. Pfeiffer CM, Rogers LM, Gregory JF. Determination of folate in cereal-grain food products using tri-enzyme extraction and combined affinity and reverse-phase liquid chromatography. J Agric Food Chem. 1997;45:407–413.
177. Seyoum E, Selhub J. Combined affinity and ion pair column chromatographies for the analysis of food folate. J Nutr Biochem. 1993;4:488–494.
178. Diaz de la Garza R, Quinlivan EP, Klaus SM, Bassett GJ, Gregory JF 3rd, Hanson AD. Folate biofortification in tomatoes by engineering the pteridine branch of folate synthesis. Proc Natl Acad Sci U S A. 2004;101:13720–13725.
179. Gregory I, Jesse F, Engelhardt R, Bhandari SD, Sartain DB, Gustafson SK. Adequacy of extraction techniques for determination of folate in foods and other biological materials. J Food Comp Anal. 1990;3:134–144.
180. Engelhardt R, Gregory JF. Adequacy of enzymatic deconjugation in quantification of folate in foods. J Agric Food Chem. 1990;38:154–158.
181. DeSouza S, Eitenmiller R. Effects of different enzyme treatments on extraction of total folate from various foods prior to microbiological assay and radioassay. J Micronutr Anal. 1990;7:37–57.
182. Martin JI, Landen WO Jr, Soliman AG, Eitenmiller RR. Application of a tri-enzyme extraction for total folate determination in foods. J Assoc Off Anal Chem. 1990;73:805–808.
183. Rader JI, Weaver CM, Angyal G. Use of a microbiological assay with tri-enzyme extraction for measurement of pre-fortification levels of folates in enriched cereal-grain products. Food Chem. 1998;62: 451–465.
184. Jacques PF, Sulsky SI, Sadowski JA, Phillips JC, Rush D, Willett NC. Comparison of micronutrient intake measured by a dietary questionnaire and biochemical indicators of micronutrient status. Am J Clin Nutr. 1993;57:182–189.
185. Rimm EB, Willett WC, Hu FB, et al. Folate and vitamin B6 from diet and supplements in relation to risk of coronary heart disease among women. JAMA. 1998;279:359–364.
186. Selhub J, Jacques PF, Wilson PW, Rush D, Rosenberg IH. Vitamin status and intake as primary determinants of homocysteinemia in an elderly population. JAMA. 1993;270:2693–2698.
187. Tucker KL, Mahnken B, Wilson PW, Jacques P, Selhub J. Folic acid fortification of the food supply. Potential benefits and risks for the elderly population. JAMA. 1996;276:1879–1885.
188. Balaghi M, Wagner C. DNA methylation in folate deficiency: use of CpG methylase. Biochem Biophys Res Commun. 1993;193:1184–1190.
189. Friso S, Choi SW, Dolnikowski GG, Selhub J. A method to assess genomic DNA methylation using high-performance liquid chromatography/electrospray ionization mass spectrometry. Anal Chem. 2002;74:4526–4531.
190. Pogribny I, Yi P, James SJ. A sensitive new method for rapid detection of abnormal methylation patterns in global DNA and within CpG islands. Biochem Biophys Res Commun. 1999;262:624–628.

# 23 Vitamin $B_{12}$

Sally P. Stabler

Vitamin $B_{12}$ (cobalamin, Cbl) holds a unique position in the science of human nutrition because there is a specific disease (pernicious anemia) that results in the isolated malabsorption of vitamin $B_{12}$ that was ultimately fatal before the development of vitamin therapy. This unique syndrome of megaloblastic anemia and demyelinating lesions of the central nervous system was recognized and described by Thomas Addison as early as 1855.[1] Pernicious anemia has such specific manifestations and such a dramatic response to the replacement of vitamin $B_{12}$ that a patient response could actually be used as a bioassay. In 1926, Minot and Murphy[2] showed that a diet containing large amounts of liver stimulated red blood cell production in patients with pernicious anemia. Their early work eventually culminated in the purification of vitamin $B_{12}$ from liver by Folkers at Merck, Sharp and Dohme in 1948 and by Smith and Parker at Glaxo in the same year.[3] During the next 50 years, the structure, X-ray crystallography, synthesis of coenzyme forms, and chemistry and biochemistry of the cobamides were elucidated.[4] Much of what we know about the role of vitamin $B_{12}$ in metabolism and the pathophysiology of the deficient state has been determined by studying patients with pernicious anemia, since this accident of nature results in a very selective model of a deficiency disease not complicated by protein-calorie malnutrition or multiple vitamin and mineral deficiencies. Nonetheless, despite 50 years of investigation of the role of vitamin $B_{12}$ in vertebrate metabolism, many unanswered questions remain, especially regarding the specific role of vitamin $B_{12}$ in myelinization of the nervous system.

## Structure of Vitamin $B_{12}$

The structure of vitamin $B_{12}$ (OH-Cbl) is shown in Figure 1. It is a very complex molecule containing a corrin ring (which coordinates a cobalt molecule), 5,6-dimethylbenzimidazole, a sugar, and an aminopropanol group. An upper axial ligand is coordinated to the cobalt and can be hydroxy, cyano, glutathonine, or the coenzyme forms methyl ($CH_3$) and adenosyl.[5] The chemistry of the carbon-cobalt bond found in the coenzyme forms is unique and has been studied extensively.[5] Only microorganisms retain the ability to synthesize cobalamins, and microbial synthesis pathways have been elucidated in a series of elegant studies.[6,7] Because plants do not use cobalamins, the source of cobalamins in all higher animals is the product of microbial synthesis. Higher animals require vitamin $B_{12}$ for only two reactions, one of which utilizes $CH_3$-Cbl and the other adenosyl-Cbl. However, analogs of Cbl with bases other than 5,6-dimethylbenzimidazole are widely found in nature, including in the human intestinal tract, but do not support coenzyme activity in higher animals, although they are utilized by various microorganisms.[8]

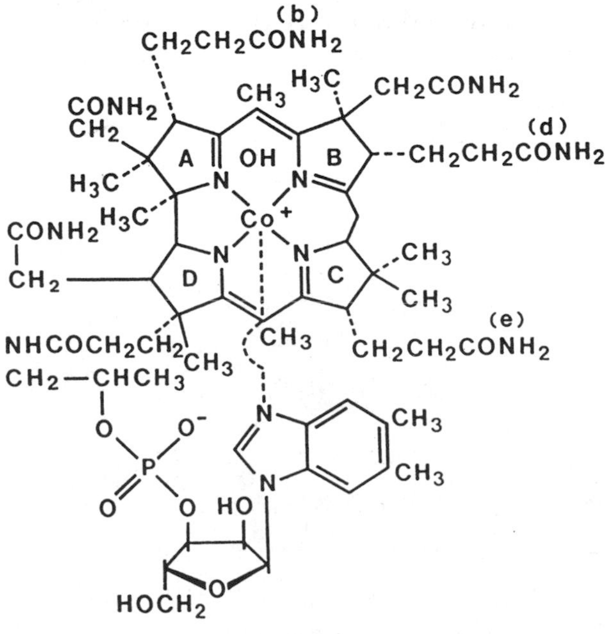

Figure 1. The structure of OH-cobalamin.

# Vitamin $B_{12}$-Dependent Enzyme Reactions

Microorganisms use various forms of vitamin $B_{12}$ in many reactions, including methionine synthesis, carbon skeleton mutation, elimination reactions, amino-mutations, and acetate and methane synthesis.[4] Higher animals require Cbl as a cofactor for only two enzymes, L-methylmalonyl-coenzyme A (CoA) mutase and methionine synthase.[9] The binding of the coenzyme forms to these two enzymes has been studied by X-ray crystallography,[10,11] and it appears that the dimethylbenzimidazole is displaced from the cobalt and a histidine residue from the enzyme coordinates at the position. Although both of these enzymes use vitamin $B_{12}$, they perform very different types of chemical reactions. During methionine synthesis and other methyl-transfer reactions, the methyl-cobalt bond undergoes heterolytic cleavage, whereas the mutase performs a homolytic cleavage of adenosyl-Cbl that results in the formation of a radical. Ludwig and Mathews[5] have described the exciting research into the enzyme mechanisms and coenzyme interactions.

# L-Methylmalonyl CoA Mutase

The pathway of propionyl-CoA metabolism is shown in Figure 2. The metabolism of amino acids such as valine and isoleucine and odd-chain fatty acids results in the formation of propionyl-CoA, which is carboxylated to form D-methylmalonyl-CoA. A racemase interconverts the two isomers, and L-methylmalonyl-CoA is a substrate for the adenosyl-Cbl-dependent enzyme L-methylmalonyl-CoA mutase.[9] D-methylmalonyl-CoA can be hydrolyzed to methylmalonic acid (MMA).[12] The mutase is a mitochondrial matrix enzyme. It has been purified from human[13] and other sources, and the genes have been cloned and sequenced, also from human[14] and bacterial sources. The enzyme is a homodimer that binds 2 mol adenosyl-Cbl per dimer. The reaction mechanisms have been intensively studied.[5,15]

The mutase is not completely saturated with adenosyl-Cbl in vivo.[16] OH-Cbl infusions in rats over 14 days increased holo L-methylmalonyl-CoA mutase activity and decreased serum MMA.[17] High-dose oral vitamin $B_{12}$ lowered mean MMA concentrations in normal subjects who had baseline concentrations over 240 nmol/L.[18] Elevated MMA is the first laboratory abnormality detected in infrequently treated subjects with pernicious anemia.[19] Also, some subjects with pernicious anemia have a marked rise in serum MMA when intramuscular injections of CN-Cbl are decreased in frequency from once a week to once every 4 weeks.[20] This exquisite sensitivity of the concentrations of MMA to the depletion or repletion of Cbl suggests that the percentage of holo-mutase must have some physiologic importance.

This pathway is an extremely important source of energy in ruminants, since the bacterial fermentation in the rumen produces large quantities of propionic acid. However, this pathway is also important in humans, because congenital defects of the mutase or of the ability to synthesize adenosyl-Cbl result in life-threatening methylmalonicaciduria, which is complicated by severe metabolic ketoacidosis.[9] Serum, urine, and cerebrospinal MMA concentrations are always increased in conditions of vitamin $B_{12}$ deficiency, such as that associated with human

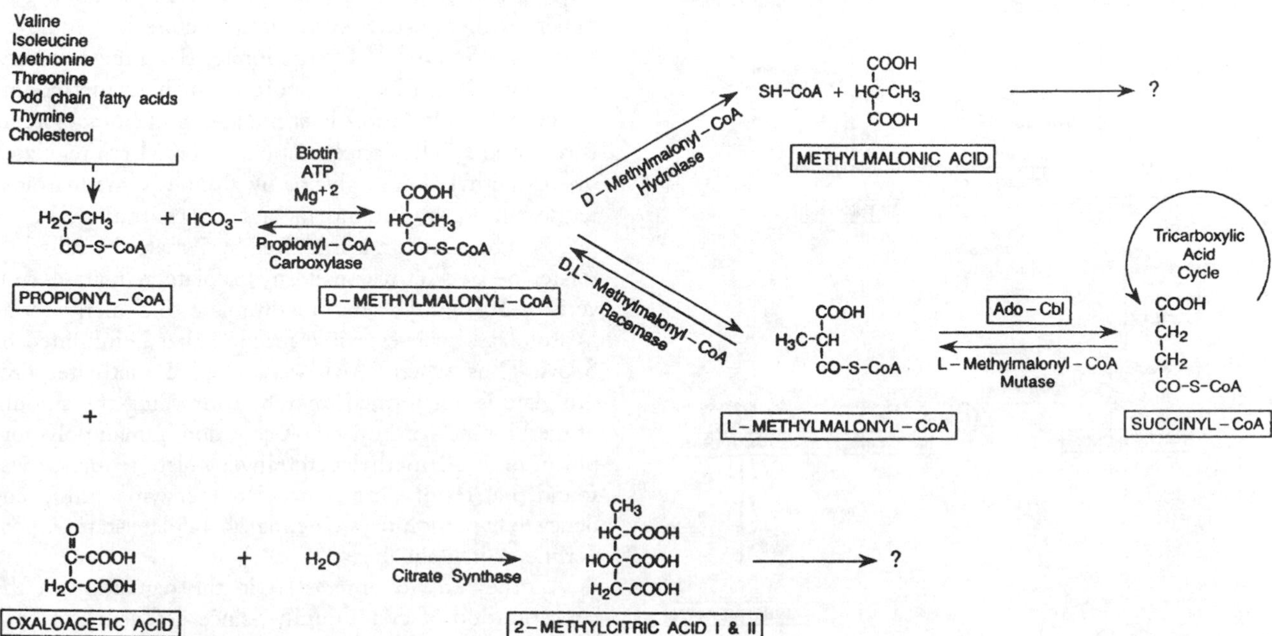


Figure 2. The pathways of propionyl-CoA and methylmalonyl-CoA. (Used with permission from Allen et al., 1993.[12])

malabsorption syndromes,[21-23] human or animal nitrous oxide-induced cobalamin inactivation,[17,23] dietary- or analog-induced animal deficiency,[17] and ruminants with cobalt deficiency.[24] Cells in tissue culture depleted of Cbl or treated with Cbl analogs also increase excretion of MMA into the media.[25] The sensitive relationship between vitamin $B_{12}$ status and quantities of MMA in body fluids has proven to be useful in investigating the pathophysiology of vitamin $B_{12}$ depletion and in the diagnosis of human or animal deficiency.

# Methionine Synthase

The pathway of methionine metabolism is shown in Figure 3.[27] Methionine is an essential amino acid that is necessary for protein synthesis but is also a crucial methyl donor after activation to S-adenosylmethionine (SAM). SAM is a source of methyl groups for the synthesis of creatine (quantitatively the most important) phospholipids and neurotransmitters, and for DNA, RNA, and protein methylation.[27] After donating the methyl group, S-adenosylhomocysteine (SAH) is formed, which is cleaved to homocysteine and adenosine by SAH-hydrolase. The homocysteine that is generated can either be remethylated to form methionine or be condensed with

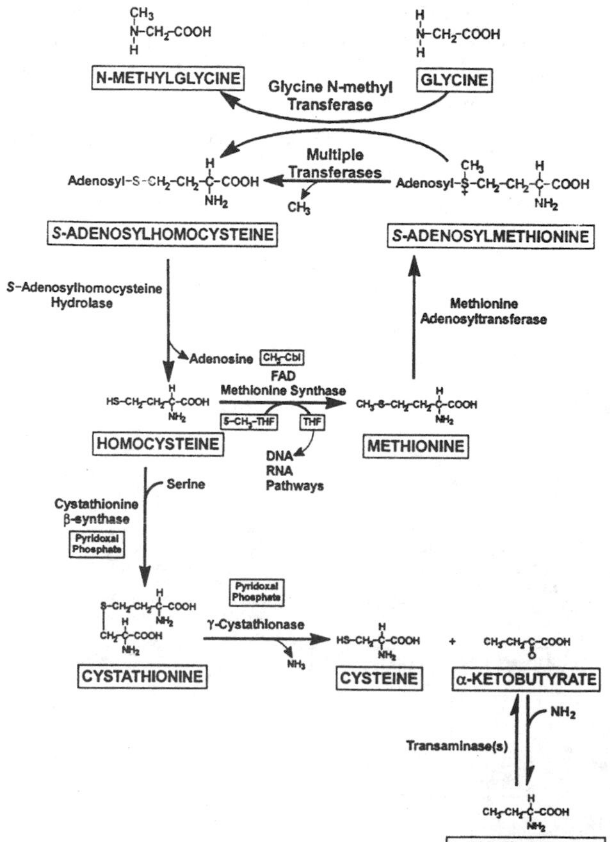


Figure 3. The pathways of methionine metabolism. (Used with permission from Allen et al., 1993.[26])

serine to form cystathionine by a vitamin $B_6$-dependent enzyme, cystathionine β-synthase. Cystathionine is further metabolized to cysteine and α-ketobutyrate by another vitamin $B_6$-dependent enzyme, γ-cystathionase.

Methionine can be synthesized by two different enzymes: Cbl-dependent methionine synthase and betaine-homocysteine methyltransferase.[28] Methionine synthase transfers a methyl group from 5-methyltetrahydrofolate to homocysteine.[5] The methyl-Cbl bound to the methionine synthase is demethylated in the reaction with the homocysteine and is then re-methylated by the reaction with 5-methyltetrahydrofolate.[5] SAM is also required because occasionally the active Cbl form, cob(1) alamin, is oxidized and must be reduced by obtaining a methyl group from SAM. Investigations show that there is also a human methionine synthase reductase that is a flavoprotein.[29] Methionine synthase is a cytoplasmic enzyme containing 1 mol Cbl/1 mol protein.[5,30]

As can be seen in Figure 3, the balance of methionine metabolism is dependent on three vitamins: vitamin $B_{12}$, folate, and vitamin $B_6$. A congenital defect of cystathionine β-synthase causes classical homocystinuria.[27] Congenital defects of methionine synthase or the synthesis of methyl-Cbl have also been described, and they cause severe hyperhomocysteinemia.[9] Deficiencies of either vitamin $B_{12}$ or folic acid also result in hyperhomocysteinemia.[21,31,32] Elevations of serum total homocysteine (tHcy) are associated with accelerated vascular disease and thrombosis, which has generated much interest in this field of congenital and acquired defects.[33]

Homocysteine is at a branch point between the re-methylation (transmethylation) to methionine and the reaction to form cystathionine, which is called transsulfuration. Transsulfuration is not reversible and eventually results in the removal of the sulfhydral group. In steady-state conditions, it appears that each homocysteine moiety is methylated several times before it is removed by transsulfuration.[34] Cystathionine β-synthase is activated by SAM; thus, in conditions of high methionine intake, transsulfuration is stimulated and homocysteine is removed.[34] The concentrations of SAM are regulated by the methylation of glycine by glycine N-methyltransferase, an enzyme found in high concentrations in the liver.[35] This reaction is inhibited by 5-methyltetrahydrofolate. 5–10-Methylenetetrahydrofolate reductase converts 5–10-methylenetetrahydrofolate to 5-methyltetrahydrofolate, an irreversible reaction that is inhibited by SAM. Thus, when SAM is abundant, 5-methyltetrahydrofolate is not formed, thereby controlling the amount of methionine synthesized. A common human polymorphism of 5–10-methylenetetrahydrofolate reductase was found that results in a thermolabile enzyme and a tendency to hyperhomocysteinemia when folate status is borderline or inadequate.[36,37]

Another area of interest is in the regulation of the concentration of cystathionine, since deficiency of both vitamin $B_{12}$ and folate causes marked rises in serum cystathionine[38] despite the fact that there is experimental evidence and theoretical reasons to believe that the deficiency of SAM in these conditions should result in a decrease in transsulfuration and the formation of cystathionine.[34]

# Metabolic Abnormalities in Vitamin $B_{12}$ Deficiency

Table 1 shows the four metabolites—MMA, homocysteine, cystathionine, and 2-methylcitric acid—that are found in elevated concentrations in body fluids (serum, urine, cerebrospinal fluid) and tissues. They occur in humans with pernicious anemia[12,21-23,38] and with other forms of vitamin $B_{12}$ deficiency, and in spontaneously occurring animal models of vitamin $B_{12}$ deficiency[24] and in experimental animal models that employ dietary means, cobalamin analogs, or nitrous oxide treatment to induce deficiency.[17] In 1962, Cox and White[22] demonstrated that 95% of symptomatic vitamin $B_{12}$-deficient humans had elevated concentrations of MMA in their urine that responded to therapy with vitamin $B_{12}$. Their work has been repeatedly confirmed over the last 40-plus years, and it is now well accepted that virtually every patient who has clinical abnormalities that respond to vitamin $B_{12}$ replacement has elevated MMA.[21,39-41] Elevations of MMA are highly specific to Cbl metabolism, with the exception of modest elevations seen in chronic renal insufficiency,[42] although these may actually respond to some degree to vitamin $B_{12}$ administration. Thus, monitoring MMA is extremely useful in diagnosing, studying treatment response, and documenting vitamin $B_{12}$ deficiency in animal or cellular models.

**Table 1.** Laboratory Abnormalities in Vitamin $B_{12}$ Deficiency

| |
|---|
| Metabolites |
| High methylmalonic acid |
| High total homocysteine |
| High cystathionine |
| High 2-methylcitric acid |
| Megaloblastic anemia |
| Peripheral blood |
| Low red blood cell count |
| Low hemoglobin and hematocrit |
| Low white blood cell count |
| Low platelet count |
| High mean cell volume |
| Hypersegmented granulocytes |
| Bone marrow |
| Hypercellularity |
| Nuclear-cytoplasmic desynchrony |
| Open nuclear chromatin pattern |
| Giant metamyelocytes and bands |
| Intramedullary cell death |
| Blood chemistry |
| Increased bilirubin |
| Increased lactate dehydrogenase |

Figure 2 shows that propionyl-CoA can be condensed with oxaloacetic acid by a mitochondrial enzyme, citrate synthase, to form 2-methylcitric acid. Elevated concentrations of 2-methylcitric acid are found in patients with inborn errors of mutase and adenosyl-Cbl synthesis, in severely affected vitamin $B_{12}$-deficient subjects, and in animal models of vitamin $B_{12}$ deficiency.[12]

Total homocysteine is frequently elevated in the serum and urine of humans with pernicious anemia[21,31,32] and other forms of vitamin $B_{12}$ deficiency and in all of the animal models of vitamin $B_{12}$ deficiency.[17] Elevated tHcy concentrations are not specific to vitamin $B_{12}$ deficiency, in contrast to MMA, since subjects with dietary folate deficiency[21,43] or defects of cystathionine β-synthase, methionine adenosyltransferase, 5–10-methylenetetrahydrofolate reductase, methionine synthase, or in the reductive pathway necessary for synthesis of methyl-Cbl may also have elevated tHcy.[9,27] The tHcy concentration is highly correlated with serum creatinine, at least partly because of the role of SAM in the formation of creatine, the precursor of creatinine.[44] However, subjects with chronic renal insufficiency and renal failure frequently have elevated tHcy concentrations that are partially responsive to large doses of vitamins, including folic acid, vitamin $B_{12}$, and possibly vitamin $B_6$.[45] The mean tHcy value of a population appears to be highly dependent on dietary and supplemental intakes of folate and vitamin $B_{12}$.[46] These additional influences make elevated tHcy less specific as a diagnostic tool for vitamin $B_{12}$ deficiency. However, it has been shown that elevated tHcy caused by vitamin $B_{12}$ deficiency is not corrected with folic acid treatment.[47]

Serum cystathionine concentration is elevated in most subjects with severe vitamin $B_{12}$ deficiency.[38] Like total homocysteine, it is not specific to vitamin $B_{12}$ deficiency, since folate deficiency and especially vitamin $B_6$ deficiency[48] also cause elevated concentrations.

Serum MMA and tHcy concentrations can reach extremely high levels in severe symptomatic vitamin $B_{12}$ deficiency, as shown in Figure 4. Only three of 313 subjects with well-documented vitamin $B_{12}$ deficiency (mostly pernicious anemia) with megaloblastic anemia had normal concentrations of both metabolites.[21] The MMA and tHcy were elevated in 121 subjects who had the neurologic syndrome of vitamin $B_{12}$ deficiency without anemia in that study.[21]

There are alterations in the total CoA pool and in carnitine metabolism as a result of the buildup of methylmalonyl-CoA in animal models of vitamin $B_{12}$ deficiency.[49,50] The increase in propionyl-CoA appears to lead to increased formation of branched-chain and odd-chain fatty acids in both inborn errors of mutase and severe vitamin $B_{12}$ deficiency.[51,52]

Figure 3 demonstrates that there are interactions between vitamin $B_{12}$ and folate metabolism. The irreversible reaction that forms 5-methyltetrahydrofolate results in a metabolically inactive form of folate unless it is demethylated by methionine synthase. 5-Methyltetrahydrofolate

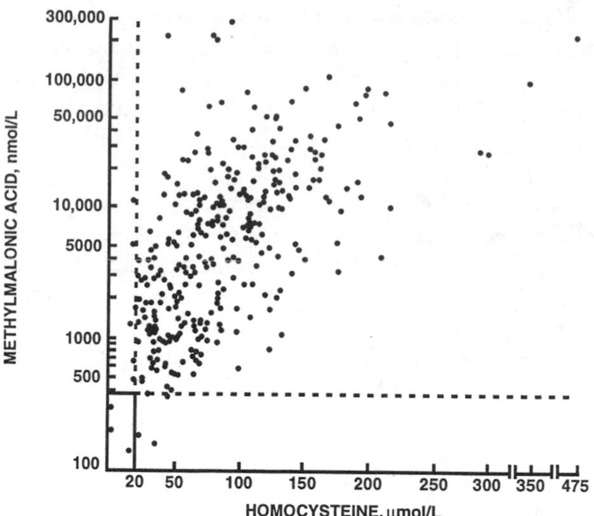


Figure 4. Serum methylmalonic acid and total homocysteine concentrations are shown in 313 episodes of cobalamin-deficient megaloblastic anemia. The dashed lines represent three standard deviations above the mean for normal controls. (From Savage et al., 1994[21] with permission from Excerpta Medica, Inc.)

is a poor substrate for folyl polyglutamate synthase and thus is not retained intracellularly and can be lost in the urine.[53] Therefore, there is "trapping" of folate as 5-methyltetrahydrofolate in severe vitamin $B_{12}$ deficiency, and this may result in secondary folate deficiency.[54] Because other forms of folate are necessary for thymidine and purine synthesis, impairments in DNA synthesis result (see below). There also are abnormalities in one-carbon metabolism in vitamin $B_{12}$ deficiency, probably because of secondary folate deficiency. For example, serum serine concentrations are elevated in animals[49] with $B_{12}$ deficiency and forminoglutamic acid in the urine[55] and formic acid in urine and blood in vitamin $B_{12}$ deficiency.[56]

# Clinical Manifestations of Vitamin $B_{12}$ Deficiency

Clinical manifestations of vitamin $B_{12}$ deficiency have been most thoroughly studied in humans with pernicious anemia. Although there are spontaneously occurring animal models of vitamin $B_{12}$ deficiency, such as ruminants pastured on cobalt-deficient soil[24] and dogs with selective malabsorption of vitamin $B_{12}$,[57] these animals do not display a syndrome similar to that of humans. The cobalamin-deficient ruminants had metabolic abnormalities such as elevated MMA similar to that in humans,[24] but they did not develop megaloblastic anemia analogous to that seen in humans and they did not develop the demyelinating lesions of the spinal cord seen in humans. Likewise, the dogs suffered severe metabolic abnormalities and failure to thrive, but they also did not have megaloblastic anemia or neurologic disease.[57] Other animal models of vitamin $B_{12}$ deficiency have also been disappointing in that dietary deficiency and nitrous oxide exposure[17] did not result in the megaloblastic anemia seen in humans. In one investigation,[58] Cbl-analog treatment of minipigs caused mild anemia and leukopenia, although the increase in mean red cell volume and morphologic changes in the bone marrow were very subtle compared with what would be expected in humans. The lack of convenient animal models has been a detriment to the study of vitamin $B_{12}$, and as a result most of the information described below comes from human studies.

## *Megaloblastic Anemia*

In humans, vitamin $B_{12}$ and folate deficiency cause identical forms of megaloblastic anemia.[59] This constellation of morphologic changes and clinical and laboratory abnormalities is due to an imbalance of decreased DNA synthesis and adequate RNA synthesis and is present in other clinical situations in which DNA synthesis is impaired. Because vitamin $B_{12}$ and folate deficiency cause identical lesions, it is thought that the secondary block in folate metabolism in vitamin $B_{12}$ deficiency is the underlying cause. The nuclei of the developing hematopoietic precursor cells in the bone marrow remain immature compared with the cytoplasm, which is maturing normally. The morphologic result is a macrocytic red blood cell (high mean cell volume) with an open chromatin pattern in the precursor nuclei. The white blood cells are enlarged and the mature granulocytes show hypersegmentation of their nuclei. Many cells die in the bone marrow, possibly by apoptosis. This is called ineffective erythropoiesis, and leads to the cellular release of bilirubin and lactate dehydrogenase into the blood.[59] When extremely severe, the profound anemia and decreased white blood cell and platelet counts combined with a cellular bone marrow packed with very immature-appearing erythroblasts have led to the mistaken diagnosis of acute leukemia. The bone marrow lesion can be completely cured with vitamin $B_{12}$ treatment. There is a rapid response with correction of hypersegmentation and the production of new red blood cells (reticulocytes). The megaloblastic anemia of vitamin $B_{12}$ deficiency can be partially corrected with folate treatment, which can lead to diagnostic errors. The results of treating vitamin $B_{12}$-deficient patients with folic acid have been thoroughly reviewed previously[54]; ultimately, many of the patients studied succumbed to rapid relapse of anemia and/or neurologic disease.

Megaloblastic anemia presents the classic picture of severe vitamin $B_{12}$-deficient anemia. More recently, many patients have only mild abnormalities of blood cells and bone marrow but may have had severe abnormalities of the nervous system.[60] Serum MMA and tHcy are markedly elevated in patients with and without megaloblastic anemia.[21] The reasons for a patient's susceptibility to megaloblastic anemia versus neurologic abnormalities are unexplained at the present time. The use of MMA and tHcy as screening tests has also led to the realization that a significant fraction of individuals with biochemically severe vitamin $B_{12}$ deficiency appear to have no signs of megaloblastic anemia or neurologic abnormalities.[61]

### *Neurologic Abnormalities*

Vitamin $B_{12}$ deficiency, whether naturally occurring or induced by nitrous oxide, leads to a demyelinating disorder of the central nervous system in humans,[60,62] nonhuman primates,[63] fruit bats,[64] and swine,[58,65] but not in other animal species. This lesion was described long before the underlying vitamin $B_{12}$ dependence was recognized. It has been termed "subacute combined degeneration" or "combined systems disease."[59] The pathology includes swelling of myelin sheaths and patchy vacuolation of myelin, with spongy degeneration of the spinal cord, starting in the thoracic and cervical dorsal columns and progressing to the lateral columns. Lesions are also seen in the brain and optic nerves and possibly the peripheral nerves. Signs and symptoms vary considerably among individuals, but the most common symptom seen in a large review of well-documented cases was painful paresthesia of the extremities.[62] The most common sign was loss of proprioception and vibration sense in the toes or ankles. One of the most intriguing discoveries has been the inverse relationship between the severity of the hematologic and neurologic abnormalities.[62] Only about one-third of patients with pernicious anemia develop neurologic abnormalities.[21] Approximately 25% of these will have almost completely normal hematologic parameters, which caused great difficulty in diagnosis in the past.[60] Serum MMA and tHcy and all of the other metabolic changes are similar in subjects with involvement of only the nervous system compared with subjects with only hematologic involvement.[21] Thus, it can be easily proved that a patient with spinal cord symptoms has vitamin $B_{12}$ deficiency even without anemia. Vitamin $B_{12}$ treatment will partially or completely correct the lesions if begun promptly.

The underlying biochemical abnormalities leading to demyelination of the central nervous system are not understood. There are intriguing negative data from observations of individuals with methylmalonicaciduria caused by mutase defects or impaired adenosyl-Cbl synthesis who do not develop the demyelinating disease of the spinal cord seen in vitamin $B_{12}$ deficiency.[9] Likewise, patients with severe folate deficiency and elevations of tHcy similar to the levels seen in vitamin $B_{12}$ deficiency do not develop myelopathy.[21] However, defects in Cbl metabolism that cause combined methylmalonicaciduria and hyperhomocysteinemia cause central nervous system disease similar to that seen in vitamin $B_{12}$ deficiency.[9] It appears that the activity of both cobalamin-dependent enzymes must be impaired to cause the demyelinating disease, although defects of methionine synthase might be an exception. There is also no explanation for why most animal species are resistant to the development of spinal cord defects.

### *Clinical Spectrum of Vitamin $B_{12}$ Deficiency*

Vitamin $B_{12}$ deficiency has a very wide spectrum of severity and manifestations.[59] The severe lesions of megaloblastic anemia and neurologic disease are discussed above. Some patients may have concentrations of MMA and tHcy as high as other patients with severe abnormalities but have no clinical symptoms.[61] Others may have additional symptoms such as glossitis of the tongue, weight loss, mental changes, and even infertility.[59] The clinical spectrum in infants is also markedly different from that in adults. Infants fed vitamin $B_{12}$-deficient breast milk develop lethargy, failure to thrive, irritability, and poor brain growth, leading to permanent developmental delay in some cases.[66]

## Causes of Vitamin $B_{12}$ Deficiency

All animals require vitamin $B_{12}$ and obtain it ultimately from the products of microbial synthesis.[8] Ruminant animals carry bacteria that synthesize cobalamins in their rumens. Herbivorous animals appear to obtain vitamin $B_{12}$ from eating feces or feces-contaminated vegetable foods. Omnivorous animals, including humans, obtain vitamin $B_{12}$ from products of animal origin, including meats, dairy products, and eggs.[67] It is possible that humans also obtain vitamin $B_{12}$ from sewage-contaminated foods. In the last 30 years, synthetic vitamin $B_{12}$ has been added to many cereals and other foods in Western countries, so fortification is also a major source of the vitamin.

### *Absorption and Intracellular Metabolism of Vitamin $B_{12}$*

Vitamin $B_{12}$ is generally bound to one of the two enzymes or other carrier proteins in food, so it must be released prior to absorption.[68] This process starts when food is chewed and mixed with saliva, which contains a Cbl-binding protein, R protein (haptocorrin). The bound Cbl is further released from the proteins in the acid environment of the stomach, where peptic digestion of proteins begins. The released vitamin $B_{12}$ is bound to R protein and carried to the duodenum. The specific Cbl-binding protein intrinsic factor (IF) is released by the gastric parietal cells, but does not bind Cbl until stomach acid is neutralized in the duodenum and digestive enzymes remove the R binder from the vitamin.[68] The binding of IF is very specific for Cbl and thus may prevent the binding and absorption of Cbl analogs also found in foods. The IF-Cbl is carried to the ileum, where a specific receptor for IF-Cbl—a complex of cubilin, amnionless, and possibly megalin[69]—has been described. During uptake, the bound IF-Cbl is internalized by receptor-mediated endocytosis. It appears that inborn errors of vitamin $B_{12}$ malabsorption and Immerslund-Gräsbeck syndrome are due to mutations in the gene for cubulin, at least in Finnish patients.[69,70]

It is not known exactly how the absorbed Cbl is then

processed so that a complex of transcobalamin II-Cbl (TCII-Cbl) is secreted into the portal blood and delivered to the liver and ultimately all tissues. TCII is the primary serum transport protein for vitamin $B_{12}$.[9,71] The TCII-Cbl is taken up by receptor-mediated endocytosis and fused to lysosomes in which the Cbl is released.[9] Defects of TCII cause severe megaloblastic anemia, elevations of MMA and tHcy, neurologic disease, and immune deficiency in the first few months of life. However, because most of the vitamin $B_{12}$ in serum is bound to other proteins—transcobalamin I (TCI) and transcobalamin III (TCIII)—these patients do not manifest a low serum vitamin $B_{12}$ concentration. There is also an inborn error in the lysosomal release of vitamin $B_{12}$, called CblF, which results in a similar syndrome.[9]

After the Cbl is released from the lysosomes, the coenzyme forms must be synthesized before they can act as cofactors. A number of defects of intracellular Cbl metabolism have been described, forming eight complementation groups with three generally similar clinical syndromes.[9] If there is a defect in synthesizing methionine or in regenerating $CH_3$-Cbl (methionine synthase, CblE, CblG), the patients have only hyperhomocysteinemia.[9] Other complementation groups have defects in L-methylmalonal-CoA mutase or in the formation of adenosyl-Cbl (mut$^o$, mut$^-$, CblA, CblB), and these patients have only methylmalonicacidemia and aciduria. However, there also are patients who have difficulty with the lysozomol release of Cbl (CblF), described above, or with a reduction step common to the synthesis of both coenzymes (CblC, CblD) who have combined hyperhomocysteinemia and methylmalonicaciduria. Patients with the combined disorders and patients with disorders that affect only the $CH_3$-Cbl synthesis or methionine synthase have megaloblastic anemia and neurologic abnormalities. Those who have defects that affect only adenosyl-Cbl or the mutase do not have megaloblastic anemia or demyelinization.[9]

## *Acquired Vitamin $B_{12}$ Deficiency*

The major causes of vitamin $B_{12}$ deficiency are shown in Table 2. The rare congenital defects involving the uptake proteins IF and cubulin, the processes involved with intracellular release and transport, and the defects of the Cbl-dependent enzymes have already been discussed. By far the most common causes of vitamin $B_{12}$ deficiency relate to acquired malabsorption.

Dietary deficiency of vitamin $B_{12}$ is rare because of the widespread consumption of foods of animal origin. The bioavailability of vitamin $B_{12}$ may vary among foods. Absolute vegetarianism, excluding even the consumption of dairy products, will lead to vitamin $B_{12}$ deficiency after 5 to 10 years.[59] However, many meat substitute foods in the United States are supplemented with vitamin $B_{12}$, so deficiency is rare if such products are consumed. Exclusively breast-fed infants of mothers with untreated pernicious anemia or who follow a vegetarian diet are at risk

**Table 2.** Causes of Vitamin $B_{12}$ Deficiency

| |
|---|
| Animals |
| Cobalt-deficient soil (ruminants only) |
| Congenital ileal malabsorption (dogs and cats) |
| Human |
| Dietary |
| Lack of foods of animal origin |
| Vitamin $B_{12}$-deficient breast milk |
| Malabsorption |
| Pernicious anemia |
| Protein-bound $B_{12}$ malabsorption |
| Pancreatic insufficiency |
| Jejunal bacterial overgrowth |
| Fish tapeworm |
| Tropical sprue |
| Total or partial gastric resection or bypass |
| Ileal disease or resection |
| Ileal-urinary conduit |
| Drugs |
| Nitrous oxide |
| Metformin |
| Stomach acid blockers |
| Congenital |
| Intrinsic factor defect |
| Transcobalamin II defect |
| Immerslund-Gräsbeck syndrome |
| Cb1A-Cb1G defects |

for deficiency, since the breast milk may be deficient in vitamin $B_{12}$ at a time when a mother is asymptomatic. Such infants display failure to thrive, with poor brain growth, developmental abnormalities, and megaloblastic anemia. The delay in diagnosis and treatment in such infants may lead to tragic neurologic consequences.[66]

Pernicious anemia, an autoimmune disease, is the most common cause of severe malabsorption of vitamin $B_{12}$.[59] Chronic autoimmune atrophic gastritis (type A atrophic gastritis) develops with antibodies to gastric parietal cells[72] and, in 50% of affected individuals, to IF.[59] The gastric parietal cell $H^+/K^+$-ATPase has been shown to be the antigen against which parietal cell antibodies are directed.[72] Because there is a complete loss of IF, vitamin $B_{12}$ malabsorption ensues. The disease is found in all races and ethnic groups throughout the world, and the prevalence increases with age and female sex.[59] Although rare, pernicious anemia occurs even in young people, and people of African origin may be at higher risk for young onset. One study found that the prevalence in people over age 65 years was 1.9%.[73] Patients with pernicious anemia have an impaired enterohepatic circulation of Cbl because the Cbl secreted in the bile cannot be bound to IF and is lost in the stool, leading to rapid depletion of Cbl when treatment is discontinued.[68]

Surgical manipulations of the gastrointestinal tract, including total and partial gastrectomy, gastric bypass operations, ileal resections, and ileal urinary conduit constructions, frequently lead to vitamin $B_{12}$ malabsorption.[68,74] Parasitic infection with the fish tapeworm and jejunal bacterial overgrowth have been shown to cause vitamin $B_{12}$ deficiency. Chronic inflammatory diseases of the ileum such as Crohn's disease or tropical sprue can also lead to vitamin $B_{12}$ deficiency.[59]

Up to 15% of elderly subjects were found to have mild to moderate vitamin $B_{12}$ deficiency documented by elevated MMA and tHcy concentrations and decreased serum Cbl levels.[61,75] Only a minority of these vitamin-deficient subjects had true pernicious anemia as documented by anti-IF antibodies or abnormal results on the classic Schilling test. The others may have had abnormalities in the release of vitamin $B_{12}$ from food and varying degrees of atrophic gastritis and achlorhydria[76] or competition for uptake of $B_{12}$ by bacterial overgrowth. Although the cause for malabsorption in these subjects remains controversial,[76] their metabolic and hematologic abnormalities improved promptly with parenteral or high-dose oral vitamin $B_{12}$ therapy.[61] Research is needed to determine adequate doses of synthetic vitamin $B_{12}$ in supplements and fortified foods for this clinical situation.

Nitrous oxide is a widely used anesthetic agent that rapidly inactivates the $CH_3$-Cbl bound to methionine synthase. Chronic intermittent abuse of nitrous oxide has been shown to cause a demyelinating nervous system disease.[23] Recent reports suggest that if borderline vitamin $B_{12}$-deficient patients are treated with nitrous oxide anesthesia, they can develop a demyelinating syndrome weeks to months postoperatively.[77] The widespread use of stomach acid blockers such as histamine blockers or proton pump inhibitors can lead to a syndrome similar to the malabsorption of protein-bound $B_{12}$.[68] Further studies of the epidemiology of this problem are needed.

## Diagnosis of Vitamin $B_{12}$ Deficiency

The mainstay of diagnosis of vitamin $B_{12}$ deficiency is a low serum Cbl level.[59] Microbial assays were initially used, which were followed by radiodilution assays using purified IF as the binder, and now there are even newer assays available. The use of serum assays for diagnosis is complicated by the fact that only about 20% of Cbl is carried on TCII, the physiologic delivery protein.[71] Also, the known roles for Cbl are all intracellular, and tissue levels may not necessarily reflect those found in plasma. In general, there is a rough correlation with serum Cbl values such that extremely low concentrations often indicate clinical deficiency and values above the mean for a population generally can be interpreted as adequate.[75] However, when serum MMA and tHcy are correlated with serum vitamin levels, there are subjects with deficiency whose Cbl levels are above the lower limit of the normal range, and many subjects with low Cbl who have normal serum metabolites, suggesting that they are not deficient.[19,61,75] Abnormalities of MMA and tHcy correlate better with response to therapy than do vitamin levels.[39] The elevated metabolites decrease promptly with vitamin $B_{12}$ therapy and rise in poorly compliant or infrequently treated patients prior to the development of anemia or, in some cases, low serum Cbl levels.[19,20,39]

A comparison of serum Cbl concentration versus serum or red cell folate concentration is frequently used to distinguish between the megaloblastic anemia resulting from deficiencies of either Cbl or folate.[54] This can also lead to diagnostic errors because red cell folate is low in subjects deficient in both vitamin $B_{12}$ and folate, and because serum folate can occasionally be low in vitamin $B_{12}$ deficiency.[54,59] It is poor medical practice to treat vitamin $B_{12}$-deficient patients with folic acid alone, since neurologic abnormalities caused by vitamin $B_{12}$ deficiency will not respond, even though megaloblastic anemia may respond to the wrong vitamin (i.e., folic acid).[54] However, because MMA concentrations are elevated only with vitamin $B_{12}$ deficiency, it is possible to at least determine that a patient with megaloblastic anemia has vitamin $B_{12}$ deficiency, although in some cases there may also be coexisting folate deficiency.[21]

In the last 100 years, the medical literature describes many subjects with severe neurologic and psychiatric abnormalities owing to vitamin $B_{12}$ deficiency in the absence of anemia, but diagnostic tests for vitamin $B_{12}$ deficiency often rely too heavily on the presence of megaloblastic anemia.[59] In fact, well-studied cohorts of vitamin $B_{12}$-deficient subjects show that there is an inverse correlation between the severity of neurologic disease and hematologic disease.[60,62]

In some cases, it will be clinically useful to determine the cause of the vitamin $B_{12}$ deficiency, since there may be a gastrointestinal pathology that needs to be treated. The presence of blocking anti-IF antibodies is diagnostic of pernicious anemia, but the test is not very sensitive.[59] The Schilling test determines the quantity of radioactive Cbl that is excreted in the urine after an oral dose of crystalline Cbl. A positive Schilling test that corrects with the addition of IF is diagnostic of pernicious anemia. Much research has been directed toward developing a protein- or food-bound Cbl absorption test, but the difference between healthy elderly and those with malabsorption appears to be so small that such a test would not be specific enough.[76] Children with metabolic Cbl deficiency clearly should be evaluated for inborn errors of metabolism or the congenital defects of malabsorption, which require lifelong surveillance and treatment as well as monitoring of siblings.

## Treatment of Vitamin $B_{12}$ Deficiency

The true vegan can be treated with small doses of oral vitamin $B_{12}$ supplements, since the daily requirement is only 2.4 μg. Parenteral vitamin $B_{12}$ is used in the United States primarily for the treatment of vitamin $B_{12}$ deficiency caused by pernicious anemia and other forms of malabsorption. A standard therapy regimen is to start with weekly intramuscular injections of 1000 μg CN-Cbl for 4 to 8 weeks until the clinical response is clearly evident, followed by monthly injections for life. An occasional patient will have serum MMA levels above the normal range on monthly injections and will require more frequent treatment.[20] High-dose daily oral therapy may be a good alternative to intermittent parenteral treatment. Investigations from 40 years ago showed that subjects with pernicious anemia absorb about 1% of a radioactively labeled oral dose.[78] It has been shown that subjects with pernicious anemia can be maintained on daily oral doses of 500 μg/d.[79] A recent investigation showed that 2000 μg/d resulted in much higher serum Cbl concentrations and lower MMA concentrations than did monthly injections of Cbl.[20] Thus, it is possible that the treatment of choice should be high-dose oral therapy. The commonly available multivitamin preparations in the United States contain much lower quantities of vitamin $B_{12}$, usually 6 to 9 μg, but some marketed to seniors contain 25 to 75 μg. Although serum Cbl concentrations are higher in seniors who take multivitamins, the serum MMA concentrations were not corrected in many individuals.[80,81] Also, subjects with pernicious anemia cannot be treated with standard multivitamin preparations containing low quantities of vitamin $B_{12}$. The efficacy of various oral vitamin $B_{12}$ doses is an area of active research. It is hoped that comparisons of pre- and post-treatment MMA and vitamin concentrations will result in the determination of an efficacious dose.

In most cases, vitamin $B_{12}$ therapy must be continued for life. It is thus imperative to fully document the deficiency prior to treatment and to convince the patient that treatment is an ongoing, lifelong necessity. Compliance with any lifetime therapy raises many issues. Some clinicians feel that requiring a patient to receive a vitamin $B_{12}$ injection by a health care provider emphasizes the importance of regular therapy. However, the pain and inconvenience of parenteral therapy, especially if not self-administered, may lead to poor compliance and cessation of treatment. A widely available and economical oral high-dose vitamin $B_{12}$ preparation would eliminate this. Another potential problem is that vitamin therapy is seen by the general public as a largely optional health-enhancing practice, whereas in pernicious anemia, vitamin $B_{12}$ replacement is necessary to sustain life. It is thus a challenge for health care providers to educate and monitor patients with pernicious anemia and other forms of vitamin $B_{12}$ deficiency if they change their therapy from parenteral to home-administered daily oral therapy. This is especially important now that the US food supply has been fortified with folic acid.

## Continuing Controversies and Future Prospects for Vitamin $B_{12}$ Nutrition

In the United States, folic acid has been added to fortified grain products since January 1998, and low serum folate concentrations have been virtually eliminated.[82,83] Serum folate levels have increased 2- to 4-fold, and serum tHcy concentrations have decreased.[82,83] The marked change in serum folate levels suggests that folate fortification has been very effective. Patients with pernicious anemia or other forms of severe vitamin $B_{12}$ deficiency may have been put at risk, however. It is possible that some individuals will consume enough folic acid in the diet to mask megaloblastic anemia caused by pernicious anemia, thus delaying diagnosis or even precipitating a vitamin $B_{12}$-deficient neurologic syndrome.

There is speculation that increased folate intake will decrease the prevalence of hyperhomocysteinemia from folate deficiency and improve the vascular health of the US population.[46] Because low serum folate levels have been almost eliminated in the United States, it appears that current hyperhomocysteinemia is due mostly to vitamin $B_{12}$ deficiency. Research into the changing causes of hyperhomocysteinemia in seniors in the United States is needed to properly assess and treat these subjects. This is particularly important because in this population, it has been shown that two-thirds of hyperhomocysteinemic subjects have elevated MMA concentrations and are thereby deficient in at least vitamin $B_{12}$.[61,84] The elderly, like everyone else, are now eating a folate-fortified diet, and it is not known whether there will be consequences from the folate treatment without adequate vitamin $B_{12}$ status.

Seniors deficient in vitamin $B_{12}$ may have impaired cognition and abnormalities with neurophysiologic testing despite no evidence of megaloblastic anemia.[85] Because it has been difficult to prove clinical benefit with vitamin $B_{12}$ treatment in many elderly subjects, there is controversy about the benefits of screening for and treating this deficiency. If clinical trials of the efficacy of lowering tHcy concentrations in vascular disease prove to be positive, it will be even more important to treat vitamin $B_{12}$-deficient subjects with vitamin $B_{12}$ and folic acid to optimize vascular health. Many of these subjects may have protein-bound vitamin $B_{12}$ malabsorption rather than pernicious anemia, and could perhaps be treated with smaller supplements of oral vitamin $B_{12}$, since IF secretion may be preserved in such individuals.[76] However, at present we do not have recommendations for a minimum effective oral dose of vitamin $B_{12}$. It would seem prudent to use the same high dose of oral vitamin $B_{12}$ used in pernicious anemia to treat this population.

The actual biochemical lesion in demyelination of the vitamin $B_{12}$-deficient nervous system continues to elude us. Further research should be directed to the role of vitamin $B_{12}$ in these processes, since the basic mechanisms may be important in other demyelinating syndromes.

## References


1. Castle WB. The history of corrinoids. In: Babior BM, ed. *Cobalamin Biochemistry and Pathophysiology*. New York: Wiley Interscience; 1975; 1–17.
2. Minot GR, Murphy WP. Treatment of pernicious anemia by a special diet. JAMA. 1926;87:470–476.
3. Folkers K. History of B12: pernicious anemia to crystalline cyanocobalamin. In: Dolphin D, ed. *B12*. New York: Wiley Interscience; 1982; 1–5.
4. Hogenkamp HPC. B12: 1948–1998. In: Banerjee R, ed. *Chemistry and Biochemistry of B12*. New York: Wiley Interscience; 1999; 3–8.
5. Ludwig ML, Mathews RG. Structure-based perspectives on B12-dependent enzymes. Annu Rev Biochem. 1997;66:269–313.
6. Battersby AR. How nature builds the pigments of life: the conquest of vitamin B12. Science. 1994;264: 1551–1557.
7. Santander PJ, Roessner CA, Stolowich NJ, et al. How corrinoids are synthesized without oxygen: nature's first pathway to vitamin B12. Chem Biol. 1997; 4:659–666.
8. Beck WS. Biological and medical aspects of vitamin B12. In: Dolphin D, ed. *B12*. New York: Wiley Interscience; 1982; 1–30.
9. Fenton WA, Rosenberg LE. Inherited disorders of cobalamin transport and metabolism. In: Scriver CR, Beaudet AL, Sly WS, Valle DR, eds. *The Metabolic and Molecular Bases of Inherited Disease*. New York: McGraw-Hill; 1995; 3129–3149.
10. Mancia F, Keep NH, Nakagawa A, et al. How coenzyme B12 radicals are generated: the crystal structure of methylmalonyl-coenzyme A mutase at 2 A resolution. Structure. 1996;4:339–350.
11. Drennan CL, Haang S, Drummond JT, et al. How a protein binds B12: A 3.0 A X-ray structure of B12-binding domains of methionine synthase. Science. 1994;266:1669–1674.
12. Allen RH, Stabler SP, Savage DG, et al. Elevation of 2-methylcitric acid I and II levels in serum, urine and cerebrospinal fluid of patients with cobalamin deficiency. Metabolism. 1993;42:978–988.
13. Kolhouse JF, Utley C, Allen RH. Isolation and characterization of methylmalonyl-CoA mutase from human placenta. J Biol Chem. 1980;255:2708–2712.
14. Jansen R, Kalousek F, Fenton WA, et al. Cloning of full-length methylmalonyl-CoA mutase from a cDNA library using the polymerase chain reaction. Genomics. 1989;4:198–205.
15. Banerjee R, Chowdhary S. Methylmalonyl-CoA mutase. In: Banerjee R, ed. *Chemistry and Biochemistry of B12*. New York: Wiley Interscience; 1999; 707–729.
16. Kondo H, Osborne ML, Kolhouse JF, et al. Nitrous oxide has multiple deleterious effects on cobalamin metabolism and causes decreases in activities of both mammalian cobalamin-dependent enzymes in rats. J Clin Invest. 1981;67:1270–1283.
17. Stabler SP, Brass EP, Allen RH, et al. Inhibition of cobalamin-dependent enzymes by cobalamin analogs in rats. J Clin Invest. 1991;87:1422–1430.
18. Rasmussen K, Moller J, Lyngbak M, et al. Age- and-gender-specific reference intervals for total homocysteine and methylmalonic acid in plasma before and after vitamin supplementation. Clin Chem. 1996;42: 630–636.
19. Lindenbaum J, Stabler SP, Allen RH. Diagnosis of cobalamin deficiency. II. Relative sensitivities of serum cobalamin, methylmalonic acid and total homocysteine concentrations. Am J Hematol. 1990;34: 99–107.
20. Kuzminski AM, Del Giacco EJ, Allen RH, et al. Effective treatment of cobalamin deficiency with oral cobalamin. Blood. 1998;92:1191–1198.
21. Savage DG, Lindenbaum J, Stabler SP, et al. Sensitivity of serum methylmalonic acid and total homocysteine determinations for diagnosing cobalamin deficiency and folate deficiencies. Am J Med. 1994; 96:239–246
22. Cox EM, White AM. Methylmalonic acid excretion: an index of vitamin B12 deficiency. Lancet. 1962;2: 853–856.
23. Stabler SP, Allen RH, Barrett RE, et al. Cerebrospinal fluid methylmalonic acid levels in normal subjects and patients with cobalamin deficiency. Neurology. 1991;41:1627–1632.
24. Rice DA, McLoughlin M, Blanchflower WJ, et al. Sequential changes in plasma methylmalonic acid and vitamin B12 in sheep eating cobalt-deficient grass. Biol Trace Elem Res. 1989;22:153–163.
25. Kolhouse JF, Stabler SP, Allen RH. Identification and perturbation of mutant human fibroblasts based on measurements of methylmalonic acid and total homocysteine in the culture media. Arch Biochem Biophys. 1993;303:355–360
26. Allen RH, Stabler SP, Lindenbaum J. Serum betaine, N-N-dimethylglycine and N-methylglycine levels in patients with cobalamin and folate deficiency and related inborn errors of metabolism. Metabolism. 1993;42:1448–1460.
27. Mudd SH, Levy HL, Skouby F. Disorders of transsulfuration. In: Scriver CR, Beaudet AL, Sly WS, Valle DR, eds. *The Metabolic and Molecular Bases of Inherited Disease*. New York: McGraw-Hill; 1995; 1279–1327.
28. Erickson LE. Betaine-homocysteine-methyl-transferases. Acta Chem Scand. 1960;14:2102–2112.
29. Leclerc D, Wilson A, Dumas R, et al. Cloning and mapping of a cDNA for methionine synthase reductase: a flavoprotein defective in patients with ho-

mocystinuria. Proc Natl Acad Sci U S A. 1998;95: 3059–3064.

30. Mathews RG. Cobalamin-dependent methionine synthase. In: Banerjee R, ed. *Chemistry and Biochemistry of B12.* New York: Wiley Interscience; 1999; 681–706.
31. Stabler SP, Marcell PD, Podell ER, et al. Elevation of total homocysteine in the serum of patients with cobalamin or folate deficiency detected by capillary gas chromatography-mass spectometry. J Clin Invest. 1988;81:466–474.
32. Brattstrom L, Israelsson B, Lindgarde F, et al. Higher total plasma homocysteine in vitamin B12 deficiency than in heterozygosity for homocystinuria due to cystathionine B-synthase deficiency. Metabolism. 1988;37:175–178.
33. Refsum H, Ueland PM, Nygard O, et al. Homocysteine and cardiovascular disease. Annu Rev Med. 1998;49:31–62.
34. Finkelstein JD. Methionine metabolism in mammals. J Nutr Biochem. 1990;1:228–237.
35. Cook RJ, Wagner C. Glycine N-methyltransferase is a folate binding protein of rat liver cytosol. Proc Natl Acad Sci U S A. 1984;81:3631–3634.
36. Frosst P, Blom HJ, Milos R, et al. A candidate genetic risk factor for vascular disease: a common mutation in methylenetetrahydrofolate reductase. Nature Genet. 1995;10:111–113.
37. Jacques PF, Bostom AG, Williams RR, et al. Relation between folate status, a common mutation in methylenetetrahydrofolate reductase and plasma homocysteine concentrations. Circulation. 1996;93: 7–9.
38. Stabler SP, Lindenbaum J, Savage DG, et al. Elevation of serum cystathionine levels in patients with cobalamin and folate deficiency. Blood. 1993;81: 3104–3113.
39. Stabler SP, Allen RH, Savage DG, et al. Clinical spectrum and diagnosis of cobalamin deficiency. Blood. 1990;76:871–881.
40. Matchar DB, Feussner JR, Millington DS, et al. Isotope dilution assay for urinary methylmalonic acid in diagnosis of vitamin B12 deficiency. Ann Intern Med. 1987;106:707–10
41. Moelby L, Rasmussen K, Jensen MK, et al. The relationship between clinically confirmed cobalamin deficiency and serum methylmalonic acid. J Intern Med. 1990;228:373–378.
42. Rasmussen K, Vyberg B, Pedersen KO, et al. Methylmalonic acid in renal insufficiency: evidence of accumulation and implications for diagnosis of cobalamin deficiency. Clin Chem. 1990;36:1523–1524.
43. Kang SS, Wong PWK, Norusis M. Homocysteinemia due to folate deficiency. Metabolism. 1987; 36:458–462.
44. Soria C, Chadefaux B, Coude M, et al. Concentrations of total homocysteine in plasma in chronic renal failure. Clin Chem. 1990;36:2137–2138.
45. Bostom AG, Lathrop L. Hyperhomocysteinemia in end-stage renal disease: prevalence, etiology, and potential relationship to arteriosclerotic outcomes. Kidney Int. 1997;52:10–20.
46. Boushey CJ, Beresford SAA, Omenn GS, et al. A quantitative assessment of plasma homocysteine as a risk factor for vascular disease: probable benefits of increasing folic acid intakes. JAMA. 1995;274: 1049–1057.
47. Allen RH, Stabler SP, Savage DG, et al. Diagnosis of cobalamin deficiency. I. Usefulness of serum methylmalonic acid and total homocysteine concentrations. Am J Hematol. 1990;34:90–98.
48. Stabler SP, Sampson DA, Wang LP, et al. Elevations of serum cystathionine and total homocysteine in pyridoxine-, folate-, and cobalamin-deficient rats. J Nutr Biochem. 1997;8:279–289.
49. Brass EP, Allen RH, Arung T, et al. Coenzyme-A metabolism in vitamin B-12-deficient rats. J Nutr. 1990;120:290–297.
50. Brass EP, Allen RH, Ruff LJ, et al. Effect of hydroxycobalamin [c-lactam] on propionate and carnitine metabolism in the rat. Biochem J. 1990;266: 809–815.
51. Coker M, de Klerk JB, The-Poll BT, et al. Plasma total odd-chain fatty acids in the monitoring of disorders of propionate, methylmalonate and biotin metabolism. J Inherit Metab Dis. 1996;19:743–751.
52. Frenkel EP. Abnormal fatty acid metabolism in peripheral nerves of patients with pernicious anemia. J Clin Invest. 1973;52:1237–1245.
53. Cichowicz DJ, Shane B. Mammalian folylpoly-γ-glutamate synthase 2: substrate specificity and kinetic properties. Biochemistry. 1987;26:530–539.
54. Savage DG, Lindenbaum J. Folate-cobalamin interactions. In: Bailey L, ed. *Folate in Health and Disease.* New York: Marcel-Dekker; 1995; 237–285.
55. Knowles JP, Prankerd TA. Abnormal folic acid metabolism in vitamin B12 deficiency. Clin Sci. 1962; 22:233–238.
56. Deacon R, Perry J, Lumb M, et al. Formate metabolism in the cobalamin-inactivated rat. Br J Haematol. 1990;74:354–359.
57. Fyfe JC, Jezyk PF, Giger U, et al. Inherited selective malabsorption of vitamin B-12 in giant Schnauzers. J Am Anim Hosp Assoc. 1989;25:533–539.
58. Stabler SP, DeMasters BK, Allen RH. Cobalamin (Cbl) analog-induced Cbl deficiency in pigs: a new model for human disease. Blood. 1991;78:253a.
59. Allen RH. Megaloblastic anemias. In: Goldman L, Bennett JC, eds. *Cecil Textbook of Medicine.* Philadelphia: WB Saunders; 2000; 859–867.
60. Lindenbaum J, Healton EB, Savage DG, et al. Neuropsychiatric disorders caused by cobalamin defi-

ciency in the absence of anemia or macrocytosis. N Engl J Med. 1988;318:1720–1728.

61. Stabler SP, Lindenbaum J, Allen RH. Vitamin B-12 deficiency in the elderly: current dilemmas. Am J Clin Nutr. 1997;66:741–749.
62. Healton EB, Savage DG, Brust JCM, et al. Neurological aspects of cobalamin deficiency. Medicine. 1991;70:229–245.
63. Scott JM, Wilson P, Dinn JJ, et al. Pathogenesis of subacute combined degeneration: a result of methyl group deficiency. J Lab Clin Med. 1985;105: 428–431.
64. Metz J. Cobalamin deficiency and the pathogenesis of nervous system disease. Annu Rev Nutr. 1992;12: 59–79.
65. Weir DG, Keating S, Molloy A, et al. Methylation deficiency causes vitamin B12 associated neuropathy in the pig. J Neurochem. 1988;51:1949–1952.
66. Graham SH, Arvela OM, Wise GA. Long term neurologic consequences of nutritional vitamin B12 deficiency in infants. J Pediatr. 1992;121:710–714.
67. Stabler SP, Allen RH. Vitamin B12 deficiency as a worldwide problem. Annu Rev Nutr. 2004;24: 299–326.
68. Fester HPM. Intrinsic factor secretion and cobalamin absorption. Scand J Gastroenterol. 1991;26 (suppl 188):1–7.
69. Moestrup SK, Verroust PJ. Mammalian receptors of vitamin B12-binding proteins. In: Banerjee R, ed. *Chemistry and Biochemistry of B12*. New York: Wiley Interscience; 1999; 475–488.
70. Fyfe JC, Madsen M, Hojrup P, et al. The functional cobalamin (vitamin B12) intrinsic factor is a novel complex of cubilin and amnionless. Blood. 2004;103: 1573–1579.
71. Allen RH. The plasma transport of vitamin B12. Br J Haematol. 1976;33:165–171.
72. Ban-Hock T, van Driel IR, Gleeson PA. Pernicious anemia. N Engl J Med. 1997;337:1441–1448.
73. Carmel R. Prevalence of undiagnosed pernicious anemia in the elderly. Arch Intern Med. 1996;156: 1097–1100.
74. Sumner AE, Chin MM, Abrahm JL, et al. Elevated methylmalonic acid and total homocysteine levels show high prevalence of vitamin B12 deficiency after gastric surgery. Ann Intern Med. 1996;124:469–476.
75. Lindenbaum J, Rosenberg I, Wilson P, et al. Prevalence of cobalamin deficiency in the Framington elderly population. Am J Clin Nutr. 1994;60:2–11.
76. Carmel R. Cobalamin, the stomach and aging. Am J Clin Nutr. 1997;66:750–759.
77. Guttormsen AA, Refsum H, Ueland PM. The interaction between nitrous oxide and cobalamin: biochemical effects and clinical consequences. Acta Anaesthesiol Scand. 1994;38:753–756.
78. Berlin R, Berlin H, Bronte G, et al. Vitamin B12 body stores during oral and parenteral treatment of pernicious anemia. Acta Med Scand. 1978;204: 81–84.
79. Waife SO, Jansen CJ, Crabtree RE, et al. Oral vitamin B12 without intrinsic factor in the treatment of pernicious anemia. Ann Intern Med. 1963;58: 810–817.
80. Koehler KM, Romero LJ, Stauber PM, et al. Vitamin supplementation and other variables affecting serum homocysteine and methylmalonic acid concentrations in elderly men and women. J Am Coll Clin Nutr. 1996;15:364–376.
81. Stabler SP, Allen RH, Fried LP, et al. Racial differences in prevalence of cobalamin and folate deficiencies in disabled elderly women. Am J Clin Nutr. 1999;70(5):911–919.
82. Lawrence JM, Petitti DB, Watkins M, et al. Trends in serum folate after food fortification. Lancet. 1999; 354:915–916.
83. Jacques PF, Selhub J, Bostom AG, et al. The effect of folic acid fortification on plasma folate and total homocysteine concentrations. N Engl J Med. 1999; 340:1449–1454.
84. Stabler SP, Lindenbaum J, Allen RH. The use of homocysteine and other metabolites in the specific diagnosis of vitamin B-12 deficiency. J Nutr. 1996; 126:1266S–1272S.
85. Carmel R, Gott PS, Waters CH, et al. The frequently low cobalamin levels in dementia usually signify treatable metabolic, neurologic and electrophysiologic abnormalities. Eur J Haematol. 1995;54: 245–253.

# 24 Biotin

Gabriela Camporeale and Janos Zempleni

## Introduction

More than 70 years ago, Boas demonstrated the requirement for the water-soluble vitamin biotin in mammals.[1] Biotin was first isolated by Kögl and Tönnies in 1932,[2] its chemical structure was determined by du Vigneaud et al. in 1942,[3] and it was chemically synthesized by Harris et al. in 1943.[4]

The route of microbial biosynthesis of biotin, largely elaborated by Eisenberg et al.[5] working with *Escherichia coli*, is depicted in Figure 1. In this pathway, dethiobiotin is formed from pimelyl-CoA (which can be synthesized from oleic acid) and carbamyl phosphate.[5] Sulfur is incorporated into dethiobiotin in a synthase-dependent step, generating biotin.[6]

Early studies of biotin catabolism were primarily conducted using microbes as model organisms. In a series of groundbreaking experiments, McCormick et al.[7] identified two pathways of biotin catabolism (Figure 2). In one pathway, biotin is catabolized by β-oxidation of the valeric acid side chain.[7] The repeated cleavage of two-carbon units leads to the formation of bisnorbiotin, tetranorbiotin, and related catabolites that are known to result from β-oxidation of fatty acids (i.e., α,β-dehydro-, β-hydroxy, and β-keto-intermediates). β-Ketobiotin and β-ketobisnorbiotin are unstable and may decarboxylate spontaneously to form bisnorbiotin methyl ketone and tetranorbiotin methyl ketone.[7,8] After degradation of the valeric acid side chain to one carbon (tetranorbiotin), microorganisms cleave and degrade the heterocyclic ring.[7] In a second pathway of biotin catabolism, the sulfur in the heterocyclic ring is oxidized to produce biotin-*l*-sulfoxide, biotin-*d*-sulfoxide, and biotin sulfone.[7] It is likely that sulfur oxidation in the biotin molecule occurs in the smooth endoplasmic reticulum in a reaction that depends on nicotinamide adenine dinucleotide phosphate.[9] Finally, biotin is catabolized by a combination of β-oxidation and sulfur oxidation, producing compounds such as bisnorbiotin sulfone.

Mammals also catabolize biotin by both β-oxidation and sulfur oxidation, producing bisnorbiotin, biotin-*d*-sulfoxide, biotin-*l*-sulfoxide, bisnorbiotin methyl ketone, biotin sulfone, and teranorbiotin-*l*-sulfoxide.[8,10] Whether the β-oxidation of biotin takes place in mitochondria or peroxisomes is uncertain.[10,11] Degradation of the heterocyclic ring is quantitatively minor in mammals.[10] Biotin catabolites and biotin each account for about half of the total biotinyl compounds in human urine and plasma.[8,12]

## Biological Functions of Biotin

It has been known for many years that biotin serves as a covalently bound coenzyme for various carboxylases.[13] More recently, evidence has emerged that biotin also plays unique roles in cell signaling, epigenetic control of gene expression, and chromatin structure.[14] The various roles of biotin in intermediary metabolism and cell biology are reviewed in this section.

### *Biotin-dependent Carboxylases*

In mammals, biotin serves as a covalently bound coenzyme for acetyl-CoA carboxylase (EC 6.4.1.2), pyruvate carboxylase (EC 6.4.1.1), propionyl-CoA carboxylase (EC 6.4.1.3), and β-methylcrotonyl-CoA carboxylase (EC 6.4.1.4).[13] The attachment of biotin to the ε-amino group of a specific lysine residue in the four apocarboxylases is catalyzed by holocarboxylase synthetase (EC 6.3.4.10); biotinylation of carboxylases requires ATP and proceeds in the following two steps[15]:

(1) ATP + biotin + holocarboxylase synthetase → biotin-AMP-holocarboxylase synthetase + pyrophosphate

(2) Biotin-AMP-holocarboxylase synthetase + apocarboxylase → holocarboxylase + AMP + holocarboxylase synthetase

(Net) ATP + biotin + apocarboxylase → holocarboxylase + AMP + pyrophosphate

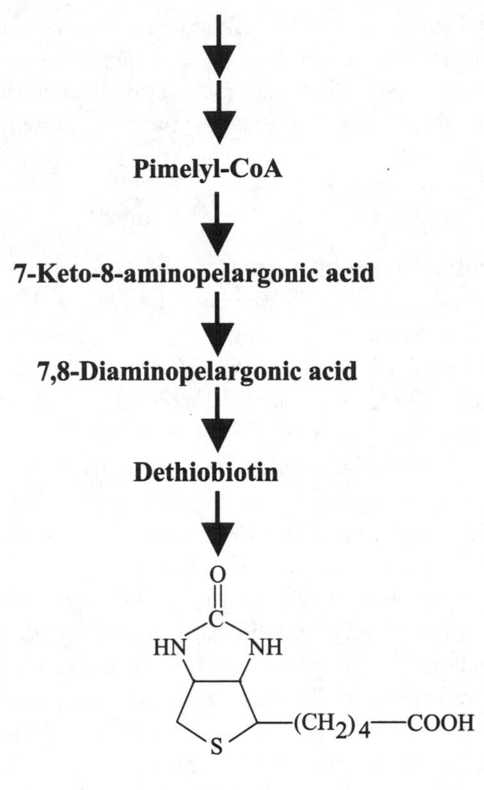


Figure 1. Pathway of biotin biosynthesis.

Biotin-dependent carboxylases mediate the covalent binding of bicarbonate to organic acids by the following carboxylation sequence: bicarbonate and ATP form carboxy phosphate, releasing ADP (line 1 in the scheme below); carboxy phosphate reacts with the 1′-N of the biotinyl moiety in holocarboxylases ("biotinyl carboxylase") to form 1′-N-carboxybiotinyl carboxylase and to release inorganic phosphate, $P_i$ (line 2). 1′-N-carboxybiotinyl carboxylase then incorporates carboxylate into an acceptor, i.e., a specific organic acid for each of the four carboxylases (line 3).

(1) $HCO_3^-$ + ATP → carboxy phosphate + ADP

(2) Carboxy phosphate + biotinyl carboxylase → 1′-N-carboxybiotinyl carboxylase + $P_i$

(3) 1′-N-carboxybiotinyl carboxylase + acceptor → biotinyl carboxylase + acceptor-$CO_2^-$

(Net) ATP + $HCO_3^-$ + acceptor → ADP + $P_i$ + acceptor-$CO_2^-$

Two isoforms of acetyl-CoA carboxylase have been identified: the cytoplasmic acetyl-CoA carboxylase α and the mitochondrial acetyl-CoA carboxylase β.[16] Both acetyl-CoA carboxylase α and acetyl-CoA carboxylase β catalyze the binding of bicarbonate to acetyl-CoA, generating malonyl-CoA (Figure 3). The two isoforms of acetyl-CoA carboxylase play distinct roles in intermediary metabolism due to their cellular localization. Acetyl-CoA carboxylase α participates in fatty acid synthesis in the cytoplasm by providing the substrate malonyl-CoA. In contrast, acetyl-CoA carboxylase β participates in the regulation of fatty acid oxidation in mitochondria. This effect of acetyl-CoA carboxylase β is also mediated by malonyl-CoA, which is an inhibitor of fatty acid transport into mitochondria.

Pyruvate carboxylase localizes to mitochondria and is a key enzyme in gluconeogenesis (Figure 3). The mitochondrial propionyl-CoA carboxylase and β-methylcrotonyl-CoA carboxylase comprise a biotin-containing α-subunit and a biotin-free β-subunit. Propionyl-CoA carboxylase catalyzes an essential step in the metabolism of isoleucine, valine, methionine, threonine, the cholesterol

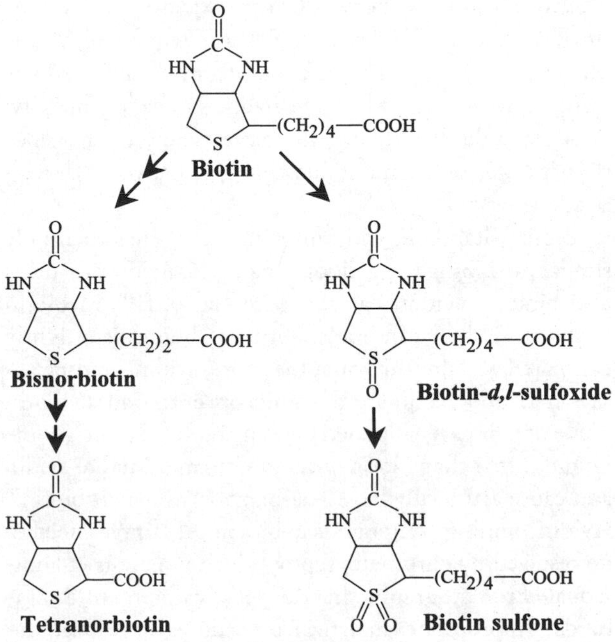

Biotin
Bisnorbiotin
Biotin-*d,l*-sulfoxide
Tetranorbiotin
Biotin sulfone

Figure 2. Pathways of biotin catabolism.

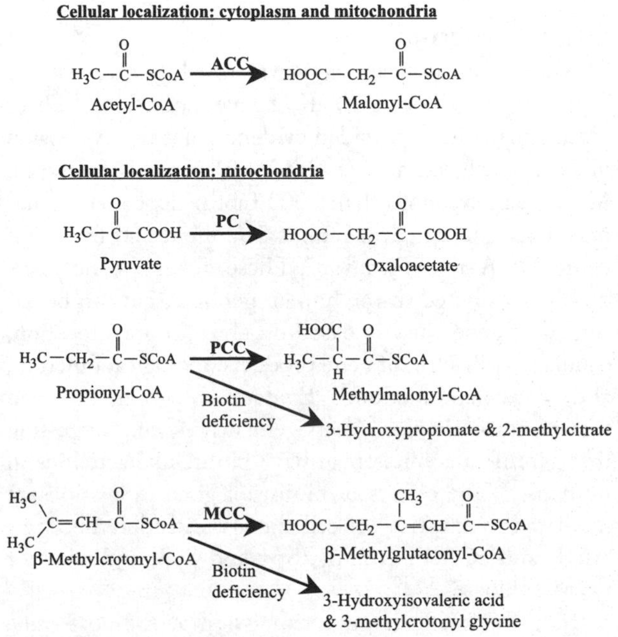

**Cellular localization: cytoplasm and mitochondria**

Acetyl-CoA —ACC→ Malonyl-CoA

**Cellular localization: mitochondria**

Pyruvate —PC→ Oxaloacetate

Propionyl-CoA —PCC→ Methylmalonyl-CoA
Biotin deficiency → 3-Hydroxypropionate & 2-methylcitrate

β-Methylcrotonyl-CoA —MCC→ β-Methylglutaconyl-CoA
Biotin deficiency → 3-Hydroxyisovaleric acid & 3-methylcrotonyl glycine

Figure 3. Biotin-dependent carboxylases.

side chain, and odd-chain fatty acids. β-Methylcrotonyl-CoA carboxylase catalyzes an essential step in leucine metabolism. Additional carboxylases have been identified in some microbes but are not discussed here.[13]

Proteolytic degradation of holocarboxylases leads to the formation of biotinyl peptides. These peptides are further degraded by biotinidase (EC 3.5.1.12) to release biotin, which is recycled in holocarboxylase synthesis.[17]

### *Biotinylation of Histones*

Evidence has been provided that histones (DNA-binding proteins) contain covalently bound biotin.[18] Evidence has been provided that both biotinidase and holocarboxylase synthetase may catalyze binding of biotin to histones.[18] All five major classes of histones in mammals are targets for biotinylation: histone H1, H2A, H2B, H3, and H4.[18] The following biotinylation sites have been identified in human histones: lysine-9 and lysine-13 in histone H2A; lysine-4, lysine-9, and lysine-18 in histone H3; and lysine-8 and lysine-12 in histone H4.[18] Binding of biotin is likely to affect the association of DNA with histones in a manner similar to other known histone modifications.[18] Evidence has been provided that biotinylation of histones might play a role in gene silencing, cell proliferation, and the cellular response to DNA damage.[18] This is consistent with a role for biotin in the epigenetic control of gene expression and genomic stability. Preliminary evidence suggests that biotinylation of histones is a reversible process, and that biotinidase may catalyze both biotinylation and debiotinylation of histones.[18] Variables such as the microenvironment in chromatin and post-translational modifications and alternate splicing of biotinidase might determine whether biotinidase acts as histone biotinyl transferase or as histone debiotinylase.

### *Gene Expression*

More than 35 years ago, evidence began to emerge suggesting that biotin may affect gene expression.[19] These pioneering studies provided evidence that the expression of rat liver glucokinase (EC 2.7.1.2) depends on biotin. More recently, more than 2000 biotin-dependent genes have been identified in human lymphoid and liver cells using DNA micro-arrays.[18] These genes are not randomly distributed in the human genome, but can be assigned to gene clusters based on chromosomal location, cellular localization of gene products, biological function, and molecular function.[18] Evidence has been provided that bisnorbiotin also affects gene expression, suggesting that biotin catabolites may have biotin-like activities in humans.[18] The effects of biotin on gene expression are mediated by a variety of cell signals, including biotinyl-AMP and cGMP, NF-κB, Sp1 and Sp3, and receptor tyrosine kinases.[18,20]

Biotin also affects gene expression at the post-transcriptional level. For example, expression of the asialoglycoprotein receptor in HepG2 hepatocarcinoma cells and propionyl-CoA carboxylase in rat hepatocytes depends on biotin; these effects are not caused by alterations in the abundance of mRNA coding for these proteins.[18]

## Methods of Biotin Analysis

### *Microbial Growth Assays*

The following microorganisms are among those that depend on biotin for growth and are commonly used in microbial growth assays: *Lactobacillus plantarum*, *Lactobacillus casei*, *Ochromonas danica*, *Escherichia coli C162*, *Saccharomyces cerevisiae*, and *Kloeckera brevis*.[21] These test organisms show variable growth responses to biotin and the various biotin precursors, catabolites, and analogs. The growth-stimulating activity of biotin is estimated by quantifying the absorbance of culture media at 610 or 660 nm, by agar plate methods, by quantifying the release of $[^{14}C]O_2$ from $[^{14}C]$methionine, by quantifying the cellular uptake of $[^{14}C]O_2$, or by titrating the lactate generated by microorganisms. For some microbes (e.g., *O. danica*, *L. plantarum*), acid or enzymatic hydrolysis of samples is required to release biotin from protein. For other organisms (e.g., *K. brevis*), the detectable biotin decreases with enzymatic hydrolysis.

### *Avidin-binding Assays*

The proteins avidin and streptavidin are widely used in biotin analysis because they bind biotin with extraordinary strength and specificity; the dissociation constant of the avidin-biotin complex is $1.3 \times 10^{-15}$ M.[21] Avidin-binding assays generally measure the ability of biotin to: 1) compete with $[^3H]$biotin or $[^{14}C]$biotin for binding to avidin (isotope dilution assays); 2) prevent binding of labeled avidin ($^{125}I$, horseradish peroxidase, etc.) to biotinylated protein adhered to plastic ("sequential, solid-phase assays"); 3) prevent the binding of biotinylated enzyme to avidin and, hence, to maintain enzyme activity; or 4) to induce a change in fluorescence, fluorescence polarization, or chemiluminescence of native or derivatized avidin.[21]

Biotin catabolites and compounds that are structurally similar to biotin (e.g., lipoic acid, hexanoic acid, urea) also bind to avidin, causing potential pitfalls in biotin analysis. First, avidin binds biotin catabolites less tightly compared with biotin[21] and, therefore, avidin-binding assays may underestimate the true concentration of biotin plus catabolites if calibrated by using biotin. Second, compounds other than biotin or catabolites may bind to avidin and cause artificially large readings for "apparent biotin." Avidin-binding compounds in biological samples need to be resolved by chromatography prior to analysis of individual chromatographic fractions against authentic standards. Appropriate analytical procedures have been reviewed elsewhere.[21]

### 4′-Hydroxyazobenzene-2-Carboxylic Acid Dye Assay

The 4′-hydroxyazobenzene-2-carboxylic acid dye assay is useful in the measurement of biotin at concentrations exceeding those typically found in biological samples, e.g., in synthetic biotinylated compounds. In the absence of biotin, 4′-hydroxyazobenzene-2-carboxylic acid forms non-covalent complexes with avidin at its biotin-binding sites to produce a characteristic absorption band at 500 nm.[21] The addition of biotin to this complex results in displacement of 4′-hydroxyazobenzene-2-carboxylic acid from the binding sites. As 4′-hydroxyazobenzene-2-carboxylic acid is displaced, the absorbance of the complex decreases proportionally.

### Biotin Analogs

Synthetic biotin analogs (e.g., biotin methyl ester, diaminobiotin, dethiobiotin, and iminobiotin) and some naturally occurring biotin metabolites (e.g., biocytin) are available commercially. Likewise, a large number of reagents are available for chemical biotinylation of amines, sulfhydryl groups, carboxyl groups, nucleic acids, and others.

## Absorption, Transport Proteins, Storage, and Excretion

### Digestion

Biotin in foods is largely protein bound.[22] Several gastrointestinal proteases may hydrolyze biotin-containing proteins to generate biotinyl peptides,[17] which are further hydrolyzed by intestinal biotinidase to release biotin. Intestinal biotinidase is found in pancreatic juice, secretions of the intestinal glands, bacterial flora, and the brush-border membranes.[17] Biotinidase activities are similar in mucosa from duodenum, jejunum, and ileum.[17] The primary site(s) for hydrolysis of biotinyl peptides is unknown. Small quantities of biotinyl peptides may be absorbed without prior hydrolysis.[23]

### Intestinal Transport and Bioavailability

Early investigations of biotin transport in rat jejunum suggested that intestinal biotin uptake is mediated by both saturable and non-saturable components.[24] At biotin concentrations less than 5 μmol/L, biotin absorption proceeds largely by the saturable process, whereas at concentrations above 25 μmol/L, non-saturable uptake predominates.[24] The saturable mechanism of biotin transport is sodium dependent.[25] Transport of biotin is faster in the jejunum than in the ileum, and is minimal in the colon (85 versus 36 versus 2.8 pmol/g tissue wet weight/25 min, respectively); the apparent $K_m$ (Michaelis-Menten constant) of the transporter for biotin in rat jejunum is 3.7 μmol/L.[25] The biotin transporter in mammalian cells has broad substrate specificity and binds biotin, pantothenic acid, and lipoic acid with similar affinity.[26] Consequently, this transporter was named the sodium-dependent multivitamin transporter (SMVT).[26] The SMVT has been detected in various species,[26-28] and its role in biotin transport was confirmed by cloning a cDNA coding for rat SMVT and expressing functional transporter in human-derived HeLa cells.[26] Likewise, rabbit intestinal SMVT was functionally expressed in human retinal pigment epithelium.[27] Four variants of SMVT transcripts have been identified in rats.[28]

The intestinal biotin uptake is regulated by protein kinase C and $Ca^{2+}$/calmodulin-mediated pathways.[29] Activation of protein kinase C inhibits biotin uptake, whereas inhibition of protein kinase C stimulates biotin uptake by Caco-2 cells. This effect of protein kinase C is mediated by alterations in the activity or abundance of biotin transporters, as opposed to alterations in transporter affinity for substrate. SMVT contains two putative protein kinase C phosphorylation sites.[29]

The 5′-regulatory regions of *SMVT* genes in rats and humans have been cloned and characterized.[30,31] The rat and human *SMVT* genes contain three and two distinct promoters, respectively. Both promoter sequences in the human gene are TATA-less, CAAT-less, contain highly GC-rich sites, and have multiple putative regulatory *cis* elements, e.g., AP-1, AP-2, C/EBP, SP1, NF1, and GATA.[31] The minimal region required for basal activity of the human SMVT promoter is encoded by a sequence between −5846 and −5313 for promoter 1 and between −4417 and −4244 for promoter 2 relative to the translation initiation codon. The three promoters in the rat SMVT gene contain *cis* elements similar to the elements observed in the human promoters, but the rat 5′-regulatory region also contains two TATA-like elements.[30]

The bioavailability of oral biotin in humans nears 100%, even if the dose administered equals about 600 times the normal dietary intake.[32] Biotin exit from the enterocyte (i.e., transport across the basolateral membrane) is carrier mediated, but is sodium independent and does not accumulate biotin against a concentration gradient.[33]

### Protein Binding in Plasma

Human albumin, α-globulin, and β-globulin bind biotin, but the binding is non-specific.[15] Biotinidase has two binding sites for biotin and might serve as a biotin-carrier protein in the plasma of normal adults.[34] One of the binding sites in biotinidase has high affinity for biotin (dissociation constant, $K_d$, = 0.5 nmol/L), whereas the other binding site has low affinity for biotin ($K_d$ = 50 nmol/L). A biotin-binding glycoprotein (MW 66,000) is present in the serum of pregnant and estrogenized female rats,[35] but not in the serum of normal male rats.[15] Immunoneutralization of the maternal biotin-binding protein decreases the transport of biotin to the embryo, resulting in early embryonic mortality.[15]

### *Biotin Uptake into Liver and Peripheral Tissues*

Uptake of biotin into liver and peripheral tissues is mediated by SMVT, as described above.[26,28] Apparent $K_m$ and $V_{max}$ (maximal transport rate) in human HepG2 hepatocarcinoma cells are 19.2 μmol/L and 6.8 nmol/mg/protein/min, respectively.[36] Both influx and efflux of biotin are mediated by the same transporter in human lymphoid cells.[37]

Both monocarboxylate transporter 1 (MCT1) and SMVT mediate biotin uptake in human lymphoid cells.[38] MCT1 is expressed ubiquitously in human tissues,[39] but it remains to be determined whether MCT1 plays a role in biotin uptake in tissues other than lymphoid cells.[38] MCT1 belongs to the family of monocarboxylate transporters. Nine MCT-related sequences have so far been identified in mammals, each having a distinct tissue distribution.[39] It is unknown if MCTs other than MCT1 play a role in biotin uptake.

### *Cell Compartments*

Biotin is distributed unequally across cellular compartments; for example, the vast majority of biotin in rat liver localizes to mitochondria and cytoplasm, whereas only a small fraction localizes to microsomes.[40] The relative enrichment of biotin in mitochondria and cytoplasm is consistent with the role of biotin as a coenzyme for carboxylases in these compartments. A quantitatively small but qualitatively important fraction of biotin localizes to the cell nucleus; about 0.7% of total biotin in human lymphoid cells can be recovered from the nuclear fraction.[18] The relative abundance of nuclear biotin increases to about 1% of total biotin in response to proliferation, which is consistent with a role for nuclear biotin-binding proteins (histones) in cell proliferation (as described above). Theoretically, the cellular partitioning of biotin is driven by binding to carboxylases in cytoplasm and mitochondria, by binding to histones in the cell nucleus, and by MCT-mediated transport across mitochondrial membranes.[18]

### *Storage*

A relatively large fraction of intravenously administered biotin accumulates in rat liver, which is consistent with a role for this organ in biotin storage.[40] Depletion and repletion experiments on biotin-dependent carboxylases in rat liver provided evidence that mitochondrial acetyl-CoA carboxylase may serve as a reservoir for biotin. Cytosolic acetyl-CoA carboxylase, the mitochondrial pyruvate carboxylase (propionyl-CoA carboxylase), and β-methylcrotonyl-CoA carboxylase do not appear to fulfill similar roles.[41]

### *Urinary Excretion*

Healthy adults excrete approximately 100 nmol/d of biotin and catabolites into urine.[8] Biotin accounts for approximately half of the total; the catabolites bisnorbiotin, biotin-*d,l*-sulfoxides, bisnorbiotin methyl ketone, biotin sulfone, and tetranorbiotin-*l*-sulfoxide account for most of the balance.[8] If physiological or pharmacological doses of biotin are administered parenterally to humans, rats, or pigs, 43% to 75% of the dose is excreted into urine.[10,32] Renal epithelia reclaim biotin that is filtered in the glomeruli in an SMVT-mediated process.[42] Biocytin is not an inhibitor of renal biotin absorption in humans.[43]

### *Biliary Excretion*

The biliary excretion of biotin and catabolites is quantitatively minor. Less than 2% of an intravenous dose of [$^{14}$C]biotin was recovered in rat bile, but more than 60% of the dose was excreted in urine.[44] The concentration ratios of biotin, bisnorbiotin, and biotin-*d,l*-sulfoxide (bile versus serum) in pigs are at least one order of magnitude smaller than the ratio measured for the cholephil compound bilirubin.[44]

## Pharmacokinetics

The mean rate constants of biotin absorption and elimination are about 2.1/h and 0.4/h, respectively, in humans[45]; the rate constant of elimination equals a half-life of 1.8 hours, which is consistent with both rapid absorption and elimination of biotin. Biotin kinetics have been studied thoroughly in cattle.[46]

[$^3$H]Biotin efflux from human lymphocytes was used to model the elimination kinetics of biotin at the cellular level.[37] Biotin efflux from lymphocytes at 37°C is fast and triphasic; the half-lives of the three elimination phases are approximately 0.2, 1.2, and 22 h. Likely, the half-life of [$^3$H]biotin during the terminal, slow phase of efflux is determined by the breakdown of biotin-dependent carboxylases to release free [$^3$H]biotin, followed by efflux of [$^3$H]biotin from lymphocytes. The half-life of [$^3$H]biotin during the terminal phase of efflux (22 h) resembles the half-lives of pyruvate carboxylase (28 h) and acetyl-CoA carboxylase (4.6 d).

## Biotin Status

### *Direct Measures*

The serum concentrations and urinary excretions of biotin and its catabolites are potential markers of biotin status. Biotin accounts for about half of the total of all biotinyl compounds in human urine and serum.[8,12] Serum concentrations and the urinary excretions of biotin and biotin catabolites in healthy adults are provided in Table 1. Tetranorbiotin-*l*-sulfoxide was detected in human urine,[8] but the avidin affinity of this compound is too low to allow meaningful quantitation.[47]

The urinary excretion of biotin and biotin catabolites decreases rapidly and substantially in biotin-deficient individuals,[48] suggesting that the urinary excretion is an early and sensitive indicator of biotin deficiency. In con-

**Table 1.** Serum Concentrations[12] and Urinary Excretions[8] of Biotin and Catabolites*

| Compound | Serum *pmol/L* | Urine *nmol/24 h* |
|---|---|---|
| Biotin | 244 ± 61 | 35 ± 14 |
| Bisnorbiotin | 189 ± 135 | 68 ± 48 |
| Biotin-*d,l*-sulfoxide | 15 ± 33 | 5 ± 6 |
| Bisnorbiotin methyl ketone | ND† | 9 ± 9 |
| Biotin sulfone | ND | 5 ± 5 |
| Total biotinyl compounds | 464 ± 178‡ | 122 ± 66 |

* Data are means ± SD ($n$ = 15 for serum; $n$ = 6 for urine).
† ND, not determined. Bisnorbiotin methyl ketone and biotin sulfone had not been identified at the time when this study of serum was conducted, so quantification of these "unknowns" was based on using biotin as a standard.
‡ Including three unidentified biotin catabolites.
Serum data used with permission from Mock, et al., 1995[12]; Urine data used with permission from Zempleni, et al., 1997[8]

trast, serum concentrations of biotin, bisnorbiotin, and biotin-*d,l*-sulfoxide do not decrease in biotin-deficient individuals[48] or in patients on biotin-free total parenteral nutrition[49] during reasonable periods of observation. Therefore, serum concentrations are not good indicators of marginal biotin deficiency.

### *Indirect Measures*

Activities of biotin-dependent carboxylases in lymphocytes are reliable markers for assessing the biotin status in humans.[50] Some investigators have modified this approach and used a "carboxylase activation index" for status assessment.[49] The carboxylase activation index equals the ratio of carboxylase activities in cells incubated with and without excess biotin. High values for the activation index suggest that a substantial fraction of a given carboxylase was present as apo-enzyme, indicating biotin deficiency. For example, in patients on biotin-free total parenteral nutrition for 24 to 40 days, the mean activation index of propionyl-CoA carboxylase was greater than 2; the activation index equaled 1 in control lymphocytes from biotin-sufficient individuals.[49]

Reduced carboxylase activities in biotin deficiency cause metabolic blocks in intermediary metabolism (Figure 3). Reduced activity of β-methylcrotonyl-CoA carboxylase impairs leucine catabolism. As a consequence, β-methylcrotonyl-CoA is shunted to alternative pathways, leading to an increased formation of 3-hydroxyisovaleric acid and 3-methylcrotonyl glycine. Biotin deficiency studies in humans suggest that the urinary excretion of 3-hydroxyisovaleric acid is an early and sensitive indicator of biotin status.[51]

Reduced activity of propionyl-CoA carboxylase causes a metabolic block in propionic acid metabolism. Consequently, propionic acid is shunted to alternative metabolic pathways. In these pathways, 3-hydroxypropionic acid and 2-methylcitric acid are formed. Recent studies in biotin-deficient individuals suggest that the urinary excretion of 3-hydroxypropionic acid and 2-methylcitric acid is not a good indicator of marginal biotin deficiency.[52] Theoretically, propionic acid may be consumed in the synthesis of odd-chain fatty acids.[53]

In severe biotin deficiency, activities of acetyl-CoA carboxylase and pyruvate carboxylase may be reduced. Reduced activities of acetyl-CoA carboxylase causes abnormal synthesis of long-chain fatty acids, including polyunsaturated fatty acids,[54] which may result in abnormal metabolism of prostaglandin and related substances. Low activities of pyruvate carboxylase may impair gluconeogenesis, but the symptoms may be too non-specific to allow for diagnosis of biotin deficiency.

## Biotin Deficiency

### *Clinical Findings of Frank Biotin Deficiency*

Signs of frank biotin deficiency have been described in patients receiving parenteral nutrition without biotin supplementation[22] and in patients with biotinidase deficiency.[55] Frank biotin deficiency may also be observed in individuals consuming large amounts of raw egg white, which contains the protein avidin. Binding of biotin to avidin in the gastrointestinal tract prevents the absorption of biotin.[56]

Clinical findings of frank biotin deficiency include periorificial dermatitis, conjunctivitis, alopecia, ataxia, hypotonia, ketolactic acidosis/organic aciduria, seizures, skin infection, and developmental delay in infants and children.[22,55] In addition, the following symptoms were observed in adults and adolescents on an egg white diet: 1) thinning hair, often with loss of hair color; 2) skin rash described as scaly (seborrheic) and red (eczematous)—in several cases the rash was distributed around the eyes, nose, and mouth; and 3) depression, lethargy, hallucinations, and paresthesias of the extremities.[22]

### *Immune System*

Biotin deficiency has adverse effects on cellular and humoral immune functions. For example, children with hereditary abnormalities of biotin metabolism developed candida dermatitis; these children also had absent delayed-hypersensitivity skin test responses, IgA deficiency, and subnormal percentages of T lymphocytes in peripheral blood.[57] Synthesis of antibodies is reduced in biotin-deficient rats.[58] Biotin deficiency in mice decreases both the number of spleen cells and the percentage of B lymphocytes in the spleen,[59] and inhibits thymocyte maturation.[60]

### *Cell Proliferation*

Biotin deficiency is associated with decreased rates of cell proliferation; for example, biotin-deficient HeLa cells arrest in the G1 phase of the cell cycle.[61] Likewise, biotin deficiency is associated with decreased proliferation rates in human lymphoid cells and choriocarcinoma cells.[62,63] There is also evidence that biotin stimulates the production of an unidentified growth factor.[64]

Human lymphoid cells respond to mitogen-induced proliferation with a 200% to 600% increase in biotin uptake compared with quiescent controls.[65] This effect is mediated by an increased expression of biotin transporters rather than by an increased affinity of transporters for biotin.[65,66] The increased biotin uptake in proliferating cells is paralleled by increased activities of β-methylcrotonyl-CoA carboxylase (180% increase compared with quiescent controls) and propionyl-CoA carboxylase (50% increase), and by increased biotinylation of histones (400% increase).[66,67] These observations are consistent with the notion that cell proliferation generates an increased demand for biotin.

### Cell Stress and Survival

Biotin deficiency causes cell stress, enhancing the nuclear translocation of the transcription factor NF-κB in human lymphoid cells.[68] NF-κB mediates activation of anti-apoptotic genes, and this is associated with enhanced survival of biotin-deficient cells in response to cell death signals compared with biotin-sufficient controls.[68] Likewise, biotin-deficient *Drosophila melanogaster* exhibit greater survival rates in response to stress than biotin-sufficient controls.[69] Finally, the relative resistance of biotin-deficient human lymphoma cells to treatment with antineoplastic drugs has been attributed to nuclear translocation of NF-κB.[70]

### Lipid Metabolism

Two biotin-dependent carboxylases are directly linked to lipid metabolism: acetyl-CoA carboxylase (fatty acid synthesis and β-oxidation) and propionyl-CoA carboxylase (metabolism of the cholesterol side chain and odd-chain fatty acids). Consistent with these roles of biotin in lipid metabolism, biotin deficiency causes alterations of the fatty acid profile in liver, skin, and serum of several animal species.[54] In particular, biotin deficiency is associated with increased abundance of odd-chain fatty acids, suggesting that this accumulation may be a marker for reduced propionyl-CoA carboxylase activity in biotin deficiency. This is consistent with observations that activities of mitochondrial carboxylases in biotin-deficient rats decrease to 3% to 18% of control values. Biotin deficiency does not affect the fatty acid composition in brain tissue to the same extent it does in liver tissue.[54]

Biotin deficiency also causes abnormalities in fatty acid composition in humans. In patients who developed biotin deficiency during parenteral alimentation, the percentage of odd-chain fatty acids (15:0, 17:0) in serum increased for each of the four major lipid classes (cholesterol esters, phospholipids, triglycerides, and free fatty acids); however, the relative changes in these lipids have not always been consistent among studies.[54]

### Teratogenic Effects of Biotin Deficiency

Biotin deficiency is teratogenic in several animal species. Hens with marginal biotin deficiency produce eggs with higher embryonic mortality, reduced hatchability, chronodystrophy ("parrot beak" deformity), perosis (an abnormality of bone tendon formation that results in a deformity similar to clubfoot), micromelia, and syndactyly.[54] In some strains of mice, biotin deficiency during pregnancy causes substantial increases in fetal malformations and mortality.[54,71] In biotin-deficient rats, the most common fetal malformations include cleft palate, micrognathia, and micromelia. Differences in teratogenic susceptibility among rodent species have been reported, and corresponding differences of biotin concentrations in fetal liver were observed. This led Watanabe et al.[72] to propose that differences in teratogenic susceptibility among rodent species are caused by differences in biotin transport from the mother to the fetus. The fetal malformations observed in biotin-deficient animals have been shown to be caused by abnormal metabolism of fatty acids and prostaglandins.[54]

### Biotin Homeostasis in the Central Nervous System

Disturbances of biotin homeostasis in the central nervous system (CNS) cause encephalopathies.[18] Factors leading to biotin imbalances in the CNS include deficiencies of biotinidase, holocarboxylase synthetase, and perhaps biotin transporters,[18] as described below. Afflicted patients typically respond to the administration of large doses of biotin by maintaining normal neurological function.[18]

Moderate dietary biotin deficiency is typically not associated with neurological symptoms, which is consistent with the hypothesis that under conditions of moderate biotin deficiency, the CNS maintains normal concentrations of biotin at the expense of other tissues. Indeed, there is evidence that biotin deficiency causes a greater than 90% decrease of biotinylated carboxylases in rat liver, whereas brain carboxylases remain unchanged.[73] Apparently, in rats, biotin deficiency decreases the expression of SMVT in the liver while maintaining normal expression of SMVT in the brain.[73]

## Disorders of Biotin Metabolism

### Biotinidase Deficiency

Biotinidase deficiency is an inborn error of metabolism in which low activities of this enzyme cause a failure to recycle biotin from degraded carboxylases, i.e., to release biotin from biocytin. Substantial amounts of biocytin are excreted into urine,[74] eventually leading to biotin deficiency. Thus, clinical and biochemical features in children with biotinidase deficiency are similar to those described above for biotin deficiency.[55] It remains uncertain if some symptoms of biotinidase deficiency can be attributed to diminished biotinylation of histones.[18]

Typically, symptoms of biotinidase deficiency appear between the ages of 1 week to 1 year.[55] Wolf proposed to distinguish between patients with profound biotinidase deficiency (less than 10% of normal serum biotinidase activity) and patients with partial deficiency (10% to 30% of normal biotinidase activity).[75] The estimated incidence of profound biotinidase deficiency is 1 in 112,271 live births, and the incidence of partial biotinidase deficiency is 1 in 129,282.[75] The combined incidence of profound and partial deficiency is 1 in 60,089, and an estimated 1 in 123 individuals is heterozygous for the disorder.[75] Most of the children in whom biotinidase deficiency has been diagnosed are Caucasian.[55] Mutations of the *biotinidase* gene have been well characterized at the molecular level.[76-78] Children with profound biotinidase deficiency are treated with 5 to 20 mg/d of biotin.[55] If identified early, symptomatic patients improve rapidly after biotin therapy is initiated, but therapy must be continued throughout life.[55]

Procedures for prenatal diagnosis of biotinidase activity in cultured amniotic fluid cells and for neonatal screening using blood samples have been proposed.[55] Biotinidase activity is measured by quantitating the release of *p*-aminobenzoic acid from *N*-biotinyl-*p*-aminobenzoate.[79] The mean (±SD) normal activity of biotinidase is 5.8 ± 0.9 nmol *p*-aminobenzoate liberated/min/mL serum.[79]

### *Carboxylase Deficiencies*

Afflicted individuals present with either isolated deficiencies of individual carboxylases or multiple deficiencies of biotin-dependent carboxylases.[80] The latter is caused by defective holocarboxylase synthetase (reducing binding of biotin to carboxylases) or by abnormal cellular uptake of biotin (reducing intracellular concentrations of biotin). Patients with multiple carboxylase deficiency characteristically exhibit low activities of all four biotin-dependent carboxylases. Wolf distinguishes two forms of multiple carboxylase deficiency: a neonatal or infantile form and a late-onset or juvenile form.[80] Mutations of the *holocarboxylase synthetase* gene have been well characterized at the molecular level.[81] It has been estimated that the incidence of holocarboxylase synthetase deficiency is less than 1 in 100,000 live births in Japan.[81] Afflicted individuals typically respond well to administration of pharmacological doses of biotin, in particular if the mutation of the gene resides in the biotin-binding region of the protein.[81] In contrast, biotin transporter deficiency is poorly characterized as a potential cause of multiple carboxylase deficiency (see below).[18]

Among the isolated carboxylase deficiencies, propionyl-CoA carboxylase deficiency is the best-characterized inborn error of metabolism. Isolated propionyl-CoA carboxylase deficiency is a rare disorder, with an estimated incidence of 1 in 350,000 individuals.[80] Afflicted individuals become symptomatic during early infancy with vomiting, lethargy, and hypotonia.[80] Treatment by administration of oral biotin may be successful. Propionyl-CoA carboxylase deficiency can be diagnosed prenatally either by demonstrating deficient enzyme activity in cultured amniotic fluid cells or by detecting the presence of elevated concentrations of methylcitrate in amniotic fluid.[80] Mutations of genes coding for the α- and β-subunits of propionyl-CoA carboxylase have been identified.[82]

A small number of patients (21 as of 1982) with isolated pyruvate carboxylase deficiency have been reported.[80] Symptoms appear in early infancy, and biotin administration has not been a successful treatment. Pyruvate carboxylase deficiency presents either as the North American phenotype (lacticacidemia, hyperalaninemia, hyperprolinemia) or the French phenotype (elevated blood levels of ammonia, citrulline, proline, and lysine).[83]

Isolated deficiencies of the two remaining carboxylases are rare. Some mutations of the genes coding for the α- and β-subunits of β-methylcrotonyl-CoA carboxylase have been identified.[84,85] One case of isolated acetyl-CoA carboxylase has been reported, in which acetyl-CoA carboxylase activity in fibroblasts was 10% of normal controls.[80]

### *Biotin Transporter Deficiency*

Recently, a case of inborn biotin transporter deficiency was identified.[18] The afflicted patient exhibited the typical signs of biotin deficiency despite normal biotin intake; transport rates of biotin in lymphoid tissues were substantially smaller compared with healthy controls. Symptoms of biotin deficiency improved in response to supplementation with pharmacological doses of biotin. Evidence was provided that biotin transporter deficiency was not caused by abnormal SMVT, but the identity of the afflicted transporter remained unknown.

## Biotin-Drug Interactions

### *Anticonvulsants*

Biotin requirements may be increased during anticonvulsant therapy. The anticonvulsants primidone and carbamazepine inhibit biotin uptake into brush-border membrane vesicles from human intestine.[22] Long-term therapy with anticonvulsants increases both biotin catabolism and urinary excretion of 3-hydroxyisovaleric acid.[22] Phenobarbital, phenytoin, and carbamazepine displace biotin from biotinidase, conceivably affecting plasma transport, renal handling, or cellular uptake of biotin,[22] all of which are associated with decreased plasma concentrations of biotin.

### *Lipoic Acid*

Lipoic acid may be administered to treat heavy metal intoxication, to reduce signs of diabetic neuropathy, and to enhance glucose disposal in patients with non-insulin-dependent diabetes mellitus.[22] Lipoic acid competes with biotin for binding to SMVT,[22] potentially decreasing the cellular uptake of biotin. Indeed, chronic administration of pharmacological doses of lipoic acid decreased the activities of pyruvate carboxylase and β-methylcrotonyl-CoA carboxylase in rat liver to 64% to 72% of that of controls.[22]

## Requirements and Recommended Intakes

### *Adequate Intakes*

The Food and Nutrition Board of the National Research Council has released recommendations for Adequate Intake (AI) of biotin (Table 2).[86] These data are based on estimated biotin intakes (not to be confused with requirements) in a group of healthy people. AIs may serve as goals for the nutrient intake of individuals. Biotin supplements may contribute substantially to biotin intake; 15% to 20% of individuals in the United States report consuming biotin-containing dietary supplements.[86]

### *Factors that Affect Biotin Requirements*

Pregnancy may be associated with an increased demand for biotin. Recent studies provide evidence for marginal biotin deficiency in human gestation, as judged by increased urinary excretion of 3-hydroxyisovaleric acid, decreased urinary excretion of biotin and bisnorbiotin, and decreased plasma concentration of biotin.[54] Pregnancy may be associated with accelerated biotin catabolism.[54] Smoking might further accelerate biotin catabolism in women.[87]

Lactation may generate an increased demand for biotin. At 8 days postpartum, biotin in human milk was approximately 8 nmol/L and accounted for 44% of biotin plus catabolites; bisnorbiotin and biotin-*d,l*-sulfoxide accounted for 48% and 8%, respectively.[88] By 6 weeks postpartum, the biotin concentration had increased to approximately 30 nmol/L and accounted for about 70% of biotin plus catabolites; bisnorbiotin and biotin-*d,l*-sulfoxides accounted for about 20% and less than 10%, respectively.

**Table 2.** Adequate Intakes of Biotin[86]

| Age | Adequate Intake μg/d |
|---|---|
| **Infants** | |
| 0–6 mo | 5 |
| 7–12 mo | 6 |
| **Children** | |
| 1–3 y | 8 |
| 4–8 y | 12 |
| **Adults** | |
| 9–13 y | 20 |
| 14–18 y | 25 |
| 19 y and older | 30 |
| Pregnant women | 30 |
| Lactating women | 35 |

Used with permission from Food and Nutrition Board, 1998[86]

## Intake and Food Sources

The majority of biotin in meats and cereals appears to be protein bound.[22] Most studies of biotin content in foods depended on the use of bioassays. Despite potential analytical limitations due to interfering endogenous compounds, protein binding, and lack of chemical specificity for biotin, there is reasonably good agreement among published reports.[22] Biotin is widely distributed in natural foods. Foods relatively rich in biotin include egg yolk, liver, and some vegetables. The dietary biotin intake in western populations is about 35 to 70 μg/d (143 to 287 nmol/d).[22]

Infants consuming 800 mL/d of mature breast milk ingest approximately 6 μg (24 nmol) of biotin.[88] It remains unclear whether biotin synthesis by gut microorganisms contributes importantly to the total biotin absorbed.[22] However, one infant reportedly developed biotin deficiency while consuming a biotin-free elemental formula.[22]

## Excess and Toxicity

Empirically, the ingestion of pharmacological doses of biotin has been considered safe. For example, lifelong treatment of biotinidase deficiency patients with biotin doses that exceed the normal dietary intake by 300 times does not produce frank signs of toxicity.[55] Likewise, no signs of biotin overdose were reported after acute oral and intravenous administration of doses that exceeded the dietary biotin intake by up to 600 times.[32] However, biotin supplementation is associated with alterations of gene expression in healthy adults and human cell culture models, as described above.[14] Some of these changes might have undesired effects in cell biology. For example, biotin supplementation increases the expression of the gene coding for cytochrome P450 1B1 in human lymphoid cells, and this is associated with increased frequency of DNA strand breaks.[89] Moreover, biotin supplementation decreases expression of the gene coding for sarco/endoplasmic reticulum ATPase 3 in human lymphoid cells, and this is associated with impaired protein folding in the endoplasmic reticulum, causing cell stress (J. B. Griffin and J. Zempleni, unpublished data).

## Future Directions

Evidence has emerged suggesting novel roles for biotin in chromatin structure and cell signaling. These functions go far beyond the classical role of biotin as a coenzyme for carboxylases. Biotin-dependent remodeling of chromatin and cell signaling offer exciting mechanistic insights into processes such as fetal development, malignant transformation of cells, gene expression, and immune function.

This is likely to be a hotbed of biotin research for years to come. In the same context, the potential participation of biotin catabolites in cell signaling has been widely ignored but deserves further investigation. Finally, it will be important to establish a database for the content of biotin and its catabolites in foods based on sound techniques such as HPLC and avidin-binding assays.

## Acknowledgments

Supported by NIH grants DK 60447 and DK 063945, and by NSF EPSCoR grant EPS-0346476.

## References

1. Boas MA. The effect of desiccation upon the nutritive properties of egg-white. Biochem J. 1927;21: 712–724.
2. Kogl F, Tonnis B. Uber das Bios-Problem. Darstellung von krystallisiertem Biotin aus Eigelb. Z Physiol Chem. 1932;242:43–73.
3. du Vigneaud V, Melville DB, Folkers K, et al. The structure of biotin: A study of desthiobiotin. J Biol Chem. 1942;146:475–485.
4. Harris SA, Wolf DE, Mozingo R, Folkers K. Synthetic biotin. Science. 1943;97:447–448.
5. Hatakeyama K, Kobayashi M, Yukawa H. Analysis of biotin biosynthesis pathway in coryneform bacteria: *Brevibacterium flavum*. In: McCormick DB, Suttie JW, Wagner C, eds. *Vitamins and Coenzymes, Part I*. San Diego: Academic Press; 1997;
6. Flint DH, Allen RM. Purification and characterization of biotin synthases. In: McCormick DM, Suttie JW, Wagner C, eds. *Vitamins and Coenzymes, Part I*. San Diego: Academic Press; 1997;.
7. McCormick DB, Wright LD. The metabolism of biotin and analogues. In: Florkin M, Stotz EH, eds. *Metabolism of Vitamins and Trace Elements*. Amsterdam: Elsevier; 1971; 81–110.
8. Zempleni J, McCormick DB, Mock DM. Identification of biotin sulfone, bisnorbiotin methyl ketone, and tetranorbiotin-l- sulfoxide in human urine. Am J Clin Nutr. 1997;65:508–511.
9. Lee YC, Hayes MG, McCormick DB. Microsomal oxidation of α-thiocarboxylic acids to sulfoxides. Biochem Pharmacol. 1970;19:2825–2832.
10. Lee HM, Wright LD, McCormick DB. Metabolism of carbonyl-labeled 14 C-biotin in the rat. J Nutr. 1972;102:1453–1463.
11. Wang KS, Mock NI, Mock DM. Biotin biotransformation to bisnorbiotin is accelerated by several peroxisome proliferators and steroid hormones in rats. J Nutr. 1997;127:2212–2216.
12. Mock DM, Lankford GL, Mock NI. Biotin accounts for only half of the total avidin-binding substances in human serum. J Nutr. 1995;125:941–946.
13. Knowles JR. The mechanism of biotin-dependent enzymes. Ann Rev Biochem. 1989;58:195–221.
14. Rodriguez-Melendez R, Zempleni J. Regulation of gene expression by biotin [review]. J Nutr Biochem. 2003;14:680–690.
15. Dakshinamurti K, Chauhan J. Biotin-binding proteins. In: Dakshinamurti K, ed. *Vitamin Receptors: Vitamins as Ligands in Cell Communication*. Cambridge, UK: Cambridge University Press; 1994; 200–249.
16. Kim KH. Regulation of mammalian acetyl-coenzyme A carboxylase. Annu Rev Nutr. 1997;17: 77–99.
17. Wolf B, Heard GS, McVoy JR, Grier RE. Biotinidase deficiency. Ann N Y Acad Sci. 1985;447: 252–262.
18. Zempleni J. Uptake, localization, and noncarboxylase roles of biotin. Annu Rev Nutr. 2005;25:175–196.
19. Dakshinamurti K, Cheah-Tan C. Liver glucokinase of the biotin deficient rat. Can J Biochem. 1968;46: 75–80.
20. Rodriguez-Melendez R, Griffin JB, Sarath G, Zempleni J. High-throughput immunoblotting identifies biotin-dependent signaling proteins in HepG2 hepatocarcinoma cells. J Nutr. 2005;135:1659–1666.
21. Zempleni J, Mock DM. Biotin. In: Song WO, Beecher GR, eds. *Modern Analytical Methodologies on Fat and Water-Soluble Vitamins*. New York, NY: Wiley & Sons; 2000; 389–409.
22. Zempleni J, Mock DM. Biotin biochemistry and human requirements. J Nutr Biochem. 1999;10: 128–138.
23. Said HM, Thuy LP, Sweetman L, Schatzman B. Transport of the biotin dietary derivative biocytin (N-biotinyl-L-lysine) in rat small intestine. Gastroenterology. 1993;104:75–80.
24. Bowman BB, Selhub J, Rosenberg IH. Intestinal absorption of biotin in the rat. J Nutr. 1986;116: 1266–1271.
25. Said HM, Redha R. A carrier-mediated system for transport of biotin in rat intestine in vitro. Am J Physiol. 1987;252(1 part 1):G52–G55.
26. Prasad PD, Wang H, Kekuda R, et al. Cloning and functional expression of a cDNA encoding a mammalian sodium-dependent vitamin transporter mediating the uptake of pantothenate, biotin, and lipoate. J Biol Chem. 1998;273:7501–7506.
27. Prasad PD, Wang H, Huang W, et al. Molecular and functional characterization of the intestinal Na+-dependent multivitamin transporter. Arch Biochem Biophys. 1999;366:95–106.
28. Said HM. Recent advances in carrier-mediated intestinal absorption of water-soluble vitamins. Annu Rev Physiol. 2004;66:419–446.

29. Said HM. Cellular uptake of biotin: mechanisms and regulation. J Nutr. 1999;129(2S suppl):490S–493S.
30. Chatterjee NS, Rubin SA, Said HM. Molecular characterization of the 5′ regulatory region of rat sodium-dependent multivitamin transporter gene. Am J Physiol Cell Physiol. 2001;280:C548–C555.
31. Dey S, Subramanian VS, Chatterjee NS, Rubin SA, Said HM. Characterization of the 5′ regulatory region of the human sodium-dependent multivitamin transporter, hSMVT. Biochim Biophys Acta. 2002; 1574:187–192.
32. Zempleni J, Mock DM. Bioavailability of biotin given orally to humans in pharmacologic doses. Am J Clin Nutr. 1999;69:504–508.
33. Said HM, Redha R, Nylander W. Biotin transport in basolateral membrane vesicles of human intestine. Gastroenterology. 1988;94(5 part 1):1157–1163.
34. Chauhan J, Dakshinamurti K. Role of human serum biotinidase as biotin-binding protein. Biochem J. 1988;256:265–270.
35. Seshagiri PB, Adiga PR. Isolation and characterisation of a biotin-binding protein from the pregnant-rat serum and comparison with that from the chicken egg-yolk. Biochim Biophys Acta. 1987;916: 474–481.
36. Said HM, Ma TY, Kamanna VS. Uptake of biotin by human hepatoma cell line, Hep G2: a carrier-mediated process similar to that of normal liver. J Cell Physiol. 1994;161:483–489.
37. Zempleni J, Mock DM. The efflux of biotin from human peripheral blood mononuclear cells. J Nutr Biochem. 1999;10:105–109.
38. Daberkow RL, White BR, Cederberg RA, Griffin JB, Zempleni J. Monocarboxylate transporter 1 mediates biotin uptake in human peripheral blood mononuclear cells. J Nutr. 2003;133:2703–2706.
39. Halestrap AP, Price NT. The proton-linked monocarboxylate transporter (MCT) family: structure, function and regulation. Biochem J. 1999;343(part 2):281–299.
40. Petrelli F, Moretti P, Paparelli M. Intracellular distribution of biotin-14C COOH in rat liver. Molec Biol Rep. 1979;4:247–252.
41. Shriver BJ, Roman-Shriver C, Allred JB. Depletion and repletion of biotinyl enzymes in liver of biotin-deficient rats: evidence of a biotin storage system. J Nutr. 1993;123:1140–1149.
42. Nabokina SM, Subramanian VS, Said HM. Comparative analysis of ontogenic changes in renal and intestinal biotin transport in the rat. Am J Physiol Renal Physiol. 2003;284:F737–F742.
43. Baur B, Baumgartner ER. Na(+)-dependent biotin transport into brush-border membrane vesicles from human kidney cortex. Pflugers Archiv. 1993;422: 499–505.
44. Zempleni J, Green GM, Spannagel AW, Mock DM. Biliary excretion of biotin and biotin metabolites is quantitatively minor in rats and pigs. J Nutr. 1997; 127:1496–1500.
45. Bitsch R, Salz I, Hötzel D. Studies on bioavailability of oral biotin doses for humans. Int J Vitam Nutr Res. 1989;59:65–71.
46. Frigg M, Hartmann D, Straub OC. Biotin kinetics in serum of cattle after intravenous and oral dosing. Int J Vitam Nutr Res. 1994;64:36–40.
47. Zempleni J, McCormick DB, Stratton SL, Mock DM. Lipoic acid (thioctic acid) analogs, tryptophan analogs, and urea do not interfere with the assay of biotin and biotin metabolites by high-performance liquid chromatography/avidin-binding assay. J Nutr Biochem. 1996;7:518–523.
48. Mock NI, Malik MI, Stumbo PJ, Bishop WP, Mock DM. Increased urinary excretion of 3-hydroxyisovaleric acid and decreased urinary excretion of biotin are sensitive early indicators of decreased status in experimental biotin deficiency. Am J Clin Nutr. 1997;65:951–958.
49. Velazquez A, Zamudio S, Baez A, Murguia-Corral R, Rangel-Peniche B, Carrasco A. Indicators of biotin status: A study of patients on prolonged total parenteral nutrition. Eur J Clin Nutr. 1990;44:11–16.
50. Mock D, Henrich C, Carnell N, Mock N, Swift L. Lymphocyte propionyl-CoA carboxylase and accumulation of odd-chain fatty acid in plasma and erythrocytes are useful indicators of marginal biotin deficiency. J Nutr Biochem. 2002;13:462–470.
51. Mock DM, Henrich CL, Carnell N, Mock NI. Indicators of marginal biotin deficiency and repletion in humans: validation of 3-hydroxyisovaleric acid excretion and a leucine challenge. Am J Clin Nutr 2002; 76:1061–1068.
52. Mock DM, Henrich-Shell CL, Carnell N, Stumbo P, Mock NI. 3-Hydroxypropionic acid and methylcitric acid are not reliable indicators of marginal biotin deficiency in humans. J Nutr. 2004;134: 317–320.
53. Mock DM, Johnson SB, Holman RT. Effects of biotin deficiency on serum fatty acid composition: Evidence for abnormalities in humans. J Nutr. 1988; 118:342–348.
54. Zempleni J, Mock DM. Marginal biotin deficiency is teratogenic. Proc Soc Exp Biol Med. 2000;223: 14–21.
55. Wolf B, Heard GS. Biotinidase deficiency. In: Barness L, Oski F, eds. *Advances in Pediatrics*. Chicago, IL: Medical Book Publishers; 1991; 1–21.
56. Spencer RP, Brody KR. Biotin transport by small intestine of rat, hamster, and other species. Am J Physiol. 1964;206:653–657.
57. Cowan MJ, Wara DW, Packman S, et al. Multiple biotin-dependent carboxylase deficiencies associated with defects in T-cell and B-cell immunity. Lancet. 1979;2:115–118.
58. Kumar M, Axelrod AE. Cellular antibody synthesis

in thiamin, riboflavin, biotin and folic acid-deficient rats. Proc Soc Exp Biol Med. 1978;157:421–423.
59. Báez-Saldaña A, Díaz G, Espinoza B, Ortega E. Biotin deficiency induces changes in subpopulations of spleen lymphocytes in mice. Am J Clin Nutr. 1998; 67:431–437.
60. Báez-Saldaña A, Ortega E. Biotin deficiency blocks thymocyte maturation, accelerates thymus involution, and decreases nose-rump length in mice. J Nutr. 2004;134:1970–1977.
61. Dakshinamurti K, Chalifour LE, Bhullar RJ. Requirement for biotin and the function of biotin in cells in culture. In: Dakshinamurti K, Bhagavan HN, eds. *Biotin*. New York: New York Academy of Science; 1985; 38–55.
62. Manthey KC, Griffin JB, Zempleni J. Biotin supply affects expression of biotin transporters, biotinylation of carboxylases, and metabolism of interleukin-2 in Jurkat cells. J Nutr. 2002;132:887–892.
63. Crisp SE, Griffin JB, White BR, et al. Biotin supply affects rates of cell proliferation, biotinylation of carboxylases and histones, and expression of the gene encoding the sodium-dependent multivitamin transporter in JAr choriocarcinoma cells. Eur J Nutr. 2004; 43:23–31.
64. Moskowitz M, Cheng DKS. Stimulation of growth factor production in cultured cells by biotin. In: Dakshinamurti K, Bhagavan HN, eds. *Biotin*. New York: New York Academy of Sciences; 1985; 212–221.
65. Zempleni J, Mock DM. Mitogen-induced proliferation increases biotin uptake into human peripheral blood mononuclear cells. Am J Physiol. 1999;276(5 part 1):C1079–C1084.
66. Stanley JS, Griffin JB, Mock DM, Zempleni J. Biotin uptake into human peripheral blood mononuclear cells increases early in the cell cycle, increasing carboxylase activities. J Nutr. 2002;132:1854–1859.
67. Stanley JS, Griffin JB, Zempleni J. Biotinylation of histones in human cells: effects of cell proliferation. Eur J Biochem. 2001;268:5424–5429.
68. Rodriguez-Melendez R, Schwab LD, Zempleni J. Jurkat cells respond to biotin deficiency with increased nuclear translocation of NF-kB, mediating cell survival. Int J Vitam Nutr Res. 2004;74:209–216.
69. Landenberger A, Kabil H, Harshman LG, Zempleni J. Biotin deficiency decreases life span and fertility but increases stress resistance in *Drosophila melanogaster*. J Nutr Biochem. 2004;15:591–600.
70. Griffin JB, Zempleni J. Biotin deficiency stimulates survival pathways in human lymphoma cells exposed to antineoplastic drugs. J Nutr Biochem. 2005;16: 96–103.
71. Mock DM, Mock NI, Stewart CW, LaBorde JB, Hansen DK. Marginal biotin deficiency is teratogenic in ICR mice. J Nutr. 2003;133:2519–2525.
72. Watanabe T, Endo A. Species and strain differences in teratogenic effects of biotin deficiency in rodents. J Nutr. 1989;119:255–261.
73. Pacheco-Alvarez D, Solorzano-Vargas RS, Gravel RA, Cervantes-Roldan R, Velazquez A, Leon-Del-Rio A. Paradoxical regulation of biotin utilization in brain and liver and implications for inherited multiple carboxylase deficiencies. J Biol Chem 2004;279: 52312–52318.
74. Suormala T, Baumgartner ER, Bausch J, Holick W, Wick H. Quantitative determination of biocytin in urine of patients with biotinidase deficiency using high-performance liquid chromatography (HPLC). Clin Chim Acta. 1988;177:253–269.
75. Wolf B. Worldwide survey of neonatal screening for biotinidase deficiency. J Inherit Metab Dis. 1991;14: 923–927.
76. Moslinger D, Muhl A, Suormala T, Baumgartner R, Stockler-Ipsiroglu S. Molecular characterisation and neuropsychological outcome of 21 patients with profound biotinidase deficiency detected by newborn screening and family studies. Eur J Pediatr. 2003; 162(suppl 1):S46–S49.
77. Laszlo A, Schuler EA, Sallay E, et al. Neonatal screening for biotinidase deficiency in Hungary: clinical, biochemical and molecular studies. J Inherit Metab Dis. 2003;26:693–698.
78. Neto EC, Schulte J, Rubim R, et al. Newborn screening for biotinidase deficiency in Brazil: biochemical and molecular characterizations. Braz J Med Biol Res. 2004;37:295–299.
79. Wolf B, Grier RE, Allen RJ, Goodman SI, Kien CL. Biotinidase deficiency: An enzymatic defect in late-onset multiple carboxylase deficiency. Clin Chim Acta. 1983;131:273–281.
80. Wolf B, Feldman GL. The biotin-dependent carboxylase deficiencies. Am J Hum Genet. 1982;34: 699–716.
81. Suzuki Y, Yang X, Aoki Y, et al. Mutations in the holocarboxylase synthetase gene. Human Mutation 2005;26:285–290.
82. Perez B, Desviat LR, Rodriguez-Pombo P, et al. Propionic acidemia: identification of twenty-four novel mutations in Europe and North America. Mol Genet Metab. 2003;78:59–67.
83. Robinson BH, Oei J, Saudubray JM, et al. The French and North American phenotypes of pyruvate carboxylase deficiency, correlation with biotin containing protein by 3H-biotin incorporation, 35S-streptavidin labeling, and northern blotting with a cloned cDNA probe. Am J Hum Genet. 1987;40: 50–59.
84. Desviat LR, Perez-Cerda C, Perez B, et al. Functional analysis of MCCA and MCCB mutations causing methylcrotonylglycinuria. Mol Genet Metab. 2003;80:315–320.
85. Baumgartner MR, Dantas MF, Suormala T, et al. Isolated 3-methylcrotonyl-CoA carboxylase defi-

ciency: evidence for an allele-specific dominant negative effect and responsiveness to biotin therapy. Am J Hum Genet. 2004;75:790–800.

86. Food and Nutrition Board, Institute of Medicine. Dietary Reference Intakes for Thiamin, Riboflavin, Niacin, Vitamin B6, Folate, Vitamin B12, Pantothenic Acid, Biotin, and Choline; 1998. Available online at: http://www.nap.edu/openbook/0309065542/html/.
87. Sealey WM, Teague AM, Stratton SL, Mock DM. Smoking accelerates biotin catabolism in women. Am J Clin Nutr. 2004;80:932–5.
88. Mock DM, Stratton SL, Mock NI. Concentrations of biotin metabolites in human milk. J Pediatr. 1997; 131:456–458.
89. Rodriguez-Melendez R, Griffin JB, Zempleni J. Biotin supplementation increases expression of the cytochrome P450 1B1 gene in Jurkat cells, increasing the occurrence of single-stranded DNA breaks. J Nutr. 2004;134:2222–2228.

# 25 Pantothenic Acid

Joshua W. Miller, Lisa M. Rogers, and Robert B. Rucker

## History

The discovery of pantothenic acid followed the same path that led to the discovery of other water-soluble vitamins: studies utilizing bacteria and single-cell eukaryotic organisms (e.g., yeast), animal models, and thoughtful chemical analysis. It was largely the efforts of research groups associated with R.J. Williams, C.A. Elvehjem, and T.H. Jukes that resulted in the identification of pantothenic acid as an essential dietary factor. Williams et al.[1] established that pantothenic acid was required for the growth of certain bacteria and yeast. Next, Elvehjem et al.[2] and Jukes et al.[3,4] demonstrated that pantothenic acid was a growth and "anti-dermatitis" factor for chickens. Williams coined the name "pantothenic" acid from the Greek meaning "from everywhere" to indicate its widespread occurrence in foodstuffs.[1,5] The eventual characterization of pantothenic acid by Williams took advantage of observations that the anti-dermatitis factor present in acid extracts of various food sources (pantothenic acid) did not bind to fuller's earth under acidic conditions. Using chromatographic and fractionation procedures that were typical of the 1930s (solvent-dependent chemical partitioning), Williams isolated several grams of pantothenic acid for structural determination from 250 kg of liver.[5] With this information, a number of research groups contributed to the chemical synthesis and commercial preparation of pantothenic acid.

In the 1950s, one of the functional forms of pantothenic acid, coenzyme A (CoA), was discovered as the cofactor essential for the acetylation of sulfonamides and choline.[6] In the mid-1960s, pantothenic acid was next identified as a component of acyl carrier protein (ACP) in the fatty acid synthesis complex.[7] These developments, in addition to a steady series of observations throughout this period on the effects of pantothenic acid deficiency in humans and other animals, provided the foundation for our current understanding of this vitamin.

## Chemistry and Nomenclature

The chemical structure of pantothenic acid consists of pantoic acid and β-alanine bound in amide linkage (Figure 1a). Metabolic processing of pantothenic acid, described in detail below, produces the important intermediate, 4′-phosphopantetheine (Figure 1b), which includes β-mercaptoethylamine (cysteamine) bound in amide linkage to the terminal carboxyl group of the molecule. 4′-Phosphopantetheine serves as a covalently linked prosthetic group for ACP (Figure 1c). Further metabolic processing with the addition of adenine and ribose 3′-phosphate produces the essential cofactor, CoA (Figure 1d).

Pure pantothenic acid is a water-soluble, viscous, yellow oil. It is stable at neutral pH, but is readily destroyed by acid, alkali, and heat. Calcium pantothenate, a white, odorless, crystalline substance, is the form of pantothenic acid usually found in commercial vitamin supplements due to its greater stability than the pure acid.[8] Early literature referred to pantothenic acid as chick anti-dermatitis factor, filtrate factor, and vitamin $B_3$. Today, it is often referred to as vitamin $B_5$, although the origin of this designation is obscure.

## Intestinal Absorption, Plasma Transport, and Excretion

The vast majority of pantothenic acid in food is present as a component of CoA or 4′-phosphopantetheine. To be absorbed, these substances must first be hydrolyzed.[9] This occurs in the intestinal lumen by the sequential activity of two hydrolases, pyrophosphatase and phosphatase, with pantetheine as the product. Pantetheine is either absorbed as is, or is further metabolized to pantothenic acid by a third intestinal hydrolase, pantetheinase.

## A. Pantothenic Acid

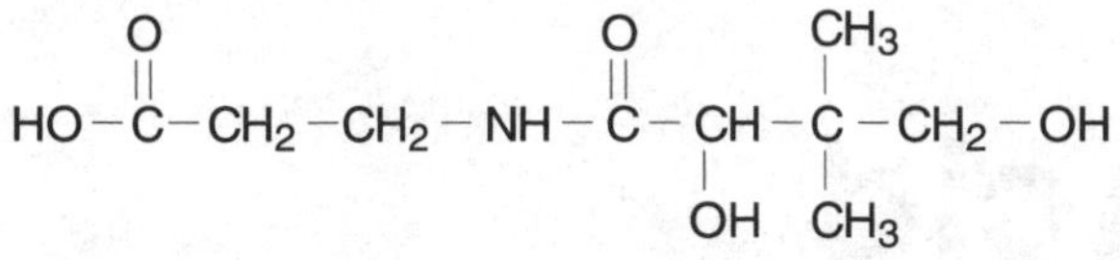

$$HO-\overset{O}{\overset{\|}{C}}-CH_2-CH_2-NH-\overset{O}{\overset{\|}{C}}-\underset{OH}{\underset{|}{CH}}-\overset{CH_3}{\overset{|}{\underset{CH_3}{\underset{|}{C}}}}-CH_2-OH$$

## B. 4'-Phosphopantetheine

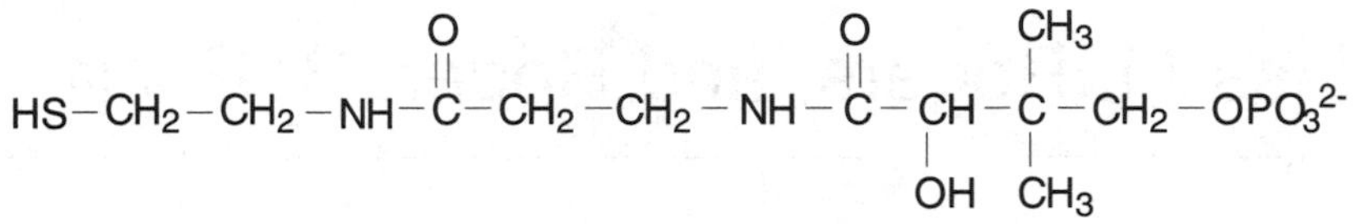

$$HS-CH_2-CH_2-NH-\overset{O}{\overset{\|}{C}}-CH_2-CH_2-NH-\overset{O}{\overset{\|}{C}}-\underset{OH}{\underset{|}{CH}}-\overset{CH_3}{\overset{|}{\underset{CH_3}{\underset{|}{C}}}}-CH_2-OPO_3^{2-}$$

## C. Acyl Carrier Protein

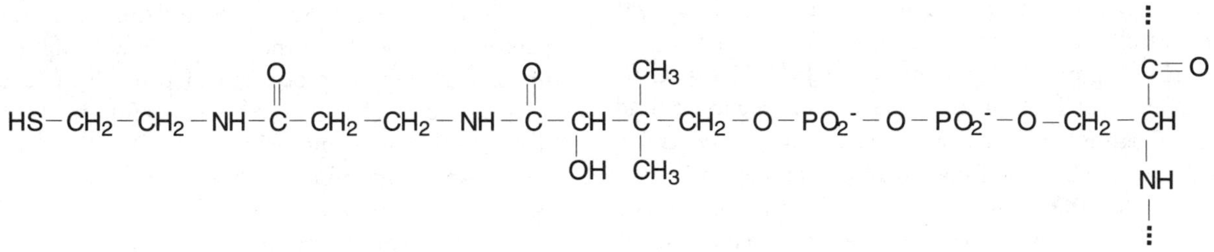

$$HS-CH_2-CH_2-NH-\overset{O}{\overset{\|}{C}}-CH_2-CH_2-NH-\overset{O}{\overset{\|}{C}}-\underset{OH}{\underset{|}{CH}}-\overset{CH_3}{\overset{|}{\underset{CH_3}{\underset{|}{C}}}}-CH_2-O-PO_2^--O-PO_2^--O-CH_2-\overset{\vdots}{\overset{|}{\overset{C=O}{\overset{|}{\underset{\vdots}{\underset{|}{\underset{NH}{\underset{|}{CH}}}}}}}}$$

## D. Coenzyme A

$$HS-CH_2-CH_2-NH-\overset{O}{\overset{\|}{C}}-CH_2-CH_2-NH-\overset{O}{\overset{\|}{C}}-\underset{OH}{\underset{|}{CH}}-\overset{CH_3}{\overset{|}{\underset{CH_3}{\underset{|}{C}}}}-CH_2-O-PO_2^--O-PO_2^--O-CH_2-\text{(ribose: H, H, H, H, OH, O}-PO_3^{2-}\text{; N-linked adenine with } NH_2\text{)}$$

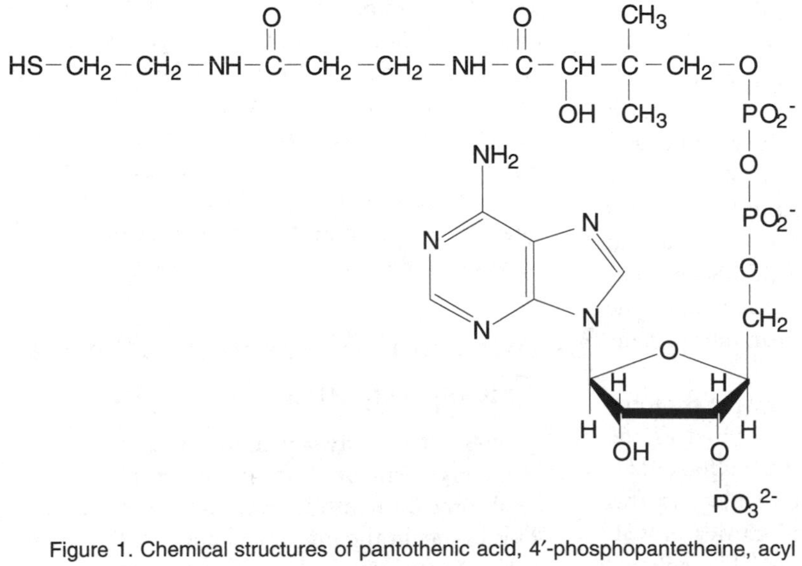

Figure 1. Chemical structures of pantothenic acid, 4′-phosphopantetheine, acyl carrier protein, and coenzyme A.

In rats, pantothenic acid absorption was initially found to occur in all sections of the small intestine by simple diffusion.[9] However, subsequent work in rats and chicks indicated that at low concentrations, the vitamin is absorbed by a saturable, sodium-dependent transport mechanism.[10] Moreover, it has been demonstrated that pantothenic acid shares a common membrane transport system in the small intestine with another vitamin, biotin. In vitro experiments utilizing Caco-2 cell mono-layers as a model of intestinal absorption established that pantothenic acid uptake is inhibited competitively by biotin and vice versa.[11] Similar observations have been made in transport experiments involving the blood-brain barrier,[12] heart,[13] and placenta.[14] After absorption, pantothenic acid enters the circulation, where it is taken up by cells in a manner similar to that of intestinal absorption (see below). The vitamin is excreted in the urine primarily as pantothenic acid. This occurs after its release from CoA by a series of hydrolysis reactions that cleave off the phosphate and β-mercaptoethylamine moieties.

# Functions and Cellular Regulation

## *Coenzyme A and Acyl Carrier Protein Synthesis*

Pantothenic acid is nutritionally essential due to the inability of animal cells to synthesize the pantoic acid moiety of the vitamin. The primary function of pantothenic acid is to serve as substrate for the synthesis of CoA and ACP (Figure 2). The first step is the phosphorylation of pantothenic acid to 4′-phosphopantothenic acid by pantothenic acid kinase.[15,16] The kinase possesses a broad pH optimum (between 6 and 9) with a $K_m$ for pantothenic acid of about 20 μM. Mg-ATP is used as the nucleotide substrate for this phosphorylation reaction with a $K_m$ of about 0.6 mM.

The pantothenic acid kinase reaction also serves as the primary control point in the synthesis of CoA and ACP. The reaction is activated and inhibited nonspecifically by various anions. More significantly, feedback inhibition of the kinase by CoA or CoA derivatives governs flux

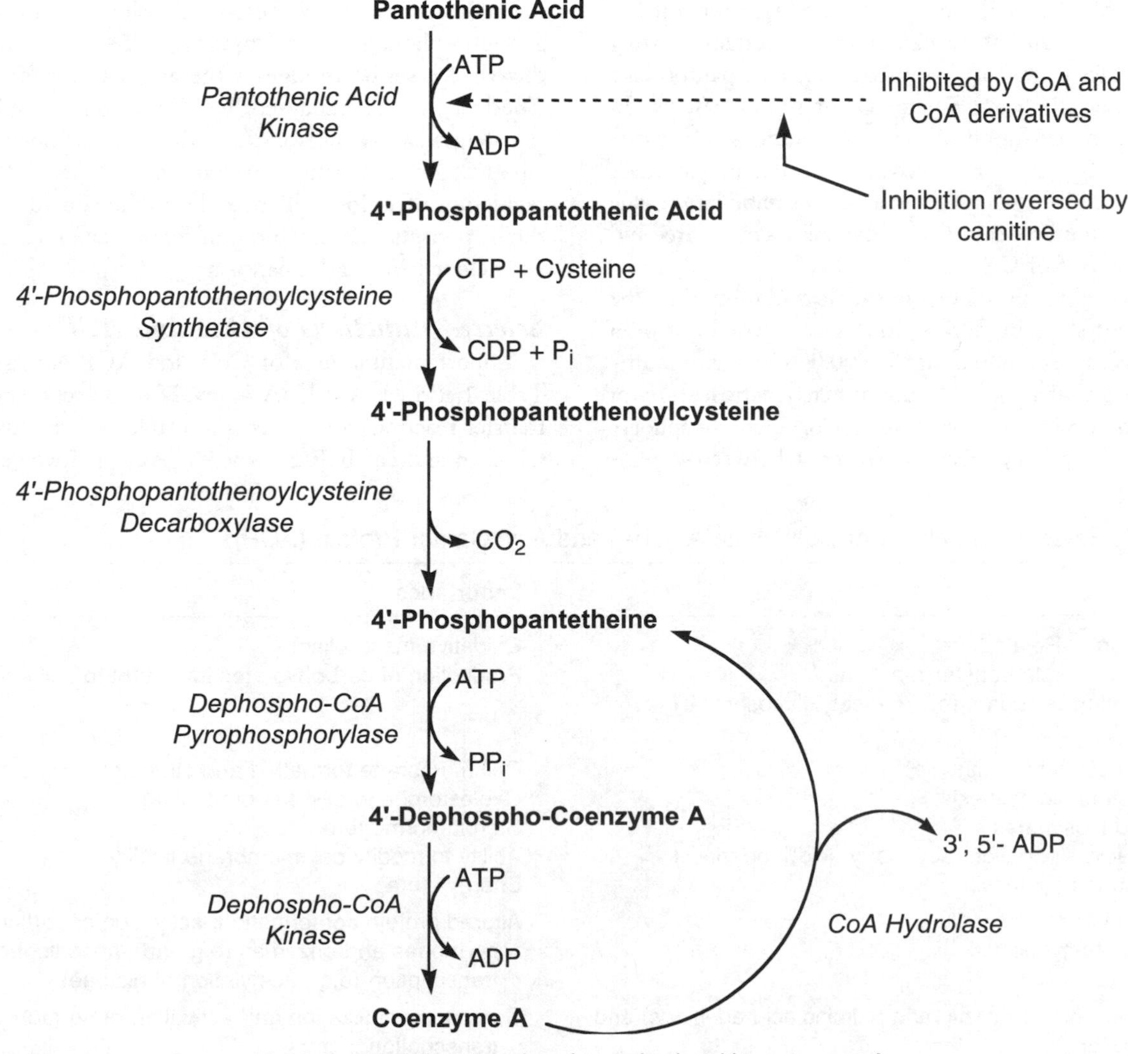


Figure 2. Metabolic conversion of pantothenic acid to coenzyme A.

through the subsequent steps in the CoA synthesis pathway and defines the upper threshold for intracellular CoA cofactor levels. Inhibition by acetyl-CoA is slightly greater than that of free CoA. The inhibition by free CoA is uncompetitive with respect to pantothenate concentration, with a $K_i$ for inhibition of 0.2 μM.

L-carnitine, which is important for the transport of fatty acids into mitochondria, is a nonessential activator of pantothenic acid kinase. Carnitine has no effect by itself, but specifically reverses the inhibition by CoA. In heart tissue, the free carnitine content varies directly with the phosphorylation of pantothenic acid. Thus, these properties of the kinase provide a potential mechanism for the control of CoA synthesis and the regulation of cellular pantothenic acid content: feedback inhibition by CoA and its acyl esters that is reversed by changes in the concentration of free carnitine. However, it is important to underscore that the free concentration of acyl CoA in cells is low and variable, because the bulk of acyl derivatives are protein bound. Moreover, similar to CoA, carnitine exists in both free and acylated forms, and reversal of kinase inhibition by CoA does not occur when carnitine is acylated.[15] The ratio of free to acylated carnitine varies considerably depending on feeding and hormonal influences, with insulin being particularly important. Fasting and diabetes (states of low insulin) increase pantothenic acid kinase activity and the total content of CoA.[17-19] In addition, the perfusion of heart preparations or incubation of liver cells with glucose, pyruvate, or palmitate markedly inhibits pantothenic acid phosphorylation, due to reduction in free carnitine and increases in the free and acylated forms of CoA.

Following 4′-phosphopantothenic acid formation, the subsequent steps in CoA synthesis are carried out on a protein complex (approximately 400,000 Da) with multifunctional catalytic sites. Important enzymatic features of this complex include dephospho-CoA-pyrophosphorylase activity, which catalyzes the reaction between 4′-phosphopantetheine and ATP to form 4′-dephospho-CoA; dephospho-CoA-kinase activity, which catalyzes the ATP-dependent final step in CoA synthesis; and CoA hydrolase activity, which catalyzes the hydrolysis of CoA to 3′,5′-ADP and 4′-phosphopantetheine. This sequence of reactions is referred to as the CoA/4′-phosphopantetheine cycle, and it provides a mechanism by which the 4′-phosphopantetheine can be recycled to form CoA. Each turn of the cycle utilizes two molecules of ATP and produces one molecule of ADP, one molecule of pyrophosphate, and one molecule of 3′,5′-ADP (Figure 2).[20]

ACP is sometimes referred to as a "macro-cofactor," because in bacteria, yeast, and plants, it is composed of a polypeptide chain (mol. wt of approximately 8500–8700 Da) to which 4′-phosphopantetheine is attached. However, in higher animals, ACP is most often associated with a fatty acid synthase complex that is composed of two very large protein subunits (mol. wt. about 250,000 Da each). The carrier segment or domain of the fatty acid synthetic complex is also called ACP, one of seven functional or catalytic domains on each of the two subunits that comprise fatty acid synthase. The inactive ACP apopolypeptide (or domain) is converted to an active holoform (or domain) by the post-translational transfer of a 4′-phosphopantetheinyl moiety to the side-chain hydroxyl of a serine residue at the active center of ACP. The reaction is catalyzed by 4′-phosphopantetheinyl transferase, which uses CoA as the 4′-phosphopantetheine substrate. Although there are few data related to the regulation of holo-ACP peptide or domain formation, the 4′-phosphopantetheine transferase gene recently has been cloned from a human source.[21]

## *Selected Functions of CoA and ACP*

Important functions of CoA and ACP are listed in Table 1. Principally, CoA is involved in acetyl and acyl transfer reactions and processes related to oxidative metabolism and catabolism, whereas ACP is involved pri-

**Table 1.** Selected Functions of Coenzyme A (CoA) and Acyl Carrier Protein (ACP)

| Function | Importance |
|---|---|
| Carbohydrate-Related | Oxidative metabolism |
| Citric acid cycle transfer reactions | Production of carbohydrates important to cell structure |
| Acetylation of sugars (e.g. N-acetylglucosamine) | |
| Lipid-Related | |
| Phospholipid biosynthesis | Cell membrane formation and structure |
| Isoprenoid biosynthesis | Cholesterol and bile salt production |
| Steroid biosynthesis | Steroid hormone production |
| Fatty acid elongation, acyl (fatty acid) and triacyl glyceride synthesis | Ability to modify cell membrane fluidity<br>Energy storage |
| Protein-related | Altered protein conformation; activation of certain hormones and enzymes (e.g., adrenocorticotropin); transcription (e.g., acetylation of histone) |
| Protein acetylation | |
| Protein acylation (myristic and palmitic acid additions) and prenylation | Compartmentalization and activation of hormones and transcription factors |

marily in synthetic reactions. The adenosyl moiety of CoA provides a site for tight binding to CoA-requiring enzymes, while allowing the phosphopantetheine portion to serve as a flexible arm to move substrates from one catalytic center to another. Similarly, when pantothenic acid (as 4′-phosphopantetheine) in ACP is used in the transfer reactions associated with the fatty acid synthase process, 4′-phosphopantetheine also functions as a flexible arm that allows for an orderly and systematic presentation of acyl derivatives to each of the active centers of the fatty acid synthase complex. A summary of catalytic sites and their functions in the fatty acid synthase complex is presented in Table 2.

In addition to fatty acid synthesis, hints that ACP-like factors may perform other functions in humans and animals come from observations that an oligosaccharide-linked ACP acts as a transmethylation inhibitor in porcine liver.[22] ACP is also structurally homologous to acidic ribosomal structural proteins, such as ribosomal protein P2.[23] Moreover, in bacteria and plants, ACP is important in a number of pathways, such as amino acid synthesis and the formation of polyketides, a remarkably diverse group of secondary metabolites that include antibiotics such as erythromycin, cholesterol-lowering drugs such as lovastatin, and putative anti-aging compounds such as resveratrol.[24]

It is also important to appreciate that intermediates arising from the transfer reactions catalyzed by CoA and 4′-phosphopantetheine in ACP may be viewed as "high-energy" compounds. CoA or ACP reacts with acetyl or acyl groups to form thioesters. Thioesters (—S—CO—R) are thermodynamically less stable than typical esters (—O—CO—R) or amides (—N—CO—R). The double-bond character of the C—O bond in —S—CO—R does not extend significantly into the C—S bond. This causes thioesters to have relatively a high energy potential, and for most reactions involving CoA or ACP, no additional energy (e.g., from ATP hydrolysis) is required for transfer of the acetyl or acyl group. For example, at pH 7.0, the $-\Delta G$ of hydrolysis is about 7.5 kcal for acetyl-CoA and 10.5 kcal for acetoacetyl-CoA compared with 7 to 8 kcal for the hydrolysis of ATP to AMP and pyrophosphate or ADP and phosphate. The terminal thiol group of CoA and ACP is also ideally suited for nucleophilic substitution reactions involving activated carboxylic acids and α- and β-carbonyl functions.[25]

## *Cellular Regulation of Pantothenic Acid and CoA Levels*

As noted above, both biotin and pantothenic acid appear to share the same transporters for cellular uptake and

**Table 2.** Catalytic Sites Associated with the Fatty Acid Synthase Complex

| Step | Action(s) |
|---|---|
| 1. Acetyl transferase | Catalyzes the transfer of an activated acetyl group on CoA to the sulfhydryl group of 4′-phosphopantetheine (ACP domain); in a subsequent step, the acetyl group is transferred to a second cysteine-derived sulfhydryl group near active site of 3-oxoacyl synthase (see step 3) leaving the 4′-phosphopantetheine sulfhydryl group free for Step 2 |
| 2. Malonyl transferase | This enzyme catalyzes the transfer of successive in-coming malonyl groups to 4′-phosphopantetheine |
| 3. 3-Oxoacyl synthetase | The first condensation reaction in the process, catalyzed by 3-oxoacyl synthase, in which attack on malonyl-ACP by the acetyl moiety (transferred in Step 1) occurs with decarboxylation and condensation to yield a 3-oxobutryl (acetoacetyl) derivative; in the second through the seventh cycles, it is the newly formed acyl moieties that attack the malonyl group added at each cycle (see Step 6) |
| 4. Oxoacyl reductase | Reductions of acetoacetyl or 3-oxoacyl intermediates involve NADPH; the first cycle of this reaction generates D-hydroxybutyrate, and in subsequent cycles, hydroxyfatty acids |
| 5. 3-Hydroxyacyl dehydratase | This enzyme catalyzes the removal of a molecule of water from the 3-hydroxyacyl derivatives produced in Step 4 to form enoyl derivatives |
| 6. Enoyl reductase | Reduction of the enoyl derivatives (Step 5) by a second molecule of NADPH generates a fatty acid; this acyl group is also transferred to the sulfhydryl group adjacent to 3-oxoacyl synthase, as described in step 1, until a 16-carbon palmitoyl group is formed; this group, still attached to the 4′-phosphopantetheine arm, is highly specific substrate for the remaining enzyme of the complex, thioester hydrolase |
| 7. Thioester hydrolase | This enzyme liberates palmitic acid (Step 6) from the 4′-phosphopantetheine arm |

ACP = acyl carrier protein; CoA = coenzyme A.

perhaps efflux.[11] Whether it is an intestinal, hepatic, or cardiac muscle cell, the process for pantothenic acid cellular uptake appears saturable, with an apparent $K_m$ of 15 to 20 μM. Transport across cell membranes appears to occur by carrier-mediated, sodium gradient-dependent, and electroneutral mechanisms.[13,26-29] Pantothenic acid cellular uptake has also been linked to protein kinase C and calmodulin-dependent regulatory and signaling pathways.[27] The dependence on protein kinase C is based on observations that pretreatment of cells with a protein kinase C activator such as phorbol 12-myristate 13-acetate or 1,2-dioctanoyl-glycerol significantly inhibits pantothenic acid uptake. If an inward sodium gradient is imposed, a rapid uptake of pantothenic acid is observed. Uptake of pantothenic acid is reduced when sodium is replaced by potassium or if external sodium is reduced below 40 mM. Ouabain, gramicidin D, cyanide, azide, and 2,4-dinitrophenol also act as inhibitors.

With regard to efflux, unlike uptake, the export of pantothenic acid is unaffected by the addition of pantothenic acid, sodium, ouabain, gramicidin D, or 2,4-dinitrophenol to the external medium. Moreover, the metabolic state also has an impact on uptake. For example, in the perfused heart, pantothenic acid transport is significantly increased when hearts are perfused and are acting as "working" hearts because of addition of a fuel source.[27]

That active uptake of pantothenic acid is underscored by the differences in cellular versus plasma concentrations of free pantothenic acid. The cellular concentration of free pantothenic acid in the liver is 10 to 15 μM and in the heart about 100 μM, compared with 1 to 5 μM observed in plasma. Similarly, the unidirectional influx of pantothenic acid across cerebral capillaries (the blood-brain barrier) occurs by a low-capacity, saturable transport system with a half-saturation concentration approximately 10 times the plasma pantothenic acid concentration.[30,31] For comparison, the concentrations of CoA and ACP are 50 to 100 μM and 10 μM, respectively, in the cytosol of typical cells. In mitochondria, the CoA concentration can be as much as 10- to 20-fold higher, or 70% to 90% of the total cellular CoA content.

In addition to cellular transport, enzymes associated with CoA synthesis also have significant impact on maintaining cellular levels of pantothenic acid and related compounds. As described above, the most important of these enzymes is pantothenic acid kinase.[15]

## Dietary Sources and Requirements

Pantothenic acid is found in a wide variety of foods of both plant and animal origin at levels ranging from 20 to 50 μg/g. Particularly rich sources of pantothenic acid include chicken, beef, liver and other organ meats, whole grains, potatoes, and tomato products.[32] Royal bee jelly and ovaries of tuna and cod also have high levels of the vitamin.[33] Because of its thermal lability and susceptibility to oxidation, significant amounts of pantothenic acid are lost from highly processed foods, including refined grains and cooked or canned meats and vegetables. Processing and refining whole grains results in a 37% to 47% loss of pantothenic acid, while canning of meats, fish, and dairy products leads to losses of 20% to 35%.[34] Greater losses of the vitamin occur during canning (46%–78%) and freezing (37%–57%) of vegetables. Pantothenic acid is also synthesized by intestinal microorganisms,[35] although the amount produced and the availability of the vitamin from this source is unknown.

The primary source of pantothenic acid in food is CoA. Intestinal phosphatases and nucleosidases are capable of very efficient hydrolysis of CoA so that near-quantitative release of pantothenic acid occurs as a normal part of digestion. Further, the overall $K_m$ for pantothenic acid intestinal uptake is 10 to 20 μM. At an intake of about 10 to 15 mg of CoA, the amount of CoA in a typical meal, the pantothenic acid concentration in luminal fluid would be about 1 to 2 μM. At this concentration, pantothenic acid would not saturate the transport system, and as a consequence, should be efficiently and actively absorbed.[11]

A dietary reference intake has yet to be established for pantothenic acid. Adequate intakes (AIs) for men and women throughout the life cycle have been suggested based on observed mean intakes and estimates of basal excretion in urine (Table 3).[36] Urinary excretion of pantothenic acid only exceeds basal levels when intakes are greater than 4 mg/d in young adult males. Thus, an intake of 4 mg/d likely reflects the level at which saturation of

**Table 3.** Adequate Intakes (AIs) for Pantothenic Acid

| Age Group | AI *(mg/d)* |
|---|---|
| Infants | |
| 0–5 months | 1.7 |
| 6–12 months | 1.8 |
| Children | |
| 1–3 years | 2.0 |
| 4–8 years | 3.0 |
| 9–13 years | 4.0 |
| Adolescents | |
| 14–18 years | 5.0 |
| Adults | |
| 19–50 years | 5.0 |
| > 50 years | 5.0 |
| Pregnant women | 6.0 |
| Lactating women | 7.0 |

Data from Food and Nutrition Board, Institute of Medicine, 1998.[36]

the body pool occurs.[37] Estimates of dietary intake in healthy adults have ranged from 4 to 7 mg/d.[37-40] There is no evidence to suggest that this range of intake is inadequate, and 5 mg/d has been set as the AI for adults. For those older than 51 years, the AI remains the same, as there is currently no basis for expecting an increased requirement in elderly individuals. During pregnancy, the AI is increased to 6 mg/d based on usual intakes of 5.3 mg/d[41] with rounding up. During lactation, the AI is increased further to 7 mg/d, accounting for additional secretion of the vitamin in human milk (1.7 mg/d) and the lower maternal blood concentrations reported when intakes are about 5 to 6 mg/d.[41-43] This is likely the result of efficient sequestering of the vitamin in human milk, estimated to be 0.4 mg for every 1 mg of pantothenic acid consumed during active lactation.[44]

The AI for infants reflects the mean intake of infants fed principally with human milk, which contains about 5 to 6 mg of pantothenic acid per 1000 kcal. Values for children and adolescents have largely been extrapolated from adult values. These values are supported by studies comparing intake and urinary excretion of the vitamin in preschool children.[45] Dietary intake of pantothenic acid was 3.8 and 5 mg/d in children of high and low socioeconomic status, respectively, and urinary excretion was 3.36 and 1.74 mg/d, respectively. In a separate study, 35 healthy girls 7 to 9 years of age were fed defined diets and urinary excretion was measured.[46] The average daily excretion was 1.3 mg/d when intake was 2.79 mg/d, and 2.7 mg/d when intake was 4.45 mg/d. Therefore, intakes of 2.8 to 4.5 mg/d exceed urinary excretion of the vitamin. In healthy adolescents (13–19 years of age), 4-day diet records indicated that the average pantothenic acid intake was 6.3 mg/d for males and 4.1 mg/d for females.[47] The average urinary excretion in this latter study was 3.3 and 4.5 mg/d for males and females, respectively, while whole blood pantothenic acid concentrations averaged 1.86 μmol/L and 1.57 μmol/L, respectively. Normal blood concentrations of the vitamin in healthy individuals have been reported to range from 1.6 to 2.7 μmol/L.[48] Taken together, these data indicate that intake of 4 mg/d is sufficient to maintain normal blood concentrations in adolescents.

Using the estimate of 20 to 50 μg pantothenic acid per gram typically found in edible animal and plant tissues, it is possible to meet the AI for adults with a mixed diet containing as little as 100 to 200 g of solid food, the equivalent of a mixed diet corresponding to 600 to 1200 kcal or 2.4 to 4.8 MJ. The typical Western diet contains 6 mg or more of available pantothenic acid.[37] For a more detailed review of the AIs for pantothenic acid, see the Dietary Reference Intakes report from the Institute of Medicine.[36]

## Deficiency and Toxicity

The essentiality of pantothenic acid has been documented in a wide variety of animal species. The classical signs of deficiency, first recognized by Elvehjem, Jukes, and colleagues[4-6] in chickens, include growth retardation and dermatitis. Many other physiological systems are affected by pantothenic acid deficiency, owing to the diversity of metabolic functions in which CoA and ACP participate. Neurological, immunological, hematological, reproductive, and gastrointestinal pathologies have been reported. The effects of pantothenic acid deficiency in different species are summarized in Table 4.[49-63]

Assuming that the human adult requirement for pantothenic acid is about 5 mg/d, it may be predicted that with a severe dietary deficiency, 5 to 6 weeks would be required before clear signs of deficiency are observed. This is based on the estimate that daily excretion of 5 mg represents a 1% to 2% loss of the total body pool of pantothenic acid. Consistent with this estimate, limited studies in humans indicate that about 6 weeks of severe depletion are

**Table 4.** Effects of Pantothenic Acid Deficiency in Selected Species

| Species | Symptoms |
|---|---|
| Chicken | Dermatitis around beak, feet, and eyes; poor feathering; spinal cord myelin degeneration; involution of the thymus; fatty degeneration of the liver[2-4,49-51] |
| Rat | Dermatitis; loss of hair color; loss of hair around the eyes; hemorrhagic necrosis of the adrenals; duodenal ulcer; spastic gait; anemia; leukopenia; impaired antibody production; gonadal atrophy with infertility[52-56] |
| Dog | Anorexia; diarrhea; acute encephalopathy; coma; hypoglycemia; leukocytosis; hyperammonemia; hyperlactemia; hepatic steatosis; mitochondrial enlargement[57,58] |
| Pig | Dermatitis; hair loss; diarrhea with impaired sodium, potassium, and glucose absorption; lachrymation; ulcerative colitis; spinal cord and peripheral nerve lesions with spastic gait[59,60] |
| Human | Numbness and burning of feet and hands; headache; fatigue; insomnia; anorexia with gastric disturbances; increased sensitivity to insulin; decreased eosinopenic response to adrenocorticotropic hormone; impaired antibody production[61-63] |

required before urinary pantothenic acid decreases to a basal level of excretion.[64-66]

Because pantothenic acid is such a ubiquitous component of foods, both animal and vegetable, deficiency in humans is very rare. If present, pantothenic acid deficiency is usually associated with multiple nutrient deficiencies, thus making it difficult to discern effects specific to a lack of pantothenic acid. What is known about pantothenic acid deficiency in humans comes primarily from two sources of information. First, during World War II, malnourished prisoners of war in Japan, Burma, and the Philippines experienced numbness and burning sensations in their feet. While these individuals suffered multiple deficiencies, this specific syndrome was only reversed upon pantothenic acid supplementation.[61] Second, experimental pantothenic acid deficiency has been induced in both animals and humans by the administration of the pantothenic acid kinase inhibitor ω-methylpantothenate, in combination with a diet low in pantothenic acid.[62,63,67] Observed symptoms in humans included numbness and burning of the hands and feet similar to that experienced by the World War II prisoners of war, as well as a myriad of other symptoms listed in Table 4. Some of the same symptoms are produced when individuals are fed a semisynthetic diet from which pantothenic acid has been essentially eliminated, but without the addition of ω-methylpantothenate.[64] Another pantothenic acid antagonist, calcium hopantenate, has been shown to induce encephalopathy with hepatic steatosis and a Reye's-like syndrome in both dogs and humans.[68,69] Oral pantothenic acid, even in doses as high as 10 to 20 g/d, is well tolerated[70,71]; however, occasional mild diarrhea may occur.

# Status Determination

Pantothenic acid status is reflected by both whole-blood concentration and urinary excretion. As cited above, whole-blood concentrations typically range from 1.6 to 2.7 μmol/L,[48] and a value under 1 μmol/L is considered low. Urinary excretion is considered a more reliable indicator of status because it is more closely related to dietary intake.[37,47,62-64] Excretion of less than 1 mg of pantothenic acid per day in urine is considered low. Plasma level of the vitamin is a poor indicator of status because it is not highly correlated with changes in intake or status.[43,72]

Pantothenic acid concentrations in whole blood, plasma, and urine are measured by microbiological assay employing *Lactobacillus plantarum*. For whole blood, enzyme pretreatment is required to convert CoA to free pantothenic acid because *L. plantarum* does not respond to CoA. Other methods that have been employed to assess pantothenic acid status include radioimmunoassay, enzyme-linked immunosorbent assay, and gas chromatography. The topic of pantothenic acid status assessment has been reviewed previously.[72]

# Health Claims

With the rapid development of the Web, information about dietary supplements and their putative health benefits can be and is disseminated to the general public with an ease and pace never before possible. However, many health claims for dietary supplements have little or no scientific basis. Although overt deficiency of pantothenic acid is extremely rare in humans, a Web search for "pantothenic acid" reveals numerous websites providing background information, health claims, and, of course, an opportunity to buy the vitamin for oral consumption. Some of the claims made on these websites are completely unwarranted. For example, the use of pantothenic acid to prevent and treat graying hair was based on the observation that pantothenic acid deficiency in rodents causes their fur to turn gray.[53] No association between graying of hair in humans and pantothenic acid status has ever been demonstrated. Moreover, although other claims for pantothenic acid have a more credible scientific basis and are summarized in the following sections, it should be noted that many such claims are based on studies that were conducted in the 1940's, 50's, and 60's and still await validation.

## *Cholesterol Lowering*

Pantothenic acid is not particularly effective in lowering serum cholesterol levels. Rather, oral doses of its metabolite, pantetheine, or more specifically the dimer, pantethine, induce favorable effects on serum cholesterol concentrations. Several studies have indicated that pantethine, in doses typically ranging from 500 to 1200 mg/d, can lower total serum cholesterol, low-density lipoprotein cholesterol, and triacylglycerols, and raise high-density lipoprotein cholesterol in individuals with dyslipidemia, hypercholesterolemia, and hyperlipoproteinemia associated with diabetes.[73-78] The effects are very favorable compared with those of the more conventional lipid-lowering drugs, such as lovastatin. Furthermore, evidence exists that pantethine therapy is more effective than dietary modification in reducing serum cholesterol and lipid concentrations.[73] The mechanism by which pantethine exerts its hypolipemic effects is unclear. A hypothesized site of action is in the regulation of liver sterol biosynthesis. Because pantethine is a coenzyme precursor, it may shunt active acetate from sterol synthesis to mitochondrial oxidative and respiratory pathways.[79] Additionally, pantethine may promote improved triacylglycerol and low-density lipoprotein cholesterol catabolism, as well as reduced cholesterol synthesis via inhibition of the enzyme hydroxymethyl glutaryl-CoA-reductase.[80-82]

## *Enhancement of Athletic Performance*

Scientific support for an effect of pantothenic acid supplements on athletic performance is also limited. Until recently, most of the potential benefit has been inferred from animal studies. More than 60 years ago, frog muscles soaked in pantothenic acid solution were shown to do twice as much work as control muscles before giving out,[83] and more than 30 years ago, rats supplemented with high doses of pantothenic acid were shown to withstand exposure to cold water longer than unsupplemented rats.[84] Moreover, rats deficient in pantothenic acid became exhausted more rapidly during exercise than did replete controls.[85] In this latter study, deficiency was associated with lower tissue CoA concentrations and greater depletion of glycogen reserves during exercise.

Studies assessing the influence of pantothenic acid on human performance are mixed. In one study, well-trained distance runners were supplemented with 2 g/d of pantothenic acid for 2 weeks.[86] These athletes outperformed other equally well-trained distance runners who received placebo. Those who received the supplements also used 8% less oxygen to perform equivalent work and had about 17% less lactic acid accumulation. However, in a separate study, no effect on performance was observed in highly conditioned distance runners after receiving 1 g/d of pantothenic acid for 2 weeks.[87] Additionally, no difference in performance was observed among highly trained cyclists given either a combination of thiamin (1 g) and pantetheine/pantothenic acid (1.9 g) or placebo. The supplement or placebo was given for 7 days before each exercise test. The investigators found no effect on any physiological or performance parameters during steady-state or high-intensity exercise.[88]

## *Rheumatoid Arthritis*

Over 50 years ago, researchers noted that young rats made acutely deficient in pantothenic acid suffered defects in growth and development of bone and cartilage that were reversed by repletion of the vitamin.[89] Subsequently, blood levels of pantothenic acid in humans with rheumatoid arthritis were found to be lower than in healthy controls. On the basis of this finding, an unblinded trial was conducted in which 20 patients with rheumatoid arthritis were injected daily with 50 mg of calcium pantothenate.[90] Blood levels of pantothenic acid increased to normal, and relief from rheumatoid symptoms was achieved in most cases. Symptoms recurred when supplementation was discontinued. Similar results were obtained in arthritic vegetarians.[90] In 1980, it was reported in a double-blind, placebo trial that oral doses of calcium pantothenate (≤2 g/d) reduced the duration of morning stiffness, degree of disability, and severity of pain in patients with rheumatoid arthritis.[91] Individuals with other forms of arthritis were not helped by the supplements, indicating that a therapeutic effect of pantothenic acid may be specific for rheumatoid arthritis. No other published studies are available to confirm this potential benefit.

## *Wound Healing*

Oral administration of pantothenic acid and application of pantothenol ointment to the skin have been shown to accelerate the closure of skin wounds and increase the strength of scar tissue in animals. Adding calcium D-pantothenate to cultured human skin cells given an artificial wound increased the number of skin cells and the distance that they migrated across the edge of the wound.[92] These effects are likely to accelerate wound healing. Little in vivo data, however, exist for humans to support the findings of accelerated wound healing in cell culture and animal studies. A randomized, double-blind study examining the effect of supplementing patients undergoing surgery for tattoo removal with 1000 mg of vitamin C and 200 mg of pantothenic acid did not demonstrate any significant improvement in the wound healing process in those who received the supplements.[93] Furthermore, no benefits were observed when the doses were increased to 3000 mg of ascorbic acid and 900 mg of pantothenic acid.[94] A topical form of pantothenic acid, panthenol or dexapanthenol, appears to play some role in the management of minor skin disorders. Dexapanthenol may help maintain skin hydration in cases of radiation dermatitis,[95] and may reduce skin irritation caused by experimental sodium lauryl sulfate exposure.[96] Dexpanthenol has also been recommended to treat cheilitis and dry nasal mucosa associated with treatment with the acne drug isotretinoin.[97]

## *Lupus Erythematosus*

It has been hypothesized by Leung[98] that lupus erythematosus, a systemic autoimmune disorder that affects the skin, joints, and various internal organ systems, may be the result of pantothenic acid deficiency. The hypothesis is based on the supposition that pantothenic acid deficiency may be induced by three drugs—procainamide, hydralazine, and isoniazid—that are also known to cause drug-induced lupus erythematosus. These drugs are metabolized via CoA-dependent acetylation, and the increased demand for CoA may cause pantothenic acid deficiency. However, no data have been generated on the effect of these drugs on cellular CoA or pantothenic acid concentrations. Leung further postulated that non-drug-induced systemic lupus erythematosus may be the consequence of an increased need for pantothenic acid in susceptible individuals with genetic polymorphisms in CoA-dependent enzymes.[98] Such polymorphisms remain to be identified. Nonetheless, Leung recommended that lupus erythematosus be treated with a combination of vitamins and minerals, including 10 g/d of pantothenic acid.[98]

Support for such pharmacological doses comes from studies carried out in the 1950s. Some, but not all, symptoms of lupus erythematosus were alleviated with high doses (8–15 g/d) of pantothenic acid derivatives (calcium pantothenate, panthenol, or sodium pantothenate) alone[99] or in combination with vitamin E supplements.[100,101] No improvements in disease symptoms were observed with lower doses (400–600 mg) of calcium pantothenate.[102] With modern technology available to probe genes for polymorphic variability, studies in lupus erythematosus patients should be repeated to test the hypothesis that a genetic-based increased requirement of pantothenic acid underlies the pathogenesis of this disease.

## Summary and Future Directions

Identified almost 60 years ago, pantothenic acid is an essential vitamin that serves as the metabolic precursor for CoA. In the form of CoA and as a component of ACP, pantothenic acid is a participant in a myriad of metabolic reactions involving lipids, proteins, and carbohydrates. Though essential, pantothenic acid deficiency in humans is rare due to its ubiquitous distribution in foods of both animal and plant origin. Pantothenic acid supplementation may have some efficacy, but further investigation into various health claims is necessary before any specific recommendations may be given.

## References


1. Williams RJ, Lyman CM, Goodyear GH, Truesdail JH, Holaday D. "Pantothenic acid", a growth determinant of universal biological occurrence. J Am Chem Soc. 1933;55:2912–2927.
2. Wooley DA, Waisman HA, Elvehjem CA. Nature and partial synthesis of the chick antidermatitic factor. J Am Chem Soc. 1939;61:977–978.
3. Jukes T.H. The pantothenic acid requirements of the chick. J Biol Chem. 1939;129:225–231.
4. Spies TD, Stanberry SR, Williams RJ, Jukes TH, Babcock SH. Pantothenic acid in human nutrition. JAMA. 1940;115:523–524.
5. Williams RJ, Majors RT. The structure of pantothenic acid. Science. 1040;91:246–248.
6. Plesofsky-Vig N, Brambi R. Pantothenic acid and coenzyme A in cellular modification of proteins. Annu Rev Nutr. 1988;8:461–482.
7. Wakil SJ. Fatty acid synthetase, a proficient multifunctional enzyme. Biochemistry. 1989;28:4523–4530.
8. Bird OD, Thompson RQ. Pantothenic acid. In: Gyorgy P, Pearson WN, eds. *The Vitamins*. 2nd ed. New York: Academic Press; 1967; 209–241.
9. Shibata K, Gross CJ, Henderson LM. Hydrolysis and absorption of pantothenate and its coenzymes in the rat small intestine. J Nutr. 1983;113:2207–2215.
10. Fenstermacher DK, Rose RC. Absorption of pantothenic acid in rat and chick intestine. Am J Physiol. 1986;250:G155–G160.
11. Said HM. Cellular uptake of biotin: mechanisms and regulation. J Nutr. 1999;129:490S–493S.
12. Spector R, Mock DM. Biotin transport through the blood-brain barrier. J Neurochem. 1987;48:400–404.
13. Beinlich CJ, Naumovitz RD, Song WO, Neely JR. Myocardial metabolism of pantothenic acid in chronically diabetic rats. J Mol Cell Cardiol. 1990; 22:323–332.
14. Grassl SM. Human placental brush-border membrane $Na^+$-pantothenate cotransport. J Biol Chem. 1992;267:22902–22906.
15. Fisher MN, Robishaw JD, Neely JR. The properties of and regulation of pantothenate kinase from rat heart. J Biol Chem. 1985;256:15745–15751.
16. Rock CO, Calder RB, Karim MA, Jackowski S. Pantothenate kinase regulation of the intracellular concentration of coenzyme A. J Biol Chem. 2000; 275:1377–1383.
17. Kirschbaum N, Climons R, Marino KA, Sheedy G, Nguygen M, Smith C. Pantothenate kinase activity in livers of genetically diabetic mice (db/db) and hormonally treated cultured rat hepatocytes. J Nutr. 1990;120:1376–1386.
18. Robishaw JD, Berkich D, Neely JR. Rate-limiting step and control of coenzyme A synthesis in cardiac muscle. J Biol Chem. 1982;257:10967–10972.
19. Reibel DK, Wyse BW, Berkich DA, Neely JR. Regulation of coenzyme A synthesis in heart muscle: effects of diabetes and fasting. Am J Physiol. 1981;240:H606–H611.
20. Bucovaz ET, MacLeod RM, Morrison JC, Whybrew WD. The coenzyme A-synthesizing protein complex and its proposed role in CoA biosynthesis in bakers' yeast. Biochimie. 1998;79:787–798.
21. Praphanphoj V, Sacksteder KA, Gould SJ, Thomas GH, Geraghty MT. Identification of the alpha-aminoadipic semialdehyde dehydrogenase phosphopantetheinyl transferase gene, the human ortholog of the yeast LYS5 gene. Mol Genet Metab. 2001;72:336–342.
22. Seo DW, Kim YK, Cho EJ, Han JW, Lee HY, Hong S, Lee HW. Oligosaccharide-linked acyl carrier protein, a novel transmethylase inhibitor from porcine liver inhibits cell growth. Arch Pharmacol Res. 2002;25:463–468.
23. Raychaudhuri S, Rajasekharan R. Nonorganellar acyl carrier protein from oleaginous yeast is a homologue of ribosomal protein P2. J Biol Chem. 2003; 278:37648–37657.
24. Khosla C, Tang Y. Chemistry: a new route to designer antibiotics. Science. 2005;308:367–368.
25. Nicholis DG, Ferguson SJ. *Bioenergetics-3*. Boston: Academic Press; 2002; 1–207.
26. Smith CM, Milner RE. The mechanism of pantothenate transport by rat liver parenchymal cells in primary culture. J Biol Chem. 1985;260:4823–4931.
27. Lopaschukf GD, Michalak M, Tsang H. Regulation of pantothenic acid transport in the heart: involvement of a $Na^+$-cotransport system. J Biol Chem. 1987;262:3615–3619.
28. Beinlich CJ, Robishaw JD, Neely JR. Metabolism

of pantothenic acid in hearts of diabetic rats. J Molec Cell Cardiol. 1989;21:641–650.
29. Said HM, Ortiz A, McCloud E, Dyer D, Moyer MP, Rubin S. Biotin uptake by human colonic epithelial NCM460 cells: a carrier-mediated process shared with pantothenic acid. Am J Physiol. 1998; 275:C1365–C1371.
30. Spector R. Development and characterization of pantothenic acid transport in brain. J Neurochem. 1987;47:563–568.
31. Spector R. Pantothenic acid transport and metabolism in the central nervous system. Am J Physiol. 1986;250:R292–R297.
32. Walsh JH, Wyse BW, Hansen RG. Pantothenic acid content of 75 processed and cooked foods. J Am Diet Assoc. 1981;78:140–144.
33. Robinson FA. *The Vitamin Co-Factors of Enzyme Systems*. Oxford: Pergamon Press; 1966.
34. Schroeder HA. Losses of vitamins and trace minerals resulting from processing and preservation of foods. Am J Clin Nutr. 1971;24:562–573.
35. Stein ED, Diamond JM. Do dietary levels of pantothenic acid regulate its intestinal uptake in mice? J Nutr. 1989;119:1973–1983.
36. Food and Nutrition Board, Institute of Medicine. Dietary Reference Intakes for Thiamin, Riboflavin, Niacin, Vitamin B6, Folate, Vitamin B12, Pantothenic Acid, Biotin, and Choline. Washington, DC: National Academies Press; 1998. Available online at: http://www.nap.edu/openbook/0309065542/html/.
37. Tarr JB, Tamura T, Stokstad EL. Availability of vitamin B6 and pantothenate in an average American diet in man. Am J Clin Nutr. 1981;34: 1328–1337.
38. Bull NL, Buss DH. Biotin, pantothenic acid and vitamin E in the British household food supply. Hum Nutr Appl Nutr. 1982;36:190–196.
39. Kathman JV, Kies C. Pantothenic acid status of free-living adolescent and young adults. Nutr Res. 1984;4:245–250.
40. Srinivasan V, Christensen N, Wyse BW, Hansen RG. Pantothenic acid nutritional status in the elderly — institutionalized and non-institutionalized. Am J Clin Nutr. 1981;34:1736–1742.
41. Song WO, Wyse BW, Hansen RG. Pantothenic acid status of pregnant and lactating women. J Am Diet Assoc. 1985;85:192–198.
42. Deodhar AD, Ramakrishnan CV. Studies on human lactation: relation between the dietary intake of lactating women and the chemical composition of milk with regard to vitamin content. J Trop Pediatr. 1961;6:44–70.
43. Cohenour SH, Calloway DH. Blood, urine, and dietary pantothenic acid levels of pregnant teenagers. Am J Clin Nutr. 1972;25:512–517.
44. Song WO, Chan GM, Wyse BW, Hansen RG. Effect of PA status on the content of the vitamin in human milk. Am J Clin Nutr. 1984;40:317–324.
45. Kerrey E, Crispin S, Fox HM, Kies C. Nutritional status of preschool children. I. dietary and biochemical findings. Am J Clin Nutr. 1968;21:1274–1279.
46. Pace JK, Stier LB, Taylor DD, Goodman PS. Metabolic patterns in preadolescent children. 5. intake and urinary excretion of pantothenic acid and folic acid. J Nutr. 1961;74:345–351.
47. Eissenstat BR, Wyse BW, Hansen RG. Pantothenic acid status of adolescents. Am J Clin Nutr. 1986;44:931–937.
48. Wittwer CT, Schweitzer C, Pearson J, Song WO, Windham CT, Wyse BW, Hansen RG. Enzymes for liberation of pantothenic acid in blood: use of plasma pantetheinase. Am J Clin Nutr. 1989;50: 1072–1078.
49. Kratzer FH, Williams DE. The pantothenic acid requirement for poults for early growth. Poult Sci. 1948;27:518–523.
50. Milligan JL, Briggs GM. Replacement of pantothenic acid by panthenol in chick diets. Poult Sci. 1949;28:202–205.
51. Gries CL, Scott ML. The pathology of thiamin, riboflavin, pantothenic acid and niacin deficiencies in the chick. J Nutr. 1972;102:1269–1285.
52. SubbaRow Y, Hitchings GH. Pantothenic acid as a factor in rat nutrition. J Am Chem Soc. 1939;61: 1615–1618.
53. Sullivan M, Nicholls J. Nutritional dermatoses in the rat: VI. the effect of pantothenic acid deficiency. AMA Archives of Dermatology and Syphilology. 1942;45:917–932.
54. Eida K, Kubato N, Nishigaki T, et al. Harderian gland: V. effect of dietary pantothenic acid deficiency on porphyrin biosynthesis in Harderian gland of rats. Chem Pharm Bull (Tokyo). 1975;23: 1–4.
55. Axelrod AE. Immune processes in vitamin deficiency states. Am J Clin Nutr. 1971;24:265–271.
56. Pietrzik K, Hesse CH, Zur Wiesch ES, Hotzel D. Urinary excretion of pantothenic acid as a measurement of nutritional requirements. Int J Vit Nutr Res. 1975;45:153–162.
57. Schaefer AE, McKibbin JM, Elvehjem CA. Pantothenic acid deficiency in dogs. J Biol Chem. 1942; 143:321–330.
58. Noda S, Haratake J, Sasaki A, Ishii N, Umezaki H, Horie A. Acute encephalopathy with hepatic steatosis induced by pantothenic acid antagonist, calcium hopantenate, in dogs. Liver. 1991;11: 134–142.
59. Wintrobe MM, Follis RH, Alcayaga R, Paulson M, Humphreys S. Pantothenic acid deficiency in swine with particular reference to the effects on growth and on the alimentary tract. Bulletin of Johns Hopkins Hospital. 1943;73:313–319.

60. Nelson RA. Intestinal transport, coenzyme A, and colitis in pantothenic acid deficiency. Am J Clin Nutr. 1968;21:495–501.
61. Glusman M. The syndrome of "burning feet" (nutritional melagia) as a manifestation of nutritional deficiency. Am J Med. 1947;3:211–223.
62. Hodges RE, Ohlson MA, Bean WB. Pantothenic acid deficiency in man. J Clin Invest. 1958;37: 1642–1657.
63. Hodges RE, Bean WB, Ohlson MA, Bleiler R. Human pantothenic acid deficiency produced by omega-methyl pantothenic acid. J Clin Invest. 1959;38:1421–1425.
64. Fry PC, Fox HM, Tao HG. Metabolic response to a pantothenic acid deficient diet in humans. J Nutr Sci Vitaminol (Tokyo). 1976;22:339–346.
65. Fox HM, Linkswiler H. Pantothenic acid excretion on three levels intake. J Nutr. 1961;75:451–454.
66. Annous KF, Song WO. Pantothenic acid uptake and metabolism by red blood cells of rats. J Nutr. 1985;125:2586–2593.
67. Drell W, Dunn MS. Production of pantothenic acid deficiency syndrome in mice with methylpantothenic acid. Arch Biochem. 1951;33:110–119.
68. Noda S, Haratake J, Sasaki A, Ishii N, Umezaki H, Horie A. Acute encephalopathy with hepatic steatosis induced by pantothenic acid antagonist, calcium hopantenate, in dogs. Liver. 1991;11: 134–142.
69. Noda S, Umezaki H, Yamamoto K, Araki T, Murakami T, Ishii N. Reye's-like syndrome following treatment with the pantothenic acid antagonist, calcium hopantenate. J Neurol Neurosurg Psychiatr. 1998;51:582–585.
70. Ralli EP, Dumm ME. Relation of pantothenic acid to adrenal cortical function. Vitam Horm. 1953;11: 133–158.
71. Tahiliani AG, Beinlich CJ. Pantothenic acid in health and disease. Vitam Horm. 1991;46: 165–228.
72. Sauberlich HE. Pantothenic acid. In: *Laboratory Tests for the Assessment of Nutritional Status*. 2nd ed. Boca Raton, FL: CRC Press; 1999; 175–183.
73. Avogaro P, Bittolo Bon G, Fusello M. Effects of pantethine on lipids, lipoproteins and apolipoproteins in man. Current Therapeutic Research. 1983; 33:488–493.
74. Gaddi A, Descovich GC, Noseda G, et al. Controlled evaluation of pantethine, a natural hypolipidemic compound, in patients with different forms of hyperlipoproteinemia. Atherosclerosis. 1984;50: 73–83.
75. Bertolini S, Donati C, Elicio N, et al. Lipoprotein changes induced by pantethine in hyperlipoproteinemic patients: adults and children. Int J Clin Pharmacol Ther Toxicol. 1986;24:630–637.
76. Arsenio L, Bodria P, Magnati G, Starta A, Trovato R. Effectiveness of long-term treatment with pantethine in patients with dyslipidemia. Clin Ther. 1986;8:537–545.
77. Miccoli R, Marchetti P, Sampietro T, Benzi L, Tognarelli M, Navalesi R. Effects of pantethine on lipids and apolipoproteins in hypercholesterolemic diabetic and nondiabetic patients. Current Therapeutic Research. 1984;36:545–549.
78. Binaghi P, Cellina G, Lo Cicero G, Bruschi F, Porcaro E, Penotti M. Evaluation of the cholesterol-lowering effectiveness of pantethine in women in perimenopausal age. Minerva Medica. 1990;81: 475–479.
79. Kameda K, Abiko Y. Stimulation of fatty acid metabolism by pantethine. In: Cavallini D, Gaull GE, Zappia V, eds. *Natural Sulfur Compounds*. New York: Plenum Press; 1980; 443–452.
80. Cighetti G, Del Puppo M, Paroni R, Galli G, Kienle MG. Modulation of HMG-CoA reductase activity by pantetheine/pantethine. Biochim Biophys Acta. 1988;963:389–393.
81. Cighetti G, Del Puppo M, Paroni R, Fiorica E, Galli G, Kienle MG. Pantethine inhibits cholesterol and fatty acid syntheses and stimulates carbon dioxide formation in isolated rat hepatocytes. J Lip Res. 1987;28:152–161.
82. Cighetti G, Del Puppo M, Paroni R, Galli G, Kienle MG. Effects of pantethine on cholesterol synthesis from mevalonate in isolated rat hepatocytes. Atherosclerosis. 1986;60:67–77.
83. Shock NW, Sebrell WH. The effect of changes in concentration of pantothenate on the work output of perfused frog muscles. Am J Physiol. 1944;142: 274–278.
84. Ralli EP. Effects of dietary supplementation on the ability of rats to withstand exposure to cold. Nutr Rev. 1968;26:124.
85. Smith CM, Narrow CM, Kendrick ZV, Steffen C. The effect of pantothenate deficiency in mice on their metabolic response to fast and exercise. Metabolism. 1987;36:115–121.
86. Litoff D, Scherzer H, Harrison J. Effects of pantothenic acid supplementation on human exercise. Med Sci Sports Exerc. 1985;17(suppl):287.
87. Nice C, Reeves A, Brinck-Johnson T, Noll W. The effects of pantothenic acid on human exercise capacity. J Sports Med Phys Fitness. 1984;24:26–29.
88. Webster MJ. Physiological and performance responses to supplementation with thiamin and pantothenic acid derivatives. Eur J Appl Physiol. 1998; 77:486–491.
89. Nelson MM, Sulon E, Becks H, Wainwright WW, Evans HM. Changes in endochondral ossification of the tibia accompanying acute pantothenic acid deficiency in young rats. Proceedings of the Society of Experimental Biology and Medicine. 1950;73: 31–36.

90. Barton-Wright EC, Elliot WA. The pantothenic acid metabolism of rheumatoid arthritis. Lancet. 1963;2:862–863.
91. U.S. General Practitioner Research Group. Calcium pantothenate in arthritic conditions. a report from the general practitioner research group. Practitioner. 1980;224:208–211.
92. Weimann BI, Hermann D. Studies on wound healing: effects of calcium D-pantothenate on the migration, proliferation and protein synthesis of human dermal fibroblasts in culture. Int J Vitam Nutr Res. 1999;69:113–119.
93. Vaxman F, Olender S, Lambert A, et al. Effect of pantothenic acid and ascorbic acid supplementation on human skin wound healing process. A double-blind, prospective and randomized trial. Eur Surg Res. 1995;27:158–166.
94. Vaxman F, Olender S, Lambert A, et al. Can the wound healing process be improved by vitamin supplementation? Experimental study on humans. Eur Surg Res. 1996;28:306–314.
95. Schmuth M, Wimmer MA, Hofer S, et al. Topical corticosteroid therapy for acute radiation dermatitis: a prospective, randomized, double-blind study. Br J Dermatol. 2002;146:983–991.
96. Biro K, Thaci D, Ochsendorf FR, et al. Efficacy of dexpanthenol in skin protection against irritation: a double-blind, placebo-controlled study. Contact Dermatitis. 2003;49:80–84.
97. Romiti R, Romiti N. Dexpanthenol cream significantly improves mucocutaneous side effects associated with isotretinoin therapy. Pediatr Dermatol. 2002;19:368–371.
98. Leung LH. Systemic lupus erythematosus: a combined deficiency disease. Med Hypotheses. 2004; 62:922–924.
99. Goldman L. Intensive panthenol therapy of lupus erythematosus. J Invest Dermatol. 1950;15:291–293.
100. Welsh, AL. Lupus erythematosus: treatment by combined use of massive amounts of calcium pantothenate or panthenol with synthetic vitamin E. AMA Archives of Dermatology and Syphilology. 1952;65:137–148.
101. Welsh AL. Lupus erythematosus: treatment by combined use of massive amounts of pantothenic acid and vitamin E. AMA Archives of Dermatology and Syphilology. 1954;70:181–198.
102. Chochrane T, Leslie G. The treatment of lupus erythematosus with calcium pantothenate and panthenol. J Invest Dermatol. 1952;18:365–367.

# 26 Carnitine

Charles J. Rebouche

## Nomenclature, Chemical, and Biochemical Properties

L-Carnitine (Figure 1) is a low-molecular-weight (161.5 g/mol), biologically active amino acid derived from the essential amino acids L-lysine and L-methionine. The optical isomer D-carnitine has no biological activity and is not produced in eukaryotic organisms. At physiological pH, L-carnitine exists as a zwitterion, containing a positively charged quaternary amine and a negatively charged carboxyl separated by a three-carbon chain. A hydroxyl group is attached to the middle carbon. This hydroxyl group is utilized biologically to form short-, medium-, and long-chain esters of organic and fatty acids with carnitine (e.g., acetyl-L-carnitine, palmitoyl-L-carnitine; Figure 1). Transfer of activated acyl moieties between carnitine and coenzyme A (CoA), catalyzed by several chain-length-specific carnitine acyltransferases, forms the core of the biological activity of carnitine.

## Methods of Analysis

### *Enzymatic/Colorimetric Methods*

Following demonstration of the function of carnitine in the import of fatty acids into mitochondria and the discovery and characterization of carnitine acetyltransferase, the spectrophotometric method of Marquis and Fritz[1] replaced the biological assay (growth of the mealworm *Tenebrio molitor*) as the standard for quantification of L-carnitine and its esters. This method is based on the reaction of L-carnitine and acetyl-CoA, catalyzed by carnitine acetyltransferase, to form acetyl-L-carnitine and CoA. The subsequent reaction between CoA and 5,5′-dithiobis-2-nitrobenzoic acid (DTNB) is quantified colorimetrically at 412 nm. This coupled assay lacks the sensitivity of the other methods now available. Nevertheless, it is used in some automated procedures for the measurement of carnitine.

An enzymatic cycling method utilizing purified bacterial carnitine dehydrogenase has been described previously.[2] Biological samples are incubated with enzyme, thio-$NAD^+$, and NADH. Carnitine dehydrogenase catalyzes conversion of L-carnitine in the sample to dehydrocarnitine with reduction of thio-$NAD^+$ to form thio-NADH. Dehydrocarnitine "cycles" back to L-carnitine with oxidation of NADH. Increase in absorbance at 415 nm due to formation of thio-NADH is used to quantify L-carnitine in the sample.

### *Radioenzymatic Method*

The radioenzymatic method, first described by Cederblad and Lindstedt,[3] is based on the same principles as the colorimetric method above utilizing carnitine acetyltransferase, except that the acetyl-CoA used in the reaction is radiolabeled. The extent of the reaction is quantified by radioactivity counting following separation by anion-exchange chromatography of radiolabeled acetyl-L-carnitine from unreacted, radiolabeled acetyl-CoA. For many years, this procedure has been the standard for most research and many clinical applications. Both the colorimetric and radioenzymatic methods suffer from interference by excess thiols in the sample, and the enzymatic reaction also is influenced by salt concentration.

### *Isotope-Dilution Tandem Mass Spectrometry*

The method of Stevens et al.[4] depends on measurement, by tandem mass spectrometry, of isotope ratios generated by carnitine in the sample and deuterium-labeled carnitine added as an internal standard. This method is more straightforward and reliable than the enzymatic methods because of its absolute molecular specificity, because the internal standard compensates for losses or variance resulting from sample preparation, and because it has no known chemical interference. Results using this procedure are reported to correlate well with the automated enzymatic/colorimetric method.[4] This method may also be used to quantify individual acylcar-

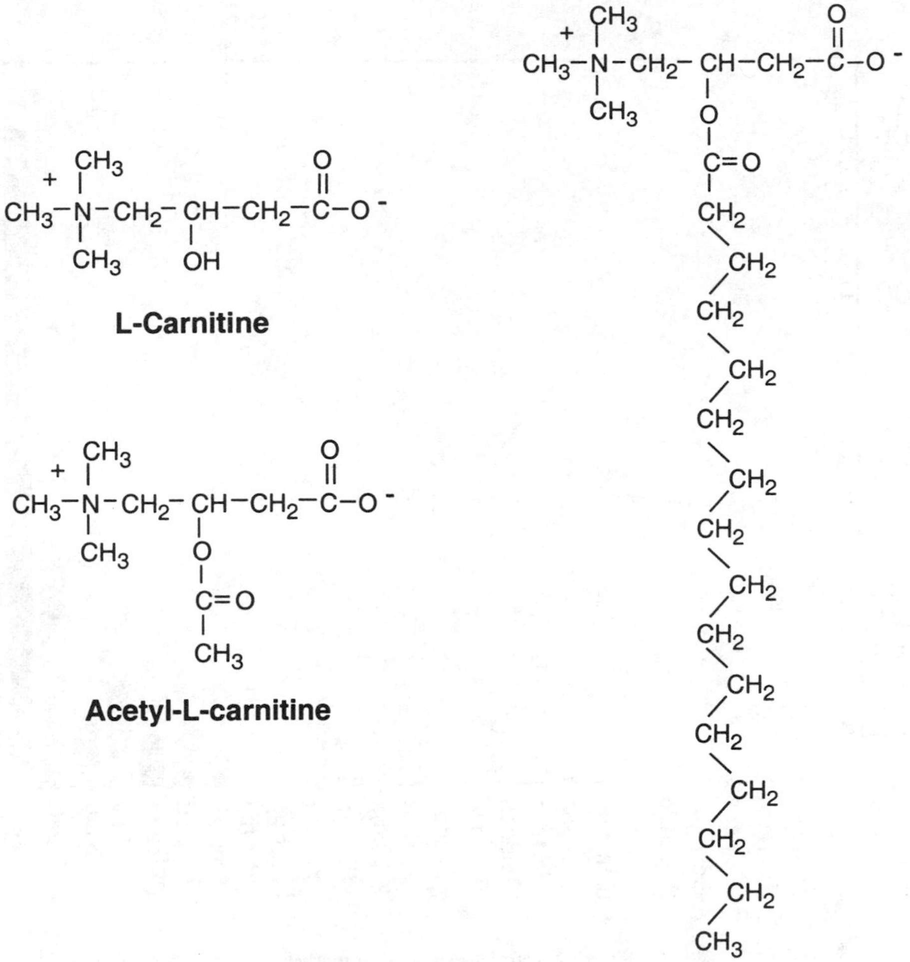

$(CH_3)_3N^+-CH_2-CH(OH)-CH_2-COO^-$

**L-Carnitine**

$(CH_3)_3N^+-CH_2-CH(O-CO-CH_3)-CH_2-COO^-$

**Acetyl-L-carnitine**

$(CH_3)_3N^+-CH_2-CH(O-CO-(CH_2)_{14}-CH_3)-CH_2-COO^-$

**Palmitoyl-L-carnitine**

Figure 1. Structures of L-carnitine and representative acylcarnitine esters.

nitine ester species in biological specimens if the corresponding isotope-labeled internal standards are available.[5]

### *Other Methods for Quantification of Carnitine and Specific Acylcarnitine Esters in Biological Specimens*

Several methods have been described to quantify carnitine and specific acylcarnitine ester species in biological specimens. These include derivatization with a chromogen followed by high-performance liquid chromatography, with spectrophotometric[6] or fluorometric[7] detection and quantification, and high-performance liquid chromatography with electrospray tandem mass spectrometric detection and quantification.[8]

## Diet, Bioavailability, and Absorption

For human adults, typical omnivorous diets provide 0.1 to 1.0 mmol of L-carnitine per day (2 to 12 μmol/kg body weight/d). Diets rich in animal products (meat, poultry, fish, and dairy products) provide almost all of the carnitine obtained from mixed diets (Figure 2). Fruits and vegetables contain very little carnitine. Vegan diets provide less than 1 μmol of carnitine/kg body weight/d. Fractional absorption of dietary carnitine is variable, generally in the range of 55% to 90%. Fractional absorption of carnitine in dietary supplements (0.5 to 4 g/d) is 15% to 25%. At low carnitine intakes, at least part of the absorption process may be facilitated or active. However, carnitine in the form of oral supplements is probably almost entirely absorbed by passive processes.

## Biosynthesis and Metabolism

### *Biosynthesis*

L-Carnitine is synthesized from ε-N-trimethyllysine, an amino acid derived from post-translational modification of lysine in a variety of proteins (Figure 3). Probably the great majority of ε-N-trimethyllysine arises from turnover of muscle proteins. Many proteins are known to contain one or a few methylated lysine residues, including actin, myosin, ATP synthase, histones, and calmodulin.

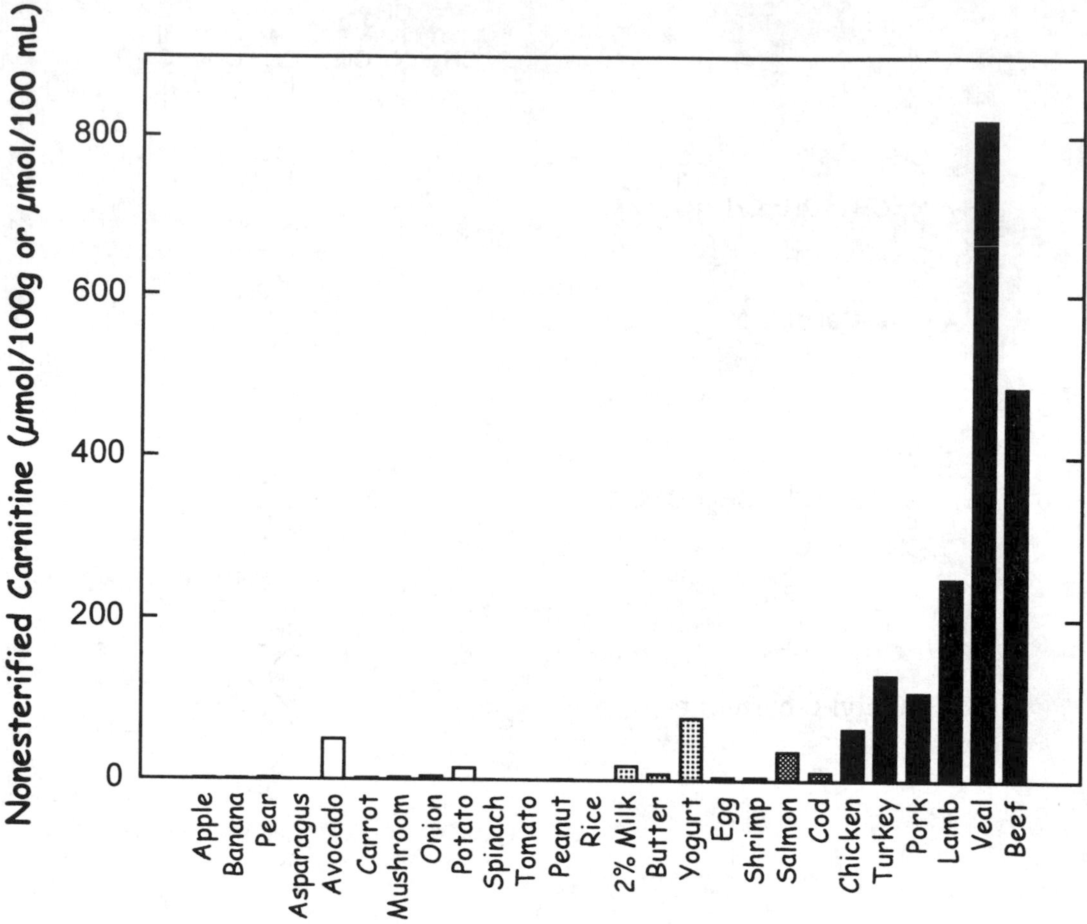


Figure 2. Carnitine content of foods.[9]

No single protein has been identified that contains a large number of these residues and/or that turns over rapidly such that it could provide a primary source of ε-N-trimethyllysine for carnitine synthesis. Rather, from an evolutionary perspective, accrual of this derivative from normal protein synthesis and degradation has been adequate for mammalian requirements for carnitine. The fungus *Neurospora crassa* is able to methylate unbound lysine,[11] but no other organism has been shown to possess this capability.

ε-N-trimethyllysine is converted to L-carnitine via a series of four enzymatic reactions, catalyzed by two dioxygenases (ε-N-trimethyllysine hydroxylase and γ-butyrobetaine hydroxylase), an aldolase (serine hydroxymethyltransferase), and a dehydrogenase (aldehyde dehydrogenase).[12] Thus the process also requires the cofactors $Fe^{2+}$, ascorbic acid, and pyridoxal phosphate, and the co-substrates α-ketoglutarate, $O_2$, and $NAD^+$. Conversion of ε-N-trimethyllysine to carnitine is not quantitative in mammals. Significant amounts of this amino acid and the penultimate precursor of carnitine, γ-butyrobetaine, are normally excreted in urine. The normal rate of carnitine synthesis in humans is estimated to be about 1.2 µmol/kg body weight/d. This estimate was obtained indirectly from rates of carnitine excretion at steady-state in the absence of significant dietary intake of carnitine. The variability among individuals or populations is not known.

## *Catabolism*

Carnitine is not degraded by enzymes of animal origin. However, degradation products of carnitine have been identified in the urine and feces of rats and humans. These arise from catabolism of carnitine by bacterial enzymes in the gastrointestinal tract. Enterobacteria metabolize L-carnitine to γ-butyrobetaine anaerobically via a two-step process (not a reverse of the single-step hydroxylation of γ-butyrobetaine in carnitine biosynthesis) (Figure 4). In these organisms, L-carnitine may serve as a growth-promoting electron acceptor in the absence of preferred substrates.[13] L-Carnitine is degraded aerobically by some organisms by carbon-nitrogen cleavage, resulting in trimethylamine and malic semialdehyde (Figure 4). Trimethylamine is absorbed from the lumen of the large intestine, and is oxidized in the liver to trimethylamine oxide.[14] Following oral administration of L-carnitine radiolabeled in the methyl groups, radiolabeled trimethylamine oxide and γ-butyrobetaine were the major degra-

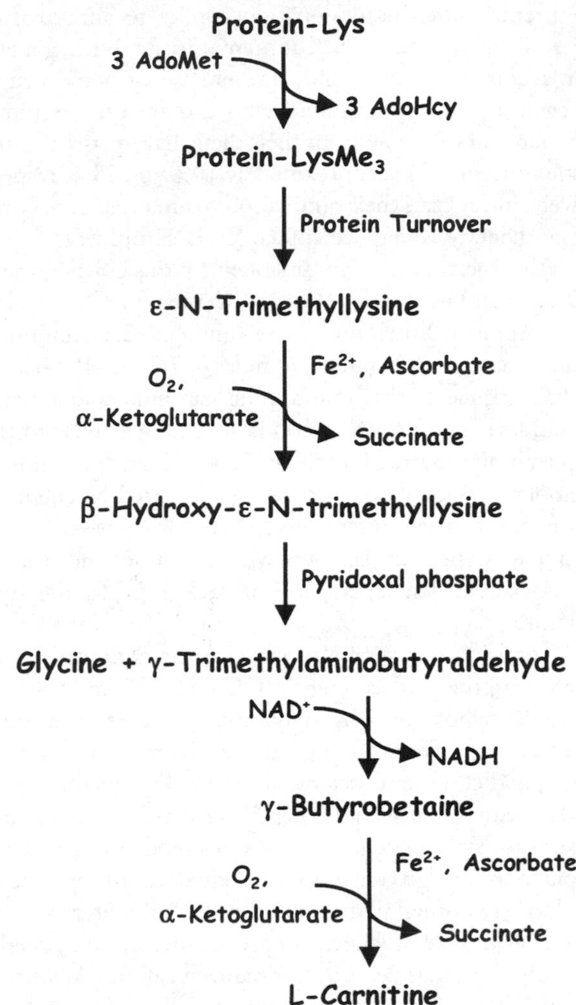


Figure 3. Pathway for carnitine biosynthesis in mammals.

dation products observed in urine and feces, respectively, in both rats and humans.

## *Kinetics and Distribution*

L-Carnitine and its esters are distributed into three kinetically defined pools in the body.[10] The largest corresponds to muscle tissues, and contains 92% to 97% of total body carnitine. A pool corresponding to other tissues including liver and kidneys contains 2% to 6% of total body carnitine. The extracellular fluid pool of carnitine accounts for the remaining 0.7% to 1.5%. Turnover of the muscle carnitine pool is relatively slow (191 hours), but because of its size, the flux of carnitine is relatively rapid (427 μmol/hour in adult humans). Collective turnover time and flux of carnitine for other tissues are 11.6 hours and 277 μmol/hour, respectively. Turnover time for the extracellular carnitine pool is 1.13 hours, and whole-body turnover of carnitine is 66 days. The total carnitine pools in tissues and extracellular fluid consist of approximately 10% to 20% esterified carnitine and 80% to 90% non-esterified carnitine. The esterified carnitine fraction consists primarily of acetyl-L-carnitine, with smaller amounts of propionyl-L-carnitine and long-chain fatty acyl carnitine esters. The concentration of carnitine is generally greater in tissues than in extracellular fluid. In skeletal muscle and liver, respectively, the total carnitine concentrations are 76 and 50 times that in extracellular fluid. The highest concentrations of carnitine and acetyl-L-carnitine (2 to 100 mmol/l) are found in epididymus.[15]

## *Transport*

Entry of L-carnitine and its short-chain acyl esters acetyl-L-carnitine and propionyl-L-carnitine into most tissues is facilitated by the organic cation transporter OCTN2. This protein has a high affinity for carnitine and its short-chain acyl esters ($K_t$ = 3 to 5 μmol/L).

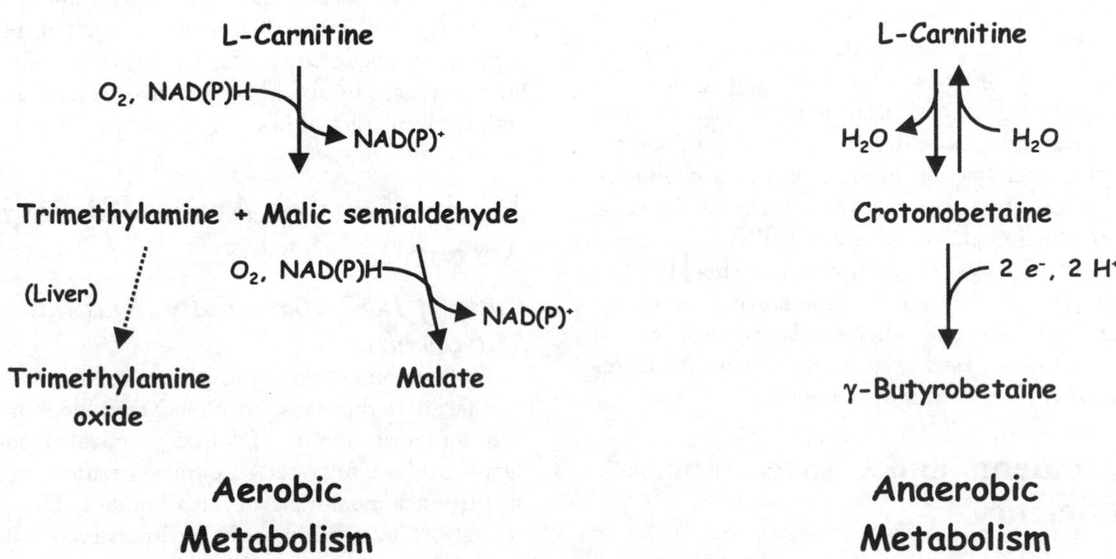


Figure 4. Catabolism of L-carnitine by microorganisms in the rat and human gastrointestinal tract.

Transport is dependent on an inwardly directed sodium-ion gradient, and sodium ions are co-transported with carnitine. This protein is highly expressed in kidney, skeletal muscle, heart, placenta, pancreas, testis and epididymus, and weakly expressed in liver, lung, and brain.[16,17] Other proteins that are capable of transporting carnitine across cell membranes include the organic cation transporters OCTN1 and OCTN3 and the amino acid transporter $ATB^{0,+}$.[18] These proteins have a lower affinity for carnitine, and their physiological roles in carnitine transport and carnitine homeostasis are unknown.

A unique carnitine transporter, designated CT-2, is specifically expressed in testes.[15] The transporter is highly specific and has high affinity ($K_T$ = 20 μmol/L) for carnitine. It is located phylogenetically between the OAT and OCT/OCTN families of organic ion transporters. CT2 protein is localized to the luminal membrane of the epididymal endothelium and within Sertoli cells.

### *Excretion and Reabsorption*

The major route for excretion of carnitine is via the kidney. Carnitine is filtered across the glomerulus. Normally, 90% to 98% of filtered carnitine is reabsorbed by humans. OCTN2 in the renal brush border membrane is primarily or totally responsible for reabsorption of carnitine and its short-chain acyl esters, and probably also the immediate precursor of carnitine, γ-butyrobetaine. Renal reabsorption of carnitine is thought to be a primary regulator of carnitine homeostasis in humans. Carnitine reabsorption is highly efficient when plasma carnitine concentrations are at or below about 60 μmol/L (normal plasma total carnitine concentration is 30 to 65 μmol/L). When the plasma carnitine concentration is increased above 60 μmol/L, by for example, intravenous infusion of carnitine or oral consumption of a carnitine supplement, the efficiency of carnitine reabsorption rapidly decreases and greater quantities are lost to urinary excretion.

Renal tubular cells secrete carnitine, short-chain acyl esters of carnitine, and γ-butyrobetaine into the tubular lumen.[19-21] Some of these are reabsorbed and some are lost in the urine. Urine total carnitine typically contains a higher percentage of acylcarnitine esters than does the circulating carnitine pool.[22] Under normal conditions, the acylcarnitine ester fraction in urine is mostly comprised of acetyl-L-carnitine. Because the affinity of the renal brush border membrane transporter OCTN2 for L-carnitine and acetyl-L-carnitine is similar, one should not be selectively reabsorbed from the glomerular filtrate over the other. Thus, the renal tubular cells may produce and secrete acylcarnitine esters selectively as a means to remove excess acyl burden from the body.

## Requirements and Consequences of Deficiency

A dietary source of carnitine is not required by normal humans. It often is described as a conditionally essential nutrient,[23] but this designation applies to abnormal or special circumstances such as prematurity at birth, genetic or acquired diseases, and chronic use of some drugs. Vegan adults and children, who acquire only minimal amounts of carnitine from their diets, have plasma carnitine concentrations approximately 10% and 25%, respectively, lower than their omnivorous counterparts.[22] There is no Dietary Reference Intake for L-carnitine.

An expert panel commissioned by the US Food and Drug Administration's (FDA's) Center for Food Safety and Applied Nutrition has recommended a minimum carnitine content in infant formulas of 7.5 μmol/100 kcal, a level similar to that found in human milk, and a maximum level of 12.4 μmol/100 kcal, a value similar to the upper limit reported for human milk.[24] These recommendations were made on the basis of reported biochemical differences when infants were fed carnitine-free diets compared with similar diets with carnitine, and despite the lack of evidence that carnitine is essential for the term infant.

Carnitine deficiency in humans occurs as a result of defects in the gene coding for OCTN2. Clinical features include hypoketotic hypoglycemia, seizures, vomiting, and lethargy, which are progressive to coma, cardiomyopathy, and chronic muscle weakness.[25] Therapeutic treatment with L-carnitine is highly successful. Plasma and liver carnitine concentrations are restored, attacks of hypoketotic hypoglycemia are prevented, and heart size is reduced to normal within months of treatment initiation. Skeletal muscle weakness improves, despite only slight increases in muscle carnitine concentration. A murine model (the *jvs* mouse) of spontaneous origin has been described.[26]

Carnitine deficiency or depletion occurs secondary to many genetic inborn errors, acquired medical conditions, and with the use of some medications. These have been reviewed extensively elsewhere.[27] In numerous case reports of low circulating carnitine concentrations, "a defect in carnitine biosynthesis" has been suggested. However, there is no documented case of carnitine deficiency in humans caused by absent or defective proteins associated with carnitine biosynthesis.

## Mechanisms of Action/Biological Activity

### *Entry of Long-chain Fatty Acids into Mitochondria*

A primary function of carnitine in cellular metabolism is to facilitate the transport of activated long-chain fatty acids into mitochondria (Figure 5). Activated long-chain fatty acids (as CoA esters) are transesterified to carnitine on the outer membrane of mitochondria. This reaction is catalyzed by carnitine palmitoyltransferase I (CPT I). Long-chain fatty acylcarnitine is transported across the mitochondrial inner membrane by carnitine-acylcarnitine

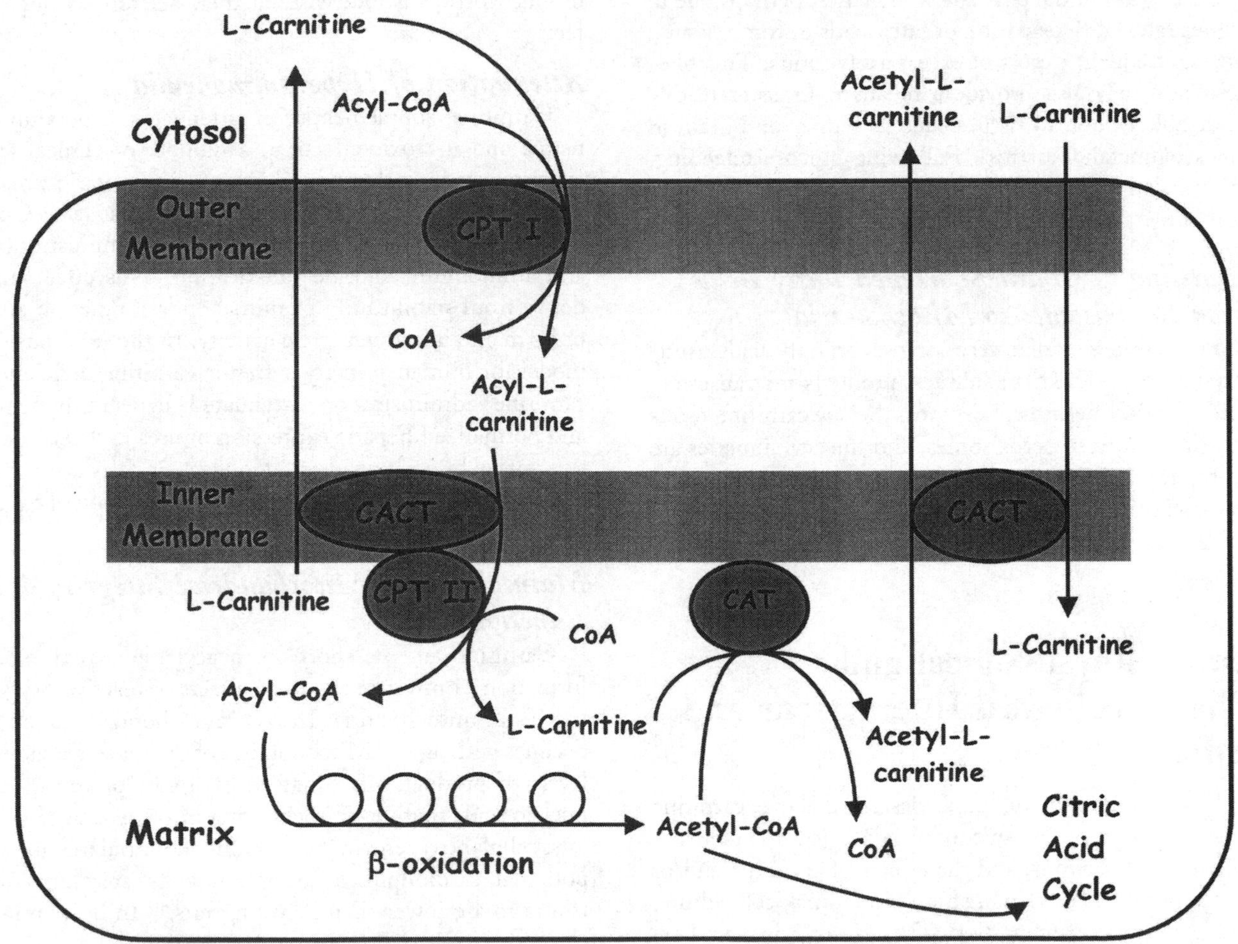


Figure 5. Facilitation of entry of long-chain fatty acids into mitochondria by carnitine. CACT = carnitine-acylcarnitine translocase; CAT = carnitine acetyltransferase; ; CoA = coenzyme A; CPT I = carnitine palmitoyltransferase I; CPT II = carnitine palmitoyltransferase II.

translocase (CACT),[28] a member of the mitochondrial metabolite carrier protein family.[29] CPT II associated with the matrix side of the mitochondrial inner membrane then catalyzes transesterification of the activated fatty acid to intramitochondrial CoA. The activated fatty acids then are oxidized through multiple cycles of the β-oxidation pathway.

CPT I is rate-controlling, although not necessarily rate-limiting, for β-oxidation of fatty acids.[30] CPT I is inhibited by malonyl-CoA and stimulated by AMP-activated protein kinase.[31] Two major forms of CPT I have been identified and are products of different genes (CPT1A and CPT1B).[32] M-CPT I is found in skeletal muscle and heart, and L-CPT I is found in liver and many other non-muscle tissues. The two forms differ in their affinity for both the inhibitor malonyl-CoA and the substrate carnitine. The carnitine concentration in tissues is not limiting for CPT I activity, unless it is abnormally low. Michaelis constants for carnitine binding to L-CPT I and M-CPT-I are 30 and 500 μmol/L, respectively.[32]

## *Maintenance of Intramitochondrial Non-Esterified Coenzyme A Availability*

Carnitine is released in the mitochondrial matrix after import of long-chain fatty acylcarnitine and transesterification of the acyl group to CoA. It can exit mitochondria via CACT, or it may be used as a reservoir for excess acetyl groups formed during β-oxidation and/or pyruvate oxidation. This process allows for the maintenance of sufficient non-esterified CoA concentration in the mitochondrial matrix to supply the β-oxidation cycle, pyruvate dehydrogenase, and the citric acid cycle. Transesterification of acetyl groups to carnitine from CoA is catalyzed by carnitine acetyltransferase. Acetyl-L-carnitine may exit the mitochondrial matrix via CACT for use in other compartments of the cell, for use by other cells or tissues, or for excretion. The ability of carnitine to act as a reservoir for activated acyl residues is also important in abnormal cellular metabolism, particularly in genetic diseases associated with defects in organic and fatty acid metabolism.[18] Experimental studies in mice, monkeys, and humans[33] show that during starvation, acetyl-L-carnitine concentration in the circulation increases, perhaps due to higher rates of β-oxidation of fatty acids in some tissues, with consequent export of excess acetyl units. This phenomenon may also provide a means to transfer readily oxidizable carbon to tissues such as kidney and brain in times of metabolic stress. Following glucose refeeding, the circulating acetyl-L-carnitine concentration decreases as this metabolite is transported into the liver.

### *Shuttling of Chain-Shortened Fatty Acids from Peroxisomes to Mitochondria*

Peroxisomes oxidize very-long-chain fatty acids. Activated medium-chain organic acid products are transesterified to carnitine in peroxisomes, the acylcarnitine esters are exported from peroxisomes, and the acyl moieties are subsequently oxidized in mitochondria. In peroxisomes, transesterification of medium-chain acyl groups from CoA to carnitine is catalyzed by carnitine octanoyltransferase.

## Other Physiological and Pharmacological Interactions and Effects

In addition to the functions described above, carnitine and its esters have a number of physiological and pharmacological interactions, and the effects of carnitine and/or its esters have been demonstrated in animal, cell culture, and in vitro experimentation. These interactions and effects may be physiological in nature, but may also be magnified by pharmacological use of these compounds.

### *Membrane Phospholipid Remodeling*

L-Carnitine and extramitochondrial carnitine palmitoyltransferase function in utilization of long-chain fatty acids for phospholipid biosynthesis and remodeling. Fatty acids bound to L-carnitine are incorporated into erythrocyte membrane phospholipids during repair after oxidative insult,[34] and into dipalmitoylphosphatidylcholine, a major component of surfactant, in lung alveolar cells.[35] L-Carnitine and acetyl-L-carnitine may increase membrane stability in mature erythrocytes, presumably by a specific interaction with cytoskeletal proteins.[36]

### *Interaction with the Glucocorticoid Receptor*

L-Carnitine at millimolar concentrations reduces binding of dexamethasone to the glucocorticoid receptor-α, while itself triggering nuclear translocation of the receptor and stimulating transcription of glucocorticoid receptor-α-responsive promoters.[37] L-Carnitine mimics several immunomodulatory effects of glucocorticoids, including suppressing lipopolysaccharide-induced cytokine production in rats, promoting fetal lung development in pregnant rats, and decreasing serum levels of tumor necrosis factor α in surgical and HIV-infected patients.[37] L-Carnitine may share some of the therapeutic properties of glucocorticoids, but without their deleterious side effects.

### *Attenuation of Hyperammonemia*

Carnitine supplementation attenuates hyperammonemia and its toxic effects in a number of clinical and experimentally induced conditions, including primary systemic carnitine deficiency, medium-chain acyl-CoA dehydrogenase deficiency, valproic acid administration, and ammonium chloride intoxication. This effect may derive from stabilization of mitochondrial function and/or by maintaining urea cycle activity. In the *jvs* mouse, a model for human primary systemic carnitine deficiency, carnitine administration attenuated hyperammonemia and normalized hepatic expression of urea cycle enzymes suppressed by accumulation of long-chain fatty acids.[38,39] These effects may be mediated by the interaction of carnitine with the glucocorticoid receptor.[37,39]

### *Maintenance of Mitochondrial Integrity and Function*

Carnitine and its short-chain acyl esters may block formation or mitigate the toxic effects of reactive oxygen species in mitochondria. In rats, mitochondrial function declines with aging. Mitochondria of old rats have higher levels of products of oxidation of lipids, proteins, and nucleic acids than do mitochondria of young rats. In old rats, cellular oxygen uptake and mitochondrial membrane potential, cardiolipin concentration, and respiratory control ratio are lower than in young rats.[40] In heart mitochondria of old rats, DNA transcription and activity of cytochrome oxidase, adenine nucleotide translocase, and CACT are reduced compared with the mitochondria of young rats.[41-43] The administration of acetyl-L-carnitine to old rats restores cardiolipin concentration and mitochondrial function to near that in young rats.[40,42,43] One mechanism proposed to explain these effects is the protection afforded by acetyl-L-carnitine on oxidative decline in activity of carnitine acetyltransferase observed in vivo and in vitro.[44] Although this effect may contribute to overall restoration of mitochondrial function, the more general effects on membrane-associated enzyme activities and transporters are probably related to the restoration of cardiolipin concentration in the mitochondrial inner membrane.

## Supplements: Health Maintenance, Performance Enhancement, and Prevention or Retardation of Aging and Chronic Disease

L-Carnitine and acetyl-L-carnitine are available commercially as dietary supplements in the United States. Propionyl-L-carnitine is available in Europe. Typical recommendations for use are 0.5 to 4 g/d. Little or no toxicity is associated with consumption of these amounts. However, occasional occurrences of diarrhea or body odor ("fish odor syndrome") have been reported.

### *Performance Enhancement*

Many commercial entities market L-carnitine as an ergogenic aid. This strategy is based on the notion that supplemental carnitine will increase oxidative metabolism of fatty acids and perhaps spare muscle glycogen. It presumes that an increase in available carnitine will increase the flux of long-chain fatty acids into mitochondria. Clinical data suggest that muscle function is sensitive to changes in carnitine content when carnitine content is less than 25% to 50% of normal, but is insensitive to changes when the carnitine concentration is normal.[45] If an increase in carnitine concentration alone is the sole factor in performance enhancement, it is unlikely that improvements would occur with carnitine supplementation, both because normal carnitine concentration is saturating for muscle CPT I kinetics, and because only a very modest increase in carnitine concentration would be expected with even the most rigorous supplementation regimen.

On the other hand, even though carnitine supplements are not likely to substantially increase muscle carnitine concentration, they may improve the efficiency of muscle metabolism by exchange of non-esterified carnitine (provided by the supplement) into muscle for excess activated acetate (as acetyl-L-carnitine) formed from β-oxidation, when the citric acid cycle and/or oxidative phosphorylation pathways are operating at maximum capacity.

Most studies of L-carnitine use to improve athletic performance have not shown any benefit. However, due to limitations in study design, the lack of evidence does not necessarily mean that L-carnitine supplements are not beneficial.[45] Particularly for elite athletes, very small increments in performance enhancement that are not quantifiable or statistically significant by standard experimental paradigms may have substantial impact on competitive outcome.

### *Weight Maintenance, Weight Reduction, and Optimization of Body Composition*

Some vendors market L-carnitine as a dietary supplement to promote weight loss. The term "fat burner" has been used to describe L-carnitine. The rationale for this claim is based mostly on animal studies carried out in very highly controlled settings. In commercial animal husbandry, the impetus for the use of L-carnitine is to partition nutrients away from fat accretion and toward muscle deposition. In growing pigs fed energy-limited, fat-containing diets with or without supplemental L-carnitine, those receiving the supplement for 10 days had improved nitrogen retention and reduced carcass fat,[46] thus supporting a role for supplemental L-carnitine to improve body composition. Obesity affects a significant proportion of domestic pets, particularly dogs and cats. L-Carnitine added to a weight reduction diet for dogs resulted in a substantially greater loss of weight (7% versus 2%) and fat mass (4% versus 2%) in those animals receiving the supplement compared with diet alone over a period of 7 weeks.[47]

Unfortunately, the success observed in animal studies has not been achieved in humans. For example, in a double-blind investigation to test the weight loss efficacy of L-carnitine, 36 moderately overweight premenopausal women were pair-matched on body mass index and randomly assigned to two groups.[48] For 8 weeks, one group ingested 2 g of L-carnitine twice daily, and the placebo group ingested the same amount of lactose. All subjects walked for 30 minutes (at 60%–70% maximum heart rate) 4 days/week. No significant changes or differences between groups in mean total body mass, fat mass, or resting lipid utilization occurred over time. The success in animals suggests that it may be possible to achieve weight reduction and more desirable body composition with the use of carnitine supplements in humans, but the regimens necessary to achieve these goals may be too rigid to be widely effective.

### *Maintenance of Mental and Physical Function and Reversal of Decline with Aging*

Administration of acetyl-L-carnitine to old rats improves ambulatory activity and restores some memory loss by improving mitochondrial function and reducing accumulation of oxidation products.[40,44] The administration of L-carnitine to old rats restores activities of citric acid cycle and electron-transferring enzymes to near those of young rats,[49] and improves ambulatory activity.[50] In one study, acetyl-L-carnitine, but not L-carnitine, attenuated the appearance of malondialdehyde, a lipid oxidation product,[50] but in another study L-carnitine supplementation increased the activities of the antioxidant enzymes superoxide dismutase and glutathione peroxidase.[51] In elderly humans, patients with depressive syndrome scored significantly lower on the Hamilton Rating Scale for Depression following supplementation with acetyl-L-carnitine.[52] Elderly subjects with mild mental impairment had better scores on cognitive performance tests following supplementation with acetyl-L-carnitine.[53] A meta-analysis of the efficacy of acetyl-L-carnitine for cognitive impairment in mild Alzheimer's disease showed a significant advantage for the supplement over placebo on both clinical scales and psychometric tests.[54] Ames[55] has advocated a "metabolic tune-up" that includes micronutrients with acetyl-L-carnitine to maintain mitochondrial function during the life cycle and prevent age-related cognitive dysfunction and other degenerative diseases associated with aging.

## Therapeutic Use and Health Claims

L-Carnitine is approved by the FDA for the treatment of primary and secondary carnitine-deficiency diseases (e.g., OCTN2 deficiency, glutaric aciduria type II, methylmalonic aciduria, propionic acidemia, and medium-

**Table 1.** Potential Therapeutic Uses* for Carnitine and/or Its Esters in Humans

| Disease or Condition | Comment | Study |
|---|---|---|
| HIV infection and antiretroviral therapy | Increase $CD4^+$ cell count, reduce lymphocyte apoptosis; improve symptoms of polyneuropathy; prevent cardiovascular damage; decrease serum triacylglycerols; treatment of antiretroviral therapy-associated lipodystrophy | Ilias et al., 2004[56] |
| Cancer chemotherapy | Alleviation of chemotherapy-induced fatigue, nephrotoxicity, cardiomyopathy | Graziano et al., 2002[57] |
| Type 2 diabetes | Improves non-oxidative glucose disposal | Mingrone, 2004[58] |
| Chronic diabetic neuropathy | Alleviates pain, improves nerve fiber regeneration and vibration perception | Sima et al., 2005[59] |
| Endothelial dysfunction associated with type 2 diabetes mellitus and/or obesity | Attenuates free-fatty-acid-induced endothelial dysfunction | Shankar et al., 2004[60] |
| Peripheral vascular disease | Improves initial and maximal treadmill walking distance | Hiatt, 2004[61] |
| Congestive heart failure | Increases exercise capacity and reduces ventricular size | Anand et al., 1998[62] |
| Angina pectoris | Increases exercise workload tolerated prior to onset of angina, and decreases ST segment depression (electrocardiographic evidence of ischemia) during exercise | The Linus Pauling Institute Micronutrient Information Center[63] |
| Long-term therapy following acute myocardial infarction | Reduction of left ventricular dilation; lowered incidence of death, congestive heart failure, and ischemic events | Iliceto et al., 1995[64] |
| Seizure disorders treated with valproic acid | Attenuates hyperammonemia; may be particularly effective with anticonvulsant polytherapy that includes valproic acid | Gidal et al., 1997[65], Coulter, 1995[66] |
| Treatment of conditions with pivoxil-containing prodrugs | Pivalate is transesterified to carnitine and is quantitatively excreted as pivaloyl-L-carnitine, which may lead to carnitine depletion if exogenous carnitine is not provided. | Brass, 2002[67] |
| Male reproductive dysfunction | Improve sperm concentration, total sperm counts, and forward motility and viability of sperm in patients with astheno- and oligoasthenozoospermia | Agarwal and Said, 2004[68] |
| Hyperthyroidism | Inhibits thyroid action by inhibiting thyroid hormone entry into the nucleus | Benvenga et al., 2003[69] |

* Some of these "therapeutic" uses may also be considered "dietary supplement" use. For example, L-carnitine is included in a formula marketed as a diet supplement to enhance fertility and improve reproductive health.

chain acyl-CoA dehydrogenase deficiency) and for end-stage renal disease patients undergoing hemodialysis. It has been suggested that L-carnitine is beneficial for relief of symptoms in a number of other diseases and medical conditions (see Table 1). In most cases, these claims are supported by experimental and/or clinical evidence, but additional clinical trials may be required to establish efficacy.

## Summary

L-Carnitine has an essential role in intermediary metabolism, but for normal humans there is no dietary requirement. L-Carnitine has been proven to be useful in treatment in several diseases of genetic and acquired origin. For a number of other conditions, L-carnitine or its acetyl or propionyl esters may prove useful in alleviation or moderation of symptoms. The use of carnitine and/or its esters as dietary supplements may prove valuable in maintaining or improving physical and mental function and slowing decline during the aging process. Many health claims for nutritional supplements have little or no scientific or medical basis. For L-carnitine and its esters, claims have been made based on studies in experimental animals, testimony, anecdotal evidence, and research studies in humans that do not meet accepted standards for proof of efficacy. For some claims, the standard placebo-controlled, double-blind paradigm would be very difficult or impossible to implement. Nevertheless, there is great promise for the use of these supplements to restore and/or maintain healthy metabolic function.

## References

1. Marquis NR, Fritz IB. Enzymological determination of free carnitine concentrations in rat tissues. J Lipid Res. 1964;5:184–187.
2. Takahashi M, Ueda S, Misaki H, et al. Carnitine determination by an enzymatic cycling method with carnitine dehydrogenase. Clin Chem. 1994;40: 817–821.
3. Cederblad G, Lindstedt S. A method for the determination of carnitine in the picomole range. Clin Chim Acta. 1972;37:235–243.
4. Stevens RD, Hillman SL, Worthy S, et al. Assay for free and total carnitine in human plasma using tandem mass spectrometry. Clin Chem. 2000;46: 727–729.
5. Vreken P, van Lint AEM, Bootsma AH, et al. Quantitative plasma acylcarnitine analysis using electrospray tandem mass spectrometry for the diagnosis of organic acidaemias and fatty acid oxidation defects. J Inher Metab Dis. 1999;22:302–306.
6. van Kempen TATG, Odle J. Quantification of carnitine esters by high-performance liquid chromatography. J Chromatogr. 1992;584:157–165.
7. Kamimori H, Hamashima Y, Konishi M. Determination of carnitine and saturated-acyl group carnitine in human urine by high-performance liquid chromatography with fluorescence detection. Anal Biochem. 1994;218:417–424.
8. Vernez L, Wenk M, Krahenbuhl S. Determination of carnitine and acylcarnitines in plasma by high-performance liquid chromatography/electrospray ionization ion trap tandem mass spectrometry. Rapid Commun Mass Spectrometry. 2004;18:1233–1238.
9. Demarquoy J, Georges W, Rigault C, et al. Radioisotopic determination of L-carnitine content in foods commonly eaten in Western countries. Food Chem. 2004;86:137–142.
10. Rebouche CJ, Engel AG. Kinetic compartmental analysis of carnitine metabolism in the human carnitine deficiency syndromes. Evidence for alterations in tissue carnitine transport. J Clin Invest. 1984;73: 857–867.
11. Borum, PR, Broquist HP. Purification of S-adenosylmethionine: ε-N-L-lysine methyltransferase. The first enzyme in carnitine biosynthesis. J Biol Chem. 1977;252:5651–5655.
12. Vaz FM, Wanders RJC. Carnitine biosynthesis in mammals. Biochem J. 2002;361:417–429.
13. Rebouche CJ, Seim H. Carnitine metabolism and its regulation in microorganisms and mammals. Annu Rev Nutr. 1998;18:39–61.
14. Higgins T, Chaykin S, Hammond KB, Humbert JR. Trimethylamine N-oxide synthesis: A human variant. Biochem Med. 1972;6:392–396.
15. Enomoto A, Wempe MF, Tsuchida H, et al. Molecular identification of a novel carnitine transporter specific to human testis. Insights into the mechanism of carnitine recognition. J Biol Chem. 2002;277: 36262–36271.
16. Wu X, Prasad PD, Leibach FH, Ganapathy V. cDNA sequence, transport function, and genomic organization of human OCTN2, a new member of the organic cation transporter family. Biochem Biophys Res Commun. 1998;246:589–595.
17. Lamhonwah AM, Skaug J, Scherer SW, Tein I. A third human carnitine/organic cation transporter (OCTN3) as a canditate for the 5q31 Crohn's disease disease locus (IBD5). Biochem Biophys Res Commun. 2003;301:98–101.
18. Rebouche CJ. Carnitine. In: Shils ME, Shike M, Ross AC, Caballero B, Weinsier RL, Cousins RJ, eds. *Modern Nutrition in Health and Disease*. 10th ed. Baltimore: Williams & Wilkins; 2006; 537–544.
19. Rebouche CJ, Engel AG. Significance of renal γ-butyrobetaine hydroxylase for carnitine biosynthesis in man. J Biol Chem. 1981;255:8700–8705.
20. Hokland BM, Bremer J. Metabolism and excretion of carnitine and acylcarnitine in the perfused rat kidney. Biochim Biophys Acta. 1986;886:223–230.
21. Mancinelli A, Longo A, Shanahan K, Evans AM. Disposition of L-carnitine and acetyl-L-carnitine in the isolated perfused rat kidney. J Pharmacol Exp Ther. 1995;274:1122–1128.
22. Lombard KA, Olson AL, Nelson SE, Rebouche CJ. Carnitine status of lactoovovegetarians and strict vegetarian adults and children. Am J Clin Nutr. 1989; 50:301–306.
23. Borum PR. Carnitine in neonatal nutrition. J Child Neurol 1995;10(suppl 2):S25–S31.
24. Raiten DJ, Talbot JM, Waters JH, eds. Assessment of nutrient requirements for infant formulas. J Nutr. 1998;128:2120S–2121S.
25. Nyhan WL, Ozand PT. *Atlas of Metabolic Diseases*. London: Chapman & Hall Medical; 1998; 212–216.
26. Hashimoto N, Suzuki F, Tamai I, et al. Gene-dose effect on carnitine transport activity in embryonic fibroblasts of JVS mice as a model of human carnitine transporter deficiency. Biochem Pharmacol. 1998; 55:1729–1732.
27. Pons R, De Vivo DC. Primary and secondary carnitine deficiency syndromes. J Child Neurol. 1995; 10(suppl 2):S8–S24.
28. Iacobazzi V, Naglieri MA, Stanley CA, et al. The structure and organization of the human carnitine/

acylcarnitine translocase (CACT) gene. Biochem Biophys Res Commun. 1998;252:770–774.

29. Palmieri F, Indiveri C, Bisaccia F, Iacobazzi V. Mitochondrial metabolite carrier proteins: purification, reconstitution, and transport studies. In: Attardi G, Chomyn A, eds. *Methods in Enzymology, Volume 260: Mitochondrial Biogenesis and Genetics, Part A.* San Diego: Academic Press; 1995; 349–369.
30. Eaton S. Control of mitochondrial β-oxidation flux. Prog Lipid Res. 2002;41:197–239.
31. Bartlett K, Eaton S. Mitochondrial β-oxidation. Eur J Biochem. 2004;271:462–469.
32. Ramsay RR, Gandour RD, van der Leij FR. Molecular enzymology of carnitine transfer and transport. Biochim Biophys Acta. 2001;1546:21–43.
33. Yamaguti K, Kuratsune H, Watanabe Y, et al. Acylcarnitine metabolism during fasting and after refeeding. Biochem Biophys Res Commun. 1996;225: 740–746.
34. Arduini A, Mancinelli G, Ramsay RR. Palmitoyl-L-carnitine, a metabolic intermediate of the fatty acid incorporation pathway in erythrocyte membrane phospholipids. Biochem Biophys Res Commun. 1990;173:212–217.
35. Arduini A, Zibellini G, Ferrari L, et al. Participation of carnitine palmitoyltransferase in the synthesis of dipalmitoylphosphatidylcholine in rat alveolar type II cells. Mol Cell Biochem. 2001;218:81–86.
36. Arduini A, Rossi M, Mancinelli G, et al. Effect of L-carnitine and acetyl-L-carnitine on the human erythrocyte membrane stability and deformability. Life Sci. 1990;47:2395–2400.
37. Manoli I, De Martino MU, Kino T, Alesci S. Modulatory effects of L-carnitine on glucocorticoid receptor activity. Ann N Y Acad Sci. 2004;1033:147–157.
38. Horiuchi M, Kobayashi K, Tomomura M, et al. Carnitine administration to juvenile visceral steatosis mice corrects the suppressed expression of urea cycle enzymes by normalizing their transcription. J Biol Chem. 1992;267:5032–5035.
39. Tomomura M, Tomomura A, Abu Musa DMA, Saheki T. Long-chain fatty acids suppress the induction of urea cycle enzyme genes by glucocorticoid action. FEBS Lett. 1996;399:310–312.
40. Ames BN, Liu J. Delaying the mitochondrial decay of aging with acetylcarnitine. Ann N Y Acad Sci. 2004;1033:108–116.
41. Gadaleta MN, Petruzzella V, Daddabbo L, et al. Mitochondrial DNA transcription and translation in aged rat. Effect of acetyl-L-carnitine. Ann N Y Acad Sci. 1994;717:150–160.
42. Paradies G, Ruggiero FM, Petrosillo G, et al. Effect of aging and acetyl-L-carnitine on the activity of cytochrome oxidase and adenine nucleotide translocase in rat heart mitochondria. FEBS Lett. 1994;350: 213–215.
43. Paradies G, Ruggiero FM, Petrosillo G, et al. Carnitine-acylcarnitine translocase activity in cardiac mitochondria from aged rats: the effect of acetyl-L-carnitine. Mech Ageing Devel. 1995;84:103–112.
44. Liu J, Killilea DW, Ames BN. Age-associated mitochondrial oxidative decay: improvement of carnitine acetyltransferase substrate-binding affinity and activity in brain by feeding old rats acetyl-L-carnitine and/ or R-α-lipoic acid. Proc Natl Acad Sci U S A. 2002; 99:1876–1881.
45. Brass EP. Carnitine and sports medicine. Use or abuse? Ann N Y Acad Sci. 2004;1033:67–78.
46. Heo K, Odle J, Han IK, et al. Dietary carnitine improves nitrogen utilization in growing pigs fed low energy, fat-containing diets. J Nutr. 2000;130: 1809–1814.
47. The Iams Company. *L-Carnitine effects in overweight dogs. Food for Thought™ Technical Bulletin No. 126R.* Available online at: http://iams.com/en_US/jhtmls/nutrition/sw_NutritionQuestions_qanswer.jhtml?speciescode=D&brandcode=I&localeid=en_US&pagetypeid=PN&questionid=380.
48. Villani RG, Gannon J, Self M, et al. L-carnitine supplementation combined with aerobic training does not promote weight loss in moderately obese women. Int J Sport Nutr. 2000;10:199–207.
49. Kumaran S, Subathra M, Balu M, Panneerselvam C. Supplementation of L-carnitine improves mitochondrial enzymes in heart and skeletal muscle of aged rats. Exp Aging Res. 2005;31:55–67.
50. Liu J, Head E, Kuratsune H, et al. Comparison of the effects of L-carnitine and acetyl-L-carnitine on carnitine levels, ambulatory activity, and oxidative stress biomarkers in the brain of old rats. Ann N Y Acad Sci. 2004;1033:117–131.
51. Juliet PAR, Joyee AG, Jayaraman G, et al. Effect of L-carnitine on nucleic acid status of aged rat brain. Exp Neurol. 2005;191:33–40.
52. Tempesta E, Casella L, Pirrongelli C, et al. L-Acetylcarnitine in depressed elderly subjects. A cross-over study vs. placebo. Drugs Exp Clin Res. 1987; XII:417–423.
53. Salvioli G, Neri M. L-Acetylcarnitine treatment of mental decline in the elderly. Drugs Exp Clin Res. 1994;XX:169–176.
54. Montgomery SA, Thal LJ, Amrein R. Meta-analysis of double blind randomized controlled clinical trials of acetyl-L-carnitine versus placebo in the treatment of mild cognitive impairment and mild Alzheimer's disease. Int Clin Psychopharmacol. 2003;18:61–71.
55. Ames BN. Delaying the mitochondrial decay of aging — a metabolic tune-up. Alzheimer Dis Assoc Disorders. 2003;17(suppl 2):S54–S57.
56. Ilias I, Manoli I, Blackman MR, et al. L-Carnitine and acetyl-L-carnitine in the treatment of complications associated with HIV infection and antiretroviral therapy. Mitochondrion. 2004;4:163–168.
57. Graziano F, Bisonni R, Catalano V, et al. Potential

role of levocarnitine supplementation for the treatment of chemotherapy-induced fatigue in non-anaemic cancer patients. Br J Cancer. 2002;86:1854–1857.

58. Mingrone G. Carnitine in type 2 diabetes. Ann N Y Acad Sci. 2004;1033:99–107.
59. Sima AAF, Calvani M, Mehra M, Amato A. Acetyl-L-carnitine improves pain, nerve regeneration, and vibratory perception in patients with chronic diabetic neuropathy. Diabetes Care. 2005;28:89–94.
60. Shankar SS, Mirzamohammadi B, Walsh JP, Steinberg HO. L-Carnitine may attenuate free fatty acid-induced endothelial dysfunction. Ann N Y Acad Sci. 2004;1033:189–197.
61. Hiatt WR. Carnitine and peripheral arterial disease. Ann N Y Acad Sci. 2004;1033:92–98.
62. Anand I, Chandrashekhan Y, De Giuli F, et al. Acute and chronic effects of propionyl-L-carnitine on the hemodynamics, exercise capacity, and hormones in patients with congestive heart failure. Cardiovasc Drugs Ther. 1998;12:291–299.
63. The Linus Pauling Institute Micronutrient Information Center. *Carnitine*. Available online at: http://lpi.oregonstate.edu/infocenter/othernuts/carnitine/.
64. Iliceto S, Scrutinio D, Bruzzi P, et al. Effects of L-carnitine administration on left ventricular remodeling after acute anterior myocardial infarction: The L-carnitine ecocardiografia digitalizzata infarto miocardico (CEDIM) trial. J Am Coll Cardiol. 1995;26:380–387.
65. Gidal BE, Inglese CM, Meyer JF, et al. Diet- and valproate-induced transient hyperammonemia: effect of L-carnitine. J Child Neurol. 1997;16:301–305.
66. Coulter DL. Carnitine deficiency in epilepsy: risk factors and treatment. J Child Neurol. 1995;10(suppl):A32–A39.
67. Brass EP. Pivalate-generating prodrugs and carnitine homeostasis in man. Pharmacol Rev. 2002;54:589–598.
68. Agarwal A, Said TM. Carnitines and male infertility. Reprod Biomed Online. 2004;8:376–384.
69. Benvenga S, Lapa D, Cannavò S, Trimarchi F. Successive thyroid storms treated with L-carnitine and low doses of methimazole. Am J Med. 2003;115:417–418.

# 27 Choline and Brain Development

Steven H. Zeisel

## Function of Choline and Its Metabolites

Choline is needed for the structural integrity and signaling functions of cell membranes, it is the major source of methyl-groups in the diet, it directly affects cholinergic neurotransmission, and it is required for lipid transport/metabolism.[1] Choline (via its metabolite, betaine) is intricately related to metabolism of folate, methionine, homocysteine, and vitamin $B_{12}$, as illustrated in Figure 1. Betaine is not only an important methyl group donor, but it is also an osmolyte used in the glomerulus of the kidney to help reabsorb water.[2] Phosphatidylcholine (lecithin) is the predominant phospholipid (>50%) in most mammalian membranes. Sphingomyelin is another important choline-phospholipid.[3] Breakdown products of these choline phospholipids are molecules that can amplify external signals or that can terminate the signaling process by generating inhibitory second messengers.[1] Acetylcholine is a neurotransmitter that is especially important in brain functions such as memory and mood,[1] but it is also the neurotransmitter most often used by neurons that interface between the brain and its periphery; the nerves controlling skeletal muscles, heart rate, breathing, sweating, and salivation all use acetylcholine. Structures of several of these important choline-containing molecules are illustrated in Figure 2.

Growing experimental evidence identifies important roles for choline in many metabolic processes such as gene expression,[4] carcinogenesis,[5] apoptosis,[6] and early brain development.[7] The human requirement for the nutrient choline was officially recognized with the establishment

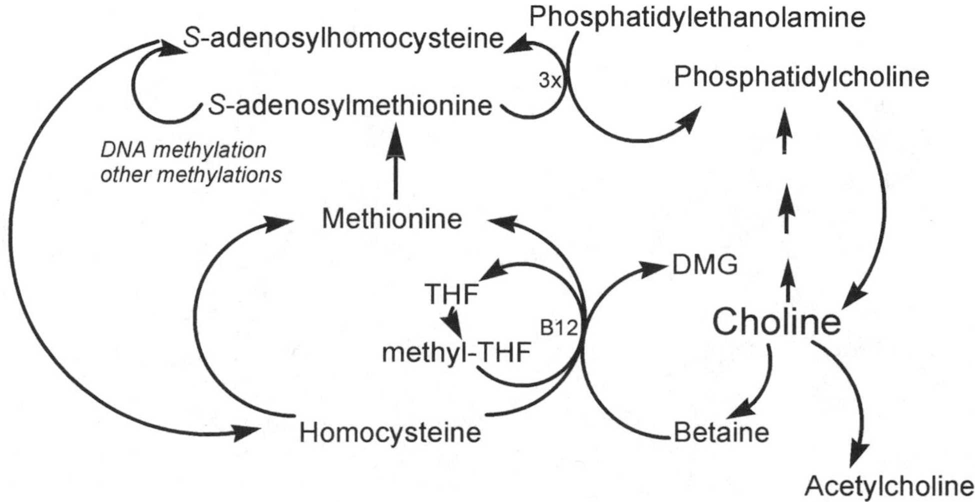


Figure 1. Choline, folate, and homocysteine metabolism are closely interrelated. The pathways for the metabolism of these three nutrients intersect at the formation of methionine from homocysteine. DMG = dimethylglycine; THF = tetrahydrofolate.

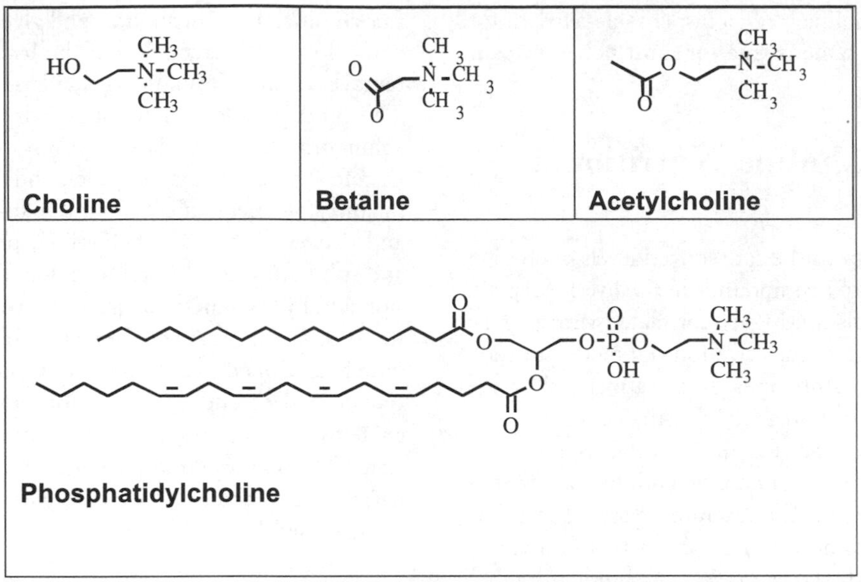

Choline Betaine Acetylcholine

Phosphatidylcholine

Figure 2. Structures of several important choline-containing molecules.

of Adequate Intake (AI) recommendations by the Food and Nutrition Board of the US Institute of Medicine in 1998.[8] In this chapter, the main focus will be on choline's role in brain development and function during the perinatal period.

# Choline Metabolism

As noted in Figure 1, choline is the precursor for the formation of a number of bioactive molecules. Acetylcholine synthesis is limited to neuronal tissue and placenta. Betaine homocysteine methyltransferase has the highest activity in the lens of the eye, in the liver, and in the kidney, but not in the brain.[9] In the predominant pathway for the synthesis of phosphatidylcholine (CDP pathway), choline is converted to CDP-choline, which then combines with diacylglycerol to form the end product. Also, sequential methylation of phosphatidylethanolamine produces phosphatidylcholine, with *S*-adenosylmethionine as the methyl donor.[1] The formation of phosphatidylcholine from choline and from phosphatidylethanolamine and *S*-adenosylmethionine are present in all tissues (though the latter pathway is most active in liver).[1] Phosphatidylcholine undergoes successive cleavage by phospholipase A2, lysophospholipase, and glycerylphosphocholine phosphodiesterase to generate free choline.[1]

# Choline and Methyl Group Metabolism

Because the metabolism of choline, folate, vitamin $B_{12}$, and methionine are interrelated (Figure 1), disturbances in one of the metabolic pathways is reflected by compensatory changes in the others. This means that the methyl groups from methyltetrahydrofolate, methionine, and choline can be interchangeable. For example, methionine can be formed via two pathways: from homocysteine using methyl groups donated by methyltetrahydrofolate, or from methyl groups donated by betaine (derived from choline).[1] Methyltetrahydrofolate synthesis also has two pathways: via one-carbon units derived from serine or from the methyl groups of choline through dimethylglycine.[9] Finally, choline can be formed from methyl groups derived from *S*-adenosylmethionine.[1] When animals and humans are fed a diet deficient in choline, dietary folate requirements increase because more methyltetrahydrofolate is used to re-methylate homocysteine in the liver.[11,12] If instead they are fed a diet deficient in folate, dietary choline requirements increase as choline becomes the primary methyl donor.[13-15] That evolution has resulted in several parallel pathways to help ensure adequate supply of methyl donors demonstrates the physiologic importance of these compounds.

# Dietary Requirements for Choline

As mentioned previously, the Institute of Medicine set an AI for choline in 1998.[8] Previously, it was not considered an essential nutrient for humans due to the endogenous pathway that exists for de novo biosynthesis of the choline moiety as part of phosphatidylcholine.[1] However, despite this capacity to synthesize some choline in liver, humans fed intravenously with solutions low in choline[16] or fed synthetic diets low in choline developed liver,[17] muscle,[18] and metabolic abnormalities (decreased clearance of homocysteine[19]), which resolved when choline was added back to their diets. Clearly, endogenous synthesis is not always adequate to prevent signs of choline deficiency, so choline is not a dispensable nutrient for some humans. The same is true for most non-ruminant species of animals.[1]

## Estimating Choline Nutritional Status

Choline deficiency in the rat reduced levels of choline and choline-containing compounds in the liver.[1] Hepatic phosphocholine levels are highly correlated with dietary choline intake, are quite sensitive to even moderate choline deficiency, and can be measured via magnetic resonance spectroscopy in humans.[19] Plasma concentrations of choline are also responsive to dietary intake: concentrations increase with intake of choline and decrease with a choline-inadequate diet.[1] Studies in humans suggest that plasma choline levels normally exhibit a two-fold variation in response to the consumption of common foods.[1] However, there appears to be an internal mechanism to keep choline concentrations above a certain minimal level, approximately 50% to 75% of normal, even after a week-long fast. Therefore, plasma choline concentrations are not the best functional indicator of choline status. Plasma choline concentration in humans ranges from 7 to 20 μmol/L, with a typical value of 10 μmol/L. Plasma phosphatidylcholine concentrations also decrease with choline deficiency and have been investigated as another possible marker. Usual levels range from 1 to 1.5 mmol/L, but are reported to be influenced by factors that change plasma lipoprotein levels. Thus, this too may not be an accurate indicator of choline status. The change in homocysteine response to a methionine load appears to be a sensitive and specific test (if folate status is normal) for choline deficiency.[19]

## Dietary Intake Recommendations for Choline

The Institute of Medicine suggests that an AI for choline in adult men is 550 mg/d and for adult women 425 mg/d.[8] Pregnancy creates increases the demands for dietary choline (see later discussion), and pregnant female rats have been shown to be susceptible to choline deficiency.[20] In rats, maternal liver choline concentration over the course of pregnancy declined from 130 μmol/L in nonpregnant adult rats to 38 μmol/L in late pregnancy.[21] The Institute of Medicine set an AI for choline of 450 mg/d for pregnant women.[8] Because lactation further consumes maternal choline stores (see later discussion), sensitivity to choline deficiency is higher in lactating rats than in non-lactating rats.[20] Thus, the AI for choline for lactating women is estimated to be 550 mg/d.[8] Although no experimental data exist, AIs for children have also been estimated.[8] There are studies under way to refine these estimates of human choline requirements.

After ingestion in foods, the water-soluble compounds free choline, phosphocholine, and glycerophosphocholine enter the portal circulation of the liver. The liver rapidly removes choline from portal circulation, acting as a sink.[1] The lipid-soluble compounds phosphatidylcholine and sphingomyelin enter via the lymph in chylomicrons and therefore miss the first-pass metabolism in the liver.[1] The majority of unesterified choline is taken up by the liver and converted to phosphocholine, phosphatidylcholine, and sphingomyelin.[1] Choline enters the tissues by diffusion and by mediated transport; nerve cells have a special transporter for choline. The genes for these transporters have been cloned.[22] In brain, a specific carrier mechanism transports free choline across the blood-brain barrier at a rate that is proportional to the serum choline concentration.[1] This choline transporter has an especially high capacity in the neonate,[1] and the significance of this will be discussed later in this review.

## Dietary Sources of Choline

Many foods contain significant amounts of choline or choline-containing compounds (www.nal.usda.gov/fnic/foodcomp/Data/Choline/Choline.html). In food, choline is found as free choline or is bound to an ester group (e.g., phosphocholine, glycerophosphocholine, sphingomyelin, or phosphatidylcholine). The best sources of choline include egg yolk, organ meats, legumes, and human milk. Food processing may also add choline, which is especially significant in the preparation of infant formula. Lecithin, a phosphatidylcholine-rich fraction prepared during commercial purification of phospholipids, is often added to foods as an emulsifying agent. It may also be taken as a dietary supplement.

The average choline intake of healthy men and women on an ad libitum diet was found to be 631 ± 157 mg/d (8.4 ± 2.1 mg/kg) in men and 443 ± 88 mg/d (6.7 ± 1.3 mg/kg) in women who were not pregnant or lactating.[23]

## Evolutionary Mechanisms for Delivering Choline to Babies

A large and growing body of evidence suggests that multiple mechanisms evolved to ensure the delivery of choline during the perinatal period. We know that circulating levels of choline in the fetus are high during normal development and progressively decrease after birth until they reach adult levels. In humans, rats, and rabbits, high perinatal serum choline concentrations persist for weeks after birth.[1] In mammals, the placenta delivers choline to the fetus by pumping it against a concentration gradient.[1] It may be that the placenta serves as a special reserve storage pool to ensure adequate delivery of choline to the fetus. The choline concentration in amniotic fluid is several times higher than that in maternal blood.[1] Presumably, these very high levels ensure enhanced availability of choline to the developing tissues. In addition, dietary supplementation of choline during the perinatal period further increases choline metabolite concentrations in both blood and brain.[1] A specific carrier mechanism that transports choline across the blood-brain barrier has an especially high capacity in the neonate.[1]

The mammary gland extracts choline from maternal blood, synthesizes phosphocholine, glycerophosphocholine, sphingomyelin, and phosphatidylcholine, and secretes all of these in milk.[1] The total choline content of human milk is approximately 1.3 to 1.5 mmol/L[24] and is likely important for sustaining tissue choline in the infant. Infant formulas differ in choline content, and many have less than is present in human breast milk.[24] When denied access to milk, rat pups had lower serum choline concentrations than their milk-fed littermates.[25]

As mentioned previously, there is an endogenous capacity to synthesize choline moiety (as apart of phosphatidylcholine) from *S*-adenosylmethionine.[1] Normally, brain has little of this activity. However, there is an isoform expressed only during the perinatal period that results in much more activity in the brains of neonates compared with adults.[1] *S*-adenosylmethionine concentrations are 40 to 50 nmol/g of tissue in newborn rat brains, and these high levels are probably sufficient to maintain high rates of choline formation.

## Choline and Embryo Development

One of the great successes of nutrition science has been the identification of the role that folate plays in normal neural tube closure: adequate dietary folate intake by the mother during pregnancy can prevent 50% or more of neural tube defects in babies.[26] As discussed previously, choline and folate metabolism are highly interrelated. Inhibition of choline uptake and metabolism was associated with the development of neural tube defects in mice.[27] Recent evidence suggests this may also be the case in humans. A retrospective case-control study (400 cases and 400 controls) of periconceptional dietary intakes of choline in women in California found that women in the lowest quartile for daily dietary choline intake had four times the risk of having a baby with a neural tube defect than did women in the highest quartile for intake.[28]

## Choline and Hippocampus Development

The perinatal period is a critical time for cholinergic organization of brain function, and substantial evidence exists to support the enduring nature of the changes induced by choline availability.[29] In rats and mice, choline availability is very important for the development of the hippocampus and septum.[7] In rodents, two sensitive periods exist during which times deficient choline retards hippocampal development and supplementary choline enhances development. These occur at days 11 to 18 of gestation and again at 16 to 30 days postnatally.[29] These two sensitive periods parallel neurogenesis (prenatal) and synaptogenesis (pre- and postnatal) in the hippocampus and basal forebrain. It is interesting that during the period that rodents are suckling and receiving milk rich in choline content from their mothers, the development of their hippocampi are not sensitive to supplemental choline.[29] In humans, hippocampal development occurs from day 56 of pregnancy through 4 years after birth. No experiments have yet been completed to determine if human hippocampal development can be influenced by dietary choline, although there is no reason to believe that it would not be. It should be noted that the hippocampus is one of the few areas of the brain in which nerve cells continue to multiply slowly in adults.

During brain development, neural progenitor cells must proliferate, migrate, differentiate, and survive to form the structures that we recognize in adult brain. Supplemental choline during fetal development increases, while choline deficiency decreases precursor cell proliferation, migration, and differentiation.[7] Not only does choline availability influence the rate at which neuronal precursor cells divide, it also alters the rate of cell death in these areas of the brain.[7] Apoptosis (cell suicide) to eliminate unwanted or damaged cells occurs as part of the normal process of brain development, and this process is modulated by choline availability in some tissues.[6] Cell death rates in fetal rodent brain on ED17 were inversely proportional to choline intake of the dams.[7]

The effects of dietary choline during embryonic brain development are detectable later in life. Neurons of the hippocampus have larger soma and an increased number of primary and secondary basal dendritic branches in rodents exposed to extra choline during the perinatal period.[30] Changes in perinatal choline availability in rodents also result in electrophysiological changes in the hippocampus that can be detected throughout life. Hippocampal long-term potentiation is an expression of synaptic plasticity, which is thought to be a potential neural substrate for learning and memory. Prenatal choline supplementation enhanced the induction of long-term potentiation in young adult rats, whereas prenatal choline deficiency diminished it.[31] The assessment of hippocampal long-term potentiation in older adult rats found similar differences.

Lifelong changes in the biochemistry of the brains of rodents occur after manipulating choline availability during the perinatal period. Perinatal choline supplementation in rats resulted in decreased choline acetyltransferase activity and increased muscarinic receptor binding (indexed by quinuclidinyl benzilate binding) in the hippocampus and frontal cortex of adult rats.[32] Phospholipase D activity in brain increased in the hippocampus of choline-supplemented rats.[33] Potassium-stimulated phosphorylation of hippocampal mitogen-activated protein kinase and cAMP-response element binding protein were enhanced in prenatally choline supplemented rodents.[34] There are a number of proteins in brain that are changed by choline availability during fetal life, and these most likely reflect changes in the composition of cells in brain. Changed proteins include calretinin, vimentin, TGFβ, p15, and p27.[35-37]

## Choline and Memory Function

Choline supplementation or deficiency in utero and/or during the early neonatal period results in permanent alteration of memory function of adult rats.[38,39] Tönjes et al.[39] showed that depriving neonatal rats (embryonic days 3–14) of maternal contact and nutrition resulted in altered memory: animals treated with supplemental choline during this time period exhibited significantly higher memory capacity in adulthood compared with animals who received choline later (embryonic days 15–28). Subsequently, Meck and Williams[38] found that choline supplementation (about three times normal dietary choline) of rat dams during pregnancy resulted in altered memory tests of their offspring on a radial maze at 60 days of age; choline-supplemented rats exhibited more accurate performance on both working and reference memory components of the task than did controls. Prenatal choline deficiency impaired memory.[29] Perinatal choline supplementation also enhanced timing and temporal memory.[40] In rats tested at 24 to 36 months of age, prenatal choline supplementation enhanced simultaneous temporal processing (i.e., the animal's ability to divide attention between multiple stimuli presented in parallel), increased attention to both the preferred and lesser preferred signal, and delayed age-related decline in simultaneous temporal processing.[41] On the other hand, while prenatal choline deficiency also increased attention to the preferred signal, it decreased attention to the lesser preferred signal and accelerated age-related decline in simultaneous temporal processing.[41]

Pups born of choline-supplemented rats used altered strategies in memory performance testing, particularly in the use of "chunking."[42] Chunking is a strategy in which elements to be remembered are grouped together into fewer, larger units to facilitate recall of more information than can be processed individually, thus allowing for more efficient processing. Investigators found significant differences related to proactive interference between perinatally choline-supplemented rats and controls.[42] Proactive interference refers to the interference of memories from previous experiences with current memory. Choline supplementation in the perinatal period resulted in rats that showed little proactive interference, while controls exhibited moderate levels and choline-deficient rats displayed high levels of proactive interference.

Perinatal choline treatment reduced the cognitive deficits associated with prenatal exposure to ethanol. Rats that had been exposed to ethanol and not treated with choline postnatally performed poorest on all tasks, while the ethanol-exposed, choline-treated animals performed significantly better.[43] Additionally, this choline-treated group's performance was similar to that of the control groups that were not exposed to ethanol. Prenatally ethanol-exposed animals were hyperactive compared with controls and performed poorly on reversal learning tasks; however, perinatal choline supplementation ameliorated hyperactivity and improved reversal learning task performance.[44] These findings suggest that perinatal choline supplementation may alter some of the structural and functional changes brought on by early alcohol exposure, and that these effects last beyond the period of supplementation.

## Proposed Mechanisms for Choline's Effects on Brain Development

A number of reasonable hypotheses exist relating to choline's mechanisms of action in the body, and particularly in the fetal brain.

### *Methyl Group Transfer*

The observed effects of dietary choline manipulation may be related to changes in gene expression.[4,45] DNA methylation occurs at cytosine bases that are followed by a guanosine (CpG sites), and influences many cellular events, including gene transcription, genomic imprinting, and genomic stability. DNA methylation also protects against fragmentation and alterations in chromatin compaction and stability in association with histone modifications. A choline-methyl-deficient diet lowered the capacity in rats to methylate DNA in brain: global DNA was significantly undermethylated.[46] Choline deficiency inhibited human neuroblastoma cell proliferation due to hypomethylation of the promoter region of the cyclin-dependent kinase inhibitor 3 gene and reduced global DNA methylation.[4] This mechanism may explain why choline availability altered the rate of neuronal stem cell proliferation, because cyclin-dependent kinase is required for completion of the cell cycle.[7] There is additional evidence that a choline-methyl-supplemented diet influences gene expression. After feeding pregnant Pseudoagouti Avy/a mice dams such a diet, offspring had permanently increased agouti/black mottling of their coats, indicating permanently altered expression of the agouti gene after exposure to dietary methyl donors in utero.[47,48] Thus, choline-methyl status directly influences gene methylation and expression in brain and other tissues.

### *Phosphatidylcholine Composition of Membranes*

Choline deficiency significantly decreases the phosphatidylcholine content of plasma membranes.[1] Membranes with decreased phosphatidylcholine are more fragile.[18] Mitochondrial membranes are similarly affected with resulting loss of mitochondrial membrane potential and leakage of reactive oxygen species.[49]

Phosphatidylcholine consists of many species that differ in fatty acid composition. Phosphatidylcholines occurring naturally in foods have a different fatty-acid composition than those endogenously synthesized.[50] Phosphatidylcholine molecules produced from choline and diacylglycerol (the CDP-choline pathway[51]) mainly contain medium-chain saturated fatty acid species. On the other hand, phosphatidylcholine molecules derived from methylation of phosphatidylethanolamine are more diverse and contain significantly more long-chain, polyunsaturated fatty acid (PUFA) species, such as arachadonic acid and docosahexaenoic acid (DHA).[50] These PUFA species of phosphatidylcholine have different packing densities in membranes and thus alter membrane properties. In addition, phosphatidylcholine is the main storage form for arachadonic acid and DHA, and it is from there that they are released to form signaling molecules and prostaglandins (this role for phosphatidylcholine as a signaling molecule is discussed later).

There are a significant number of studies suggesting that DHA availability to brain modulates brain development,[52] and this DHA is mainly present in phosphatidylcholine molecules. In PEMT knockout mice (which cannot form phosphatidylcholine by methylation of phosphatidylethanolamine), PUFA species of phosphatidylcholine are greatly diminished in liver and in plasma.[53] Choline-deficient mice have a two-fold increased formation of phosphatidylcholine by methylation of phosphatidylethanolamine in the liver compared with controls.[54] In brain, choline deficiency increased this activity in females, but not in males.[55] Female mice produce more phosphatidylcholine via this pathway than do male mice.[56] Estimates of the amount of increased activity in female humans vary between 10% and 50%.[57,58] Thus, differences in the pathways used to make phosphatidylcholine are common, are sensitive to dietary choline, and result in changes in membrane composition that have important physical and functional consequences.

### *Changes in Phosphatidylcholine-Derived Signaling Molecules*

The hydrolysis of phosphatidylcholine generates phosphocholine and diacylglycerol, while the hydrolysis of sphingomyelin generates ceramide.[1] Phosphocholine is a signal that increases cell division after stimulation by specific growth factors.[1] Diacylglycerol is an important activator of protein kinase C, which phosphorylates proteins in the signaling pathways controlling cell growth.[1] Ceramide activates cell suicide (apoptosis).[59] Choline-deficient cells die by apoptosis because of increased ceramide signaling and because of decreased survival-factor signals.[60]

### *Acetylcholine*

Choline is a precursor for the formation of acetylcholine, and this molecule is not only a neurotransmitter, but is also a direct modulator of brain development.[1] Though changes in the acetylcholine concentrations of whole fetal brain are not detected when pregnant rats are supplemented with dietary choline, it is possible that changes in acetylcholine concentrations in specific regions of the brain do occur and modulate neuronal development. Supplemental choline accelerates the synthesis and release of acetylcholine in the brains of adult rodents.[61] Increased plasma choline may augment acetylcholine synthesis only if there is simultaneous activation of cholinergic neurons or if acetylcholine stores have already been depleted.[62]

## Summary

Humans require choline in their diets, and adequate dietary intakes have been formulated that are similar to estimated dietary intake by humans. Choline is intricately involved in one-carbon metabolism and is the precursor for many important compounds, including phospholipids, acetylcholine, and the methyl donor betaine. Choline is essential for transport of lipoproteins from the liver, myelination of nervous tissue, synthesis of lung surfactant, and in neurodevelopment. Perinatal supplementation of choline enhances memory and learning functions and these changes endure across the lifespan. Conversely, choline deficiency during this period results in memory and cognitive deficits that also persist. Studies suggest that perinatal choline supplementation can reduce the behavioral effects of prenatal stress and the cognitive effects of prenatal alcohol exposure in offspring.

## Acknowledgements

This work was funded by grants from the National Institutes of Health (DK55865, AG09525, ES012997) and by a grant from the Gerber Foundation. Support for this work was also provided by grants from the NIH to the UNC Clinical Nutrition Research Unit (DK56350).

## References

1. Zeisel SH, Blusztajn JK. Choline and human nutrition. Annu Rev Nutr. 1994;14:269–296.
2. Burg M. Molecular basis of osmotic regulation. Am J Physiol. 1995;268:F983–F996.
3. Diringer H, Koch MA. Biosynthesis of sphingomyelin. Transfer of phosphorylcholine from phosphatidylcholine to erythro-ceramide in a cell-free system. Hoppe Seylers Zeitschrift Fur Physiologische Chemie [JC:gb3]. 1973;354:1661–1665.
4. Niculescu MD, Yamamuro Y, Zeisel SH. Choline availability modulates human neuroblastoma cell proliferation and alters the methylation of the promoter region of the cyclin-dependent kinase inhibitor 3 gene. J Neurochem. 2004;89:1252–1259.
5. Zeisel SH, Albright CD, Shin O-K, Mar M-H, Salganik RI, da Costa K-A. Choline deficiency selects for resistance to p53-independent apoptosis and

causes tumorigenic transformation of rat hepatocytes. Carcinogenesis. 1997;18:731–738.

6. Albright CD, Lui R, Bethea TC, da Costa K-A, Salganik RI, Zeisel SH. Choline deficiency induces apoptosis in SV40-immortalized CWSV-1 rat hepatocytes in culture. FASEB J. 1996;10:510–516.
7. Craciunescu CN, Albright CD, Mar MH, Song J, Zeisel SH. Choline availability during embryonic development alters progenitor cell mitosis in developing mouse hippocampus. J Nutr. 2003;133:3614–3618.
8. Food and Nutrition Board, Institute of Medicine. Dietary Reference Intakes for Thiamin, Riboflavin, Niacin, Vitamin B6, Folate, Vitamin B12, Pantothenic Acid, Biotin, and Choline. Washington, DC: National Academies Press; 1998. Available online at: http://www.nap.edu/openbook/0309065542/html/.
9. Delgado-Reyes CV, Wallig MA, Garrow TA. Immunohistochemical detection of betaine-homocysteine S-methyltransferase in human, pig, and rat liver and kidney. Arch Biochem Biophys. 2001;393: 184–186.
10. Gregory JF, 3rd, Cuskelly GJ, Shane B, Toth JP, Baumgartner TG, Stacpoole PW. Primed, constant infusion with [$^2H_3$]serine allows in vivo kinetic measurement of serine turnover, homocysteine remethylation, and transsulfuration processes in human one-carbon metabolism. Am J Clin Nutr. 2000;72: 1535–1541.
11. Selhub J, Seyoum E, Pomfret EA, Zeisel SH. Effects of choline deficiency and methotrexate treatment upon liver folate content and distribution. Cancer Res. 1991;51:16–21.
12. Varela-Moreiras G, Selhub J, da Costa K, Zeisel SH. Effect of chronic choline deficiency in rats on liver folate content and distribution. J Nutr Biochem. 1992;3:519–522.
13. Jacob R, Jenden D, Okoji R, Allman M, Swendseid M. Choline status of men and women is decreased by low dietary folate. FASEB J. 1998;12:A512.
14. Jacob RA, Jenden DJ, Allman-Farinelli MA, Swendseid ME. Folate nutriture alters choline status of women and men fed low choline diets. J Nutr. 1999; 129:712–717.
15. Kim Y-I, Miller JW, da Costa K-A, et al. Folate deficiency causes secondary depletion of choline and phosphocholine in liver. J Nutr. 1995;124: 2197–2203.
16. Buchman AL, Ament ME, Sohel M, et al. Choline deficiency causes reversible hepatic abnormalities in patients receiving parenteral nutrition: proof of a human choline requirement: a placebo-controlled trial. J Parenter Enteral Nutr. 2001;25:260–268.
17. Zeisel SH, daCosta K-A, Franklin PD, et al. Choline, an essential nutrient for humans. FASEB J. 1991;5:2093–2098.
18. da Costa KA, Badea M, Fischer LM, Zeisel SH. Elevated serum creatine phosphokinase in choline-deficient humans: mechanistic studies in C2C12 mouse myoblasts. Am J Clin Nutr. 2004;80: 163–170.
19. da Costa KA, Gaffney CE, Fischer LM, Zeisel SH. Choline deficiency in mice and humans is associated with increased plasma homocysteine concentration after a methionine load. Am J Clin Nutr 2005;81: 440–4.
20. Zeisel SH, Mar M-H, Zhou Z-W, da Costa K-A. Pregnancy and lactation are associated with diminished concentrations of choline and its metabolites in rat liver. J. Nutr. 1995;125:3049–3054.
21. Gwee MC, Sim MK. Free choline concentration and cephalin-N-methyltransferase activity in the maternal and foetal liver and placenta of pregnant rats. Clin. Exper. Pharmacol. Physiol. 1978;5:649–53.
22. Yuan Z, Wagner L, Poloumienko A, Bakovic M. Identification and expression of a mouse muscle-specific CTL1 gene. Gene 2004;341:305–12.
23. Fischer L, Scearce J, Mar, et al. Ad libitum choline intake in healthy individuals meets or exceeds the proposed Adequate Intake level. J. Nutr 2005;in press.
24. Holmes-McNary M, Cheng WL, Mar. MH, Fussell S, Zeisel SH. Choline and choline esters in human and rat milk and infant formulas. Am. J. Clin. Nutr. 1996;64:572–576.
25. Zeisel SH, Wurtman RJ. Developmental changes in rat blood choline concentration. Biochem. J. 1981; 198:565–570.
26. Shaw GM, Schaffer D, Velie EM, Morland K, Harris JA. Periconceptional vitamin use, dietary folate, and the occurrence of neural tube defects. Epidemiology 1995;6:219–26.
27. Fisher MC, Zeisel SH, Mar MH, Sadler TW. Inhibitors of choline uptake and metabolism cause developmental abnormalities in neurulating mouse embryos. Teratology 2001;64:114–22.
28. Shaw GM, Carmichael SL, Yang W, Selvin S, Schaffer DM. Periconceptional dietary intake of choline and betaine and neural tube defects in offspring. Am J Epidemiol 2004;160:102–9.
29. Meck WH, Williams CL. Metabolic imprinting of choline by its availability during gestation: Implications for memory and attentional processing across the lifespan. Neurosci. Biobehav. Rev. 2003;27: 385–399.
30. Li Q, Guo-Ross S, Lewis DV, et al. Dietary prenatal choline supplementation alters postnatal hippocampal structure and function. J Neurophysiol 2004;91: 1545–55.
31. Pyapali G, Turner D, Williams C, Meck W, Swartzwelder HS. Prenatal choline supplementation decreases the threshold for induction of long-term po-

tentiation in young adult rats. J. Neurophysiol. 1998; 79:1790–1796.

32. Meck WH, Smith RA, Williams CL. Organizational changes in cholinergic activity and enhanced visuospatial memory as a function of choline administered prenatally or postnatally or both. Behav. Neurosci. 1989;103:1234–1241.
33. Holler T, Cermak J, Blusztajn J. Dietary choline supplementation in pregnant rats increases hippocampal phospholipase D activity of the offspring. FASEB J 1996;10:1653–1659.
34. Mellott TJ, Williams CL, Meck WH, Blusztajn JK. Prenatal choline supplementation advances hippocampal development and enhances MAPK and CREB activation. Faseb J 2004;18:545–7.
35. Albright CD, Mar MH, Friedrich CB, Brown EC, Zeisel SH. Maternal choline availability alters the localization of p15Ink4B and p27Kip1 cyclin-dependent kinase inhibitors in the developing fetal rat brain hippocampus. Dev Neurosci 2001;23:100–6.
36. Albright CD, Siwek DF, Craciunescu CN, et al. Choline availability during embryonic development alters the localization of calretinin in developing and aging mouse hippocampus. Nutr Neurosci 2003;6: 129–34.
37. Albright CD, Tsai AY, Mar M-H, Zeisel SH. Choline availability modulates the expression of TGFβ1 and cytoskeletal proteins in the hippocampus of developing rat brain. Neurochem. Res. 1998;23: 751–758.
38. Meck WH, Smith RA, Williams CL. Pre- and postnatal choline supplementation produces long-term facilitation of spatial memory. Dev. Psychobiol. 1988;21:339–353.
39. Tonjes R, Hecht K, Brautzsch M, Lucius R, D:orner G. Behavioural changes in adult rats produced by early postnatal maternal deprivation and treatment with choline chloride. Experimental & Clinical Endocrinology 1986;88:151–7.
40. Meck W, Williams C. Characterization of the facilitative effects of perinatal choline supplementation on timing and temporal memory. Neuroreport 1997;8: 2831–5.
41. Meck W, Williams C. Simultaneous temporal processing is sensitive to prenatal choline availability in mature and aged rats. Neuroreport 1997;8:3045–51.
42. Meck WH, Williams CL. Choline supplementation during prenatal development reduces proactive interference in spatial memory. Brain Res Dev Brain Res 1999;118:51–9.
43. Thomas JD, La Fiette MH, Quinn VR, Riley EP. Neonatal choline supplementation ameliorates the effects of prenatal alcohol exposure on a discrimination learning task in rats. Neurotoxicol Teratol 2000; 22:703–11.
44. Thomas JD, Garrison M, O'Neill TM. Perinatal choline supplementation attenuates behavioral alterations associated with neonatal alcohol exposure in rats. Neurotoxicol Teratol 2004;26:35–45.
45. Niculescu M, Craciunescu N, Zeisel S. Gene expression profiling of choline deficient neural precursor cells isolated from mouse brain. Brain Research 2005: in press.
46. Alonso-Aperte E, Varela-Moreiras G. Brain folates and DNA methylation in rats fed a choline deficient diet or treated with low doses of methotrexate. Int J Vitam Nutr Res 1996;66:232–6.
47. Waterland RA, Jirtle RL. Transposable elements: targets for early nutritional effects on epigenetic gene regulation. Mol Cell Biol 2003;23:5293–300.
48. Wolff GL, Kodell RL, Moore SR, Cooney CA. Maternal epigenetics and methyl supplements affect agouti gene expression in Avy/a mice. Faseb J 1998; 12:949–57.
49. Albright CD, Salganik RI, Craciunescu CN, Mar MH, Zeisel SH. Mitochondrial and microsomal derived reactive oxygen species mediate apoptosis induced by transforming growth factor-beta1 in immortalized rat hepatocytes. J Cell Biochem 2003;89: 254–61.
50. DeLong CJ, Shen YJ, Thomas MJ, Cui Z. Molecular distinction of phosphatidylcholine synthesis between the CDP- choline pathway and phosphatidylethanolamine methylation pathway. J Biol Chem 1999; 274:29683–8.
51. Kennedy EP, Weiss SB. The function of cytidine coenzymes in the biosynthesis of phospholipids. J. Biol. Chem. 1956;222:193–214.
52. Uauy R, Peirano P, Hoffman D, Mena P, Birch D, Birch E. Role of essential fatty acids in the function of the developing nervous system. Lipids 1996;31 Suppl:S167–76.
53. Watkins SM, Zhu X, Zeisel SH. Phosphatidylethanolamine-N-methyltransferase activity and dietary choline regulate liver-plasma lipid flux and essential fatty acid metabolism in mice. J Nutr 2003;133: 3386–91.
54. Ridgway ND, Yao Z, Vance DE. Phosphatidylethanolamine levels and regulation of phosphatidylethanolamine N-methyltransferase. J. Biol. Chem. 1989; 264:1203–7.
55. Johnson PI, Blusztajn JK. Sexually dimorphic activation of liver and brain phosphatidylethanolamine N-methyltransferase by dietary choline deficiency. Neurochem Res 1998;23:583–7.
56. Noga AA, Vance DE. A gender-specific role for phosphatidylethanolamine N-methyltransferase-derived phosphatidylcholine in the regulation of plasma high density and very low density lipoproteins in mice. J Biol Chem 2003;278:21851–9.
57. Bjornstad P, Bremer J. In vivo studies on pathways for the biosynthesis of lecithin in the rat. J. Lipid Res. 1966;7:38–45.
58. Lyman RL, Sheehan G, Tinoco J. Diet and 14CH3-methionine incorporation into liver phosphatidyl-

choline fractions of male and female rats. Can. J. Biochem. 1971;49:71–9.

59. Obeid L, Hannun Y. Ceramide: a stress signal and mediator of growth suppression and apoptosis. J Cell Biochem 1995;58:191–198.
60. Albright CD, da Costa KA, Craciunescu CN, Klem E, Mar MH, Zeisel SH. Regulation of choline deficiency apoptosis by epidermal growth factor in CWSV-1 rat hepatocytes. Cell Physiol Biochem 2005;15:59–68.
61. Cohen EL, Wurtman RJ. Brain acetylcholine: increase after systemic choline administration. Life Sci. 1975;16:1095–102.
62. Wecker L. Neurochemical effects of choline supplementation. Can. J. Physiol. Pharmacol. 1986;64: 329–33.

# 28
# Dietary Flavonoids

Jeffrey B. Blumberg and Paul E. Milbury

## Introduction

Flavonoids (or bioflavonoids) are a subclass of plant polyphenols with over 6000 compounds identified to date. Ubiquitous in plant foods and phytomedicines, flavonoids are secondary metabolites of the shikimic acid pathway and act as phytoalexins to protect the plant from predators and environmental stresses. In addition to providing aroma, color, and/or taste to several foods, many flavonoids are bioavailable and bioactive and may contribute to the health benefits associated with the consumption of fruits, vegetables, and whole grains.

The conservation of flavonoids over a billion years of evolution indicates their importance to plant survival, helps to explain their great diversity, and suggests their influence on the evolution of vascular plants and animal species.[1] In addition to their role as phytoalexins, some flavonoids serve as pigments to screen ultraviolet light and are also involved in photosensitization, energy transfer, and photosynthesis.[2] Further, flavonoids may modulate the activity of plant enzymes, growth hormones, morphogenesis, respiration, and sex determination. Flavonoids can also activate the bacterial *Rhizobium* genes involved in nitrogen fixation, suggesting that these phytochemicals may also have the potential to influence the expression of mammalian genes.[3]

## Nomenclature and Structure

Flavonoids possess two or more aromatic rings linked by an oxygenated heterocyclic bridge containing one oxygen and three carbon atoms (Figure 1). The major classes of dietary flavonoids are the anthocyanidins, flavanols (or catechins), flavanones, flavones, flavonols, and isoflavones, and are defined by six basic ring structures and hydroxylation patterns with methyl groups and a variety of mono- and disaccharides responsible for the vast number of individual flavonoids (Figure 2). The isoflavones are often referred to as phytoestrogens due to hydroxyl groups in the 7 and 4′ ring positions and their affinity to estrogen receptors. Anthocyanins exist as glycosides of polyhydroxy and polymethoxy derivatives of the 2-phenylbenzopyrylium cation, so they are distinct from the other classes with an electron deficiency in their ring structure. The structural differences between the flavonoid classes can account for the differences observed in their bioavailability and bioactivity (Table 1).

Some flavonoids may form oligomers and polymers of their basic structure to produce high-molecular weight compounds called tannins. Tannins contain many hydroxyl and carboxyl groups capable of forming strong complexes with proteins and other macromolecules. Hydrolyzable tannins, as found in pomegranate and raspberries, contain non-aromatic polyol carbohydrate moieties esterified with phenolics such as gallic acid (gallotannins) or ellagic acid (ellagitannins) and are easily hydrolyzed with acids or bases to liberate carbohydrate and phenolic acids. Condensed tannins (or proanthocyanidins) are polymers of flavanols joined by carbon-carbon bonds and are not susceptible to hydrolysis. Derived tannins are formed during food processing (e.g., the theaflavins and thearubigns

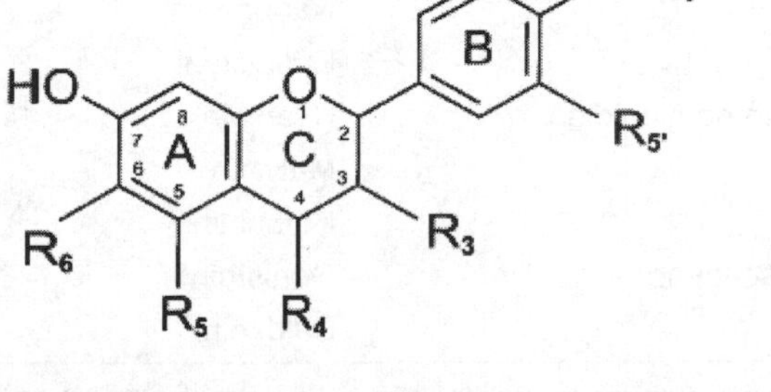

Figure 1. Basic structure and numbering system of flavonoids. Flavonoids contain two aromatic rings (A and B) linked by an oxygenated heterocycle (ring C). R substitutions include hydroxy, methyl, and mono- or disaccharide groups.

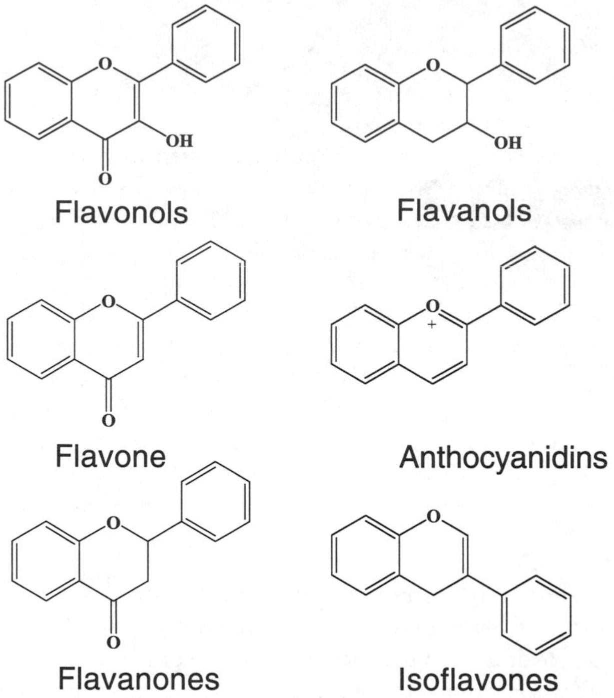

Flavonols | Flavanols | Flavone | Anthocyanidins | Flavanones | Isoflavones

Figure 2. Flavonoid classes and core structures. Flavonoids within each class are structurally distinct due to different patterns of hydroxylation, methylation and conjugation with mono- and disaccharides.

in black and oolong tea), and are usually absent from healthy, intact plant tissue.

# Food Sources

Flavonols, particularly kaempferol, isorhamnetin, myricetin, and quercetin, are the most ubiquitous flavonoids in plant foods. Flavonol-rich vegetables (15–40 mg/100 g) include broccoli, kale, leeks, and onions. Fruits, including apples, blueberries, grapes, and tomatoes, also contain flavonols, although they are found predominantly in the skin. Flavonol biosynthesis is stimulated by ultraviolet light, which may explain their higher concentration in plant parts with the greatest light exposure.

Flavanols are found in a wide variety of fruits and seeds, including apples, apricots, and red grapes, which are good sources (2–20 mg/100 g), and green tea and dark chocolate (containing proanthocyanidins) among the richest sources (40–65 mg/100 g), in part because they represent extracted and/or concentrated natural products. In contrast to other flavonoids, flavanols exist as aglycones (absent sugar substitutions) and are quite stable during cooking and processing.[4] The predominant flavanols are catechin, epicatechin, epicatechin-3-gallate, epigallocatechin, and epigallocatechin-3-gallate.

Flavones, such as apigenin and luteolin, are found in

**Table 1** Structures of Individual Flavonoids*

| Flavonoid Subclass | Flavonoid | Substituents | | | | | |
|---|---|---|---|---|---|---|---|
| | | 3 | 5 | 7 | 3′ | 4′ | 5′ |
| Flavonols | Quercetin | OH | OH | OH | OH | OH | H |
| | Kaempferol | OH | OH | OH | H | OH | H |
| | Myricetin | OH | OH | OH | OH | OH | OH |
| Flavones | Apigenin | H | OH | OH | H | OH | H |
| | Luteolin | H | OH | OH | OH | OH | H |
| Flavan-3-ols | Catechin | OH | OH | OH | OH | OH | H |
| | Epigallocatechin | OH | OH | OH | OH | OH | OH |
| | Epigallocatechin gallate | G | OH | OH | OH | OH | OH |
| Flavanones | Hesperetin | H | OH | OH | OH | $OCH_3$ | H |
| | Naringenin | H | OH | OH | H | OH | H |
| | Eriodictyol | H | OH | OH | OH | OH | H |
| Anthocyanidins | Cyanidin | OH | OH | OH | OH | OH | H |
| | Malvidin | OH | OH | OH | $OCH_3$ | OH | $OCH_3$ |
| | Petunidin | OH | OH | OH | $OCH_3$ | OH | OH |
| Isoflavones | Genistein | H* | OH | OH | H | OH | H |
| | Daidzein | H* | H | OH | H | OH | H |

*Individual molecular structures of flavonoids are determined by the addition of hydroxyl, methyl, and methoxy groups, most commonly at position 3, 5, 7, 3′, 4′ or 5′ on the flavonoid nucleus. The number and positioning of hydroxyl groups together with the degree of saturation of the C-ring determine the antioxidant capacity of individual flavonoids. G = gallate. H* indicates the hydrogen is attached to position 2 because of the connection of the C and B rings at position 3 in isoflavones.

celery and cereals (approximately 20 mg/100 g) and at high concentrations in parsley (635 mg/100 g). Polymethoxylated flavones, such as tangeretin, are found concentrated in the rinds of citrus fruit.

Flavanones, including eriodictyol, hesperidin, and narigenin, are found primarily in citrus fruit (15–50 mg/100 g), with the highest concentrations in the membraneous parts and peel. Grapefruit and orange juice with pulp can provide up to 140 mg flavanone glycosides per serving, although estimated mean daily intakes in the United States are less than 1 mg.

Isoflavones are unique to legumes such as soy, and include daidzein, genistein, and glycitein. The isoflavones in soy occur as glycosides, but some fermented products contain free aglycones. The aglycones are quite stable during processing and, thus, can be found in high concentrations in foods such as tofu, tempeh, and some soy flours (28, 53, and 200 mg/100 g, respectively).[5]

About 400 anthocyanins, many as blue and red pigments, have been found in nature, but their distribution in foods is more limited, with good sources (50–150 mg/100 g) found in cherries, radishes, red cabbage, red onions, and red wine.[6] The richest sources of anthocyanins are black, blue, and red berries (100–600 mg/100 g). The major anthocyanin aglycones (anthocyanindins) include cyanidin, delphinidin, malvidin, pelargonidin, peonidin, and petunidin. Unlike the flavanols, anthocyanins are relatively unstable compounds and can be destroyed during food processing.

## Dietary Intake

Determination of flavonoid intakes has only recently been attempted, and, partly due to the analytical challenge of characterizing so many individual compounds, databases are incomplete and typically describe these phytochemicals only in their aglycone form. Some reports have estimated daily flavonoid intake at 10 to 100 mg, but typically focus on only one or two of the six classes and thus greatly underestimate actual total flavonoid consumption. Estimates of intake are also imprecise because current databases do not fully account for factors that can markedly affect flavonoid content, including agricultural practices, cultivars, ripeness, and season, as well as post-harvest processing, storage, and cooking.[7] Nonetheless, differences in flavonoid intake can vary markedly between population groups due to dietary patterns and the availability of particular fruits and vegetables. Thus, isoflavone intake at about 50 mg/d is greatest in Asian countries where soy foods are prevalent and flavanol intake at about 70 mg/d is greatest in countries such as the Netherlands, where tea is a popular beverage. Individual foods may play a disproportionate role in contributing to specific flavonoid intake when they are available only in a specific season, though the ready availability of frozen fruits and vegetables in some countries can mitigate this influence.

## Bioavailability

Early reports suggested that flavonoid glycosides were not absorbed because of their size, polarity, and avid binding to dietary proteins. Others speculated that bioavailability would only be achieved following hydrolysis to their aglycones by enzymes from the gut wall or microflora. However, the demonstration of some flavonoids and their metabolites reaching plasma concentrations of about 10 μmol/L have confirmed their bioavailability, although the fraction absorbed usually ranges from 1% to 10%, depending upon the compound studied.[8] The extent and pattern of flavonoid bioavailability is affected by the presence of lipids, emulsifiers, and other food matrix parameters, as well as the number and position of glycosyl groups. For example, quercetin-4′-glucoside from fried onions is absorbed in the small intestine and reaches peak concentrations in plasma after about 45 minutes, while quercetin-3-β-O-rhamnosylglucoside (rutin) from buckwheat tea is absorbed in the colon after deglycosylation, and peak plasma concentrations are reached after about 4 hours.

Studies in rats and ileostomy patients reveal that quercetin glucosides may be absorbed intact through the small intestine, possibly via the $Na^+$-dependent D-glucose transporter-1 (SGLT-1), into plasma.[9] However, experiments in human intestinal Caco-2 cells indicate that the apical transporter multi-drug resistance-associated protein-2 (MRP-2) may counter absorption carrying flavonoid glucosides back into the intestinal lumen.[10] While quercetin noncompetitively and reversibly inhibits the sodium-dependent vitamin-C transporter 1 (SVCT-1), studies have shown that it is not transported by this system.[11] Importantly, flavonoid glucosides are generally hydrolyzed by lactase phlorizin hydrolase on the enterocyte brush border and/or by cytosolic β-glucosidase in gastrointestinal tissues during absorption.[12] However, anthocyanins also appear to be absorbed intact and have been detected in blood and tissue, both as the parent molecule and as glucuronide and methyl-glucuronide derivatives.[13] Little data are available regarding potential changes in bioavailability following long-term consumption.

## Metabolism

During and after absorption, flavonoid aglycones undergo extensive conjugation by phase II enzymes, producing methoxylated, glucuronidated, and sulfated compounds. Though deconjugation may occur in some tissues, the extent of this biotransformation suggests that flavonoid bioactivity may be due largely to metabolites rather than to the free form or the parent glucoside. However, due to the analytical difficulty of determining each metabolite, flavonoid status is generally expressed as aglycone equivalents following treatment of plasma and tissue with β-glucoronidase and sulfatase. For example, throughout its 11- to 28-hour half-life, over 95% of quercetin in plasma circulates as methyl, sulfate, or glucuronic acid conjugates, with little of the total (1–5 μmol/L aglycone equivalents in clinical trials) found in free or glucoside forms.[14] Interventions with flavanols generally achieve a markedly lower plasma status (0.1–0.2 μmol/L) than flavonols and are characterized by a shorter half-life of 2 to 3 hours. Interestingly, flavanols such as (–)-epicatechin are found exclusively as conjugates in plasma, while epigallocatechin gallate remains primarily in its unconjugated form. The half-life of isoflavones is typically intermediate between flavonols and flavanols, although their plasma concentrations, principally as glucuronides or sulfates, are comparable to that of flavonols.[15] Following the consumption of cocoa or grape seeds, plasma procyanidin concentrations are less than 50 nmol/L, suggesting that their bioactivity results from unknown metabolites or monomeric flavanols.

Flavonoids are excreted principally via bile and urine. Flavanols and isoflavones can undergo extensive enterohepatic cycling, with a significant portion of these compounds being excreted in the bile. The range of flavonoid elimination via urine is substantial and dependent upon the compound, its food source, bioavailability, and dose.[16] For example, the mean urinary excretion of naringenin following consumption from grapefruit juice was found to be 30.2%, in contrast to 1.1% from orange juice, despite similar ratios between dose and maximal plasma concentrations.[17] In addition to marked inter-individual differences in urinary excretion, this variability suggests that urinary flavonoids are not a good biomarker of dietary intake.

Intestinal biotransformation of flavonoids by microflora, principally in the colon, includes dehydroxylation, reduction, C-ring cleavage, and demethylation, and appears to play an important role in their metabolism and conversion to bioactive compounds. After microbial enzyme-catalyzed deconjugation, flavonoids may be absorbed or further metabolized to simpler phenolic compounds such as homovanillic acid. In vitro incubation of flavonoids with human colonic microflora results in the production of hydroxylated derivatives of phenylacetic, phenylpropionic, and phenylvaleric acids. Gut microflora are responsible for the metabolism of quercetin to catechuic acid by oxidases and of daidzein to equol by specific bacterial hydrolases. Studies of isoflavone metabolism suggest that about 30% of women can metabolize daidzein to equol, and that these "equol producers" are the ones showing the benefits from isoflavones on measures of bone mineral density.[18] The differences in absorption, distribution, metabolism, and elimination between individual flavonoids vary substantially and can confound simple correlations between flavonoid intake, status, and bioactivity or health outcomes.[19]

## Antioxidant Activity

In 1936, Szent-Gyorgyi and his colleagues first identified the ability of a lemon juice extract to decrease capillary wall permeability and called the active ingredient "vitamin P" (later identified as hesperidin and eriodictiol glycoside). Though flavonoids were later found to be nonessential and, thus, not candidates as vitamins, this early work did note a synergy between flavonoids and vitamin C and suggested their activity as antioxidants. In vitro, flavonoid aglycones are potent antioxidants due to their degree of hydroxylation and the presence of a B-ring catechol group. However, the B-ring catechol can be metabolized in vivo, principally by *O*-glucuronidation and the formation of sulfate esters.[20] Little information is available on the antioxidant capacity of flavonoid conjugates in vitro, although these metabolites predominate in vivo and have different properties than their parent compounds. The non-catechol hydroxyl groups on flavonoids can chelate transition minerals such as copper and iron to inhibit Fenton-Weiss-Haber reactions and the generation of reactive oxygen species. Some dietary flavonoids may be sufficiently effective chelators of non-heme iron in the gut to aggravate or precipitate iron-deficiency anemia.[21] However, flavonoids may provide a benefit to people with high iron status because plasma ferritin has been proposed as a risk factor for cardiovascular disease and colon cancer.

While interventions with some flavonoid-rich foods have revealed an increase in plasma measures of "total antioxidant capacity" (e.g., by using the ferric reducing antioxidant power and oxygen radical absorbance activity assays) and a reduction in biomarkers of oxidative stress (e.g., phospholipid peroxides, malondialdehyde, and $F_{2\alpha}$-isoprostanes in plasma and 8-OH-deoxyguanosine in leukocytes), other studies have not found a significant antioxidant action of these compounds in vivo.[22-24] Such contrasting reports may reflect differences in the specific flavonoids being tested, as well as differences in the health or oxidative stress status of the subjects and the dose and duration of treatment. Nonetheless, the direct stoichiometric contribution of intracellular flavonoids to quenching reactive species in vivo appears small relative to the higher concentration of other dietary antioxidants. For example, supplementation with 50 mg of epigallocatechin gallate results in peak plasma concentrations of about 0.15 μmol/L, while the usual status of ascorbate is 3 to 7 mmol/L. However, a marked synergy between flavonoids and other components of the antioxidant defense network, including vitamins C and E via mutual recycling, sparing, or other mechanisms, may result in a significant impact on the quenching of reactive oxygen and nitrogen species.[25] Flavonoids may act indirectly to substantially increase antioxidant defenses and redox status by inducing phase II enzymes, including those regulating glutathione synthetase, peroxidase, and S-transferase.[26] For example, using transgenic mice, berry fruit flavonoids have been found to increase the activity of the heavy subunit promoter (GCSh) of γ-glutamylcysteine synthetase, the rate-limiting step in the synthesis of glutathione.[27]

Flavonoids may act as pro-oxidants by reducing $Fe^{+3}$

to $Fe^{+2}$ to yield hydroxyl radicals, although no such effects have been demonstrated in vivo. While flavonoid catechols can be oxidized to quinones, which may generate reactive species through redox cycling, enzymes such as quinone reductase and catechol-O-methyltransferase would limit their formation in tissue.

## Influence on Enzyme Activity and Cell Signaling

In addition to their action as antioxidants, a key factor in the bioactivity of flavonoids may be their ability to modulate enzyme activity and affect cell signaling events.[28] Flavonoids have been shown to interact with all the major enzyme classes, including hydrolases, isomerases, ligases, lyases, oxidoreductases, and transferases, although the majority of these investigations have been conducted in vitro.[29] Flavonoids can selectively inhibit a number of kinases by binding directly to the enzymes or to associated membrane receptors and thereby influencing signal transduction pathways.[30]

Flavonoids may induce phase II detoxification enzymes such as glutathione S-transferase, UDP-glucuronosyltransferase, NAD(P)H:quinone oxidoreductase 1, and epoxide hydrolase.[31] The promoter regions of the genes for these enzymes are transcriptionally regulated by several xenobiotic response elements, including the antioxidant and electrophile response elements (ARE and EpRE, respectively).[32] Upstream regulation of ARE and EpRE is partly coordinated through binding of the transcription factor Nrf2. Translocation of Nrf2 from cytosol to nucleus is inhibited by the cytoskeleton-associated protein Keap1. Binding of Nrf2 is critically dependent on thiols in Keap1 and, thus, under feedback control of ARE- and EpRE-regulated enzyme systems. Flavonoid oxidation products such as quinones and quinone methides that are not recycled by ascorbate or other antioxidants may arylate protein thiols and thereby affect the expression of these enzymes.

In addition to their potential for quenching reactive oxygen species, flavonoids can affect cellular redox status via other mechanism. For example, flavonoids with a B-ring catechol moiety can inhibit succinoxidase and promote a mitochondrial respiratory burst of hydrogen peroxide and superoxide anion. Flavonoids with a 2,3 double bond/3-OH, in conjugation with the 4-oxo function on the C-ring, can reduce mitochondrial membrane fluidity and cause uncoupling or, especially in compounds with a B-ring *o*-di-OH, inhibit the respiratory chain.[33] Other flavonoids may induce mitochondrial permeability transition and release of $Ca^{2+}$.

Isoflavones appear to influence several facets of estrogen activity by inhibiting its synthesis via 17β-steroid oxidoreductase and transactivating estrogen receptors α and β to modulate signal transduction pathways, including phosphatidylinositol-3-kinase, mitogen-activated protein kinase, and other tyrosine kinase cascades.[34] Genistein has also been reported to affect phosphoinositide turnover via its action on topoisomerase II activity and transforming growth factor β signaling.

## Anti-Inflammatory Actions

The effect of flavonoids on tyrosine and serine-threonine protein kinases and other elements of signal transduction pathways suggest a potentially beneficial anti-inflammatory action.[29] In vitro, flavanols and procyanidins modulate the transcription of interleukins in activated peripheral blood mononuclear cells and inhibit mitogen-induced proliferation of T-cells and polyclonal Ig production by B-cells.[35] Kaempferol is a potent inhibitor of lipopolysaccharide-stimulated prostaglandin $E_2$, a key inflammatory eicosanoid, in human whole blood cultures.[36] Apigenin and luteolin can inhibit the expression of cellular adhesion molecules for leukocytes via antagonizing the activation of nuclear factor κB,[37] while quercetin has a similar effect via modulation of the c-Jun $NH_2$-terminal kinase pathway and activator protein-1 activation.[38] Flavonoids and other polyphenols from red wine inhibit platelet-derived growth factor-induced vascular smooth muscle cell migration through the inhibition of signaling cascades involving phosphatidylinositol-3 kinase and p38 mitogen-activated protein kinase, actions that may also affect inflammatory responses.[39] Like other flavonoids, the isoflavones also inhibit tyrosine kinases, though an untoward immunosuppressive effect of phytoestrogens has been suggested to increase the risk of autoimmune diseases, particularly in infants fed soy-based formulas.[40]

## Flavonoids and Chronic Disease

Research with cell cultures and animal models suggests that flavonoids may play a role in promoting human health and reducing the risk of some chronic diseases. Flavonoids have been proposed to have a beneficial affect on cardiovascular disease, cancer, neurodegenerative diseases, diabetes, and osteoporosis, as well as having anti-bacterial, anti-cariogenic, anti-inflammatory, diuretic, and immunostimulatory actions. Some acute and short-term clinical interventions have indicated that flavonoids can affect putative intermediary biomarkers of chronic diseases, and observational studies have associated the intake of flavonoids and flavonoid-rich foods with specific conditions. While observational studies of the relationship between flavonoids and health represent an important research approach, they are limited due in part to incomplete nutrient databases and the absence of biomarkers reflecting long-term exposure. Randomized, controlled trials with flavonoids examining chronic disease outcomes have not yet been undertaken.

### *Cardiovascular Disease*

The oxidative modification of low-density lipoprotein (LDL) appears as an early event in the pathogenesis of atherosclerosis. While most flavonoids can potently increase the resistance of LDL to oxidation in vitro, ex vivo investigations in human studies provide only equivocal evidence, perhaps because the polar flavonoid conjugates in plasma are removed or degraded during the isolation of LDL. However, flavonoids may have other actions relevant to slowing the formation of atheromatous lesions, such as the inhibition of smooth muscle cell proliferation by flavanols and the reduction of blood lipids by flavanones.[41] Flavonoid-rich cocoa, grape juice, and red wine have been shown to exert anti-thrombotic effects via inhibition of platelet aggregation or changes in bleeding time,[42] although no such effect has been found with citrus juices, onion, or tea.[43] Also, flavonoids in black tea, cocoa, red wine, and soy have been found to promote endothelial-dependent vasodilation and improve vascular dysfunction via actions on nitric oxide production or oxidation[44] (Table 2A).

Several prospective, observational studies have revealed an inverse relationship between flavonoid intake and cardiovascular disease.[45] For example, in the Zutphen Elderly Study, examining approximately 800 men followed for 10 years for coronary artery disease (CAD), high flavanol intake (124.0 vs. 25.3 mg/d) was associated with a relative risk (RR) of 0.49, with a 95% confidence interval (CI) of 0.27, 0.88, and high flavonol and flavone intake (41.6 vs. 12.0 mg/d) with a RR of 0.47 (95% CI = 0.27,0.82) (46). Similarly, the Iowa Women's Health Study, a cohort of 34,492 postmenopausal subjects also followed for 10 years, found that flavonol and flavone intake (28.6 vs. 4.0 mg/d) reduced CAD risk (RR = 0.62; 95% CI = 0.44, 0.87).[47] In contrast, the 6-year Health Professionals Follow-up Study of 38,036 American men found no significant effect of flavonol and flavone intake (40.0 vs. 7.1 mg/d) on CAD (RR = 0.77; 95% CI = 0.45, 1.35), although a reduction in coronary mortality rates was observed in those with a history of CAD.[48] Fewer reports on flavonoids and stroke are available, although 28-year follow-up data from the Finnish Mobile Clinic Health Examination Survey of 9131 people showed higher intakes of flavonols, flavones, and flavanones (>26.9 vs. <4.3 mg/d in men and >39.5 vs. <8.5 mg/d in women) associated with a reduction in risk for incident stroke (RR = 0.79; 95% CI = 0.64, 0.98).[49]

**Table 2.** Putative Anti-Atherosclerosis and Anti-Cancer Mechanisms of Flavonoids

| Anti-Atherosclerosis | |
|---|---|
| **Observed Effects** | **Potential Mechanisms** |
| ↓ Platelet aggregation | ↓ Cyclooxygenase, ↓ thromboxane |
| ↓ Plaque formation | ↓ LDL oxidation, ↓ PDGF |
| ↓ Anti-inflammation | ↓ Prostaglandin $E_2$ |
| ↓ Cellular adhesion molecules | ↓ NF-κB, ↓ c-Jun $NH_2$-terminal kinase, ↓ AP-1 |
| ↑ Vascular responsiveness | ↑ NO bioavailability |
| ↓ Plasma lipids | ↓ Hepatic cholesterol absorption, ↓ triglyceride assembly and secretion |
| **Anti-Cancer** | |
| **Observed effects** | **Potential Mechanisms** |
| ↓ Carcinogen formation | ↓ Activation enzymes, ↑ detoxification enzymes |
| ↓ DNA mutation | ↓ DNA oxidation |
| ↓ Cell proliferation | ↑ Apoptosis, ↓ AP-1, ↓ protein kinase C, ↑ G1 phase arrest |
| ↓ Metastasis | ↓ Cell migration, ↑ DNA repair |

## *Cancer*

The anticarcinogenic efficacy of flavonoids in reducing the number of chemically induced tumors and the growth of implanted cancer cell lines has been well-established in a number of rodent studies.[50] The mechanisms proposed for this chemopreventive action include modulating cytochrome P450 enzymes to prevent carcinogen activation and increasing the expression of phase II conjugating enzymes to facilitate carcinogen excretion.[51] In addition, some flavonoids reduce cell proliferation by inhibiting protein kinase C and activator protein-1-dependent transcriptional activity to block growth-related signal transduction.[52] Some flavonoids appear to limit the formation of initiated cells by stimulating DNA repair systems[53] (Table 2B).

The association between flavonoids and cancer risk has been examined in about a dozen prospective and case-control studies in Finland, the Netherlands, and the United States, with no consistent trend observed either for specific forms of cancer or total cancers.[45] However, it is worth noting that the 24-year follow-up data from the Finnish Mobile Clinic Health Examination Survey of 9959 people showed a reduction in risk for lung cancer (RR = 0.53; 95% CI = 0.29, 0.97) in those with high flavonol and flavone intakes (>4.8 vs. <2.1 mg/d for men and >5.5 vs. <2.4 mg/d for women).[49] Consistent with this finding, after 6.1 years of follow-up, the Alpha-Tocopherol, Beta-Carotene Cancer Prevention Study of 27,110 Finnish men also found a significant reduction in lung cancer risk (RR = 0.56; 95% CI = 0.45, 0.69) among those with the highest flavonol and flavone intake (16.3 vs. 4.2 mg/d).[55] The Iowa Women's Health Study observed a decline in rectal cancer (RR = 0.55; 95% CI = 0.32, 0.95) with flavanol intake (75.1 vs. 3.6 mg/d) among its cohort of 34,651 subjects, but no association with colon cancer.[55]

## *Other Chronic Diseases*

Some studies suggest a role for flavonoids in neurodegenerative diseases. In vitro, physiologically relevant concentrations of flavanols protect neuronal cells against the toxic effects of β-amyloid, 6-hydroxydopamine, and oxidized LDL (though not $H_2O_2$) by modulating cell proliferation and apoptosis via increasing protein kinase C activity or inhibiting nuclear factor κB translocation.[56] However, little is known about flavonoid concentrations in the brain, although they appear quite low compared with plasma levels due to the poor permeability of the blood-brain barrier to anionic conjugates.[57] Nonetheless, old rats fed aqueous extracts of blueberry, spinach, or strawberry showed a reduction in age-related declines of motor behavior, cognitive function, and neuronal signal transduction, suggesting that effective concentrations of flavonoids can reach the brain.[58] Similarly, in rats, dietary supplementation with grape polyphenols protected synaptic protein functions against injury from chronic ethanol consumption,[59] and epigallocatechin gallate restored dopaminergic activity following administration of a neurotoxin used to induce a Parkinsonian syndrome.[60] While the potential for unknown confounding is always present, a few observational studies have found inverse correlations between the intake of flavonols and flavones or wine consumption and the risk of age-related dementia.[61]

Traditional phytomedicines containing flavonoids have long been used in the treatment of diabetes, although research results indicating such a benefit are contradictory. In vitro studies in rat tissues show acylated anthocyanins inhibit intestinal α-glucosidase[62] and quercetin monoglucosides inhibit the SGLT1 transporter in everted gut sacs,[63] suggesting that flavonoids may inhibit glucose absorption. Flavonoids may also affect glucose uptake by tissues, because tea flavanols have been found to promote glucose absorption into rat adipocytes.[64] In contrast, quercetin inhibits glucose uptake in rat adipocytes[65] and non-competitively inhibits the glucose transporter GLUT2 in hamster ovary cells.[66] Genistein has been found to augment insulin release by pancreatic β-cells,[67] but inhibits glucose uptake in human erythrocytes by interacting directly with the glucose transporter GLUT1.[68] Epigallcatechin gallate has been shown to inhibit gluconeogenesis by increasing several insulin-activated kinases (albeit with slower kinetics than insulin) and regulate genes encoding gluconeogenic enzymes by modulating cellular redox status in rat H4IIE hepatoma cells,[69] but quercetin inhibits insulin receptor function in rat adipocytes.[65]

While these in vitro studies suggest flavonoid-specific effects on insulin activity, it is important to note that many employed supra-physiologic concentrations of these nutrients. Perhaps more compelling evidence for flavonoid efficacy comes from in vivo studies in both healthy and diabetic mice and in rats showing that anthocyanins and flavanols improve glucose tolerance.[70,71] However, the very limited data available from short-term human studies show no effect on glycemic profiles of a daily 50 mg supplement of a red-orange extract containing anthocyanins and flavanones in type 2 diabetics[72] or diosmin (1800 mg/d) plus hesperidin (200 mg/d) in type 1 diabetics, though the latter treatment did reduce glycated hemoglobin.[73] No relationship was found between the intake of flavonols, flavones, and/or flavanones and the risk for type 2 diabetes in the prospective Finnish Mobile Clinic Health Examination Survey.[49]

The similar structure of the isoflavones to estradiol and their relatively selective binding to the estrogen receptor β suggests a potential role in bone remodeling and the prevention of osteoporosis. In vitro, daidzein down-regulates osteoclast differentiation via caspase 3 and reduces resorption activity.[74] In vivo studies in rodent models indicate that dietary isoflavones given at 10 to 50 mg/kg body weight reduce ovariectomy-induced loss of bone mineral density and trabecular volume, although they did not reverse established osteopenia.[75,76] Interventions with soy-rich diets in postmenopausal women have been shown to increase increase osteoblastic activity, as indicated by increases in serum osteocalcin.[77,78] A few clinical trials with isoflavone supplementation at 37 to 62 mg/d demonstrate that such interventions can increase serum bone-specific alkaline phosphatase and bone γ-carboxyglutamate [AU: CORRECT FOR "Gla"?] protein and reduce urinary pyridinoline and deoxypyridinoline, biomarkers of bone resorption, and improve bone density.[79,80] Very limited evidence suggests that some flavanols and flavonols may also have a beneficial effect on bone health.

## Conclusion

Flavonoids can make a substantial contribution to nutrient intake, but nutrient databases remain incomplete in their characterization of these phytochemicals, so the accuracy of dietary assessment is still far from precise. Our knowledge of the biological actions of flavonoids is still in its infancy. In vitro studies have suggested several mechanisms of action of these compounds pertinent to health outcomes, but mostly have not been conducted with the flavonoid metabolites that are actually presented to cells in vivo. Many flavonoids are bioavailable, though with a low fractional absorption, and extensively metabolized both by gut microflora and body tissue, but our characterization of these processes is still being established and little is known about the subsequent distribution of these compounds. Observational studies of large cohorts have generated exciting hypotheses about the putative health benefits of flavonoid-rich foods, though by their nature are confounded both by the other ingredients in these foods and unknown interactions with other dietary and environmental factors. Recent research suggests new studies examine not only single foods or flavonoids, but the potential for antagonism or synergy when they are consumed as complex mixtures with other foods/nutrients. While many studies in humans have been published, most have been of short duration and conducted with small sample sizes, so caution is warranted when trying to extrapolate their findings to the promotion of health and the prevention of disease.

## Acknowledgements

We thank Brigitte A. Graf for her thoughtful suggestions. This work was supported by the US Department of Agriculture, Agricultural Research Service under Cooperative Agreement No. 58-1950-4-401

## References

1. Koes RE, Quattrocchio F, Joseph NM. The flavonoid biosynthetic pathway in plants: Function and evolution. Mol Biol Essays. 1994;16:123–132.
2. Smith DA, Banks SW. Biosynthesis, elicitation and biological activity of isoflavonoid phytoalexins. Phytochemistry. 1986;25:979–995.
3. Zaat SAJ, Wijffelman CA, Spaink HP, et al. Induction of the nodA promoter of Rhizobium leguminosarum symplasmid pRLIJI by plant flavanones and flavones. J Bacteriol. 1987;169:198–204.
4. Zhu QY, Zhang, AQ, Tsang D, et al. Stability of green tea catechins. J Agric Food Chem. 1997;45: 4624–4628.
5. Coward L, Smith M, Kirk M, Barnes S. Chemical modification of isoflavones in soyfoods during cooking and processing. Am J Clin Nutr. 1998;68: 1486S–1491S.
6. Harborne JB, Williams CA. Anthocyanins and other flavonoids. Natural Product Report. 2001;18: 310–333.
7. Price KR, Bacon JR, Rhodes MJC. Effect of storage and domestic processing on the content and composition of flavonol glucosides in onion (*Allium cepa*). J Agric Food Chem. 1997;45:938–942.
8. Williamson G, Manach C. Bioavailability and bioefficacy of polyphenols in humans. II. Review of 93 intervention studies. Am J Clin Nutr. 2005;81: 243S–255S.
9. Wolffram S, Block M, Ader P. Quercetin-3-glucoside is transported by the glucose carrier SGLT1 across the brush border membrane of rat small intestine. J Nutr. 2002; 132:630–635.
10. Walgren RA, Karnaky KJ Jr, Lindenmayer GE, Walle T. Efflux of dietary flavonoid quercetin 4′-beta-glucoside across human intestinal Caco-2 cell monolayers by apical multidrug resistanceassociated protein-2. J Pharmacol Exp Ther. 2000;294: 830–836.
11. Song J, Kwon O, Chen S, et al. Flavonoid inhibition of sodium-dependent vitamin C transporter 1 (SVCT1) and glucose transporter isoform 2 (GLUT2), intestinal transporters for vitamin C and glucose. J Biol Chem. 2001;277:15252–15260.
12. Day AJ, Gee JM, DuPont MS, et al. Absorption of quercetin-3-glucoside and quercetin-4′-glucoside in the rat small intestine: the role of lactase phlorizin hydrolase and the sodium-dependent glucose transporter. Biochem Pharmacol. 2003;65:1199–1206.
13. Kay CD, Mazza GJ, Holub BJ. Anthocyanins exist in the circulation primarily as metabolites in adult men. J Nutr. 2005;135:2582–2588.
14. Day AJ, Mellon FA, Barron D, et al. Human metabolism of dietary flavonoids: identification of plasma metabolites of quercetin. Free Radic Res. 2001;212: 941–952.
15. Setchell KD, Brown NM, Desai P, et al. Bioavailability of pure isoflavones in healthy humans and analysis of commercial soy isoflavone supplements. J Nutr. 2001;131:1362S–1375S.
16. Manach C, Williamson G, Morand C, Scalbert A, Rémés y C. Bioavailability and bioefficacy of polyphenols in humans. I. Review of 97 bioavailability studies. Am J Clin Nutr. 2005;81:230S–242S.
17. Erlund I, Meririnne E, Alfthan G, Aro A. Plasma kinetics and urinary excretion of the flavanones naringenin and hesperetin in humans after ingestion of orange juice and grapefruit juice. J Nutr. 2001;131: 235–241.
18. Setchell KD, Brown NM, Lydeking-Olsen E. The clinical importance of the metabolite equol: a clue to the effectiveness of soy and its isoflavones. J Nutr. 2002;132:3577–3584.
19. Manach C, Scalbert A, Morand C, et al. Polyphenols: food sources and bioavailability. Am J Clin Nutr. 2004;79:727–747.
20. Bors W, Michel C, Stettmaier K. Structure-activity relationships governing antioxidant capacities of plant polyphenols. Meth Enzymol. 2001;335: 166–180.
21. Zijp IM, Korver O, Tijburg LBM. Effect of tea and other dietary factors on iron absorption. Crit Rev Food Sci Nutr. 2000;40:371–398.
22. Widlansky ME, Duffy SJ, Hamburg NM, et al. Effects of black tea consumption on plasma catechins and markers of oxidative stress and inflammation in patients with coronary artery disease. Free Radic Biol Med. 2005;38:499–506.
23. Wiswedel I, Hirsch D, Kropf S, et al. Flavanol-rich cocoa drink lowers plasma F2-isoprostane concentrations in humans. Free Radic Biol Med. 2004;37: 411–421.
24. Lean ME, Noroozi M, Kelly I, et al. Dietary flavonols protect diabetic human lymphocytes against oxidative damage to DNA. Diabetes. 1999;48:176–181.
25. Chen C-Y, Milbury PE, Lapsley K, Blumberg JB. Flavonoids from almond skins are bioavailable and act synergistically with vitamins C and E to enhance hamster and human LDL resistance to oxidation. J Nutr. 2005;135:1366–1373.
26. Kong AN, Owuor E, Yu R, et al. Induction of xenobiotic enzymes by the MAP kinase pathway and the

antioxidant or electrophile response element (ARE/EpRE). Drug Metab Rev. 2001;33:255–271.

27. Carlsen H, Myhrstad MC, Thoresen M, et al. Berry intake increases the activity of the gamma-glutamylcysteine synthetase promoter in transgenic reporter mice. J Nutr. 2003;133:2137–2140.
28. Williams RJ, Spencer JPE, Rice-Evans C. Flavonoids: Antioxidants or signaling molecules? Free Radic Biol Med. 2004;36:838–849.
29. Middleton E Jr, Kandaswami C, Theoharides TC. The effects of plant flavonoids on mammalian cells: implications for inflammation, heart disease, and cancer. Pharmacol Rev. 2000;52:673–751.
30. Hollosy F, Keri G. Plant-derived protein tyrosine kinase inhibitors as anticancer agents. Curr Med Chem Anti-Canc Agents. 2004;4:173–197.
31. Zhang Y, Gordon GB. A strategy for cancer prevention: Stimulation of the Nrf2-ARE signaling pathway. Mol Cancer Ther. 2004;3:885–893.
32. Nguyen T, Sherratt PJ, Pickett CB. Regulatory mechanisms controlling gene expression mediated by the antioxidant response element. Annu Rev Pharmacol Toxicol. 2003;43:233–260.
33. Dorta DJ, Pigoso AA, Mingatto FE, et al. The interaction of flavonoids with mitochondria: effects on energetic processes. Chemico-Biol Interact. 2005; 152:67–78.
34. Polkowski K, Mazurek AP. Biological properties of genistein. A review of in vitro and in vivo data. Acta Pol Pharm. 2000;57:135–155.
35. Sanbongi C, Suzuki N, Sakane T. Polyphenols in chocolate, which have antioxidant activity, modulate immune functions in humans in vitro. Cell Immunol. 1997;177:129–136.
36. Miles EA, Zoubouli P, Calder PC. Differential anti-inflammatory effects of phenolic compounds from extra virgin olive oil identified in human whole blood cultures. Nutrition. 2005;21:389–394.
37. Choi J-S, Choi Y-J, Park SH, et al. Flavones mitigate tumor necrosis factor-α-induced adhesion molecule upregulation in cultured human endothelial cells: Role of nuclear factor-κB. J Nutr. 2004;134: 1013–1019.
38. Kobuchi H, Roy S, Sen CK, et al. Quercetin inhibits inducible ICAM-1 expression in human endothelial cells through the JNK pathway. Am J Physiol. 1999; 277:C403–C411.
39. Iijima K, Yoshizumi M, Hashimoto M, et al. Red wine polyphenols inhibit vascular smooth muscle cell migration through two distinct signaling pathway. Circulation. 2002;105:2404–2410.
40. Yellayi S, Naaz A, Szewczykowski MA, et al. The phytoestrogen genistein induces thymic and immune changes: A human health concern? Proc Natl Acad Sci U S A. 2002;99:7616–7621.
41. Maeda K, Kuzuya M, Cheng XW, et al. Green tea catechins inhibit the cultured smooth muscle cell invasion through the basement barrier. Atherosclerosis. 2003;166:23–30.
42. Rein D, Paglieroni TG, Wun T, et al. Cocoa inhibits platelet activation and function Am J Clin Nutr. 2000;72:30–35.
43. Keevil JG, Osman HE, Reed JD, Folts JD. Grape juice, but not orange juice or grapefruit juice, inhibits platelet aggregation. J Nutr. 2000;130:53–56.
44. Duffy SJ, Keaney JF, Jr, HHolbrook M, et al. Short- and long-term black tea consumption reverses endothelial dysfunction in patients with coronary artery disease. Circulation. 2001;104:151–156.
45. Arts ICW, Hollman PCH. Polyphenols and disease risk in epidemiologic studies. Am J Clin Nutr. 2005; 81:317S–325S.
46. Arts ICW, Hollman PCH, Feskens EJM, et al. Catechin intake might explain the inverse relation between tea consumption and ischemic heart disease: the Zutphen Elderly Study. Am J Clin Nutr. 2001; 74:227–232.
47. Yochum L, Kushi LH, Meyer K, Folsom AR. Dietary flavonoid intake and risk of cardiovascular disease in postmenopausal women. Am J Epidemiol. 1999;149:943–949.
48. Rimm EB, Katan MB, Ascherio A, et al. Relation between intake of flavonoids and risk for coronary heart disease in male health professionals. Ann Intern Med. 1996;125:384–389.
49. Knekt P, Kumpulainen J, Jarvinen R, et al. Flavonoid intake and risk of chronic diseases. Am J Clin Nutr. 2002;76:560–568.
50. Yang CS, Landau JM, Huang MT, Newmark HL. Inhibition of carcinogenesis by dietary polyphenolic compounds.1 Annu Rev Nutr. 2001;21:381–406.
51. Suschetet M, Siess MH, Le Bon AM, Canivenc-Lavier MC. Anticarcinogenic properties of some flavonoids. In: Vercauteren J, Cheze, Triaud J, eds. *Polyphenols.* Paris: INRA Editions; 1997; 165–204.
52. Barthelman M, Bair WB, Strickland KK, et al. (–)-Epigallocatechin-3-gallate inhibition of ultraviolet B-induced AP-1 activity. Carcinogensis. 1998;19: 2201–2204.
53. Webster RP, Gawde MD, Bhattacharya RK. Protective effect of rutin, a flavonol glycoside, on the carcinogen-induced DNA damage and repair enzymes in rats. Cancer Lett. 1996;109:185–191.
54. Hirvonen T, Virtamo J, Korhonen P, et al. Flavonol and flavone intake and the risk of cancer in male smokers (Finland). Cancer Causes Control. 2001;12: 789–796.
55. Arts IC, Jacobs DR Jr, Gross M, Harnack LJ, Folsom AR. Dietary catechins and cancer ncidence among postmenopausal women: the Iowa Women's Health Study (United States). Cancer Causes Control. 2002;13:373–382.
56. Levites Y, Amit T, Youdim MB, Mandel S. Involvement of protein kinase C activation and cell survival/

cell cycle genes in green tea polyphenol, (−)-epigallocatechin-3-gallate neuroprotective action. Attentuation of 6-hydroxydopamine (6-OHDA)-induced nuclear factor-kappaB (NF-kappaB) activation and cell death by tea extracts in neuronal cultures. J Biol Chem. 2002;63:21–29.

57. Mullen W, Graf BA, Caldwell ST, et al. Determination of flavonol metabolites in plasma and tissues of rats by HPLC-radiocounting and tandem mass spectrometry following oral ingestion of [2($^{14}$)C]quercetin-4′-glucoside. J Agric Food Chem. 2002;50: 6902–6909.
58. Joseph JA, Shukitt-Hale B, Denisova NA, et al. Reversals of age-related declines in neuroal singal transduction, cognitive, and motor behavioral deficits with blueberry, spinach, or strawberry dietary supplementation. J Neurosci. 1999;19:8114–8121.
59. Sun GY, Xia J, Draczynska-Lusiak B, et al. Grape polyphenols protect neurodegenerative changes induced by chronic ethanol administration. Neuroreport. 1999;10:93–96.
60. Levites Y, Weinreb O, Maor G, et al. Green tea polyphenol (−)-epigallocatechin-2-gallate prevents N-methyl-4-phenyl-1,2,3,6-tetrahydropyridine-induced dopaminergic neurodegeneration. J Neurochem. 2001;78:1073–1082.
61. Commenges D, Scotet V, Renaud S, et al. Intake of flavonoids and risk of dementia. Eur J Epidemiol. 2000;16:357–363.
62. Matsui T, Ueda T, Oki T, et al. Alpha-glucosidase inhibitory action of natural acylated anthocyanins. 2. alpha-Glucosidase inhibition by isolated aclated anthocyanins. J Agric Food Chem. 2001;49:1952–1956.
63. Gee JM, DuPont MS, Day AJ, et al. Intestinal transport of quercetin glycosides in rats involves both deglycosylation and interaction with the hexose transport pathway. J Nutr. 2000;130:2765–2771.
64. Anderson RA, Polansky MM. Tea enhances insulin activity. J Agric Food Chem. 2002;50:7182–7186.
65. Shisheva A, Shechter Y. Quercetin selectively inhibits insulin receptor function in vitro and the bioresponses of insulin and insulinomemetic agents in rat adipocytes. Biochemistry. 1992;31:8059–8063.
66. Song J, Kwon O, Chen S, et al. Flavonoid inhibition of sodium-dependent vitamin C transporter 1 (SVCT1) and glucose transporter 2 (GLUT2), intestinal transporters for vitamin C and glucose. J Biol Chem. 2002;277:15252–15260.
67. Ohno T, Kato N, Ishii C, et al. Genistein augments cyclic adenosine 3′5′-monophosphate (cAMP) accumulation and insulin release in MIN6 cells. Endocr Res. 1993;19:273–285.
68. Vera JC, Reyes AM, Carcamo JG, et al. Genistein is a natural inhibitor of hexose and dehydroascorbic acid transport through the glucose transporter, GLUT1. J Biol Chem. 1996;271:8719–8724.
69. Waltner-Law ME, Wang XL, Law BK, et al. Epigallocatechin gallate, a constituent of green tea, represses hepatic glucose production. J Biol Chem. 2002;277:34933–34940.
70. Matsui T, Ebuchi S, Kobayashi M, et al. Antiphyperglycemic effect of diacylated anothcyanin derived from Ipomoea batatas cultivar Ayamuraski can be achieved through the alpha-glucosidase inhibitory action. J Agric Food Chem. 2002;50:7244–7248.
71. Shenoy C. Hypoglycemic activity of bio-tea in mice. Indian J Exp Biol. 2000;38:278–279.
72. Bonina FP, Leotta C, Calia G, et al. Evaluation of oxidative stress in diabetic patients after supplementation with a standardized red orange extract. Diabetes Nutr Metab. 2002;15:14–19.
73. Manuel y Keenoy B, Vertommen J, De Leeuw I. The effect of flavonoid treatment on the glycation and antioxidant status in Type 1 diabetic patients. Diabetes Nutr Metab. 1999;12:256–263.
74. Rassi CM, Lieberherr M, Chaumaz G, et al. Down-regulation of osteoclast differentation by daidzein via caspase 3. J Bone Miner Res. 2002;17:630–638.
75. Nakajima D, Kim CS, Oh TW, et al. Suppressive effects of genistein dosage and resistance exercise on bone loss in ovariectomized rats. J Physiol Anthropol Appl Human Sci. 2001;20:285–291.
76. Picherit C, Bennetau-Pelissero C, Chanteranne B, et al. Soybean isoflavones dose-dependently reduce bone turnover but do not reverse established osteopenia in adult ovariectomized rats. J Nutr. 2001;131: 723–728.
77. Chiechi LM, Secreto G, D'Amore M, et al. Efficacy of a soy rich diet in preventing postmenopausal osteoporosis: The Menfis randomized trial. Maturitas. 2002;42:295–300.
78. Scheiber MD, Liu JH, Subbiah MT, et al. Dietary inclusion of whole soy foods results in significant reductions in clinical risk factors for osteoporosis and cardiovascular disease in normal postmenopausal women. Menopause. 2001;8:384–392.
79. Yamori Y, Moriguchi EH, Teramoto T, et al. Soybean isoflavones reduce postmenopausal bone resorption in female Japanese immigrants in Brazil: A ten week study. J Am Coll Nutr. 2002;21:560–563.
80. Morabito N, Crisafulli A, Vergara C, et al. Effects of genistein and hormone-replacement therapy on bone loss in early postmenopausal women: A randomized double-blind placebo-controlled study. J Bone Miner Res. 2002;17:1904–1912.

# VI Minerals and Trace Elements

# 29

# Calcium

Connie M. Weaver

## Introduction

Calcium is the most abundant mineral in the body. It forms a functional reserve during mineralization of bone, and is required by essentially all body processes. Thus, finely tuned homeostatic control mechanisms to maintain constant blood levels of calcium have evolved, as have complex cellular mechanisms to control movement of intracellular calcium. Inadequate dietary calcium is associated with an increased risk of a number of diseases.

## Distribution and Function in Body

### *Bone*

Of the 23 to 25 moles (920–1000 g) calcium in the adult female and the 30 moles (1200 g) calcium in the adult male, over 99% exists in the skeleton. This calcium exists mainly as hydroxyapatite: $Ca_{10}(PO_4)_6(OH)_2$. Therefore, bone is a large reserve of calcium ready to be drawn on in times of inadequate intakes. Calcium is unusual in that the storage form is also functional. Calcium status can be assessed by measuring bone mineral content (BMC) by bone densitometry, because it is present in a constant ratio (39% of total body BMC).

With the exception of the teeth, bone remodeling occurs throughout life. Bone resorption initiated by osteoclasts (bone-resorbing cells) results in microscopic pits on bone surfaces. This is necessary for modeling changes in bone size during growth, repairing microarchitectural damage, and maintaining serum calcium levels. Bone formation under the control of osteoblasts fills in the pits. Bone formation exceeds resorption during growth and often lags behind resorption later in life, resulting in age-related bone loss.

Skeleton growth across childhood is not uniform. Adolescence is a period of rapid skeletal growth. The window of opportunity to build bone ends for important skeletal sites by the end of adolescence. Approximately 90% of total body BMC in girls is achieved by age 16.9 ± 1.3 years, and 99% is achieved by age 26.2 ± 3.7 years.[1] Peak BMC accretion occurs 1.5 years later in boys than in girls[2]; however, the hip achieves its peak by the age of 16 to 18 years.[3] The onset of bone loss occurs in women at age 48 for the spine and at age 37 for the femoral neck.[4] Maximal loss occurs at ages 54 and 58 for the spine and hip, respectively. Rates of bone loss in women at least 5 years postmenopausal are comparable to elderly men. Better lifestyle choices influence rates of loss; for example, energy-adjusted calcium intake was associated with reduced hip bone loss in perimenopausal women.[5] A national survey showed that low milk intake in childhood was associated with lower bone mass and a doubling of hip fractures in postmenopausal women.[6]

### *Extracellular Fluid Calcium*

Calcium concentrations in blood and extracellular fluids are maintained under tight regulation at 2.5 mM/L. About half of the calcium plasma exists in the free ionized form and is functionally available. Most of the rest is bound to albumin, some to globulin, and less than 10% to phosphate, citrate, and other anions.

Extracellular calcium levels can be perceived by a surface $Ca^{2+}$ sensing receptor (CaR), a member of the superfamily of G-protein-coupled receptors in parathyroid, kidney, intestine, lung, brain, skin, bone marrow, osteoblasts, breast, and other cells.[7] The CaR permits $Ca^{2+}$ to act as an extracellular first messenger in the manner of calciotropic hormone. For example, parathyroid glands detect small changes in extracellular concentrations of $Ca^{2+}$, which regulates the release of parathyroid hormone (PTH) into the circulation. Similarly, CaR allows minute-to-minute regulation of renal tubular $Ca^{2+}$ reabsorption. The role of these actions in calcium homeostasis is described below. Extracellular calcium serves mainly as a source of $Ca^{2+}$ to the skeleton and cells, but essential functions in its own right including participating in blood clotting and intercellular adhesion.

### *Intracellular Calcium*

Intracellular calcium concentrations, at 100 nmol/M, are about 10,000-fold less than extracellular calcium concentrations. In response to a chemical, electrical, or physical stimulus interaction with a cell surface receptor, intracellular calcium concentrations rise from an influx of extracellular calcium or from internal calcium stores such as the endoplasmic or sarcoplasmic reticulum. The rise in intracellular calcium triggers a specific cellular response, usually through activating one or more kinases to phosphorylate one or more proteins. Thus, calcium acts as a second messenger to activate a wide range of physiological responses, including muscle contractions, hormone release, neurotransmitter release, vision, glycogen metabolism, cellular differentiation, proliferation, and motility. A number of enzymes are activated or stabilized by $Ca^{2+}$, a function unrelated to changes in intracellular calcium concentration. These include several proteases and dehydrogenases.

### *Calcium Homeostasis*

Blood calcium levels are almost invariant. Thus, serum calcium concentrations do not reflect nutritional status. The homeostatic regulation of serum calcium to ensure a constant supply to tissues is complex and incompletely understood. When calcium levels fall even slightly, levels are returned to normal by a PTH/vitamin D-controlled increase in calcium absorption, increase in renal tubular reabsorption, and bone resorption (Figure 1). Elevated levels of extracellular $Ca^{2+}$ inhibit secretion of PTH and production of calcitriol (1,25 dihydroxy vitamin D) and stimulate the secretion of calcitonin, a peptide hormone produced in the thyroid gland. This results in decreased calcium absorption, increased urinary calcium excretion, and decreased bone resorption. Extracellular $Ca^{2+}$ binds to CaR on the surface of parathyroid cells, which stimulates a conformational change in the receptor, leading to an inhibition of PTH secretion from the parathyroid.[8] CaR has also been located on the calcitonin-secreting c-cells of the thyroid gland, the calcitriol-producing cells of the renal proximal tubule, the intestine, and osteoblast cell lines,[7] suggesting that it plays a similar role in monitoring $Ca^{2+}$ levels at these sites to normalize serum calcium levels.

The intestine is the dominant site of adaptation to dietary calcium deficiency. Calcium absorption efficiency (fractional absorption) is influenced by calcium status. However, prolonged calcium deficiency is not completely corrected by an increase in absorption efficiency, so bone loss ensues to maintain serum calcium concentration. Calcium absorption occurs by two routes. The vitamin D-PTH-dependent transcellular route is subject to homeostatic regulation. Calcium absorption by this route is upregulated when calcitriol (increased when serum calcium levels fall, as shown in Figure 1) interacts with the vitamin D receptor in the enterocyte and stimulates the synthesis of calcium-binding proteins. Epithelial calcium channels (e.g., $TRPV_6$) mediate calcium entry into the cell, and calcium transporters (e.g., calbindin 9K) shuttle $Ca^{2+}$ across the intestinal epithelial cell.[9] Calcium absorption by the paracellular route (i.e., the passive diffusion that occurs between cells) is not under homeostatic control.

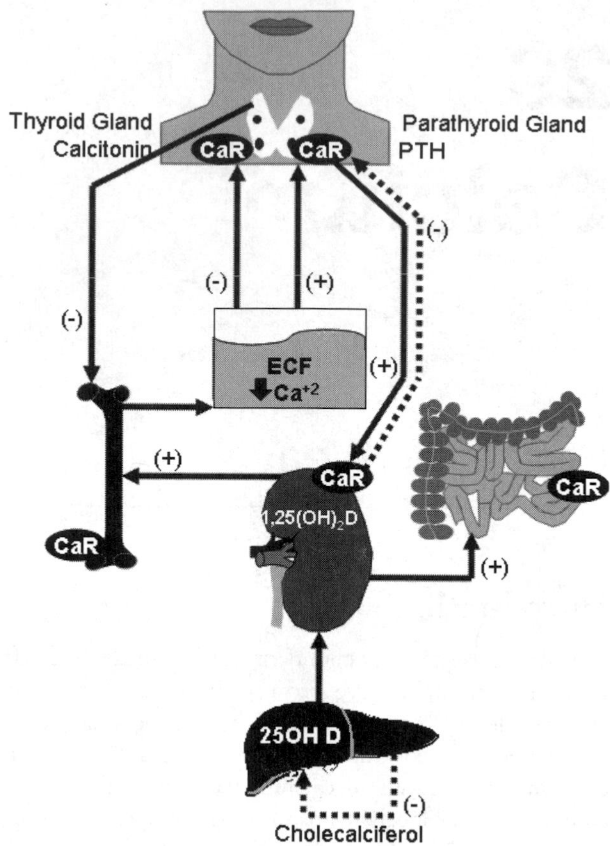


Figure 1. Homeostatic regulation of calcium. The + and − signs indicate the stimulatory and inhibitory responses to a fall in serum or extracellular fluid (ECF) $Ca^{2+}$ below 2.5 mM. The $Ca^{2+}$-sensing receptor, CaR, has been localized in each of the cells depicted, but its direct role in calcium homeostasis at the intestine has not been demonstrated.

Calcium absorption is also influenced by the calcium content of the meal. As the calcium load increases, absorption efficiency decreases,[10] although the net calcium absorbed increases (Figure 2). Practically, calcium absorption will be more efficient if consumed in divided doses throughout the day.

## Calcium Requirements

The 1997 Adequate Intakes (AIs) for calcium for North America are listed in Table 1. The requirements were determined, where possible, as the intakes that resulted in maximal calcium retention. Balance studies on a range of calcium intakes, randomized clinical trials of the effect of calcium supplementation on bone density and fracture incidence, and epidemiological and retro-

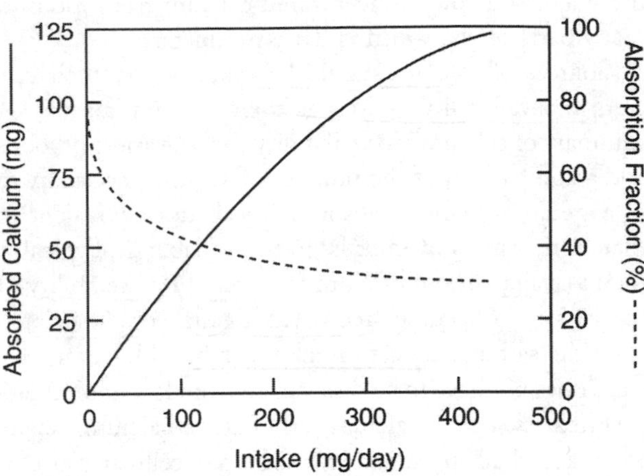


Figure 2. Theoretical relationship between calcium intake and net calcium absorbed (solid line) and absorption efficiency (dashed line). To convert grams to moles, multiply by 0.023.

spective studies were all considered. The 1997 requirements were the first time that intake for achieving maximal calcium retention was applied to data in the literature to determine requirements for people in North America. An upward trend in calcium requirements has occurred in Europe and North America in the last 15 years. The range in calcium recommendations around the world is large; for example, calcium requirements for adolescents

**Table 1.** Adequate Intakes (AI) for Calcium by Life-Stage Group for the United States and Canada

| Life-Stage Group | AI *mg/d* |
|---|---|
| 0–6 months | 210 |
| 6–12 months | 270 |
| 1–3 years | 500 |
| 4–8 years | 800 |
| 9–13 years | 1300 |
| 14–18 years | 1300 |
| 19–30 years | 1000 |
| 31–50 years | 1000 |
| 51–70 years | 1200 |
| >70 years | 1200 |
| Pregnant women | |
| ≤18 years | 1300 |
| 19–50 years | 1000 |
| Lactating women | |
| ≤ 18 years | 1300 |
| 19–50 years | 1000 |

Data from Food and Nutrition Board, Institute of Medicine, 1997.[11]

range between 500 and 1300 mg/d. In addition to assumed differences in peoples, differences in calcium requirements occur through aiming for preventing deficiencies as opposed to aiming for optimal health and preventing chronic disease, with different end points from maximal retention to replacing losses, and using different assumptions for absorption efficiency and losses. Many countries simply adopt the requirements determined by North America, the United Kingdom, or authoritative bodies such as the Food and Agriculture Organization of the United Nations (FAO) or the World Health Organization (WHO).

During growth, it is desirable to maximize calcium retention in order to maximize the acquisition of peak bone mass, although it is debated whether recommending an intake to achieve 100% of the maximum is practical. The relationship between calcium intakes and calcium retention is illustrated in Figure 3. Maximal calcium retention occurs at approximately the onset of menarche in women. After peak bone mass has been achieved, calcium intakes required to achieve maximal retention remained at 32.5 mmol/d (1300 mg/d), but net retention decreases with age postmenarche as absorption efficiency and renal tubular reabsorption efficiency decline.[12] In the years when bone density is generally at a plateau, calcium balance is expected to be zero. In later years, calcium intake should not be the limiting factor in minimizing age-related bone loss. Requirements after age 50 are higher because of declining calcium absorption with age.

Recommended calcium intakes for women were not increased for pregnancy and lactation in North America, in contrast to the increased requirement during lactation established by the United Kingdom.[13] Calcium supplementation does not prevent lactation-induced bone loss, but the bone is regained upon weaning.[14] Calcium absorption efficiency is enhanced during the third trimester of pregnancy, when fetal demand for calcium is greatest. Generally, fetal skeletons are protected at all but excep-

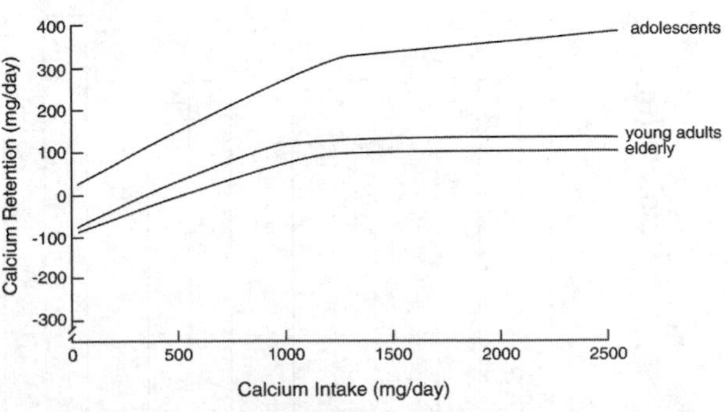


Figure 3. Predicted relationship between calcium intakes and retention illustrating higher intakes for maximal retention during rapid growth and again during later years, but decreasing ability to retain calcium with age. The figure is based on relationships determined from data in the literature.[11] To convert grams to moles, multiply by 0.023.

tionally low calcium intakes of mothers, and there is no association between pregnancy, lactation, and risk of fracture.[15] A longitudinal study showed some compromise of pelvic and spine bone mineral density (BMD) despite an increase in arm and leg BMD,[16] and low dairy intake was associated with decreased fetal femur length in pregnant African-American adolescents.[17] The additional allowance for lactation (17.5 mmol for non-lactating women vs. 30 mmol for lactating women) in the United Kingdom brings their requirements closer to and even higher than the recommendation for adult women in North America.

# Achieving Adequate Dietary Calcium

## *Calcium Intakes*

Calcium intakes of most populations, especially adolescent females, are generally below the calcium requirements established by each country. Generally, calcium intakes are highest in Scandinavian countries and lowest in Asian countries. The gap between recommended intakes and actual mean intakes in the United States is shown in Figure 4. The current trend of marketing so many calcium-fortified foods and supplements suggests that future estimates of calcium intakes should include these calcium sources. However, it is unlikely that many adolescents and elderly have corrected the daily shortfall of hundreds of milligrams of calcium depicted in Figure 4.

## *Calcium Sources*

Calcium intakes have declined because cultivated cereal grains have become the staple plants in the diets of most of the world's population, and the calcium content of grains and fruits are typically quite low. Consequently, the major source of concentrated calcium from foods in many parts of the world is dairy products.

Sources of calcium should be evaluated by their calcium bioavailability as well as their calcium content. A summary of calcium bioavailability from a variety of foods and a comparison of the number of servings necessary to provide an amount of absorbable calcium equivalent to that from a glass of milk is given in Table 2. Typically, the bioavailability of calcium is dictated by the ability of the cation to become free of its ligands or dissociated from the salt and then to remain soluble. However, calcium does not have to be dissociated from low-molecular-weight salts such as calcium carbonate or calcium oxalate to be absorbed, presumably by the paracellular route or by pinocytosis.[18] That low-molecular-weight calcium salts can be absorbed without the aid of a vitamin D-inducible calcium transporter, as is required in active calcium absorption, suggests possible treatments for individuals with impaired kidney function who cannot synthesize calcitriol. Solubility of calcium salts in water over the wide range of 0.1 to 10.0 mmol/L did not influence calcium absorption.[19] One study showed that the condition of achlorhydria does not reduce calcium absorption as long as the salt is consumed with food.[20] Not considered in that study[20] is the possibility that appreciable quantities of calcium carbonate were absorbed intact in patients with achlorhydria. Thus, either the pH of the intestinal milieu is an important factor in calcium bioavailability or the understanding of calcium absorption needs to be revised, because it appears that solubility of a calcium source may be less important than traditionally thought.

Calcium absorption can be inhibited by some ligands and enhanced by others. The strongest known inhibitor of calcium absorption, oxalate, forms a salt with calcium

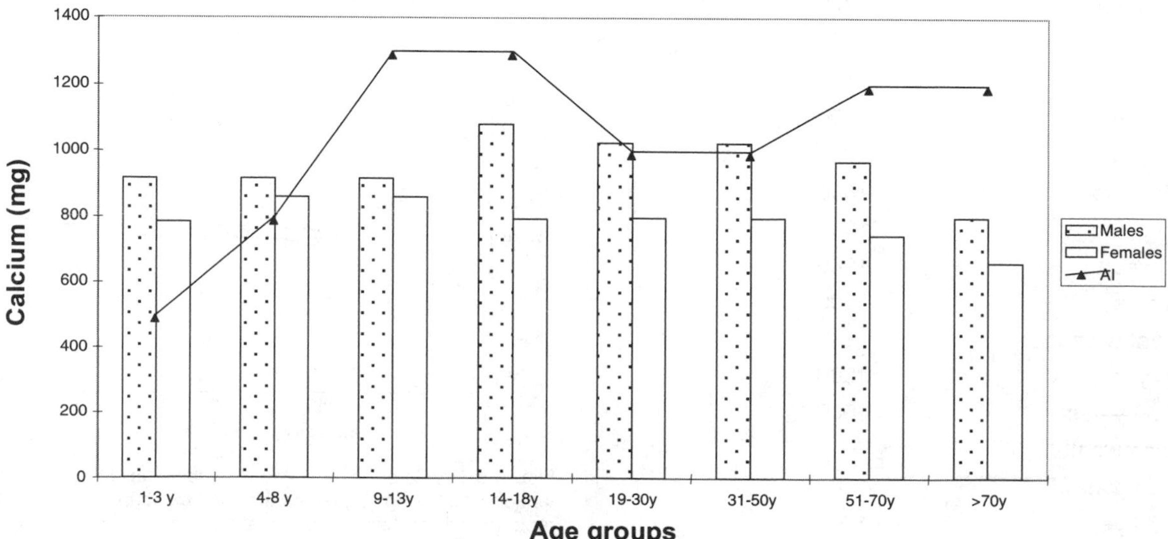


Figure 4. Adequate intakes for calcium with age (line) compared to mean intakes of calcium for men and women in the United States (bars). Mean intakes for calcium are from the NHANES 1999–2000 data.

**Table 2.** Comparing Food Sources for Absorbable Calcium

| Food | Serving Size g | Calcium Content mg | Fractional Absorption % | Estimated Absorbable Ca/serving mg | Servings needed to = 1 cup milk |
|---|---|---|---|---|---|
| Milk | 240 | 300 | 32.1 | 96.3 | 1.0 |
| Beans, pinto | 86 | 44.7 | 26.7 | 11.9 | 8.1 |
| Beans, red | 172 | 40.5 | 24.4 | 9.9 | 9.7 |
| Beans, white | 110 | 113 | 21.8 | 24.7 | 3.9 |
| Bok choy | 85 | 79 | 53.8 | 42.5 | 2.3 |
| Broccoli | 71 | 35 | 61.3 | 21.5 | 4.5 |
| Cheddar cheese | 42 | 303 | 32.1 | 97.2 | 1.0 |
| Chinese mustard greens | 85 | 212 | 40.2 | 85.3 | 1.1 |
| Juices, fortified with most calcium salts | 240 | 300 | 32.1 | 96.3 | 1.0 |
| Juices, fortified with calcium citrate malate | 240 | 300 | 52.0 | 15.6 | 0.62 |
| Kale | 85 | 61 | 49.3 | 30.1 | 3.2 |
| Soymilk, fortified with tricalcium phosphate | 240 | 300 | 23.7 | 71.1 | 1.35 |
| Spinach | 85 | 115 | 5.1 | 5.9 | 16.3 |
| Sweet potatoes | 164 | 44 | 22.2 | 9.8 | 9.8 |
| Rhubarb | 120 | 174 | 8.54 | 10.1 | 9.5 |
| Yogurt | 240 | 300 | 32.1 | 96.3 | 1.0 |

Adapted from Weaver et al., 1999[26] with permission from *The American Journal of Clinical Nutrition.* Copyright Am J Clin Nutr. American Society for Nutrition.

that has a solubility (0.04 mmol/L) considerably below the solubility range discussed above.[19] Other modest inhibitors to calcium absorption form salts that cannot be completely dissociated in the gut and are too large to be absorbed intact by the paracellular route. Phytic acid is such an inhibitor. A three-fold difference in phytic acid content in soybeans reduced calcium absorption by 25%.[21] Although phytate is a more modest inhibitor of calcium absorption than oxalate, it is consumed in higher amounts. However, in developed countries, phytate consumption is less detrimental where bread is leavened and phytate complexes are hydrolyzed by enzymes in yeast during fermentation.

Fiber was once thought to inhibit calcium absorption, but it is now considered to be more likely that the phytate associated with fibers in seeds is the inhibitor. Purified fibers have little effect on 5-hour calcium absorption.[22] Enhancers of calcium absorption are extremely soluble salts that either prevent precipitation of calcium by phosphates in the gut or alter the calcium absorption capacity of the intestinal epithelium. Calcium citrate malate, with a solubility of 80 mmol/L, is the best-studied example of a salt with superior calcium absorption.[19] Some casein and whey peptides prevent precipitation of calcium by phosphates.[23] Inulin and fructooligosaccharides have been shown to increase calcium absorption and improve accretion during growth and inhibit bone resorption later in life.[24,25] As a rule, calcium absorption determined on the same calcium intake or load is similar for most dairy foods, salts used to fortify foods, and supplements that provide the major contributors of calcium to the diet. Consequently, when assessing dietary calcium, it is appropriate to ensure adequate total intake without undue focus on bioavailability. However, if alternatives to dairy products are selected as the primary source of calcium, it is important to ensure that nutrients other than calcium provided by dairy products—including magnesium, vitamin D (fluid milk), riboflavin, and vitamin $B_{12}$—are also adequate.

## *Interactions of Calcium with Other Nutrients*

Some dietary constituents an important role in calcium retention. Urinary calcium excretion accounts for about 50% of the variability in calcium retention. Ironically, calcium intake has less influence than other dietary factors on urinary calcium output. Calcium intake explains only 6% of the variation in urinary calcium.[12] Dietary sodium is the key dietary factor influencing urinary calcium loss. Every additional 43 mmol (1 g) of sodium results in an additional loss of about 0.66 mmols (26.3 mg) of calcium in adults.[26] The effect of sodium on urinary calcium loss and net calcium retention is greater in white than in black children.[27] A longitudinal study in postmenopausal women illustrated the negative consequences of high salt intakes on bone density.[28] No bone loss occurred with calcium intakes as high as 44.2 mmol/d (1768 mg/d) or on urinary sodium excretion (reflecting dietary intakes) as low as 92 mmol/d (2115 mg/d). Dietary protein also increases urinary calcium loss, but does not decrease net calcium retention because of offsetting changes in endogenous secretion or calcium absorption.[29] In fact, bone loss and fractures in the elderly is reduced by higher protein intakes.[30]

## Calcium and Disease Prevention

Low calcium intake has been associated with a multitude of disorders. When the functional reserve (skeleton) is depleted chronically to maintain normal serum calcium levels, low bone mass ensues and can lead to osteoporosis. Low amounts of calcium reaching the lower bowel (unabsorbed calcium) can increase vulnerability to colon cancer and kidney stones. Failure to maintain extracellular calcium concentrations may increase risk of hypertension, pre-eclampsia, premenstrual syndrome, obesity, polycystic ovary syndrome, and hyperparathyroidism.

### *Osteoporosis*

Of the relationships between dietary calcium and disease prevention, osteoporosis is the most studied (see Chapter __). Connecting calcium intake to skeletal health is obvious, given that 99% of the body's calcium resides in the skeleton. Osteoporosis is characterized by reduced bone mass, which results in increased skeletal fragility and susceptibility to fractures.

Calcium is not the only nutrient important to bone health, but it is the one most likely to be deficient. Good nutrition is not the only requisite for good bone health. Also important are physical activity, especially weight-bearing exercise and not smoking. Hormonal sufficiency promotes bone maintenance, but estrogen therapy after menopause has also been associated with increased risk of breast cancer and stroke.[31] Adequate calcium intake can potentiate the advantage of physical activity[32] and estrogen[33] on bone. The primary strategies for reducing the risk of osteoporosis are to maximize development of peak bone mass during growth and to reduce bone loss later in life. Adequate calcium intakes are important for both of these aims. Maximizing peak bone density protects against fracture at any age. Children who avoid milk had a fracture rate 1.75 times higher than expected from their birth cohort.[34] Calcium intake has been associated with decreased fracture risk in postmenopausal women: a 4% decrease for each 300 mg increase in calcium intake in one meta-analysis,[35] and odds ratios of 0.77 (95% CI 0.54–1.09) for vertebral fractures and 0.86 (95% CI 0.43–172) for non-verbal fractures in another.[36]

The benefit of calcium on skeletal health has been reviewed previously.[37] In all but two of 52 randomized, controlled intervention trials, increasing calcium intake either increased calcium balance, increased bone gain during growth, reduced bone loss in later years, or reduced fracture incidence. Furthermore, in almost 75% of 86 observational studies, calcium intakes were positively related to bone health. Low fractional calcium absorption has been associated with increased risk of hip fracture.[38]

Calcium enhances skeletal strength both as the principal constituent of mineralization and by lowering bone turnover rate through reduction of serum PTH.[39] A meta-analysis of 15 trials reported calcium supplementation reduced bone loss by an average of 2.02% after 2 or more years compared with placebo.[36]

On cessation of calcium supplementation, the skeletal advantage gained during treatment in randomized, controlled trials disappears with follow-up in most trials,[40] unless the subjects were on low habitual calcium intakes when the trial began.[41] In children habitually consuming approximately 850 mg/d, skeletal advantages in the radius and total body BMD with calcium supplementation compared with the placebo group gained during puberty generally disappeared in spite of continued supplementation post puberty.[42] However, the ability for girls to exhibit "catch-up" skeletal growth was size dependent, as those who were taller at peak bone mass had reduced bone accretion at the forearm if on placebo compared with calcium treatment from the ages of 10 to 18 years. Furthermore, other skeletal sites such as the hip failed to exhibit complete catch-up growth.[43] At this time, the best recommendation is to maintain adequate calcium intakes throughout life to optimize the development of peak bone mass during growth and to minimize bone loss later in life.

A future area of investigation is the role of genetics in determining the responsiveness of calcium absorption and bone parameters to dietary calcium. Vitamin D polymorphisms have been associated with fractional calcium absorption in some studies.[44] Dietary calcium gene interactions have been reported. Further insights into genetics and nutrition are likely to help explain racial and sex differences in calcium absorption and identify individuals who can benefit by rigorous interventions.

### *Hypertension and Cardiovascular Disease*

The ability of calcium supplementation to control hypertension has been controversial. However, ensuring adequate calcium intake, particularly through dairy products, is a primary non-pharmacologic strategy for the reduction of high blood pressure recommended by the Joint Committee on Prevention, Detection, Evaluation, and Treatment of High Blood Pressure.[45] Meta-analyses of randomized, controlled calcium supplement trials show that blood pressure reduction is greater in persons with low habitual calcium intakes[46] and during pregnancy.[47]

More recently, increasing attention has been given to the influence of dietary patterns rather than on individual nutrients on disease prevention. The Dietary Approaches to Stop Hypertension (DASH) study showed an impressive and quick response of lowered blood pressure on a diet rich in fruits and vegetables and an even greater reduction if three servings of low-fat dairy foods were consumed daily.[48] Approximately 70% of subjects who would have required antihypertension drug therapy experienced normalization of blood pressure on the DASH diet. Calcium may influence blood pressure by reducing sympathetic nervous system activity or through its role in intracellular signaling.

A number of cardiovascular benefits have been associated with a calcium-rich diet, including effects on plasma lipids and insulin resistance.[49] Furthermore, in 85,764 women participating in the Nurses' Health Study, those who had calcium intakes in the lowest quintile had a significantly greater incidence of ischemic stroke than those in the highest quintile.[50]

### *Cancer*

Increasing calcium and dairy food intakes appears to reduce the risk of colon cancer, particularly that of the distal colon.[51] Calcium may lower fecal free bile acid and free fatty acid concentrations, thereby lowering cytotoxicity and/or through direct effects on the colorectal epithelium.[52] Holt[53] analyzed the trials to date on the ability of calcium supplementation to decrease cell proliferation, which have not yielded consistent results. He concluded that negative results were observed when the incidence of cell proliferation at baseline was low and when preparation of patients were not standardized across centers. In a randomized, controlled trial that provided 1.2 g/d of calcium, recurrent adenomas were decreased.[54]

Dietary calcium and vitamin D might also protect against breast and other cancers.[55] The relationship of dietary calcium or dairy consumption and risk of prostate cancer is controversial. The only randomized, controlled trial to address this showed a trend ($P = 0.09$) toward a decreased incidence, but the trial was too short to evaluate late-stage cancer.[56]

### *Kidney Stones*

Observational studies suggest that adequate dietary calcium decreases the incidence of kidney stones.[57] A controlled trial demonstrated that increased calcium intake reduced kidney stone incidence by half and was associated with a decreased urinary oxalate excretion.[58] In the gut, calcium combines with oxalate from dietary sources. The rather insoluble calcium oxalate salt is poorly absorbed,[18] and oxalic acid is less available for stone formation. However, when calcium supplements are not consumed with meals, they have no opportunity to bind with dietary oxalate and may increase urinary calcium levels, which are often already high in people who form stones, further aggravating stone formation.[59] People who form kidney stone are often characterized by a renal leak of calcium that reduces skeletal mass.[60] Lowering calcium intake in such individuals would not likely correct their kidney stone problem, but would undoubtedly further compromise their skeletal health.

### *Other Disorders*

Adequate calcium intake may be associated with protection against several other disorders. One multicenter trial showed that calcium supplementation at 30 mmol/d (1200 mg/d) of calcium for 3 months significantly reduced symptoms of premenstrual syndrome by 48% compared to 30% in the placebo group.[61] An observational study showed a protective effect of calcium and vitamin D against polycystic ovarian syndrome, a common cause of menstrual dysfunction and infertility.[62] Dietary calcium adjusted for energy may have a protective role in weight management.[63] All of these relationships may work through regulation of parathyroid hormone levels.

## Potential Problems of Excessive Calcium Intake

Tolerable Upper intakes Levels (ULs) for calcium were established by the Food and Nutrition Board of the US Institute of Medicine in 1997.[11] Little evidence exists suggesting that excessive calcium intakes pose harm in healthy individuals. A consensus view was that 2500 mg/d is safe for all population subcategories. This upper limit for calcium has also been adopted by the European Community, Japan, the Nordic countries, and Taiwan.

Hypercalcemia from excessive calcium intake is rare but has been associated with the ingestion of large quantities of supplements taken with absorbable alkali (milk alkali syndrome). Symptoms include lax muscle tone, constipation, large urine volumes, nausea, and ultimately, confusion, coma, and death.

Some concern about calcium supplementation and reduced absorption of trace elements has been raised, especially regarding iron. However, Minihane and Fairweather-Tate[64] showed that although calcium at 10 mmol (400 mg) can significantly reduce iron absorption in a single meal, chronic calcium supplementation at 30 mmol/d (1200 mg/d) does not decrease iron status. Presumably, iron absorption is up-regulated as stores decrease. The risks of excessive calcium intakes in healthy individuals are poorly defined. Individuals who consume liberal quantities of dairy products need not consume large quantities of calcium-fortified foods and supplements. With the advent of so many calcium-rich choices on the market, nutrition education will be necessary to avoid exceeding the UL of 62.5 mmol/d (2500 mg/d). However, at present, inadequate calcium intake is still the primary concern for optimizing calcium nutrition for most individuals.

## Future Directions

More is known about the relationship between calcium and bone health than for any other disorder, yet several questions remain. The 2004 Surgeon General's Report on Bone Health and Osteoporosis emphasized the role of good nutrition, and calcium and vitamin D in particular, for normal bone growth and osteoporosis prevention and treatment. Important areas for future research include strategies to maximize peak bone mass in boys and girls in ethnically diverse populations.

The prevention and reversibility of calcium and vitamin D deficiency in disease states also needs to be better understood. For each of the calcium nutrition-related disorders outlined above, additional research including randomized, controlled trials is needed to establish the importance of dietary calcium. We are gaining information on the relationship between calcium intake and cancer, but we need to better understand its importance in late-stage cancers. A new area of active research stemming from increased incidence of obesity is the consequence of bone loss accompanying weight loss. The Surgeon General's report identified finding mechanisms and interventions to preserve bone during weight loss as an important area of future research. Adequate dietary calcium has been shown to be a useful countermeasure.[65] Epidemiological studies would become more useful in identifying the relationship of calcium intake and disease once more accurate means for assessing calcium intake are developed. For each calcium-related disease and metabolic parameter, the interaction between diet and genetics will be a dominant area of investigation in the coming decades.

## References


1. Teegarden D, Proulx WR, Martin BR, et al. Peak bone mass in young women. J Bone Min Res. 1995; 10:711–715.
2. Bailey DA, McKay HA, Mirwald RL, Crocker PR, Faulkner RA. A six-year longitudinal study of the relationship of physical activity to bone mineral accrual in growing children: the university of Saskatchewan bone mineral accrual study. J Bone Miner Res. 1999;14:1672–1679.
3. Matkovic V, Jelic T, Wardlaw GM, et al. Timing of peak bone mass in Caucasian females and its implications for the prevention of osteoporosis. J Clin Invest. 1994;93:799–808.
4. Hui SL, Zhou L, Evans R, et al. Rates of growth and loss of bone mineral in the spine and femoral neck in white females. Osteoporosis. 1999;9: 200–205.
5. MacDonald HM. Nutritional associations with bone loss during the menopausal transition: Evidence of a beneficial effect of calcium, alcohol, and fruit and vegetable nutrients and of a detrimental effect of fatty acids. Am J Clin Nutr. 2004;79:155–165.
6. Kalkwarf HJ, Khoury JC, Lamphear BP. Milk intake during childhood and adolescence, adult bone density, and osteoporotic fractures in US women. Am J Clin Nutr. 2003;77:257–265.
7. Brown EM. Physiology and pathophysiology of the extracellular calcium-sensing receptor. Am J Med. 1999;106:238–253.
8. Pearce S. Extracellular "calcistat" in health and disease. Lancet. 1999;353:831.
9. Song Y, Peng X, Porta A, et al. Calcium transporter and epithelial calcium channel messenger ribonucleic acid are differentially regulated by 1,25 dihydroxyvitamin $D_3$ in the intestine and kidney of mice. Endocrinology. 2003;144:3885–3894.
10. Heaney RP, Weaver CM, Fitzimmons ML. Influence of calcium load on absorption fraction. J Bone Min Res. 1990;5:1135–1138.
11. Food and Nutrition Board, Institute of Medicine. Dietary Reference Intakes for Calcium, Phosphorus, Magnesium, Vitamin D, and Fluoride. Washington, DC: National Academies Press; 1997. Available online at: http://www.nap.edu/books/0309063507/html.
12. Jackman LA, Millane SS, Martin BR, Wood OB, McCabe GP, Peacock M, Weaver CM. Calcium retention in relation to calcium intake and post-menarcheal age in adolescent females. Am J Clin Nutr. 1997;66:327–333.
13. Department of Health Report on Health and Social Subjects 49 Nutrition and Bone Health: with particular reference to calcium and vitamin D. Report of the Subgroup on Bone Health, Working Group on the Nutritional Status of the Population of the Committee on Medical Aspects of Food and Nutrition Policy. London: The Stationery Office, 1998.
14. Kalkwarf HJ, Specker BL, Bianchi C, Ranz J, Ho M. The effect of calcium supplementation on bone density during lactation and after weaning. N Engl J Med. 1997;337:523–528.
15. Kalkwarf HJ, Specker BL. Bone mineral changes during pregnancy and lactation. Endocrine. 2002;17: 49–53.
16. Naylor KE, Igbal P, Fledelius C, et al. The effect of pregnancy on bone density and bone turnover. J Bone Min Res. 2000;15:129–137.
17. Chang SC, O'Brien KO, Nathansen MS, Caulfield LA, Mancini J, Witter FR. Fetal femur length is influenced by maternal dairy intake in pregnant African American adolescents. Am J Clin Nutr. 2003; 77:1248–1254.
18. Hanes DA, Weaver CM, Heaney RP, Wastney ME. Absorption of calcium oxalate does not require dissociation in rats. J Nutr. 1999;129:170–173.
19. Heaney RP, Recker RR, Weaver CM. Absorbability of calcium sources: The limited role of solubility. Calcif Tissue Int. 1990;46:300–304.

20. Recker RR. Calcium absorption and achlorhydria. N Engl J Med. 1985;313:70–73.
21. Heaney RP, Weaver CM, Fitzsimmons ML. Soybean phytate content: effect and calcium absorption. Am J Clin Nutr. 1991;53:745–747.
22. Heaney RP, Weaver CM. Effect of psyllium on absorption of co-ingested calcium. J Am Geriatr Soc. 1995;43:1–3.
23. Mykkanen HM, Wasserman RH. Enhanced absorption of calcium by casein phosphopeptides in rachitic and normal chicks. J Nutr. 1980;110:2141–2148.
24. Zafar TA, Weaver CM, Zhao Y, Martin BR, Wastney ME. Nondigestible oligosaccharides increase calcium absorption and suppress bone resorption in ovariectomized rats. Am J Clin Nutr. 2004;123: 399–402.
25. Abrams SA, Griffin IJ, Hawthorne KM, Liang L, Gunn SK, Darlington G, Ellis KJ. A combination of prebiotic short- and long-chain inulin-type fructans enhances calcium absorption and bone mineralization in young adolescents. Am J Clin Nutr. 2005;82: 471–476.
26. Weaver CM, Proulx WR., Heaney RP. Choices for achieving dietary calcium within a vegetarian diet. Am J Clin Nutr. 1999;70:543S–548S.
27. Wigertz K, Palacios C, Jackman LA, et al. Racial differences in calcium retention in response to dietary salt in adolescent girls. Am J Clin Nutr. 2005;81: 845–850.
28. Devine A, Criddle RA, Dick IM, Kerr DA, Price RL. A longitudinal study of the effect of sodium and calcium intakes on regional bone density in postmenopausal women. Am J Clin Nutr. 1995;62: 740–745.
29. Kerstetter JE, O'Brien KO, Caseria DM, et al. The impact of dietary protein on calcium absorption and kinetic measures of bone turnover in women. J Clin Endocrinol Metab. 2005;90:26–31.
30. Dawson-Hughes B. Interaction of dietary calcium and protein in bone health in humans. J Nutr. 2003; 133:852S–854S.
31. Writing Group for the Women's Health Initiative Investigators. Risks and benefits of estrogen plus progestin in healthy postmenopausal women. JAMA. 2002;288:321–333.
32. Specker BL. Evidence for an interaction between calcium intake and physical activity on changes in bone mineral density. J Bone Min Res. 1996;11: 1539–1544.
33. Nieves JW, Komar L, Cosman F, Lindsay R. Calcium potentiates the effect of estrogen and calcitonin on bone mass: review and analysis. Am J Clin Nutr. 1998;67:18–24
34. Goulding A, Rochell JEP, Black RE, et al. Children who avoid drinking cow's milk are at increased risk for prepubertal bone fractures. J Am Diet Assoc. 2004:104:250–253.
35. Cumming RG, Nevitt MC. Calcium for prevention of osteoporotic fractures in postmenopausal women. J Bone Miner Res. 1997;12:321–329.
36. Shea B, Wells G, Cranney A et al. Meta-analysis of therapies for postmenopausal osteoporosis. VII. Meta-analysis of calcium supplementation for the prevention of postmenopausal osteoporosis. Endocr Rev. 2002;23:552–559.
37. Heaney RP. Calcium, dairy products, and osteoporosis. J Am Coll Nutr. 2000;19:83S–99S.
38. Ensrud KE, Duong T, Cauley JA et al. Low fractional calcium absorption increases the risk for hip fracture in women with low calcium intake. Study of Osteoporosis Fracture Research Group. Ann Intern Med. 2000;132:345–353.
39. Heaney RP, Weaver CM. Newer perspective on calcium nutrition and bone quality. Am J Clin Nutr. 2006; In press.
40. Dawson-Hughes B, Harris SS, Krall EA, Dallal GE. Effect of withdrawl of calcium and vitamin D supplements on bone mass in elderly men and women. Am J Clin Nutr. 2000:72:745–750.
41. Dodink-Gad R, Rozen GS, Reunert G, Rennert HS, Ish-Shalom S. Sustained effect of short term calcium supplementation on bone mass in adolescent girls with low calcium intake. Am J Clin Nutr. 2005;81: 168–174.
42. Matkovic V, Goel PK, Badenhop-Stevens NE, et al. Calcium supplementation and bone mineral density in females from childhood to young adulthood: a randomized controlled trial. Am J Clin Nutr. 2005;81: 175–188.
43. Matkovic V, Landoll JD, Badenhop-Stevens NE, et al. Nutrition influences skeletal development from childhood to adulthood: A study of hip, spine, and forearm in adolescent females. J Nutr. 2004;134: 701S–705S.
44. Ames SK, Ellis KJ, Gunn SR, Copeland K, Abrams SA. Vitamin D receptor gene $F_{ok1}$ polymorphism predicts calcium absorption and bone mineral density in children. J Bone Min Res. 1999;14:740–746.
45. Chobanian AV, Bakris GL, Black HR et al. The Seventh Report of the Joint National Committee and Prevention, Detection, Evaluation, and Treatment of High Blood Pressure: the JNC 7 report. JAMA. 2003;289:2560–2571.
46. Bucher HC, Cook RJ, Guyatt GH, Lang JD, Cook DJ, Hatala R, Hunt DL. Effects of dietary calcium supplementation on blood pressure: a meta-analysis of randomized controlled trials. JAMA. 1996;275: 1016–1022.
47. Bucher HC, Guyatt GH, Cook RJ, et al. Effect of calcium supplementation on pregnancy-induced hypertension and preeclampsia: a meta-analysis of randomized clinical trials. JAMA. 1996;275: 1113–1117.
48. Appel LJ, Moore TJ, Obarzanek E, et al. A clinical

trial of the effects of dietary patterns of blood pressure. N Engl J Med. 1997;336:1117–1124.
49. Pereira MA, Jacobs DR, Van Horn L, Slattery ML, Kartashov AI, Ludwig DS. Dairy consumption, obesity, and the insulin resistance syndrome in young adults. JAMA. 2002;287:2081–2089.
50. Iso H, Stampfer MJ, Manson JE, et al. Prospective study of calcium, potassium, and magnesium intake and risk of stroke in women. Stroke. 1999;30: 1772–1779.
51. Wu K, Willett WC, Fuchs CS, Colditz GA, Giovanucchi EL. Calcium intake and risk of colon cancer in women and men. J Natl Cancer Inst. 2002;94: 437–446
52. Lamprecht SA, Lipkin M. Chemoprevention of colon cancer by calcium, vitamin D and folate: Molecular mechanisms. Nat Rev Cancer. 2003;3: 601–614.
53. Holt PR. Studies of calcium in food supplements in humans, cancer prevention. Ann N Y Acad Sci. 1999; 889:128–137
54. Baron JA, Beach M, Mandel JS, et al. A randomized trial of calcium supplementation to prevent colorectal adenomas. N Engl J Med. 1999;340:101–107.
55. Lipkin M, Newmark HL. Vitamin D, calcium and prevention of breast cancer: A review. Am J Coll Nutr. 1999;18:392S–397S.
56. Wallace K, Pearson LH, Beach ML, Mott LA, Baron JA. Calcium supplementation and prostate cancer risk: a randomized analysis (abstract 2479). Proc Am Assoc Cancer Res. 2001;260
57. Curhan GC, Willett WC, Rumm EB, et al. A protective study of dietary calcium and other nutrients and the risk of symptomatic kidney stones. N Engl J Med. 1993;328:833–838.
58. Borghi L, Schianchi T, Meschi T, et al. Comparison of two diets for the prevention of recurrent stones in idiopathic hypercalciuria. N Engl J Med. 2002;346: 77–84.
59. Curhan GC, Willett WC, Speizer FE, et al. Comparison of dietary calcium with supplemental calcium and other nutrients are factors affecting the risk of kidney stones in women. Ann Intern Med. 1997;126: 497–504.
60. Heller JH. The role of calcium in the prevention of kidney stones. J Am Coll Nutr. 1999;18:373S–378S.
61. Thys-Jacobs S, Starhey P, Bernstein D, Tian J. Calcium carbonate and premenstrual syndrome: Effects on premenstrual and menstrual symptoms. Am J Obstet Gynecol. 1998;179:444–452.
62. Thys-Jacobs S, Donovan D, Papadopoulos A, Sarrel P, Bilezikian JP. Vitamin D and calcium dysregulation in the polycystic ovarian syndrome. Steroids. 1999;64:430–435.
63. Zemel MB, Richards J, Mathis S, Milstead A, Gebhardt L, Silva E. Dairy augmentation of total and central fat loss in obese subjects. Int J Obes Relat Metab Disord. 2005;29:391–397.
64. Minihane AM, Fairweather-Tate M. Effect of calcium supplementation on daily nonheme-iron absorption and long-term iron status. Am J Clin Nutr. 1998;68:96–102.
65. Shapses SA, Heshka S, Heymsfield SB. Effect of calcium supplementation on weight and fat loss in women. J Clin Endocrinol Metab. 2004;89: 632–637.

# 30 Phosphorus

John J.B. Anderson, Philip J. Klemmer, Mary Lee Sell Watts, Sanford C. Garner, and Mona S. Calvo

## Introduction

Phosphorus, one of the most abundant elements on earth, exists in plant and animal foods and biological fluids as phosphate ions, the most common being $HPO_4^{2-}$. A maximum of about 850 g of elemental phosphorus is present in the adult human body at any point in time—85% in the skeleton, 14% in the soft tissues, and 1% in the extracellular fluids, intracellular structures, and cell membranes. From infancy to adulthood, the percent total body phosphorus content increases from 0.5% to 0.65%–1.1%.[1] The percentage in extracellular fluids is small, but this compartment is where dietary phosphorus, as phosphate ions, first enters and from which urinary inorganic phosphorus (Pi) is cleared. A balanced exchange of Pi occurs between the extracellular fluid compartment and bone: the bone fluid compartment. Pi transferred from the bone fluid compartment and from resorbed bone also enters this fraction.[1]

The body pool of Pi is maintained by intestinal absorption and parathyroid hormone-mediated renal excretion. Phosphate anions participate in numerous cellular reactions and physiological processes and are key components of essential molecules such as the phospholipids, adenosine triphosphate, and the nucleic acids DNA and RNA. Serum Pi and calcium ions are under the control of parathyroid hormone (PTH) and the active metabolite of vitamin D, 1,25-dihydroxyvitamin D, also known as $1,25(OH)_2D$ or calcitriol. Clearly, Pi ions are essential to life for both their cellular roles, such as the cell's energy cycle, and for their extracellular uses, such as for the mineralization of bones and teeth.

The critical interrelationships between the calcium and phosphate ions in body fluids are affected by the dietary intake of both minerals. Studies of whole-body phosphate metabolism have been limited by the lack of both a safe radioactive isotope and a stable isotope of phosphorus. The phosphorus content of the US food supply is growing, as more highly processed snack and convenience foods are consumed.[2,3] It is important to address, separately from calcium, the new findings that enhance our understanding of how serum Pi levels influence the endocrine and autocrine regulation that impact skeletal and renal tissues. Topics covered here include biochemical processes within the cells and mineralized tissues, physiological processes involving PTH and vitamin D, food sources, actual intakes, dietary phosphorus recommendations, and potential problems with high phosphorus intakes that may contribute to or exacerbate disease states.

## Biochemistry of Phosphate-Containing Molecules

Phosphorus has numerous roles in cells and in extracellular fluids. A few phosphate-containing molecules are reviewed in the context of their roles in cellular functions or in mineralization.

### *Cells*

Organic phosphates are so widely used in key roles in cellular biochemistry that life on earth could not exist without them. The membranes that surround all cells and separate the intracellular organelles from cytoplasm consist primarily of a bilayer of phospholipids. The genetic material of the cell, both DNA and RNA, contains phosphate groups linking the deoxyribose and ribose sugars along the backbone of the molecule. Phosphates are components of the intracellular structure, and also function in the metabolic reactions that occur within the cells. Several important molecules that contain phosphorus are illustrated in Figure 1.

Glucose, the ultimate energy source for most cellular activities, must be phosphorylated inside the cell before entering into the glycolytic pathway. The energy derived

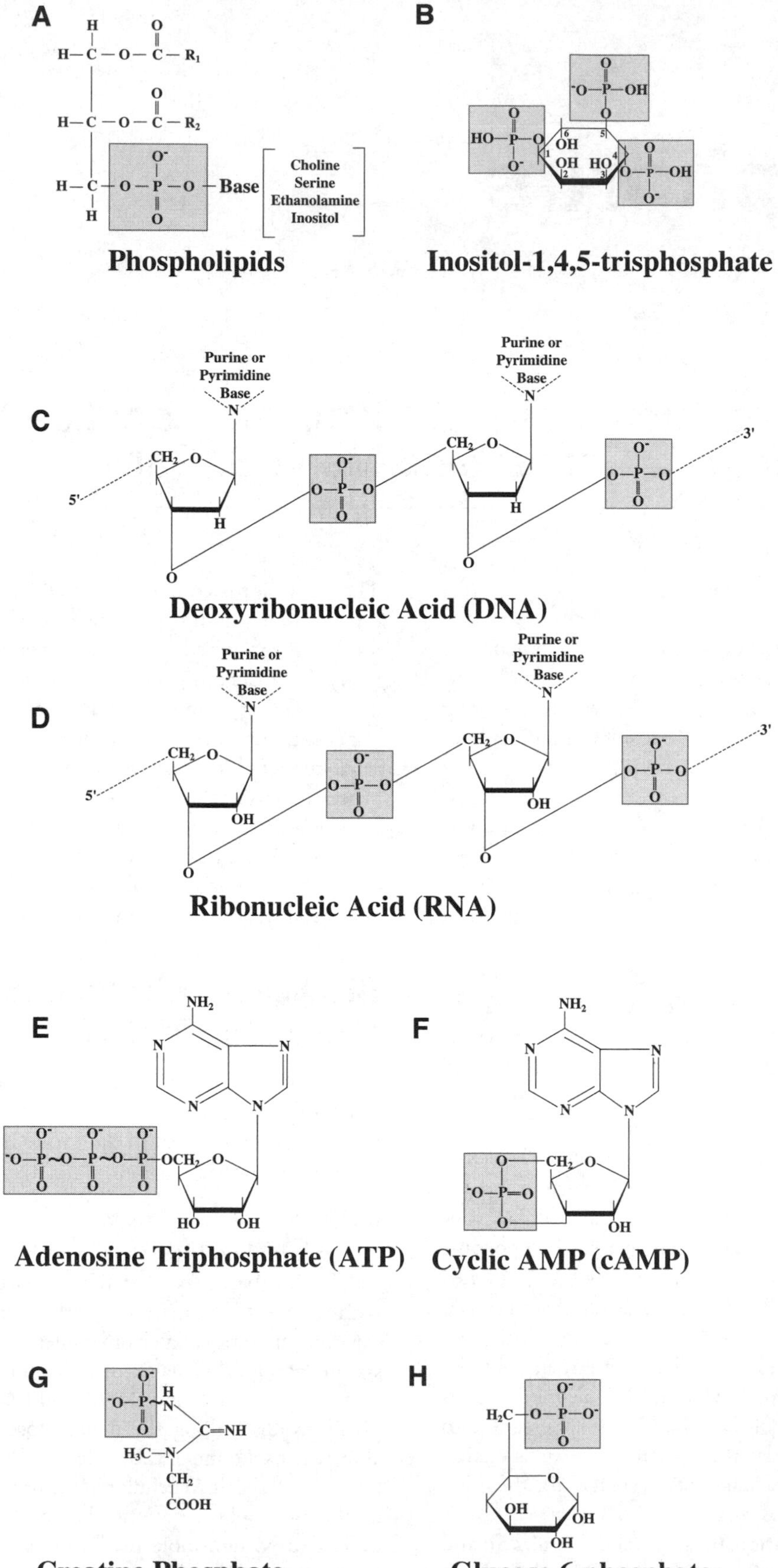

**A**

Base
Choline
Serine
Ethanolamine
Inositol

**Phospholipids**

**B**

**Inositol-1,4,5-trisphosphate**

**C**

Purine or Pyrimidine Base

5'

3'

**Deoxyribonucleic Acid (DNA)**

**D**

Purine or Pyrimidine Base

5'

3'

**Ribonucleic Acid (RNA)**

**E**

**Adenosine Triphosphate (ATP)**

**F**

**Cyclic AMP (cAMP)**

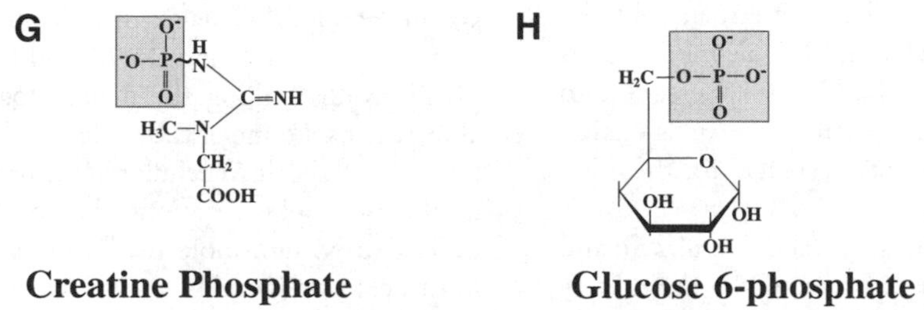


**Creatine Phosphate**

**Glucose 6-phosphate**

Figure 1. Chemical structures of important phosphorus (P)-containing molecules that represent various aspects of phosphate metabolism.

from both anaerobic and aerobic glycolysis is stored in the form of high-energy pyrophosphate bonds in adenosine triphosphate (ATP). In muscle cells, some energy storage also involves creatine phosphate. ATP can also be converted to cyclic adenosine monophosphate (cAMP) by the enzyme adenyl cyclase. Cyclic AMP (cAMP) is an intracellular second messenger through which many hormones signal changes in cellular activity. For example, glucagon, which acts in part to oppose the effects of insulin by increasing blood glucose levels, binds to cell-surface receptors on liver cells, and increases intracellular cAMP.

The cAMP-dependent protein kinase activates phosphorylase, the enzyme that degrades glycogen to release glucose molecules by adding phosphate groups to specific amino acids. Thus, both the cAMP molecule, which transmits the intracellular message, and the activated phosphorylase enzyme require phosphate derived from ATP. Another membrane-derived signal is inositol phosphate ($IP_3$), which is released from the structure enveloping the cell into the intracellular compartment, the cytoplasm. In the cytoplasm, inositol phosphate releases calcium from intracellular stores to activate calcium-calmodulin-dependent protein kinase.

### *Bone*

The mineral phase of skeletal tissues consists of hydroxyapatite crystals that contain a constant ratio of calcium-to-phosphate of approximately 2:1 and trace amounts of other minerals. Pi moves in and out of bone mineral by two processes: ionic exchange and active bone resorption. Bone tissue typically has a slow rate of turnover (remodeling) in adults, but its dynamic ion exchange permits the maintenance of Pi concentration as well as that of the ionic calcium in blood serum and extracellular fluids. During the growth periods of life, Pi turnover is generally higher than at other times. In growing skeletal tissue, the supply of Pi from dietary sources becomes potentially limiting, but because of the abundance of phosphorus in the diet, this risk is never as rate-limiting as for dietary calcium.

## Physiological Aspects of Phosphate Regulation

Human blood contains two fractions of phosphate: organic (70%) and inorganic (30%).[4] The phospholipid components of blood, especially those of lipoproteins, contain most of the organic phosphorus. The inorganic phosphates exist in three distinct forms, with three, two, or one negative charge. Although these forms are interconvertible, the predominant form is $HPO_4^{2-}$. This divalent anion is more soluble in blood than the others, and it constitutes almost 50% of the free Pi at a physiologic pH of 7.40, with 10% as monovalent anion and less than 0.01% as the trivalent anion ($PO_4^{3-}$).[4] The remaining 40% of the Pi, mainly $HPO_4^{2-}$, is complexed as sodium, calcium, and magnesium salts in blood. Within the blood compartment, Pi ions serve both as very effective buffers of blood pH and as regulators of whole-body acid-base balance by aiding in the renal excretion of hydrogen ions as they take on an additional proton (i.e., shift from $HPO_4^{2-}$ to $H_2PO_4^{-}$).[5] Phosphate ions contribute to approximately 50% of the daily urinary hydrogen ion excretion, or titratable acidity.

### *Overall Phosphate Balance*

The whole-body balance of phosphorus and calcium is maintained through the actions of the two major input and output components—the small intestine and the kidneys—whereas bone acts as the reservoir for exchangeable phosphate ions (Figure 2). Figure 2 shows a simplified schematic of phosphorus fluxes into and out of the plasma. In addition to the two major components and bone, the plasma Pi pool is in equilibrium with the soft tissue pools (not shown in diagram). Both Pi and calcium are in balance when the output (losses via urine, sweat, and fecal endogenous loss) is equal to the absorbed input (net intestinal absorption). At balance, net loss from the skeleton (resorption) also equals net gain in bone (accretion). An uncompensated change in any of the two input-output components or in exchange with bone mineral will result in an imbalance in these minerals, leading to either hypophosphatemia or hyperphosphatemia. In infants and children, phosphorus balance can be achieved despite differences in bone resorption or accretion, because substantial amounts of Pi exist in soft tissues,[6] as well as because of a higher serum Pi concentration resulting from an increase in renal tubular Pi reabsorption (transport maximum for Pi, or "TmPi").

Hypophosphatemia can also result from the redistribu-

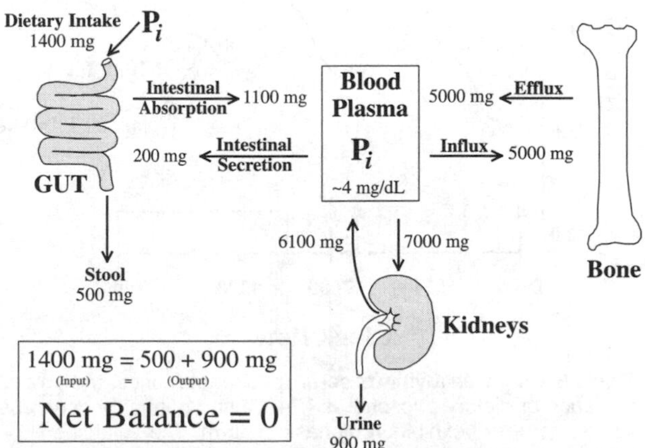


Figure 2. Phosphorus homeostasis and balance. The intestine, kidneys, and bone are organs involved in phosphate homeostasis. Fluxes of phosphate ions between blood and these organs are shown. Note the high fluxes in and out of bone each day. Pi, inorganic phosphate. To convert phosphorus values from mg to mmol, multiply by 32.29; from mg/dL to mmol/L, multiply by 0.3229. (Data from Lobaugh 1996.[4])

tion of Pi from extracellular fluids, especially blood, to intracellular stores, a process that occurs with exercise, changes in arterial blood acid-base status (i.e., alkalemia), or excessive glucose infusion. Serum Pi is therefore not a very good indicator of body stores, because concentrations may appear normal when some body stores are depleted[4] and serum Pi may be low when total body Pi is normal. Serum Pi values vary with age and are approximately two-fold higher in young children than in adults; consequently, two reference intervals (normal ranges) for serum phosphate values are used in clinical evaluations.[7] The reference interval for serum phosphate in adults is 2.5 to 4.5 mg/dL of Pi expressed as phosphorus (0.81–1.45 mmol/L) and for children is 4.0 to 7.0 mg/dL (1.29–2.26 mmol/L).[8] With increasing age, serum phosphate levels do not change in women, but they decrease in elderly men.[8,9] Serum Pi and PTH are reported to be significantly higher in women who are more than 10 years post menopause.[7,10]

Serum Pi follows pronounced, characteristic post-absorptive and circadian rhythms in old and young women (Figure 3),[11] with peak concentrations occurring in the late afternoon and in the evenings after meals. Dietary intake does not disrupt the overall biphasic diurnal rhythm, but a high phosphorus intake does accentuate peak height, as shown in Figure 3.[12] The integrated 24-hour serum Pi concentrations closely reflect the absorbed phosphorus that is derived from meals and correlate with tissue exposures, but most studies that only examine fasting serum Pi levels have not observed the dietary effect.[1] In contrast, serum calcium concentrations, both total and ionized, do not show the wide diurnal excursions seen for serum Pi levels.[11]

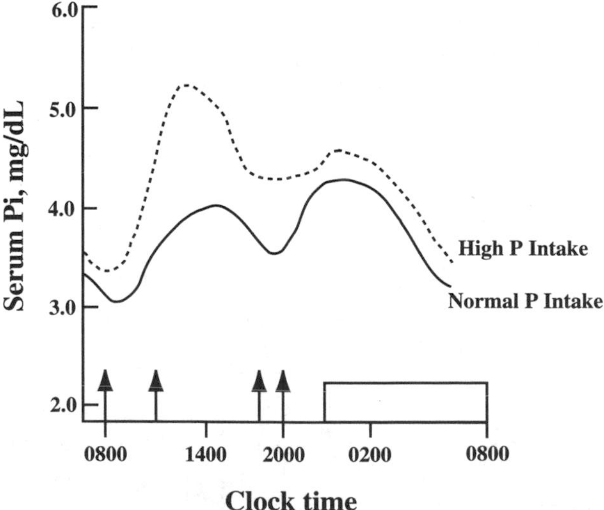


Figure 3. Circadian rhythm of serum phosphate concentration and influence of dietary phosphorus (Pi). During normal phosphorus intake, serum Pi exhibits a biphasic pattern. The solid line illustrates rises in serum Pi with peaks in the very early morning hours and afternoon. Meals and snacks are marked by arrows along the timeline, and a period of recumbent posture is marked by a rectangle on the timeline. After a high phosphorus intake, an exaggerated rise in serum Pi concentration occurs in the early phase (dashed line), but the basic diurnal rhythm is maintained. To convert phosphorus values from mg/dL to mmol/L multiply by 0.3229. (Data from Calvo et al., 1991[11] and Portale et al., 1989.[12])

The homeostatic system, which evolved to maintain blood calcium and Pi concentrations within their respective limits, is a classic endocrine feedback loop system primarily involving PTH and 1,25(OH)$_2$D. These two hormones modulate the processes of gastrointestinal absorption, renal tubular reabsorption, and accretion over a wide range of dietary calcium and phosphorus.[13] In addition to PTH and PTH-related peptide, other factors are now recognized as being involved in phosphate homeostasis.[14] PTH is the principle endocrine regulator of minute-to-minute extracellular fluid concentrations of calcium and Pi, whereas 1,25(OH)$_2$D facilitates long-term adaptation to calcium and phosphorus intakes. Other humoral factors, namely the phosphatonins, are now recognized as having important roles in the regulation of phosphate homeostasis, especially renal phosphaturia.[14] Inadequate or excessive phosphorus intake may perturb Pi homeostasis, especially if excretory and bone-buffering mechanisms are perturbed. For example, renal failure results in hyperphosphatemia because of decreased renal excretion of phosphate. In extreme cases, inadequate phosphorus intake may cause hypophosphatemia. The law of mass action governs the shifts in the two ions, Pi and calcium, thereby allowing the product of the two ion concentrations in blood to remain constant. Therefore, an increase in dietary phosphorus leads to an increase in Pi concentration in blood, and this in turn results in a decrease in the calcium ion concentration, with the calcium-phosphate product remaining constant. Therefore, PTH secretion is stimulated by the low calcium ion concentration and, perhaps, hyperphosphatemia per se to readjust both the serum calcium and phosphate concentrations to their normal physiologic set points. This self-correcting feedback system requires normal renal function.

## *Intestinal Absorption of Phosphates*

Pi ions, derived from either an inorganic form in foods or from the digestion of organic molecules, are absorbed by epithelial cells of the small intestine, primarily by facilitated diffusion rather than by an active process.[15] A high efficiency of Pi absorption exists in the range of 60% to 70% in adults over a wide range of intakes.[15,16] The linear relationship between absorption and intake holds across the broad range of intakes, and the rise in serum Pi concentration follows within 1 hour after ingestion, as shown with radioactive phosphate in an animal model.[15] The ability of the gut to absorb Pi ions by an active transport process springs into action only when phosphorus intake is low or the demand for it is greatly increased.[17] The hormonal form of vitamin D, 1,25(OH)$_2$D, may further enhance the intestinal absorption of phosphate ions when intakes of phosphorus have been low, but the evidence for this action remains limited.[17]

Variations in phosphorus intake, examined over a wide range, have little to no effect on calcium absorption, even when the calcium intake is low.[18,19] Net calcium balance is also not affected by dietary phosphorus intake.[19,20] Variations in phosphorus intake are reported to influence calcium flux into bone without affecting net balance. Higher phosphorus intakes have been reported to decrease urinary calcium excretion while increasing intestinal (endogenous) calcium secretion, with no net change in calcium balance.[20]

## *Hormonal and Renal Regulation of Phosphate Homeostasis*

Although the skeleton contains most of the phosphorus in the body, the release of Pi ions into blood from skeletal tissues is secondary to the regulation of blood calcium concentration, the primary role of PTH. Normal limits of serum Pi concentration for adults range from 0.97 to 1.45 mmol/L (3.0 to 4.5 mg/dL) (Figure 3).[4] As mentioned above, serum Pi may vary significantly throughout the day according to circadian rhythms (Figure 3).[11]

In addition to PTH, $1,25(OH)_2D$, and the humoral phosphaturic factors known as phosphatonins, Pi ions in body fluids are regulated by insulin, growth hormone, and steroid hormones. All of these act on the kidney, the main regulatory organ of extracellular Pi homeostasis, to either increase or decrease the kidney's capacity to reabsorb filtered Pi.[21] The kidneys reclaim about 80% of the filtered Pi load, with 60% reabsorbed in the proximal convoluted tubule, 15% to 20% in the proximal straight tubule, and less than 10% in the more distal segments of the nephron.[21] A limit to the renal transport capacity for Pi is reached at a filtered load equal to the maximal tubular capacity (TmPi). A useful index for renal Pi handling is the theoretical renal phosphate threshold, which is obtained by dividing TmPi by the glomerular filtration rate (GFR).

Pi uptake at the apical cell surface (luminal or brush-border membrane) in the proximal tubule is the rate-limiting step and the major site of hormonal regulation for phosphate reabsorption, as well as the main site of action of the phosphatonins in response to dietary changes in phosphorus intake.[22] Phosphatonins also act primarily at proximal tubular cell apical membranes to inhibit renal Pi reabsorption in response to changes in dietary phosphorus.[21,22] Both the phosphatonins and PTH act on the Pi transporters in luminal membranes of the proximal tubule.[23-25] Pi transport is driven by an $Na^+$-dependent Pi-transporter protein that resides in the brush-border membrane; this transport is the principal step in the regulation of Pi homeostasis. When serum concentrations of Pi deviate from the range of normality, the rate (TmPi) of proximal tubular Pi reabsorption is adjusted through the direct action of various hormones on the $Na^+$-Pi cotransport proteins.[5]

Most proximal tubular Pi reabsorption is thought to occur via the type IIa cotransporter (NPT2 cotransporter) based on evidence from the type IIa-knockout mouse model in which $Na^+$-Pi cotransport in brush-border membrane vesicles was reduced by 70%.[25] New evidence suggests that the phosphaturic effect of PTH may be attributed to changes in the amount of type IIa cotransporters inserted into the apical membrane of proximal tubular cells.[26-28]

Dietary phosphorus intake also regulates renal Pi excretion rates. A chronic high-phosphorus diet results in down-regulation of type IIa cotransporters by internalizing the $Na^+$-Pi cotransporter proteins in endocytic vacuoles.[28] Murer et al.[24] postulate a novel cellular and molecular mechanism of action in which both PTH and high phosphorus intake regulate a cascade of events leading to the removal of the cotransporter from the membrane and, ultimately, lysosomal degradation (Figure 4).[21,25,28] They also showed that the inhibition of renal Pi reabsorption is irreversible and requires de novo synthesis of the cotransporter proteins to restore it.

Hypophosphatemia or low phosphorus intake directly increases TmPi/GFR, which in turn can be attributed to an acute increase in the amount of $Na^+$-Pi cotransporter in the brush-border membrane.[28] Many of the genetic disorders characterized by hypophosphatemia, such as the X-linked hypophosphatemia and hereditary hypophosphatemic rickets with hypercalciuria (Dent's disease or syndrome), involve impaired renal Pi reabsorption arising from defects in the proximal tubular $Na^+$-Pi cotransporters or to abnormal PTH removal and recycling from its tubular receptor.[21,29]

Dent's disease is an example of a rare, X-linked hypophosphatemic syndrome whose molecular details have recently been elucidated.[29] Patients with Dent's disease have defective endocytosis in their proximal tubular endothelial cells arising from mutations in the voltage-gated chloride channel. Defective endocytosis results in failure to clear PTH from its tubular receptor, leading to a progressive increase in PTH at its tubular receptor. This continuous PTH-receptor binding results in a form of hyperparathyroidism limited to renal phosphate effects only, and develops in the absence of an elevation in serum PTH concentration (Figure 4D). The physiological consequences of this excessive tubular action of PTH are predictable: renal Pi wastage, hypophosphatemia, high production rate of $1,25(OH)_2D$, enteric hypercalciuria, renal stones, and renal calcification.

Phosphatonins (also known as phosphotonins) are newly discovered phosphaturic factors that have been studied in various disorders of the kidney that result in both phosphate wasting and rare cases of oncogenic osteomalacia.[30-31] These molecules, especially fibroblast growth factor 23 (FGF23) and PHEX,[30-34] promote tubular excretion of phosphate ions. FGF-23 is released from bone and other tissues, whereas circulating PHEX is a protease enzyme that inactivates circulating FGF-

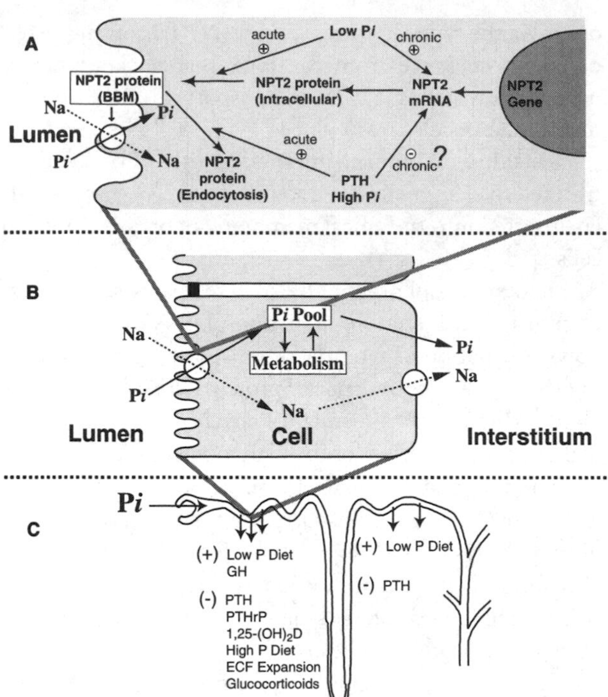


Figure 4. Regulation of renal phosphate transport. Three levels of organization are detailed: in A, the subcellular level of a proximal renal tubular cell, in B, the brush border of a renal cell, and in C, the level of an entire nephron unit of the kidney. A, Renal phosphate transport is regulated at the molecular level by changes in the number of sodium (Na)-phosphate type 2 cotransporter (NPT2) protein molecules in the brush-border membranes (BBM). NPT2 mRNA stability is up-regulated by chronically low dietary Pi and may be down-regulated by high dietary Pi and elevated parathyroid hormone (PTH). Deprivation of Pi in the diet increases the amount of NPT2 protein in the BBM. Conversely, a high-phosphorus diet decreases the amount of NPT2 protein in the BBM by increasing internalization of the protein by endocytosis, which is followed by degradation. B, The movement of sodium and phosphate from the lumen of the nephron into the cell is mediated by the BBM cotransporter. Intracellular Pi may be used in cellular metabolism or the anion may be transported to the extracellular fluid (interstitium) as a counter ion for sodium, which is actively extruded from the cell. C, Reabsorption of Pi takes place in both the proximal and distal tubule of the nephron segments. Reabsorption in the proximal tubule is stimulated by a low-Pi diet and by growth hormone (GH), whereas PTH, PTH-related peptide (PTHrP), 1,25-dihydroxyvitamin D (1,25(OH)$_2$D), high-Pi diet, expansion of extracellular fluid (ECF) volume, or glucocorticoids inhibit the reabsorption of Pi. In the distal tubule, Pi reabsorption may be stimulated by a low-Pi diet or inhibited by PTH. (Panel A data from Tennenhouse 1997[21]; panel B data from Breslau 1996[15]; panel C data from Lemann 1993.[36])

23 in healthy individuals. Circulating concentrations of FGF23 fluctuate with dietary phosphorus intake in young adults, and the highest concentrations occur after phosphorus loading and in the early stages of chronic renal failure.[22] The pathways through which these proteins operate, as well as the identification of new phosphaturic factors, are still unfolding so that a full understanding is not yet available.[35] Figure 5 illustrates that FGF23 operates at the luminal membrane of proximal renal tubular cells in the regulation of serum Pi concentration. FGF-23 and PHEX, the most studied phosphatonins, help regulate phosphate homeostasis by acting on NaPiII cotransporter protein in proximal renal tubular cells. PHEX, a metalloprotease, enzymatically degrades circulating FGF-23 in healthy individuals (Figure 5).[30]

Patients with X-linked hypophosphatemia (XLH) have elevated serum concentrations of PHEX, but are not able to degrade FGFR-23 because of a genetically altered amino acid sequence. Therefore, XLH patients have high circulating levels of FGF-23 with concomitant hypophosphatemia.[30,32-35] FGF-23 not only causes a reduction in serum phosphate but also a decline in serum 1,25(OH)$_2$D because of a down-regulation of RNA-directed synthesis of the vitamin D hormone.[33] Therefore, FGF-23 regulates phosphate reabsorption via the NaPiII transporter by a mechanism independent of PTH, and also suppresses serum 1,25(OH)$_2$D concentrations by altering renal expression of the critical enzyme needed for renal synthesis of the vitamin D hormone.

# Dietary Sources of Phosphorus

As a vital constituent of cell membranes, plant cell walls, and structural and soluble cellular proteins, virtually all foods consumed contain some phosphorus. Phosphorus, primarily in the form of phosphate, is found in three major dietary sources: foods containing natural phosphorus, foods processed with phosphate salts (additives), and dietary supplements containing phosphorus. Phosphorus deficiency is extremely rare in normal, healthy individuals, because it is found in all tissues of both plants and animals. Those rare cases of phosphorus depletion are usually associated with metabolic or genetic disorders, such as syndromes of renal phosphate wasting, diabetic ketoacidosis, hypophosphatemic rickets,[30,36-37] or Dent's syndrome.[29]

In the United States, phosphorus intake is consistently higher than calcium intake when calcium supplements are not consumed. The importance of the size of this imbalance between calcium and phosphorus intake and whether physiologic responses to higher phosphorus intake adversely affect skeletal or renal health remain controversial. The dietary imbalance of these two nutrients—which may be as great as 1 calcium to 4 Pi—has been attributed partly to an ubiquitous distribution of phosphorus but a limited distribution of calcium in foods; increased consumption of highly processed foods containing phosphate additives; increased consumption of soft drinks containing phosphoric acid coupled with reduced intakes of milk and dairy products; and increased use of phosphate-containing supplements.[38,39]

## *Natural Foods*

Although dietary calcium is limited to a few foods, phosphorus is found in practically all foods. Approxi-

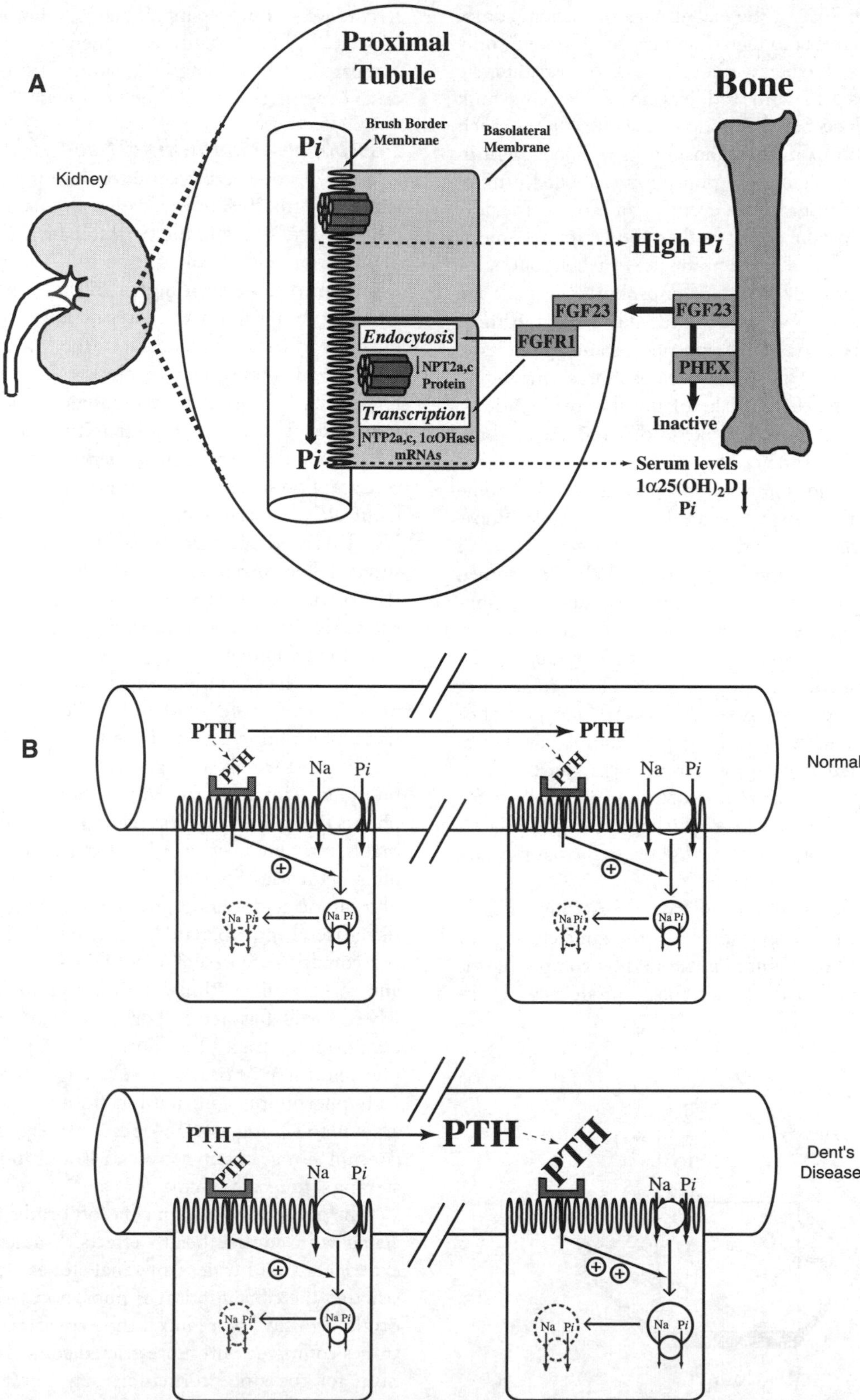


Figure 5. A, In addition to the classical control by PTH on the proximal tubule, renal phosphate homeostasis is also regulated by FGF 23, one of several phosphatonins. High serum Pi concentrations stimulate the production of FGF 23 from skeletal or other sites, which act on the FGFR 1 receptor on the proximal tubule to increase urinary Pi excretion by promoting endocytotic loss of NPT2a channels. (FGF 23 also decreases 1,25 dihydroxy vitamin D formation by inhibition of mitochondrial 1 alpha hydroxylase.[24]) B, Insufficient removal of PTH from its brush-border membrane receptor. The humoral regulation of Pi homeostasis by the phosphatonin FGF23 in conjunction with PHEX results in insufficient degradation (by endocytosis) of the NPT2 cotransporter protein, resulting in a persistent PTH stimulation and chronic renal Pi loss, as well as excessive mitochondrial production of 1,25$(OH)_2$D (not shown). Hyperphosphaturia becomes continuous and inappropriately high, characteristics of Dent's disease.

mately 60% to 70% of the daily intake of calcium comes from milk and milk products, but dairy foods provide only 20% to 30% of the dietary phosphorus for most adult age and sex groups. In infants, toddlers, and adolescents, milk and milk products have been shown to contribute as much as 32% to 48% of dietary phosphorus.[40] Foods high in protein are as a rule high in phosphorus: about 15 mg of phosphorus is consumed for every 1 g of protein. In addition to dairy products, two other food groups—meat, poultry, and fish and grain products—each accounts for 20% to 30% of daily intake of phosphorus in most age and sex groups.[38] Soft drinks and soda ranked 10th in the order of food sources of phosphorus among adults in the United States. This source of phosphorus contributed 2.1% of the total daily intake of phosphorus by adults, whereas milk and cheeses ranked no. 1 (16.2%) and no. 2 (9.7%).[30,41] For infants, the specific category of infant foods was the major source of phosphorus (31%).[40] Some forms of natural phosphorus are less bioavailable. Phosphorus is present as phytic acid in the outer coating of cereal grains such as the bran portion. When consumed with other minerals such as calcium, zinc, and iron, phytates form complexes that can bind these cations (Figure 6), forming a cation-phytate complex and rendering the mineral unavailable for absorption.[42] The formation of the mineral-phytate complex also makes dietary phosphorus less bioavailable. The total phosphorus content of grain-based diets may be measurably high, but the bioavailable phosphorus content is considerably lower if the foods are not prepared in ways that lower the phytate content, such as leavening bread with yeasts that produce phytase.

The phosphorus content of food is also influenced by the amount of processing involved in manufacturing the food product. This point is illustrated by comparing the levels of phosphorus in various cheese products with different levels of processing. The phosphorus content of 1 ounce (28 g) of naturally aged cheddar cheese is 145 mg compared with 211 mg in 1 ounce of processed cheese or 257 mg in 1 ounce of cheese spread.[43]

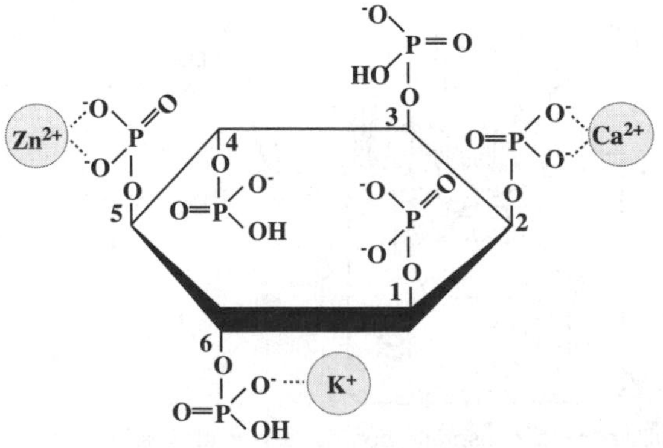

Figure 6. Complexation of mineral cations by phosphate groups of phytate, which make these mineral ions unavailable for intestinal absorption. Phosphate groups of phytates may therefore adversely affect the bioavailability of mineral cations. (Data from Anderson and Garner, 2000.[42])

## *Phosphorus-Containing Food Additives*

In 1979, food additive use was estimated to contribute about 20% to 30% of adult phosphorus intake or about 320 mg/d[2,3]; by 1990, the per capita availability of phosphorus from additives had risen to 470 mg/d,[44-45] and it is presumed to be even higher in the early 21st century. Nutrient composition databases do not reflect the current practices of food additive use in food processing; therefore, actual intakes of phosphorus are almost certainly higher than reported, as estimated by Oenning et al.[46] Estimates of nationally representative nutrient intakes of the US population are usually derived from national food consumption surveys such as the joint Centers for Disease Control/National Center for Health Statistics (CDC/NCHS) and the US Department of Agriculture (USDA) surveys. The current system for estimating nutrient content of survey foods in the national food consumption surveys is not capable of capturing the phosphorus intake from food additive use.[38]

Among the 45 or more direct food additives containing phosphorus that are listed in the Code of Federal Regulations, phosphoric acid and the polyphosphate molecules are the most widely used and the greatest contributors to phosphorus intake in the United States.[38,45] Annual phosphorus use in food-processing applications in the United States, estimated between 1980 and 1990, showed a doubling in the use of phosphoric acid.[47] The increased use of phosphoric acid in food processing is consistent with the rising trend in carbonated soft drink consumption. The cola soft drinks represent 66% of the soft drinks consumed and contain 44 to 70 mg of Pi per 12-oz (354-mL) can, whereas fruit-flavored soft drinks that are acidulated with citrate rather than phosphoric acid contain little or no phosphorus.[48,49] For a large percentage of consumers, total daily phosphorus contribution from cola beverages may amount to 120 mg (two 12-oz cans per day), although some consumers may obtain between 240 and 360 mg from consuming 4 to 6 cans of cola per day.[39]

The phosphoric acid in cola soft drinks has been associated with adverse health effects. Studies in men who experienced an incident of renal stones showed that restricting the consumption of phosphorus-containing soft drinks significantly reduced the 3-year recurrence rate of stones compared with unrestricted controls. The mechanism for the stone formation may result from the increased acid load that in turn increases urinary calcium excretion. In contrast, men who restricted citric acid-containing soft drinks experienced similar stone recurrence rates as their own controls.[50] A recent clinical study reported that acute cola consumption caused changes in urinary biochemical and physicochemical risk factors associated with calcium oxalate stone formation.[51] A case-controlled study in Mexican children assessed whether the intake of soft drinks containing phosphoric acid was a risk factor in the development of hypocalcemia.[52] A similar study examined the relationship between phosphoric acid-containing soft drinks and hypocalcemia in postmenopausal women.[53] Both studies found that cola consumption was associated with reduced ionic calcium (i.e., hypocalcemia).[52,53] Women who consumed noncarbonated beverages did not show declines in hip bone mineral density (BMD). In contrast to these findings, no association was found between cola intake and BMD in older women,[54] but high soft drink consumption has been linked to higher incidence of bone fracture even in adolescents.[55] Whether adverse skeletal effects of cola-type beverages are related to the hypocalcemia resulting from the phosphorus content or to the metabolic release of hydrogen ions from the phosphoric acid is not clear.

### *Dietary Supplements*

Phosphorus supplements are not widely used by healthy individuals in the United States.[1] The phosphorus content in multiple vitamin preparations varies, but is usually under 150 mg and is often present as the anion component of the salt of another nutrient such as di- and tri-calcium phosphate, ferric phosphate, or potassium phosphate. Therefore, in contrast to calcium, significant contributions of phosphorus by dietary supplement use have not been an important consideration in establishing the safe upper limit of phosphorus intake.[1] However, new categories of dietary supplements, such as high-energy bars and shakes or creatinine monophosphate supplements used to enhance athletic performance and build muscle mass, may contribute significantly to daily phosphorus intake in users. Phosphorus is critical for glucose utilization by muscle and for creatine to function within the muscle fiber. Consequently, a large amount of phosphorus as phosphates may be assumed to be a desired feature of ergogenic and muscle-building dietary supplement products. According to the phosphorus content displayed in the nutrition facts panel and the manufacturer's recommended daily dose, some products currently on the market provide up to 3000 mg/d of phosphorus. The safe use of such products merits further study, considering that this phosphate load would be in addition to the usual dietary contribution of 1200 to 1600 mg for young men. This scenario could result in daily intakes in excess of the Tolerable Upper Intake Level (UL) of 4000 mg/d.[1] Finally, ingredients lists on foods must include the names of any phosphorus additives, but amounts of these additives do not need to be disclosed.

## Dietary Phosphorus Intakes and Dietary Reference Intakes

The most recent estimates of phosphorus and calcium intakes in the United States are shown in Figure 7. The 1997 Dietary Reference Intakes (DRIs) for phosphorus, which include the Estimated Average Requirement (EAR), Recommended Dietary Allowances (RDA), Adequate Intake (AI), and UL, are presented in Table 1.[1] The EAR is defined as the dietary intake level estimated to meet the requirement for phosphorus in 50% of a lifestage or gender-specific group. The EAR is used in setting the RDA and in assessing the adequacy of dietary

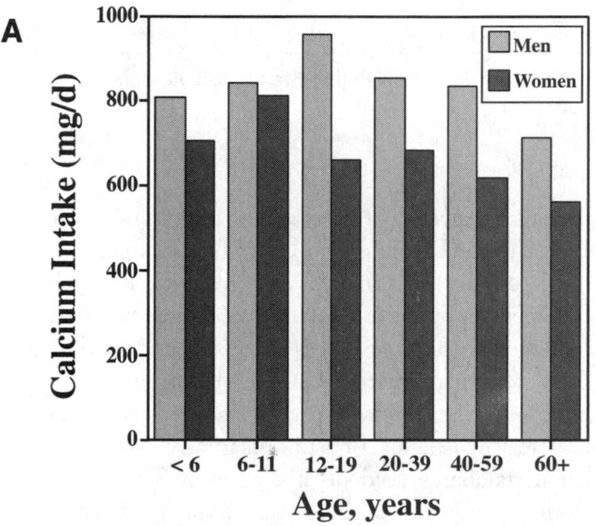


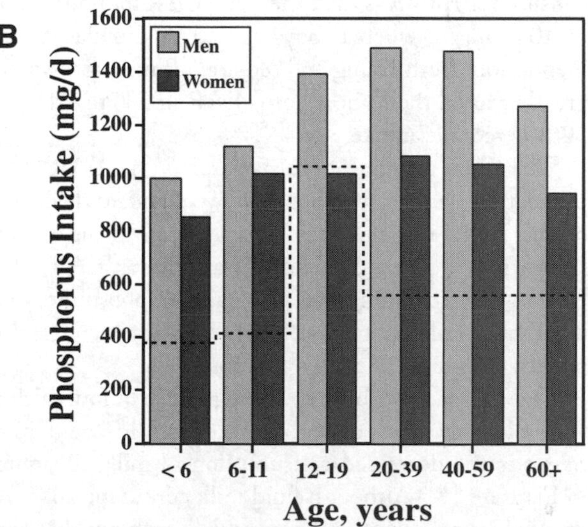


Figure 7. Phosphorus (A) and calcium (B) intakes by females and males compared with the Estimated Average Requirements (EARs). Median (50th percentile) intakes for phosphorus by age and sex from estimates of one 24-hour dietary recall interview from the National Health and Nutrition Examination Survey 1999–2000 for the US population (Data from Ervin et al., 2004.[88]) Population medians are weighted to produce national estimates and are presented by sex and age groups. The 1997 EARs for phosphorus for all age groups are shown by the horizontal dashed line. No EARs for calcium were established in 1997. (Data from Food and Nutrition Board, Institute of Medicine, 1997.[1])

**Table 1.** Dietary Reference Intakes for Phosphorus for Males and Females: Recommended Dietary Allowances (RDAs), Estimated Average Requirements (EARs), and Tolerable Upper Intake Levels (UL)

| Age (years) | RDA | EAR | UL |
|---|---|---|---|
| 1–3 | 460 | 380 | — |
| 4–8 | 500 | 405 | — |
| 9–18 | 1250 | 1055 | 4000 |
| 19–50 | 700 | 580 | 4000 |
| 51–70 | 700 | 580 | 4000 |
| >70 | 700 | 580 | 3000 |

Data from Food and Nutrition Board, Institute of Medicine, 1997.[1]

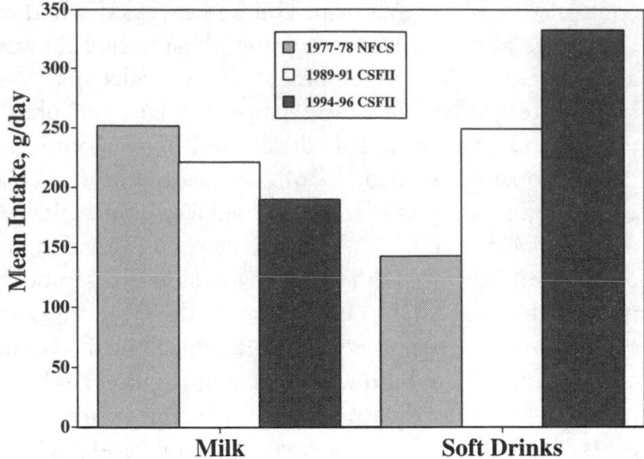


Figure 8. Changing trends in the consumption of milk and carbonated soft drinks showing the mean intake of fluid milk and carbonated beverages by the total US population based on day-1 data from the food intake surveys conducted by the US Department of Agriculture: Nationwide Food Consumption Survey (NFCS 1977–78), provided by Y.K. Park of the Food and Drug Administration, and the Continuing Survey of Food Intakes by Individuals (US Department of Agriculture. Continuing Survey of Food Intakes by Individuals (CSFII): Diet and Health Knowledge Survey 1989. Springfield, VA: US Department of Commerce, National Technical Information Service (PB93500411: machine readable data set); 1993 and US Department of Agriculture. Continuing Survey of Food Intakes by Individuals (CSFII): Diet and Health Knowledge Survey 1990. Springfield, VA: U.S. Department of Commerce, National Technical Information Service (PB93504843: machine readable data set); 1993.) Fluid milk includes whole, low-fat, skim, and acidophilus milk; buttermilk; reconstituted dry milk; evaporated milk; and sweetened condensed milk. Carbonated soft drinks include regular and low-energy carbonated soft drinks and sweetened and unsweetened carbonated water. Prepared by Y.K. Park and M.S. Calvo of the Food and Drug Administration.

intakes of specific groups, and it is therefore compared with the median phosphorus intakes in Figure 7B, but not in Figure 7A, since EARs across the life cycle have not been set by the US Institute of Medicine. In general, median phosphorus intakes in the United States exceed DRIs for both genders by 300 to 600 mg/d.[56] An important point that should not be overlooked is that these data underestimate actual phosphorus intakes, because the nutrient databases used do not account for contributions from phosphorus additive use in the foods consumed. At the 50th percentile intake, teen and adolescent girls consume slightly less than the 1997 EAR for phosphorus of 1055 mg/d, whereas boys exceed this intake recommendation. Both young and older adult men and women greatly exceed their phosphorus EAR of 580 mg/d at the 50th percentile intake.

The RDA for phosphorus is based on the EAR of the population plus a safety factor of two standard deviations of the EAR, whereas the AI is used when insufficient scientific evidence is available to calculate an EAR.[1] The UL is the maximum level of intake of phosphorus per day that is unlikely to result in risk of adverse effects to healthy members of the population.[1]

One factor contributing to the pattern of low calcium and relatively high phosphorus intakes in the United States is the decreased consumption of milk, illustrated in Figure 8.[39,45] Although fluid milk consumption, a traditional source of both calcium and phosphorus, has consistently decreased, soft drink consumption has steadily increased. During the past two decades, the percentage of people drinking fluid milk has decreased by 18%, whereas the percentage of people drinking soft drinks has increased by 32%. Most of the different types of soft drinks, about 66%, supply phosphorus but none contains calcium.[48] The decrease in milk, and therefore calcium, consumption coupled with the high consumption of soft drinks that is prevalent in teens and adolescents has raised concerns about bone health.[55]

# Potential Problems of Excessive Phosphorus Intakes

Two potential problems of Pi metabolism related to excessive consumption of phosphorus—and usually accompanied by inadequate intake of calcium—are insufficient bone accretion and direct stimulation of PTH secretion by phosphorus. Renal failure resulting in renal osteodystrophy is covered in Chapter 54.

## *Insufficient Bone Accretion*

Experimental studies of phosphorus loading and investigations using diets reflecting typical consumption patterns (i.e., low calcium and high phosphorus) have induced hormonal changes that are not conducive to the development or even maintenance of optimal peak bone mass in young adults. Most clinical studies of acute and longer exposures to phosphorus loading in the presence or absence of adequate levels of calcium show an increase in PTH levels.[57-68] The acute rise in PTH is considered to be secondary to a decrease in serum ionized calcium concentration, as demonstrated by an abrupt increase in serum Pi after an oral load.[16] The mechanism is accepted to be an increase in the formation of the calcium-phosphate complex in serum that decreases the ionic calcium concentration according to the law of mass action. In one study, several days of high dietary phosphorus intake resulted in an increase in the circadian peak height of serum Pi and an elevation in serum PTH levels over the entire circadian pattern.[12,61] When high-phosphorus diets were fed for 4 weeks, serum Pi levels showed remarkable adaptation, returning to baseline levels across the circadian pattern, whereas PTH levels remained elevated.[62]

For both short-[61] and long-term[62] exposure to low-calcium, high-phosphorus diets, a moderate elevation of PTH has been observed; however, $1{,}25(OH)_2D$ levels were shown to be significantly increased in young adults.[61] This increase is to be expected, because PTH is the strongest stimulus for $1{,}25(OH)_2D$ synthesis. On the other hand, when this type of diet was fed to young women for 4 weeks, no significant increase in $1{,}25(OH)_2D$ levels was observed.[50] Others have shown that high levels of dietary phosphates can attenuate the PTH-induced stimulation of $1{,}25(OH)_2D$ synthesis.[58,60,67,69] The important adaptive response to low calcium intake, namely, the increase in $1{,}25(OH)_2D$ synthesis, that was observed in short-term feeding studies appears to be impaired with slightly longer studies.[61,62] The implication of these findings is that in growing young adults who are still accruing peak bone mass, a chronic high phosphorus intake may impair the adaptive mechanism needed for adequate calcium absorption and optimal bone accretion.

Biochemical markers of bone turnover have been used in phosphorus feeding studies to determine whether bone resorption increases with the observed increase in PTH. Single oral loads (1500 mg) stimulated a rise in PTH, and markers of bone formation either declined[64] or showed no change.[65] When phosphorus salts were added to diets and fed for at least a week, no changes were observed in resorptive markers of bone turnover despite observed increases in serum PTH.[66] Other studies have failed to demonstrate significant changes in markers of bone resorption, such as free deoxypyridinoline[64,65] or hydroxyproline,[60,62,69] despite evidence of PTH stimulation. Clinical evidence in support of PTH-induced bone loss in individuals with healthy kidneys on high phosphorus intakes is lacking. Nevertheless, the observed poor response with resorptive markers of bone turnover does not preclude the possibility that bone accretion may be impaired. In contrast to an increase of dietary phosphorus, resorptive markers of bone turnover respond as predicted to depletion of dietary calcium.[70]

No prospective study in humans has demonstrated bone loss with the consumption of a diet with a low calcium-to-phosphorus ratio. A cross-sectional study in Danish perimenopausal women, however, reported a significant positive relationship between BMD and the dietary calcium-to-phosphorus ratio.[71] In that study, the dietary calcium-to-phosphorus ratio showed a stronger positive relation to bone mass and a stronger negative association to $1{,}25(OH)_2D$ than did calcium intake. The possibility that a lifetime of intake with a low calcium-to-phosphorus ratio resulted in poor bone accretion and lower bone mass may also be considered in interpreting these results.

In the absence of long-term clinical studies examining effects on bone, animal models can be used to resolve whether adverse health effects result from low calcium intake alone or from the prevalent pattern of combined low calcium intake and high phosphorus intake. Secondary hyperparathyroidism and increased bone resorption have been demonstrated in several animal models in response to a low dietary calcium-to-phosphorus ratio when calcium intake was adequate or deficient.[38,72] To date, only one study has attempted to discriminate between the effects of a low-calcium diet and those of a low-calcium, high-phosphorus diet. Pettifor et al.[73] fed diets with various calcium and phosphorus contents for 16 months to young vitamin D-replete baboons. The phosphorus content of the four experimental diets was adequate and constant in all but one, and the calcium content was high, medium, or low. After 16 months, the baboons fed the low-calcium, normal-phosphorus diet showed histological evidence of increased bone resorption and lower femoral ash content, whereas those fed the low-calcium, low-phosphorus diet showed only histological features of osteomalacia.[73] In these growing primates, the diet with the lower calcium-to-phosphorus ratio appeared to be more harmful to bone than calcium inadequacy alone.

### *Direct Stimulation of Parathyroid Hormone Secretion*

Phosphorus retention plays a key role in both the development of hyperplasia of the parathyroid glands and increased circulating levels of PTH that characterize the altered mineral metabolism in advanced chronic renal failure.[74] Growing evidence suggests that a direct effect of phosphorus on parathyroid gland function is probably independent of changes in ionized calcium and $1{,}252D_3$.[74-77] The magnitude of hyperphosphatemia needed to stimulate PTH secretion directly in the in vivo experiments is well above the normal physiological range. Further study is needed to determine whether this direct effect of serum Pi on PTH secretion is influenced by renal retention of phosphorus. It is, therefore, not clear whether dietary phosphorus levels are sufficiently high to stimulate PTH secretion directly in humans. The direct stimulatory effect of a high serum concentration of Pi, as mediated by the $Na^+$-dependent Pi cotransporters in the plasma membrane of parathyroid cells, may, however, increase

PTH secretion.[78] Previously, the only clear evidence of a secondary stimulation of PTH secretion was through lowering of the serum ionized calcium level.[57,62]

## Role of Phosphorus in Chronic Renal Failure

The kidney is the major organ system in the regulation of phosphorus homeostasis; consequently, the most damaging effects of excess phosphorus intake occur when renal function is diminished. Renal failure may be characterized by an acute or chronic decline in the GFR. Although acute episodes are often reversible, chronic renal failure is progressive, permanent, and ultimately requires dialysis or transplantation. One consequence of renal failure is the derangement of calcium and Pi homeostasis that may lead over long periods to a bone disease known as renal osteodystrophy. Recently, a relationship between renal osteodystrophy and vascular calcification (mineralization) has been established.[79]

The homeostasis of both calcium and Pi is affected rather early in the process of renal failure (Figure 9A); however, clinical signs and symptoms usually do not manifest until later in the development of the disease (Figure 9B). As the GFR decreases, the serum concentration of Pi increases, because the kidneys can not excrete phosphate. Progressive Pi retention leads to hyperphosphatemia, which affects serum calcium directly and indirectly. Elevated serum Pi concentrations depress serum ionic calcium concentrations because of increasing formation of calcium phosphate complexes. Hyperphosphatemia also indirectly contributes to hypocalcemia by diminishing renal $1,25(OH)_2D$ production, which reduces intestinal calcium absorption. Lower serum ionized calcium initially signals the parathyroid gland to secrete PTH, which acts

Level of Renal Function Adaptation

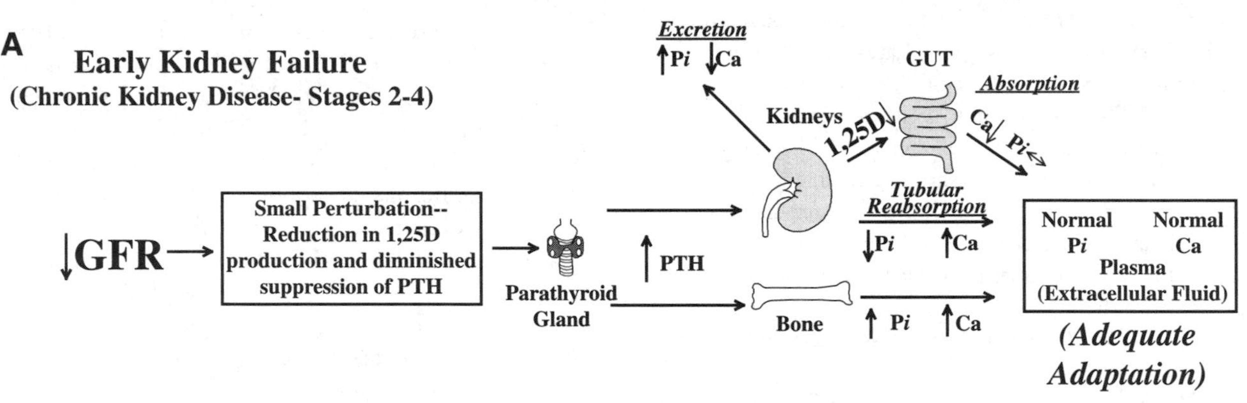


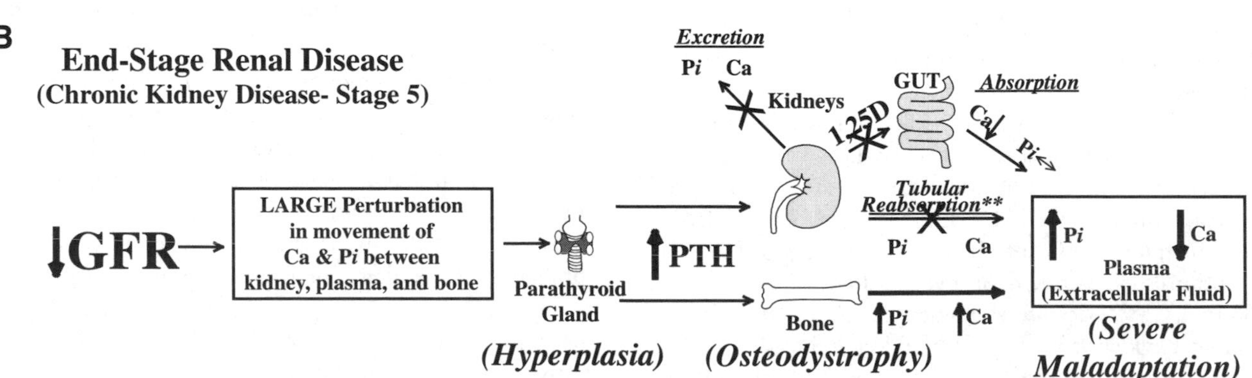


**Zero Reabsorption

Figure 9. Development of renal secondary hyperparathyroidism and osteodystrophy. A, Early changes in chronic kidney failure (stages 2–4) include a notable increase in serum Pi concentration, but hormonal adaptations correct this short-lived elevation after meals. The hormonal adaptations are an increase in serum PTH concentration and a decrease in serum $1,25(OH)_2D$ concentration. B, End-stage renal failure (chronic renal failure stage 5). Elevated serum Pi concentration cannot be corrected, and serum calcium concentration also becomes chronically depressed. The low calcium signals for continuous PTH secretion and higher than normal levels of PTH circulate in blood. The kidneys can no longer excrete adequate amounts of Pi and calcium ions, and the constant elevation of PTH causes excessive bone turnover and loss of mineral, a condition known as renal osteodystrophy. GFR, glomerular filtration rate; PTH, parathyroid hormone. (Data from Anderson and Garner, 1996.[5])

on the renal proximal tubules to decrease the rate of Pi reabsorption. To restore serum calcium (ionized calcium) concentration to its normal set point, PTH stimulates calcium and Pi release from bone as well as 1,25$(OH)_2D$ synthesis by the kidney; the newly synthesized 1,25 $(OH)_2D$ facilitates the active absorption of calcium by the intestine. As renal failure progresses, 1,25$(OH)_2D$ synthesis is impaired and low serum calcium levels resulting from poor intestinal absorption stimulate a sustained PTH secretion and further promote parathyroid gland hyperplasia. As discussed earlier, recent evidence exists for a direct effect of Pi on parathyroid gland stimulation, but this appears to be dependent on supraphysiologic levels of Pi, such as the Pi retention experienced in chronic renal failure.[75]

Several studies demonstrate that dietary phosphorus restriction, independent of serum levels of ionized calcium and 1,25$(OH)_2D$, attenuate parathyroid hyperplasia and prevent secondary hyperparathyroidism in patients with chronic renal failure[81-83] and in experimental animal models of renal failure.[84] Phosphorus-restricted diets are usually prescribed for patients with chronic renal failure, with the goal being to limit phosphorus intake to 800 to 1000 mg/d. Because all foods contain phosphorus, this dietary goal is difficult to achieve. Since protein malnutrition is an independent predictor of death in advanced chronic kidney disease patients, it is important that dietary protein intake be maintained at a high level (1.2 g/kg body weight), even though it contributes to the Pi load. This protein-derived Pi can largely be bound to oral phosphate-binders taken at meal times and is not absorbed. Phosphate-rich processed foods and dairy products, on the other hand, should be restricted. Food labeling regulations currently do not require that the phosphorus content of a food be listed, which makes it difficult to estimate total phosphorus intake from both foods and additives. In end-stage renal disease, phosphate binders—molecules that bind and, thus, prevent intestinal absorption of phosphorus—are prescribed in conjunction with a low-phosphorus diet. Examples of these phosphate binders include aluminum hydroxide, aluminum carbonate, aluminum sucrafate, calcium acetate, calcium carbonate, lanthanum carbonate, and sevelamer hydrochloride.[85,86] It is important to note that the use of metal-based phosphate binders may have serious side effects, including calcium loading, accelerated vascular calcification,[79] and, in the case of aluminum salts, neurologic and skeletal toxicities. Early intervention with dietary phosphorus restriction and appropriate use of safe phosphate binders is needed to prevent the vascular and skeletal effects of the elevated calcium-phosphate complex (product) and hypersecretion of PTH. Accurate information on the phosphorus content of foods is needed to achieve a low phosphorus intake and effectively manage chronic renal failure.[87]

# Concluding Remarks

Phosphorus is ubiquitous in its distribution in the body, and is critical for all its cellular processes. Phosphate ions are involved in virtually every metabolic function, from membrane lipid-protein interfaces to enabling glucose to enter the glycolytic pathway and the storage of the resulting energy in pyrophosphate bonds. Phosphate ions become components of the backbone of DNA and RNA, as well as a major component of hydroxyapatite, which provides structure and rigidity to bone. Hormones and enzymes regulate energy flow (and therefore Pi flow) through biochemical pathways by the simple addition or removal of a phosphate group on a protein or nucleotide. At least in part, phosphorus intake even regulates its own rates of excretion and elimination, maintaining serum Pi within fairly normal limits. Because of its widespread distribution in foods, it is not surprising that severe phosphorus deficiency is rare.

Recent evidence suggests a trend toward increasing consumption of phosphorus in the US population with increasing intakes of convenience and prepared processed foods. High phosphorus consumption may contribute to the progression of renal stones, the progression of renal failure, and suboptimal gain in bone mass during adolescence that could increase the risk of bone fracture with age. Investigations of phosphate regulation have revealed new information relating to renal tubular reabsorption. The adverse effects of high dietary phosphorus intake in chronic renal failure are well established. Whether diets with a low calcium-to-phosphorus ratio adversely affect the maintenance of skeletal mass and density or the development of renal stones in the normal population remains to be established. A number of rare genetic disorders ("experiments in nature") have advanced our knowledge and understanding of normal physiological control mechanisms of serum phosphate concentration.

# Acknowledgment

The authors wish to acknowledge the assistance of Agna Boass, PhD, in the preparation of this manuscript.

# References

1. Food and Nutrition Board, Institute of Medicine. Dietary Reference Intakes for Calcium, Phosphorus, Magnesium, Vitamin D, and Fluoride. Washington, DC: National Academies Press; 1997. Available online at: http://www.nap.edu/books/0309063507/html.
2. Bell RR, Draper HH, Tzeng DYM, et al. Physiological responses of human adults to foods containing phosphate additives. J Nutr. 1977:107:42–50.
3. Greger JL, Krystofiak M. Phosphorus intake of Americans. Food Technol. 1982;36:78–84.
4. Lobaugh B. Blood calcium and phosphorus regula-

tion. In: Anderson JJB, Garner SC, eds. *Calcium and Phosphorus in Health and Disease*. Boca Raton, FL: CRC Press; 1996; 27–43.

5. Anderson JJB, Garner SC. Dietary issues of calcium and phosphorus. In: Anderson JJB, Garner SC, eds. *Calcium and Phosphorus in Health and Disease*. Boca Raton, FL: CRC Press; 1996; 7–23.
6. Lolitch G, Halstead AC, Albersheim S, et al. Age- and sex-specific pediatric reference intervals for biochemistry analytes as measured with the Ektachem-700 analyzer. Clin Chem. 1988;34:1622–1625.
7. Endres, DB, Morgan CH, Gary PJ, Omdahl JL. Age-related changes in serum immunoreactive parathyroid hormone and its biologic action in healthy men and women. J Clin Endocrinol Metab. 1987; 65:724–731.
8. Endres DB, Rude RK. Mineral and bone metabolism. In: Burtis CA, Ashwood EK, eds. *Teitz Clinical Chemistry*. 2nd ed. Philadelphia, PA: WB Saunders; 1996; 1887–1972.
9. Sherman SS, Hollis BW, Tobin JB. Vitamin D status and related parameters in a healthy population: the effects of age, sex and season. J Clin Endocrinol Metab. 1990;71:405–413.
10. Prince RL, Dick I, Devine A, et al. The effects of menopause and age on calcitropic hormones: a cross sectional study of 655 healthy women aged 35 to 90. J Bone Miner Res. 1995;10:835–842.
11. Calvo MS, Eastell R, Offord KP, et al. Circadian variations in ionized calcium and intact parathyroid hormone: evidence for sex differences in calcium homeostasis. J Clin Endocrinol Metab. 1991;72:69–76.
12. Portale AA, Halloran BP, Morris RC Jr. Physiologic regulation of the serum concentration of 1,25-dihydroxyvitamin D by phosphorus in normal men. J Clin Invest. 1989;83:1494–1499.
13. Garner SC. Parathyroid hormone. In: Anderson JJB, Garner SC, eds. *Calcium and Phosphorus in Health and Disease*. Boca Raton, FL: CRC Press; 1966; 157–175.
14. Quarles LD. Evidence for a bone-kidney axis regulating phosphate homeostasis. J Clin Invest. 2003; 112:642–646.
15. Breslau NA. Calcium, magnesium, and phosphorus: intestinal absorption. In: Favus MJ, ed. *Primer on the Metabolic Bone Diseases and Disorders of Mineral Metabolism*. 3rd ed. Philadelphia: Lippincott-Raven Publishers; 1996; 41–49.
16. Anderson JJB. Nutritional biochemistry of calcium and phosphorus. J Nutr Biochem. 1991;2:300–309.
17. Peterlik M, Wasserman RH. Effect of vitamin D on transepithelial phosphate transport in chicken intestine. Am J Physiol. 1978;244:E379–E388.
18. Spencer H, Menczel J, Lewin I, Samachson I. Effect of high phosphorus intake on calcium and phosphorus metabolism in man. J Nutr. 1965;86:125–132.
19. Spencer H, Kramer L, Osis D, Norris C. Effect of phosphorus on the absorption of calcium and on the calcium balance in man. J Nutr. 1978;108:447–457.
20. Heaney RP, Recker R. Effects of nitrogen, phosphorus, and caffeine on calcium balance in women. J Lab Clin Med. 1982;99:46–55.
21. Tennenhouse HS. Cellular and molecular mechanisms of renal phosphate transport. J Bone Miner Res. 1997;12:159–164.
22. Ferrari SL, Bonjour J-P, Rizzoli R. Fibroblast growth factor-23 relationship to dietary phosphate and renal phosphate handling in healthy young men. J Clin Endocr Metab 2005;90:1519–1524.
23. Saito H, Kusano K, Kinosaki M, et al. Human fibroblast growth factor-23 mutants express $Na^+$-dependent phosphate co-transport activity and 1□,25-dihydroxyvitamin D3 production. J Biol Chem 2003; 278:2206–2211.
24. Takeda E, Yamamoto H, Nashiki K, et al. Inorganic phosphate homeostasis and the role of dietary phosphorus. J Cell Mol Med 2004;8:191–200.
25. Murer H, Forster I, Hernando N, et al. Posttranscriptional regulation of proximal tubule NaPi-II transporter in response to PTH and dietary Pi. Am J Physiol 1999;277:F676–F684.
26. Beck LA, Karaplis AC, Amizuga N, et al. Targeted inactivation of NPT2 in mice leads to severe renal phosphate wasting. Hypercalciuria, and skeletal abnormalities. Proc Natl Acad Sci USA 1998;95: 5372–7.
27. Traebert M, Roth J, Biber J, et al. Internalization of proximal tubular type II Na-Pi cotransporter by PTH: immunogold electron microscopy. Am J Physiol 2000;278:F148–54.
28. Tennenhouse HS. Regulation of phosphorus homeostasis by Type IIa Na/phosphate cotransporter. Annu Rev Nutr 2005;10:1–18.
29. Jentsch TJ, Poet M, Fuhrmann JC, Zdebik AA. Physiological functions of CLC Cl-channels gleaned from human genetic disease and mouse models Annu Rev Physiol 2005;67:779–807.
30. Calvo MS, Carpenter TO. Influence of phosphorus on the skeleton. In: New SI, Bonjour J-P, eds. Nutritional Aspects of Bone Health. Royal Chemistry Society, Cambridge, UK, 2004:229–265.
31. Kumar R. New insights into phosphate homeostasis: fibroblast growth factor 23 and frizzled-related protein-4 are phosphaturic factors derived from tumors associated with osteomalacia. Curr Opin Nephrol Hypertens 2002;11:577–583.
32. Quarles LD. FGF 23, PHEX, and MEPE regulation of phosphate homeostasis and skeletal mineralization. Am J Physiol 2003;285:E1–E9.
33. Shimada T, Hasegawa H, Yamazaki Y, et al. FGF-23 is a potent regulator of vitamin D metabolism and phosphate homeostasis. J Bone Miner Res. 2004;19: 429–435.

34. Carpenter TO. Oncogenic osteomalacia: a complex dance of factors. N Engl J Med 2002;348:1705–1708.
35. Carpenter TO, Ellis BK, Insogna KL, et al. Fibroblast growth factor 7: an inhibitor of phosphate transport derived from oncogenic osteomalacia causing tumors. J Clin Endocr Metab. 2005;90:1012–1020.
36. Lemann J Jr. Urinary excretion of calcium, magnesium, and phosphorus. In: Favus MJ, ed. *Primer on the Metabolic Bone Diseases and Disorders of Mineral Metabolism.* 2nd ed. New York: Raven Press; 1993; 50–54.
37. Weisinger JR, Bellorin-Font E. Electrolyte quintet: magnesium and phosphorus. Lancet 1998;352: 391–396.
38. Calvo MS, Park YK. Changing phosphorus content of the U.S. diet: Potential for adverse effects on bone. J Nutr. 1996;126:1168S–1180S.
39. Harnack L, Stang J, Story M. Soft Drink consumption among US children and adolescents: Nutritional consequences. J Am Diet Assoc. 1999;99:436–441.
40. Hunt C, Meacham S. Aluminum, boron, calcium, copper, iron, magnesium, manganese, molybdenum, phosphorus, potassium, sodium, and zinc: Concentrations in common Western foods and estimated daily intakes by infants; toddlers; and male and female adolescents, adults and seniors in the United States. J Am Diet Assoc. 2001;101:1058–1060.
41. Subar AF, Krebs-Smith SM, Cook A, et al. Dietary sources of nutrients among adults, 1989–1991. J Am Diet Assoc. 1998;98:537–547.
42. Anderson JJB, Garner SC. The soybean as a source of bioactive molecules. In: Schmidl MK, Labuza TP, eds. *Functional Foods.* Gaithersburg, MD: Aspen Publishers; 2000; 239–269.
43. Louie DS. Intestinal bioavailability and absorption of calcium. In: Anderson JJB, Garner SC, eds. *Calcium and Phosphorus in Health and Disease.* Boca Raton, FL: CRC Press; 1996; 45–62.
44. ESHA Research. Food processor network version software, 1999 update. Salem, OR: ESHA Research; 1999.
45. Calvo MS. Dietary phosphorus, calcium metabolism, and bone. J Nutr. 1993;123: 1627–1633.
46. Oenning LJ, Vogel J, Calvo MS. Accuracy of methods estimating calcium and phosphorus intake in daily diets. J Am Diet Assoc. 1988;88:1076–1078.
47. International Food Additives Council. *Disappearance of Phosphorus in U.S. Food Applications.* Atlanta: International Food Additives Council; 1992.
48. Pao EM, Fleming KH, Guenther PM, Mickle SJ. Foods commonly eaten by individuals: amount per eating occasion. USDA Human Nutrition Services Home Economics Research Report No. 44. Washington, DC: U.S. Government Printing Office; 1982.
49. Massey LK, Strang MM. Soft drink consumption, phosphorus intake and osteoporosis. J Am Diet Assoc. 1982;80:581–583.
50. Shuster J, Jenkins A, Logan C, et al. Soft drink consumption and urinary stone recurrence: a randomized prevention trial. J Clin Epidemiol. 1992;45:911–916.
51. Rodgers A. Effect of cola consumption on urinary biochemical and physicochemical risk factors associated with calcium oxalate urolithiasis. Urol Res. 1999;27:77–81.
52. Mazariegos-Ramos E, Guerro-Romero F, Rodriguez-Moran M, et al. Consumption of soft drinks with phosphoric acid as a risk factor for development of hypocalcemia in children: A case control study. J Pediatr. 1995;126:940–942.
53. Guerro-Romero F, Rodriguez-Moran, M, Reyes, E. Consumption of soft drinks with phosphoric acid as a risk factor for the development of hypocalcemia in postmenopausal women. J Clin Epidemiol. 1999;52: 1007–1010.
54. Kim SH, Morton DJ, Barrett-Connor E. Carbonated beverage consumption and bone mineral density among older women: the Rancho Bernardo Study. Am J Public Health. 1997;87:276–279.
55. Whyshak G, Frisch RE. Carbonated beverages, dietary calcium, the dietary calcium/phpsphorus ratio, and bone fractures in girls and boys. J Adolesc Health. 1994;15:210–215.
56. US Department of Agriculture. Data tables: results from USDA's 1994–96 Continuing Survey of Food Intakes by Individuals and 1994–96 Diet and Health Knowledge Survey. Washington, DC: US Government Printing Office; 1997; 29–32.
57. Reiss E, Canterbury JM, Bercovitz MA, Kaplan EL. The role of phosphate in the secretion of parathyroid hormone in man. J Clin Invest. 1970;49:146–149.
58. Van den Berg CJ, Kumar R, Wilson DM, et al. Orthophosphate therapy decreases urinary calcium excretion and serum 1,25-dihydroxyvitamin D concentrations in idiopathic hypercalciuria. J Clin Endocrinol Metab. 1980;51:99–101.
59. Silverberg SJ, Shane E, Clemens TL,et al. The effect of oral phosphate administration on major indices of skeletal metabolism in normal subjects. J Bone Miner Res. 1986;1:383–388.
60. Silverberg S J, Shane E, Luz de la Cruz RN, et al. Abnormalities in parathyroid hormone secretion and 1,25-dihydroxyvitamin D3 formation in women with osteoporosis. N Engl J Med. 1989;320:277–281.
61. Calvo MS, Kumar R, Heath H III. Elevated secretion and action of serum parathyroid hormone in young adults consuming high phosphorus, low calcium diets assembled from common foods. J Clin Endocrinol Metab. 1988;66:823–829.
62. Calvo MS, Kumar R, Heath H III. Persistently elevated parathyroid hormone secretion and action in young woman after four weeks of ingesting high

phosphorus low calcium diets. J Clin Endocrinol Metab. 1990;70:1334–1340.

63. Brixen K, Nielsen HK, Charles P, Mosekilde L. Effects of a short course of oral phosphate treatment on serum parathyroid hormone (1–84) and biochemical markers of bone turnover: A dose response study. Calcif Tissue Int. 1992;51:276–281.
64. Karkkainen M, Lamberg-Allardt C. An acute intake of phosphate increases parathyroid hormone secretion and inhibits bone formation in young women. J Bone Miner Res. 1996;11:1905–1912.
65. Bizik BK, Ding W, Cerklewski FL. Evidence that bone resorption of young men is not increased by high dietary phosphorus obtained from milk and cheese. Nutr Res. 1996;16:1143–1146.
66. Whybro A, Jager H, Barker M, Eastell, R. Phosphate supplementation in young men: Lack of effect on calcium homeostasis and bone turnover. Eur J Clin Nutr. 1998;52:29–33.
67. Portale AA, Halloran BP, Murphy MM, Morris RC Jr. Oral intake of phosphorus can determine the serum concentration of 1,25-dihydroxyvitamin D by determining its production rate in humans. J Clin Invest. 1986;77:7–12.
68. Portale AA, Halloran BH, Morris RC Jr. Dietary intake of phosphorus modulates the circadian rhythm in serum concentration of phosphorus. J Clin Invest. 1987;80:1147–1154.
69. Zemel MB, Linkswiler HM. Calcium metabolism in the young adult male as affected by level and form of phosphorus intake and level of calcium intake. J Nutr. 1981;111:315–324.
70. Akesson K, Lau K-H, Johnston P, et al. Effects of short-term calcium depletion and repletion on biochemical markers of bone turnover in young adult women. J Clin Endocrinol Metab. 1998;83:1921–1927.
71. Brot C, Jorgensen N, Jensen LB, Sorensen OH. Relationships between bone mineral density, serum vitamin D metabolites and calcium:phosphorus intake in healthy perimenopausal women. J Intern Med. 1999;245:509–516.
72. Anderson JJB. Calcium, phosphorus and human bone development. J Nutr. 1996;126:1153S–1158S.
73. Pettifor, JM, Marie PJ, Sly MR, et al. The effects of differing dietary calcium and phosphorus contents on mineral metabolism and bone histomorphometry in young vitamin D-replete baboons. Calcif Tissue Int. 1984;36:668–676.
74. Slatopolsky E, Brown A. The role of phosphorus in the development of secondary hyperparathyroidism and parathyroid cell proliferation in chronic renal failure. Am J Med Sci. 1999;317:370–376.
75. Almaden Y, Canalejo A, Hernandez A, et al. Direct effect of phosphorus on PTH secretion from whole rat parathyroid glands in vitro. J Bone Miner Res. 1996;11:970–976.
76. Almaden Y, Hernandez A, Torregrosa V, et al. High phosphate level directly stimulates parathyroid hormone secretion and synthesis by human parathyroid tissue in vitro. J Am Soc Nephrol. 1998;9:1845–1852.
77. Canalejo A, Hernandez A, Almaden Y, et al. The effect of a high phosphorus diets on parathyroid cell cycle. Nephrol Dial Transplant. 1998;13(suppl 3): 19–22.
78. Tatsumi S, Segawa H, Morita R, et al. Molecular cloning and hormonal regulation of PiT-1, a sodium-dependent phosphate cotransporter from rat parathyroid glands. Endocrinology. 1998;139:1692–1699.
79. Chertow GM, Burke SK, Raggi P. Sevelamer attenuates the progression of coronary and aortic vascular calcification in hemodialysis patients. Kidney Int. 2002;62:245–252.
80. Slatopolsky E, Brown A, Dusso A. Pathogenesis of secondary hyperparathyroidism. Kidney Int. 1999; 73(suppl):514–519.
81. Portale AA, Booth BE, Halloran BP, Morris RC Jr. Effect of dietary phosphorus on circulating concentrations of 1,25-dihydroxyvitamin D and immunoreactive parathyroid hormone in children with moderate renal insufficiency. J Clin Invest. 1984;73: 1580–1589.
82. Lopez-Hilker S, Dusso A, Rapp N. Phosphorus restriction reverses hyperparathyroidism in uremia independent of changes in calcium and calcitriol. Am J Physiol. 1990;259:F432–F437.
83. Slatopolsky E, Finch J, Dendra M, et al. Phosphorus restriction prevents parathyroid gland growth. Phosphorus directly stimulates secretion in vitro. J Clin Invest. 1996;97:2534–2540.
84. Dendra M, Finch J, Slatopolsky E. Phosphorus accelerates the development of parathyroid hyperplasia and secondary hyperparathyroidism in rats with renal failure. Am J Kidney Dis. 1996;28:596–602.
85. Goodman, WG, Coburn JW, Slatopolsky E, Salusky IB. Renal osteodystrophy in adults and children. In: Favus M, ed. *Primer on the Metabolic Bone Diseases and Disorders of Mineral Metabolism.* 3rd ed. Philadelphia: Lippincott-Raven; 1996; 341–360.
86. Sheikh MS, Maruire JA, Emmet M, et al. Reduction of dietary phosphorus absorption by phosphorus binders. J Clin Invest. 1989;83:66–73.
87. Uribarri J, Calvo MS. Hidden sources of phosphorus in the typical American diet: does it matter in nephrology? Semin Dial. 2003;16:186–188.
88. Ervin RB, Wang C-Y, Wright J, et al. Dietary intake of selected minerals for the United States population: 1999–2000. In: *Advance Data from Vital and Health Statistics No. 341, April 27, 2004.* Washington, DC: Centers for Disease Control and Prevention, National Center for Health Statistics, US Public Health Service; 2004.

89. US Department of Agriculture. Continuing Survey of Food Intakes by Individuals (CSFII): Diet and Health Knowledge Survey 1989. Springfield, VA: US Department of Commerce, National Technical Information Service (PB93500411: machine readable data set); 1993.

90. US Department of Agriculture. Continuing Survey of Food Intakes by Individuals (CSFII): Diet and Health Knowledge Survey 1990. Springfield, VA: U.S. Department of Commerce, National Technical Information Service (PB93504843: machine readable data set); 1993.

# 31 Magnesium

Stella Lucia Volpe

## Introduction

Magnesium is an essential mineral and a cofactor for over 300 enzymatic reactions in the body.[1] These reactions include: deoxyribonucleic acid (DNA) and ribonucleic acid (RNA) synthesis, protein synthesis, cell growth and reproduction, adenylate cyclase synthesis, cellular energy production and storage, preservation of cellular electrolyte composition, and stabilization of mitochondrial membranes.[3-6] Magnesium also plays a fundamental role in controlling nerve transmission, cardiac excitability, neuromuscular conduction, muscular contraction, vasomotor tone, and blood pressure.[3-6]

## Distribution

The body consists of about 25 g of magnesium, with about 50% to 60% in the bone, and the other 50% in soft tissue.[1,5] Less than 1% of total body magnesium is in the blood.[1] Note that most of the clinical laboratory data are derived from the assessment of serum magnesium concentrations,[1] although this has changed in the last several years with other methods of magnesium assessment evolving, such as evaluating plasma ionized magnesium.

Approximately one-third of skeletal magnesium is exchangeable, and acts as a pool for sustaining normal extracellular magnesium levels[7] (Table 1). Normal serum magnesium concentrations range from 1.8 to 2.3 mg/dL,[8] and this concentration is tightly regulated. Wary et al.[9] reported that 30 healthy male volunteers showed no significant change in plasma magnesium levels after one month of supplementation with 12 mmol/d of magnesium lactate.

## Chemistry and Functions

Magnesium ($Mg^{+2}$) is a divalent metal ion. It is the fourth most abundant cation in the body after calcium, potassium, and sodium.[10] Magnesium is the most prevalent intracellular divalent cation and the second most abundant intracellular cation after potassium.[2,7] It is usually bound to ligands and forms comparatively stable complexes.[1,10] Ionized magnesium represents the physiologically active form of the mineral; however, the protein-bound and the chelated forms of magnesium act as buffers for the ionized pool.[1]

There are a minimum of three different body pools of magnesium in the human body: one with a quick turnover (from about 1.6 to 28 hours), which is largely comprised of extracellular magnesium; a second with a turnover rate of half of the first pool, principally consisting of intracellular magnesium (about 11 days); and a third pool containing skeletal magnesium with a slow turnover rate (over 11 days).[11-13] Approximately 30% of serum magnesium is bound to protein, while the majority of the residual portion is ionized and filtered through the kidney. Intracellular magnesium is bound chiefly to protein and energy-rich phosphates.[4,11] The primary role of magnesium in the body is to complex highly charged anions, such as polyphosphates and nucleic acids, to support enzyme-substrate interactions, or to stabilize the conformation of polymers.[4,10]

Magnesium is required for a number of metabolic reactions, including aerobic and anaerobic metabolism, gly-

**Table 1.** Distribution of Magnesium in the Body

| | |
|---|---|
| Bone | 0.5% of bone ash |
| Muscle | 9 mmol/kg wet weight |
| Soft tissue | 9 mmol/kg wet weight |
| Adipose tissue | 0.8 mmol/kg wet weight |
| Serum magnesium (free) | ~0.56 mmol/L |
| Saliva, gastric, bile | 0.3 to 0.7 mmol/L |
| Sweat | 0.3 mmol/L |

Used with permission from Newhouse and Finstad, 2000.[3]

colysis (both directly as an enzyme activator and indirectly as part of the magnesium-adenosine triphosphate (ATP) complex), and in oxidative phosphorylation.[7] Magnesium is also required for the adequate supply of purines and pyrmidines for RNA and DNA synthesis. Magnesium may directly augment adenylate cyclase activity, as well as sodium, potassium-ATPase activity,[14] which is required for the active transport of potassium.[15]

Magnesium has been called "nature's physiological calcium channel blocker,"[16,17] because during magnesium depletion, intracellular calcium increases. It has been well documented that calcium plays an important role in skeletal and smooth muscle contraction; therefore, magnesium depletion can lead to muscle cramps, hypertension, and coronary and cerebral vasospasms.[8] Indeed, magnesium therapy may show promise as an important adjuvant therapy for acute myocardial infarction.[19-21] Because magnesium is an inorganic calcium channel blocker,[16,22] its ability to decrease infarct size may be a result of magnesium's calcium channel-blocking action at the level of the plasma membrane or an intracellular site.[21]

## Absorption and Homeostasis

Like most minerals, the amount of magnesium absorbed is inversely proportional to the amount ingested. Although magnesium is absorbed throughout the intestinal tract, the greatest amount is absorbed in the distal jejunum and ileum,[23] with about a 40% to 60% net absorption rate from food. Magnesium is absorbed via active transport and passive diffusion; active transport accounts for a greater fractional absorption of calcium at low dietary intakes, while passive diffusion occurs at higher dietary intakes, resulting in lower fractional absorption.[24,25] Calbindin-D9k may play a role in magnesium absorption,[8] but its role has not been clearly defined.

The kidney is the primary organ regulating magnesium homeostasis.[26] About 65% of filtered magnesium is reabsorbed at the loop of Henle via active transport.[26] Approximately 20% to 30% of magnesium is reabsorbed via passive diffusion in the proximal convoluted tubule of the kidney, which is associated with calcium, sodium, and water transport.[23,26] Though excessive magnesium is almost entirely excreted, during magnesium deficiency, the kidney excretes less than 12 to 24 mg/d.[23] Renal magnesium excretion is augmented by diets high in sodium, calcium, and protein, as well as by caffeine and alcohol consumption.[27-30]

The method(s) of magnesium transport in the intestine and kidney have not been elucidated, and at present, there have not been any specific hormones or other compounds that have been designated to play a major role.[23]

## Factors Affecting Absorption

A dietary intake averaging about 300 to 350 mg/d of magnesium will typically result in a fractional absorption rate between 30% and 50%.[31] A number of factors can decrease magnesium absorption, including: fiber, phytates and oxalates from fruits, vegetables, and grains; excessive alcohol intake; and medications such as diuretics.

Phosphorus, calcium, and protein have been shown to decrease magnesium absorption. It appears that the phytate in high-fiber foods results in binding magnesium to the phosphate groups on the phytates, resulting in decreased magnesium absorption.[32-34]

Several researchers have reported no effects of either high-calcium diets (up to 2000 mg/d) on magnesium absorption, or high magnesium intakes (up to 826 mg/d) on calcium absorption.[35,36] Nonetheless, because many calcium channels are dependent on magnesium, intracellular calcium levels increase with magnesium deficiency.[37] Furthermore, individuals who have low serum magnesium levels and are also calcium deficient do not respond to calcium supplementation until the magnesium deficiency has been corrected.[38,39] Parathyroid hormone (PTH) is most likely the principal reason for this, because magnesium deficiency impairs PTH release and its uptake by bone.[38-41]

Protein has also been associated with magnesium absorption, which is lower when dietary protein is less than 30 g/d.[42] Higher protein intakes of more than 94 g/d may result in increased renal magnesium excretion due to the increased acid load; however, magnesium retention has been shown to remain the same on higher-protein diets.[43,44] Others have reported that magnesium absorption and maintenance were better with higher protein intakes (93 g/d) than with lower protein intakes (43 g/d).[45]

Though there is no definitive research on how boron may affect magnesium absorption, there does appear to be an interaction between the two.[46-48] It appears that, when boron concentrations are low, magnesium may be the mineral called upon to take over boron's roles in the body.[46] Furthermore, it appears that boron supplementation may increase serum magnesium concentrations over time.[47,48]

## Magnesium Transport

Magnesium transport in and out of cells requires carrier-mediated transport systems.[49,50] Magnesium efflux from the cell is associated with sodium transport, while magnesium influx is associated with sodium and bicarbonate transport, although by a different method than that of magnesium efflux.[8,49,50]

## Magnesium Requirements

The Dietary Reference Intakes (DRIs) for magnesium are listed in Table 2. These represent the most recent DRIs established in 1997. The indicators used to establish the Estimated Average Requirements (EAR) for magnesium were based upon magnesium balance studies, because there were not sufficient data to determine an ad-

**Table 2.** Dietary Reference Intakes for Magnesium

| Age & Sex | AI | EAR | RDA *mg/d* | UL* |
|---|---|---|---|---|
| Infants | | | | Unable to establish for magnesium supplementation |
| (Boys & Girls) | | | | |
| 0 to 6 months | 30 | NA | NA | |
| 7 to 12 months | 75 | NA | NA | |
| Children | | | | |
| (Boys & Girls) | | | | |
| 4 to 8 years | NA | 65 | 80 | 65 |
| 4 to 8 years | NA | 110 | 130 | 110 |
| 9 to 13 years | NA | 200 | 240 | 350 |
| Males | | | | |
| 14 to 18 years | NA | 340 | 410 | 350 |
| 19 to 30 years | NA | 330 | 400 | 350 |
| 31 to >70 years | NA | 350 | 420 | 350 |
| Females | | | | |
| 14 to 18 years | NA | 300 | 360 | 350 |
| 19 to 30 years | NA | 255 | 310 | 350 |
| 31 to >70 years | NA | 265 | 320 | 350 |
| Pregnant Females | | | | |
| 14 to 18 years | NA | 335 | 400 | 350 |
| 19 to 30 years | NA | 290 | 350 | 350 |
| 31 to 50 years | NA | 300 | 360 | 350 |
| Lactating Females | | | | |
| 14 to 18 years | NA | 300 | 360 | 350 |
| 19 to 30 years | NA | 255 | 310 | 350 |
| 31 to 50 years | NA | 265 | 320 | 350 |

AI = Adequate Intake; EAR = Estimated Average Requirement; RDA = Recommended Dietary Allowance; UL = Tolerable Upper Intake Levels
*Only includes intake from supplements, not food and water
NA = Not applicable
Data from Food and Nutrition Board, Institute of Medicine, 1997.[8]

vantage for maximal magnesium retention.[8] Because magnesium intake from foods has not been shown to result in adverse effects, the Tolerable Upper Intake Level (UL) of magnesium was established by assessing pharmacological doses of magnesium (e.g., magnesium salts), which have resulted in adverse outcomes.[8]

## Food Sources of Magnesium

Magnesium is a rather ubiquitous mineral, found in a number of foods. Good food sources of magnesium include green, leafy vegetables, unpolished grains, and nuts. Intermediate sources of magnesium include meats, starches, and milk. Refined foods are poor sources of magnesium. Table 3 lists several sources of magnesium.[51,52]

## Magnesium Deficiency

Magnesium deficiency may be caused by excessive alcohol intake, certain medications (e.g., diuretics), malabsorption (typically resulting from short bowel syndrome, celiac disease [gluten-sensitive enteropathy], or Crohn's disease), and/or insufficient intake of magnesium.[8] Loss of appetite, nausea, vomiting, fatigue, and weakness are early signs of magnesium deficiency. As magnesium deficiency is exacerbated, such symptoms as numbness, tingling, muscle contractions and cramps, seizures, personality changes, and coronary spasms (angina pectoris) can transpire.[8,23] Magnesium deficiency has been shown to lead to hypocalcemia, neuromuscular excitability, osteoporosis, diabetes mellitus, and cardiac complications such as hypertension, dysrhythmias, angina pectoris, acute

**Table 3.** Food Sources of Magnesium

| Food | Milligrams (mg) |
|---|---|
| Halibut, cooked, 3 ounces | 90 |
| Almonds, dry roasted, 1 ounce | 80 |
| Cashews, dry roasted, 1 ounce | 75 |
| Soybeans, mature, cooked, 1/2 cup | 75 |
| Spinach, frozen, cooked, 1/2 cup | 75 |
| Nuts, mixed, dry roasted, 1 ounce | 65 |
| Cereal, shredded wheat, 2 rectangular biscuits | 55 |
| Oatmeal, instant, fortified, prepared w/ water, 1 cup | 55 |
| Potato, baked w/ skin, 1 medium | 50 |
| Peanuts, dry roasted, 1 ounce | 50 |
| Peanut butter, smooth, 2 tablespoons | 50 |
| Wheat bran, crude, 2 tablespoons | 45 |
| Black-eyed peas, cooked, 1/2 cup | 45 |
| Yogurt, plain, skim milk, 8 fluid ounces | 45 |
| Bran flakes, 3/4 cup | 40 |
| Vegetarian baked beans, 1/2 cup | 40 |
| Rice, brown, long-grained, cooked, 1/2 cup | 40 |
| Lentils, mature seeds, cooked, 1/2 cup | 35 |
| Banana, raw, 1 medium | 30 |
| Milk, reduced fat (2%) or fat-free, 1 cup | 27 |
| Bread, whole wheat, commercially prepared, 1 slice | 25 |
| Whole milk, 1 cup | 24 |

Used with permission from Gunther 1993.[49]

myocardial infarction, and dyslipidemias.[53] Magnesium supplementation will reverse most of these conditions. Normen et al.[54] assessed whether magnesium (and calcium and sulfate) would be absorbed from mineral water in subjects who had had an ileostomy. The main purpose of conducting their study was to assess if the mineral water would provide an alternative for individuals at risk for developing a deficiency due to low intakes. This was a randomized, controlled cross-over study. Compared with the control period, participants absorbed 30% more magnesium with the mineral water, with consumption during meals showing greater absorption.[54] Therefore, supplementation with magnesium in the form of mineral water appears to be a viable method of increasing intake and absorption.

## Effects of Deficiency

Severe hypomagnesemia (< 12.3 mg/dL) has been associated with increased mortality rates (41%) in patients admitted to postoperative ICUs compared to patients in ICUs with normal serum magnesium concentrations (13%).[55] Low serum magnesium levels, though not a sensitive or precise predictor of patient survival, was frequent among postoperative ICU patients, and patients with severe hypomagnesemia had more cases of hypokalemia (which can lead to dysrhythmias) and greater mortality rates than patients with comparable illnesses who had normal serum magnesium concentrations.[55]

### *Cardiovascular System*

Magnesium may play a role in the management of acute myocardial infarction and atherosclerosis.[1] Because cardiovascular disease typically does not manifest itself until later in life, it is important that there is an improved understanding of ionized magnesium metabolism, which will lead to a better comprehension of the chronic changes of magnesium status that may be dormant.[1] Rosenlund et al.[56] did not find a protective effect against myocardial infarction in individuals who consumed drinking water that had higher levels of magnesium.

"Idiopathic mitral valve prolapse (IMVP) refers to the systolic displacement of one or both mitral leaflets into the left atrium, with or without mitral regurgitation."[57] IMVP is most commonly seen among young women and may be caused by latent tetany due to magnesium deficiency (either by insufficient intake or excessive urinary loss). Because normal plasma magnesium levels are not indicative of magnesium deficiency, Bobkowski et al.[57] recommend that laboratory evaluation include assessment of plasma, erythrocyte, and urinary magnesium concentrations, as well as blood and urinary markers of calcium. Furthermore, correction of the symptoms by the oral magnesium load test (5 mg of magnesium/kg/d) is indicative that the cause was a due to magnesium deficiency. Finally, the authors state that it is necessary to combine magnesium-sparing diuretics or physiological doses of vitamin D with oral magnesium supplementation to sustain the positive results.[57]

### *Blood Pressure*

One of the recommendations from the Canadian Hypertension Education Program is to "follow a reduced fat, low cholesterol diet with an adequate intake of potassium, magnesium and calcium."[58] It appears that diets high in calcium, magnesium, and potassium help to manage hypertension, though the results of epidemiological studies have provided stronger evidence for this[59,60] than magnesium supplementation trials.[61,62] Nevertheless, as is often the case with nutritional studies, more than one nutrient may play a role. Appel et al.[63] reported a significant reduction in blood pressure in non-hypertensive adults who increased their dietary intake of magnesium by approximately 247 mg/d, through increased consumption of fruits and vegetables. These individuals also increased their potassium intake and calcium intake through non-fat dairy consumption[63]; both minerals positively influence blood pressure.

### *Body Mass Index*

Though there is no direct link between magnesium and body mass index (BMI), there may be a correlation between the two. Wang et al.[64] assessed calcium, copper, iron, magnesium, potassium, sodium, and zinc concentrations in the hair samples of women 20 to 50 years of age (N = 392). The women were separated into four groups based upon their BMI: 1) BMI $< 18$ kg/m$^2$, 2) BMI $= 18$ to 25 kg/m$^2$, 3) BMI $= 26$ to 35 kg/m$^2$, and 4) BMI $>$ 35 kg/m$^2$. Group 1 had the highest ratios for calcium-to-magnesium, iron-to-copper, and zinc-to-copper, but the lowest ratio for potassium-to-sodium.[64] In contrast, Group 4 had the highest ratio for potassium-to-sodium, but the lowest for iron-to-copper and zinc-to-copper.[64] There were significant differences between the groups in hair magnesium concentrations. Although these data only show correlations, more research is needed to assess if there are implications to the differences in magnesium status.

### *Osteoporosis*

Magnesium deficiency has been shown to be a risk factor for osteoporosis.[65,66] Stendig-Linberg et al.[67] reported a significant increase in radial bone mineral density (BMD) in women after 750 mg/d of magnesium supplementation for 6 months, followed by 250 mg/d of magnesium for 18 months. Ohgitani et al.[68] found a negative correlation between fingernail magnesium concentration and lumbar BMD.

There is a need for prospective clinical trials to elucidate the effects of magnesium intake (via supplementation and/or increased dietary intake) on the prevention of osteoporosis.[69] Possible mechanisms of how magnesium deficiency may result in osteoporosis include impaired production of PTH and 1,25-dihydroxyvitamin D3, and a compound P-stimulated release of inflammatory cytokines.[69]

### *Calcium Stones*

One of the effects of magnesium deficiency is hypocalcemia, which then can lead to calcium urolithiasis (calcium stones). Johannsson et al.[70] reported that in 56 individuals given magnesium hydroxide, 45 were free of recurrences of new calcium stones, and those who did have recurrences only had 0.03 stones per year during a two-year follow-up period, compared with 0.8 stones per year prior to the magnesium treatment. Of the 34 individuals who had no prophylactic magnesium therapy, 15 had experienced calcium stones after two years.

Conversely, in a retrospective study of 7000 patients suffering from calcium oxalate stones, Schwartz et al.[71] reported that calcium stone formation was slightly, but not significantly, increased in patients with hypomagnesuria. They stated that "the beneficial effects of urinary magnesium on stone formation may be less than previously reported. The role of oral magnesium supplementation and the subsequent increase in urinary magnesium in calcium urinary stone formation remains unknown... If magnesium has a protective effect, it may work through pathways that enhance citrate excretion."[71]

### *Diabetes Mellitus*

It has been reported that magnesium deficiency can lead to insulin resistance and impaired insulin secretion.[8] Magnesium supplementation can improve glucose tolerance and insulin response in elderly individuals with type 2 diabetes mellitus.[72,73]

Diabetes mellitus can lead to long-term complications, such as angiopathy (cardiovascular disease), neuropathy (nerve damage), nephropathy (kidney disease), and retinopathy (retinal problems with the eye). Because of the high rate of cardiovascular disease that occurs with diabetes mellitus, Soltani et al.[74] studied oral magnesium administration to prevent vascular complications in diabetic rats.

The rats were separated into 6 groups: 2 groups received tap water for 8 weeks (control), 2 groups (made diabetic by injection of STZ) were treated with magnesium sulfate (10 g/L) added to the drinking water, and 2 groups (made diabetic by injection of STZ) received tap water only. Mean arterial blood pressure and mean perfusion pressure of the mesenteric vascular bed were significantly lower in the magnesium-treated rats than in the non-treated rats. The authors concluded that magnesium sulfate supplementation was effective in preventing vascular complications associated with diabetes mellitus.[74]

## Magnesium Supplementation

Magnesium supplementation may be required in specific conditions that may decrease magnesium absorption or result in excessive loss.[75-77] As previously discussed, some medications may result in magnesium deficiency, such as some diuretics, antibiotics, and anti-cancer medications.[5,78,79]

Hypomagnesemia occurs in approximately 30% to 60% of individuals with alcoholism; low serum magnesium concentrations occur in about 90% of individuals who are going through withdrawal from alcohol.[80,81]

Those with Crohn's disease, gluten-sensitive enteropathy (celiac disease), regional enteritis, intestinal surgery, or other chronic malabsorptive problems may lose magnesium through diarrhea and fat malabsorption.[82] These individuals may be candidates for magnesium supplementation.

It has been shown that individuals who have poorly managed diabetes mellitus may require supplementation. This is due to the fact that they have increased urinary magnesium excretion coupled with hyperglycemia.[83]

As previously stated, magnesium interacts with calcium and potassium. Therefore, persons with persistently low blood calcium and potassium concentrations may actually have a fundamental problem with magnesium deficiency. Supplements with magnesium may help to alleviate the calcium and potassium deficiencies.[5]

Another group of individuals who may require magnesium supplementation are older adults. The National Health and Nutrition Examination Surveys (NHANES) (both 1999 to 2000 and 1998 to 1994) have shown that older individuals have lower dietary magnesium intakes than do younger individuals.[84,85] Furthermore, older individuals have a greater rate of renal magnesium excretion and a lower rate of intestinal magnesium absorption, exacerbating the problem of a low intake.[8] Many older adults are on multiple medications, which can also lead to a drug-magnesium interaction, further aggravating the decreased intake and absorption and increased renal excretion.[8]

## Effects of Magnesium Excess

Magnesium intake from food substances has not been shown to be harmful; however, magnesium intake from excess supplement intakes has.[8] The main initial effect of excess magnesium intake is diarrhea; magnesium is known for its cathartic effect.[86,87] Nausea and abdominal cramping may also occur.[88]

High serum magnesium concentrations can result in renal failure, which is typically accompanied by high intakes of non-food sources of magnesium.[89,90] For example, high doses of magnesium-containing laxatives and antacids have been shown to cause toxicity.[91]

Signs of excess magnesium can be similar to magnesium deficiency and include changes in mental status, nausea, diarrhea, appetite loss, muscle weakness, difficulty breathing, extremely low blood pressure, and irregular heartbeat.[92-95]

## Methods for Assessing Magnesium Status in Individuals

Serum magnesium is perhaps the most common and straightforward method of assessing magnesium status. An atomic absorption spectrophotometer is used to evaluate magnesium concentration; a serum magnesium concentration under 1.8 mg/dL is indicative of magnesium depletion.[7] Nonetheless, plasma-ionized magnesium may be a better method of assessing magnesium status.[8] Other techniques to assess magnesium status include: clinical evaluation, blood mononuclear cells, magnesium excretion, intracellular magnesium assessment, red blood cell magnesium concentration determined by nuclear magnetic resonance, magnesium balance studies, magnesium tolerance test, and epidemiological studies and meta-analysis.[5,8] The magnesium tolerance test has been used for a number of years, and is considered the "gold standard" for assessing magnesium status in adults, but not infants and children.[8] In the magnesium tolerance test, the renal excretion of magnesium is assessed, and is based on magnesium that has been supplied through a parenteral route.[8] Although the magnesium tolerance test may be a good indicator of hypomagnesemia, it does not appear to be sensitive enough to sense changes in magnesium status in healthy individuals who have been given magnesium supplementation.[8]

Approximately 99% of the body magnesium is intracellular, and therefore, assessment of intracellular ionized magnesium is physiologically appropriate.[96] Malon et al.[96] examined ionized magnesium in erythrocytes to establish reliable methodology in the evaluation of functional magnesium status. The authors also assessed ionized magnesium and total serum magnesium (by atomic absorption spectrometry). The aforementioned measurements were conducted in critically ill postoperative patients. They reported hypomagnesemia in 15.9% of the patients using total serum magnesium, compared with 22.2% using ionized magnesium and 36.5% using ionized magnesium in erythrocytes. The authors concluded that ionized magnesium in erythrocytes may be the best method to detect hypo- or hypermagnesemia.

## Future Research Directions

Due to magnesium's role in many reactions in the body, there are a number of research areas that could be pursued, especially those that may help to prevent disease. It is clear that magnesium benefits the cardiovascular system; however, the main question that comes to mind is the exact mechanism through which magnesium plays a role in diabetes mellitus, cardiovascular disease, and hypertension. Basic scientific research needs to be conducted to ascertain the mechanisms involved. In addition, longitudinal studies in humans are required to evaluate the levels of magnesium necessary to prevent chronic disease. These need to be followed by magnesium supplementation studies to evaluate the effectiveness of supplementation on the prevention of disease, and the effects it may have on exercise performance.

## References


1. Elin RJ. Magnesium: the fifth but forgotten electrolyte. Am J Clin Pathol. 1994;102:616–622.
2. Rude RK, Oldham SB. Disorders of magnesium metabolism. In: Cohen RD, Lewis B, Alberti KG, Denman AM, eds. *The Metabolic and Molecular Basis of Acquired Disease*. London: Bailliere Tindall; 1990; 1124–1148.
3. Newhouse IJ, Finstad EW. The effects of magnesium supplementation on exercise performance. Clin J Sport Med. 2000;10:195–200.
4. Bohl CH, Volpe SL. Magnesium and exercise. Crit Rev Food Sci Nutr. 2002;42:533–563.
5. Shils ME. Magnesium. In: Shils ME, Olson JA,

Shike M, Ross AC, eds. *Modern Nutrition in Health and Disease.* 9th ed. Baltimore: Lippincott Williams & Wilkins; 1999; 169–192.

6. Chubanov V, Gudermann T, Schlingmann KP. Essential role for TRPM6 in epithelial magnesium transport and body magnesium homeostasis. Pflugers Arch. 2005;Jun 17:[Epub ahead of print].
7. Elin RJ. Assessment of magnesium status. Clin Chem. 1987;33:1965–1970.
8. Food and Nutrition Board, Institute of Medicine. Dietary Reference Intakes for Calcium, Phosphorus, Magnesium, Vitamin D, and Fluoride. Washington, DC: National Academies Press; 1997. Available online at: http://www.nap.edu/books/0309063507/html.
9. Wary C, Brillault-Salvat C, Bloch G, et al. Effect of chronic magnesium supplementation on magnesium distribution in healthy volunteers evaluated by $^{31}$P-NMRS and ion selective electrodes. Br J Clin Pharmacol. 1999;48:655–662.
10. Frausto da Silva JJR, Williams RJ. The biological chemistry of magnesium: phosphorus metabolism. In: *The Biological Chemistry of the Elements.* Oxford: Oxford University Press; 1991; 241–267.
11. Wester PO. Magnesium. Am J Clin Nutr. 1987; 45(suppl):1305–1312.
12. Feillet-Coudray C, Coudray C, Tressol JC, et al. Exchangeable magnesium pool masses in healthy women: effects of magnesium supplementation. Am J Clin Nutr. 2002;75:72–78.
13. Feillet-Coudray C, Coudray C, Brule F, et al. Exchangeable magnesium pool masses reflect the magnesium status of rats. J Nutr. 2000;130:2306–2311.
14. Maguire ME. Hormone-sensitive magnesium transport and magnesium regulation of adenylate cyclase. Trends Pharmacol Sci. 1984;5:73–77.
15. Dorup I, Clausen T. Correlation between magnesium and potassium contents in muscle: Role of $Na(^{+})$-$K(^{+})$ pump. Am J Physiol. 1993;264: C457–C463.
16. Iseri LT, French JH. Magnesium: nature's physiologic calcium blocker. Am Heart J. 1984;108: 188–193.
17. White RE, Hartzell HC. Magnesium ions in cardiac function. Biochem Pharmacol. 1989;38:859–867.
18. Teo KK, Yusuf S. Role of magnesium in reducing mortality in acute myocardial infarction. Drugs. 1993;46:347–359.
19. Horner SM. Efficacy of intravenous magnesium in acute myocardial infarction in reducing arrhythmias and mortality. Circulation. 1992;86:774–779.
20. Herzog WR, Schlossberg ML, MacMurdy KS, et al. Timing of magnesium therapy affects experimental infarct size. Circulation. 1995;92:2622–2626.
21. Sadeh M. Action of magnesium sulfate in the treatment of preeclampsia-eclampsia. Stroke. 1989;20: 1273–1275.
22. White RE, Hartzell HC. Magnesium ions in cardiac function. Biochem Pharmacol. 1989;38:859–867.
23. Rude RK. Magnesium deficiency: A cause of heterogeneous disease in humans. J Bone Miner Res. 1998; 13:749–758.
24. Kayne LH, Lee DBN. Intestinal magnesium absorption. Miner Electrolyte Metab. 1993;19:210–217.
25. Fine KD, Santa Ana CA, Porter JL, Fordtran JS. Intestinal absorption of magnesium from food and supplements. J Clin Invest. 1991;88:396–402.
26. Quamme GA, Dirks JH. The physiology of renal magnesium handling. Renal Physiol. 1986;9:257–269.
27. Mahalko JR, Sandstead HH, Johnson LK, Milne DB. Effect of a moderate increase in dietary protein on the retention and excretion of Ca, Cu, Fe, Mg, P, and Zn by adult males. Am J Clin Nutr. 1983;37: 8–14.
28. Martinez ME, Salinas M, Miguel JL, et al. Magnesium excretion in idiopathic hypercalciuria. Nephron. 1985;40:446–450.
29. Massey LK, Whiting SJ. Caffeine, urinary calcium, calcium metabolism and bone. J Nutr. 1993;123: 1611–1614.
30. Abbott L, Nadler J, Rude RK. Magnesium deficiency in alcoholism: Possible contribution to osteoporosis and cardiovascular disease in alcoholics. Alcohol Clin Exp Res. 1994;18:1976–1082.
31. Schwartz R, Spencer H, Welsh JJ. Magnesium absorption in human subjects from leafy vegetables, intrinsically labeled with stable $^{26}$Mg. Am J Clin Nutr. 1984;39:571–576.
32. Brink EJ, Beynen AC. Nutrition and magnesium absorption: A review. Prog Food Nutr Sci. 1992;16: 125–162.
33. Franz KB. Influence of phosphorus on intestinal absorption of calcium and magnesium. In: Itokawa Y, Durlach J, eds. *Magnesium in Health and Disease.* London: John Libbey & Co.; 1989; 71–78.
34. Wisker E, Nagel R, Tanudjaja TK, Feldheim W. Calcium, magnesium, zinc, and iron balances in young women: Effects of a low-phytate barley-fiber concentrate. Am J Clin Nutr. 1991;54:553–559.
35. Spencer H, Fuller H, Norris C, Williams D. Effect of magnesium on the intestinal absorption of calcium in man. J Am Coll Nutr. 1994;13:485–492.
36. Andon MB, Ilich JZ, Tzagournis MA, Matkovic V. Magnesium balance in adolescent females consuming a low- or high-calcium diet. Am J Nutr. 1996;63: 950–953.
37. Dacey MJ. Hypomagnesemic disorders. Crit Care Clin. 2001;17:155–173.
38. Al-Ghamdi SM, Cameron EC, Sutton RA. Magnesium deficiency: Pathophysiology and clinical overview. Am J Kidney Dis. 1994;24:737–752.
39. Dhupa N, Proulx J. Hypocalcemia and hypomagne-

semia. Vet Clin North Am Small Anim Pract. 1998; 28:587–608.

40. Estep H, Shaw WA, Watlington C, et al. Hypocalcemia due to hypomagnesemia and reversible parathyroid hormone unresponsiveness. J Clin Endocrinol Metab. 1969;29:842–848.
41. Freitag JJ, Martin KJ, Conrades MB, et al. Evidence for skeletal resistance to parathyroid hormone in magnesium deficiency: Studies in isolated perfused bone. J Clin Invest. 1979:64:1238–1244.
42. Hunt MS, Schofield FA. Magnesium balance and protein intake level in adult human female. Am J Clin Nutr. 1969;22:367–373.
43. Mahalko JR, Sandstead HH, Johnson LK, Milne DB. Effect of a moderate increase in dietary protein on the retention and excretion of Ca, Cu, Fe, Mg, P, and Zn by adult males. Am J Clin Nutr. 1983;37: 8–14.
44. Wong NL, Quamme GA, Dirks JH. Effects of acid-base disturbances on renal handling of magnesium in the dog. Clin Sci. 1986;70:277–284.
45. Schwartz R, Walker G, Linz MD, MacKellar I. Metabolic responses of adolescent boys to two levels of dietary magnesium and protein. I. Magnesium and nitrogen retention. Am J Clin Nutr. 1973;26: 510–518.
46. Volpe SL, Taper LJ, Meacham SL. The relationship between boron and magnesium status, and bone mineral density in humans: A review. Magnes Res. 1993; 6:291–296.
47. Meacham SL, Taper LJ, Volpe SL. The effect of boron supplementation on blood and urinary calcium, magnesium, phosphorus, and urinary boron in female athletes. Am J Clin Nutr. 1995;61:341–345.
48. Meacham SL, Taper LJ, Volpe SL. The effects of boron supplementation on bone mineral density, dietary, blood and urinary calcium, phosphorus, magnesium, and boron in female athletes. Environ Health Perspectives (NIEHS Publication: Proceedings of the 1st International Symposium on the Health Effects of Boron and its Compounds). 1994; 102(suppl 7):79–82.
49. Gunther T. Mechanisms and regulation of $Mg^{2+}$ efflux and $Mg^{2+}$ influx. Miner Electrolyte Metab. 1993;19:259–265.
50. Romani A, Marfella C, Scarpa A. Cell magnesium transport and homeostasis: role of intracellular compartments. Miner Electrolyte Metab. 1993;19: 282–289.
51. U.S. Department of Agriculture, Agricultural Research Service. 2003. USDA National Nutrient Database for Standard Reference, Release 16. Nutrient Data Laboratory Home Page, http://www.nal.usda.gov/fnic/foodcomp.
52. National Institutes of Health, Office of Dietary Supplements. Retrieved August 14, 2005 http://ods.od.nih.gov/factsheets/magnesium.asp, updated January 30, 2005
53. Gums JG. Magnesium in cardiovascular and other disorders. Am J Health-Syst Pharm. 2004;61: 1569–1576.
54. Normen L, Arnaud MJ, Carlsson NG, Andersson H. Small bowel absorption of magnesium and calcium sulphate from a natural mineral water in subjects with ileostomy. Eur J Nutr. 2005;Jul 15:[Epub ahead of print].
55. Chernow B, Bamberger S, Stoiko M, et al. Hypomagnesemia in patients in postoperative intensive care. Chest. 1989;95:391–397.
56. Rosenlund M, Berglind N, Hallqvist J, et al. Daily intake of magnesium and calcium from drinking water in relation to myocardial infarction. Epidemiol. 2005;16:570–576.
57. Bobkowski W, Nowak A, Durlach J. The importance of magnesium status in the pathophysiology of mitral valve prolapse. Magnes Res. 2005;18:35–52.
58. Khan NA, McAlister FA, Lewanczuk RZ, et al. The 2005 Canadian Hypertension Education Program recommendations for the management of hypertension: Part II - Therapy. Can J Cardiol. 2005;21: 657–672.
59. Ascherio R, Rimm EB, Giovannucci EL, et al. A prospective study of nutritional factors and hypertension among U.S. men. Circulation. 1992;86: 1475–1484.
60. Ma J, Folsom AR, Melnick SL, et al. Associations of serum and dietary magnesium with cardiovascular disease, hypertension, diabetes, insulin, and carotid arterial wall thickness: The ARIC study. Atherosclerosis Risk in Community Study. J Clin Epidemiol. 1995;48:927–940.
61. Sacks FM, Brown LE, Appel L, et al. Combinations of potassium, calcium, and magnesium supplements in hypertension. Hypertension. 1995;26:950–956.
62. Yamamoto ME, Applegate WB, Klag MJ, et al. Lack of blood pressure effect with calcium and magnesium supplementation in adults with high-normal blood pressure. Results from Phase I of the Trials of Hypertension Prevention (TOPH). Trials of Hypertension Prevention (TOPH) Research Group. Ann Epidemiol. 1995;5:96–107.
63. Appel LJ, Moore TJ, Obarzanek E, et al. A clinical trial of the effects of the dietary patterns on blood pressure. N Engl J Med. 1997;336:1117–1124.
64. Wang CT, Chang WT, Zeng WF, Lin CH. Concentrations of calcium, copper, iron, magnesium, potassium, sodium and zinc in adult female hair with different body mass indexes in Taiwan. Clin Chem Lab Med. 2005;43:389–393.
65. Stendig-Lindberg G, Koeller W, Bauer A, Rob PM. Prolonged magnesium deficiency causes osteoporosis in the rat. J Am Coll Nutr. 2004;23:704S–711S.
66. Saito N, Tabata N, Saito S, et al. Bone mineral den-

sity, serum albumin and serum magnesium. J Am Coll Nutr. 2004;23:701S–703S.
67. Stendig-Lindberg G, Tepper R, Leichter I. Trabecular bone density in a two year controlled trial of peroral magnesium in osteoporosis. Magnes Res. 1993; 6:155–163.
68. Ohgitani S, Fujita T, Fujii Y, Hayashi C, Nishio H. Nail calcium and magnesium content in relation to age and bone mineral density. J Bone Miner Metab. 2005;23:318–322.
69. Rude RK, Gruber HE. Magnesium deficiency and osteoporosis: animal and human observations. J Nutr Biochem. 2004;15:710–716.
70. Johansson G, Backman U, Danielson BG, Fellstrom B, Ljunghall S, Wikstrom B. Biochemical and clinical effects of the prophylactic treatment of renal calcium stones with magnesium hydroxide. J Urol. 1980;124:770–774.
71. Schwartz BF, Bruce J, Leslie S, Stoller ML. Rethinking the role of urinary magnesium in calcium urolithiasis. J Endourol. 2001;15:233–235.
72. Paolisso G, Sgambato S, Gambardella A, et al. Daily magnesium supplements improve glucose handling in elderly subjects. Am J Clin Nutr. 1992;55: 1161–1167.
73. Paolisso G, Passariello N, Pizza G, et al. Dietary magnesium supplements improve B-cell response to glucose and arginine in elderly non-insulin-dependent diabetic subjects. Acad Endocrinol Copenh. 1989;121:16–20.
74. Soltani N, Keshavarz M, Sohanaki H, et al. Oral magnesium administration prevents vascular complications in STZ-diabetic rats. Life Sci. 2005;76: 1455–1464.
75. Vormann J. Magnesium: nutrition and metabolism. Molec Aspects Med. 2003;24:27–37.
76. Ladefoged K, Hessov I, Jarnum S. Nutrition in short-bowel syndrome. Scand J Gastroenterol Suppl. 1996;216:122–131.
77. Kelepouris E, Agus ZS. Hypomagnesemia: renal magnesium handling. Semin Nephrol. 1998;18: 58–73.
78. Ramsay LE, Yeo WW, Jackson PR. Metabolic effects of diuretics. Cardiology. 1994;84(suppl 2): 48–56.
79. Lajer H, Daugaard G. Cisplatin and hypomagnesemia. Ca Treat Rev. 1999;25:47–58.
80. Elisaf M, Bairaktari E, Kalaitzidis R, Siamopoulos K. Hypomagnesemia in alcoholic patients. Alcohol Clin Exp Res. 1998;22:244–246.
81. Abbott L, Nadler J, Rude RK. Magnesium deficiency in alcoholism: Possible contribution to osteoporosis and cardiovascular disease in alcoholics. Alcohol Clin Exp Res. 1994;18:1076–1082.
82. Rude RK, Olerich M. Magnesium deficiency: Possible role in osteoporosis associated with gluten-sensitive enteropathy. Osteoporos Int. 1996;6: 453–461.
83. American Diabetes Association. Nutrition recommendations and principles for people with diabetes mellitus. Diabetes Care. 1999;22:542–545.
84. Ford ES, Mokdad AH. Dietary magnesium intake in a national sample of U.S. adults. J Nutr. 2003;133: 2879–2882.
85. Bialostosky K, Wright JD, Kennedy-Stephenson J, et al. *Dietary Intake of Macronutrients, Micronutrients and Other Dietary Constituents: United States 1988–1994. Vital Heath Stat. 11(245).* Washington, DC: National Center for Health Statistics; 2002; 168.
86. Rude RK, Singer FR. Magnesium deficiency and excess. Ann Rev Med. 1980;32:245–259.
87. Fine KD, Santa Ana CA, Fordtran JS. Diagnosis of magnesium-induced diarrhea. N Engl J Med. 1981; 324:1012–1017.
88. Ricci JM, Hariharan S, Helfott A. Oral tocolysis with magnesium chloride: A randomized controlled prospective clinical trial. Am J Obstet Gynecol. 1991; 165:603–610.
89. Mordes JP, Wacker WE. Excessive magnesium. Pharmacol Rev. 1978;29:273–300.
90. Randall RE, Cohen D, Spray CC, Rossmeisl EC. Hypermagnesemia in renal failure. Ann Intern Med. 1964;61:73–88.
91. Xing JH, Soffer EE. Adverse effects of laxatives. Dis Colon Rectum. 2001;44:1201–1209.
92. Jaing TH, Hung IH, Chung HT, et al. Acute hypermagnesemia: A rare complication of antacid administration after bone marrow transplantation. Clinica Chimica Acta. 2002;326:201–203.
93. Whang R. Clinical disorders of magnesium metabolism. Compr Ther. 1997;23:168–173.
94. Ho J, Moyer TP, Phillips S. Chronic diarrhea: The role of magnesium. Mayo Clin Proc. 1995;70: 1091–1092.
95. Nordt S, Williams SR, Turchen S, et al. Hypermagnesemia following an acute ingestion of Epsom salt in a patient with normal renal function. J Toxicol Clin Toxicol. 1996;34:735–739.
96. Malon A, Brockmann C, Fijalkowska-Morawska J, et al. Ionized magnesium in erythrocytes—the best magnesium parameter to observe hypo- or hypermagnesemia. Clin Chim Acta. 2004;349:67–73.

# 32 Electrolytes: Sodium, Chloride, and Potassium

Harry G. Preuss

## *General Background*

Life is estimated to have begun 2 billion years ago in the Precambrian seas[1] because they provided mobility, richness in dissolved substances, and stability of physicochemical conditions.[1-7] The presence of oceans and seas is unique in our solar system. It is generally believed that no other planet possesses liquid water, although speculation exists that Mars may have had some in the past. Many scientists believe that the existence of ancient oceans and seas on earth were essential for the development of life as we know it. It is further postulated that terrestrial life emerged from the early Ordovician seas 360 million years ago.[1] In order to live on land, the various forms of life retained their own sea in the form of extracellular and intracellular body fluids.[7,8] Considering the above overall time frame for the emergence of various forms of life, the existence of man is relatively short; man probably came upon the scene 2 million years ago.[9]

The proportions of sodium, chloride, and potassium in the ancient seas has been closely linked with the development of life. Table 1 compares the estimated concentrations of many constituents in seawater during various geological periods with that of human plasma and muscle water.[2,3,5,6,8] It is interesting to speculate whether life could have evolved from ancient oceans had they possessed the current distributions of electrolytes that have changed significantly over time. Over the centuries, the amount of sodium and chloride in the oceans has steadily increased. In contrast, the potassium content has decreased. An interesting hypothesis concerning the evolution of life is based upon the knowledge that the potassium content of the Precambrian seas was much higher with respect to sodium concentration than it is now. Many relate this observation to the high potassium concentrations within cells. Later, with the emergence of life from seas having higher sodium content, this became the basis for the high levels of sodium in extracellular fluid.[10] Regardless of whether these suppositions are real, cells could grow, function, and survive by retaining a friendly environment via tight regulation of their "internal seas."

Kidneys played a major role in the emergence of terrestrial life. Homer Smith[4,8] and later Robert Pitts[9] discussed the crucial role of kidneys in regulating ions and fluid in the body, which allowed vertebrates to leave the sea. The regulation of sodium, chloride, and potassium in both the intracellular and extracellular body fluid compartments by kidneys is especially crucial, because the presence of these cations and anions dictate the size of the body fluid compartments via effects on osmolality and play a significant role in the acid-base balance of the organism. A major difference between plasma and the past and current oceans is the presence of a substantial concentration of proteins in the former. Proteins occupy about 6% of the blood plasma volume, but all of the ions in the blood reside in the remaining 94% of water. Healthy kidneys protect the circulating concentrations of proteins by preventing renal losses. Bernard referred to the precise renal regulation of fluid and solutes as homeostasis of the "milieu interieur."[1]

The regulation of sodium, potassium, and chloride in the human body also depends largely on both the intake of these micronutrients and their eventual loss.[11] Dietary intake has changed over the years and continues to change. These changes play a prominent role in the overall health of numerous modern countries, because nutritional intake can strongly influence the development of many prevalent current health problems, especially cardiovascular and metabolic disorders.[12-14] Cordain et al.[15] noted seven crucial areas in modern diets that may relate to the prevalence of the modern diseases: 1) glycemic load, 2) fatty acid composition, 3) macronutrient compo-

**Table 1.** Ion Concentrations in the Oceans at Various Geological Periods and in Vertebrate Extracellular Fluid

| Ion | Precambrian Sea* | Early Ordovician Sea† | Ocean Today *mmol/L* | Human Plasma | Human Muscle‡ |
|---|---|---|---|---|---|
| Sodium | 298 | 379 | 478 | 142 | 10 |
| Potassium | 104 | 51 | 10 | 4 | 160 |
| Calcium | 2 | 7 | 11 | 5 | |
| Magnesium | 11 | 38 | 55 | 3 | 17.55 |
| Chloride | 298 | 441 | 559 | 103 | 2 |
| Sulfate | 54 | 40 | 29 | 1 | |
| Phosphate | | | Trace | 2 | 140 |
| Protein § | | | | 16 | 55 |

* Approximate time of the development of unicellular organisms.
† Time of emergence of vertebrates.
‡ Per liter of water.
§ Expressed as mEq/L.

sition, 4) micronutrient density, 5) acid-base balance, 6) sodium-potassium ratio, and 7) fiber content. Cardiovascular diseases (CVD) are the most significant cause of death in the industrialized world, including the United States, accounting for approximately 50% of mortality beyond age 65.[16,17] With the emergence of the modern Western diet, in contrast to that of many non-acculturated societies, many cardiovascular and metabolic disorders have become more common. The disorders include obesity, insulin resistance, hypertension, and lipid perturbations. The collection of these risk factors is often referred to as the metabolic syndrome.[18]

It is generally accepted that earlier diets and those from non-acculturated diets contained a higher proportion of potassium than sodium.[19] The reversal of potassium and sodium concentrations in human diets is relatively new in the history of mankind, and unfortunately may play an integral role in the development of modern chronic diseases.[15] Between 1994 and 1996, the typical US diet had a reported average sodium content of 3.27 g/d, an amount that significantly exceeds the average potassium content of 2.62 g/d according to the US Department of Agriculture.[20] The addition of manufactured salt to the food supply and the displacement of traditional potassium-rich foods by foods introduced during the Neolithic and industrial periods caused a 400% decline in the potassium intake while simultaneously initiating a 400% increase in sodium ingestion.[12,21,22] To obtain a better understanding, sodium and potassium as nutrients will be described separately.

# Sodium

## *Facts about Sodium*

To gain a better understanding of sodium balance, it is necessary to differentiate between sodium and salt. Sodium is an essential mineral (micronutrient) that is vital in the balance of body fluids. Dietary sodium is usually measured in grams, but sometimes also in millequivalents or millimoles. The most common source of dietary sodium is table salt, sodium chloride. Because table salt is only 40% sodium, it is necessary to discern whether any reference to mass is discussing grams of sodium or grams of salt. One teaspoon of table salt contains 5.75 g of salt, equivalent to 2.3 g of sodium. A realistic intake of salt is roughly 6.0 ± 1.0 g/d of salt or roughly 2.4 ± 0.4 g of sodium (close to a teaspoonful).

It is generally recognized that most people consuming a modern diet ingest more than the dietary allowances recommended by most groups. The current Recommendation Daily Allowance (RDA) for sodium in the United States is to consume less than 2.4 g/d. The United Kingdom Recommended Nutritional Intake (RNI) advocates an upper limit of 1.6 g. The National Research Council of the National Academy of Sciences suggests a daily range of 1.1 to 3.3 g of sodium for adults. The American Heart Association recommends that 2.3 g/d not be exceeded. However, in those individuals with hypertension, many believe that a daily intake not to exceed 1.5 g of sodium is more appropriate. In contrast to too much sodium, sodium deficiency is uncommon. However, the latter may occur due to loss in sweat during heavy exertion and/or associated with high external temperatures. Not infrequently, physicians treating renal patients with hypertension and congestive heart failure by reducing the body content of sodium are surprised by the elevation of blood urea, which indicates that too much sodium has been removed. Signs of sodium deficiency include: thirst, nausea, weakness, fatigue, and cramps.

## *Salt Intake and Requirements*

In the early half of the 20th century, the widespread use of table salt received little attention from nutritionists, but with the recognition of the association of salt and hypertension, focus on evaluating salt consumption increased considerably.[11] French authors first proposed that exclusion of salt from the diet reduced elevated blood pressure.[23] Early on, the chloride moiety was assumed to be responsible for the blood pressure perturbations—possibly because the measurement of chloride was much more accurate than that of sodium and afforded better evaluation.[24] Later, the development of the flame photometer led to more emphasis on the sodium moiety as the major cause for the significant elevation of blood pressure by salt. However, the two ions seem to work together to control extracellular volume and blood pressure. Sodium coupled to chloride—not to other anions such as bicarbonate—affects fluid distribution in the extracellular compartment.[25] Therefore, although most references here are to sodium, it is important to remember that sodium and chloride are coupled most of the time in the actions—both good and bad—discussed below.

Primal herbivorous humans probably consumed ≤10 mmol/d (0.2–0.3 g/d) of sodium.[11,26] On a successful hunting day, carnivorous humans might even have consumed as much as 60 mmol (1.4 g) of sodium. Over the ensuing years, however, humans developed a significant salt appetite that brought about an estimated increase in sodium intake of 87 to 260 mmol/d (2.0–6.0 g/d). Sodium intake varies greatly among countries. In 1988, Simpson[27] found that the daily intake was ≥300 mmol (6.9 g) in some Japanese men; 235 mmol (5.4 g) in Finland; 150 to 170 mmol (3.5–3.9 g) in the United States, Thailand, and New Zealand; 62 mmol (1.4 g) in a Polynesian island; and <30 mmol (0.69 g) in the Amazon jungle, New Guinea highlands, and Kalahari desert.[28] The values for the United States are slightly higher than the average daily intake reported 10 years later by the US Department of Agriculture.[20]

A difficult-to-answer question often arises concerning whether humans have adapted adequately to the drastic increase in dietary sodium over their 2 million years of existence. It is generally agreed that the intake of sodium by most people exceeds the amount necessary to maintain the balance for healthy existence.[29] How do we handle this? Little sodium appears in the feces, whereas >90% of intake is excreted in the urine. In addition to excreting the usual excesses, the healthy kidney can also conserve sodium at the expense of hydrogen and potassium when necessary. The renal conservation of sodium is so efficient that, if necessary, an intake of only a few millimoles is required to balance the small, non-urinary losses of sodium. To give an example, an average balance of sodium chloride might be a dietary intake of 10.5 g/d in foods and a dietary output of 10.5 g/d: 10.0 g/d in urine, 0.25 g/d in sweat, and 0.25 g/d in the feces.[30]

Recent changes in intake have taken place, because the public has become aware of some of the consequences of "too much salt." Overall consumption of sodium in the United States has declined since 1980 despite the previous steady increase in salt consumption over the last century.[31] The major decrease in sodium intake between 1980 and 1990 was in the discretionary sodium intake from salt shakers—0.06 vs. 0.02 mmol (1.4 vs. 0.5 g)—and not the sodium intake directly from foods, which has remained fairly steady at 0.12 mmol (2.7 g). Data from the Third Health and Nutrition Examination Survey show an average sodium intake of 170 mmol/d (3.9 g/d) for males and 120 mmol/d (2.8 g/d) for females.[32] Most of the sodium in the diet comes from processed foods. A survey of the daily intake of 25 nutrients by 4000 American households conducted by General Mills found that about 70% of sodium consumed in food sources is from meat, fish, poultry, and eggs, mixed dishes, and grain products.[31] The mixed-dish group is divided into soups, grain-based dishes such as macaroni and cheese, and meat-based dishes. Greater interest in the sodium content of the general diet is expected in the future because of access to values on new food labels and the campaign by the National Heart, Lung, and Blood Institute to reduce sodium intake.

Individual minimum daily requirements for salt are difficult to establish. In the Intersalt Study,[33] sodium excretion data from 52 centers throughout the world were examined. There was a wide range of disparity in the excretion used to estimate intake. The ranges of intake, adjusted for body mass index and alcohol intake, were roughly 50 to 250 mmol (1.2 to 5.8 g) sodium over 24 hours.[33] Interestingly, the four centers with the lowest sodium excretion also had the lowest average systolic and diastolic blood pressures. One assumption based on these and other data is that a sodium intake of under 100 mmol/d (2.3 g/d) would lead to a healthful reduction in blood pressure even in individuals without hypertension.

## *Sodium and Chloride in the Body*

The total body sodium of a normal adult averages about 60 mmol/kg body weight.[34] For the typical 70-kg person, this is 4200 mmol, or almost 100 g of sodium. Bone contains 1800 mmol: 40% to 45% of the total sodium. Approximately 2000 to 2200 mmol of the remaining sodium resides in the extracellular fluid. Rounding gives 50% of total sodium as extracellular, 40% associated with bone, and 10% as intracellular.

Sodium stores can be classified as exchangeable and non-exchangeable.[34] Measurements using radioactive isotopes have estimated exchangeable sodium at 42 mmol/kg body weight. Exchangeable sodium consists of all extracellular sodium, all intracellular sodium, and a little less than half of the bone sodium. Essentially, all non-exchangeable sodium is in bone, where it is buried within the bone structure. Exchangeable sodium is important because when sodium is lost from the blood plasma into the urine or feces, it can be replaced rapidly from other compartments via diffusion. In turn, sodium retained in edema is also spread out among these various compartments.

Total body chloride averages 33 mmol/kg body weight; therefore, a 70-kg person has 2310 mmol of chloride.[23] The majority of the chloride (about 70%) is distributed in the extracellular fluid. Much of the remaining chloride is localized in the collagen of connective tissue, which is largely exchangeable.

## *Sodium Homeostasis in the Body*

Over 40 years ago, Dahl[11] remarked, "This widespread use of salt has received little attention from nutritionists." This certainly is not the case today. It is now generally recognized that a substance in such common use as table salt might be noxious when consumed in amounts determined by dietary customs and taste. It is further recognized that potential adverse effects from salt consumption are also influenced by genetic factors and the simultaneous intake of other nutrients, such as potassium, magnesium, and calcium.[35] Although much emphasis has recently been placed on the potential toxicities that could emanate from excess salt consumption, certainly less emphasis has been placed on the perturbations that could occur with too little salt.[36] In examining salt balance and its role in volume control, water homeostasis must also be considered.

As indicated above, the amount of sodium consumed (intake) must equal the amount of sodium lost (output) to maintain balance. Calculating intake is fairly simple. Sodium is essentially absorbed completely in the small intestine. Therefore, if 4 g of sodium is ingested, 4 g is delivered to the body. Salt intake can be influenced by salt appetite, and the brain renin-angiotensin system is important in this respect. We know this because intracerebral injection of angiotensin II stimulates salt appetite, whereas blocking the formation of angiotensin II via central administration of captopril diminishes salt appetite.[37,38] Thirst also plays a significant role in the regulation of volume and body space size. Changes in osmolality related to sodium and chloride homeostasis affect the thirst mechanism and the release of vasopressin, which affects the handling of water in the renal collecting duct.[39]

In contrast to calculating input, calculating output can be difficult because a number of routes must be considered in the estimate. Normal losses of sodium occur through the skin, feces, and urine. In the absence of considerable physical effort or heat stress, only small amounts are lost via the skin, mainly by sweating, with lesser losses through skin sloughing. In subjects who were ambulatory but not actively working or sweating, daily consumption of 100 to 150 mg of sodium led to average daily losses of under 25 mg. The investigators attributed this small loss to desquamation of epithelial cells, sebaceous secretions, unnoticed sweat, and possibly some insensible perspiration.[36] Changing the production of salt-retaining hormones such as aldosterone can regulate losses of sodium in sweat. Conn[40] demonstrated that healthy individuals sweating as much as 5 to 9 L/d could decrease sodium concentrations in sweat to as little as 0.1 g/L after acclimation. Under normal conditions skin losses are small, but substantial amounts of sodium can be removed through excess sweating.

As mentioned above, loss of sodium via feces is small even when sodium intake is high.[41] On a daily sodium intake ranging widely from 0.05 to 4.1 g/d, only 10 to 125 mg appeared in stools.[42,43] Cases of severe diarrhea may result in substantial losses. Potential losses via hair, nails, saliva, semen, and menstruation are too negligible in the overall picture to be considered.

More than 90% of sodium removal is via the kidneys. When sodium intake is acutely reduced to an extremely low value, urinary sodium excretion decreases exponentially over 4 to 5 days; excess sodium intake above a certain level results in the excretion of the excess.[29] As mentioned above, the intake of sodium is accurately estimated by the amount present in urine in the absence of gross sweating. Pragmatically, the small amounts in the sweat and feces can be ignored in the overall calculations of balance, because the amount of sodium in the modern Western diet is relatively large.

The overall control of body sodium homeostasis via the interplay of various factors on the kidneys is incompletely understood. Both intra- and extra-renal factors are involved. Extra-renal mechanisms working interdependently associated with sodium homeostasis are plasma renin activity[44]; plasma angiotensin II[45]; aldosterone production[45]; atrial natriuretic peptide[46]; catecholamines such as adrenaline, noradrenaline, and dopamine[47]; hormones such as vasoactive intestinal peptide[48]; and possibly $Na^+,K^+$-ATPase inhibitors.[49,50]

## *Maintenance of Body Fluid Compartments*

The total body water content of an individual varies roughly between 45% and 70% of body weight, with a range of 50% to 60% being most representative of normal adults.[9,34] Infants have proportionately more water, whereas the elderly have less. Females have proportionately less water than do males. As illustrated in Figure 1, body water is divided into extracellular and intracellular compartments: one-third is extracellular and two-thirds is intracellular. The extracellular compartment is further divided into plasma and interstitial fluid. The latter is roughly three times larger than the former, that is, 1/12 and 1/4 of the total body water.

Sodium and chloride, being the most important electrolytes of the extracellular compartment, to a great extent determine the extracellular volume. Circulating proteins also influence the relationship between the plasma and interstitial fluid volumes. Endothelium of the capillaries allows rapid distribution of diffusable ions and water, but restricts the passage of protein between the plasma and interstitial fluid. Interstitial fluid, therefore, is an ultrafiltrate of plasma. Because of the virtual absence of protein with its negative charge on one side of the capillary wall (1% vs. 6%), diffusable ions distribute themselves according to the Gibbs-Donnan rule: more anions such as chlo-

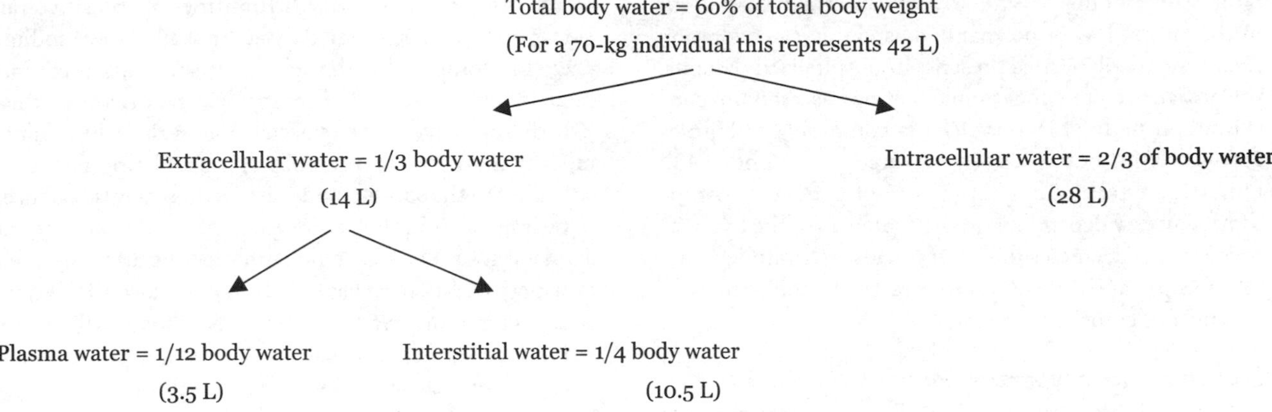


Figure 1. Body fluid compartments.

ride and bicarbonate will be on the relatively protein-free side of the membrane.[9] Nevertheless, the sum of the cations and anions must be equal on each side of the membrane. The presence of the non-penetrable protein also causes a slight increase in oncotic pressure on the plasma side that is balanced by the hydrostatic pressure developed by the heart. Sodium is maintained in the extracellular compartment and potassium in the intracellular compartment, mainly through the actions of the $Na^+,K^+$-ATPase exchange pump. Accordingly, sodium is the major cation in the extracellular fluid and the major osmotic particle outside the borders of the cell, whereas potassium is concentrated within the cells.

In the above discussion, sodium and chloride have been considered together. Total amounts of both sodium and chloride determine the size of the extracellular space. Restriction of dietary chloride without the restriction of sodium prevents expansion, whereas it is well-recognized that the administration of sodium coupled to other anions such as bicarbonate has a negligible effect on expansion of the extracellular body space.[49] The average concentration of sodium, as estimated via specific electrodes or flame photometry, is 135 to 145 mmol/L, and that of chloride, as estimated by titration and specific electrodes, is 98 to 108 mmol/L. Because of various forces maintaining high sodium concentration in the extracellular fluid, infusions of normal saline result predominantly in expansion of the extracellular space. Infusions of dextrose solutions result in the fluid distribution between intracellular and extracellular water compartments.

## *Perturbations Associated with Volume Control*

Edema, the accumulation of excess fluid in the body, can lead to symptoms such as swelling of a part or all of the body.[51] Accumulation of fluid in the lungs leads to difficulty in breathing. Causes of generalized edema are listed in Table 2; the major causes can be related to cardiac, renal, or hepatic perturbations. Sodium chloride retention may indicate a physiological response of the kidneys to what is perceived as inadequate arterial blood volume, or it may reflect an abnormal renal response to internal damage or hormonal perturbations. In addition to treating the major cause of the edema, excess fluid is often treated by limiting the intake of salt or removing excess sodium by using diuretics.[52] Too small a circulating volume can cause symptoms and signs ranging from tiredness and low blood pressure to outright disorientation and shock. Judicious replacement of salt and water often overcomes this status.

The subject of hyponatremia (low serum sodium) and hypernatremia (high serum sodium) is beyond the scope of this chapter.[53] Suffice it to say that hyponatremia can be associated with an excess of total body sodium, as well as an excess of water, because the overall water volume is important in the disturbance. Thus, a patient with hyponatremia may not be depleted of body sodium, but instead may have an excess of intravascular water (e.g., if an increase in water volume exceeds an increase in sodium, hyponatremia will develop despite the increase in

**Table 2.** Causes of Generalized Edema

| |
|---|
| Cardiac |
| Congestive heart failure |
| Pericardial disease |
| Renal |
| Nephrotic syndrome |
| Renal insufficiency |
| Hepatic |
| Cirrhosis |
| Hepatic venous disease |
| Endocrine |
| Myxedema |
| Hyperaldosteronism |
| Pharmaceuticals that Cause Fluid Retention |
| Nonsteroidal anti-inflammatory drugs |
| Chlorpropamide |
| Tolbutamide |
| Hormones |
| Idiopathic Edema |

total body sodium).[54] Similarly, hypernatremia can occur in the face of low or normal body sodium if dehydration (i.e., water depletion) is present. In hospitalized patients, the prevalence of hyponatremia (defined as a sodium concentration under 135 mmol/L) is commonly as high as 15% to 22%, but more severe dilutions of under 130 mmol/L are seen in only 1% to 4% of patients.[55] Symptoms may vary depending on the acuteness of the hyponatremia; slow decreases in sodium (nausea, lassitude, muscle cramps) are usually less severe than rapid decreases (confusion, coma, convulsions).

## *Sodium and Hypertension*

Many observation and clinical studies over the past century implicated salt (sodium and chloride) intake with hypertension.[56,57] Around 1900, French workers proposed that hypertension arose from a failure of kidneys to adapt to excess dietary salt.[23] In support of this theory, Allen[58] showed that severe restriction of dietary salt in many hypertensive patients reduced blood pressure, which he believed was due to an unknown renal defect in sodium excretion. The beneficial effects of the famous Kempner rice diet were attributed to low sodium content.[59] Hypertension in the elderly and in blacks is generally characterized by low plasma renin activity, suggesting volume expansion, and less sodium excretion when challenged with this cation.[56] Furthermore, the elevated blood pressure of blacks responds especially well to treatment with diuretics.[60] However, studies limited to industrialized societies have often failed to find a conclusive relationship between blood pressure and sodium excretion.[61] Stamler[33] reported that the prevalence of hypertension was 1.7% in non-obese subjects consuming a low-sodium diet compared with 11.9% for non-obese subjects consuming a high-sodium diet. Although the recent Intersalt Study shows a positive correlation between blood pressure and sodium ingestion from 52 participating centers,[33] the removal of data from the four centers reporting the lowest sodium intake lessens the significance of the correlation. Tobian[62] believes the reason behind this is that persons genetically resistant to hypertension outnumber those genetically susceptible, and a correlation between sodium intake and blood pressure is only apparent in those who are susceptible.

What is known about the genetic component of sodium-induced hypertension? Laboratory studies provide evidence that Allen[58] could be correct—that a genetic component works through kidneys. Dahl[63] developed two rat substrains—one exquisitely sensitive to salt and one very resistant—and showed that the expression of the genetic defect in salt-sensitive rats was in the kidneys. The salt-resistant rats were nephrectomized and then received kidneys from the salt-sensitive rats; hypertension developed when these rats ate high-salt diets (4%–8% by weight). In contrast, nephrectomized, salt-sensitive rats receiving kidneys from resistant rats did not develop hypertension while eating high-salt diets. Experiments using isolated kidneys from the salt-sensitive rats confirmed an intrinsic renal defect that allows less sodium excretion compared with the salt-resistant rats at comparable inflow pressures.[64] Tobian[64] also reported that thiazide diuretics overcame hypertension in the salt-sensitive rats. In addition, the presence of a circulating factor responding to the sodium and water status was also believed to be important in the pathogenesis.[64] Earlier work found an association between circulating factors affecting renal transport and hypertension.[65-67] Salt-induced hypertension occurs more readily in animals when renal mass is reduced by surgical extirpation or renal failure,[64] and circulating factors correlating with hypertension have also been reported to occur under similar conditions.[68,69]

How could sodium retention lead to blood pressure elevation? Although the pathogenic mechanisms are uncertain, Haddy et al.[56,70] pointed out that retention of sodium causes water retention, which releases a digitalis-like substance that increases contractile activity of heart and blood vessels. An alternative explanation is that sodium itself penetrates the vascular smooth muscle, causing it to contract. In salt-induced hypertension in humans, accumulation of sodium and water with expansion of the extracellular volume seems to precede the development of hypertension whether the defect is intrinsic to kidneys, secondary to circulating factors, or both.[70]

## *Salt Sensitivity*

Over recent years, less emphasis has been placed on avoiding dietary salt. Factors such as loss of excess body weight could prove to be as important or more important in the future.[71,72] A plausible explanation for the difficulty in associating sodium consumption with blood pressure may be that the connection between salt and high blood pressure pertains only to those individuals who are "salt sensitive." Many recent studies examined the pros and cons of the association of sodium with hypertension.[12,14,73-75] Most individuals can consume large amounts of sodium without its affecting blood pressure markedly, because they excrete excess sodium adequately. Others do not excrete sodium as quickly, and blood pressure increases. These individuals, like those with kidney disease, are salt sensitive. More than half of those with hypertension have a marked increase in blood pressure in response to a sodium challenge.[57] These individuals tend to retain sodium, because they excrete the sodium load more slowly. Normotensive relatives of hypertensive subjects, especially older individuals, have a blunted natriuretic effect. Supporting the contention that sodium retention is important in the pathogenesis of hypertension is that acculturated people have extracellular fluid volume 15% greater than non-acculturated people who exhibit less hypertension.[70] Many believe that blood pressure rises to compensate for sodium and water retention, because elevated blood pressure allows the kidney to excrete more sodium and water to maintain balance.[76] In general, more blacks than whites have difficulty handling a sodium challenge,[77] and hypertension is more prevalent in the black population, suggesting a genetic predisposition. Other factors associated with salt sensitivity include female gender, aging, obesity, insulin resistance, and a positive history of hypertension.[13] Thus, inappropriate renal sodium handling can occur via many initiating causes: for example, inheritance of inborn renal transport defects, the presence of circulating factors influencing renal reabsorption, and decreasing renal mass. None of these is mutually exclusive.

# Potassium

## *General Background*

To clearly understand potassium in a dietary sense, one must recognize the various facets of overall potassium balance and the plethora of conditions and drugs affecting that balance.[78-80] Potassium is the major intracellular cation and plays a significant role in several physiological processes. Circulating potassium enters all tissue and has profound effects on the function of some organs, particularly depolarization and contraction of the heart. A number of organ systems are involved in maintaining potassium balance. Ninety percent of ingested potassium is absorbed via the gastrointestinal tract for use in the body, leaving 10% to be excreted in stool. Potassium is readily absorbed in the small intestine in proportion to the presented load. Under normal circumstances, circulating concentrations are relatively stable, because cells immediately take up most potassium entering the body. Cellular uptake is facilitated by insulin, catecholamines, and aldosterone. The kidney is the principal excretory organ, and decreased renal function from any cause may result in excess potassium retention and excess circulating concentrations. Usually, it takes several days to as much as 3 weeks for the kidney to adapt to excess potassium intake. In cases of renal dysfunction when the kidneys cannot respond appropriately, the gastrointestinal tract can reestablish balance, at least in part, by eliminating increased amounts of potassium (i.e., 30%–40% of daily intake).[81]

## *Facts about Potassium*

The total body potassium of a normal adult male averages 45 mmol/kg body weight.[34] The body of a 70-kg person has 3150 mmol (1230 g) of potassium. Only 60 mmol or about 2% of potassium is distributed in the extracellular fluid. Virtually all body potassium is labile and exchangeable. The circulating potassium concentrations are low, about 3.5 to 5.0 mmol/L, and the plasma concentration of potassium is often a poor indicator of tissue potassium stores. Intracellular potassium is maintained at 140 to 150 mmol/L.[82,83] Potassium status not only depends on the intake and output of potassium but on its distribution as well.[78] Distribution depends on the energy-consuming processes at the cell membranes, where sodium extrusion is coupled to entry of potassium. Although the kidneys can adapt to high and low potassium intake over 2 to 3 weeks, the minimum rate of excretion is 5 mmol/d, which, taken together with obligatory extra renal losses, implies that potassium balance cannot be achieved on intakes of less than 10 to 20 mmol/d.[78]

## *Sources*

Because potassium is the principal cation of the intracellular fluid, the major source of dietary potassium is the cellular materials consumed in foodstuffs (Table 3). Potassium is a major constituent of meats, vegetables, and fruits. Consequently, a potassium-free diet is virtually impossible to devise. The potassium content of the average American diet ranges between 50 and 100 mmol/d. Only a small portion of oral potassium absorbed remains in the extracellular compartment. Normal rates of dietary intake cause only negligible changes in plasma levels. At high intakes (200–300 mmol/d), patients unaccustomed to large loads may develop a significant elevation in circulating potassium despite normal renal function.[78] Secretion of insulin, catecholamines, and aldosterone is augmented by potassium loads that helps maintain the "milieu interior."

## *Functions within the Body*

Potassium has a crucial role in energy metabolism and membrane transport. A major function of potassium is membrane polarization, which depends on the concentrations of internal and external potassium (on either side of the membrane). The major clinical features of disordered potassium homeostasis relate to perturbations in membrane function, especially noted in the neuromuscular and cardiac conduction systems. Accordingly, both deficient and excess circulating potassium concentrations can lead to disorders in cardiac, muscle, and neurological function.

**Table 3.** Approximate Values for Potassium Content in Some Common Foods

| | Potassium | |
|---|---|---|
| **Food** | ***mmol*** | ***mg*** |
| Apple, raw, with skin | 3.4 | 133 |
| Asparagus, raw, 5–6 spears | 7.0 | 273 |
| Avocado (1/2) | 15.0 | 585 |
| Banana | 19.2 | 749 |
| Beef patty (113 g, or 1/4 lb) | 10.0 | 390 |
| Beer (237 mL, or 8 oz) | 1.0 | 39 |
| Butter, salted (5 g, or 1 tsp) | 0.08 | 3 |
| Celery, raw (1 large stalk) | 4.0 | 156 |
| Chicken (98 g, or 3.5 oz) | 8.0 | 312 |
| Egg | 1.8 | 70 |
| Frankfurter | 3.0 | 117 |
| Whole milk (237 mL, or 8 oz) | 9.0 | 351 |
| Sweet potato (1 small) | 6.2 | 242 |
| Tomato juice (237 mL, or 8 oz) | 14.0 | 546 |

## *Potassium and Blood Pressure*

In contrast to the deleterious effects of high sodium intake that frequently increase blood pressure, ingestion of more potassium may influence blood pressure favorably by lowering any elevations.[84-86] Many studies have shown that potassium has a good blood pressure-lowering effect, especially in salt-sensitive individuals.[87,88] The beneficial effects of potassium (and even magnesium and calcium) work, at least in part, through an effect on sodium balance: potassium is more effective in salt-sensitive individuals.

A high intake of potassium has been reported to protect against increased blood pressure and other cardiovascular risks.[84,85,87-90] Analysis of results from the Intersalt Study shows a lowering of systolic blood pressure at higher potassium excretory rates, presumably reflecting higher intakes.[33] Various clinical trials suggest a lowering of blood pressure in persons taking potassium supplements.[91,92] One meta-analysis reviewed 19 clinical trials involving a total of 586 participants.[85] Results showed that oral potassium supplements significantly lowered systolic blood pressure (by 5.9 mmHg) and diastolic blood pressure (by 3.4 mmHg). In mildly hypertensive individuals, a low-potassium diet can augment the already elevated systolic and diastolic pressures but also causes sodium retention.[93] In healthy individuals, dietary potassium depletion also can cause sodium retention and augmented blood pressure[94]; however, persons with hypertension are more likely to benefit from potassium supplementation than normotensive persons.[95]

Low intake of potassium rather than excess sodium consumption may be more important in the prominence of severe hypertension among blacks.[96,97] A small trial suggested a particular benefit to blacks from potassium supplementation.[98] In addition to benefiting hypertensive individuals,[99,100] potassium supplementation of diabetics could appreciably check the negative effects of diabetic vascular disease by enhancing vascular perfusion and improving carbohydate metabolism.[101] Over and above the natriuretic effects of potassium, increased urinary kallikrein[102] and stimulation of the sodium-potassium ATPase in vascular smooth muscle cells and adrenergic nerve terminals[103,104] may be important in blood pressure lowering.

The DASH (Dietary Approaches to Stop Hypertension) diet seems particularly effective in lowering blood pressure (see Chapter __). Results from two DASH studies have been published thus far.[105-107] The basic diet resulted in a marked reduction of blood pressure. Although many nutrients are responsible for the overall effect, potassium probably is most important in producing the beneficial effects. In the second trial, the DASH-Sodium Trial, salt intake was monitored at three different levels, with the greatest effects on blood pressure being seen with the lowest sodium intake. A 12-month follow-up study was instituted to determine the effects of the DASH diet with sodium reduction after discontinuation of the feeding intervention.[108] Compared with control participants, DASH diet participants ate more fruit and vegetables and maintained reduced blood pressure even though their sodium intake increased.

## *Safety and Toxicity*

Total body potassium can be decreased and lead to decreased serum concentration of potassium, a condition called hypokalemia.[78,79,109] However, hypokalemia can also result from shifts of potassium out of the blood and into the cells, even though total body potassium is normal. Common causes of hypokalemia include increased renal excretion (poor renal tubular function, diuretic drugs), adrenal disorders (hyperaldosteronism), increased gastrointestinal losses (vomiting, diarrhea), increased uptake by cells (insulin, beta adrenergic agonists), and decreased intake (chronic alcoholism, anorexia nervosa). Mild hypokalemia may be asymptomatic or may be accompanied by muscle weakness, constipation, fatigue, and malaise. Patients with underlying cardiac diseases are prone to arrhythmias. Moderate hypokalemia may result in more severe constipation, an inability to concentrate urine accompanied by polyuria, and a tendency for the development of encephalopathy in patients with concomitant renal disease. Severe hypokalemia can result in muscular paralysis and even in poor respiration because of immobilization of the diaphragm and decreased blood pressure.

When high circulating concentrations of potassium are present (hyperkalemia), it is important to differentiate between pseudohyperkalemia and laboratory error and the actual increases in total body potassium. Pseudohyperkalemia is not a real increase in circulating potassium, but rather a response to a condition that should be recognized. Pseudohyperkalemia may arise from hemolysis of red blood cells, causing potassium release into the serum, which can also be caused by massive leukocytosis or thrombocytosis. In the case of true hyperkalemia, the most important clinical manifestation is cardiac arrest caused by perturbations in electrical (membrane) conduction. Various characteristic changes in the electrocardiogram assessment aid in the diagnosis. Neuromuscular symptoms of too much potassium include tingling, paresthesia, weakness, and flaccid paralysis. In addition to spurious hyperkalemia caused by hemolysis or too many blood cells in the specimen, as mentioned above, common causes of true hyperkalemia are decreased renal excretion; adrenal disorders; and use of medications such as spironolactone, triamterene, amiloride, angiotensin-converting enzyme inhibitors, nonsteroidal anti-inflammatory drugs, and heparin.

## *Efficacy*

The major use of potassium in therapy is to replace a deficit. However, there is some evidence that potassium supplementation may be helpful in lowering elevated blood pressure. In this case, most physicians would prefer replacement using foods rich in potassium.

Diuretic usage is the most common cause of hypokalemia in United States. Elderly women using long-acting thiazides or loop diuretics are at increased risk. A low-sodium, high-potassium diet, lower doses of diuretic agents, and substitution of different antihypertensive drugs may ameliorate the problem. Patients with normal renal function who receive diuretics and digitalis-type compounds may need potassium supplementation or an agent lessening potassium loss via the kidneys (e.g., aldactone, triamterene, and amiloride). Laxative abuse often leads to hypokalemia and can be overcome by ceasing to use the causative agent.

Replacement therapy with potassium salts can be effective. The major risk factor with potassium replacement is going too far and producing hyperkalemia. Gastrointestinal bleeding is a not infrequent complication of oral potassium replacement, as many potassium salts are harsh in regards to the gastrointestinal lining. Severe systemic depletion of potassium may necessitate the use of intravenous preparations for replacement.

Hyperkalemia is, of course, treated by eliminating excess intake and reversing the other causes mentioned above. When the problem is severe and immediate action must be taken, several therapeutic choices exist. First, one can antagonize the membrane effects by giving calcium gluconate or hypertonic saline. Second, cellular uptake of potassium can be stimulated by giving sodium bicarbonate, glucose, or insulin. Finally, potassium can be removed from the body by using certain diuretics (thiazides), cation-exchange resins (Kayexalate®), and dialysis (peritoneal or hemodialysis).

### *Dosage*

Oral replacement in potassium deficiency states is generally preferable to intravenous administration, and the amount given depends on the body deficit. A rough rule is that a 1 mmol/L decrease in circulating levels is equivalent to 200 to 300 mmol of body potassium stores. Oral or intravenous potassium at a dose of 40 to 120 mmol/d generally improves all symptoms of hypokalemia. Any intravenous fluid should contain ≤40 mmol/L and administration should be <10 mmol/hour. If more rapid administration is necessary, it should be performed with electrocardiogram monitoring.

### *Cofactors and Interactions*

Chronic hyperkalemia is treated by eliminating excess potassium from the extracellular space and reversing the primary cause of the disturbance and any cofactors that would increase potassium retention. Many drugs and conditions accentuate potassium retention. Drugs causing hyperkalemia include β-adrenergic blocking agents, digitalis, arginine succinylcholine, potassium penicillin, potassium salts, angiotensin-converting enzyme inhibitors, and potassium-retaining diuretics (e.g., aldactone, triamterene, and amiloride). Acidosis, insulinemia, low levels of catecholamines, and hypoaldosteronism may contribute to high levels of circulating potassium.

Hypokalemia is often associated with metabolic alkalosis. Therefore, replacement of potassium in the form of potassium chloride may ameliorate the alkalosis more effectively. Hypomagnesemia is somehow related to hypokalemia. The latter may prove resistant to replacement until the magnesium deficiency is corrected. Drugs causing hypokalemia include diuretics, antibiotics (e.g., carbenicillin, penicillin, polymyxin B, and gentamicin), drugs causing magnesium wasting, and drugs causing metabolic alkalosis.

### *Contraindications*

Potassium supplementation must be considered carefully in the face of evident renal failure, because kidneys are the major regulator of potassium homeostasis. Patients with severe gastrointestinal stress, such as previous history of ulcers and bleeding, should be considered carefully before instituting oral potassium replacement.

## Summary

Important to note is that when life emerged from the safe confines of the relatively stable seas, it became necessary to retain at all times a similar internal sea-like environment (extracellular and intracellular body fluid) within acceptable limits. Falling short or exceeding the acceptable range would lead to disaster. This meant that the intake of salts and electrolytes had to equal losses and vice versa—that is, the intake and output of sodium, potassium, and chloride over a finite period of time had to equal each other. It is obvious that any phenomenon necessary for life, such as maintaining the "milieu interior," has to be controlled by more than one mechanism, with checks and balances regulating intake and output. Therefore, when symptoms occur because the acceptable limits for a healthy existence have not been maintained, more than one mechanism is involved. Further, adaptations to change often occur gradually. Accordingly, attempts to treat perturbations are more successful when they can be instituted gradually, either by correcting the major pathological processes involved or by carefully replacing deficits or correcting excesses of fluids and electrolytes. A rational therapeutic approach to ameliorate or overcome perturbations in fluid and electrolyte balance mandates a solid knowledge of pertinent physiology and pathophysiology.

## References


1. Battarbee HD, Meneely GR. Nutrient toxicities in animal and man: sodium. In: Rechcigl M Jr, ed. *Handbook Series in Nutrition and Food.* Boca Raton, FL: CRC Press; 1978; 119–140.
2. Bernard C. *An Introduction to the Study of Experi-*

*mental Medicine*. New York: Dover Publications; 1957.

3. Conway EJ. Mean geochemical data in relation to oceanic evolution. Proc R Irish Acad. 1942;48: 119–152.
4. Conway EJ. The chemical evolution of the ocean. Proc R Irish Acad. 1943;48:161–212.
5. Smith HW. The evolution of the kidney. In: *Lectures on the Kidney, Porter Lectures, Series IX*. Lawrence, KS: University of Kansas Press; 1943.
6. Conway EJ. Exchanges of K, Na and H ions between the cell and the environment. Irish J Med SC. 1947;263:654–680.
7. Elkinton JR, Danowsky TS. *The Body Fluids: Basic Physiology and Practical Therapeutics*. Baltimore: Williams & Wilkins; 1955.
8. Smith HW. *From Fish to Philosopher*. Boston: Little, Brown; 1953.
9. Pitts RF. *Physiology of the Kidney and Body Fluids*. 3rd ed. Chicago: Year Book Medical Publishers; 1974; 11–35.
10. Macallum AB. The paleochemistry of the body fluids and tissues. Physiol Rev. 1926;6:316–357.
11. Dahl LK. Salt intake and salt need. N Engl J Med. 1958;258:1152–1157.
12. Hooper L, Bartlett C, Davey SG, Ebrahim S. Advice to reduce dietary salt for prevention of cardiovascular disease. Cochrane Database Syst Rev. 2003;CD003656.
13. Suter PM, Sierro C, Vetter W. Nutritional factors in the control of blood pressure and hypertension. Nutr Clin Care. 2002;5:9–19.
14. Weinberger MH. Sodium and blood pressure 2003. Curr Opin Cardiol. 2004;19:353–356.
15. Cordain L, Eaton SB, Sebastian A, Mann N, Lindeberg S, Watkins BA, O'Keefe JH, Brand-Miller JB. Origins and evolution of the Western diet: health implications for the 21st century. Am J Clin Nutr. 2005;81:341–354.
16. Braunwald E. Shattuck Lecture: Cardiovascular medicine at the turn of the millennium: Triumphs, concerns and opportunities. N Engl J Med. 1997; 337:1360–1369.
17. Kotchen TA, Kotchen JM. Nutrition and cardiovascular health. In: *Nutritional Aspects and Clinical Management of Chronic Disorders and Diseases*. Boca Raton, FL: CRC Press; 2003; 23–43.
18. Reaven GM: Role of insulin resistance in human disease (Banting Lecture 1988). Diabetes. 1988;37: 1595–1607.
19. Frassetto L, Morris RC Jr, Sellmeyer DE, Todd K, Sebastain A. Diet, evolution and aging—the pathophysiologic effects of the post-agricultural inversion of the potassium-to-sodium and base-to-chloride ratios in the human diet. Eur J Nutr. 2001;40: 200–213.
20. US Department of Agriculture, Agricultural Research Service, ARS Food Surveys Research Group. *Data Tables: Results from USDA's 1994–96 Continuing Survey of Food Intakes by Individuals and 1994–96 Diet and Health Knowledge Survey*. Washington, DC: USDA; 1997.
21. Eaton SB, Konner MJ. Paleolithic nutrition. A consideration of its nature and current implications. N Engl J Med. 1985;312:283–289.
22. Cordain L. The nutritional characteristics of a contemporary diet based upon Paleolithic food groups. J Am Nutraceutical Assoc. 2002;5:15–24.
23. Ambard L, Bedaujard E. Causes de l'hypertension arterielle. Arch Intern Med. 1904;1:520–533.
24. Kaunitz H. Toxic and nontoxic effects of chloride in animals and man. In: Rechcigl M Jr, ed. *Handbook Series in Nutrition and Food*. Boca Raton, FL: CRC Press; 1978; 141–145.
25. Luft FC. Salt, water, and extracellular volume regulation. In: Ziegler EE, Filer LJ Jr, ed. *Present Knowledge in Nutrition*. 7th ed. Washington, DC: ILSI Press; 1996; 265–271.
26. Meneely GR, Dahl LK. Electrolytes in hypertension: the effects of sodium chloride. Med Clin North Am. 1961;45:271–283.
27. Simpson FO. Sodium intake, body sodium, and sodium excretion. Lancet. 1988;2:25–28.
28. Simpson FO. Blood pressure and sodium intake. In: Bulpitt CJ, ed. *Handbook of Hypertension, Volume 6: Epidemiology of Hypertension*. Amsterdam: Elsevier; 1985; 175–190.
29. Strauss MB, Lamdin E, Smith WP, Bleifer DJ. Surfeit and deficit of sodium. Arch Intern Med. 1958;102:527–536.
30. Vander AJ. Basic renal processes for sodium, chloride and water. In: *Renal Physiology*. 5th ed. New York: McGraw-Hill; 1995.
31. Engstrom A, Tobelmann RC, Albertson AM. Sodium intake trends and food choices. Am J Clin Nutr. 1997;65(suppl):704S–707S.
32. Alaimo K, McDowell MA, Briefel RR, et al. *Dietary Intake of Vitamins, Minerals, and Fiber of Persons Ages 2 Months and over in the United States: Third National Health and Nutrition Examination Survey, Phase 1, 1988–1991*. Hyattsville, MD: National Center for Health Statistics; 1994; 1–28.
33. Intersalt Cooperative Research Group. Intersalt: an international study of electrolyte excretion and blood pressure. Results for 24 hour urinary sodium and potassium excretion. Br Med J. 1988;297: 319–328.
34. Pitts RF. Ionic composition of body fluids. In: *The Physiological Basis of Diuretic Therapy*. Springfield, IL: Charles C. Thomas Publishers; 1959.
35. Nurminen ML, Korpela R, Vapaatalo H. Dietary

factors in the pathogenesis and treatment of hypertension. Ann Med. 1998;30:143–150.
36. Dahl LK, Stall BG, Cotzias GC. Metabolic effects of marked sodium restriction in hypertensive patients: skin electrolyte losses. J Clin Invest. 1955; 34:462–470.
37. Fitzsimmons JT. Angiotensin stimulation of the central nervous system. Rev Physiol Biochem Pharmacol. 1980;87:117–167.
38. Robertson JLS. The Franz Gross memorial lecture: the renin-aldosterone connection: past, present, and future. J Hypertens. 1984;2(suppl 3):1–14.
39. Robertson JLS. Salt, volume, and hypertension: causation or correlation: Kidney Int. 1987;32: 590–602.
40. Conn JW. Mechanism of acclimatization to heat. Adv Intern Med. 1949;3:373–393.
41. Baldwin D, Alexander RW, Warner EG Jr. Chronic sodium chloride challenge studies in man. J Lab Clin Med. 1960;55:362–375.
42. Dole VP, Dahl LK, Cotzias GC, et al. Dietary treatment of hypertension: clinical and metabolic studies of patients on rice-fruit diets. J Clin Invest. 1950;29:1189–1206.
43. Henneman PH, Dempsey EF. Factors determining fecal electrolyte excretion [abstract]. J Clin Invest. 1956;35:711.
44. Laragh JH, Baer L, Brunner HR, et al,. Renin, angiotensin, and aldosterone system in pathogenesis and management of hypertensive vascular disease. Am J Med. 1972;52:633–652.
45. Brown JJ, Lever AF, Morton JJ, Fraser R, Love DR, Robertson JI. Raised plasma angiotensin II and aldosterone during dietary sodium restriction in man. Lancet. 1972;7787:1106–1107.
46. Sagnella GA, Markandu ND, Shore AC, MacGregor GA. Plasma immunoreactive atrial natriuretic peptide and changes in dietary sodium intake in man. Life Sci. 1987;40:139–143.
47. Romoff MS, Keusch G, Campese VM, et al. Effect of sodium intake on plasma catecholamines in normal subjects. J Clin Endocrinol Metab. 1979;48: 26–31.
48. Duggan KA, Macdonald GJ. Vasoactive intestinal peptide: a direct natriuretic substance. Clin Sci. 1987;72:195–200.
49. deWardener HE, Macgregor GA. The relation of a circulating sodium transport inhibitor (the natriuretic hormone?) to hypertension. Medicine. 1983; 62:310–326.
50. Blaustein MP. How salt causes hypertension: the natriuretic hormone–Na/Ca exchange–hypertension hypothesis. Klin Wochenschr. 1985;63(suppl III):82–85.
51. Michelis MF, Rakowski TA. Edema and diuretic therapy. In: Preuss HG, ed. *Management of Common Problems in Renal Disease*. Philadelphia: Field and Wood; 1988; 109–117.
52. Ellison DH. Clinical use of diuretics: therapy of edema. In: *Primer on Kidney Diseases*. San Diego, CA: Academic Press; 1994; 324–332.
53. Michelis MF, Davis BB. Hypo and hypernatremia. In: Preuss HG, ed. *Management of Common Problems in Renal Disease*. Philadelphia: Field and Wood; 1988; 118–127.
54. DeVita MV, Michelis MF. Perturbations in sodium balance: hyponatremia and hypernatremia. In: Preuss HG, ed. *Clinics in Laboratory Medicine: Renal Function*. Philadelphia: WB Saunders; 1993; 135–148.
55. Verbalis JG. Hyponatremia and hypoosmolar disorders. In: *Primer on Kidney Diseases*. San Diego, CA: Academic Press; 1994; 361–367.
56. Haddy FJ, Pamnani MB. Role of dietary salt in hypertension. J Am Coll Nutr. 1995;14:428–438.
57. Sullivan JM. Salt sensitivity. Hypertension. 1991; 17(suppl 1):61–68.
58. Allen FM. *Treatment of Kidney Disease and High Blood Pressure*. Morristown, NJ: The Psychiatric Institute; 1925.
59. Kempner W. Treatment of hypertensive vascular disease with rice diet. Am J Med. 1948;4:545–577.
60. Fries ED. Salt in hypertension and the effects of diuretics. Annu Rev Pharmacol Toxicol. 1979;19: 13–23.
61. Pickering G. Salt intake and essential hypertension. Cardiovasc Rev Rep. 1980:1:13–17.
62. Tobian L. Human essential hypertension: Implications of animal studies. Ann Intern Med. 1983;98: 729–734.
63. Dahl LK, Heine M, Tassinari L. Effects of chronic salt ingestion: evidence that genetic factors play an important role in susceptibility to experimental hypertension. J Exp Med. 1962;115:1173–1190.
64. Tobian L, Pumper M, Johnson S, Iwai JA. A circulating humoral pressor agent in Dahl S rats with salt hypertension. Clin Sci Mol Med. 1979;57: 345S–347S.
65. Preuss HG, Grant K, Parris R, Zmudka M. Effects of sera and sera fractions from spontaneously hypertensive rats on renal organic anion and cation transport. Proc Soc Exp Biol Med. 1974;145:397–402.
66. Gharib N, Gao CY, Areas J, et al. Correlation of organic anion and cation transport with blood pressure. Clin Nephrol. 1991;36:87–92.
67. Preuss HG, Al-Karadaghi P, Yousufi A, MacArthy P. Effects of canrenone on RRM-sucrose hypertension in WKY. Clin Exp Hypertens. 1991;A13: 917–923.
68. Razavi H, Schubert P, Areas J, Preuss HG. Presence of a serum vasoconstrictive factor following

unilateral nephrectomy. Am J Hypertens. 1988;1: 915–955.

69. Preuss HG. Renotropin: a possible association with hypertension. In: Brenner B, Kaplan N, Laragh J, eds. *Endocrine Mechanisms of Hypertension*. Vol. 2. New York: Raven Press; 1989; 335–341.
70. Haddy FJ, Overbeck HW. The role of humoral agents in volume expanded hypertension. Life Sci. 1976;19:935–948.
71. Hart KE, Warriner EM. Weight loss and biomedical health improvement on a very low calorie diet: the moderating role of history of weight cycling. Behav Med. 2005;30:161–170.
72. Aucott L, Poobalan A, Smith WC, Avenell A, Jung R, Broom J. Effects of weight loss in overweight/obese individuals and long-term hypertension outcomes: a systematic review. Hypertension. 2005;45: 1035–1041.
73. McCarron DA. The dietary guideline for sodium: Should we shake it up? Yes! Am J Clin Nutr. 2000; 71:1013–1019.
74. Kaplan NM. The dietary guideline for sodium: Should we shake it up? No! Am J Clin Nutr. 2000; 71:1020–1026.
75. Luft FC. Salt and hypertension at the close of the millennium. Wien Klin Wochenschr. 1998;110: 459–466.
76. Guyton AC, Coleman TG, Cowley AW, et al. Arterial pressure regulation: overriding dominance of the kidneys in long-term regulation and in hypertension. Am J Med. 1972;52:584–594.
77. Flack JM, Ensrud KE, Mascioli S, et al. Racial and ethnic modifiers of salt-blood pressure response. Hypertension. 1991;17(suppl 1):115–121.
78. Perez G, Delaney VB, Bourke E. Hypo and hyperkalemia. In: Preuss HG, ed. *Management of Common Problems in Renal Disease*. Philadelphia: Field and Wood; 1988; 109–117.
79. Latta K, Hisano S, Chan JCM. Perturbations in potassium balance. In: Preuss HG, ed. *Clinics in Laboratory Medicine: Renal Function*. Philadelphia: WB Saunders; 1993; 149–156.
80. Halperin ML, Kamel KS. Potassium. Lancet. 1998; 352:235–140.
81. Brown RS. Extrarenal potassium homeostasis. Kidney Int. 1986;30:116–127
82. Brenner BM, Berliner RW. The transport of potassium. In: Orloff J, Berliner RW, eds. *Renal Physiology*. Washington, DC: American Physiological Society; 1973; 497–520.
83. Hayslett JP, Binder HJ. Mechanism of potassium adaptation. Am J Physiol. 1982;243:F103–F112.
84. Langford HG. Dietary potassium and hypertension: epidemiologic data. Ann Intern Med. 1983; 98(part 2):770–772.
85. Cappuccio FP, MacGregor GA. Does potassium supplementation lower blood pressure? A meta-analysis of published trials. J Hypertens. 1991;9: 465–473.
86. Bari YM, Wingo CS. The effects of potassium depletion and supplementation on blood pressure: a clinical review. Am J Med Sci. 1997;314:37–40.
87. Suter PM. Potassium and hypertension. Nutr Rev. 1998;56:151–153.
88. He FJ, MacGregor GA. Beneficial effects of potassium. Br Med J. 2001;323:497–501.
89. Nowsom CA, Morgan TO, Gibbons C. Decreasing dietary sodium while following a self-selected potassium-rich diet reduces blood pressure. J Nutr. 2003;133:4118–4123.
90. Demigne C, Houda S, Remesy C, Meneton P. Protective effects of high dietary potassium: nutritional and metabolic aspects. J Nutr. 2004;134: 2903–2906.
91. Siani A, Strazzullo P, Giacco A, et al. Increasing the dietary potassium intake reduces the need for antihypertensive medication. Ann Intern Med. 1991;115:753–759.
92. Linas SL. The role of potassium in the pathogenesis and treatment of hypertension. Kidney Int. 1991; 39:771–786.
93. Krishna GG, Kapoor SC. Potassium depletion exacerbates essential hypertension. Ann Intern Med. 1991;115:77–93.
94. Krishna GG, Cushid P, Hoeldtke ED. Mild potassium depletion provides renal sodium retention. J Lab Clin Med. 1987;109:724–730.
95. Siani A, Strazzullo P, Russo L, et al. Control of long-term oral potassium supplements in patients with mild hypertension. Br Med J. 1987;294: 1453–1456.
96. Weinberger MG. Racial differences in renal sodium excretion: relationship to hypertension. Am J Kidney Dis. 1993;21(suppl 1):41–45.
97. Langford HC, Watson RL. Potassium and calcium intake, excretion, and homeostasis in blacks and their relation to blood pressure. Cardiovasc Drugs Ther. 1990;4(suppl 2):403–406.
98. Obel AO. Placebo-controlled trial of potassium supplements in black patients with mild essential hypertension. J Cardiovasc Pharmacol. 1989;14: 294–296.
99. Koneth I, Suter PM, Vetter W. Schweiz Rundsch Med Prax. 2000;89:1499–1505.
100. He FJ, Markandu ND, Coltart R, Barron J, MacGregor GA. Effect of short-term supplementation of potassium chloride and potassium citrate on blood pressure in hypertensives. Hypertension. 2005;45:571–574.
101. Whang R, Sims G. Magnesium and potassium supplementation in the prevention of diabetic vascular disease. Medical Hypotheses. 2000;55:263–265.
102. Valdes G, Bio CP, Montero J, Abedano R. Potas-

sium supplementation lowers blood pressure and increases urinary kallikrein in essential hypertensives. J Hum Hypertens. 1991;5:91–96.
103. Haddy FJ. Ionic control of vascular smooth muscle cells. Kidney Int. 1988;346(suppl 25):S2–S8.
104. Haddy FJ. Potassium effects on contraction in arterial smooth muscle mediated by $Na^+,K^+$-ATPase. Fed Proc. 1983;42:239–245.
105. Appel LJ, Moore TJ, Obarzanek E, et al. A clinical trial of the effects of dietary patterns on blood pressure. DASH Collaborative Research Group. N Engl J Med. 1997;336:1117–1124.
106. Sack FM, Svetkey LP, Vollmer WM, et al. Effects on blood pressure of reduced dietary sodium and the Dietary Approaches to Stop Hypertension (DASH) diet. DASH-Sodium Collaborative Research Group. N Engl J Med. 2001;344:3–10.
107. Bray GA, Vollmer VM, Sack FM, Obarzanek E, Svetkey LP, Appel LG; DASH Collaborative Research Group: A further subgroup analysis of the effects of the DASH diet and three dietary sodium levels on blood pressure: results of the DASH-Sodium Trial. Am J Cardiol. 2004;94:222–227.
108. Ard JD, Coffman CJ, Lin PH, Svetkey LP. One-year follow-up study of blood pressure and dietary patterns in dietary approaches to stop hypertension (DASH)-sodium participants. Am J Hypertens. 2004;17:1156–1162.
109. Gennari FJ. Hypokalemia. N Engl J Med. 1998; 339:451–458.

# 33 Human Water and Electrolyte Balance

Scott J. Montain, Samuel N. Cheuvront, Robert Carter III, and Michael N. Sawka

## Introduction

Humans demonstrate a remarkable ability to regulate daily body water and electrolyte balance so long as food and fluid are readily available.[1] The imposition of exercise and environmental stress can, however, challenge this ability. Most circumstances involving physical exercise require the formation and vaporization of sweat as the principle means of heat removal in man. Sweat losses, if not replaced, reduce body water volume and electrolyte content. Excessive body water or electrolyte losses can disrupt physiological homeostasis and threaten both health and performance.[1]

Persons often dehydrate during physical activity or exposure to hot weather because of fluid non-availability or because of a mismatch between thirst and body water losses.[2] In these instances, the person begins the task with normal total body water, and dehydrates over a prolonged period. This scenario is common for most athletic and occupational settings; however, in some situations the person might begin exercise with a body water deficit. For example, in several sports (e.g., boxing, power lifting, wrestling) athletes frequently dehydrate to compete in lower weight classes. Also, persons medicated with diuretics may be dehydrated prior to initiating exercise. If sodium chloride deficits occur, then the extracellular fluid volume will contract and cause "salt depletion dehydration." A sodium chloride deficit usually occurs due to sweat sodium losses combined with excessive water consumption, but a sodium deficit can also occur without excessive water intake owing to high sweat sodium losses. Both of these scenarios produce sodium dilution, which is more commonly known as hyponatremia or "water intoxication."[3,4]

This chapter reviews the physiology, needs, and assessment of human water and electrolyte balance. The extent to which water and electrolyte imbalances affect temperature regulation and exercise performance are also considered. Throughout the chapter, the term euhydration refers to normal body water content, hypohydration refers to a body water deficit, and hyperhydration refers to increased body water content. Dehydration refers to the dynamic loss of body water.

## Physiology of Water and Electrolyte Balance

Net body water balance (loss = gain) is generally regulated well as a result of thirst and hunger drives coupled with free access to food and beverage.[1] This is accomplished by neuroendocrine and renal responses[5] to body water volume and tonicity changes, as well as non-regulatory social-behavioral factors.[6] These homeostatic responses collectively ensure that small degrees of over- and underhydration are readily compensated for in the short term. Using water balance studies, Adolph[7,8] found that daily body water varied narrowly between 0.22% and 0.48% in temperate and warm environments, respectively. However, exercise and environmental insult often pose a greater acute challenge to fluid balance homeostasis.

Water (total body water) is the principal chemical constituent of the human body. For an average young adult male, total body water is relatively constant and represents 50% to 70% of body weight.[9] Variability in total body water is primarily due to differences in body composition.[1,9] Total body water is distributed into intracellular fluid (ICF) and extracellular fluid (ECF) compartments. The ICF and ECF contain about 65% and 35% of total body water, respectively. The ECF is further divided into the interstitial and plasma spaces. Water balance represents the net difference between water intake and loss. When losses exceed intakes, total body water is decreased.

When body water deficits occur from sweat losses, a hypertonic hypovolemia generally results. Plasma volume decreases and plasma osmotic pressure increases in proportion to the decrease in total body water. Plasma volume decreases because it provides the fluid for sweat, and osmolality increases because sweat is ordinarily hypotonic relative to plasma. Resting plasma osmolality increases in a linear manner from about 283 mosmol/kg when euhydrated, to more than 300 mosmol/kg when hypohydrated by 15% of total body water.[1] The increase in osmotic pressure is primarily due to increased plasma sodium and chloride. with no consistent effect on potassium concentration.[10-12]

Incomplete fluid replacement decreases total body water, and as a consequence of free fluid exchange, affects each fluid space.[13-16] For example, Nose et al.[15] determined the distribution of body water loss among fluid spaces as well as among different body organs during hypohydration. They thermally dehydrated rats by 10% of body weight, and after the animals regained their normal core temperature, the body water measurements were obtained. The fluid deficit was apportioned between the intracellular (41%) and extracellular (59%) spaces. Regarding organ fluid loss, 40% came from muscle, 30% from skin, 14% from viscera, and 14% from bone. Neither the brain nor liver lost significant water content. They concluded that hypohydration results in water redistribution largely from the intra- and extracellular spaces of muscle and skin in order to maintain blood volume.

Different methods of dehydration are known or suspected to affect the partitioning of body water losses differently than those just described. For example, diuretics increase urine formation and generally result in the loss of both solutes and water. Diuretic-induced hypohydration generally results in an iso-osmotic hypovolemia, with a much greater ratio of plasma loss to body water loss than either exercise or heat-induced hypohydration.[10,17] As a result, relatively less intracellular fluid is lost after diuretic administration, since there is not an extracellular solute excess to stimulate redistribution of body water. In contrast, several studies[13,18,19] report substantial decreases in skeletal muscle intracellular water content following prolonged exercise without fluid replacement glycogen.

Exercise-induced hypohydration may result in a greater intracellular water loss than simple sweat-induced hypohydration (passive thermal dehydration). Kozlowski and Saltin[20] reported data to support this view, but Costill and Saltin[18] found no difference between exercise and thermal dehydration for the partitioning of water between the fluid compartments. It is therefore clear that the ratio of intracellular to extracellular water losses that occur with dehydration from sweating and diuretic use are different, but any difference between active and passive sweating remains unresolved. Other factors such as heat acclimatization status, posture, climate, mode, and intensity of exercise can also produce significant variability in the responses described above.[21,22]

## Water and Electrolyte Needs

Human water and electrolyte needs should not be based on a "minimal" intake, as this might eventually lead to a deficit and possible adverse performance and health consequences. Instead, the Food and Nutrition Board of the Institute of Medicine bases water needs on Adequate Intake (AI). The AI is based on experimentally derived intake levels that are expected to meet nutritional adequacy for essentially all members of a healthy population. The AI level for water is 2.7 to 3.7 L/d for sedentary women and men over age 19, respectively.[1] These values represent total water intake from all fluids (80%) and foods (20%). The AI for sodium is 1.5 g/d or 3.8 g/d sodium chloride.[1] The report also indicates that athletes and workers performing stressful exercise in the heat can exceed the AI for water and sodium.

Table 1[23] illustrates the wide variability in hourly sweat losses observed both within and between sports. Depending upon the duration of activity and heat stress exposure, the impact of these elevated hourly sweat rates on daily water requirements will vary. Figure 1 depicts generalized modeling approximations for daily water requirements based upon calculated sweating rates as a function of daily energy expenditure (activity level) and air temperature.[1] Applying this prediction model, it is clear that daily water requirements can increase two- to six-fold from baseline by simple manipulation of either variable. For example, daily water requirements for any given energy expenditure in temperate climates (20°C) can triple in very hot weather (40°C). In addition to air temperature, other environmental factors also modify sweat losses; these include relative humidity, air motion, solar load, and choice of clothing for protection against

**Table 1.** Sweating Rates for Different Sports

| Sport | Mean | Range |
|---|---|---|
| | *L/h* | |
| Water polo | 0.55 | 0.30–0.80 |
| Cycling | 0.80 | 0.29–1.25 |
| Running | 1.10 | 0.54–1.83 |
| Basketball | 1.11 | 0.70–1.60 |
| Soccer | 1.17 | 0.70–2.10 |

Data from Rehrer and Burke 1996.[23]

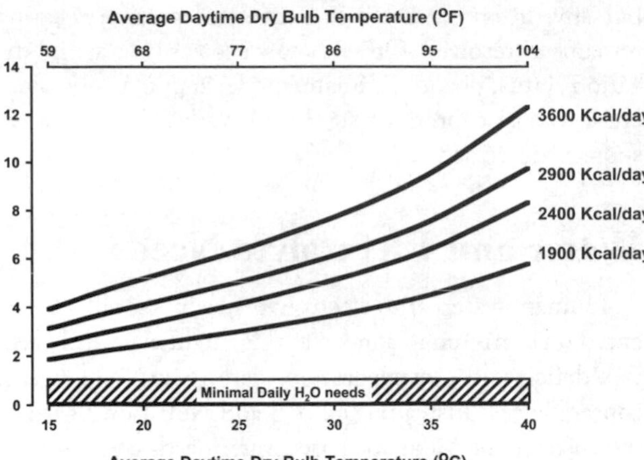


Figure 1. Daily water needs (l/d) estimated from sweat loss predictions due to changes in physical activity and air temperature. Daily energy expenditures of 1900, 2400, 2900 and 3600 kcal correspond to sedentary, low activity, active, and very active, respectively. (Data from Food and Nutrition Board, Institute of Medicine, 2004.[1])

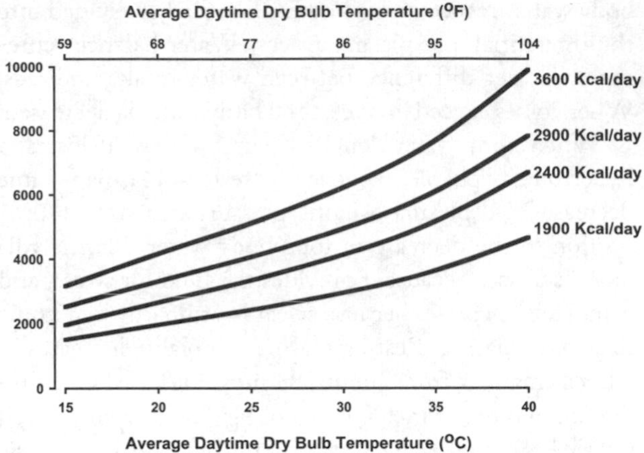


Figure 2. Daily sodium needs (mg/d) estimated from sweat loss predictions due to changes in physical activity and air temperature. Daily energy expenditures of 1900, 2400, 2900, and 3600 kcal correspond to sedentary, low activity, active, and very active, respectively. (Data from Food and Nutrition Board, Institute of Medicine, 2004.[1])

environmental elements.[24] Therefore, it is expected that water losses, and therefore water needs, will vary considerably among moderately active people based on changing extraneous influences.

Sweat is hypotonic to extracellular fluid, but contains electrolytes, primarily sodium chloride and, to a lesser extent, potassium, calcium, and magnesium.[25-27] Sweat sodium concentration averages 35 mEq/L (range 10–70 mEq /L) and varies depending upon diet, sweating rate, hydration level, and heat acclimation state.[25,28,29] Sweat potassium concentration averages 5 mEq/L (range 3–15 mEq /L), calcium 1 mEq/L (range 0.3–2 mEq/L), magnesium 0.8 mEq /L (range 0.2–1.5 mEq /L), and chloride 30 mEq/L (range 5–60 mEq/L).[29] Neither gender nor aging seem to have marked effects on sweat electrolyte concentrations.[30,31] Sweat glands reabsorb sodium by active transport, but the ability to reabsorb sweat sodium does not increase proportionally with the sweating rate. As a result, the concentration of sweat sodium increases at high sweating rates.[25,28] Heat acclimation improves the ability to reabsorb sodium, so heat-acclimated persons have lower sweat sodium concentrations (>50% reduction) for any given sweating rate.[28]

Figure 2 depicts generalized modeling approximations for daily sodium needs based upon calculated sweating rates as a function of daily energy expenditure (activity level) and air temperature.[1] This analysis assumes that persons are heat acclimated and have a sweat sodium concentration of 25 mEq/L (about 0.6 g/L). The average American diet contains about 4 g/d of sodium,[1] but this varies greatly depending upon ethnic preferences for food. Increases or decreases in sodium stores are usually corrected by adjustments in a person's salt appetite. In addition, when physical activity increases, the additional caloric intake associated with increased activity usually covers the additional sodium required.[1] Therefore, sodium supplementation is generally not necessary (unless subjects are performing very heavy activity) for the first several days of heat exposure, as normal dietary sodium intake appears adequate to compensate for sweat sodium losses.[2,32] If persons need additional sodium, this can be achieved by salting their food to taste. Another strategy is to rehydrate with fluids containing about 20 mEq/L of sodium. Most commercial sports beverages approximate this concentration.[2,32]

## Hydration Assessment

Although plasma osmolality is the criterion used as the hydration assessment measure for large-scale fluid needs assessment surveys,[1] the optimal choice of method for assessing hydration, particularly in sport, is limited by the circumstances and intent of the measurement. Popular hydration assessment techniques vary greatly in their applicability to laboratory or field use due to methodological limitations, which include the necessary circumstances for accurate measurement, ease of application, and sensitivity for detecting small, but meaningful changes in hydration status.[33]

Although there is presently no consensus for using one assessment approach over another, in most athletic arenas, the use of first morning body mass measurements in combination with some measure of urine concentration should allow ample sensitivity (low false negative) for detecting deviations in fluid balance. When more precision of acute hydration changes is desired, plasma osmolality and isotope dilution provide for gradations in measurement.[33] However, the simplest way to track acute hydration changes is to measure body mass before and after exercise using the reasonable assumption that 1 g of lost

**Table 2.** Hydration Assessment Indices

| Measure | Practicality | Validity (Acute vs. Chronic) | Euhydration Cutoff |
|---|---|---|---|
| Total body water | Low | Acute and chronic | < 2% |
| Plasma osmolality | Medium | Acute and chronic | < 290 mOsmol |
| Urine specific gravity | High | Chronic | < 1.020 g/ml |
| Urine osmolality | High | Chronic | < 700 mOsmol |
| Urine color | High | Chronic | < 4 |
| Body mass | High | Acute and chronic* | < 1% |

* Potentially confounded by changes in body composition during very prolonged assessment periods.

mass is equivalent to 1 mL of lost fluid. In fact, if proper controls are made, body mass changes can provide a more sensitive estimate of acute total body water changes than repeat measurements by dilution methods.[34] For longer periods (1–2-weeks), body mass may even remain stable enough to be a reliable hydration measure during periods of hard exercise and acute fluid flux whether in temperate[35,36] or hot[37] climates. Table 2 provides definable thresholds from the literature,[1,37-43] which can be used as a guide to detect a negative body fluid balance. Fluid intakes should be considered adequate when any two assessment outcomes are consistent with euhydration.

# Fluid Balance, Temperature Regulation, and Exercise Performance

The difficulty encountered when trying to match fluid consumption to sweat losses during exercise can produce hypohydration by 2% to 6% of body weight.[44] Although this is more common in hot environments, similar losses are observed in cold climates when working in heavy clothing.[45] The mismatch between intakes and losses is due to physiological and behavioral factors.

## *Hypohydration*

Hypohydration increases core temperature responses during exercise in temperate and hot climates.[46] In fact, a deficit of only 1% of body weight elevates core temperature during exercise.[47] As the magnitude of water deficit increases, the magnitude of core temperature elevation ranges from 0.1 to 0.23°C for every percent body weight lost,[1,46] but the core temperature elevation may be greater during exercise in hot compared with temperate climates.[48] In addition, altering the time of fluid ingestion (early or late into the exercise bout) does not modify the core temperature elevation from progressive dehydration.[49] Hypohydration not only elevates core temperature, but also negates the core temperature advantages conferred by high aerobic fitness and heat acclimation.[46]

When hypohydrated, elevated core temperature responses result from a reduction in the capacity for heat dissipation. The relative contributions of evaporative and dry heat loss during exercise depend upon the specific environmental conditions,[50] but both avenues of heat loss are adversely affected by hypohydration.[1] Local sweating and skin blood flow responses are both reduced for a given core temperature,[46,48] and whole-body sweating is usually either reduced[51] or unchanged[52] during exercise at a given metabolic rate in the heat. However, even when hypohydration is associated with no change in whole-body sweating rate, core temperature is usually elevated, so that whole-body sweating rate for a given core temperature is lower. Both the singular and combined effects of plasma hyperosmolality and hypovolemia have been suggested as mediating the reduced heat loss response during exercise-heat stress.[48] Figure 3 summarizes the relative contributions of hyperosmolality and hypovolemia to adverse thermoregulatory responses during exercise in temperate and hot climates.[48] These effects are noticeably smaller in cooler environments.[48,53,54]

Hypohydration can decrease dynamic exercise performance.[1] Dehydration by more than 2% of body weight degrades endurance exercise, especially in hot environments.[1,55] The magnitude of the performance decrement is variable, and probably depends on the individual, on environmental conditions, and on exercise mode differences. However, for a given person and event, the greater the dehydration level (after achieving the threshold for performance degradation) the greater the performance

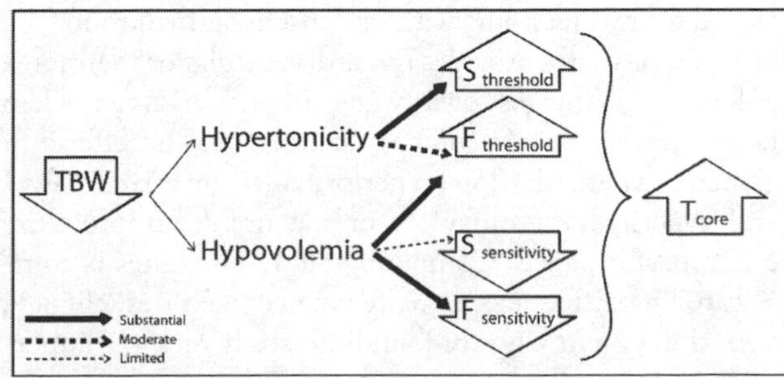


Figure 3. Effects of reducing total body water (TBW) on sweating (S) and skin blood flow (F) thresholds and sensitivities. Substantial, moderate, and limited descriptors are based on amount of supporting data. (Used with permission from Cheuvront et al. 2004.[48])

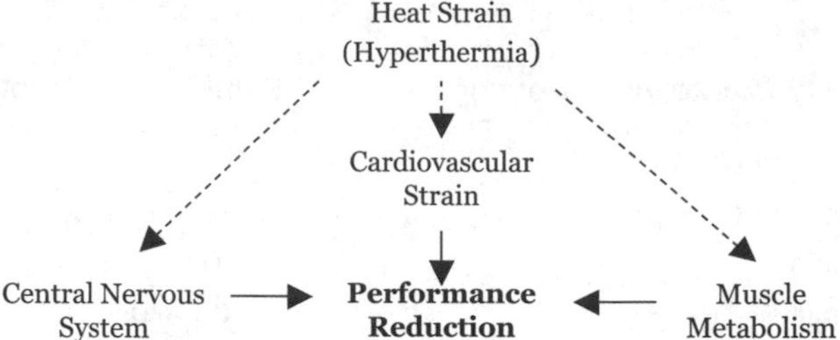


Figure 4. Physiologic factors that contribute to dehydration-mediated performance decrements. (Used with permission from Cheuvront et al. 2003.[55])

decrement. Dehydration probably does not alter muscle strength,[56] but sometimes has been reported to reduce dynamic small muscle endurance.[57,58] In addition, dehydration of over 2% often adversely influences cognitive function in the heat; however, this area requires more research.[1]

Physiologic factors that contribute to dehydration-mediated performance decrements include hyperthermia,[59,60] increased cardiovascular strain,[61,62] altered metabolic function,[63] or perhaps via events originating in the central nervous system[55,58] (Figure 4). Though each factor is unique, evidence suggests that they interact to contribute in concert, rather than in isolation, to degrading exercise performance. The relative contribution of each factor may differ depending on the event, environmental conditions, and athletic prowess, but elevated hyperthermia probably acts to accentuate the performance decrement.[55,64,65]

### *Hyperhydration*

Hyperhydration is not easy to sustain, since overdrinking of water or carbohydrate- electrolyte solutions produce a fluid overload that is rapidly excreted by the kidneys.[66] Greater fluid retention can be achieved with an aqueous solution containing glycerol,[66,67] which increases fluid retention by reducing free water clearance.[66] However, both exercise and heat stress decrease renal blood flow and free water clearance and therefore negate glycerol's effectiveness as a hyperhydrating agent if ingested during exercise.[68] Studies demonstrate that total body water can be increased by approximately 1.5 L and sustained for several hours with glycerol hyperhydration[66,68]; however, glycerol provides no cardiovascular or thermoregulatory advantages over water ingestion alone when taken during exercise or heat stress.[68-70] The effects of glycerol hyperhydration on performance are mixed. Glycerol hyperhydration may[71-73] or may not[69,70] improve exercise performance. Comparing study outcomes is complicated by differences in performance measures, climate, and the potentially confounding study design limitations.[68]

### *Hyponatremia*

Symptomatic hyponatremia (typically associated with serum sodium concentrations of less than 125–130 mEq/L) has been observed during marathon and ultramarathon competition,[74-76] military training,[77,78] and recreational activities.[79] In athletic events, the condition is more likely to occur in females and slower competitors. The severity of the symptomatology is related to the magnitude that the serum sodium concentration falls and the rapidity with which it develops.[80] If hyponatremia develops over many hours, it might cause less brain swelling and fewer adverse symptoms.[80] The hyponatremia associated with prolonged exercise develops primarily because individuals drink excessively large quantities of hypotonic fluids (relative to sweating rate) for many hours.[3,76,77] Unreplaced sodium losses contribute to the rate and magnitude of sodium dilution. Additionally, nausea (which increases vasopressin levels) and heat/exercise stress (which reduce renal blood flow and urine output) can negatively affect the ability of the kidney to rapidly correct the fluid-electrolyte imbalance.[81] The syndrome can be prevented by not drinking in excess of the sweating rate, and by consuming salt-containing fluids or foods when participating in exercise events that produce multiple hours of continuous or near-continuous sweating.

## Summary

Among the greatest challenges to body water homeostasis is exercise and environmental stress. Sweating results in water and electrolyte losses. Because sweat output often exceeds water intake, there is an acute water deficit that results in a hypertonic hypovolemia and intracellular and extracellular fluid contraction. Although water and electrolyte needs increase as a result of exercise, eloquent physiological and behavioral adaptations allow humans to regulate daily body water and electrolyte balance so long as food and fluid are readily available. Although there is presently no consensus for choosing one hydration assessment approach over another, deviations in daily fluid balance can be determined with ample sensitivity using a combination of any two common assessment measures. Hypohydration increases heat storage by reducing sweating rate and skin blood flow responses for a given core temperature. Aerobic exercise tasks can be adversely affected if hypohydration exceeds about 2% of normal body mass, with the potential effect greater in warm environments. Hyperhydration provides no thermoregulatory or exercise performance advantages over euhydration in the heat. Excessive consumption of hypotonic fluid over many hours can lead to hyponatremia. Marked electrolyte losses can accelerate the dilution and exacerbate the problem. Hyponatremia can be avoided by proper attention to diet and fluid needs.

## Acknowledgments

The authors would like to thank Rob Demes for technical assistance in preparing this manuscript. The views, opinions, and/or findings contained in this report are those of the authors and should not be construed as an official Department of the Army position, or decision, unless so designated by other official documentation. Approved for public release; distribution unlimited.

## References


1. Food and Nutrition Board, Institute of Medicine. Dietary Reference Intakes for Water, Potassium, Sodium, Chloride, and Sulfate. Washington, DC: National Academies Press; 2005. Available online at: http://www.nap.edu/books/0309091691/html.
2. Marriott BM. *Fluid Replacement and Heat Stress*. Washington, DC: National Academies Press; 1994.
3. Montain SJ, Sawka MN, Wenger CB. Exertional hyponatremia: risk factors and pathogenesis. Exerc Sports Sci Rev. 2001;29:113–117.
4. Vrijens DMJ, Rehrer NJ. Sodium-free fluid ingestion decreases plasma sodium during exercise in the heat. J Appl Physiol. 1999;86:1847–1851.
5. Andreoli T, Reeves W, Bichet D. Endocrine control of water balance. In: Fray J, Goodman H, eds. *Handbook of Physiology, Section 7, Volume III: Endocrine Regulation of Water and Electrolyte Balance*. New York: Oxford University Press; 2000; 530–569.
6. Rolls B, Rolls E. *Thirst*. Cambridge: Cambridge University Press; 1982.
7. Adolph EF, DB Dill. Observations on water metabolism in the desert. Am J Physiol. 1938;123: 369–378.
8. Adolph EF. *Physiological Regulations*. Lancaster, PA: Jacques Cattell Press; 1943; 100.
9. Sawka MN, Coyle EF. Influence of body water and blood volume on thermoregulation and exercise performance in the heat. In: Hollozsy JO, ed. *Exercise and Sport Sciences Reviews*. Baltimore: Williams & Wilkins; 1999; 167–218.
10. Kubica R, Nielsen B, Bonnesen A, et al. Relationship between plasma volume reduction and plasma electrolyte changes after prolonged bicycle exercise, passive heating and diuretic dehydration. Acta Physiol Pol. 1983;34:569–579.
11. Montain SJ, Laird JE, Latzka WA, Sawka MN. Aldosterone and vasopressin responses in the heat: hydration level and exercise intensity effects. Med Sci Sports Exerc. 1997;29:661–668.
12. Senay LC. Relationship of evaporative rates to serum [Na+], [K+], and osmolality in acute heat stress. J Appl Physiol. 1968;25:149–152.
13. Costill DL, Coté R, Fink W. Muscle water and electrolytes following varied levels of dehydration in man. J Appl Physiol. 1976;40:6–11.
14. Durkot MJ, Martinez O, Brooks-McQuade D, Francesconi R. Simultaneous determination of fluid shifts during thermal stress in a small animal model. J Appl Physiol. 1986;61:1031–1034.
15. Nose H, Morimoto T, Ogura K. Distribution of water losses among fluid compartments of tissues under thermal dehydration in the rat. Jpn J Physiol. 1983;33:1019–1029.
16. Singh MV, Rawal SB, Pichan G, Tyagi AK. Changes in body fluid compartments during hypohydration and rehydration in heat-acclimated tropical subjects. Aviat Space Environ Med. 1993;64: 295–299.
17. O'Brien C, Young AJ, Sawka MN. Hypohydration and thermoregulation in cold air. J Appl Physiol. 1998;84:185–189.
18. Costill DL, Saltin B. Muscle glycogen and electrolytes following exercise and thermal dehydration. In: Howald H, Poortmans JR, eds. *Metabolic Adaptations to Prolonged Physical Exercise*. Basel: Birkhaiser Verlag; 1975; 352–360.
19. Costill DL, Cote R, Fink WJ, van Handel P. Muscle water and electrolyte distribution during prolonged exercise. Int J Sports Med. 1981;2:130–134.
20. Kozlowski S, Saltin B. Effect of sweat loss on body fluids. J Appl Physiol. 1964;19:1119–1124.
21. Harrison, M.H. Effects on thermal stress and exercise on blood volume in humans. Physiol Rev. 1985; 65:149–209.
22. Sawka, M.N. Body fluid responses and hypohydration during exercise-heat stress. In: Pandolf KB, Sawka, MN, and Gonzalez, RR, eds. *Human Performance Physiology and Environmental Medicine at Terrestrial Extremes*. Indianapolis, IN: Benchmark Press; 1988; 227–266.
23. Rehrer N, Burke L. Sweat losses during various sports. Aust J Nutr Diet. 1996;53:S13–S16.
24. Latzka WA, Montain SJ. Water and electrolyte requirements for exercise. Clin Sports Med. 1999;18: 513–524.
25. Costill DL, Cote R, Miller E, Miller T, Wynder S. Water and electrolyte replacement during repeated days of work in the heat. Aviat Space Environ Med 1975;46(6):795–800.
26. Costill DL. Sweating: its composition and effects on body fluids. Ann N Y Acad Sci. 1977;301:160–173.
27. Verde T, Shephard RJ, Corey P, Moore R. Sweat composition in exercise and in heat. J Appl Physiol. 1982;53:1540–1545.
28. Allan JR, Wilson CG. Influence of acclimatization on sweat sodium concentration. J Appl Physiol. 1971; 30:708–712.
29. Brouns F. Heat-sweat-dehydration-rehydration: a praxis oriented approach. J Sports Sci. 1991;9: 143–152.
30. Meyer F, Bar-Or O, MacDougal D, Heigenhauser GJF. Sweat electrolyte loss during exercise in the heat: effects of gender and maturation. Med Sci Sports Exerc. 1992;24:776–781.
31. Morimoto T, Slabochova Z, Naman RK, Sargent F. Sex differences in physiological reactions to thermal stress. J Appl Physiol. 1967;22:526–532.

32. Convertino VA, Armstrong LE, Coyle EF, et al. American College of Sports Medicine Position Stand: exercise and fluid replacement. Med Sci Sports Exerc. 1996;28:i–vii.
33. Oppliger, RA, Bartok, C. Hydration testing for athletes. Sports Medicine. 2002;32:959–971.
34. Gudivaka R, Schoeller DA, Kushner RF, Bolt MJG. Single- and multifrequency models for bioelectrical impedance analysis of body water compartments. J Appl Physiol. 1999;87:1087–1096.
35. Leiper J, Carnie A, Maughan R. Water turnover rates in sedentary and exercising middle aged men. Br J Sports Med. 1996;30:24–26.
36. Leiper J, Pitsiladis Y, Maughan R. Comparison of water turnover rates in men undertaking prolonged cycling exercise and sedentary men. Int J Sports Med. 2001;22:181–185.
37. Cheuvront SN, Carter III R, Montain SJ, and Sawka, MN. Daily body mass variability and stability in active men undergoing exercise-heat stress. Int J Sport Nutr Exerc Metab. 2004;14:532–540.
38. Armstrong LE, Maresh JW, Castellani MF, et al. Urinary indices of hydration status. Int J Sport Nutr. 1994;4:265–279.
39. Bartok C, Schoeller DA, Sullivan JC, et al. Hydration testing in collegiate wrestlers undergoing hypertonic dehydration. Med Sci Sports Exerc. 2004;36: 510–517.
40. Popowski LA, Oppliger RA, Lambert GP, et al. Blood and urinary measures of hydration during progressive acute dehydration. Med Sci Sports Exerc. 2001;33:747–753.
41. Ritz P. Methods of assessing body water and body composition. In: *Hydration Throughout Life*. Arnaud MJ, ed. Vittel, France: Perrier Vittel Water Institute; 1998; 63–74.
42. Senay LC. Effects of exercise in the heat on body fluid distribution. Med Sci Sports Exerc. 1979;11: 42–48.
43. Shirreffs SM, Maughan RJ. Urine osmolality and conductivity as indices of hydration status in athletes in the heat. Med Sci Sports Exerc. 1998;30: 1598–1602.
44. Sawka MN, Cheuvront SN, Carter R 3rd. Human water needs. Nutr Rev. 2005;63(6 part 2):S30–S39.
45. O'Brien C, Freund BJ, Sawka MN, et al. Hydration assessment during cold-weather military field training exercises. Arct Med Res. 1996;55:20–26.
46. Sawka MN. Physiological consequences of hydration: exercise performance and thermoregulation. Med Sci Sports Exerc. 1992;24:657–670.
47. Ekblom B, Greenleaf CJ, Greenleaf JE, Hermansen L. Temperature regulation during exercise dehydration in man. Acta Physiol Scand. 1970;79:475–483.
48. Cheuvront SN, Carter III R, Montain SJ, et al. Influence of hydration and airflow on thermoregulatory control in the heat. J Therm Biol. 2004;29:471–477.
49. Montain SJ, Coyle EF. Influence of the timing of fluid ingestion on temperature regulation during exercise. J Appl Physiol. 1993;75:688–695.
50. Sawka MN, Wenger CB, Pandolf KB. Thermoregulatory responses to acute exercise-heat stress and heat acclimation. In: Fregly MJ, Blatteis CM, eds. *Handbook of Physiology, Section 4, Environmental Physiology*. New York: Oxford University Press; 1996; 157–185.
51. Sawka MN, Young AJ, Dennis RC, et al. Human intravascular immunoglobulin responses to exercise: heat and hypohydration. Aviat Space Environ Med. 1989;60:634–638.
52. Armstrong LE, Maresh CM, Gabaree CV, et al. Thermal and circulatory responses during exercise: effects of hypohydration, dehydration, and water intake. J Appl Physiol. 1997;82:2028–2035.
53. Sawka MN, Toner MM, Francesconi RP, Pandolf KB. Hypohydration and exercise: effects of heat acclimation, gender, and environment. J Appl Physiol. 1983;55:1147–1153.
54. Nielsen B. Effect of changes in plasma $Na^+$ and $Ca^{2+}$ ion concentration on body temperature during exercise. Acta Physiol Scand. 1974;91:123–129.
55. Cheuvront SN, Carter III R, Sawka MN. Fluid balance and endurance exercise performance. Curr Sports Med Rep. 2003;2:202–208.
56. Greiwe JS, Staffey KS, Melrose DR, Narve M, Knowlton RG. Effects of dehydration on isometric muscular strength and endurance. Med Sci Sports Exerc. 1998;30:284–288.
57. Bigard A H, Sanchez G Claveyrolas, S Martin, et al. Effects of dehydration and rehydration on EMG changes during fatiguing contractions. Med Sci Sports Exerc. 2001;33:1694–1700.
58. Montain SJ, Smith SA, Matott RP, et al. Hypohydration effects on skeletal muscle performance and metabolism: A 31P MRS study. J Appl Physiol. 1998;84:1889–1894.
59. Nielsen B, Hyldig T, Bidstrup F, et al. Brain activity and fatigue during prolonged exercise in the heat. Pflugers Arch. 2001;442:41–48.
60. Gonzalez-Alonso J, Teller C, Andersen SL, et al. Influence of body temperature on the development of fatigue during prolonged exercise in the heat. J Appl Physiol. 1999;86:1032–1039.
61. Gonzalez-Alonso J, Mora-Rodriguez R, Below P, Coyle E. Dehydration reduces cardiac output and increases systemic and cutaneous vascular resistance during exercise. J Appl Physiol. 1995;79:1487–1496.
62. Montain SJ, Coyle EF. Influence of graded dehydration on hyperthermia and cardiovascular drift during exercise. J Appl Physiol. 1992;73:1340–1350.
63. Febbraio MA. Does muscle function and metabolism affect exercise performance in the heat? Exerc Sport Sci Rev. 2000;28:171–176.
64. Gonzalez-Alonso J, Mora-Rodriguez R, Below P,

Coyle E. Dehydration markedly impairs cardiovascular function in hyperthermic endurance athletes during exercise. J Appl Physiol. 1997;82:1229–1236.
65. Gonzalez-Alonso J, Mora-Rodriguez R, Coyle EF. Stroke volume during exercise: interaction of environment and hydration. Am J Physiol Heart Circ Physiol. 2000;278:H321–H330.
66. Freund BJ, Montain SJ, Young AJ, et al. Glycerol hyperhydration: hormonal, renal, and vascular fluid responses. J Appl Physiol. 1995;79:2069–2077.
67. Riedesel ML, Allen DY, Peake GT, Al-Qattan K. Hyperhydration with glycerol solutions. J Appl Physiol. 1987;63:2262–2268.
68. Latzka WA, Sawka MN. Hyperhydration and glycerol: Thermoregulatory effects during exercise in hot climates. Can J Appl Physiol. 2000;25:536–545.
69. Magal M, Webster MJ, Sistrunk LE, et al. Comparison of glycerol and water hydration regimens on tennis related performance. Med Sci Sports Exerc. 2003; 35:150–156.
70. Marino FE, Kay D, Cannon J. Glycerol hyperhydration fails to improve endurance performance and thermoregulation in humans in a warm humid environment. Pflugers Arch. 2003;446:455–462.
71. Anderson MJ, Cotter JD, Garnham AP, et al. Effect of glycerol-induced hyperhydration on thermoregulation and metabolism during exercise in the heat. Int J Sport Nutr Exerc Metab. 2001;11:315–333.
72. Coutts A, Reaburn P, Mummery K, Holmes M. The effect of glycerol hyperhydration on Olympic distance triathlon performance in high ambient temperatures. Int J Sport Nutr Exerc Metab. 2002;12: 105–119.
73. Hitchins S, Martin DT, Burke L, et al. Glycerol hyperhydration improves cycle time trial performance in hot humid conditions. Eur J Appl Physiol. 1999;80:494–501.
74. Davis DP, Videen JS, Marino A, et al. Exercise-associated hyponatremia in marathon runners: a two-year experience. J Emerg Med. 2001;21:47–57.
75. Hew TD, Chorley JN, Cianca JC, Divine JG. The incidence, risk factors, and clinical manifestations of hyponatremia in marathon runners. Clin J Sport Med. 2003;13:41–47.
76. Speedy DB, Noakes TD, Schneider C. Exercise-associated hyponatremia. Emerg Med. 2001;13: 17–27.
77. Garigan T, Ristedt DE. Death from hyponatremia as a result of acute water intoxication in an Army basic trainee. Mil Med. 1999;164:234–237.
78. O'Brien KK, Montain SJ, Corr WP, et al. Hyponatremia associated with overhydration in U.S. Army trainees. Mil Med. 2001;166:405–410.
79. Backer HD, Shopes E, Collins SL. Hyponatremia in recreational hikers in Grand Canyon National Park. J Wild Med. 1993;4:391–406.
80. Knochel JP. Clinical complications of body fluid and electrolyte balance. In: Buskirk ER, Puhl SM, eds. *Body Fluid Balance: Exercise and Sport*. Boca Raton, FL: CRC Press; 1996; 297–317.
81. Zambraski EJ. The kidney and body fluid balance during exercise. In: Buskirk ER, Puhl SM, eds. *Body Fluid Balance*. Boca Raton: CRC Press; 1996; 75–95.

# 34 Iron

John Beard

## History and Introduction

Iron has been an integral component of biologic systems since the beginning of life on this planet. There have been arguments that without iron, life could not exist as we conceive of it at this time.[1] Iron therapeutics were used in ancient China 2000 years B.C. and have also been used in chemical treatments for various physical and health aliments by most of the great cultures of our world. Thomas Sydenham (1624–1689) treated chlorosis with oral iron, while Nicholas Lemery (1645–1715) first observed the presence of iron in blood that had been ashed.[2] Iron was identified as a constituent of animal liver and blood in the early 18th century, with Boussingalut being the first to describe the essentiality of iron in 1872.[3] Biologists progressed with the identification of specific forms of iron in mammalian systems over the next several decades with the identification of the roles of these essential and non-essential iron compounds in human biology.

Iron is a component of every known living organism, with very few exceptions. It is both an essential nutrient and a potential toxicant to cells, and as such requires a highly sophisticated and complex set of regulatory approaches to meet the demands of cells and to prevent excess accumulation. A sufficient supply is essential for the functioning of many biochemical processes, which include electron transfer reactions, gene regulation, binding and transport of oxygen, and regulation of cell growth and differentiation. This homeostasis involves the regulation of iron entry into the body, the regulation of iron entry into cells, the storage of iron in ferritin, the incorporation of iron into proteins, and the regulation of iron release from cells for transport to other cells and organs.

## Chemistry

Iron is element number 26 in the periodic table and has an atomic weight of 55.85. It is the fourth most abundant element and the second most abundant metal in the earth's crust. In simple aqueous solutions, iron exists in two principle oxidation states: ferrous iron ($Fe^{+2}$) and ferric iron ($Fe^{+3}$). The two forms of iron in solution are interchanged by the addition or subtraction of an electron. Many common reducing agents (e.g., ascorbic acid) will convert ferric iron to ferrous iron, while simple exposure to oxygen in solution will convert ferrous back to ferric iron. The amount of "free" iron within cells or in the fluid spaces of the body is quite low, since iron can easily participate in redox reactions that underlie the inherent toxicity of excess free iron within cells. This well-known Haber-Weiss-Fenton reaction is illustrated below:

$$Fe^{+2} + O_2 \Rightarrow Fe^{+3} + O_2$$
$$2O_2 + 2H^+ \Rightarrow H_2O_2 + O_2$$
$$Fe^{+2} + H_2O_2 \Rightarrow OH\bullet + \bullet OH^- + Fe^{+3}$$

The hydroxyl radical, OH•, is capable of attacking most proteins, nucleic acids, and carbohydrates, and initiating lipid peroxidation reactions.[4] The vast majority of iron within cells of plants and animals is: 1) stored within large complex proteins such as hemosiderin or ferritin; 2) contained as an essential component with proteins and enzymes and critical for their functioning; or 3) contained in proteins of iron transport that move iron from one cellular organelle to another, from one cell to another cell, or between organs (transferrin is an example of this iron-protein complex).

The interconversion of iron oxidation states is not only a mechanism whereby iron participates in electron transfer, but it is also a mechanism whereby iron can reversibly bind ligands. Iron can bind to many ligands by virtue of its unoccupied *d* orbitals. The preferred biological ligands for iron are oxygen, nitrogen, and sulfur atoms. The electronic spin state and biological redox potential (from +1000 mV for some heme proteins to −550 mV for some bacterial ferredoxins) of iron can change according to the ligand to which it is bound. By exploiting the oxidation state, redox potential, and electron spin state of iron, nature can precisely adjust iron's chemical reactivity. Thus, iron is particularly suited to participate in a large number of useful biochemical reactions.[5] The general classification of these reactions is oxygen transport and storage, electron transfer, and substrate oxidation-reduction. It is important to note that the activity of many of these enzymes decreases during tissue iron deficiency. Only rarely, however, have direct connections between biochemical events and clinical manifestations been firmly established.

## Biochemistry and Metabolism

Four major classes of iron-containing proteins carry out these reactions in the mammalian system: iron-containing non-enzymatic proteins (hemoglobin and myoglobin), iron-sulfur enzymes, heme-containing enzymes, and iron-containing enzymes that are non-iron-sulfur, non-heme enzymes (Table 1). In principal oxygen transport, a non-enzymatic protein (hemoglobin or myoglobin) functions as a critical ligand for the binding of dioxygen. In iron-sulfur enzymes, iron participates in single electron-transfer reactions, primarily in energy metabolism. In the third category, iron is bound to various forms of heme and participates again in electron-transfer reactions when associated with various cofactors (e.g., cytochrome P450 complexes). The final group of iron-containing enzymes is a catch-all grouping in which iron is not bound to a porphyrin ring structure or in iron-sulfur complexes.

### *Oxygen Transport and Storage*

The movement of oxygen from the environment to terminal oxidases is one of the key functions of iron. Oxygen is bound to porphyrin ring iron-containing molecules, either as part of the prosthetic group of hemoglobin within red blood cells or as myoglobin, the facilitator of oxygen diffusion in tissue.

Hemoglobin is a tetrameric protein with two pairs of identical subunits ($\alpha 2$ and $\beta 2$, with a molecular weight of 64,000). Each subunit has one prosthetic group, iron-protoporphyrin-IX, whose ferrous iron reversibly binds dioxygen. The synthesis of erythroid heme is partially controlled by the availability of iron to maturing erythroblasts, as iron regulates the initial rate-limiting step in heme biosynthesis by altering the stability of the specific ($\delta$-amino-levulinic acid synthetase) mRNA. The four subunits are not covalently attached to each other, but do react cooperatively with dioxygen with specific modulation by pH, $CO_2$ pressure ($pCO_2$), organic phosphates, and temperature. These modulators of the affinity of hemoglobin for iron determine the efficiency of the transport of oxygen from the alveoli capillary interface in the lung to the red cell/capillary tissue interface in peripheral tissues.

The allosteric effect of decreasing pH, the well-known Bohr effect, decreases the binding affinity of heme iron for dioxygen via protonation of His-146 on $\beta$-chains and Val-1 on $\alpha$-chains in the presence of $Cl^{-1}$ and $CO_2$. $CO_2$ forms a Schiff base with the terminal amino acids of each chain and decreases dioxygen affinity. This favors the unloading of oxygen in tissues in which the pH is lower and the $pCO_2$ is higher than in arterial blood. 2,3-Diphosphoglycerate is a product of a side pathway within erythrocytes and binds to a specific region of the $\beta$-chain to decrease hemoglobin-oxygen binding affinity. Homeostasis with respect to oxygen transport is evident in iron-deficient anemic individuals. There is usually a rightward shift of the dissociation curve with anemia, where the blood content of hemoglobin is significantly reduced and there is an increased cardiac output that is only partially compensatory. The increase in cardiac output is the result of an increase in both stroke volume and heart rate, with a resulting hypertrophy of the ventricular muscle wall that is concentric in nature.[6] There may also be physiological conditions that increase the demand for oxygen transport, such as high physical exertion rates (discussed later in this review), with a resulting decreased maximal aerobic capacity because of limitations in oxygen transport ability. It is uncommon, however, to find significant arterial desaturation unless very high rates of oxygen transport are required.

Myoglobin is the single-chain hemoprotein in cyto-

**Table 1.** Categories of Iron-Containing Proteins in Mammalian Metabolism

| Iron-Sulfur Enzymes | Iron Storage and Transport Proteins | Hemoproteins | Other Iron-Dependent Enzymes |
|---|---|---|---|
| Flavoproteins | • Transferrin<br>• Lactoferrin<br>• Uteroferin<br>• Transferrin-like proteins | Hemoglobin | Iron-activated enzymes |
| Heme flavoproteins<br>• 1Fe-1S<br>• 2Fe-2S<br>• 4Fe-4S | Ferritin<br>Hemosiderin | Myoglobin<br>Cytochromes | |

plasm (molecular weight 17,000) that increases the rate of diffusion of dioxygen from capillary red cells to cytoplasm and mitochondria. The concentration of myoglobin in skeletal muscle is drastically reduced (40%–60%) in tissue iron deficiency, thus limiting the rate of diffusion of dioxygen from erythrocytes to mitochondria.[7] The sensitivity of myoglobin concentration to iron status has not been established in other tissues.

### *Electron Transport*

The second group of iron-containing proteins comprise heme enzymes that use iron within the porphyrin ring structure and are usually coupled with other enzymes in integrated electron transport processes. The overall scheme of the electron transport chain and the forms of iron that participate in electron transport are summarized elsewhere.[8] This family of cytochromes contains heme as the active site with the iron-porphyrin ring functioning to reduce ferrous iron to ferric iron with the acceptance of electrons.

The third group of iron-containing proteins, the iron sulfur enzymes, also act as electron carriers via the action of iron bound to either two or four sulfur atoms and cysteine side chains. The 40 different proteins that constitute the respiratory chain contain six different heme proteins, six iron sulfur centers, two copper centers, and ubiquinone to connect NADH to oxygen. There are numerous examples of these proteins and enzymes, which are summarized in Table 2. Although the sensitivity of many of these enzymes to iron depletion has been observed, the systematic evaluation of tissue sensitivity for this modest list is lacking.

## Inter-Organ Iron Exchange

### *Overview*

The dynamics of iron movement from dietary intake to inter-organ distribution are well described by scientists in the fields of clinical science, nutrition, and iron biology.[9-14] The regulation of iron movement across the enterocyte optimizes iron assimilation into the body when an individual is iron depleted and limits iron absorption when iron stores are replete. The exact nature of the feedback signal from body iron status to the enterocyte is now being elucidated, with a putative signal protein, hepcidin, being recently described (see more detailed description below). A prolonged negative iron balance or an acute rapid blood loss both ultimately lead to a depletion of the storage iron pool, which can contain as much as 2000 to 3000 mg of iron (Figure 1). The storage iron bound into tissue ferritin is used to meet the daily requirements not provided by the diet. Nearly all cells contain ferritin, although the bulk of the body's storage iron pool is in the liver and spleen.[9] Iron mobilized from tissue iron is transported by the iron transporter transferrin, and comprises a small pool of iron (under 5 mg typically) that is very labile. This plasma transport protein is normally only 25% to 50% saturated with iron bound to its two identical

**Table 2.** Newly Discovered Iron Proteins

| Name(s) | Characteristics | Predominant Function |
|---|---|---|
| IREG-1 (ferroportin 1) | 570 amino acids, 5′-IRE, 10 transmembrane-spanning domains, no homology with other known proteins | Located on the basolateral membrane of the enterocyte and acts as an metal exporter |
| Dcytb (duodenal cytochrome B) | 286 amino acids, 50% homology with Cyt B5, no IRE, six transmembrane domains | Ferroxidase protein on apical enterocyte membrane; reductase activity is greater than the iron absorption rate |
| DMT-1,2 (divalent metal transporter, NRAMP2) | 561 amino acids, 12 trans-membrane regions. 3′-IRE on one isoform; DMT-2 is a splice variant with a missing 16 to 18 amino acids at C terminus, no IRE, different cellular distribution than DMT-1 | Functions to move divalent metals from endosomes to cytoplasmic space and is coupled with the TfR recycling endosome to deliver iron to cellular spaces |
| Hepcidin (LEAP1-liver expressed antimicrobial peptide) | 86 amino acids with a signal peptide and reduced to 20 amino acids in plasma; 8 disulfide linkages | Plasma protein from hepatocytes that associates with ferroportin to regulate iron release from macrophages and enterocytes |
| HFE (hemochromatosis gene) | Class-1 MHC protein that binds to a β2-microglobular protein on basolateral membrane of enterocytes | Competitive binding with iron and ferroportin-hepciden complex to regulate iron release from enterocytes |

IRE = Iron-response element; MHC = major histocompatibility complex.

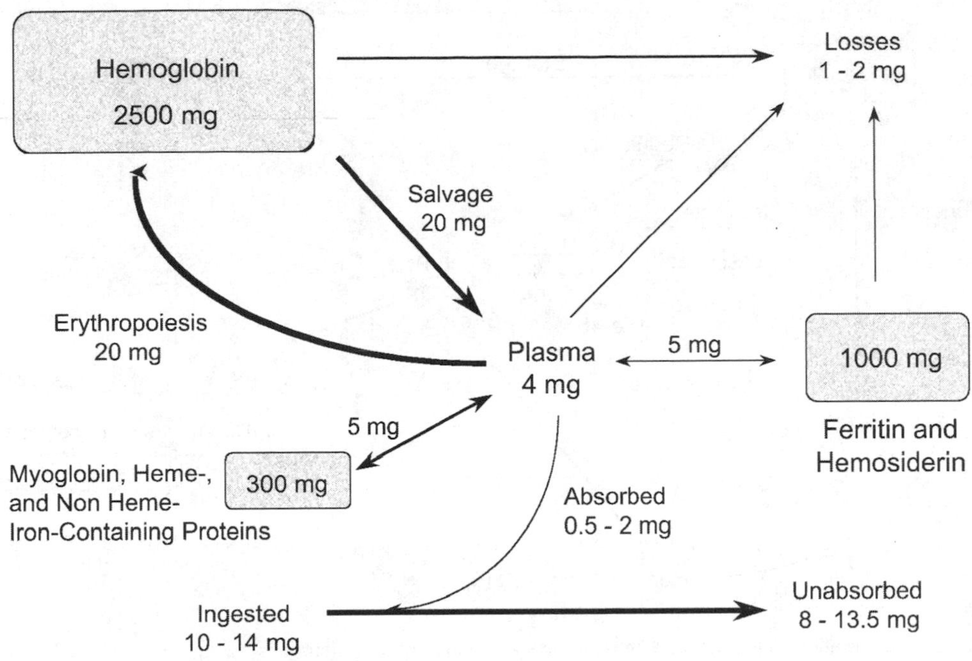


Figure 1. Body iron metabolism reflecting limiting efficiency of iron absorption, high quantitative movement to bone marrow, recycling from senescent red cells, and other essential iron pools.

binding sites.[15] A negative iron balance will eventually lead to the depletion of the storage iron pools, with a resulting decline in the transferrin saturation to less than 15%, meaning that less than adequate iron is available for delivery to essential body iron proteins.[9]

The commonly accepted primary route of iron uptake into cells is mediated by the transferrin receptor on the cell surface,[16] the amount of which is influenced by the cellular iron status, with the ultimate regulation exerted by iron-response proteins (IRPs) binding to mRNA iron-response elements (IREs).[17] Thus, as the cellular pool of low-molecular-weight iron decreases, there is an up-regulation of iron intake into cells and a down-regulation of the synthesis of the iron storage proteins. This influence is exerted via the existence of iron-regulatory proteins (IRP-1, IRP-2) and their role in the regulation of mRNA translation (Figure 2).[16-18]

## *Iron Turnover and Redistribution*

Plasma iron turnover is primarily mediated by the destruction of senescent erythrocytes by the reticuloendothelial system.[19] For example, in a 70-kg individual with a normal iron status, about 35 mg/d of iron is turned over in the plasma. Erythrocytes, which contain about 80% of the body's functional iron, have a mean functional lifetime of 120 days in humans. About 85% of the iron derived from hemoglobin degradation is re-released to the body in the form of iron bound to transferrin or ferritin. Each day, 0.66% of the body's total iron content is recycled in this manner. Smaller contributions are made to plasma iron turnover by the degradation of myoglobin and iron-containing enzymes.

## *Storage and Mobilization of Iron*

The concentration of iron in the body is approximately 30 to 40 mg/kg body weight. However, that concentration varies as a function of age and sex and the specific tissues and organs being examined. About 85% to 90% of non-storage iron is found in the erythroid mass.[9] The storage iron concentration in the body varies from 0 to 15 mg/kg body weight depending on the sex and iron status of the individual. The distribution of this stored iron is not uniform, because the liver contains about 60% of the ferritin in the body. The remaining 40% is found in muscle tissues and cells of the reticuloendothelial system. Normally, 95% of the stored iron in liver tissue is found in hepatocytes as ferritin. Hemosiderin constitutes the remaining 5% and is found predominately in Kupffer cell lysosomal remnants. However, during iron overload, the mass of hemosiderin in the liver accumulates at 10 times the rate of ferritin.[20]

## *Ferritin*

The overall structure of ferritin is conserved among higher eukaryotes, and in humans is composed of 24 polypeptide subunits.[21] At least two distinct isoforms of the polypeptide subunits exist, and combinations of these subunits allow for considerable heterogeneity in the structure of the full protein. The isoform designated H ferritin is a 22-kD protein composed of 182 amino acids; the

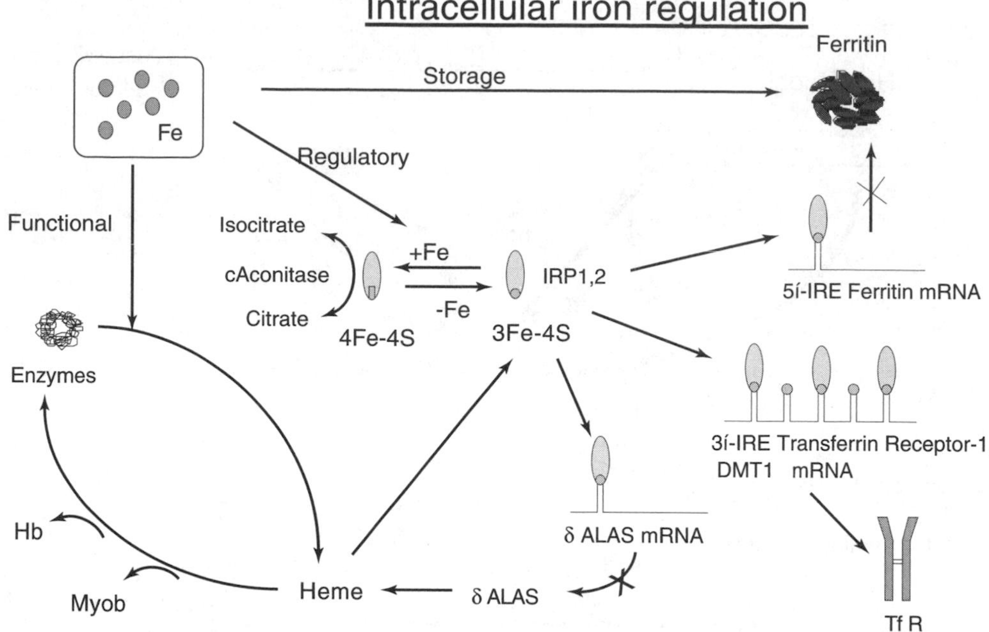


Figure 2. Intracellular iron metabolism indicating primary known functions of iron within cells.

L-isoform is a 20-kD protein containing 174 amino acids. The subunit composition of ferritin seems to be tissue specific. Theoretically, up to 4500 ferric iron atoms can be stored in ferritin.[22] In vivo, ferritin is normally about 20% saturated (800 out of 4500 iron sites occupied), with a variable ratio of H- to L-subunits.[23] The structure and composition of the mineralized core is analogous to a polymer of ferrhydrite ($5Fe_2O_3 \bullet 9H_2O$) with a variable amount of phosphate.[22] H-chain ferritin possesses a distinct ferroxidase site, which can quickly move iron into and out of the core.[24] The L-chain of ferritin lacks this ferroxidase site, and L-chain-predominant ferritin is viewed as a longer-term storage pool of iron.[17,25] The regulation of the synthesis of ferritin is primarily through the IRE-IRP binding motifs. An elevation in cellular iron concentration shifts the cytoplasmic aconitase-IRP1 equilibrium toward IRP-1 (Figure 2). The increased levels of the IRP stabilize the mRNA for ferritin by binding to the IRE and allowing greater amounts of ferritin protein production.[11]

### *Intracellular Regulation*

The intracellular regulation of iron flux is an evolving story, given the identification of new iron importers and exporters and their regulation by cytoplasmic iron concentrations. The amount of ferritin that is synthesized by a cell is under the regulation of the mRNA-binding protein IRP, which binds with high affinity at an IRE located in the 5′-untranslated end of the ferritin mRNA.[10,16] There is a similar set of IREs on the 3′ end of the mRNA for transferrin receptor and DMT-1 (divalent metal transporter-1) that allows for a reciprocal regulation of iron storage and iron uptake. This IRE-IRP system of regulation, however, is also susceptible to oxidative control because nitric oxide alters the affinity of this regulator of protein translation.[11,26] The amount of IRP1 is in turn dependent on the cytosolic free iron concentration; in the presence of cytosolic iron, IRP1 becomes cytoplasmic aconitase with the iron in a 4Fe-4S complex.

In the absence of iron, the IRP1 (now a 3Fe-4S complex) binds to the IREs of various iron proteins to regulate the translation of the mRNA transcripts. IRP2, a second isoform, appears to primarily be an oxygen sensor that is also sensitive to cytosolic free iron and has somewhat different binding affinities to IREs than does IRP1.[11] IRP2 is produced in a distinctly different fashion than the aconitase-related IRP1, and appears to be the predominant regulator of IRE binding at the partial pressure of most mammalian cells in vivo.[26] Thus, the observation that hypoxia increases iron absorption[27] independently of erythropoiesis can be explained by the binding of IRP2 to IRE on the mRNA of ferritin and transferrin receptors.

There are clinically relevant examples in the hemochromatosis literature of IRPs being the principal iron sensors in the enterocytes and determining the fate of iron movement for export or storage in ferritin.[28-30] Concentrations of mucosal cell ferritin mRNA and ferritin protein in patients with familial hemochromatosis are lower than those of patients with secondary iron overload.

## Iron Homeostasis

### *Dietary Forms of Iron*

Iron occurs in two fundamental forms in the human diet: heme iron and non-heme iron.[9,31] Heme iron refers to all forms of iron from plant and animal sources in which the iron molecule is tightly bound within the porphyrin ring structure, as is found in both myoglobin and hemoglobin. Non-heme iron refers to all other forms of iron. Contaminant iron that is derived from dust and soil iron is relatively unavailable to the absorptive cells, but may constitute a significant amount of iron intake in developing countries. There is substantial evidence that nearly all non-heme dietary iron mixes in a luminal "pool" of iron in the upper gastrointestinal tract because of acidification in the stomach and then exposure to pancreatic and gastrointestinal enzymes. Inorganic iron is solubilized and ionized by gastric acid juices, reduced to the ferrous form, and kept soluble in the upper gastrointestinal tract by chelation to compounds such as citrate and ascorbic acid. The type and amount of other materials such as ascorbic acid that can chelate iron to keep it in solution also determine the amount of non-heme iron in a soluble luminal pool (Figure 3).

The number of "inhibitors" of non-heme iron absorption is substantial, with phytate, polyphenols, and tannins leading the list. These inhibitors typically bind either ferric or ferrous iron in a tight complex in the lumen of the gut and make it unavailable for the absorptive proteins. Thus, a diet containing a large amount of unrefined grains and non-digestible fibers will have poor bioavailability. In contrast, a diet that is highly refined and contains little roughage and substantial portions of meat will have a greater iron bioavailability regardless of other factors. The American diet typically contains about 50% of its iron from grain products in which the iron concentration is between 0.1 and 0.4 mg per serving. Some fortified cereals, however, may contain as much as 24 mg of iron in a single serving. Heme iron is more highly bioavailable than non-heme iron, and its bioavailability is less affected by other components of the diet than is the non-heme iron. Heme iron represents only about 10% of total dietary iron intake in many Western countries. A large number of studies have examined the chemical characteristics of iron salts, iron-containing meals, and food items in an attempt to create optimal combinations of materials that would maintain the solubility of iron in the basic pH of the upper bowel but yet make it available for absorptive processes. Thorough reviews on this have been published.[31,32]

## Regulation of Absorption

As noted previously, there are fundamental regulators of the amount of iron absorbed in humans. The first is the total amount and form of iron compounds ingested, which reflects the physio-chemical properties of the diet (discussed elsewhere), and the second is the iron status of the individual.[13] Individuals with a high iron status will absorb proportionally less of any amount of iron consumed than will an iron-deficient individual. Individuals with a lower iron status will absorb more of any dietary intake. This process of selective absorption is the funda-

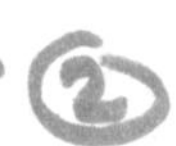

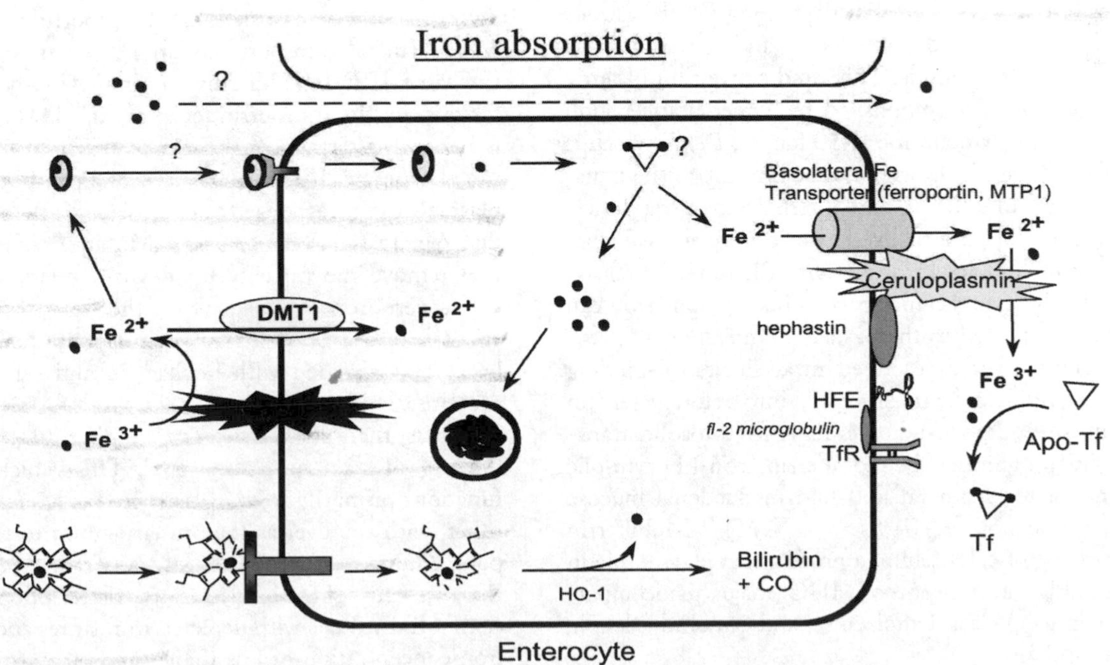


Figure 3. Putative mechanism for the absorption of iron in enterocytes of the upper gastrointestinal tract in humans. On the left side of the diagram is the putative heme iron transporter DMT-1 (divalent metal transporter 1), which mediates uptake coupled to a ferroxidase, and a poorly described non-heme iron transporter independent of DMT1. Soluble intracellular iron can be inserted into ferritin (in the center of the cell) or exported through the MTP-1 (metal transport protein 1) shuttle system located in close proximity to copper-containing hepastin or ceruloplasmin. The hemochromatosis gene product HFE is likely to exert its influence at this site of iron export from the absorptive cell.

mental mechanism whereby humans regulate iron balance[9] (Figure 3). Iron uptake by enterocytes at normal dietary levels is mediated by a series of receptors and binding proteins that distinguish between heme and non-heme iron.

### *Heme Iron Absorption*

Heme iron is soluble in an alkaline environment, so no binding proteins are necessary for its luminal absorption. Specific transporters exist for heme on the surface of enterocytes, and efforts are being made to characterize these.[33] After binding to its receptor, the heme molecule is then internalized and acted upon by HOX1 (heme oxygenase 1) to release the iron to the soluble cytoplasmic pool.[34] HOX1 is not induced by oral administration of hemoglobin (a source of heme), but is induced by iron deficiency, suggesting some form of feedback regulation from the iron stores "signal." The distribution in the intestine is identical to the areas of maximal heme iron absorption, and is far more efficient at absorption than in the non-heme iron pathway.[35] In a typical American diet, it is reasonable to expect that overall dietary non-heme iron is absorbed at approximately 5% to 10% efficiency and heme iron at nearly 40%.

### *Non-Heme Iron Absorption*

DMT is a trans-membrane protein that resides on the luminal membrane, has a strong preference for divalent metals, and exists in several isoforms (including DMT1 and DMT2).[13,36] The non-heme iron in the lumen of the gut has variable solubility depending on the various amounts of ferric and ferrous iron and the amount of iron-binding compounds. The rapid conversion of ferric to ferrous iron is accomplished by a membrane-bound member of the cytochrome P450 family, *Dcytb*, which is in sufficient abundance as to not be limiting to the transport capacity of DMT1 and internalization via vesicle endocytosis. The internalized vesicle undergoes further modification and acidification, with the resulting release of iron to the cytoplasmic space. This cytosolic iron can then be transported to the basolateral membrane for export by some as yet undescribed intracellular iron-binding protein(s), or it can be incorporated into a storage ferritin molecule.[11,23] One candidate for this cytosolic transferrin-like protein may be mobilferrin, a 56-kD cytosolic protein isolated from rat and human duodenal mucosa that can bind iron ($K_d = 9 \times 10^{-5}$ M).[33] Mobilferrin is a homolog of calreticulin, a protein that plays a role in the assembly and transport of MHC (major histocompatibility complex) class-1 molecules, and can bind calcium, copper, and zinc.

Given the frequent observation of increased efficiency of iron absorption in individuals with low iron stores and decreased efficiency with high iron stores, it has long been predicted that some sort of plasma-borne signal communicates to enterocytes as part of this homeostatic control loop.[37] This signal compound could tell the basolateral membrane to export iron (or not), signal internal iron-binding proteins to preferentially move iron to ferritin within the enterocyte, or somehow communicate with the luminal membrane to change the amount of iron imported into the cell. It is now clear that the signal is the newly described protein hepcidin.[38] This protein was first identified as a small peptide with antimicrobial activity and is classified as a type II acute-phase protein.[39] Mice that lack the hepcidin gene accumulate toxic amounts of iron in liver, while overexpressing mice develop iron deficiency.[38] The amount of hepcidin in the plasma is in proportion to the amount of liver iron stores. Other target tissues for this secreted protein appear to be macrophages, renal epithelial cells, and placenta.[38-40] Hepcidin binds to receptors, which in turn alters the release of iron from the target cells. The production of hepcidin is influenced by inflammation markers such as interleukin-1 (IL-1) and IL-6, which may explain why inflammation is associated with a reduced release of iron from macrophages and a reduced absorption of dietary iron.[37]

### *Basolateral Membrane Iron Export*

Hepcidin, the putative plasma protein regulator of iron absorption, is released from liver and its plasma concentration is proportional to the amount of liver iron stores and cytokine regulation.[38] This secreted protein appears to have two primary targets: the macrophage and the basolateral membrane of the enterocyte. On the basolateral membrane of the enterocyte, hepcidin becomes associated with an iron "exporter" ferroportin, with a resulting internalization and its destruction.[39] Ferroportin is also called MTP1 (metal transport protein 1), and is regulated by the same IRE-IRP binding motif previously described for ferritin, the transferrin receptor, and DMT-1. There is a prompt alteration in the release of iron from the abluminal enterocyte surface as hepcidin concentrations in plasma vary in response to the onset of inflammation or due to increased liver iron stores. Mutations of ferroportin that remove the capacity for down-regulation result in very severe iron overload. Once the ferroportin protein releases ferrous iron into the plasma pool, the iron likely becomes associated with hephaestin and ceruloplasmin proteins, which act in a redox couple to form ferric iron. There is then high-efficiency binding to transferrin-binding sites in the plasma pool. This vehicle for iron functions primarily to move iron from one organ to another, with the liver as the primary donor to the plasma pool. The rate of production of transferrin is affected by the iron status of the individual via transcriptional regulation.[13] Individuals with depleted iron stores and a plasma iron concentration of less than 40 to 60 μg/dL will increase transferrin production and increase the plasma transferrin concentration by nearly 100%. The two binding sites on transferrin are nearly identical in binding affinity for iron ($K_d = 10^{-22}$ M). In vivo, transferrin is normally 25% to 50% saturated with iron, but in extreme iron deficiency, it can be less than 5%.[27] One of the criteria for establishing iron deficiency is for the transferrin saturation to be under 15%.[9] At this level of saturation, there is insufficient delivery of iron to bone marrow to maintain normal rates of erythropoiesis. Thus, under normal physiological circumstances, the iron-binding capacity of plasma is always in excess of the iron concentration. The rate and location of the uptake of iron from the plasma pool is proportional to the number of transferrin receptors expressed on plasma membranes.

### *Iron Losses*

The low solubility of iron precludes excretion as a major mechanism of maintaining homeostasis, which is the method used by most other trace minerals. The primary mechanism of maintaining whole-body iron homeostasis is to regulate the amount of iron absorbed so that it approximates iron losses.[32] Iron losses can vary considerably with the sex of the individual and with pathologies that have blood loss as a significant component. In male humans, total iron losses from the body have been calculated to be approximately 0.8 to 0.9 mg/d. For premenopausal female humans, this loss is slightly higher. The predominant route of loss is from the gastrointestinal tract and amounts to 0.6 mg/d in adult males.[19,20] Fecal iron losses result from shed enterocytes, extravasated red blood cells, and biliary heme breakdown products that are poorly absorbed. Urogenital and integumental iron losses have been estimated to be greater than 0.1 and 0.3 mg/d, respectively, in adult males.[20] Menstrual iron loss, estimated from an average blood loss of 33 mL/month, equals 1.5 mg/d but may be as high as 2.1 mg/d.[41] Oral contraceptives reduce this loss and intrauterine devices increase it.

A number of clinical and pathological conditions are accompanied by variable amounts of blood loss. These include hemorrhage, hookworm infestation, peptic gastric or anastomotic ulceration, ulcerative colitis, colonic neoplasia, cow's milk feeding to infants, aspirin, nonsteroidal anti-inflammatory drugs or corticosteroid administration and hereditary hemorrhagic telangiectasia. Blood loss through donation contains 210 to 240 mg of Fe per unit of blood donated. Thus, regular blood donation can rapidly deplete iron stores. It is estimated that it takes 6 to 8 months of consuming a typical Western diet to restore the iron lost in one unit of donated blood.

## Iron Requirements

Iron deficiency can be defined as the state when body stores of iron (iron contained bound to the storage proteins ferritin and hemosiderin) become depleted of iron and a restriction of supply of iron to various tissues becomes apparent[20] (Figure 4). The Recommended Dietary Allowances (RDAs) and the Estimated Average Requirements (EARs) have been recently recomputed for the US population, and are separated by age and sex groups (Table 3).[41] The higher requirements during periods of growth and development and during pregnancy reflect the increased need for iron in those periods of life. The very dramatic elevation in RDA for iron in reproductive-

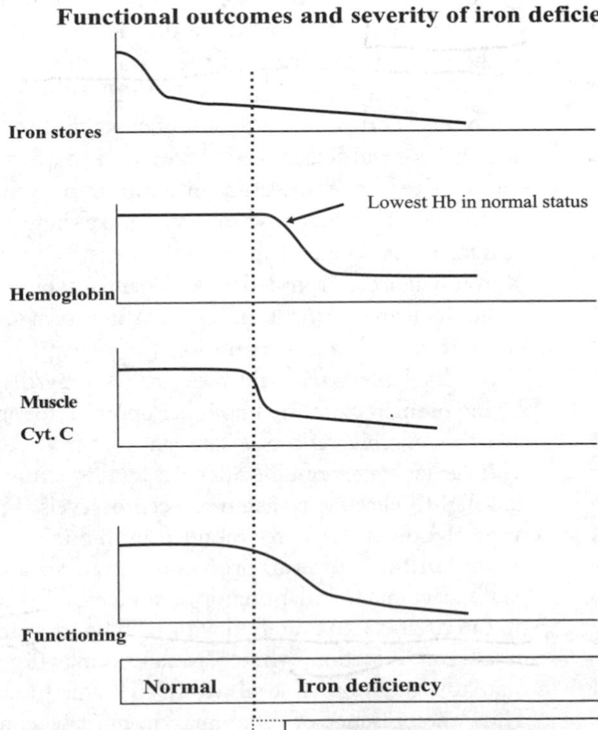

Functional outcomes and severity of iron deficiency
Iron stores
As iron stores declines with a negative iron balance, serum ferritin continues to drop. There are few known functional consequences until stores are depleted.
Lowest Hb in normal status
Hemoglobin
Once iron stores fall below approximately 100 mg (ferritin <10-15 ug/L), the transferrin saturation fall below 15%, and iron deficiency erythropoiesis results.
Muscle
Cyt. C
Muscle Fe-sulfur and heme iron enzymes begin to decline in content and activity due to a deficit in iron delivery to tissue.
Immunologic, exercise, and neural functioning begin to decline in performance with the deficit in iron delivery to tissue.
Functioning
Normal
Iron deficiency
Iron deficiency anemia

Figure 4. Iron stores depletion and functional changes as iron stores become depleted.

**Table 3.** Recommended Daily Allowances (RDA) and Estimated Average Requirements (EAR) for Iron Consumption

| Age | EAR | RDA |
|---|---|---|
| | *mg Fe/d* | |
| 7–12 mo* | 6.9 | 11 |
| 1–3 yr | 2.9 | 7 |
| 4–8 yr | 4.1 | 9 |
| 9–13 yr (boys) | 6.6 | 11 |
| 14–18 yr (boys) | 7.8 | 11 |
| 9–13 yr (girls) | 6.4 | 11 |
| 14–18 yr (girls) | 8.3 | 16 |
| Adult men | 6 | 8 |
| Adult women 19–50 years† | 8.1 | 19 |
| Adult women >51 years | 5 | 8 |
| Pregnant women‡ | 22.6 | 27 |
| Lactating women | 6.3 | 9 |

* Before 6 months of age, only Adequate Intakes (AIs) can be estimated (0.27 mg/d).
† Values are estimates for reproductive-age women.
‡ This is an overall estimate for the entire pregnancy, but iron requirements vary by trimester; the estimate is slightly higher for teenage pregnancy (EAR of 22.8 mg/d and RDA of 27 mg/d).
Data from Food and Nutrition Board, Institute of Medicine, 2001.[41]

age females reflects the additional iron requirements associated with menstruation and the fact that blood iron losses in this group can be quite significant.

The process of depletion of iron stores can occur rapidly or very slowly, and is dependent on the balance between iron intake (or stores) and iron requirements. The concept was converted to a quantitative relationship via the computation of "body iron"[42] by using the serum ferritin and serum transferrin receptor concentrations. Serial phlebotomy was performed in a small number of subjects, allowing the quantification of the exact relationship between changes in serum ferritin and transferrin receptors and the amount of iron removed from the body. The utility of this approach is that individuals in a sample or population are viewed in a "continuum" of iron status instead of being categorized as iron-deficient anemic, iron-deficient non-anemic, mildly iron deficient, or iron sufficient. The next task is to identify at which level of negative body iron there are functional deficits. Surveillance programs can also utilize this approach to monitor the extent of iron deficiency (negative body iron), as well as to index the response to intervention programs.

The greater prevalence of iron deficiency in women is due to this shift in the balance equation and not due to "femaleness" or "maleness." Requirements for iron in pregnancy are increased dramatically to approximately 4 mg/d and perhaps even higher if the pregnancy occurs in adolescents still having some significant growth spurt.[41] The requirements for iron are of course higher in the growing child and give rise to the concept of "critical periods" during both prenatal and post-natal growth.[42] The rate at which individual tissues and cellular organelles within those tissues develop a true "deficit" in iron is dependent on the rate of turnover of these iron-containing proteins, as well as the intracellular mechanisms for recycling the iron.[43] The manifestations of this depletion of essential body iron have profound effects in skeletal muscle, with a significant decrease in mitochondrial iron-sulfur content, mitochondrial cytochrome content, and total mitochondrial oxidative capacity.[7] The activity of tricarboxylic acid (TCA) cycle enzymes and the oxidative capacity of mitochondria from other organs is less strongly affected.[44] An additional caveat is the difference between enzymes that require soluble iron as a cofactor and those that require iron to be present during their synthesis. Since the red cell has a lifetime of approximately 120 days in humans and shorter times in other species, it is apparent that certain tissues and organelles may actually experience some functional lack of iron prior to our capacity to measure a significant change in hematological parameters. There is little or no information relating neurological function or changes in brain iron metabolism to changes in iron status in this early stage of iron deficiency.

## Iron Status Assessment

Iron deficiency has traditionally been separated into iron deficiency anemia and tissue iron deficiency, also referred to as "depleted iron stores," and has been diagrammatically represented this way for more than two decades. The most common indicator of iron stores is serum ferritin, with a public health derived cutoff value of 12 μg/L indicating sufficient iron stores (approximately 100 mg of storage iron).[7,9] All other indicators are in their normal range. Iron-deficient erythropoiesis is defined as insufficient iron delivery to marrow, and is characterized by an elevation in serum transferrin receptors, a slight lowering in serum iron, and a slight elevation in transferrin. The end stage of the negative progression in iron balance is iron deficiency anemia, which is diagnosed as a low serum transferrin saturation (<15%), a low serum ferritin concentration (< 12 μg/L), and an elevated soluble transferrin receptor (>6 mg/dL) in the setting of microcytic anemia. It is important to remember that this anemia reflects a late stage of iron depletion, with earlier stages often evidenced by low serum ferritin and slightly elevated transferrin receptor levels. The diagnosis of iron status is confounded by the fact that both serum ferritin and serum iron concentrations are acute-phase reactants to inflammatory cytokines.[45] Serum ferritin can rise two- to four-fold within 72 hours of the onset of an acute infection, while plasma iron may drop to less than 50% of a normal level within the same time period. Thus, the presence of inflammation must be considered in a diagnosis of iron deficiency either at the clinical level or at the population level of analysis.

## *Iron Deficiency*

*Clinical symptoms*: The overt physical manifestations of iron deficiency include the generic symptoms of anemia: tiredness, lassitude, and general feelings of lack of energy. Clinical manifestations of iron deficiency are glossitis, angular stomatitis, koilonchyia (spoon nails), blue sclera, esophageal webbing (Plummer-Vinson syndrome), and microcytic hypochromic anemia. Behavioral disturbances such as pica, which is characterized by abnormal consumption of non-food items such as dirt (geophagia) and ice (pagophagia), are often present in iron deficiency, but clear biological explanations for these abnormalities are lacking.

*Functional changes*: There is a significant amount of scientific literature documenting alterations in immune function, exercise and endurance capacity, and behavior and cognitive function with iron deficiency.[12] Because nearly all of the functional consequences of iron deficiency are strongly related to the severity of anemia, the challenge of separating oxygen transport events from tissue iron deficits looms large. However, this is largely an academic question because tissue iron deficits occur simultaneously with deficits in oxygen transport in naturally occurring iron deficiency anemia. A good example of this is that there is a 50% decrease in muscle myoglobin content, cytochrome oxidase activity, and electron transport capacity in skeletal muscle with iron deficiency at the same time the subjects have a 50% decreased oxygen transport capacity due to anemia.[46] Thus, although it is convenient at times to categorize individuals as iron-deficient anemic versus iron-deficient non-anemic, this is not biological reality. Instead, it is more accurate to consider individuals along a continuum of iron nutriture, with different functional consequences arising at different stages of severity. Studies performed two decades ago demonstrated that iron deficiency alters both endurance and maximum aerobic capacity in humans, with resulting changes in worker productivity on both sugarcane plantations and tea plantations.[47,48] More recently, studies in factories demonstrate a reduction in output in individuals with iron deficiency.[49]

*Immune function*: Although most pathogens require iron and other micronutrients and have evolved sophisticated strategies for acquiring them, iron is also required by the host for mounting an effective immune response. In a conceptual model of nutritional immunity, the host must effectively sequester iron from pathogens and simultaneously provide a supply of iron that is not limiting to its immune system.[45] Many unicellular organisms, as well as humans, share a common lineage of metal transporters.[50] These DMTs have been identified and cloned in both bacteria and humans and are used to internalize iron from extracellular spaces. NRAMP1 (natural resistance associated macrophage protein 1) and NRAMP2 transport iron, zinc, copper, manganese, and other divalent metals from endosomal vesicles into the cytoplasmic space.[16] Bacterial virulence is associated with the genes that code for iron acquisition in both *Escherichia coli* and *Vibrio*.[50] Thus, the acquisition of iron from biological fluids by siderophores secreted by bacteria is one of their routes of obtaining this essential nutrient. In vitro studies show that the provision of iron to rodents increases the pathogenicity of a number of bacteria.[51] Data showing that this is also the case for humans are far less convincing. An often-quoted study of Murray et al.[52] examined Somali nomads with iron deficiency anemia. Oral iron therapy led to a 12-fold increase in infections compared with no therapy. Replication of such a powerful effect of iron status has not been seen in other studies.[53]

*Immunity during iron deficiency*: Experimental and clinical evidence suggests that within the context of poverty, malnutrition, and poor access to health care, iron deficiency may be associated with an impaired immune system.[45] Iron is an important component of peroxide-generating enzymes and nitrous oxide-generating enzymes that are critical for the proper enzymatic functioning of some immune cells and cell signaling pathways.[54] Non-specific immunity is affected by iron deficiency in several ways. Macrophage bactericidal activity is attenuated, neutrophils have a reduced activity of the iron-containing enzyme myeloperoxidase, and there is a decrease in both T-lymphocyte number and T-lymphocyte blastogenesis and mitogenesis.[55,56] In iron-deficient humans, however, antibody production in response to immunization with most antigens is preserved.[54,55] Galen et al.[57] reported a reduction in IL-2 production by activated lymphocytes in iron-deficient subjects. The release of IL-2 is fundamental to communication between lymphocyte subsets and natural killer cells, but it does not appear to be the only cytokine that is altered by iron status.[51] There is a feedback loop from activation of cytokine release on iron metabolism by the regulation of iron transport proteins.[16] Tumor necrosis factor, IL-1, and interferon-δ work in a coordinated fashion to reduce the size of the intracellular labile iron pool by reducing the amount of transferrin receptor on the cell surface, increasing the synthesis of ferritin for iron storage, and activating nitric oxide systems.[50,51,53] Thus, sequestration of iron seems to be an important part of the host response to infection and a route of reducing the pathogenicity of invading microorganisms.

*Muscle and metabolic function*: It is not uncommon for individuals with iron deficiency to complain of lethargy, apathy, and listlessness. Some portion of these complaints is no doubt related to the changes in central nervous system functioning, but a portion might also be attributable to true reductions in muscle functioning and abnormalities in fuel metabolism.[7,12,46] Decreased exercise capacity is related to diminished oxygen transport, oxygen diffusion within the exercising tissue, and oxidative capacity of muscle.[58] As would be expected from the previous discussion regarding the essential iron pool in tissues, there is a significant decrease in mitochondrial iron-sulfur content,[58] mitochondrial cytochrome content, and total mitochondrial oxidative capacity with iron deficiency. The metabolic adaptation or perhaps the consequence of this reduced mitochondrial capacity is an alteration in glucose and lactate metabolism.[7,8]

Animal studies, but not human studies, show alterations in glucose and lactate metabolism consistent with a limitation in mitochondrial aerobic functioning and altered sensitivity to insulin. Although the efficiency of oxygen extraction is improved by the hemoglobin-oxygen saturation curve shifts, maximal oxygen consumption is still decreased by 30% to 50% in both animals and humans. Human studies demonstrate a reduction in endurance capacity in laboratory testing as well as in the real-world outcomes of agricultural output.[47,48] Most of the effects are seen in anemic individuals, but more recent work shows alterations in metabolic efficiency in iron deficiency without anemia.[49] The public health importance of this could be quite large, as the prevalence of iron deficiency is about twice that of iron deficiency anemia. Economic implications for developing countries with a high prevalence of iron deficiency and a large manual workforce are obvious and of great consequence.

*Central nervous system functioning*: Animal studies have for more than three decades demonstrated that iron deficiency inducted in utero and during lactation reduces iron content by over 30% in many parts of the brain.[58] When rats are given low-iron diets post-weaning, there is over a 50% decline in iron content in some brain regions, which can be restored to normal levels with dietary rehabilitation. Autopsy studies in human infants who are iron deficient show similar levels of decline in brain iron content. The areas of the brain that are sensitive to iron depletion in early life are often co-localized with dopaminergic regions of the brain and differ from the regions rich in iron in adulthood.[59]

Functionally, iron is required for proper myelination of the white matter tracts.[60,61] It is also a cofactor for a number of enzymes involved in neurotransmitter synthesis, including tryptophan hydroxylase (serotonin) and tyrosine hydroxylase (norepinephrine and dopamine) and ribonucleotide reductase.[58] The failure to deliver iron to neural cells such as the oligodendrocytes that produce myelin during particular periods of early brain development could be causally related to delayed motor maturation and perhaps behavioral alterations in young humans.[62] Roncagliolo et al.[62] demonstrated a slowed nerve conduction velocity during an auditory evoked potential test. Alternatively, the slower nerve conduction velocity may be attributed to alterations in dopamine metabolism, as a number of animal studies have documented changes in dopamine transporters and in receptor, uptake, and release biology.[58,63-65] Others have noted alterations in γ-aminobutyric acid (GABA) metabolism, but little substantive biochemical work has been done with the GABA system, especially with regard to its regulatory role on dopaminergic system functioning. The substantial work in dopamine in rodent models has great importance with regard to the alterations seen in human functioning. For instance, attentional processing of environmental information is highly dependent on appropriate rates of dopamine clearance from the interstitial space, a process known to be slowed in the iron-deficient brain. Alterations in dopamine metabolism in the mesolimbic and nigrostriatal tracts are associated with changes in motor control (e.g., tardive dyskinesia), as well as altered perception, memory, and motivation (Parkinson's disease). A recently described alteration in motor control in human, "restless legs syndrome," is believed to be related to brain iron deficiency.[67] Treatment of these patients with iron and L-DOPA are the most effective strategies, which strongly suggests that this disease of aging is related to alterations in brain iron metabolism.

In studies of human infants, there is the disturbing observation that iron deficiency in the first year or so of life results in irreversible developmental delays.[68,69] Blinded clinical intervention trials of several months or longer demonstrate lower developmental test scores in iron-deficient anemic infants. One study showed a dramatic improvement after iron treatment, while others only showed a modest response or no improvement. Some of these individuals have now been examined more than 10 to 15 years later, and have persistent deficits in cognitive and behavioral functioning.[68] This suggests long-term persistent deficits in neural functioning despite improvement in systemic iron status at an early age. Infants from 12 to 24 months of age appear to be the most vulnerable, but studies in 2- to 5-year-old children, pre-adolescents, adolescents, and adults all demonstrate that iron deficiency during any time in life can affect both behavioral and cognitive functioning.[58,68] In many of these studies of functioning in older children and adults, attention, vigilance, and learning are adversely affected by poor iron status. Iron intervention in the older groups often "normalizes" functioning in the individuals who respond to iron therapy, implying a causal and non-irreversible role for iron in brain biology.

## Treatment of Iron Deficiency

A normal treatment protocol after the diagnosis of true iron deficiency is the oral administration of 125 to 250 mg/d of ferrous sulfate. This dose of the salt will deliver 39 to 72 mg of highly bioavailable iron per day and will typically return an anemic person to iron sufficiency in 8 to 12 weeks. While there is some evidence that doses greater than 250 mg ferrous sulfate convey additional benefits, there is emerging evidence that gastrointestinal distress occurs at these higher doses. There is a high prevalence of complaints of gastrointestinal distress, constipation, and blackened stools at these higher doses, as well as much poorer compliance.

In 2001, the US Food and Nutrition Board of the National Academy of Sciences released the current evaluation of recommended intakes and upper limits of safe intakes.[41] That committee had the perspective that functional consequences of iron deficiency occurs only when there are depleted iron stores and there is insufficient delivery of iron to the essential iron pools in all tissues. In the evaluation of assessment of iron status, the review panel utilized the following indicators: 1) serum or plasma ferritin as an indicator of iron storage pool size; 2) plasma-soluble transferrin receptor as an indicator of adequacy of iron delivery to rapidly growing cells; 3) plasma or serum transferrin saturation as an indicator of iron transport; and 4) hemoglobin concentration, hematocrit, or red cell counts as an indication of the existence of anemia. The need to utilize all of these indicators is well justified given the impact that acute and chronic infections have on the evaluation of iron status.[70] The discovery of the serum transferrin receptor is relatively recent, but this receptor is not sensitive to inflammation, so there is great promise that it will prove to be a valuable indicator of iron status in complicated clinical and nutritional diagnosis. The suggested levels of intake represent the required intakes to ensure adequate nutrition in 95% to 97.5% of the population, and are an overestimation of the level needed for most people in any given group. Individuals who do not routinely consume the suggested level of iron from foods should be encouraged to supplement their diets with iron compounds.

## Approaches to Preventative Iron Supplementation

One of the great concerns regarding iron deficiency anemia is the adequacy of iron intake during periods of high iron losses. This has led to a re-evaluation of the concept of "daily iron supplements."[71,72] At issue is the relative effectiveness of daily therapeutic doses of iron compared with the administration of lower "preventative intermittent" iron doses. The concept is that since the gastrointestinal enterocyte will "reset" its set point for iron absorption every 3 to 4 days as a new crop of crypt cells migrate up to the tip of the villus, the large doses of iron given on days 2 and 3 is wasted and may in fact result in oxidative damage and mucosal injury. To test this hypothesis, a number of studies in developing countries have compared the efficacy of daily doses compared with intermittent doses in correcting iron deficiency anemia in adolescents, reproductive-age women, pregnant women, and children. The daily dosage approach had a faster response but lower compliance than the intermittent dose approach. The end result in terms of correcting the anemia was similar in nearly all populations, with the exception of pregnant women, in whom daily iron therapy clearly provided a greater benefit.[42] Blood loss from the body is the single largest cause of increased or altered iron requirements. Bleeding ulcers, lesions, and leaking inflammatory states in the gut are all associated with a decreased iron status due to increased rates of blood and iron loss.

Doses of iron near 180 mg may be lethal in adults.[73] High acute intakes of iron may be associated with necrotizing gastritis and enteritis, pallor, lassitude, and frequent diarrhea. The rapid rise in the plasma iron concentration within 60 minutes to levels in excess of 500 ug/dL is common and is likely related to the pathology. Rapid treatment with iron chelators such as desferrioxamine will rapidly decrease plasma iron concentration; gastric lavage improves recovery rates.

There are a number of iron compounds on the market that can effectively and safely supplement dietary iron to bring individuals back into iron balance. There is risk, however, that overzealous use of supplements can lead to gastrointestinal distress and, in some individuals with genetic mutations, toxic iron overload and even death. New understanding of the genetic causality of iron overload syndromes will provide greater avenues for preventing accidental iron overload in the near future.

## Iron Overload

Iron overload diseases have received much attention in the last decade, especially in the last 5 years, with the discovery of the gene associated with hereditary hemochromatosis. One in 200 to 400 individuals of Anglo-Saxon ancestry are affected by an autosomal recessive gene mutation that results in the iron overload disease called hereditary hemochromatosis.[3] The mutation of the HFE gene in position C282Y accounts for the vast majority of the cases of hemochromatosis in individuals of Celtic origin. Various other mutations have also been described. The current thinking is that mutations in the HFE protein are associated with a failure of the HFE protein to bind effectively with the β2 microglobulin protein and the transferrin receptor-1 protein at the plasma membrane. The failure of the association is related to the lack of control of iron flux across the enterocyte. Hereditary hemochromatosis is thus characterized by an inability to control iron absorption in the enterocyte, with a resulting accumulation of iron in iron storage pools, primarily in cells of the reticuloendothelial system. Without treatment, clinical signs of iron toxicity occur in homozygous individuals in their 40s or earlier, at which time their total body iron content is more than 20 g. Lack of treatment by chelation and phlebotomy results in cirrhosis of the liver, hepatocellular carcinoma, myocardial pathology, and damage to the pancreatic function. This accumulation of iron in the liver appears to be causal by being linked to the accompanying hepatic fibrosis and cirrhosis. The evidence for iron accumulation in heterozygous individuals is less clear, and the role of dietary iron bioavailability in body iron accumulation in these individuals is still being debated.[74] At the time, it appears prudent for known heterozygous individuals to limit their consumption of iron supplements.

Other forms of iron overload due to chronic excessively high iron intakes have been reported, but these intakes of approximately 200 to 1200 mg/d of iron for long periods are unusual. Bantu siderosis in Africa is an additional example of iron toxicity due to excessively high iron intakes for prolonged periods of time.[74] Home brewing of beer in large iron pots was associated with an intake of iron in excess of 50 to 100 mg/d of iron, with resulting iron overload disease. There is also some evidence that there is a genetic component to this disease.

Transfusional iron overload may result from the accumulation of iron after senescent transfused red cells are metabolized in the reticuloendothelial system. Since each unit of blood contains approximately 225 mg of iron, there is a real danger of hepatic iron overload with repeated transfusions. Individuals with disorders in effective erythropoiesis who receive transfusions have the additional iron burden of excessive iron absorption—that is, iron accumulation in the reticuloendothelial system occurs due to both high rates of red cell turnover and high rates of iron absorption.

## Future Directions

Our knowledge of the cell biology of iron has increased exponentially in the last 5 to 8 years with the identification of hepcidin, haephestin, DMT-1, ferroportin, and other iron-related proteins and their molecular regulation. There is an emerging understanding of hemochromatosis and the causes of this dysregulation of iron absorption. There are new insights relative to understanding the changes in iron absorption and hypoferremia in the presence of infection, which will open new avenues for both the assessment and treatment of poor iron status during chronic inflammation. However, there are still great challenges that span the public health, clinical, and cellular realms of iron biology. The prevalence of iron deficiency in children and pregnant women has not changed in a decade despite great efforts to implement fortification and supplementation programs. New approaches that more fully integrate iron into the food supply are needed, and perhaps the new initiative in "biofortification" of staple foods can shift significant portions of undernourished populations toward iron sufficiency.[75] The identification of the role of iron in the pathogenesis of chronic diseases such as cancer and cardiovascular disease is forefront to issues in the clinical domain. Does iron fortification of our food supply in the United States increase our risk of these diseases? The proof does not exist yet, but it is premature to exclude that possibility. Finally, the effects of iron deficiency on neural development and the potential irreversible nature of this alteration in infants need to be resolved.

## References

1. de Duve C. Prelude to a cell. The Sciences. 1990; 30:22–28.
2. Eaton SB, Konner M. Paleolithic nutrition. A consideration of its nature and current implications. N Engl J Med. 1985;312:283–289.
3. Boussingault JB. Du fer contenu dans le sang et dans les aliments. Acad Sci Paris, Comptes Rendus. 1872; 74:1353–1359.
4. Gutteridge JM, Halliwell B. Free radicals and antioxidants in the year 2000. A historical look to the future. Ann N Y Acad Sci. 2000;899:136–147.
5. Webb EC. *Enzyme Nomenclature*. San Diego: Academic Press; 1992.
6. Medeiros D, Beard JL Dietary iron deficiency results in cardiac eccentric hypertrophy in rats. Proc Soc Exp Biol Med. 1998;218:370–375.
7. Dallman PR. Biochemical basis for the manifestations of iron deficiency. Annu Rev Nutr. 1986;6: 13–40.
8. Beard JL, Dawson H, Pinero D. Iron metabolism: a comprehensive review. Nutr Rev. 1996;54:295–317.
9. Bothwell TH, Charlton RW, Cook JD, Finch CA. *Iron Metabolism in Man*. Oxford: Blackwell Scientific Publications; 1979.
10. Hentze MW, Kuhn LC. Molecular control of vertebrate iron metabolism: mRNA-based regulatory circuits operated by iron, nitric oxide, and oxidative stress. Proc Natl Acad Sci U S A. 1996;93: 8175–8182.
11. Eisenstein RS. Iron regulatory proteins and the molecular control of mammalian iron metabolism. Annu Rev Nutr. 2000;20:627–662.
12. Beard JL. Iron biology in immune function, muscle metabolism and neuronal functioning. J Nutr. 2001; 131:568S–580S.
13. Aisen P, Listowsky I. Iron transport and storage proteins. Annu Rev Biochem. 1980;49:357–393.
14. Andrews NC. Iron metabolism: iron deficiency and iron overload. Annu Rev Genomics Hum Genet. 2000;1:75–98.
15. Princiotto JV, Zapolski EJ. Functional heterogeneity and pH-dependent dissociation properties of human transferrin. Biochim Biophys Acta. 1976;428: 766–771.
16. Ponka P, Beaumont C, Richardson DR. Function and regulation of transferrin and ferritin. Semin Hematol. 1998;35:35–54.
17. Casey JL, Hentze MW, Koeller DM, et al. Iron-responsive elements: regulatory RNA sequences that control mRNA levels and translation. Science. 1988; 240:924–928.
18. Rao K, Harford JB, Rouault T, McClelland A, Ruddle FH, Klausner RD. Transcriptional regulation by iron of the gene for transferrin receptor. Mol Cell Biol. 1986;6:236–240.
19. Finch CA, Deubelbeiss K, Cook JD, et al. Ferrokinetics in man. Medicine (Baltimore). 1970;49: 17–53.
20. Green R, Charlton R, Seftel H, et al. Body iron ex-

cretion in man: a collaborative study. Am J Med. 1968;45:336–53.
21. Theil EC, Eisenstein RS. Combinatorial mRNA regulation: iron regulatory proteins and iso-iron-responsive elements (Iso-IREs). J Biol Chem. 2000; 275:40659–40662.
22. Fischbach FA, Anderegg JW. An x-ray scattering study of ferritin and apoferritin. J Mol Biol. 1965; 14:458–473.
23. Crichton RR, Ward RJ. An overview of iron metabolism: molecular and cellular criteria for the selection of iron chelators. Curr Med Chem. 2003;10: 997–1004.
24. Levi S, Luzzago A, Cesareni G, et al. Mechanism of ferritin iron uptake: activity of the H-chain and deletion mapping of the ferro-oxidase site. A study of iron uptake and ferro-oxidase activity of human liver, recombinant H-chain ferritins, and of two H-chain deletion mutants. J Biol Chem. 1988;263: 18086–18092.
25. Levi S, Salfeld J, Franceschinelli F, Cozzi A, Doerner MH, Arosio P. Expression and structure and functional properties of human ferritin L-chain from *Escherichia coli*. Biochemistry. 1989;28:5179–5185.
26. Meyron-Holtz EG, Ghosh MC, Rouault RA. Mammalian tissue oxygen levels modulate iron-regulatory protein activities in vivo. Science. 2004; 306:2087–2090.
27. Mendel GA. Studies on iron absorption. I: The relationships between the rate of erythropoiesis, hypoxia and iron absorption. Blood. 1961;18:727–736.
28. Rouault T, Klausner R. Regulation of iron metabolism in eukaryotes. Curr Top Cell Regul. 1997;35: 1–19.
29. Rouault TA. Post-transcriptional regulation of human iron metabolism by iron regulatory proteins. Blood Cells Mol Dis. 2002;29:309–314.
30. Pietrangelo A, Trautwein C. Mechanisms of disease: the role of hepcidin in iron homeostasis: implications for hemochromatosis and other disorders. Nature Clinical Practice. 2004;1:39–45.
31. Hurrell R. Improvement of trace element status through food fortification: technological, biological and health aspects. Bibl Nutr Dieta. 1998;54:40–57.
32. Hallberg L, Hulthen L. Prediction of dietary iron absorption: an algorithm for calculating absorption and bioavailability of dietary iron. Am J Clin Nutr. 2000;71:1147–1160.
33. Conrad ME, Burton BI, Williams HL, Foy AL. Human absorption of hemoglobin-iron. Gastroenterology. 1967;53:5–10.
34. Raffin SB, Woo CH, Roost KT, Price DC, Schmid R. Intestinal absorption of hemoglobin heme iron cleavage by mucosal heme oxygenase. J Clin Invest. 1974;54:1344–1352.
35. Raja KB, Simpson RJ, Pippard MJ, Peters TJ. In vivo studies on the relationship between intestinal iron (Fe3+) absorption, hypoxia, and erythropoiesis in the mouse. Br J Haematol. 1988;68:373–378.
36. Canonne-Hergaux F, Gruenheid S, Ponka P, Gros P. Cellular and subcellular localization of the Nramp2 iron transporter in the intestinal brush border and regulation by dietary iron. Blood. 1999;93: 4406–4417.
37. Lee P, Gelbart T, West C, Halloran C, Beutler E. Seeking candidate mutations that affect iron homeostasis. Blood, Cells, Molecules and Diseases. 2002; 29:471–487.
38. Nicolas, G, Bennoun M, Porteu A, et al. Severe iron deficiency anemia in transgenic mice expressing liver hepcidin. Proc Natl Acad Sci U S A. 2002;98: 4596–4601.
39. Nemeth E, Tuttle MS, Powelson J, et al. Hepcidin regulates cellular iron efflux by binding to ferroportin and inducing its internalization. Science. 2004;306: 2090–2093.
40. Kulaksiz H, Theilig F, Bachmann S, et al. The iron-regulatory peptide hormone hepcidin: expression and cellular localization in the mammalian kidney. J Endocrinol. 2005;184:361–370.
41. Food and Nutrition Board, Institute of Medicine. Dietary Reference Intakes for Vitamin A, Vitamin K, Arsenic, Boron, Chromium, Copper, Iodine, Iron, Manganese, Molybdenum, Nickel, Silicon, Vanadium, and Zinc. Washington, DC: National Academies Press; 2001. Available online at: http://www.nap.edu/books/0309072794/html/.
42. Beaton GH, Statistical approaches to establish mineral element recommendations. J Nutr. 1996; 126(suppl 9):2320S–2328S.
43. Cook JD, Flowers CH, Skikne BS. The quantitative assessment of body iron. Blood. 2003;101: 3359–3364.
44. Willis WT, Gohil K, Brooks GA, Dallman PR. Iron deficiency: improved exercise performance within 15 hours of iron treatment in rats. J Nutr. 1990;120: 909–916.
45. Hershko C. Iron and infection. Iron Nutr Health Dis. 1996;22:231–238.
46. Davies KJ, Maguire JJ, Brooks GA, Dallman PR, Packer L. Muscle mitochondrial bioenergetics, oxygen supply, and work capacity during dietary iron deficiency and repletion. Am J Physiol. 1982;242: E418–E427.
47. Edgerton VR, Ohira Y, Hettiarachchi J, Senewiratne B, Gardner GW, Barnard RJ. Elevation of hemoglobin and work tolerance in iron-deficient subjects. J Nutr Sci Vitaminol (Tokyo). 1981;27:77–86.
48. Viteri FE. & Torun B. Anemia and physical work capacity. In: Garby L, ed. *Clinics in Haematology*. London: WB Sanders; 1974; 609–626.
49. Brownlie T 4th, Utermohlen V, Hinton PS, Giordano C, Haas JD. Marginal iron deficiency without

anemia impairs aerobic adaptation among previously untrained women. Am J Clin Nutr. 2002;75: 734–742.

50. Fishbane S. Review of issues relating to iron and infection. Am J Kidney Dis. 1999;34(4 suppl 2): S47–S52.
51. Sussman M. Iron and infection. In: Jacobs A, Worwood AM, eds. *Iron in Biochemistry and Medicine*. New York: Academic Press; 1974; 649–679.
52. Murray MJ, Murray AB, Murray MB, Murry CJ. The adverse effect of iron repletion on the course of certain infections. Br Med J. 1978;2:1113–1115.
53. Damodaran M, Naidu AN, Sarma KV. Anemia and morbidity in rural preschool children. Indian J Med Res. 1979;69:448–456.
54. Spear AT, Sherman AR. Iron deficiency alters DMBA-induced tumor burden and natural killer cytotoxicity rats. J Nutr. 1992;122:46–55.
55. Hallquist NA, McNeil LK, Lockwood JF, Sherman AR. Maternal-iron-deficiency effects on peritoneal macrophage and peritoneal natural-killer-cell cytotoxicity in rat pups. Am J Clin Nutr. 1992;55: 741–746.
56. Kuvibidila SR, Kitchens D, Baliga BS. In vivo and in vitro iron deficiency reduces protein kinase C activity and translocation in murine splenic and purified T cells. J Cell Biochem. 1999;74:468–478.
57. Galan P, Thibault H, Preziosi P, Hercberg S. Interleukin 2 production in iron-deficient children. Biol Trace Elem Res. 1992;32:421–426.
58. Beard JL, Connor JR. Iron deficiency and neural functioning. Annu Rev Nutr. 2003;23:41–58.
59. Hill JM. The distribution of iron in the brain. In: Youdim MBH, ed. *Brain Iron: Neurochemistry and Behavioural Aspects*. London: Taylor and Francis; 1988; 1–24.
60. Larkin EC, Rao GA. Importance of fetal and neonatal iron: Adequacy for normal development of central nervous system. In: Dobbing J, ed. *Brain, Behavior and Iron in the Infant Diet*. London: Springer-Verlag; 1990; 43–63.
61. Ortiz E, Pasquini JM, Thompson K, Felt B, Butkus G, Beard J, Connor JR. Effect of manipulation of iron storage, transport, or availability on myelin composition and brain iron content in three different animal models. J Neurosci Res. 2004;77:681–689.
62. Roncagliolo M, Garrido M, Walter T, Peirano P, Lozoff B. Evidence of altered central nervous system development in infants with iron deficiency anemia at 6 mo: delayed maturation of auditory brainstem responses. Am J Clin Nutr. 1998;68:683–690.
63. Youdim MB. Neuropharmacological and neurobiochemical aspects of iron deficiency. In: Dobbing J, ed. *Brain, Behavior and Iron in the Infant Diet*. London: Springer-Verlag; 1990; 83–106.
64. Youdim MB, Ben-Shachar D, Yehuda S. Putative biological mechanisms on the effects of iron deficiency on brain biochemistry. Am J Clin Nutr. 1989; 50(suppl 3):607S–617S.
65. Yehuda S. Neurochemical basis of behavioral effects of brain iron deficiency in animals. In: Dobbing J, ed. *Brain, Behavior and Iron in the Infant Diet*. London: Springer-Verlag; 1990; 63–82.
66. Taneja V, Mishra K, Agarwal KN. Effect of early iron deficiency in the rat on gamma aminobutyric acid shunt in brain. J Neurochem. 1986;46: 1670–1674.
67. Earley CJ, Allen RP, Beard JL, Connor JR. Insight into the pathophysiology of restless legs syndrome. J Neurosci Res. 2000;62:623–628.
68. Lozoff B, De Andraca I, Castillo M, Smith JB, Walter T, Pino P. Behavioral and developmental effects of preventing iron deficiency anemia in healthy full-term infants. Pediatrics. 2003;112:846–854.
69. Pollitt E. Iron deficiency and educational deficiency. Nutr Rev. 1997;55:133–141.
70. Schumann K. Safety aspects of iron in food. Ann Nutr Metab. 2001;45:91–101.
71. Hallberg L. Combating iron deficiency: daily administration of iron is far superior to weekly administration. Am J Clin Nutr. 1998;68:213–217.
72. Beard JL. Effectiveness and strategies of iron supplementation during pregnancy. Am J Clin Nutr. 2000; 71(suppl 5):1288S–1294S.
73. Ellenhorn MJ, Barceloux DG, eds. Iron. In: *Medical Toxicology*. New York: Elsevier; 1988; 1023–1030.
74. Gordeuk VR, Caleffi A, Corradini E, et al. Iron overload in Africans and African-Americans and a common mutation in the SCL40A1 (ferroportin 1) gene. Blood Cells Mol Dis. 2003;31:299–304.
75. Bouis H. Micronutrient fortification of plants through plant breeding: can it improve nutrition in man at low cost? Proc Nutr Soc. 2003;62:403–411.

# 35 Zinc

Robert J. Cousins

There are many centers of activity providing new information about the nutritional significance of zinc. These include molecular approaches to zinc status assessment, molecular characterization of cellular zinc transport systems, the role of zinc in cognition and central nervous system activity, zinc as a determinant of immune system development and maintenance of host defense (including nitric oxide and oxygen radical protection), zinc and apoptotic cell death, and the molecular biology of zinc (including transcriptional control of specific genes and zinc finger proteins associated with cellular proliferation and differentiation and intracellular signaling).

## Chemistry

Details of the chemistry of and analytical methods for zinc were reviewed in an earlier volume.[1] Zinc is a strong Lewis acid (electron acceptor). Zn(II) does not exhibit redox chemistry. Nevertheless, $Zn^{2+}$ thiolate clusters, which are abundant in biology, may serve as redox centers where $Zn^{2+}$ release caused by oxidants leads to an oxidized disulfide. Recently, the use of fluorescent probes to measure free zinc abundance within cells during altered physiologic conditions has increased.[2] These probes, upon excitation, emit fluorescence when Zn(II) is bound. Many of the probes are available as cell-permeant ester forms and cell-impermeant forms. They are amenable to experiments using spectrofluorometric analysis and fluorescence microscopy. Fluorescent probes may replace $^{65}Zn$ as a tracer in cell-level experiments.[3]

## Zinc Transporters

Dramatic improvements in understanding zinc metabolism have evolved with the identification and characterization of zinc transporter genes. These are within two families: *SLC30A* or *ZnT* genes and *SLC39A* or *Zip* genes.[4] These groups are comprised of 10 and 14 members, respectively. Topology and some experimental data suggest that the ZnT transporters lower intracellular $Zn^{2+}$ concentrations, either through efflux at the plasma membrane or by influx into vesicles. Conversely, Zip transporters may raise intracellular $Zn^{2+}$, either through influx across the plasma membrane from the extracellular fluid or efflux from intracellular vesicles. These genes display wide differences in tissue expression and responsiveness to dietary zinc intake, hormones, cytokines, and other mediators, suggesting specific individual functions for the transporter proteins produced. A number of the transporter genes have metal response elements, which accounts for their responsiveness to zinc levels in the diet. Some of the zinc transporters may also transport other metals such as iron and manganese. Putative functions of some zinc transporters, based primarily on integrative approaches, are presented in Table 1.

## Absorption

The zinc content of the human body (1.5–2.5 g) approaches that of iron.[1] This level is maintained with absorption of about 5 mg/d. Zinc is absorbed from the small intestine, primarily the duodenum and jejunum but also the ileum.[11] Absorption may also occur from the colon. Lumen perfusion studies in humans suggest the jejunum exhibits the highest zinc absorption rate.[12] The anatomical region that is quantitatively most important is not clear. Under controlled conditions, apparent absorption of zinc is about 33%.[13] The extent of digestion, transit time, and binding to specific factors in the diet (e.g., phytic acid) influence the quantitative significance of each region in the absorption process.

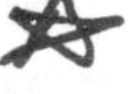

Homeostatic control of zinc metabolism involves a balance between absorption of dietary zinc and endogenous secretions through adaptive regulation programmed by the dietary zinc supply. The intestine is the key organ in maintaining that balance. When isolated from systemic influences and pancreatic secretions, the intestine retains evidence of adaptation to absorption programmed by previous dietary intake.[14] This suggests that some adaptation

**Table 1.** Transporters and Integrative Zinc Metabolism

| Transporter | Tissue/Cell | Proposed Function | Regulating Agent (Response) | References |
|---|---|---|---|---|
| ZnT1 | Enterocytes (basolateral) | Zinc absorption and cell export | High zinc intake (up-regulation) | McMahon and Cousins, 1998[8] |
| ZnT1 | Placenta (villus yolk sac) | Maternal/fetal zinc transport | Low zinc intake (down-regulation) | Langmade et al., 2000,[15] Liuzzi et al., 2003,[9] Andrews et al.[10] |
| ZnT1, ZnT2 | Exocrine pancreas (acinar cells) | Endogenous zinc loss through export | Low zinc intake (down-regulation) | Liuzzi et al., 2004[7] |
| ZnT1* | Total leukocytes | Zinc export | Zinc intake above RDA (up-regulation) | Aydemir et al., 2006[16] |
| ZnT1* | Monocytes<br>T lymphocytes<br>Granulocytes | Zinc export | Immune activation (down-regulation) | Aydemir et al., 2006[16] |
| Zip3* | Total leukocytes | Unknown | Zinc intake above RDA (down-regulation) | Aydemir et al., 2006[16] |
| Zip4* | Enterocytes (apical) | Zinc absorption (acrodermatitis enteropathica gene) | Low zinc intake (up-regulation) | Wang et al., 2002,[5] Dufner-Beattie et al., 2003,[6] Liuzzi et al., 2004[7] |
| Zip14 | Liver parenchymal cells (apical) | Hepatic zinc accumulation (hypozincemia of inflammation) | Interleukin-6 (up-regulation) | Liuzzi et al., 2005[3] |

* Data are from human cells. All other data were obtained from rodent studies.

of absorption to dietary zinc intake is controlled at the intestinal level. When true absorption is measured, which eliminates endogenous zinc as a factor in calculations, low zinc intake increases the efficiency of absorption.[17,18] This suggests that up-regulation of zinc uptake upon zinc restriction also occurs at the intestinal level in humans, as in experimental animals. The origin of endogenous zinc is not known, but most likely is a mixture of secretions from the pancreas and intestinal cells.

Experimental approaches to elucidate the mechanism of zinc absorption have been directed at brush border uptake, intracellular diffusion, basolateral transport, and plasma (corporeal) phases. A seminal discovery was the recent identification of the acrodermatitis enteropathica gene, i.e., the zinc transporter Zip4 (SLC39A4), as the factor responsible for this zinc malabsorption syndrome.[5] In mice, dietary zinc deficiency causes upregulation of Zip4 expression.[6,7] Zip4 is increasingly localized to the apical membrane of enterocytes from zinc-deficient mice. Except for decreases in intestinal ZnT and ZnT expression in zinc-deficient mouse intestine, Zip4 is the only transporter gene, from a survey of 15 zinc transporter genes that responds to a reduction in the dietary zinc supply,[7] suggesting that Zip4 is a key regulated component of the zinc absorptive pathway.[7] Remission of signs of zinc deficiency in acrodermatitis enteropathica patients upon zinc supplementation[19] suggests that other zinc transporters, perhaps of lower affinity, contribute to the absorption process.

Repeatedly, zinc absorption kinetics have been shown to involve a mediated (saturable) component and a non-mediated (non-saturable) component. These appear to be a function of the luminal zinc concentration.[11] Without a doubt, Zip4 is a primary factor responsible for the saturable kinetics of the mediated component. In rats, kinetic evidence suggests that the velocity of transfer, rather than a differing $K_m$ (affinity), produces the increased zinc absorption when a zinc-deficient diet is fed. Increased Zip4 abundance at the apical membrane of enterocytes may yield the increase in velocity of zinc transfer. In humans, the rate of zinc absorption from perfused jejunum is proportional to the luminal zinc concentration over the range 0.1 to 1.8 mM, but is saturable above 1.8 mM.[12] Measurement of zinc transport across the apical membrane of enterocytes is difficult to approach experimentally, so the form of zinc transported by Zip4 and perhaps other transporters is not known. Zinc transporter proteins usually have a histidine-rich loop, which might help to facilitate zinc release from zinc-binding ligands in the intestinal lumen.[4] It is possible that specific ligands are required for zinc transport. However, cumulative data in many model systems showing that zinc transport occurs without specific factors argues against such a requirement.

The intracellular phase of zinc absorption (transcellular movement) has been extensively studied. Zinc newly acquired from the intestinal lumen is bound to many different molecular species based on chromatographic evidence. The most widely studied has been metallothionein.[11] Metallothionein (MT) expression in intestine is directly correlated to dietary zinc intake. Zinc absorption declines as metallothionein synthesis is elevated in response to dietary zinc. Metallothionein is envisioned by some investigators as an expandable zinc pool within enterocytes that impedes zinc movement by acting as a transient intracellular buffer.[11,14] It is also possible that metallothionein provides a zinc sequestration role, wherein it helps to facilitate zinc acquisition from the diet.[20] A vesicular mechanism for transcellular zinc movement has been proposed that is similar to one proposed for calcium. This model is based on decreased zinc transport by Caco-2 cells treated with quinacrine, a lysosome-disrupting agent.[21] Recent studies of zinc transporter localization in the mouse intestine have also shown vesicular orientation,[7,9] suggesting that zinc movement across enterocytes involves vesicular transport.

Extrusion of zinc from enterocytes appears as a linear function of the luminal zinc concentration.[11] The first zinc transporter discovered, ZnT1 (SLC30A1),[22] has been localized primarily to the basolateral membrane of rat intestine.[8] This suggests an efflux role for ZnT1 in zinc transfer from enterocytes to the portal supply. Zinc transport in the serosal to mucosal direction has been reported[11] and may contribute to the endogenous zinc secretions necessary for fecal zinc loss and homeostatic control.

The non-mediated (non-saturable) component of zinc absorption is observed at higher luminal zinc concentrations.[11] While this mode of luminal-to-vascular zinc transport could represent a linear phase of transcellular movement, it more likely represents paracellular diffusion between enterocytes. It may be by this route that zinc in high amounts and some zinc chelates are absorbed. Albumin appears to be the major portal carrier for newly absorbed zinc.[1,11] Changes in the systemic level of albumin do not appear to alter zinc absorption.

As components of the diet are degraded, zinc is presented to enterocytes as smaller zinc-binding ligands (primarily peptides, amino acids, and nucleotides) and, perhaps to a limited extent, as free zinc.[11] Solubility may be an important factor determining zinc uptake by enterocytes in these situations.[23] Many factors have been reported to promote or antagonize zinc absorption.[1,19] For example, inhibition of gastric acid secretion may lower zinc absorption in man.[24] Phytate has been shown to reduce zinc absorption by a variety of experimental techniques and in actual feeding situations, probably by reducing the solubility of zinc in forms needed for brush border uptake.[25] Phytate was a contributing factor in human zinc deficiency reported in the Middle East in the 1960s.[26] It may account for the lower zinc bioavailability from some soy-based products. The absorption of zinc chelates has not been well studied. The binding constants of some may be such that $Zn^{2+}$ is not available. For example, the zinc-picolinic acid complex may promote urinary zinc excretion and lead to negative zinc balance.[27,28] In other cases, zinc consumed as a chelate may be highly available.[23]

Some minerals in the diet may alter zinc absorption. Inorganic iron in pharmacological doses may decrease zinc uptake.[29] This could result from an interaction between high concentrations of $Fe^{2+}$ and a critical zinc transporter such as Zip4, or between $Fe^{2+}$ and $Zn^{2+}$ for DMT1 (divalent metal transporter 1), since the latter may transport multiple cations.[30] Other studies suggest that heme iron has an inhibitory effect, but the capacity to absorb iron does not influence zinc uptake.[31] Copper appears to have little direct effect on zinc absorption. Evidence suggests that calcium and zinc are transported by distinctly different mechanisms. Calcium supplements, however, have been shown to have both positive and negative effects on zinc absorption.[32,33] High intakes of calcium cause parakeratosis in pigs, a skin disorder related to concomitant zinc restriction.

## Metabolism

Plasma zinc comprises 0.1% of the body's zinc.[1,19] Normally, in animals and humans, plasma zinc concentrations are maintained within strict limits at about 1 μg/mL. Albumin and $\alpha_2$-macroglobulin comprise most of the plasma zinc (70% and 20%–40%, respectively). There is a large molar excess of albumin compared with zinc. Albumin has a low association constant for $Zn^{2+}$, which is consistent with rapid exchange by cells. This is commonly referred to as "loosely bound" zinc. Less than 1% of the plasma zinc is bound to low-molecular weight complexes (primarily with cysteine and histidine). These complexes may have roles in cellular zinc uptake. Over 80% of blood zinc is found in cells, mostly in erythrocytes. In red cells, carbonic anhydrases account for most of the zinc (>85%), with about 5% as Cu/Zn-superoxide dismutase.[19] Reticulocytes contain some metallothionein, in amounts that reflect zinc intake.[34,35] In human blood, erythrocytes contain about 1 mg zinc/$10^6$ cells, while mononuclear and polynuclear cells have more, up to 6 mg zinc/$10^6$ cells.[36]

The plasma zinc level responds markedly to external stimuli, including fluctuations in zinc intake, fasting, and a variety of acute stresses such as infection.[37] These responses are frequently dramatic in studies with rodents. A reproducible reduction in the level (15%) occurs postprandially, and is perhaps related to meal-induced changes in insulin and glucose.[38] These transient reductions in plasma zinc levels are believed to reflect hepatic zinc uptake, perhaps resulting from hormonal control. The increase in plasma zinc upon fasting results from hormonally regulated catabolic changes wherein a portion of the large reserve of the zinc in muscle (57% of body zinc) is mobilized.[39] In experimental zinc depletion of human subjects, plasma zinc levels are reduced with severe restriction[40] but not with moderate restriction.[1,19]

Kinetic modeling experiments with human subjects and animals have provided valuable data on how zinc metabolic compartments are utilized. Using $^{65}Zn$ as a tracer, two phases of turnover, rapid (approx. 12.5 days) and slow (approx. 300 days), were detected in humans.[41] Very reactive tissues are liver, followed by pancreas, kidney, and spleen, while tissues with slow turnover are the central nervous system and bone. A similar kinetic model developed in rats documented high metabolic activity of zinc in bone marrow.[42] These kinetic models respond to metabolic changes produced by specific hormones. There appears to be little zinc available as a stored reserve, so when adaptation to intake fails, deficiency occurs rapidly.[43]

Considerable evidence from tracer studies and isolated cells suggest that the zinc-binding protein metallothionein is a factor in influencing zinc metabolism. Included in this concept is that metallothionein is inducible by dietary zinc[44] via the metal response element (MRE) and metal-binding transcription factor (MTF-1) mechanism of transcriptional regulation described in a later section. Dietary regulation of metallothionein expression appears to constitute an autoregulation cycle, wherein increased metallothionein synthesis is linked to increased zinc binding (retention) within cells. Metallothionein may act as a Zn(II) buffer, controlling the free Zn(II) level or participating in the regulation and coordination of intracellular distribution, which is responsive to both hormones and diet. Reduction in plasma zinc has been shown by kinetic modeling to coincide with metallothionein synthesis and zinc binding by the metallothionein kinetic compartment.[42] Transgenic mice have been developed in which the MT gene has been inactivated (knockout, null mutation) by homologous recombination techniques.[44] These animals develop normally, but are sensitive to cadmium toxicity and some forms of stress. This suggests that metallothionein is not necessary for development but may be important for homeostatic responses to stresses and/or processing of a fluctuating dietary zinc supply.

Zinc transporters that regulate influx or efflux may allow cells to adapt further to differences in zinc intake independent of metallothionein. Upon dietary zinc restriction of mice, there is a marked upregulation of intestinal Zip4 expression and downregulation of the pancreatic transporters ZnT1 and ZnT2.[7] These changes have been proposed as contributing to homeostatic control by increasing zinc absorption and decreasing endogenous loss. Similar mechanisms likely are operative in humans. At zinc intakes of 7, 15, and 30 mg/d, human subjects have fecal zinc losses of 6.8, 14.4, and 30.1 mg/d, respectively.[45] Reduction in fecal zinc as a function of duration of depletion is observed within days.[46] The endogenous losses of zinc in feces are a mix of pancreatic and intestinal secretions. Renal zinc loss is low, and is not significantly influenced by zinc intake.[45,46] Urinary zinc responds to changes in muscle catabolism.[47]

Cytokines, primarily interleukins-1 (IL-1) and -6 (IL-6), have been shown to influence zinc metabolism. It is believed that a stress, such as an acute infection in which endotoxins are produced, leads to secretion of cytokines, which have multiple effects, including activation of immune cells. Tracer studies show that IL-1 causes $^{65}Zn$ redistribution to liver, bone marrow, and thymus, with less going to bone, skin, and intestine.[48] IL-6, a major regulator of the acute-phase response, has been shown to mediate the hypozincemia associated with infection and inflammation.[3] IL-6 specifically upregulates hepatic Zip14 expression and localization to the plasma membrane of hepatocytes, which increases $Zn^{2+}$ influx from the plasma. IL-1 administered to pregnant rats produces zinc-related changes in fetal metallothionein expression.[49] This may have implications for zinc-related defects in fetal development caused by disease incidence during pregnancy. In this regard, ZnT1 has been shown to be highly expressed in the villous visceral membrane,[10,50] and a ZnT1 null mutation is lethal to the embryo.[10] A number of zinc transporters are expressed in the placenta, and some are responsive to dietary zinc intake.[4] Successful fetal development, therefore, depends on both an adequate maternal zinc supply and efficient maternal/fetal zinc transporter activity.

## Physiologic (Biochemical) Function

The biochemical functions of zinc that determine physiologic effects have received extensive study. However, the signs of altered zinc status are diverse and have not been assigned to a defect in a specific function. The ubiquitous distribution of zinc among cells, coupled with the fact that zinc is the most abundant intracellular trace element, points to very basic functions. Three different functions define the role of zinc in biology: catalytic, structural, and regulatory.

Catalytic roles are found in enzymes from all six classes of enzymes.[51] Examples are the RNA nucleotide transferases (RNA polymerases I, II, and III), alkaline phosphatase, and the carbonic anhydrases. While well over 200 zinc metalloenzymes have been characterized, when the same enzyme from different sources (plant, microbial, and animal) are counted only once, over 50 enzymes are found to contain zinc. An enzyme is generally considered as a zinc metalloenzyme if removal of the zinc causes a reduction in activity without affecting the enzyme protein irreversibly, and if reconstitution with zinc restores activity. How zinc is donated to apo-metalloenzyme proteins is not known. It may involve posttranslational modification (metal donation), perhaps coordinated within vesicular zinc compartments.

The literature is filled with examples of zinc metalloenzymes that are influenced by the dietary zinc supply. However, unequivocal evidence of a direct link between zinc deficiency/toxicity signs and individual enzymes in complex organisms is still lacking. A physiologic defect will only occur if the zinc-requiring enzyme is acting at a rate-limiting step in a critical biochemical pathway/process. The relationship of zinc nutrition to alcoholic liver disease has focused on the zinc metalloenzyme alcohol dehydrogenase (EC 1.1.1.1), which serves as a historical example of a proposed zinc metalloenzyme/disease relationship. The growth response seen in zinc-supplemented children serves as a more recent example where a metalloenzyme defect may produce a decrease in function, perhaps via augmented RNA polymerase activity.

The structural function of zinc is a rapidly expanding area of biological investigation. Structure roles for zinc in metalloenzymes exist. The cytosolic enzyme CuZn-superoxide dismutase is an example. Copper serves at the catalytic site, while zinc serves a role in structure. The zinc finger motif in proteins represents an extremely important structural role. These have the following general structure: $-C-X_2-C-X_n-C-X_2-C-$, where C designates cysteine and X other amino acids. Zinc fingers (where some histidines replace cysteine) are the most abundant. First identified in 1985 in frog (*Xenopus*) oocyte transcription factor TFIIIA, estimates reveal that at least 3% of the human genome code is for zinc finger proteins.[52] It has been estimated that, of the 1960 transcription factors in eukaryotic cells, there are approximately 762 zinc finger proteins.[53]

Classic examples of zinc finger transcription factors are the retinoic acid and calcitriol receptors. Originally considered as DNA-binding domains of transcription factors in the cell nucleus, further study has indicated a broader cellular distribution and biochemical role of zinc finger domains of proteins. Some zinc finger proteins are involved in functions requiring protein-protein interactions. Most of these appear to have some effect on signal transduction modulating cellular differentiation, proliferation, and adhesion. Evidence suggests that zinc is redistributed within cellular sites during signal transduction.[54] Zinc can be removed from finger motifs by nitrosative or oxidative stress and by electrophilic attack. These usually result in loss of function, but in some cases may have regulatory functions.[55] Interest in zinc finger motifs is intense because they are potential targets for therapeutic intervention with drugs.

The influence of zinc nutrition on cellular components containing zinc fingers needs to be defined. However, three points are clear: 1) considering their abundance, zinc fingers contribute to the overall zinc requirement; 2) zinc fingers provide a rationale for the tight homeostatic control of zinc metabolism; and 3) zinc fingers may provide an explanation for divergent biological effects of zinc deprivation. Binding constants for zinc finger motifs vary widely, but it is generally believed that $Zn^{2+}$ insertion into these cysteine thiol/histidine imidazole sites is a coordinated process.[56] This could be via a zinc-trafficking protein, such as metallothionein,[56] and/or within zinc-rich vesicles with high zinc transporter activity.[4] The extent to which dietary zinc intake influences the function of specific zinc finger proteins has not been widely investigated.

A third generalized biochemical role for zinc is through binding to transacting factors responsible for regulating the expression of specific genes. The only well-studied example of this role is in the expression of the MT gene. The basic components are a MTF protein and an MRE protein, a unique, 7-bp core nucleotide sequence found in the regulatory sequence of genes. The most likely mechanism for this on/off switch for transcription is that zinc ions, originally derived from the diet, upon transport into cells can interact with the MTF facilitating translocation to the nucleus for MRE binding to stimulate transcription. MTF-1 is the only MTF that has been characterized.[57] The distribution of MRE sequences is widespread in the genomes of mice and humans. The ubiquitous distribution of MREs is suggestive of regulatory functions for zinc beyond the scope of metal metabolism. Two lines of evidence support a wider role in biology. First, MTF-1 binding to MREs is influenced by the cellular redox state.[58] Furthermore, MTF-1 expression is regulated by nitric oxide[59] and lipopolysaccharide.[60] Secondly, homozygous MTF-1 knock out mice die by day 9 of gestation, with evidence of dysregulation of numerous genes found in their livers.[61] Alternatively, lethality could result from the defective regulation of placental/fetal ZnT1 expression which requires MTF-1.[10] Consequently, MTF-1 may regulate numerous genes associated with the biology of zinc. In this regard, global gene profiling has shown that there are populations of genes that are negatively or positively responsive to cellular zinc status.[61,62] Another MTF, distinct from MTF-1, may become active when zinc status is low,[62] or MTF-1 without zinc bound may activate some genes during zinc depletion conditions.

Despite the detailed knowledge of biochemical functions, how these functions directly influence physiology and contribute to pathology associated with low zinc intake remain elusive. The effects of zinc on lipid peroxidation, protein oxidation, nitrosative stress, apoptosis, proliferation, and differentiation at the cellular level have been widely described. At the integrative level, control of nitrosative/oxidative stress and regulation of immune cell function and turnover have been under investigation.

Beneficial effects of zinc as a protective agent against various noxious agents (including organic compounds), reactive oxygen species, and x- and gamma-radiation have been widely demonstrated. Such actions extend to nitrosative stress associated with inflammation and events required for normal cell signaling. Early biochemical evidence for a cytoprotective effect of zinc was the hydroxyl radical scavenging role of metallothionein.[63] Zinc-sulfhydryl clusters, such as those of metallothionein, are viewed as reductants that, upon interaction with an oxidant, undergo sulfhydryl oxidation and concomitant $Zn^{2+}$ release.[64] This release could also be induced by nitrosative stress, which causes $Zn^{2+}$ release from the β-Zn cluster of metallothionein, the weaker of the two metal-binding domains.[65] These events could be envisioned as a "metallothionein cycle," in which pro-inflammatory cytokines upregulate both expression of the metallothionein gene and cellular events leading to increased nitrosative/oxidative stress. The latter initiates $Zn^{2+}$ release from the metalloprotein, which is simultaneously nitrosated or oxidized in the process. Cyclooxygenase-2 (COX-2) expression is upregulated in lingual and esophageal epithelia of zinc-deficient rats, possibly reflecting another anti-inflammatory role for zinc.[66]

Zinc may act as a regulator of apoptotic cell death. Such a basic function could explain why prime cellular targets of zinc deficiency are immune cells and epithelial cell barriers, both of which are systems in which cell turnover is very rapid. The outcomes of these defects have been well described at the cellular level. Zinc chelation has been shown to result in apoptosis, and zinc supplementation at high levels (>500 μM) may inhibit apoptosis.[67,68] Experiments with zinc fluorophores suggest that intracellular zinc fluxes are correlated with apoptosis.[54] The underlying mechanism for the anti-apoptotic role of zinc may involve control of caspase-3 activity,[69] but this has not been universally observed. Similarly, regulation of DNA-binding activity of nuclear factor kappaβ (NF-κβ) by changes in intracellular zinc fluxes could influence apoptosis.[70] Physiologic changes that influence intracellular zinc fluxes through metallothionein expression, such as specific cytokines, may regulate apoptosis in specific cell populations. The plethora of zinc transporter genes, their cell-specific expression, and responsiveness to specific stimuli suggest that they influence these fluxes of intracellular zinc. Such specificity may have clinical relevance. Expression profiling of zinc responsive genes of murine thymocytes and human mononuclear cells reveal many that are involved in the apoptotic process.[70,71]

## Deficiency

Overt signs of zinc deficiency have been well documented in animals and in man.[13,19,72] These include retarded growth, depressed immune function, skin lesions, depressed appetite, skeletal abnormalities, and impaired reproductive ability. Classic studies have documented diet-related zinc deficiency in humans, and growth reduction (to the point of dwarfism), infections, and sexual immaturity in males are among the findings.[26] These signs diminish upon zinc supplementation, which also increases serum alkaline phosphatase (a zinc metalloenzyme) activity. Nevertheless, human zinc deficiency has been a challenge to clearly define.

Zinc deficiency is a type II nutritional deficiency in which the first response is a reduction in growth without an apparent reduction in tissue concentration.[43] In some experimental animals, a reduction in food intake appears to be a sensitive response to a reduction in the dietary zinc supply.[19] Poor appetite tends to be a clinical feature of zinc deficiency in children.[19,72] The mechanism responsible for the zinc-related anorexia is complex, but may include release of opiates, cholecystokinin, and/or neuropeptide Y, with sites of action in the brain (possibly hypothalamic) and/or intestine.[72] The function of the reduction in energy intake may be for adaptation, since by limiting growth tissue zinc levels are conserved for critical functions.

The reduction in growth with reduced zinc in the diet is coincident with a reduction in endogenous losses.[13,19,72] As tissues conserve zinc, it has been suggested that only a small cellular pool of zinc is exchangeable. Data obtained with stable zinc isotopes as tracers support the concept of a labile, exchangeable zinc pool.[73] Such a pool may function to help control intracellular processes and thus contribute to zinc homeostasis. Perhaps when that pool is depleted, signs of deficiency occur. In rodents, the plasma zinc concentration drops rapidly when zinc is removed from the diet. Simultaneously, tissue-specific changes in zinc transporter expression and the amount of metallothionein-bound zinc change markedly.[4,7,19] Clinical manifestations of zinc deficiency result when altered zinc metabolism is drastic enough that homeostatic controls cannot supply the various body pools necessary to maintain biochemical functions. The large number of zinc transporter proteins associated with vesicles suggests that these are the intracellular sites where zinc is available for specialized functions.[4] Ordinarily, fluctuations in the dietary zinc supply may be compensated for using the reserves from muscle, where over 50% of the body zinc in humans is located. Fasting increases plasma zinc in humans and rodents, and may be a reflection of this redistribution.[39,48]

The exact biochemical basis for compromised immunity in zinc-deficient subjects has not been established.[13,19,72] Reduced zinc intake clearly results in thymus atrophy in pigs and cattle and reduced T-helper cell function in mice. Mutations in the *Zip4* gene cause zinc malabsorption and are responsible for acrodermatitis enteropathica in humans[5] and probably Adema disease in cattle.[19] These conditions result in skin lesions and impaired immunity, exhibited as susceptibility to infection.[19] Both are reversible by zinc supplementation. Adema disease produces thymic atrophy and acrodermatitis enteropathica is associated with *Candida albicans* infections.[19] These inherited disorders demonstrate a link between zinc deficiency and immune function.

Total parenteral nutrition (TPN) without adequate zinc leads to decreased natural killer cell activity.[1,19] A hypothesis that zinc may be needed for structure/activity of thymulin, a nine-amino acid peptide found in plasma that requires zinc for stimulation of T-cell development, has not received considerable support. More likely, zinc increases peripheral blood mononuclear cell synthesis of interferon-gamma (INF$\gamma$), IL-1 and IL-6, tumor necrosis factor-alpha (TNF$\alpha$), and the IL-2 receptor.[68,74] Zinc within physiologic concentrations may control the secretion/production of these immune regulators and could have therapeutic applications requiring monocyte activation.[16,68] The molecular mechanism(s) responsible could relate to any of the three basic functions of zinc (catalytic, structural, and regulatory). As mentioned above, evidence suggests that intracellular zinc may alter the cell selection process through apoptosis. For example, flow cytometry has clearly shown that early B-cells in bone marrow are depleted in nutritional zinc deficiency,[75] and this could occur though increased apoptosis signaled by zinc deficiency. Other mechanisms could explain altered immune cell growth found in zinc deficiency. Attempts to augment immunocompetence in elderly subjects without signs of zinc deficiency have not always had beneficial outcomes. In such situations, supplemental zinc may only be beneficial where there is a preexisting dietary or laboratory evidence of zinc deficiency.[76]

Globally, the prevalence of low zinc intake could be as high as 50%.[77] Intervention studies in many geographical regions have shown that zinc supplements improve immune function in malnourished children.[78] A dramatic reduction in diarrhea incidence upon zinc supplementation has been a consistent finding. Stunting, diminished cognitive ability, and reduced activity levels tend to reverse with zinc supplementation in similar populations.[79] Beneficial effects of zinc supplementation for subjects with HIV, tuberculosis, and shigellosis have not been universally found.[78] Always an issue in such intervention studies is the actual zinc status of the study populations.

Apart from the marked growth reduction and immune dysfunction defining human zinc deficiency, other clinical manifestations may be less pronounced. The clinical literature is abundant with descriptions of a more subjective nature describing dysfunctions that may have zinc-dependent components or be in some way zinc related. Reduced plasma zinc concentrations are common in inflammatory bowel disease, which may indicate reduced zinc absorption or increased zinc losses and may respond to zinc therapy. Alternatively, such observations may be manifestations of the hypozincemia that occurs with inflammation.[19] The relationship between gut microflora and inflammatory responses of the intestine share many mediators also commonly known to influence zinc metabolism.[1] These include TNF$\alpha$, IFN-$\gamma$, and IL-6. Diets low in zinc content, coupled with intestinal infections (e.g., HIV) or high alcohol consumption, could disturb such balances, cause intestinal inflammation, and lead to endogenous zinc losses.

Alcoholism, perhaps accompanied by pancreatic or liver disease, may result in marginal zinc deficiency due to reduced absorption or retention.[1,19] Zinc-related responses to taste and smell dysfunction and skin disorders have been reported. If truly zinc responsive, these may be explained on the same basis of a preexisting marginal zinc deficiency.

## Requirements, Recommended Daily Allowance, Upper Limits, and Status Assessment

It has been estimated that, worldwide, about one-half of the human population is at risk of low zinc intake.[77] In the United States, the median intake is at the Recommended Daily Allowance (RDA), but 10% may consume less than one-half of the RDA.[13] These numerical values can be misleading, however, because zinc bioavailability is highly variable. Limitation of meat intake with greater amounts of phytate-rich foods from plants may yield a diet with little absorbable zinc.

Age, gender, pregnancy, and lactation are factors that contribute to the RDA calculation for zinc. Numerous studies with isotopic zinc tracers (particularly stable isotopes) have shown that fecal endogenous zinc output is a function of dietary intake. These were used to calculate the most recent RDA for zinc.[13] Tracer data were used to calculate the intestinal endogenous zinc losses over a range of absorbed zinc. Those values, when added to other losses of endogenous zinc (through the urine, skin, sweat, semen, or menstruation) represented total endogenous losses. Urinary zinc levels are not markedly influenced by the dietary supply. The amount of absorbed zinc needed to balance those total losses was then fitted to an asymptotic function of absorbed zinc versus ingested zinc to determine the Estimated Average Requirement (EAR). A coefficient of variation of 10% for the EAR was used to derive the RDA. This factorial approach produced the RDA values shown in Table 2. Guidelines for zinc intake during TPN are available.[80] Zinc as zinc sulfate is preferred for infusion solutions that contain less than 10 mg Zn/L. Requirements are 2.5 to 4 mg Zn/d for adult TPN and 100 to 300 μg Zn/kg body weight for pediatric TPN.

The assessment of zinc status in human subjects has proven to be a difficult undertaking. The development of atomic absorption spectrometry has made the measurement of plasma zinc concentrations a standard practice for most surveys. Normally, plasma zinc is maintained at 0.8 to 1.2 μg/mL (12–18 μmol/L). However, as indicated above, physiological changes can influence this parameter. Nevertheless, dietary zinc restriction has been shown to reduce plasma zinc levels by up to 50% under

**Table 2.** Dietary Reference Intake Recommendations for Zinc

| Age Group | Criterion | RDA mg/d Males | RDA mg/d Females | UL |
|---|---|---|---|---|
| 0–6 mo | Zinc from milk only | 2 AI* | 2 AI | 4 |
| 7–12 mo | Factorial analysis | 3 | 3 | 5 |
| 1–3 y | Factorial analysis | 3 | 3 | 7 |
| 4–8 y | Factorial analysis | 5 | 5 | 12 |
| 9–13 y | Factorial analysis | 8 | 8 | 23 |
| 14–18 y | Factorial analysis | 11 | 9 | 34 |
| ≥ 19 y | Factorial analysis | 11 | 8 | 40 |
| Pregnant Women | | | | |
| 14–18 y | EAR plus fetal accumulation | | 12 | 34 |
| 19–50 y | EAR plus fetal accumulation | | 11 | 40 |
| Lactating Women | | | | |
| 14–18 y | EAR plus zinc secreted in milk | | 13 | 34 |
| 19–50 y | EAR plus zinc secreted in milk | | 12 | 40 |

*The average intake (AI) is not equivalent to the RDA. The AI was calculated from the zinc content of human milk consumed at 0.78 L per day.
EAR = Estimated Average Requirement; RDA = Recommended Daily Allowance; UL = Tolerable Upper Intake Level.
Data from Food and Nutrition Board, Institute of Medicine, 2001.[13]

experimental conditions.[1,19] In extensive experiments with human subjects under controlled and field conditions, plasma zinc has been shown to be a poor index of zinc status.[13] Leukocyte zinc, erythrocyte zinc, hair zinc, and saliva zinc are among the parameters that have also been suggested as indices, but are not viewed as good indicators.[13] A zinc tolerance test was proposed as a method to detect low zinc status.[81] The basis of this assessment method is to observe the increase in plasma zinc concentration within hours after consumption of an oral dose of zinc (25–50 mg). A lower response curve is presumed as indicative of better zinc status (low absorption). The method is not recognized as a method of choice for status assessment.

An alternative approach to assessment is to use a functional outcome, i.e., metalloenzyme activity or zinc-induced processes. Plasma alkaline phosphatase (EC 3.1.3.1) has been the most commonly used enzyme for zinc status assessment,[13,19] particularly in survey conditions. The angiotensin-converting enzyme (EC 3.4.15.1) has shown some value as an index. Overall, zinc metalloenzymes have not proven to be indicative of dietary zinc status.[13] Synthesis of metallothionein, which is zinc dependent, has been shown to reflect zinc intake in both rats and humans. The mechanistic basis for this was presented in a previous section. In rats, zinc deficiency markedly reduced plasma[82] and erythrocyte[34] metallothionein levels measured by radioimmunoassay. In human subjects, zinc depletion or supplementation produced the response of erythrocyte metallothionein expected of zinc-dependent events programmed during reticulocyte development in the bone marrow.[35,83] Monocyte metallothionein mRNA levels have been shown to be responsive to zinc supplementation, and may provide an alternative method of assessment using quantitative reverse transcriptase polymerase chain reaction (RT-PCR).[83] Expression of some zinc transporter genes has been shown to be zinc responsive and holds promise for use in status assessment.[62]

## Food and Other Sources

Foods vary greatly in their inherent zinc content, with red meat and shellfish being the best sources. Foods of vegetable origin tend to be low in zinc, with the exception of the embryo portion of grains, such as wheat germ. The presence of phytic acid in plant products is a major factor that limits zinc bioavailability from these sources (discussed earlier).[13] On this basis, it has been argued that vegetarians are more likely to have a compromised zinc supply. The zinc/phytic acid complex is insoluble and poorly absorbed from the gastrointestinal tract. Under experimental conditions, a diet with high phytate content can rapidly reduce plasma zinc concentrations in humans.[40] Certain food preparation practices, such as leavening of bread through the action of yeast, allows phytase activity to substantially lower the phytate content of breads and similar products.[19] Phytate in unleavened bread was believed to be a contributing factor to the development of human zinc deficiency described in the Middle East.[26] Zinc bioavailability is greater from human milk than from cow's milk or soy protein. Proteins in human milk, which bind most of the zinc, are believed to be more easily digestible than casein, the major protein in cow's milk.[1] This difference may explain the higher zinc bioavailability from human milk.

Total zinc content of the diet provides only a gross estimate of zinc intake. Bioavailable zinc is that portion from the diet that is absorbed and utilized. The majority of zinc in foods is bound to proteins and nucleic acids. In most cases, these associations are stable complexes that require substantial digestive activity to render zinc in a readily available form.[11] Numerous other components in foods provide ligands for zinc binding; some improve zinc absorption while others do not. Since the mechanism of zinc absorption is not fully understood, the mode of action of these factors is not clear. Some zinc complexes, particularly when consumed in large amounts, may be absorbed by the paracellular route, which would bypass transcellular absorptive mechanisms. Inhibitory factors in zinc absorption are found in some soy products (high phytate content), wheat and corn flour, coffee, tea, various beans, cheeses, and cow's milk. Calcium supplements have an equivocal influence on zinc absorption.[32,33]

Methods to assess zinc bioavailability include metabolic studies with foods intrinsically or extrinsically labeled with stable or radioactive isotopes, intestinal lavage, balance studies, zinc tolerance tests, growth measurements, and slope ratio assay.[1] In some studies, the method of expression (i.e., true absorption versus apparent absorption) can produce differing results. As an example, using true absorption as a measure, the absorption of zinc from beef was 55%, and from high fiber cereal it was 15%. Under the same conditions, calculated apparent absorption was 15% and −25%, respectively.[84] Accounting for endogenous zinc losses provides a more realistic estimate of bioavailability.

Sources of zinc used as supplements, either alone or combined in mineral/vitamin preparations, vary widely in bioavailability. Imbalances created by the addition of other trace elements such as iron may interfere with zinc absorption.[1] Information on zinc bioavailability is more abundant in the animal literature than in that for humans. Zinc in the form of organic acids (acetate and gluconate), amino acid chelates (with methionine), or zinc sulfate is more soluble than zinc oxide and hence has higher bioavailability.[22] Unfortunately, because zinc oxide has a high percentage of zinc (80%) by weight, it is frequently the choice for mineral/vitamin supplement formulations.

## Excess and Toxicity

Acute zinc toxicity results in gastric distress, dizziness, and nausea.[85] This can be a complicating factor in zinc supplementation studies, with an emetic effect occurring at much over 150 mg Zn/d. Gastric problems are observed in chronic toxicity. Among other chronic effects are a reduction in immune function (i.e., a decrease in lymphocyte stimulation to phytohemagglutinin) and a reduction in HDL cholesterol, which have been reported with very high supplements (300 mg Zn/d). A depression in lymphocyte stimulation was not observed at 100 mg Zn/d. In contrast, supplementation at 150 mg Zn/d decreased LDL and lowered serum ceruloplasmin ferroxidase activity. No significant changes in HDL were found.[13] In elderly subjects, 100 mg Zn/d did not improve immunocompetence and did not alter total serum cholesterol or HDL cholesterol.[86] Feeding zinc to chickens at 100 mg/kg diet produced pancreatic acinar cell exocrine dysfunction.[87] The mechanisms for these effects are unknown.

Hypocupremia, observed when sickle cell anemia patients were treated with 150 mg/d of zinc, results from a zinc-induced copper deficiency.[88] This effect has been used as a way to decrease copper absorption in Wilson's disease, a copper accumulation disorder. Presumably, zinc-induced intestinal metallothionein binds copper preferentially and leads to copper loss via desquamation of enterocytes.[89] Copper-zinc superoxide dismutase activity is decreased in erythrocytes when excess zinc is consumed.[13] Because the effect was detected at zinc intakes as low as 60 mg/d,[90] the reduction in activity was used as the basis for the lowest observed adverse effect level (LOAEL) to establish a tolerable upper intake level (UL). An uncertainty factor of 1.5 was selected, thus placing the UL for adults at 40 mg/d (Table 2). The induction of metallothionein mRNA in monocytes occurs at 15 mg/d,[16,83] which is well below the UL.

A number of emerging issues relate to zinc toxicity via supplementation. The first is that metallothionein induction by zinc in bone marrow cells may have a protective effect for stem cells from some chemotherapeutic agents.[91] Secondly, as more becomes known about zinc responsive stress genes, focused therapeutic uses of zinc may develop. For example, age-related macular degeneration, a photic injury to the zinc-rich retinal pigment epithelium in the macular region, may lead to oxidative damage and cause degeneration. Of particular interest is the decreased mortality in age-related macular degeneration patients who received supplemental zinc oxide.[92] Finally, zinc is found in abundance in the central nervous system.[72] Accounting for 1.5% of total body zinc, turnover of brain zinc is slow. Regional areas of high zinc content, such as the hippocampus, occur through specific zinc transporter activity. Synaptic vesicles of nerve terminals actively take up zinc. Stimulation of nerve fibers, particularly in the hippocampus, where much zinc is stored, causes release of zinc. High concentrations of zinc may produce neuronal death.[93]

Based upon current knowledge, zinc should be considered as a relatively nontoxic micronutrient in moderate supplementation levels. The concern is that nutrient imbalances and interactions due to individual selective supplementation may produce toxicity not encountered with usual dietary practices.

## Summary

Zinc nutrition is a very active area of research. State-of-the-art methods are being applied toward the goal of improving our understanding of absorption mechanisms, cellular transport and metabolism, functional targets, and biomarkers for status assessment. Intake data suggest that the consumption of zinc in amounts needed to meet dietary reference recommendations is geographically diverse. Differences in bioavailability from complex diets may produce vast differences in actual amounts of zinc absorbed. Successful zinc intervention therapy in developing countries suggests that zinc deficiency remains of current medical interest. Newer biochemical evidence suggests that zinc supplementation may have beneficial consequences; specifically, the influence of zinc in gene regulation and cellular responses to stress suggests a wide range of functions for this micronutrient.

## References

1. Cousins RJ. Zinc. In: Filer LJ, Ziegler EE, eds. *Present Knowledge in Nutrition.* 7th ed. Washington, DC: International Life Sciences Institute; 1996;293–306.
2. Chang CJ, Jaworski J, Nolan EM, Sheng M, Lippard SJ. A tautomeric zinc sensor for ratiometric fluorescence imaging: application to nitric oxide-induced release of intracellular zinc. Proc Natl Acad Sci U S A. 2004;101:1129–1134.
3. Liuzzi JP, Lichten LA, Rivera S, et al. Interleukin-6 regulates the zinc transporter Zip14 in liver and contributes to the hypozincemia of the acute phase response. Proc Natl Acad Sci U S A. 2005;102: 6843–6848.
4. Liuzzi JP, Cousins RJ. Mammalian zinc transporters. Annu Rev Nutr. 2004;24:151–172.
5. Wang K, Zhou B, Kuo YM, Zemansky J, Gitschier J. A novel member of a zinc transporter family is defective in acrodermatitis enteropathica. Am J Hum Genet. 2002;71:66–73.
6. Dufner-Beattie J, Langmade SJ, Wang F, Eide D, Andrews GK. Structure, function, and regulation of a subfamily of mouse zinc transporter genes. J Biol Chem. 2003;278:50142–50150.
7. Liuzzi JP, Bobo JA, Lichten LA, Samuelson DA, Cousins RJ. Responsive transporter genes within the murine intestinal-pancreatic axis form a basis of zinc homeostasis. Proc Natl Acad Sci U S A. 2004;101: 14355–14360.
8. McMahon RJ, Cousins RJ. Regulation of the zinc transporter ZnT1 by dietary zinc. Proc Natl Acad Sci U S A. 1998;95:4841–4846.
9. Liuzzi JP, Bobo JA, Cui L, McMahon RJ, Cousins RJ. Zinc transporters 1, 2 and 4 are differentially expressed and localized in rats during pregnancy and lactation. J Nutr. 2003;133:342–351.
10. Andrews GK, Wang H, Dey SK, Palmiter RD. Mouse zinc transporter 1 gene provides an essential function during early embryonic development. Genesis. 2004;40:74–81.
11. Cousins RJ. Theoretical and practical aspects of zinc uptake and absorption. In: Laszlo JA, Dintzis FR, eds. *Mineral Absorption in the Monogastric GI Tract: Chemical, Nutritional and Physiological Aspects.* New York: Plenum Publishing; 1989; 312.
12. Lee HH, Prasad AS, Brewer GJ, Owyang C. Zinc absorption in human small intestine. Am J Physiol. 1989;256(1 part 1):G87–G91.
13. Food and Nutrition Board, Institute of Medicine. *Dietary Reference Intakes for Vitamin A, Vitamin K, Arsenic, Boron, Chromium, Copper, Iodine, Iron, Manganese, Molybdenum, Nickel, Silicon, Vanadium, and Zinc.* Washington, DC: National Academies Press; 2001. Available online at: http://www.nap.edu/books/0309072794/html/.
14. Hoadley JE, Leinart AS, Cousins RJ. Kinetic analysis of zinc uptake and serosal transfer by vascularly perfused rat intestine. Am J Physiol. 1987;252(6 part 1): G825–G831.
15. Langmade SJ, Ravindra R, Daniels PJ, Andrews GK. The transcription factor MTF-1 mediates metal regulation of the mouse ZnT1 gene. J Biol Chem. 2000; 275:34803–34809.
16. Aydemir TB, Blanchard RK, Cousins RJ. Zinc supplementation of young men alters metallothionein, zinc transporter, and cytokine gene expression in leukocyte populations. Proc Natl Acad Sci USA. 2006; 103:1699–1704.
17. Ziegler EE, Serfass RE, Nelson SE, et al. Effect of low zinc intake on absorption and excretion of zinc by infants studied with $^{70}Zn$ as extrinsic tag. J Nutr. 1989;119:1647–1653.
18. Lee D Y, Prasad AS, Hydrick-Adair C, Brewer G, Johnson PE. Homeostasis of zinc in marginal human zinc deficiency: role of absorption and endogenous excretion of zinc. J Lab Clin Med. 1993;122: 549–556.
19. Mills CF, ed. *Zinc in Human Biology.* New York: Springer-Verlag; 1989.
20. Coyle P, Philcox JC, Rofe AM. Metallothionein-null mice absorb less Zn from an egg-white diet, but a similar amount from solutions, although with altered intertissue Zn distribution. J Nutr. 1999;129: 372–379.
21. Fleet JC, Turnbull AJ, Bourcier M, Wood RJ. Vitamin D sensitive and quinacrine sensitive zinc transport in human intestinal cell line Caco-2. Am J Physiol. 1993;264(6 part 1):G1037–G1045.
22. Palmiter RD, Findley SD. Cloning and functional characterization of a mammalian zinc transporter

that confers resistance to zinc. EMBO J. 1995;14: 639–649.

23. Allen LH. Zinc and micronutrient supplements for children. Am J Clin Nutr. 1998;68(suppl 2): 495S–498S.
24. Sturniolo GC, Montino MC, Rossetto L, et al. Inhibition of gastric acid secretion reduces zinc absorption in man. J Am Coll Nutr. 1991;10:372–375.
25. Han O, Failla ML, Hill AD, Morris ER, Smith JC Jr. Inositol phosphates inhibit uptake and transport of iron and zinc by a human intestinal cell line. J Nutr. 1994;124:580–587.
26. Prasad AS. *Zinc in Human Nutrition.* Boca Raton, FL: CRC Press; 1979.
27. Roth HP, Kirchgessner M. Utilization of zinc from picolinic or citric acid complexes in relation to dietary protein source in rats. J Nutr. 1985;115:1641–1649.
28. Seal CJ, Heaton FW. Effect of dietary picolinic acid on the metabolism of exogenous and endogenous zinc in the rat. J Nutr 1985;115:986–993.
29. Solomons NW, Cousins RJ. Zinc. In: Solomons NW, Rosenberg IH, eds. *Absorption and Malabsorption of Mineral Nutrients.* New York: Alan R. Liss; 1984; 125–197.
30. Gunshin H, Mackenzie B, Berger UV, et al. Cloning and characterization of a mammalian proton-coupled metal-ion transporter. Nature. 1997;388:482–488.
31. Valberg LS, Flanagan PR, Chamberlain MJ. Effects of iron, tin, and copper on zinc absorption. Am J Clin Nutr. 1984:40:536–541.
32. McKenna AA, Ilich JZ, Andon MB, Wang C, Matkovic V. Zinc balance in adolescent females consuming a low- or high-calcium diet. Am J Clin Nutr. 1997;65:1460–1464.
33. Wood RJ, Zheng JJ. High dietary calcium intakes reduce zinc absorption and balance in humans. Am J Clin Nutr. 1997;65:1803–1809.
34. Robertson A, Morrison JN, Wood AM, Bremner I. Effects of iron deficiency on metallothionein I concentrations in blood and tissues of rats. J Nutr. 1989; 119:439–445.
35. Grider A, Bailey LB, Cousins RJ. Erythrocyte metallothionein as an index of zinc status in humans. Proc Natl Acad Sci U S A. 1990;87:1259–1262.
36. Milne DB, Ralston NV, Wallwork JC. Zinc content of cellular components of blood: methods for cell separation and analysis evaluated. Clin Chem. 1985;31: 65–69.
37. Cousins RJ. Absorption, transport and hepatic metabolism of copper and zinc: special reference to metallothionein and ceruloplasmin. Physiol Rev. 1985; 65:238–309.
38. King JC, Hambidge KM, Westcott JL, Kern DL, Marshall G. Daily variation in plasma zinc concentrations in women fed meals at six hour intervals. J Nutr. 1994;124:508–516.
39. Henry RW, Elmes ME. Plasma zinc in acute starvation. Br Med J. 1975;4:625–626.
40. Gordon PR, Woodruff CW, Anderson HL, O'Dell BL. Effect of acute zinc deprivation on plasma zinc and platelet aggregation in adult males. Am J Clin Nutr. 1982;35:113–119.
41. Wastney ME, Aamodt RL, Rumble WF, Henkin RI. Kinetic analysis of zinc metabolism and its regulation in normal humans. Am J Physiol. 1986;251(2 part 2):R398–R408.
42. Dunn MA, Cousins RJ. Kinetics of zinc metabolism in the rat: effect of dibutyryl cAMP. Am J Physiol. 1989;256(3 part 1):E420–E430.
43. Golden MN. The diagnosis of zinc deficiency. In: Mills CF, ed. *Zinc in Human Biology.* New York: Springer-Verlag; 1989;323–333.
44. Davis SR, Cousins RJ. Metallothionein expression in animals: a physiological perspective on function. J Nutr. 2000;130:1085–1088.
45. Jackson MJ, Jones DA, Edwards RH, Swainbank IG, Coleman ML. Zinc homeostasis in man: studies using a new stable isotope dilution technique. Br J Nutr. 1984;51:199–208.
46. Baer MT, King JC. Tissue zinc levels and zinc excretion during experimental zinc depletion in young men. Am J Clin Nutr. 1984;39:556–570.
47. Fell GS, Fleck A, Cuthbertson DP, et al. Urinary zinc levels as an indication of muscle catabolism. Lancet. 1973;1:280–282.
48. Cousins RJ, Leinart AS. Tissue specific regulation of zinc metabolism and metallothionein genes by interleukin 1. FASEB J. 1988;2:2884–2890.
49. Huber KL, Cousins RJ. Maternal zinc deprivation and interleukin 1 influence metallothionein gene expression and zinc metabolism of rats. J Nutr. 1988; 118:1570–1576.
50. Cousins RJ, McMahon RJ. Integrative aspects of zinc transporters. J Nutr. 2000;130(suppl 5S): 1384S–1387S.
51. Vallee BL, Galdes A. The metallobiochemistry of zinc enzymes. In Meister A, ed. *Advances in Enzymology.* New York: John Wiley and Sons; 1984; 283–429.
52. Lu D, Searles MA, Klug A. Crystal structure of a zinc-finger-RNA complex reveals two modes of molecular recognition. Nature. 2003;426:96–100.
53. Messina DN, Glasscock J, Gish W, Lovett M. An ORFeome-based analysis of human transcription factor genes and the construction of a microarray to interrogate their expression. Genome Res. 2004;14: 2041–2047.
54. Truong-Tran AQ, Ho LH, Chai F, Zalewski PD. Cellular zinc fluxes and the regulation of apoptosis/gene-directed cell death. J Nutr. 2000;130(suppl 5S): 1459S–1466S.
55. Kroncke KD, Klotz LO, Suschek CV, Sies H. Comparing nitrosative versus oxidative stress toward zinc

finger-dependent transcription. Unique role for NO. J Biol Chem. 2002;277:13294–13301.

56. Roesijadi G, Bogumil R, Vasak M, Kagi JH. Modulation of DNA binding of a tramtrack zinc finger peptide by the metallothionein-thionein conjugate pair. J Biol Chem. 1998;273:17425–17432.
57. Saydam N, Adams TK, Steiner F, Schaffner W, Freedman JH. Regulation of metallothionein transcription by the metal-responsive transcription factor MTF-1: identification of signal transduction cascades that control metal-inducible transcription. J Biol Chem. 2002;277:20438–20445.
58. Dalton TP, Li Q, Bittel D, Liang L, Andrews GK. Oxidative stress activates metal-responsive transcription factor-1 binding activity. Occupancy in vivo of metal response elements in the metallothionein-I gene promoter. J Biol Chem. 1996;271: 26233–26241.
59. Lichten LA, Cousins RJ. Metallothionein may protect hepatocytes from nitrosative stress through metallothionein recycling and interaction with metal responsive transcription factor 1. FASEB J. 2005;19: A458.
60. Huang Q, Liu D, Majewski P, et al. The plasticity of dendritic cell responses to pathogens and their components. Science. 2001;294:870–875.
61. Wimmer U, Wang Y, Georgiev O, Schaffner. Two major branches of anti-cadmium defense in the mouse: MTF-1/metallothioneins and glutathione. Nuc Acids Res 2005;33:5715–5727.
62. Cousins RJ, Blanchard RK, Popp MP, et al. A global view of the selectivity of zinc deprivation and excess on genes expressed in human THP-1 mononuclear cells. Proc Natl Acad Sci U S A. 2003;100: 6952–6957.
63. Thornalley PJ, Vasak M. Possible role for metallothionein in protection against radiation induced oxidative stress. Biochem Biophys Acta. 1985;827:36–44.
64. Maret W. Zinc and sulfur: a critical biological partnership. Biochemistry. 2004;43:3301–3309.
65. Zangger K, Oz G, Haslinger E, Kunert O, Armitage IM. Nitric oxide selectively releases metals from the amino terminal domain of metallothioneins: potential role at inflammatory sites. FASEB J. 2001;15: 1303–1305.
66. Fong LY, Zhang L, Jiang Y, Farber JL. Dietary zinc modulation of COX-2 expression and lingual and esophageal carcinogenesis in rats. J Natl Cancer Inst. 2005;97:40–50.
67. Kimura E, Aoki S, Kikuta E, Koike T. A macrocyclic zinc(II) fluorophore as a detector of apoptosis. Proc Natl Acad Sci U S A. 2003;100:3731–3736.
68. Ibs KH, Rink L. Zinc-altered immune function. J Nutr. 2003;133(5 suppl 1):1452S–1456S.
69. Kondoh M, Tasaki E, Takiguchi M, Higashimoto M, Watanabe Y, Sato M. Activation of caspase-3 in HL-60 cells treated with pyrithione and zinc. Biol Pharm Bull. 2005;28:757–759.
70. Kim CH, Kim JH, Lee J, Ahn YS. Zinc-induced NF-κB inhibition can be modulated by changes in the intracellular metallothionein level. Toxicol Appl Pharmacol. 2003;190:189–196.
71. Moore JB, Blanchard RK, Cousins RJ. Dietary zinc modulates gene expression in murine thymus: results from a comprehensive differential display screening. Proc Natl Acad Sci U S A. 2003;100:3883–3888.
72. Hambidge M, Cousins RJ, Costello RB. Introduction. J Nutr. 2000;130(suppl 5):1341S–1343S.
73. Miller LV, Hambidge KM, Naake VL, Hong Z, Westcott JL, Fennessey PV. Size of the zinc pools that exchange rapidly with plasma zinc in humans: alternative techniques for measuring and relation to dietary zinc intake. J Nutr. 1994;124:268–276.
74. Prasad AS. Zinc and immunity: molecular mechanisms of zinc action on T helper cells. Journal of Trace Elements in Experimental Medicine. 2003;16: 139–163.
75. Fraker PJ, King LE. Reprogramming of the immune system during zinc deficiency. Annu Rev Nutr. 2004; 24:277–298.
76. Life Sciences Research Office. *Zinc and Immune Function in the Elderly.* Bethesda, MD: Federation of American Societies for Experimental Biology; 1991.
77. Brown KH, Wuehler SE, ed. *Zinc and Human Health: the Results of Recent Trials and Implications for Program Interventions and Research.* Ottawa, Ontario, Canada: Micronutrient Initiative; 2000.
78. Walker CF, Black RE. Zinc and the risk for infectious disease. Annu Rev Nutr. 2004;24:255–275.
79. Black MM. The evidence linking zinc deficiency with children's cognitive and motor functioning. J Nutr. 2003;133(5 suppl 1):1473S–1476S.
80. Solomons NW. Zinc. In Baumgartner TG, ed. *Clinical Guide to Parenteral Micronutrition.* 2nd ed. Deerfield, IL: Fujisawa USA; 1991; 215–233.
81. Sullivan JF, Jetton MM, Burch RE. A zinc tolerance test. J Lab Clin Med. 1979;93:485–492.
82. Sato M, Mehra RK, Bremner I. Measurement of plasma metallothionein-I in the assessment of the zinc status of zinc-deficient and stressed rats. J Nutr. 1984;114:1683–1689.
83. Cao J, Cousins RJ. Metallothionein mRNA in monocytes and peripheral blood mononuclear cells and in cells from dried blood spots increases after zinc supplementation of men. J Nutr. 2000;130: 2180–2187.
84. Zheng JJ, Mason JB, Rosenberg IH, Wood RJ. Measurement of zinc bioavailability from beef and a ready-to-eat high-fiber breakfast cereal in humans: application of whole-gut lavage technique. Am J Clin Nutr. 1993;58:902–907.
85. Fosmire G. Zinc toxicity. Am J Clin Nutr. 1990;51: 225–227.

86. Bogden JD, Oleske JM, Lavenhar MA, et al. Zinc and immunocompetence in elderly people: effects of zinc supplementation for 3 months. Am J Clin Nutr. 1988;48:655–663.
87. Lü J, Combs GF. Effect of excess dietary zinc on pancreatic exocrine function in the chick. J Nutr. 1988;118:681–689.
88. Prasad AS, Brewer GJ, Schoomaker EB, Rabbani P. Hypocupremia induced by zinc therapy in adults. JAMA. 1978;240:2166–2168.
89. Yuzbasiyan Gurkan V, Grider A, Nostrant T, Cousins RJ, Brewer GJ. Treatment of Wilson's disease with zinc: X. Intestinal metallothionein induction. J Lab Clin Med. 1992;120:380–386.
90. Yadrick MK, Kenney MA, Winterfeldt EA. Iron, copper, and zinc status: response to supplementation with zinc or zinc and iron in adult females. Am J Clin Nutr. 1989;49:145–150.
91. Doz F, Berens ME, Deschepper CF, et al. Experimental basis for increasing the therapeutic index of cis-diamminedicarboxylatocyclobutaneplatinum(II) in brain tumor therapy by a high-zinc diet. Cancer Chemother Pharmacol. 1992;29:219–226.
92. Clemons TE, Kurinij N, Sperduto RD; AREDS Research Group. Associations of mortality with ocular disorders and an intervention of high-dose antioxidants and zinc in the Age-Related Eye Disease Study: AREDS Report No. 13. Arch Ophthalmol. 2004;122:716–726.
93. Canzoniero LM, Manzerra P, Sheline CT, Choi DW. Membrane-permeant chelators can attenuate $Zn^{2+}$-induced cortical neuronal death. Neuropharmacology. 2003;45:420–428.

# 36 Copper

Joseph R. Prohaska

## Introduction

Copper was thought to be essential for humans since the middle of the nineteenth century, but was proven to be essential through careful experimental work in the 1920s. Organisms use either protein-bound, oxidized cupric ion ($Cu^{2+}$) or reduced cuprous ion ($Cu^{1+}$) for a number of single-electron transfer reactions involving oxygen. Sophisticated mechanisms for the regulated acquisition, tissue distribution, utilization, and excretion exist to prevent deleterious reactions from copper excess. Major advances in our understanding of copper homeostasis have evolved through the use of molecular genetics. This chapter summarizes many of these new insights, especially as they relate to human health and disease. Dietary Reference Intakes (DRIs), first established in 2001, will also be discussed. Apologies are extended to the many investigators whose efforts and discoveries have contributed to the advancement of the copper field but are not referenced because of space limitations.

## Biological Functions of Copper

Humans contain just over 1 mg of copper per kilogram body weight. This copper has no known structural role, nor is there a major copper storage reservoir. Rather, copper serves as an essential catalytic cofactor for about a dozen mammalian cuproenzymes (Table 1). The metal centers in these proteins binds oxygen and produce water, superoxide, or hydrogen peroxide in addition to various organic products. Although limited in number, compared with other essential metal-dependent enzymes that require iron or zinc, these cuproenzymes are involved in such fundamental processes as energy production, iron utilization, maturation of the extracellular matrix, activation of neuropeptides, and neurotransmitter synthesis. The physical properties of these enzymes have been reviewed elsewhere.[1]

Mammalian copper-dependent amine oxidases (EC 1.4.3.6) include a group of enzymes found in plasma and tissues as dimers, which deaminate monoamines and diamines, releasing aldehydes, ammonia, and hydrogen peroxide. They are inhibited by semicarbazide and contain the cofactor 2,4,5-trihydroxyphenylalanine quinone, the synthesis of which is also copper dependent.[2] They may also function in the metabolism of certain amines or may be involved in intracellular signaling by generation of hydrogen peroxide. One such example is vascular adhesion protein-1 (VAP-1) a copper amine oxidase that is involved in leukocyte trafficking.[3] Absence of the protein, also called amine oxidase copper-containing-3 (AOC3), decreased both leukocyte and lymphocyte homing and attenuated inflammatory responses.[4]

Ceruloplasmin is a blue copper oxidase (also known as ferroxidase) that oxidizes ferrous iron with the production of water rather than reactive oxygen species such as superoxide or hydrogen peroxide. Ceruloplasmin is an abundant, 132-kD plasma glycoprotein made and secreted by liver. Ceruloplasmin expression, once thought to be limited to hepatocytes, is now evident in many cell types. For example, brain expresses a glycosyl phosphatidylinositol (GIP)-anchored form of ceruloplasmin. Furthermore, there are ceruloplasmin-like proteins that also function to catalyze the oxidation of ferrous ion to facilitate iron efflux. Discovery and characterization of individuals with aceruloplasminemia, an autosomal recessive disorder, has clearly demonstrated an essential function of ceruloplasmin.[5] Individuals with this disorder are characterized by low serum iron, high iron deposits in liver, brain, and pancreas, and the development of insulin-dependent diabetes, dementia, and other neurological disorders. However, copper metabolism remains normal in aceruloplasminemic patients. Studies with ceruloplasmin-null mice confirm the impairment in iron mobilization and normal copper metabolism.[6] Thus, former hypotheses suggesting that the main function of ceruloplasmin was to transport copper are likely false.

**Table 1.** Mammalian Copper-Dependent Enzymes

| Enzyme | Function | Other Cofactors |
|---|---|---|
| Amine Oxidases | Amine oxidative deamination | Topaquinone |
| Ceruloplasmin | $Fe^{2+}$ oxidation | |
| Cytochrome *c* oxidase | Oxygen electron transfer | Heme $Fe^{2+}$, $Zn^{2+}$, $Mg^{2+}$ |
| Dopamine-β-monooxygenase | Norepinephrine synthesis | |
| Extracellular superoxide dismutase | Superoxide disproportionation | $Zn^{2+}$ |
| Hephaestin | $Fe^{2+}$ oxidation | |
| Lysyl oxidase | Elastin and collagen crosslinking | Lysyl tyrosyl quinone |
| Peptidylglycine α-amidating monooxygenase | Peptide C-terminal α-amidation | |
| Superoxide dismutase 1 | Superoxide disproportionation | $Zn^{2+}$ |
| Tyrosinase | DOPA quinone synthesis | |

Cytochrome *c* oxidase (CCO), also known as complex IV, contains 13 protein subunits, two heme groups, zinc, magnesium, and three copper ions located in the inner mitochondrial membrane. CCO catalyzes the reduction of molecular oxygen to water and generates a proton gradient that is necessary for ATP synthesis. The assembly of CCO is dependent on additional accessory proteins, some of which are involved in copper delivery and insertion into subunits I and II. Adequate dietary copper is necessary to support the activity of CCO. Mutations resulting in total loss of CCO are likely lethal. Mutations in the assembly proteins affect CCO and result in pathophysiology.[7]

Dopamine-β-monooxygenase (DBM) requires copper in each of its four subunits and ascorbate as a cosubstrate to convert dopamine to norepinephrine. DBM is expressed in adrenal medulla, sympathetic neurons of the peripheral nervous system, and noradrenergic and adrenergic neurons in brain. Deletion of the DBM gene is lethal for mouse embryos, suggesting a critical role of norepinephrine during development.[8]

Mammals have three separate genes that produce proteins that catalyze dismutation of superoxide, the univalent reduction product of molecular oxygen. Two of these proteins, Cu,Zn-superoxide dismutase (SOD1) and extracellular SOD (EC-SOD), require copper. The other protein, manganese SOD (SOD2), is located in the mitochondrial matrix. Both SOD1 and EC-SOD also contain zinc as a cofactor. SOD1 is a homodimer of subunit size 16 kD. EC-SOD is a tetramer of subunit size 135 kD that functions as an antioxidant in the extracellular matrix and is the predominant dismutase in extracellular fluids such as lymph, synovial fluid, and plasma.[9] Studies with EC-SOD knockout mice support a role for this protein and extracellular superoxide in modulating vascular tone by interacting with nitric oxide.[10]

Hephaestin is protein 50% identical to ceruloplasmin that was discovered as the defective gene in sex-linked anemia in mice. The mutation deleted a portion of the protein that causes failure to migrate to the plasma membrane, thus impairing location of its ferroxidase activity, resulting in iron retention in the intestine, a tissue enriched in this protein.[11] There appears to be a ceruloplasmin homolog in placenta that also functions in iron efflux.[12] It is also likely that a similar, if not identical, protein exists in mammary tissue, since iron efflux to milk is also copper dependent. Thus, one important biological function of copper is to serve as a catalyst for proper iron efflux and homeostasis.

Lysyl oxidase (LO) (EC 1.4.3.13) is another copper-dependent amine oxidase. It contains a unique cofactor, lysyl tyrosyl quinone, which is required for the oxidative deamination of specific lysine residues in the extracellular matrix.[13] This reaction initiates the formation of cross-links that stabilize elastin and collagen. The discovery of at least four additional genes expressing proteins related to LO (LOXL1–LOXL4) with conserved catalytic domain, copper and cofactor binding sites that are highly expressed in specific tissues is opening new avenues in the investigation of the functions of these cuproenzymes.[14]

Peptidylglycine α-amidating monoxygenase (PAM), like DBM, requires both copper and ascorbate as cofactors. PAM is required for post-translational modification of many peptides to their bioactive forms. Representative α-amidated peptides include α-melanocyte stimulating hormone, cholecystokinin, gastrin, neuropeptide Y, substance P, vasoactive intestinal peptide, and vasopressin. There are two distinct catalytic domains required for covalent modification. Copper and ascorbate are required for monooxygenase activity to convert C-terminal glycine residues to hydroxyglycyl residues that are subsequently hydrolyzed by a lyase domain to produce α-amidated peptides and glyoxylate.[15] PAM is especially enriched in the nervous and endocrine system, with very high levels in the pituitary and cardiac atria. The importance of PAM has recently been documented by demonstrating embryonic lethality in mice following gene ablation.[16]

Tyrosinase (monophenol oxidase) performs a highly specialized function. This enzyme begins melanin biosynthesis in melanocytes. Mutational loss of catalytic function leads to albinism. Copper restriction confirms an important role of tyrosinase in pigmentation, because achromotrichia is observed in domestic and laboratory animals consuming diets low in copper.

There are a number of copper-binding proteins in mammals that function as transport proteins and copper chaperones to maintain copper homeostasis,[17,18] and these will be discussed later. There are a number of enzymes whose activity either increases or decreases in response to changes in nutritional copper intake, however, these changes do not necessarily mean that these are cuproenzymes.[19] There are other proteins that may have catalytic properties dependent on copper but are less well established, including clotting factors V and VIII, S-adenosylhomocysteine hydrolase, prion protein, and many others.[19] Many of the pathophysiological consequences of dietary copper deficiency can be related to the known biological functions of copper as a cofactor in specific enzymes.

# Copper Homeostasis

## *Whole Body Metabolism*

Tracer studies have contributed markedly to our present understanding of mammalian copper metabolism. Ingested food and digestive secretory fluids (salivary, pancreatic, and biliary) all contribute to the copper pool present in the intestinal lumen. Copper likely enters small intestinal epithelial cells by a facilitated process that involves a specific cuprous ion carrier, Ctr1, or non-specific divalent metal ion transporters located on the brush-border surface (Figure 1).[17,18] The tissue acquisition of newly absorbed copper occurs in two phases. The first involves vectorial transport of copper across the basolateral membrane of the enterocyte into portal circulation, where it is transported to liver in association with albumin and macroglobulins. However, results showing that absorption and tissue distribution of copper are normal in analbuminemic rats indicate that albumin is not essential for the delivery of the copper to liver.[20] Copper is secreted into plasma bound to ceruloplasmin; this is the major pool of this metal in blood plasma. As discussed above, the lack of disturbances in copper metabolism in aceruloplasminemia patients and mice clearly demonstrate that the primary function of plasma ceruloplasmin is not to mediate cellular acquisition of copper. Plasma has a small non-ceruloplasmin component made up largely of amino acid complexes; however, the mechanisms by which protein-bound or amino acid-bound copper is transported from plasma into cells remain unknown.

Copper concentration varies with tissue[1]: liver, brain, and kidney contain higher quantities per unit weight than muscle and other tissues. Generally, copper is not stored in tissues, suggesting that differences in concentrations of the metal may reflect relative quantities of cuproenzymes.

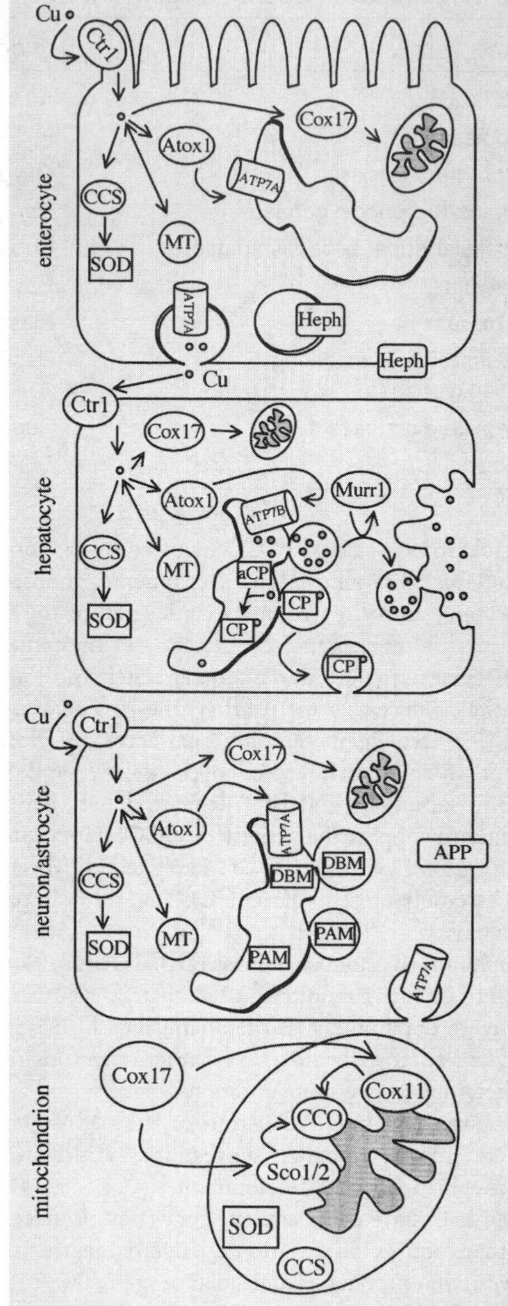


Figure 1. Model of cellular copper transport and homeostasis from intestine to liver to brain. Cuprous ion is transferred across the enterocyte plasma membrane by Ctr1. Copper binds to a group of chaperones: Atox1, Cox17, and the copper chaperone for superoxide dismutase (CCS) that deliver copper to the targeted cuproenzymes cytochrome *c* oxidase (CCO) and superoxide dismutase-1 (SOD1) or copper-translocating ATPases (ATP7A and ATP7B). Usually, these energy-dependent pumps transfer copper into the trans-Golgi network for incorporation into apo-cuproenzymes that are secreted from the cell such as ceruloplasmin (Cp) or peptidylglycine α-amidating monoxygenase (PAM) or are bound to the plasma membrane. When intracellular concentrations of copper are elevated, the copper-translocating ATPases are redistributed to cytoplasmic vesicles. Exocytosis of copper-loaded vesicles mediates copper efflux, thereby preventing accumulation of toxic concentrations of copper. Copper pools are also associated with metallothionein (MT). Specialized copper binding proteins function in the intestine (hephaestin), liver (Murr1), and brain (amyloid precursor protein).

Transport of copper from the liver into the bile represents the primary route for excretion of endogenous copper. This pathway is immature in fetal and neonatal liver, thereby accounting for the storage of hepatic copper at these early stages of development. Likewise, cholestasis can result in the accumulation of hepatic copper after the neonatal period. Copper of biliary origin and nonabsorbed oral copper are eliminated from the body in feces. Daily losses of copper in urine are minimal in healthy individuals.

Stable isotope studies with healthy human subjects under controlled conditions have shown that both absorption and retention of copper readily respond to wide fluctuations in dietary copper intake. Under normal copper intake conditions, it has been estimated that true copper absorption is about 10%, since there is a 30% loss of newly absorbed copper via the endogenous secretion pathway involving active biliary excretion.[21] The apparent percentages of ingested copper absorbed when dietary intakes were 0.8, 1.7, and 7.5 mg/d were 56%, 36%, and 12%, respectively.[22] This adaptation in the efficiency of absorption, as well as modulation of retention in endogenous copper, resulted in restoration of normal balance after relatively short periods and maintenance of normal levels of copper and cuproenzyme activities in plasma and blood cells. Likewise, copper retention in many organs, particularly in brain and heart, is markedly increased in response to restricted copper intake in the rat.[23] However, the ability of these adaptive mechanisms to maintain normal copper status in humans is exceeded when chronic dietary copper intake is less than 0.7 mg/d. It is important to note that such low levels of dietary copper are below that present in typical Western diets.[24]

## *Cellular Homeostasis*

It is essential that cells adapt to obtain adequate but not excessive amounts of copper. Recent exciting discoveries are helping to elucidate this complex process (Figure 1, Table 2). Luminal copper must be reduced to cuprous ion for uptake by Ctr1. This reduction process has not been elucidated. Silver ion but not divalent ions inhibit copper uptake by Ctr1. Despite this specificity, interesting data suggest that Ctr1 mediates the uptake of cisplatin, a potent and common cancer chemotherapeutic drug.[25] Ctr1 is a transmembrane protein essential for copper distribution to the organism, as deletion is lethal to embryos and surviving heterozygous knockout mice ($Ctr1^{+/-}$) have reduced copper content and function in selected organs.[26,27] If a redundant copper transport system does exist, as suggested from in vitro cell culture studies with immortalized cell lines and studies in Caco-2 cells, it must be weak, since it cannot replace Ctr1 function in the whole animal. There is evidence in certain cell lines that Ctr1 is imported by endocytosis rather than by pumping copper through a pore.[28] However, this concept has been challenged.[29] It will be important to determine

**Table 2.** Mammalian Copper-Binding Proteins

| Protein | Putative Copper Function | Location |
|---|---|---|
| Albumin | Transport | Portal blood plasma |
| Amyloid precursor protein | Transport | Brain |
| Atox1 | Chaperone | Cytoplasm |
| ATP7A | Efflux | TGN, plasma membrane |
| ATP7B | Efflux | Liver TGN, vesicle membrane |
| CCS | Chaperone | Cytoplasm, mitochondria |
| Clotting factors V, VIII | Unknown | Plasma |
| Cox11 | Chaperone | Mitochondria |
| Cox17 | Chaperone | Cytoplasm |
| Ctr1 | Transport | Plasma membrane |
| Ctr2 | Transport | Vesicles |
| Doppel | Reproduction (?) | Heart, testis |
| Macroglobulin | Transport | Portal blood plasma |
| Metallothionein | Storage | Cytoplasm |
| Monooxygenase X | Unknown | Endoplasmic reticuluum |
| Murr1 | Biliary excretion | Vesicle membrane |
| Prion protein | Unknown | Membranes |
| Sco1 | Chaperone | Mitochondria |
| Sco2 | Chaperone | Mitochondria |

CCS = copper chaperone for superoxide dismutase; TGN = trans-Golgi network which mechanism exists for mammalian enterocytes in vivo and if copper regulates Ctr1 expression and/or distribution.

Imported cytoplasmic copper binds to a group of ubiquitous copper chaperone proteins and perhaps other copper-binding species such as metallothionein (MT) I and MT II. MTs are a family of cysteine-rich proteins with high affinity for heavy metal ions. They provide cells with a secondary system of detoxification when copper efflux process is either not operational (e.g., during early stages of development and when efflux is defective) or when activity of the efflux pump becomes inadequate during acute exposure to high amounts of copper. Chaperones deliver copper directly to target proteins in cytoplasm and in membranes of organelles for incorporation of the metal to apo-cuproproteins.[17]

The copper chaperone for SOD, CCS, transfers copper to cytoplasmic and intermitochondrial membrane space SOD1. Deletion of CCS results in low SOD1 activity, a phenotype similar to SOD1-knockout mice.[30] Cox17 is necessary to deliver cytoplasmic copper to the mitochondria for CCO assembly. Deletion of Cox17 results in embryonic lethality in a temporal pattern similar to Ctr1-knockout mice.[31] Within the mitochondria, additional chaperones are necessary to deliver copper to CCO subunits I and II. These chaperones are Cox11 and Sco1 and Sco2, and are described in greater detail elsewhere.[17,18] Atox1 is another key chaperone that delivers copper to P-type ATPases that mediate energy-dependent transport of the metal to the lumen of the trans-Golgi network for incorporation of the metal into secretory copper-dependent proteins such as ceruloplasmin, DBM, LO, PAM, and tyrosinase. Deletion of Atox1 results in perinatal mortality with symptoms consistent with copper deficiency.[32]

Two distinct copper-translocating, P-type ATPases have been identified.[33] Hepatocytes, mammary tissue, and certain neurons express the copper-translocating ATPase referred to as ATP7B, whereas other cells have a highly homologous ATPase referred to as ATP7A. It is now recognized that ATP7A and ATP7B cycle between the trans-Golgi network and cytoplasmic vesicles. ATP7A is the protein missing in humans with Menkes' syndrome, which results in copper deficiency. ATP7B is the protein mutated in Wilson's disease, and leads to hepatic copper overload toxicity. When intracellular copper is low or normal, copper ATPases are localized predominantly in the trans-Golgi network to facilitate the delivery of the metal to secretory apo-cuproproteins. As cellular copper increases, the ATPases are redistributed into cytoplasmic vesicles.[34] The vesicles presumably contain the pool of copper destined for efflux. For example, fusion of copper-loaded cytoplasmic vesicles with the canicular membrane of the hepatocyte is required for biliary copper excretion (Figure 1). This process requires another protein, Murr1, which interacts with ATP7B and is missing in canine toxicosis, a disorder of liver copper overload.[35] Fusion of copper-loaded vesicles with the basolateral surface of enterocyte and placental trophoblast are likely to facilitate copper efflux to plasma and transfer of placental copper to the fetal compartment, respectively. The high efficiency of the copper efflux pathway is supported by minimal binding of copper to cytoplasmic MT after weaning.

Recent evidence suggests there may be a copper storage pool. Some have suggested that MT might provide a buffer for copper during times when the metal is limiting.[36] Perhaps copper is stored in a vesicular compartment and transported by Ctr2, a protein homologous to Ctr1, which provides this function in budding yeast.[37]

There have been many copper-binding proteins reported for which functions remain unknown or copper dependence has not been confirmed.[19] Recent candidates include proteins important to human health, including the prion protein PrPC and amyloid precursor protein (APP). Some suggest that the function of PrPC, a copper-binding protein, is to transport copper into brain and serve as another SOD or as a chaperone for SOD1.[38] However, others have not found any changes in brain copper or SOD1 activity in PrPC-knockout mice or transgenic mice overexpressing this protein 10-fold.[39] Stronger evidence exists for APP. APP null mice have increased brain copper levels[40]; in contrast, mice overexpressing APP have reduced brain copper levels.[41] These observations suggest a role for APP in the regulation of brain copper content. Since APP is expressed in all major tissues, it may function elsewhere in modulating copper homeostasis. Recent studies indicate that APP expression may be regulated by copper.[42]

# Factors Affecting Copper Status

There are thresholds at the lower and upper ends of copper exposure for which the adaptive responses are insufficient to prevent the development of copper deficiency and toxicity, respectively. In addition to the obvious importance of copper intake, other dietary components and physiological factors can affect the bioavailability and tissue distribution of copper.

## *Copper Intake*

The copper content of the typical diet in the United States provides the majority of adults with the lower limit of the current Recommended Dietary Allowance (RDA) of 0.9 mg.[24] There are certain gender and age groups, however, that appear to consume less than their specific RDA.[43] Absorption efficiency can range between 50% and 25% when diets contain 1 to 7 mg of copper, respectively. The richest food sources of copper include shellfish, nuts, seeds, organ meats, wheat bran cereals, whole grain products, and chocolate foods. Vegetarian diets generally contain a generous supply of copper, although the efficiency of copper absorption seems lower.[44] Multimineral and vitamin supplements represent another potential source of copper intake. Copper is often also present in adult, pediatric, and prenatal formulations as cupric oxide, which is very poorly absorbed.[45] Drinking water can be an additional source of copper. Although fresh drinking water generally contains very low levels of copper, widespread use of copper pipes for household plumbing can lead to leaching of the metal under some conditions. Thus, copper-contaminated water may serve as an important source of the metal when copper in foods becomes limiting or when considering total copper intake as a detriment to health.

### *Copper Bioavailability*

Adverse effects of certain proteins, zinc, iron, molybdenum, ascorbic acid, certain amino acids, and certain saccharides on copper absorption and utilization have been reported.[46] Some interactions have been studied only in animal models. It is clear that administration of high doses of zinc will induce copper deficiency signs in both infants and adults. Perhaps even low intake of dietary zinc can impact the copper status of humans.[47] Dietary fiber appears to have minimal impact on copper absorption by adults in contrast to effects on zinc and iron availability. Infants may be particularly vulnerable to the influences of various minerals, fiber, and protein source on copper absorption and excretion, since digestive processes and the regulation of copper absorption and excretion are not fully mature.

### *Physiological Conditions*

Hepatic levels of copper bound to MT are elevated markedly during the final trimester of fetal development, presumably as a storage pool of copper in this organ to provide the rapidly growing newborn with a supply of the metal. However, the susceptibility of infants fed only cow's milk, known to be low in copper, of developing copper deficiency suggests that an exogenous source of the metal is required. Gender, age, and pregnancy may have some impact on copper absorption and retention.[48] Plasma levels of copper increase transiently during episodes of inflammation and infection, since ceruloplasmin synthesis and secretion is stimulated by proinflammatory cytokines. Similarly, plasma copper and ceruloplasmin are elevated in response to increased plasma estrogen.[1] The significance, if any, of changes in plasma copper on whole body metabolism, utilization, and requirement is unknown. Studies in rats following copper injection show that lactation markedly enhances the avidity of the mammary gland for copper.[49] These studies collectively illustrate that copper requirements and metabolism are impacted by physiological state.

### *Genetic Controls*

It seems very likely that copper requirements will be influenced by genetic factors that determine the expression of copper homeostatic genes. The susceptibility of various mouse strains to copper depletion supports this notion, however, molecular confirmation is not yet available. In elegant studies in fungi, many of the genetic details of copper homeostasis have been described.[50] Transport, storage, and protection from excess copper are under transcriptional control in budding yeast by two major regulators, Mac1 and Ace1, that respond to low and high cellular copper, respectively. There are functional orthologs of these transcription factors in other fungi. Thus far, no copper-responsive mammalian transcription factors have been discovered. Steady-state mRNA levels of Ctr1, ATP7A, and ATP7B are not altered by copper deficiency in mammals.[17] Rather, transport and efflux are regulated by copper-dependent post-translational trafficking. Perhaps copper-binding protein expression is influenced by cellular copper levels through a degradation pathway. Genetic aberrations in copper metabolism in humans are evident due to loss of ATP7A (Menkes' syndrome) or a mutation in ATP7B (Wilson's disease), two genes coding for copper efflux transporters.

## Copper Requirement

Dietary Reference Intakes for copper were established in 2001.[51] The RDA for adult males and females was set at 0.9 mg. This is approximately a 1.8 mg/kg copper diet based on a 2000 kcal and 500 g dry weight estimate. Prior to 2001, the recommended "Estimated Safe and Adequate Daily Dietary Intake" of copper for adults was 1.5 to 3.0 mg/d. The RDA for pregnant women set in 2001 is 1 mg and for lactating women 1.3 mg. Recent work with mice suggests the possibility that the human RDA for pregnancy/lactation may be set too low.[52] The same dietary level of copper that was lethal to pups during mid-lactation produced no discernible changes in copper status to non-lactating adult females. The Tolerable Upper Intake Level (UL) for copper is 10 mg.

## Copper Deficiency

Common characteristics of severe copper deficiency in mammals include hypochromic anemia that is refractory to iron supplementation, neutropenia, thrombocytopenia, and hypopigmentation, plus anatomical and functional abnormalities in the skeletal, cardiovascular, and immune systems.[53] Copper deprivation during the fetal and neonatal periods also causes neurological abnormalities. Although many of these diverse effects seem to be associated with decreased activities of known cuproenzymes (Table 1), unequivocal evidence that the decline in catalytic activity actually alters the metabolic flux and generation of products in specific pathways remains somewhat elusive. Novel roles for copper remain to be discovered. Inadequate tissue levels of copper result from insufficient absorption of exogenous copper and excessive losses of endogenous copper. The pleiotropic effects of defective cellular copper transport in individuals with Menkes' syndrome are consistent with tissue copper deficiency observed in experimental animals.

Acquired copper deficiency is relatively rare in humans, although reports of copper deficiency in infants, children, and adults continue to appear in the clinical literature. Groups that are susceptible to developing copper deficiency include: individuals at any age receiving total parenteral nutrition without supplemental copper for extended periods; preterm infants fed milk-based formula without adequate copper; infants recovering from malnutrition or chronic diarrhea; patients undergoing chronic peritoneal dialysis; severe burn patients; ambulatory renal dialysis patients; and individuals consuming excessive doses of zinc, antacids, or copper chelators.

Copper deficiency can also develop in humans with malabsorption syndromes. Examples of conditions that can compromise copper status include: celiac disease, cystic fibrosis, surgical resection of the short-bowel, and sprue. The RDA intake may be too low under these conditions. Impact of copper deficiency, regardless of its etiology, can have a major impact on several biological systems.

## *Cardiovascular System*

Anatomical, electrical, mechanical, and biochemical abnormalities are evident in hearts of young animals fed diets severely restricted in copper. Severely copper-deficient young rats often die of ventricular rupture. Many of the defects generally are assumed to result from decreased activities of various cardiac cuproenzymes, including CCO, DBM, LO, PAM, and SOD1. Systematic investigations have yielded a detailed characterization of the sequence of events leading to cardiac dysfunction in the rat, and are reviewed elsewhere.[54] Notable observations are that cardiac hypertrophy in copper-deficient rats is not dependent on anemia; marginally copper-deficient diets also induce cardiac abnormalities; and adult rats fed a copper-deficient diet develop cardiovascular defects but not hypertrophy.

The development of cardiovascular abnormalities in animals fed low-copper diets and the possibility that the typical Western diet lacks adequate copper provide the conceptual basis for speculation that copper deficiency contributes to the incidence of ischemic heart disease in humans. Although cardiac arrhythmias were experienced by several subjects ingesting low-copper diets in metabolic trials, healthy adults in other studies in which low copper diets were fed for extended periods had normal cardiac function. Individuals with Menkes' syndrome exhibit pathology in major vessels but not in the heart.[55]

Copper status can also impact the circulatory system. Proper cross-linking in large vessels, as well as vasoactivity in arterioles, capillaries, and venules are copper dependent.[56] Dietary copper deficiency increases histamine-mediated protein leakage in venules by increasing the numbers of localized mast cells, inhibits platelet interactions that lead to thrombogenesis, and decreases nitric oxide-induced relaxation of arteriolar smooth muscle cells. Copper status also has an impact on the acute inflammatory response, including vasodilation, protein extravasation from microvascular leakage, and neutrophil adhesion and diapedesis. These lines of investigation are expected to uncover specific roles for copper in the regulation of peripheral blood flow and hemostasis.

Altered blood lipid profiles, blood pressure, and anemia can all impact the cardiovascular system and are known to be impacted by copper status. Hypertriglyceridemia and hypercholesterolemia are frequently observed in severe copper deficiency. Studies suggest that the abnormalities may be due to changes in hepatic thiol redox status induced by a lack of copper. Increased activity of $\gamma$-glutamylcysteine synthetase, the rate-limiting enzyme for glutathione synthesis, in copper-deficient rat liver is associated with an elevated concentration of reduced, but not oxidized, glutathione in the tissue.[57] When activity of the synthetase was partially inhibited to reduce the concentration of reduced glutathione in the copper-deficient liver to that in copper-adequate tissue, activities of fatty acid synthase and hydroxymethylglutaryl coenzyme A (HMG-CoA) reductase were similar in the two groups. These observations suggest that increased levels of reduced glutathione in copper-deficient liver alters expression of a variety of genes that are regulated by activities of redox-sensitive transcription factors that influence lipid metabolism. Copper deficiency also increases plasma HDL protein levels in rats. This change appears to be due to enhanced transcription of the genes for apolipoproteins or A1 in liver.[58] Gel-shift assay suggested that binding of hepatocyte nuclear factor 4 and other undefined nuclear proteins to oligonucleotides containing one of the regulatory sites in the promoter of the ApoA1 gene is enhanced by copper deficiency.

## *Hemopoietic System*

It is likely that copper plays a fundamental role in myeloid progenitor cell differentiation, as a prominent feature of copper deficiency is alterations in erythrocyte (lower), neutrophil (lower), and platelet (higher) levels. The anemia of copper deficiency is a consequence of both fewer red blood cells and less hemoglobin content per cell. Some believe that the primary determinant of anemia is a failure to absorb and retain dietary iron following dietary copper deficiency.[59] Others believe it is related to a failure to mobilize iron from tissue stores such as liver because ceruloplasmin (ferroxidase) is copper dependent. However, ceruloplasmin-null mice and aceruloplasminemia in humans does not result in pronounced anemia. A direct role of copper in hemoglobin synthesis and/or hemopoiesis should not be ruled out.

## *Immune System*

Clinical and experimental reports indicate that inherited and acquired copper deficiencies often are associated with increased risk of infection.[60] Severe copper deficiency generally changes the phenotypic profiles of immune cells in blood, bone marrow, and lymphoid tissues.

It also suppresses a number of activities of lymphocytes and phagocytic cells. Growth and tissue levels of copper (except in brain) and cuproenzymes were similar for adult rats chronically fed a diet with either adequate (6.7 mg Cu/kg) or marginally low (2.8 mg Cu/kg) copper. However, in vitro DNA synthesis and IL-2 secretion by mitogen-treated splenic T-lymphocytes and respiratory burst activity of neutrophils were markedly impaired in cells from animals fed diet with marginally low copper.[61]

Neutropenia is a hallmark of copper deficiency in humans. Several recent studies have suggested that moderate and even marginal copper deficiency also affect some activities of T-lymphocytes and phagocytic cells adversely. In vitro responsiveness of T-lymphocytes to mitogenic activation was decreased after adult males were fed a diet with 0.38 mg/d copper for 6 weeks. This alteration was associated with a reduction in plasma copper and activities of several cuproenzymes, but not hematologic indices.[62] Similarly, IL-2 synthesis by a human T-cell line and bactericidal activity and secretion of proinflammatory cytokines TNF-alpha, IL-1, and IL-6 by a human monocytic cell line were decreased after inducing moderate copper deficiency with a copper chelator.[63] These changes were eliminated by supplementation of the medium with copper, but not with iron or zinc, and were not associated with alterations in cellular iron status or general metabolic activities.

The decreased synthesis of IL-2 in low-copper T-cells results from decreased transcription of the IL-2 gene in activated cells. Although these results support a direct role for copper in the ability of defense cells to respond to stimuli, the unique roles that copper plays in the maturation, activation, and effector activities of immune cells remain unknown. Likewise, the link between suppressed activities of immune cells in copper-deficient humans and increased susceptibility to infection remains weak, partly because of the inability to accurately assess marginal and moderate deficiencies of this micronutrient.

## *Nervous System*

The essentiality of adequate copper intake and utilization for the normal development of the brain is well recognized. Domestic animals grazing on pastures low in copper produced offspring that exhibited ataxia and severe neuronal pathology.[64] Neuronal pathology is a salient feature of infants who die of Menkes' syndrome. Copper accumulates in the brain during late gestation and lactation. Thus, restricted intake of copper by pregnant and lactating individuals has severe consequences for offspring. In fact, rats that experienced copper deficiency during the perinatal period exhibited permanent behavioral abnormalities, even after ingesting a copper-adequate diet for 6 months.[65,66] Even marginal copper deficiency can impact brain. Brain copper was significantly lower in rats fed a diet containing moderate copper (2.8 mg/kg) than in those fed adequate copper (6.7 mg/kg) for 6 months postnatally; whereas growth and copper concentrations in liver, lung, and bone were similar for the two dietary groups.[61] Similarly, maturation of hippocampus and dentate gyrus was impaired in rats subjected to moderate copper deficiency during gestation and lactation.[67] These studies underscore the importance of adequate copper during perinatal development.

The blood-brain barrier restricts entry of copper from plasma. Brain copper increased only 30% after suckling mice were injected subcutaneously with 10 mg Cu/kg, whereas supplementation elevated liver copper severalfold.[68] Transfer of copper from plasma to neurons and delivery to cuproenzymes requires Ctr1, Atox1, ATP7A, and perhaps ATP7B. $Ctr1^{+/-}$ mice and $atox1^{-/-}$ mice have lower brain copper levels and decreased CCO activity.[26,32] Brindled mice that have a non-functional ATP7A protein have altered PAM activity, as evidenced by peptide amidation defects.[69]

The neurochemical functions of copper are thought to be associated with the cuproenzymes that are present in most tissues (Table 1), and several unique cuproproteins. Copper deficiency alters the enzyme activity and protein level of rodent brain CCO, DBM, SOD1, and PAM.[70] Perhaps altered enzyme activity and levels are responsible for the altered neuropathology and behavior. A glycosylphosphatidylinositol-anchored form of ceruloplasmin that is synthesized from an alternatively spliced RNA variant has been identified in brain.[71] Ablation of the ceruloplasmin gene in mice is associated with iron overload in brain. In contrast, dietary copper deficiency and lower ceruloplasmin activity are associated with lower brain iron.[72] Brain ferroxidase has not been evaluated following copper deficiency. Judicious use of gene-knockout techniques are expected to reveal unique neurochemical roles of copper and elucidate mechanisms of neuronal pathology that accompany imbalances in copper homeostasis.

Although it is generally believed that copper is most critical during brain development, other neurological functions depend on adequate copper throughout life. Recently, several cases of adult myelopathy have been characterized and associated with low serum copper and ceruloplasmin, implying a relationship with a copper-deficient state.[73]

## *Skeletal and Integumentary System*

There is a well-established association between decreased LO activity, connective tissue disorders, generalized osteoporosis, and bone defects that occur in dietary and inherited copper deficiency in humans and other species.[55] LO and perhaps LOXL proteins are involved in cross-linking of collagen. Dietary recommendations for prevention of osteoporosis focus on optimizing bone mineralization by increasing the intakes of calcium and vitamin D. However, collagen rather than bone mineral is the primary determinant of the rigidity, mechanical strength, and biomechanical competence of bone.

Bone abnormalities are common in copper-deficient infants, and resemble features observed following vitamin

C deficiency.[53] Changes include osteoporosis, bone fractures, spur formation, and subperiostal new bone formation. Relationships between copper and bone health exist in adults as well. Long-term studies suggest that copper supplementation may decrease bone loss. Reduction of copper intake from 1.6 to 0.7 mg/d for 8 weeks increased the rate of bone resorption as assessed by urinary excretion of pyridinium cross-links in healthy adult males; this change was reversed after restoration of dietary copper to 1.6 mg/d.[74] However, supplementation of healthy males and females 22 to 46 years of age with 3 and 6 mg copper/d for 6 weeks did not affect biochemical markers of bone formation or resorption. The possibility that long-term supplementation of aging males and females with copper may retard net losses of bone merits further investigation.

## Copper Toxicity

Considering the homeostatic regulation of copper absorption and excretion, it is not surprising that the incidence of copper toxicity is quite low in the general population. Copper, like inorganic iron, can participate in Fenton chemistry and generate reactive oxygen species.[75] Symptoms associated with the ingestion of fluids and foods contaminated with high quantities of copper usually include metallic taste and gastrointestinal distress. Copper was used historically to induce vomiting. Recall that the recent UL established for copper is 10 mg. Results from a multicenter (Chile, Northern Ireland, United States) study indicated that the No Adverse Effect Level (NOAEL) in drinking water was about 5 mg copper/L. Taste of copper in water was detected at about half this level.[76] WHO guidelines indicate a provisional safety of 2 mg copper/L. The reaction of test subjects to copper depends on the liquid vehicle, as tolerance was greater with an orange drink than with water.

The inclusion of copper in micronutrient and complete nutritional supplements does not seem to pose any adverse effects. Supplementation of adults with 10 mg copper daily as cupric gluconate for 12 weeks did not cause gastrointestinal difficulties or liver damage in a double-blind study.[77] There is a need for standard assessment of liver damage and recording of reported incidence of other symptoms of copper toxicity, such as gastrointestinal distress, in all human studies involving copper supplementation to establish a more complete database. Moreover, some groups are predisposed to accumulation of toxic levels of copper in liver when intake is elevated chronically. Immaturity of biliary excretion and increased efficiency of copper absorption suggest a potential risk of copper toxicity in infants. The accumulation of toxic levels of copper in livers of children diagnosed with Indian childhood cirrhosis, certain infants in Austrian Tyrol, and those with idiopathic copper toxicosis is often associated with the use of copper-contaminated water to prepare infant formula and other foods that were stored or prepared in brass vessels.[76] Public health programs aimed at changing practices associated with infant feeding and genetic dilution have largely eliminated the incidence of these diseases. Obviously, individuals with Wilson's disease and other inherited or acquired disorders that impair elimination of excess copper via the biliary route should avoid ingestion of copper-fortified products and copper-contaminated water.

Copper in brain can also act as a pro-oxidant that leads to neurological dysfunction.[75] Certain mutations in the SOD1 gene produce an abnormal protein that has peroxidase activity and results in Lou Gehrig's disease. The APP of Alzheimer's disease catalyzes the reduction of cupric ion, thus generating a potential reactant to produce the hydroxyl radical.

## Assessment of Copper Status

The identification of copper status biomarkers that are sensitive, noninvasive and reliable indicators continues to be problematic.[78] Experimental studies with young animals show that moderate to severe reductions of the copper content of standard formulations of nutritionally adequate, semipurified diets usually induces a relatively rapid decline in plasma copper and ceruloplasmin activity. The impact of dietary treatment on the concentration of the metal and cuproenzyme activities in cells and tissues is dependent on numerous factors, including severity of the reduction in dietary copper, species, strain, organ, and gender. The traditional approach in human studies has been to examine the level of copper and activities of cuproenzymes in plasma and blood cells. Reductions of plasma copper and ceruloplasmin often are observed in individuals with diagnosed copper deficiency. However, estrogen status and conditions such as pregnancy, infection, inflammation, and some cancers increase plasma ceruloplasmin and copper levels, thereby compromising their utility as reliable indicators for screening copper status. Even under well-controlled conditions, dietary copper must be reduced to 0.6 mg copper/d or less for periods of at least 6 weeks for healthy adults before markers decline. Other potential markers that have been monitored in various human studies include copper content in platelets and mononuclear cells and activities of SOD1 in erythrocytes and CCO in platelets and mononuclear cells. Influences of factors other than copper, required sample volume, wide variations within individuals, and technical difficulties represent difficulties for using these markers as reliable indicators for assessing copper status.

Other cuproenzymes deserve further evaluation as possible indicators of copper status. Serum and tissue activity of PAM in rats are correlated with dietary copper intake.[70] Also, the addition of copper to serum from rats fed copper-restricted diets restored activity to control levels, suggesting that copper status might be assessed by quantifying enzyme activity in the presence and absence of exogenous copper. Preliminary tests using plasma from several subjects with a mild variant of Menkes' syndrome and from an individual with acquired copper deficiency suggest that the assay may be a useful marker of copper status in humans.[79] Moreover, the assay requires very small volumes of plasma and is not altered by endocrine changes in rats.

Studies in rats have reported that activity of plasma diamine oxidase is decreased in response to marginal and moderate changes in copper status. Studies in an adult subject with acquired copper deficiency and response to copper supplementation suggest further work on this enzyme as a biomarker is needed.[80,81] The utility of this enzyme as a marker of copper status may be limited, since a number of pathological conditions of the intestine or kidney, as well as pregnancy, affect plasma activity.[78] Furthermore, there was a major rise in plasma diamine oxidase when subjects were given a 3-mg copper supplement to a diet containing adequate copper. Does the enzyme elevation reflect a response to suboptimal copper status or an adverse reaction to the copper supplement? Another potential assessment tool has been recently proposed. Following copper deficiency, the immunoreactive content of SOD1 is lower and that of its specific chaperone, CCS, is markedly higher in rodents.[17,18] Thus the ratio of CCS to SOD1 protein is markedly higher in copper-deficient tissues, including erythrocytes.[82]

Although functional and behavioral activities in animals and in vitro cellular assays have been shown to be responsive to marginal and moderate reductions in copper, their potential utility for evaluating copper status in humans remains unknown.

## Future Directions

Research during the past five years has provided new and exciting insights about copper homeostasis at the cellular level. Ongoing investigations employing the tools of molecular genetics and confocal microscopy are certain to identify additional genes and proteins required for the transport of copper across membranes and its utilization within various cellular compartments. Elucidation of the direct and indirect roles of copper in the development and degeneration of the nervous system, the integrity of the cardiovascular and skeletal systems, and the activities of the immune system certainly will be facilitated by judicious use of molecular techniques such as gene knockout, overexpression, functional genomics, and proteomics. Stable isotope technology has provided an understanding of whole-body copper metabolism in healthy adults. Continued application of this methodology and increased use of mathematical modeling are expected to provide new information about copper metabolism and requirements for selected populations, and especially those likely to be at higher risk of developing copper deficiency. These include premature and term infants, pregnant malnourished adolescents, the institutionalized elderly, and individuals with chronic diseases such as cystic fibrosis, Crohn's disease, and other malabsorption syndromes. Studies in animals suggest the possibility that marginal copper deficiency, though difficult to diagnose, may compromise our ability to adapt metabolically to various physiological, pathophysiological, and emotional stresses. Development of a panel of sensitive biochemical and functional indices for the accurate assessment of copper status represents an important challenge for investigators interested in the biology and nutrition of copper.

## Acknowledgement

The insightful organization of the previous version of the copper chapter by lead author Mark L. Failla is appreciated.

## References

1. Linder MC, Hazegh-Azam M. Copper biochemistry and molecular biology. Am J Clin Nutr 1996;63; 797S–811S.
2. Brazeau BJ, Johnson BJ, Wilmot CM. Copper-containing amine oxidases. Biogenesis and catalysis; a structural perspective. Arch Biochem Biophys 2004; 428;22–31.
3. Salmi M, Jalkanen S. VAP-1: an adhesin and an enzyme. Trends Immunol 2001;22;211–216.
4. Stolen CM, Marttila-Ichihara F, Koskinen K, et al. Absence of the endothelial oxidase AOC3 leads to abnormal leukocyte traffic in vivo. Immunity 2005; 22;105–115.
5. Gitlin JD. Aceruloplasminemia. Pediatr Res 1998; 44;271–276.
6. Meyer LA, Durley AP, Prohaska JR, Harris ZL. Copper transport and metabolism are normal in aceruloplasminemic mice. J Biol Chem 2001;276; 36857–61.
7. Hamza I, Gitlin JD. Copper chaperones for cytochrome c oxidase and human disease. J Bioenerg Biomembr 2002;34;381–388.
8. Thomas SA, Matsumoto AM, Palmiter RD. Noradrenaline is essential for mouse fetal development. Nature 1995;374;643–646.
9. Fattman CL, Schaefer LM, Oury TD. Extracellular superoxide dismutase in biology and medicine. Free Radic Biol Med 2003;35;236–256.
10. Jung O, Marklund SL, Geiger H, et al. Extracellular superoxide dismutase is a major determinant of nitric oxide bioavailability: in vivo and ex vivo evidence from ecSOD-deficient mice. Circ Res 2003;93; 622–629.
11. Kuo YM, Su T, Chen H, et al. Mislocalisation of hephaestin, a multicopper ferroxidase involved in basolateral intestinal iron transport, in the sex linked anaemia mouse. Gut 2004;53;201–206.
12. Danzeisen R, Fosset C, Chariana Z, et al. Placental ceruloplasmin homolog is regulated by iron and cop-

per and is implicated in iron metabolism. Am J Physiol 2002;282;C472–C478.
13. Kagan HM, Li W. Lysyl oxidase: properties, specificity, and biological roles inside and outside of the cell. J Cell Biochem 2003;88;660–672.
14. Molnar J, Fong KS, He QP, et al. Structural and functional diversity of lysyl oxidase and the LOX-like proteins. Biochim Biophys Acta 2003;1647; 220–224.
15. Eipper BA, Stoffers DA, Mains RE. The biosynthesis of neuropeptides: peptide alpha-amidation. Annu Rev Neurosci 1992;15;57–85.
16. Czyzyk TA, Morgan DJ, Peng B, et al. Targeted mutagenesis of processing enzymes and regulators: implications for development and physiology. J Neurosci Res 2003;74;446–455.
17. Prohaska JR, Gybina AA. Intracellular copper transport in mammals. J Nutr 2004;134;1003–1006.
18. Bertinato J, L'Abbe MR. Maintaining copper homeostasis: regulation of copper-trafficking proteins in response to copper deficiency or overload. J Nutr Biochem 2004;15;316–322.
19. Prohaska JR. Biochemical functions of copper in animals. In: A.S. Prasad, EditorEssential and Toxic Trace Elements in Human Health and Disease, New York, NY: Alan R. Liss, Inc., 1988:105–124.
20. Vargas EJ, Shoho AR, Linder MC. Copper transport in the Nagase analbuminemic rat. Am J Physiol 1994; 267;G259–G269.
21. Harvey LJ, Dainty JR, Hollands WJ, et al. Use of mathematical modeling to study copper metabolism in humans. Am J Clin Nutr 2005;81;807–13.
22. Turnlund JR, Keyes WR, Peiffer GL, Scott KC. Copper absorption, excretion, and retention by young men consuming low dietary copper determined by using the stable isotope 65Cu. Am J Clin Nutr 1998;67;1219–1225.
23. Levenson CW, Janghorbani M. Long-term measurement of organ copper turnover in rats by continuous feeding of a stable isotope. Anal Biochem 1994; 221;243–249.
24. Pennington JA, Schoen SA. Total diet study: estimated dietary intakes of nutritional elements, 1982–1991. Int J Vitam Nutr Res 1996;66;350–362.
25. Ishida S, Lee J, Thiele DJ, Herskowitz I. Uptake of the anticancer drug cisplatin mediated by the copper transporter Ctr1 in yeast and mammals. Proc Natl Acad Sci U S A 2002;99;14298–14302.
26. Lee J, Prohaska JR, Thiele DJ. Essential role for mammalian copper transporter Ctr1 in copper homeostasis and embryonic development. Proc Natl Acad Sci USA 2001;98;6842–6847.
27. Kuo YM, Zhou B, Cosco D, Gitschier J. The copper transporter CTR1 provides an essential function in mammalian embryonic development. Proc Natl Acad Sci USA 2001;98;6836–6841.
28. Petris MJ, Smith K, Lee J, Thiele DJ. Copper-stimulated endocytosis and degradation of the human copper transporter, hCtr1. J Biol Chem 2003;278; 9639–9646.
29. Eisses JF, Chi Y, Kaplan JH. Stable plasma membrane levels of hCTR1 mediate cellular copper uptake. J Biol Chem 2005;280;9635–9639.
30. Wong PC, Waggoner D, Subramaniam JR, et al. Copper chaperone for superoxide dismutase is essential to activate mammalian Cu/Zn superoxide dismutase. Proc Natl Acad Sci USA 2000;97;2886–2891.
31. Takahashi Y, Kako K, Kashiwabara S, et al. Mammalian copper chaperone Cox17p has an essential role in activation of cytochrome C oxidase and embryonic development. Mol Cell Biol 2002;22; 7614–7621.
32. Hamza I, Faisst A, Prohaska J, et al. The metallochaperone Atox1 plays a critical role in perinatal copper homeostasis. Proc Natl Acad Sci USA 2001;98; 6848–6852.
33. Camakaris J, Voskoboinik I, Mercer JF. Molecular mechanisms of copper homeostasis. Biochem Biophys Res Commun 1999;261;225–232.
34. Lutsenko S, Petris MJ. Function and regulation of the mammalian copper-transporting ATPases: insights from biochemical and cell biological approaches. J Membr Biol 2003;191;1–12.
35. Tao TY, Liu F, Klomp L, et al. The copper toxicosis gene product Murr1 directly interacts with the Wilson disease protein. J Biol Chem 2003;278; 41593–41596.
36. Suzuki KT, Someya A, Komada Y, Ogra Y. Roles of metallothionein in copper homeostasis: responses to Cu-deficient diets in mice. J Inorg Biochem 2002; 88;173–182.
37. Rees EM, Lee J, Thiele DJ. Mobilization of intracellular copper stores by the ctr2 vacuolar copper transporter. J Biol Chem 2004;279;54221–54229.
38. Brown DR. Copper and prion disease. Brain Res Bull 2001;55;165–173.
39. Waggoner DJ, Drisaldi B, Bartnikas TB, et al. Brain copper content and cuproenzyme activity do not vary with prion protein expression level. J Biol Chem 2000;275;7455–7458.
40. White AR, Reyes R, Mercer JF, et al. Copper levels are increased in the cerebral cortex and liver of APP and APLP2 knockout mice. Brain Res 1999;842; 439–444.
41. Maynard CJ, Cappai R, Volitakis I, et al. Overexpression of Alzheimer's disease amyloid-beta opposes the age-dependent elevations of brain copper and iron. J Biol Chem 2002;277;44670–44676.
42. Bellingham SA, Lahiri DK, Maloney B, et al. Copper depletion down-regulates expression of the Alzheimer's disease amyloid-beta precursor protein gene. J Biol Chem 2004;279;20378–20386.
43. Hunt CD, Meacham SL. Aluminum, boron, calcium, copper, iron, magnesium, manganese, molyb-

denum, phosphorus, potassium, sodium, and zinc: concentrations in common western foods and estimated daily intakes by infants; toddlers; and male and female adolescents, adults, and seniors in the United States. J Am Diet Assoc 2001;101;1058–60.
44. Hunt JR, Matthys LA, Johnson LK. Zinc absorption, mineral balance, and blood lipids in women consuming controlled lactoovovegetarian and omnivorous diets for 8 wk. Am J Clin Nutr 1998;67; 421–430.
45. Baker DH. Cupric oxide should not be used as a copper supplement for either animals or humans. J Nutr 1999;129;2278–2279.
46. Lonnerdal B. Copper nutrition during infancy and childhood. Am J Clin Nutr 1998;67;1046S–1053S.
47. Milne DB, Davis CD, Nielsen FH. Low dietary zinc alters indices of copper function and status in postmenopausal women. Nutrition 2001;17;701–708.
48. Johnson PE, Milne DB, Lykken GI. Effects of age and sex on copper absorption, biological half-life, and status in humans. Am J Clin Nutr 1992;56;917–925.
49. Donley SA, Ilagan BJ, Rim H, Linder MC. Copper transport to mammary gland and milk during lactation in rats. Am J Physiol Endocrinol Metab 2002; 283;E667–E675.
50. Rutherford JC, Bird AJ. Metal-responsive transcription factors that regulate iron, zinc, and copper homeostasis in eukaryotic cells. Eukaryot Cell 2004;3; 1–13.
51. Trumbo P, Yates AA, Schlicker S, Poos M. Dietary reference intakes: vitamin A, vitamin K, arsenic, boron, chromium, copper, iodine, iron, manganese, molybdenum, nickel, silicon, vanadium, and zinc. J Am Diet Assoc 2001;101;294–301.
52. Prohaska JR, Brokate B. The timing of perinatal copper deficiency in mice influences offspring survival. J Nutr 2002;132;3142–3145.
53. Uauy R, Olivares M, Gonzalez M. Essentiality of copper in humans. Am J Clin Nutr 1998;67; 952S–959S.
54. Medeiros DM, Wildman RE. Newer findings on a unified perspective of copper restriction and cardiomyopathy. Proc Soc Exp Biol Med 1997;215; 299–313.
55. Danks DM. Copper deficiency in humans. Annu Rev Nutr 1988;8;235–257.
56. Saari JT, Schuschke DA. Cardiovascular effects of dietary copper deficiency. Biofactors 1999;10; 359–375.
57. Kim S, Chao PY, Allen KG. Inhibition of elevated hepatic glutathione abolishes copper deficiency cholesterolemia. Faseb J 1992;6;2467–2471.
58. Wu JY, Zhang JJ, Wang Y, et al. Regulation of apolipoprotein A-I gene expression in Hep G2 cells depleted of Cu by cupruretic tetramine. Am J Physiol 1997;273;C1362–C1370.
59. Reeves PG, Demars LC, Johnson WT, Lukaski HC. Dietary copper deficiency reduces iron absorption and duodenal enterocyte hephaestin protein in male and female rats. J Nutr 2005;135;92–98.
60. Prohaska JR, Failla ML. Copper and Immunity. In: D.M. Klurfield, EditorHuman Nutrition-A Comprehensive Treatise, New York: Plenum Press, 1993: 309–332.
61. Hopkins RG, Failla ML. Chronic intake of a marginally low copper diet impairs in vitro activities of lymphocytes and neutrophils from male rats despite minimal impact on conventional indicators of copper status. J Nutr 1995;125;2658–2668.
62. Kelley DS, Daudu PA, Taylor PC, et al. Effects of low-copper diets on human immune response. Am J Clin Nutr 1995;62;412–416.
63. Hopkins RG, Failla ML. Transcriptional regulation of interleukin-2 gene expression is impaired by copper deficiency in Jurkat human T lymphocytes. J Nutr 1999;129;596–601.
64. Smith RM. Copper and the developing brain. In: I.E. Dreosti and R.M. Smith, EditorsNeurobiology of the Trace Elements, Clifton, New Jersey: Humana Press, 1983:1–40.
65. Prohaska JR, Hoffman RG. Auditory startle response is diminished in rats after recovery from perinatal copper deficiency. J Nutr 1996;126;618–627.
66. Penland JG, Prohaska JR. Abnormal motor function persists following recovery from perinatal copper deficiency in rats. J Nutr 2004;134;1984–1988.
67. Hunt CD, Idso JP. Moderate copper deprivation during gestation and lactation affects dentate gyrus and hippocampal maturation in immature male rats. J Nutr 1995;125;2700–2710.
68. Prohaska JR. Repletion of copper-deficient mice and brindled mice with copper or iron. J Nutr 1984;114; 422–430.
69. Steveson TC, Ciccotosto GD, Ma XM, et al. Menkes protein contributes to the function of peptidylglycine alpha-amidating monooxygenase. Endocrinology 2003;144;188–200.
70. Prohaska JR, Gybina AA, Broderius M, Brokate B. Peptidylglycine-alpha-amidating monooxygenase activity and protein are lower in copper-deficient rats and suckling copper-deficient mice. Arch Biochem Biophys 2005;434;212–220.
71. Patel BN, Dunn RJ, Jeong SY, et al. Ceruloplasmin regulates iron levels in the CNS and prevents free radical injury. J Neurosci 2002;22;6578–6586.
72. Prohaska JR, Gybina AA. Rat brain iron concentration is lower following perinatal copper deficiency. J Neurochem 2005;93;698–705.
73. Kumar N, Crum B, Petersen RC, et al. Copper deficiency myelopathy. Arch Neurol 2004;61;762–766.
74. Baker A, Harvey L, Majask-Newman G, et al. Effect of dietary copper intakes on biochemical markers of bone metabolism in healthy adult males. Eur J Clin Nutr 1999;53;408–412.

75. Prohaska JR. Neurochemical roles of copper as antioxidant or prooxidant. In: J.R. Connor, EditorMetals and Oxidative Damage in Neurological Disorders, New York, NY: Plenum Press, 1997: 57–75.
76. Araya M, Koletzko B, Uauy R. Copper deficiency and excess in infancy: developing a research agenda. J Pediatr Gastroenterol Nutr 2003;37;422–429.
77. Pratt WB, Omdahl JL, Sorenson JR. Lack of effects of copper gluconate supplementation. Am J Clin Nutr 1985;42;681–682.
78. Failla ML. Considerations for determining 'optimal nutrition' for copper, zinc, manganese and molybdenum. Proc Nutr Soc 1999;58;497–505.
79. Prohaska JR, Tamura T, Percy AK, Turnlund JR. In vitro copper stimulation of plasma peptidylglycine alpha-amidating monooxygenase in Menkes disease variant with occipital horns. Pediatr Res 1997;42; 862–865.
80. DiSilvestro RA, Jones AA, Smith D, Wildman R. Plasma diamine oxidase activities in renal dialysis patients, a human with spontaneous copper deficiency and marginally copper deficient rats. Clin Biochem 1997;30;559–563.
81. Kehoe CA, Turley E, Bonham MP, et al. Response of putative indices of copper status to copper supplementation in human subjects. Br J Nutr 2000;84; 151–156.
82. West EC, Prohaska JR. Cu,Zn-superoxide dismutase is lower and copper chaperone CCS is higher in erythrocytes of copper-deficient rats and mice. Exp Biol Med 2004;229;756–764.

# 37 Iodine and the Iodine Deficiency Disorders

Michael B. Zimmermann

## Introduction

Iodine (atomic weight 126.9 g/atom) is an essential component of the hormones produced by the thyroid gland. Thyroid hormones, and therefore iodine, are essential for mammalian life. In 1811, Courtois discovered iodine as a violet vapor arising from seaweed ash while manufacturing gunpowder for Napoleon's army. Gay-Lussac identified it as a new element and named it iodine from the Greek word for "violet."[1] Iodine was found in the thyroid gland by Baumann in 1895. In 1907, Marine showed that thyroid enlargement (goiter) was caused by iodine deficiency and could be prevented by iodine supplementation. Goiter prophylaxis through salt iodization was first introduced in Switzerland and the United States in the early 1920s.[1]

## Ecology

Iodine (as iodide) is widely but unevenly distributed in the earth's environment. In many regions, leaching from glaciation, flooding, and erosion have depleted surface soils of iodide, and most iodide is found in the oceans. The concentration of iodide in sea water is about 50 μg/L. Iodide ions in seawater are oxidized to elemental iodine, which volatilizes into the atmosphere and is returned to the soil by rain, completing the cycle.[2] However, iodine cycling in many regions is slow and incomplete, leaving soils and drinking water iodine depleted. Crops grown in these soils will be low in iodine, and humans and animals consuming food grown in these soils become iodine deficient. In plant foods grown in deficient soils, iodine concentrations may be as low as 10 μg/kg dry weight, as opposed to about 1 mg/kg in plants from iodine-sufficient soils.

Iodine deficient soils are common in mountainous areas (e.g., the Alps, Andes, Atlas, and Himalaya ranges) and areas of frequent flooding, especially in south and southeast Asia (e.g., the Ganges River plain of northeastern India). Many inland areas, including central Asia and Africa and central and eastern Europe are iodine deficient. Iodine deficiency in populations residing in these areas will persist until iodine enters the food chain through the addition of iodine to foods (e.g. iodization of salt) or dietary diversification introduces foods produced outside of the iodine-deficient area.

## Dietary Sources

The native iodine content of most foods and beverages is low. In general, commonly consumed foods provide 3 to 80 μg per serving.[3,4] Foods of marine origin have higher iodine content because marine plants and animals concentrate iodine from seawater. Iodine in organic form occurs in high amounts in certain seaweeds. Inhabitants of the coastal regions of Japan, whose diets contain large amounts of seaweed, have remarkably high iodine intakes: 50,000 to 80,000 μg/d. In the United States, the median intake of iodine from food in the mid-1990s was estimated to be 240 to 300 μg/d for men and 190 to 210 μg/d for women.[5] Major dietary sources of iodine in the United States are bread and milk.[6] In Switzerland, based on direct food analysis, mean intake of dietary iodine is about 140 μg/d, mainly from bread and dairy products.[4] In many countries, the use of iodized salt in households for cooking and at the table provides additional iodine. Boiling, baking, and canning of foods containing iodated salt cause only small losses (≤10%) of iodine content.[7]

The iodine content of foods is also influenced by iodine-containing compounds used in irrigation, fertilizers, and livestock feed. Iodophors used for cleaning milk cans and cow teats can increase the native iodine content of dairy products. Traditionally, iodate was used in bread making as a dough conditioner, but it is being replaced by non-iodine-containing conditioners. Erythrosine is a red coloring agent high in iodine that is widely used in foods, cosmetics, and pharmaceuticals. Dietary supplements often contain iodine. Based on data from the Third National Health and Nutrition Examination Survey (NHANES III), 12% of men and 15% of non-pregnant women took supplements containing iodine, and the median intake of iodine from supplements was about 140 μg/d for adults.[5] Other sources of iodine include water purification tablets, radiographic contrast media, medicines (e.g., amiodarone, an antiarrhythmic drug, contains 75 mg/tablet), and skin disinfectants (e.g., povidone iodine contains about 10 mg/mL).

## Absorption and Bioavailability

Iodine is ingested in several chemical forms. Iodide is rapidly and nearly completely absorbed in the stomach and duodenum. Iodate, widely used in salt iodization, is reduced in the gut and absorbed as iodide. In healthy adults, the absorption of iodide is more than 90%.[5] Organically bound iodine is typically digested and the released iodide absorbed, but some forms may be absorbed intact. For example, about 75% of an oral dose of thyroxine, the thyroid hormone, is absorbed intact.

Iodine deficiency is the main cause of endemic goiter (see below), but other dietary substances that interfere with thyroid metabolism, called "goitrogens," can aggravate the effect.[8] A well-known example is linamarin, a thioglycoside found in cassava, a staple food in many developing counties. If cassava is not adequately soaked or cooked to remove the linamarin, it is hydrolyzed in the gut to release cyanide, which is metabolized to thiocyanate. Thiocyanate blocks thyroidal uptake of iodine. Other goitrogenic substances are found in millet, sweet potato, beans, and cruciferous vegetables (e.g., cabbage). Soy-based flour can inhibit iodine absorption, and the use of soy-based formula without added iodine can produce goiter and hypothyroidism in infants. Unclean drinking water may contain humic substances that block thyroidal iodination. Industrial pollutants, including resorcinol, perchlorate, and phthalic acid, may also be goitrogenic. Most of these substances do not have a major clinical effect unless there is coexisting iodine deficiency.

Deficiencies of selenium, iron, and vitamin A exacerbate the effects of iodine deficiency. Glutathione peroxidase and the deoidinases are selenium-dependent enzymes. In selenium deficiency, accumulated peroxides may damage the thyroid, and deiodinase deficiency impairs thyroid hormone synthesis.[9] These effects have been implicated in the etiology of myxedematous cretinism (see below). Iron deficiency reduces heme-dependent thyroperoxidase activity in the thyroid and impairs production of thyroid hormone. In goitrous children, iron deficiency anemia blunts the efficacy of iodine prophylaxis, while iron supplementation improves the efficacy of iodized oil and iodized salt.[9] Vitamin A deficiency in iodine-deficient children increases thyroid-stimulating hormone (TSH) and risk for goiter, probably through decreased vitamin A-mediated suppression of the pituitary TSHβ gene.[10]

## Metabolism and Excretion

The distribution space of absorbed iodine is nearly equal to the extracellular fluid volume. Iodine is cleared from the circulation mainly by the thyroid and kidney, and while renal iodine clearance is fairly constant, thyroid clearance varies with iodine intake. In conditions of adequate iodine supply, ≤10% of absorbed iodine is taken up by the thyroid. In chronic iodine deficiency, this fraction can exceed 80%.[11] During lactation, the mammary gland concentrates iodine and secretes it into breast milk to provide for the newborn. The salivary glands, gastric mucosa, and choroid plexus also take up small amounts of iodine. Iodine in the blood is turned over rapidly; under normal circumstances, plasma iodine has a half-life of about 10 hours, but this is shortened if the thyroid is overactive, as in iodine deficiency or hyperthyroidism.

The body of a healthy adult contains 15 to 20 mg of iodine, of which 70% to 80% is in the thyroid. In chronic iodine deficiency, the iodine content of the thyroid may decrease to under 20 μg. In iodine-sufficient areas, the adult thyroid traps about 60 μg/d of iodine to balance losses and maintain thyroid hormone synthesis. A transmembrane protein in the basolateral membrane, the sodium/iodide symporter (NIS), transfers iodide into the thyroid at a concentration gradient 20 to 50 times that of plasma.[12] The human NIS gene is located on chromosome 19 and codes for a protein of 643 amino acids. The NIS concentrates iodine by an active transport process that couples the energy released by the inward translocation of sodium down its electrochemical gradient to the simultaneous inward translocation of iodine against its electrochemical gradient.

Thyroglobulin, a large glycoprotein (molecular weight 660,000), is the carrier of iodine in the thyroid (Figure 1). At the apical surface of the thyrocyte, the enzymes thyroperoxidase (TPO) and hydrogen peroxide oxidize iodide and attach it to tyrosyl residues on thyroglobulin, to produce monoiodotyrosine (MIT) and diiodotyrosine (DIT), the precursors of thyroid hormone. TPO then catalyzes the coupling of the phenyl groups of the iodotyrosines through a di-ether bridge to form the thyroid hormones.[11] Linkage of two DIT molecules produces tetraiodothyronine or thyroxine (T4), and linkage of a MIT and DIT produces triiodothyronine (T3). Thus, T3 is structurally identical to T4 but has one less iodine (at the 5′ position on the outer ring). Iodine comprises 65% and 59% of the weights of T4 and T3, respectively. In the thyroid, mature thyroglobulin, containing 0.1% to 1.0% of its weight as iodine, is stored extracellularly in the lumi-

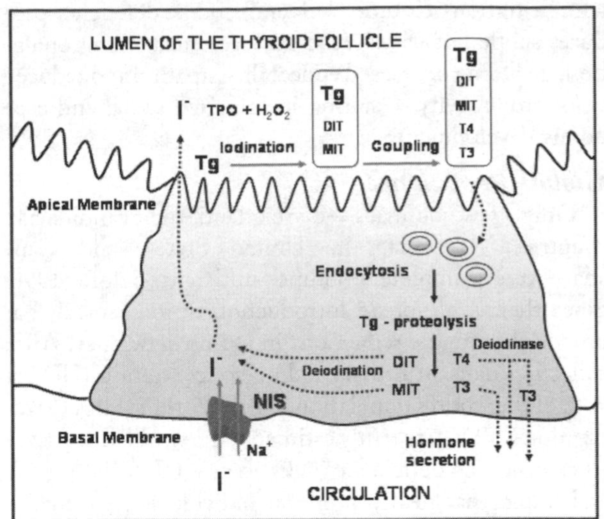


Figure 1. Iodine pathway in the thyroid cell. Iodide ($I^-$) is transported into the thyrocyte by the sodium iodide symporter (NIS) at the basal membrane and migrates to the apical membrane. The $I^-$ is oxidized by the enzymes thyroperoxidase (TPO) and hydrogen peroxidase ($H_2O_2$), and attached to tyrosyl residues in thyroglobulin (Tg) to produce the hormone precursors iodotyrosine (MIT) and diiodotyrosine (DIT). The residues then couple to form thyroxine (T4) and triiodothyronine (T3) within the Tg molecule in the follicular lumen. Tg enters the cell by endocytosis and is digested. T4 and T3 are released into the circulation, and non-hormonal iodine on MIT and DIT is recycled within the thyrocyte.

nal colloid of the thyroid follicle. After endocytosis, endosomal and lysosomal proteases digest thyroglobulin and release T4 and T3 into the circulation. MIT and DIT are not normally released into the blood. Iodine is removed from their tyrosines by a selenium-dependent deiodinase, and is then recycled for use within the thyroid, conserving iodine.[11]

In the circulation, thyroid hormone is bound noncovalently to carrier proteins, mainly thyroxine-binding globulin, but also to transthyretin and albumin. In target tissues—liver, kidney, heart, muscle, pituitary, and the developing brain—T4 is deiodinated to T3, the main physiologically active form of thyroid hormone, and binds to nuclear receptors. The thyroid hormone receptors have been cloned and regulatory DNA elements identified in thyroid hormone-responsive genes.[13] Hormone-receptor interactions stimulate several pathways, including the adenosine triphosphate (ATP) and inositol phosphate-$Ca^{2+}$ cascades, which in turn stimulate or inhibit protein synthesis.

Both T4 and T3 are degraded through a complex series of pathways, and their turnover is relatively slow: the half-life of T4 is about 5 days and for T3, 1.5 to 3 days.[14] The released iodine enters the plasma iodine pool and can be taken up again by the thyroid or excreted by the kidney. More than 90% of ingested iodine is ultimately excreted in the urine, with only small amounts appearing in the feces.

The principal regulator of thyroid hormone metabolism is TSH, a protein hormone (molecular weight about 28,000) secreted by the pituitary. TSH secretion is controlled through negative feedback by the level of circulating thyroid hormone, modulated by TSH-releasing hormone from the hypothalamus. In the thyroid, TSH increases iodine uptake through the stimulation of NIS expression. TSH exerts its action at the transcription level of the NIS gene through a thyroid-specific enhancer that contains binding sites for the transcription factor Pax8 and a cAMP response element-like sequence.[15] TSH also stimulates breakdown of thyroglobulin and release of thyroid hormone into the blood, but does not influence iodine absorption from the gut or renal iodide excretion. Because the primary stimulus to TSH secretion is circulating thyroid hormone, an elevated serum TSH concentration generally indicates primary hypothyroidism, while a low concentration indicates primary hyperthyroidism.

# Physiologic Function

Thyroid hormone regulates a variety of physiologic processes, including reproductive function, growth, and development. During pregnancy, thyroid hormone crosses the placenta to the fetus early in the first trimester, before the fetal thyroid is functioning. In the developing brain, it influences cell growth and migration.[16] It also promotes growth and maturation of peripheral tissues and the skeleton. Thyroid hormone increases energy metabolism in most tissues, and raises the basal metabolic rate. Other physiologic functions of iodine are less well defined: it may influence fibrocystic breast disease, play a role in immune response, and modify risk for gastric cancer.[5]

# Deficiency

Iodine deficiency has multiple adverse effects on growth and development in animals and humans. These are collectively termed the iodine deficiency disorders, and are one of the most important and common human diseases.[17] They result from inadequate thyroid hormone production due to lack of sufficient iodine.

## *Goiter*

Thyroid enlargement (goiter) is the classic sign of iodine deficiency. It is a physiologic adaptation to chronic iodine deficiency. As iodine intake decreases, the secretion of TSH increases in an effort to maximize uptake of available iodine, and TSH stimulates thyroid hypertrophy and hyperplasia. Initially, goiters are characterized by diffuse, homogeneous enlargement, but over time, thyroid follicles may fuse and become encapsulated, a condition termed nodular goiter. Large goiters may be cosmetically unattractive, can obstruct the trachea and esophagus, and may damage the recurrent laryngeal nerves and cause hoarseness. Surgery to reduce goiter has significant risks, including bleeding and nerve damage, and hypothyroidism may develop after removal of thyroid tissue.

### *Neurocognitive Impairment*

Although goiter is the most visible effect of iodine deficiency, the most serious adverse effect is damage to reproduction. Severe iodine deficiency during pregnancy is associated with a greater incidence of stillbirths, abortions, and congenital abnormalities. Iodine prophylaxis with iodized oil in pregnant women in areas of severe deficiency reduces fetal and perinatal mortality.[18] The fetal brain is particularly vulnerable to iodine deficiency. The most critical period is from the second trimester of pregnancy to the third year after birth.[17] Normal levels of thyroid hormones are required for neuronal migration and myelination of the central nervous system.[19] The most severe form of neurological damage from fetal hypothyroidism is termed cretinism. It is characterized by gross mental retardation along with varying degrees of short stature, deaf mutism, and spasticity. Two distinct types have been described. The more common, neurologic cretinism, has specific neurologic deficits that include spastic quadriplegia with sparing of the distal extremities. The myxedematous form is seen most frequently in central Africa, and has the predominant finding of profound hypothyroidism, with thyroid atrophy and fibrosis. Up to 10% of populations with severe iodine deficiency may be cretinous. Iodine prophylaxis has completely eliminated the appearance of new cases of cretinism in previously iodine-deficient Switzerland and other countries.[18]

Although new cases of cretinism are now rare, mild-to-moderate iodine deficiency affects up to 30% of the global population (see below), and can impair cognitive development and school performance in children. A meta-analysis of 18 studies concluded that iodine deficiency reduces mean IQ scores by 13.5 points.[20] Iodine deficiency is thus considered the most common cause of preventable mental retardation worldwide. In school-age children born and raised in areas of iodine deficiency, cognitive impairment is at least partially reversible by the administration of iodine.[21] Overall, iodine deficiency produces subtle but widespread adverse effects in a population, including decreased educability, apathy, and reduced work productivity, resulting in impaired social and economic development.

### *Global Prevalence*

Only a few countries—Switzerland, the Scandinavian countries, Australia, the United States, and Canada—were completely iodine sufficient before 1990. Since then, widespread introduction of iodized salt has produced dramatic reductions in iodine deficiency. After collecting data on urinary iodine concentration (UI) for 92% of the world's population,[22] the World Health Organization (WHO) recently estimated the worldwide prevalence of iodine deficiency (defined as a UI <100 μg/L), and found that nearly 2 billion individuals have inadequate iodine nutrition, of whom 285 million are school-aged children (Table 1). The prevalence of iodine deficiency in school-aged children is 36.4%.[23] The lowest prevalence of iodine deficiency is found in the Americas (10.1%), where the proportion of households consuming iodized salt is the highest in the world (90%). Surprisingly, the highest prevalence of iodine deficiency is in Europe (59.9%), where the proportion of households consuming iodized salt is the lowest (27%), and most countries have weak or non-existent national programs. In Australia and the United States, two countries previously iodine sufficient, iodine intakes are falling. Australia is now mildly iodine deficient, and in the United States, the median UI is 145 μg/L, still adequate but half the median value of 321 μg/L found in the 1970s.[24] These changes emphasize the importance of regular monitoring of iodine status in all countries.

## Requirements

The Food and Nutrition Board of the US National Academy of Sciences has set an Adequate Intake (AI) for

**Table 1.** Prevalence of Iodine Deficiency in the General Population (All Age Groups) and in School-Age Children (6–12 Years) in 2003

| | Population with Urinary Iodine <100μg/L | |
|---|---|---|
| **WHO Regions*** | **General Population** | **School-age Children** |
| Africa | 260,325,000 (42.6%) | 49,465,000 (42.3%) |
| Americas | 75,081,000 (9.8%) | 9,955,000 (10.1%) |
| Eastern Mediterranean | 228,451,000 (54.1%) | 40,224,000 (55.4%) |
| Europe | 435,452,000 (56.9%) | 42,215,000 (59.9%) |
| Southeast Asia | 624,013,000 (39.8%) | 95,628,000 (39.9%) |
| Western Pacific | 365,332,000 (24.0%) | 47,056,000 (25.7%) |
| Total | 1,988,654,000 (35.2%) | 284,543,000 (36.4%) |

* 192 WHO Member States.
† Based on population estimates for 2002 (United Nations, Population Division, World Population Prospects: the 2002 revision).
Data from de Benoist et al., 2003.[23]

**Table 2.** Recommendations for Iodine Intake by Age or Population Group

| Age or Population Group | Iodine Recommendation µg/d |
|---|---|
| Infants 0–6 months | |
| Adequate Intake | 110 |
| Infants 7–12 months | |
| Adequate Intake | 130 |
| Children 1–8 years | |
| Estimated Average Requirement | 65 |
| Recommended Dietary Allowance | 90 |
| Children 9–13 | |
| Estimated Average Requirement | 73 |
| Recommended Dietary Allowance | 120 |
| Adults ≥14 years | |
| Estimated Average Requirement | 95 |
| Recommended Dietary Allowance | 150 |
| Pregnancy | |
| Estimated Average Requirement | 160 |
| Recommended Dietary Allowance | 220 |
| Lactation | |
| Estimated Average Requirement | 209 |
| Recommended Dietary Allowance | 290 |

Data from Food and Nutrition Board, Institute of Medicine, 2001.[5]

iodine in infancy and a Recommended Dietary Allowance (RDA) for children, adults, and pregnant and lactating women (Table 2).[5] The WHO recommends a daily intake of iodine of 90 µg for preschool children (0 to 59 months), 120 µg for schoolchildren (6 to 12 years), 150 µg for adults (above 12 years),[17] and 250 µg for pregnant and lactating women.[25]

## Status Assessment

Several methods are available for assessment of iodine nutrition. The most commonly used are measurement of thyroid size and concentration of UI.[17] Additional indicators include newborn thyrotropin (TSH), and blood concentrations of thyroglobulin, thyroxine (T4) or triiodothyronine (T3). As discussed below, UI is a sensitive indicator of recent iodine intake (days) and serum thyroglobulin shows an intermediate response (weeks to months), whereas changes in the goiter rate reflect long-term iodine nutrition (months to years).

### *Thyroid Size*

Two methods are available for measuring goiter: neck inspection/palpation and thyroid ultrasonography. Goiter surveys are usually done in school-age children. By palpation, a thyroid is considered goitrous when each lateral lobe has a volume greater than the terminal phalanx of the thumbs of the subject being examined. In the classification system of WHO,[17] grade 0 is defined as a thyroid that is not palpable or visible, grade 1 is a goiter that is palpable but not visible when the neck is in the normal position (i.e., the thyroid is not visibly enlarged), and grade 2 is a thyroid that is clearly visible when the neck is in a normal position.

In areas of mild to moderate iodine deficiency, where goiters are small, measurement of thyroid size by ultrasonography is a more objective and precise method, and is preferable to palpation. Portable ultrasound equipment can be used in the field, and goiter classified according to international reference criteria for iodine-sufficient children by age, gender, and body surface area.[26] The total goiter rate is used to define severity using the following criteria: <5% = iodine sufficiency; 5.0%–19.9% = mild deficiency; 20.0%–29.9% = moderate deficiency; and >30% = severe deficiency.[17]

In areas of endemic goiter, although thyroid size predictably decreases in response to increases in iodine intake, thyroid size may not return to normal for months or years after correction of iodine deficiency.[27] During this transition period, the goiter rate is difficult to interpret, because it reflects both a population's history of iodine nutrition and its present status.[17] Despite this lag period, a sustained salt iodization program will decrease the goiter rate to under 5% in school-age children, and this indicates disappearance of iodine deficiency as a significant public health problem.[17]

### *Urinary Iodine Concentration*

Because over 90% of ingested iodine is excreted in the urine, UI is an excellent indicator of recent iodine intake. Most methods of measuring UI are based on the Sandell-Kolthoff reaction, in which iodide catalyzes the reduction of yellow ceric ammonium sulfate to the colorless cerous form in the presence of arsenious acid.[28] UI can be expressed as a concentration (in micrograms per liter), in relationship to creatinine excretion (in micrograms of iodine per gram of creatinine), or as 24-hour excretion (in micrograms per day). To estimate iodine intakes in individuals, 24-hour collections are preferable. For populations, because it is impractical to collect 24-hour samples in field studies, UI can be measured in spot urine specimens from a representative sample of the target group, and expressed as the median, in micrograms per liter[17] (Table 3). Variations in hydration among individuals generally even out in a large number of samples, so

**Table 3.** Epidemiological Criteria for Assessing Iodine Nutrition Based on Median Urinary Iodine Concentrations in School-aged Children

| Median Urinary Iodine μg/L | Iodine Intake | Iodine Nutrition |
|---|---|---|
| <20 | Insufficient | Severe iodine deficiency |
| 20–49 | Insufficient | Moderate iodine deficiency |
| 50–99 | Insufficient | Mild iodine deficiency |
| 100–199 | Adequate | Optimal |
| 200–299 | More than adequate | Risk of iodine-induced hyperthyroidism in susceptible groups |
| >300 | Excessive | Risk of adverse health consequences (iodine-induced hyperthyroidism, autoimmune thyroid disease) |

Data from the World Health Organization, 2001.[17]

that the median UI in spot samples correlates well with that from 24-hour samples.[28] Creatinine may be unreliable for estimating daily iodine excretion from spot samples, especially in malnourished subjects, in whom creatinine concentration is low.[17] UI measurements from populations should be properly interpreted. Individual spot UI concentrations are highly variable over time, and a common mistake is to assume that all subjects with a spot UI of under 100 μg/L are iodine deficient. However, in a population with a median of 100 μg/L (indicating iodine sufficiency), then by definition, half of the values will be below this level.

Daily iodine intake for population estimates can be extrapolated from UI using estimates of mean 24-hour urine volume and assuming an average iodine bioavailability of 92%. This can be done using the following formula[5]:

Urinary iodine (μg/L) × 0.0235 × body weight (kg) = daily iodine intake.

Using this formula, a UI of 100 μg/L in an average adult corresponds roughly to a daily intake of 150 μg.

### *Thyroid Stimulating Hormone*

Because serum TSH is determined mainly by the level of circulating thyroid hormone (which in turn reflects iodine intake), TSH can be used as an indicator of iodine nutrition. However, in older children and adults, although serum TSH may be slightly increased by iodine deficiency, values often remain within the normal range. TSH is therefore a relatively insensitive indicator of iodine nutrition in adults.[17] In contrast, TSH is a sensitive indicator of iodine status in the newborn period.[29] Compared with the adult, the newborn thyroid contains less iodine but has higher rates of iodine turnover. Particularly when the iodine supply is low, maintaining high iodine turnover requires increased TSH stimulation. Serum TSH concentrations are therefore increased in iodine-deficient infants for the first few weeks of life, a condition called "transient newborn hypothyroidism." In areas of iodine deficiency, an increase in transient newborn hypothyroidism, indicated by more than 3% of newborn TSH values above the threshold of 5 mU/L whole blood, suggests iodine deficiency in the population.[30] TSH is used in many countries for routine newborn screening to detect congenital hypothyroidism. If already in place, such screening offers a sensitive indicator of iodine nutrition.[31] Newborn TSH is an important measure because it reflects iodine status during a period when the developing brain is particularly sensitive to iodine deficiency.

### *Thyroglobulin*

Thyroglobulin is synthesized only in the thyroid, and is the most abundant intrathyroidal protein.[11] In iodine sufficiency, small amounts of thyroglobulin are secreted into the circulation, and serum thyroglobulin is normally under 10 μg/L.[30] In areas of endemic goiter, serum thyroglobulin increases due to greater thyroid cell mass and TSH stimulation. Serum thyroglobulin is well correlated with the severity of iodine deficiency as measured by UI,[32] and is a more sensitive indicator of iodine repletion than serum TSH or T4.[17] Thyroglobulin can also be assayed on dried blood spots taken by a finger prick,[33] simplifying collection and transport. In a prospective study in goitrous children, dried blood spot thyroglobulin was a sensitive measure of iodine status before and after introduction of iodized salt.[33] In contrast, thyroid hormone concentrations are poor indicators of iodine status. In iodine-deficient populations, serum T3 increases or remains unchanged, and serum T4 usually decreases. However, these changes are often within the normal range, and the overlap with iodine-sufficient populations is large enough to make thyroid hormone levels an insensitive measure of iodine nutrition.[17]

## Prophylaxis and Treatment

There are two methods commonly used to correct iodine deficiency in a population: iodized oil and iodized salt. In nearly all regions affected by iodine deficiency, the most effective way to control iodine deficiency is through salt iodization.[17] All salt for human consumption, including salt used in the food industry, should be iodized. In Switzerland, a country previously affected by endemic goiter and cretinism, a monitored national program in place for over half a century has effectively eliminated iodine deficiency.[31] Iodine can be added to salt in the form of potassium iodide (KI) or potassium iodate ($KIO_3$). Because $KIO_3$ has higher stability in the presence of salt impurities, humidity, and porous packaging,[34] it is the recommended form.[17] Iodine is usually added at a level of 20 to 40 mg iodine/kg salt, depending on local salt intake.

Due to a major international effort led by WHO, the United Nations Childrens Fund (UNICEF), and the International Council for the Control of Iodine Deficiency Disorders (ICCIDD), 68% of households in the 130 countries having iodine deficiency had access to iodized salt in 1999, compared with under 10% in 1990.[17] However, when coverage is not complete, iodized salt use is often lowest in the poorest socioeconomic classes, typically the population most affected by iodine deficiency.[35] For a national program to succeed, ≥95% of salt for human consumption should be iodized according to government standards at the production or importation site. Worldwide, sustainability of iodized salt programs has become a major focus. These programs are fragile, and require a long-term commitment from national governments, donors, consumers, and the salt industry. In several countries where iodine deficiency had been eliminated, salt iodization programs fell apart, and iodine deficiency recurred.[36] Children in iodine-deficient areas are vulnerable to even short-term lapses in iodized salt programs.[37]

In some regions, iodization of salt may not be practical for control of iodine deficiency, at least in the short term. This may occur in remote areas where communication is poor or where there are numerous very small-scale salt producers. In these areas, other options for correction of iodine deficiency should be considered, such as iodized oil,[38] which is prepared by esterification of the unsaturated fatty acids in seed or vegetable oils and adding iodine to the double bonds. It can be given orally or by intramuscular injection. The intramuscular route has a longer duration of action, but oral administration is more common because it is simpler. Iodized oil is recommended for populations with moderate to severe iodine deficiency that do not have access to iodized salt,[17] and may be targeted to women of child-bearing age, pregnant women, and children. Usual doses are 200 to 400 mg iodine/year.[38] Iodine can also be given as potassium iodide or iodate as drops or tablets and in drinking or irrigation water.[39] Iodine supplements (about 150 μg/d) are recommended for pregnant and lactating women residing in areas of mild-to-moderate iodine deficiency.[40]

## Excess and Toxicity

Acute iodine poisoning caused by the ingestion of many grams of iodine causes gastrointestinal irritation, abdominal pain, nausea, vomiting, and diarrhea, as well as cardiovascular symptoms, coma, and cyanosis.[41] Excess iodine intake may very rarely precipitate iodermia, a skin disorder consisting of acneiform eruptions, pruritic rash, and urticaria.[42]

Most people are remarkably tolerant to high dietary intakes of iodine.[41] The U.S. Food and Nutrition Board of the National Academy of Sciences has set a Tolerable Upper Intake Level (UL) for iodine.[5] The UL is the highest level of daily intake that is likely to pose no risk of adverse health effects in almost all individuals. The UL is 200 μg/d for ages 1 to 3 years, 300 μg/d for ages 4 to 8 years, 600 μg/d for ages 9 to 13 years, 900 μg/d for ages 14 to 18 years, and 1100 μg/d thereafter.[5] Individuals with autoimmune thyroid disease or chronic iodine deficiency may respond adversely to intakes lower than these.

In iodine-sufficient individuals, the earliest effect of high iodine intakes is typically an increase in serum TSH without a decrease in serum T4 or T3, a condition called "subclinical hypothyroidism." Large excesses of iodine inhibit thyroid hormone production, leading to increased TSH stimulation, thyroid growth, and goiter. A clinical trial in healthy adults found that TSH concentrations were increased by total iodine intakes of ≥750 μg/d.[43] In children, chronic intakes of ≥500 μg/d are associated with increased thyroid volume, an early sign of thyroid dysfunction.[44] Doses of ≥18,000 μg/d can produce goiter in adults.[45] Iodine-induced goiter and hypothyroidism can occur in newborns due to high maternal intakes or through exposure to excess iodine at delivery from the use of antiseptics containing beta-iodine.[46] It is unclear if risk of thyroid papillary cancer[47] or thyroid autoimmunity[48] is increased by high iodine intakes. Incidence of Graves' disease and Hashimoto's disease appears not to be affected by high dietary iodine.

A rapid increase in iodine intake of populations with chronic iodine deficiency may precipitate iodine-induced hyperthyroidism.[49] This is more likely to occur if the iodine is given in excess, for example, if the iodine content of iodized salt is too high, or when iodine-containing medication is given. Iodine-induced hyperthyroidism occurs mainly in older people with nodular goiter. Thyrocytes in nodules often become insensitive to TSH control, and if the iodine supply is suddenly increased, these autonomous nodules may overproduce thyroid hormone.[50] Symptoms of iodine-induced hyperthyroidism include weight loss, tachycardia, muscle weakness, and skin warmth, without the ophthalmopathy of Graves' disease. Iodine-induced hyperthyroidism is dangerous when superimposed on underlying heart disease, and may be lethal. The introduction of iodine prophylaxis has been associated with increased hospitalizations for iodine-induced hyperthyroidism in Europe, the United States, and several African countries.[49] The incidence tends to gradually abate, but may rise again when the level of iodine in salt is increased. Its occurrence should not be an argument against salt iodization, as the underlying cause of most autonomous nodules and iodine-induced hyperthyroidism is chronic iodine deficiency. To reduce risk for iodine-induced hyperthyroidism, the iodine level in salt should be monitored and reduced if too high.

## References

1. Merke F. *History and Iconography of Endemic Goiter and Cretinism*. Bern: Hans Huber; 1984.
2. Goldschmidt VW. *Geochemistry*. Oxford: Oxford University Press; 1954.
3. Pennington JAT, Schoen SA, Salmon GD, et al. Composition of core foods in the U.S. food supply, 1982–1991. J Food Comp Anal. 1995;8:171–217.
4. Haldimann M, Alt A, Blanc A, Blondeau K. Iodine content of food groups. J Food Comp Anal. 2005; 18:461–471.
5. Food and Nutrition Board, Institute of Medicine. Dietary Reference Intakes for Vitamin A, Vitamin K, Arsenic, Boron, Chromium, Copper, Iodine, Iron, Manganese, Molybdenum, Nickel, Silicon, Vanadium, and Zinc. Washington, DC: National Academies Press; 2001. Available online at: http://www.nap.edu/books/0309072794/html/.
6. Pearce EN, Pino S, He X, et al. Sources of dietary iodine: bread, cows' milk, and infant formula in the Boston area. J Clin Endocrinol Metab. 2004;89: 3421–3424.
7. Chavasit V, Malaivongse P, Judprasong K. Study on stability of iodine in iodated salt by use of different cooking model conditions. J Food Comp Anal. 2002; 15:265–276.
8. Gaitan E. *Environmental Goitrogenesis*. Boca Raton: CRC Press; 1989.
9. Zimmermann MB, Köhrle J. The impact of iron and selenium deficiencies on iodine and thyroid metabolism: biochemistry and relevance to public health. Thyroid. 2002;12:867–878.
10. Zimmermann MB, Wegmueller R, Zeder C, et al. The effects of vitamin A deficiency and vitamin A supplementation on thyroid function in goitrous children. J Clin Endocrinol Metab. 2004;89:5441–5447.
11. Rousset BA, Dunn JT. Thyroid hormone synthesis and secretion. In: DeGroot LE, Hannemann G, eds. *The Thyroid and Its Diseases*. Available at: http://www.thyroidmanager.org/Chapter2/2-frame.htm.
12. Eskandari S, Loo DD, Dai G, et al. Thyroid $Na^+$/$I^-$ symporter. Mechanism, stoichiometry, and specificity. J Biol Chem. 1997;272:27230–27238.
13. Yen PM. Physiological and molecular basis of thyroid hormone action. Physiol Rev. 2001;81: 1097–1142.
14. Oppenheimer JH, Schwartz HL, Surks MI. Determlnatlon of common parameters of iodothyronine metabolism and distribution in man by noncompartmental analysis. J Clin Endocrinol Metab. 1975;41: 319–324.
15. Taki K, Kogai T, Kanamoto Y, et al. A thyroid-specific far-upstream enhancer in the human sodium/iodide symporter gene requires Pax-8 binding and cyclic adenosine 3′,5′-monophosphate response element-like sequence binding proteins for full activity and is differentially regulated in normal and thyroid cancer cells. Mol Endocrinol. 2002;16:2266–2282.
16. Morreale de Escobar G, Obregon MJ, Escobar del Rey F. Role of thyroid hormone during early brain development. Eur J Endocrinol. 2004;151(suppl 3): U25–U37.
17. World Health Organization/International Council for the Control of the Iodine Deficiency Disorders/United Nations Childrens Fund. *Assessment of the Iodine Deficiency Disorders and Monitoring their Elimination. WHO/NHD/01.1*. Geneva: WHO; 2001.
18. Delange F, Hetzel B. The iodine deficiency disorders. In: DeGroot LE, Hannemann G, eds *The Thyroid and Its Diseases*. Available at: http://www.thyroidmanager.org/Chapter20/20-frame.htm.
19. Auso E, Lavado-Autric R, Cuevas E, et al. A moderate and transient deficiency of maternal thyroid function at the beginning of fetal neocorticogenesis alters neuronal migration. Endocrinology. 2004;145: 4037–4047.
20. Bleichrodt N, Born MP. A metaanalysis of research on iodine and its relationship to cognitive development. In: Stanbury JB, ed. *The Damaged Brain of Iodine Deficiency*. New York: Cognizant Communication; 1994; 195–200.
21. Zimmermann MB, Connolly K, Bozo M, Bridson J, Rohner F, Grimci L. Iodine supplementation improves cognition in iodine-deficient schoolchildren in Albania: a randomized, controlled, double-blind study. Am J Clin Nutr. 2006;83:108–114.
22. World Health Organization. *Global Database on Iodine Deficiency*. Available at: http://www3.who.int/whosis/menu.cfm?path = whosis,mn,mn_iodine& language = english.
23. de Benoist B, Andersson M, Takkouche B, Egli I. Prevalence of iodine deficiency worldwide. Lancet. 2003;362:1859–1860.
24. Hollowell JG, Staehling NW, Hannon WH, et al. Iodine nutrition in the United States. Trends and public health implications : iodine excretion data from National Health and Nutrition Examination Surveys I and III (1971–1974 and 1988–1994). J Clin Endocrinol Metab. 1998;83:3401–3408.
25. World Health Organization. Recommendations of a WHO Technical Consultation: The prevention and control of iodine deficiency in pregnant and lactating women and in children less than two years old. Geneva: WHO. 2006; In press.
26. Zimmermann MB, Hess SY, Molinari L, et al. New reference values for thyroid volume by ultrasound in

iodine-sufficient schoolchildren: a WHO/NHD Iodine Deficiency Study Group Report. Am J Clin Nutr. 2004;79:231–237.

27. Zimmermann MB, Hess SY, Adou P, et al. Thyroid size and goiter prevalence after introduction of iodized salt: a 5-yr prospective study in schoolchildren in Côte d'Ivoire. Am J Clin Nutr. 2003;77: 663–667.
28. Bier D, Rendl J, Ziemann M, Freystadt D, Reiners C. Methodological and analytical aspects of simple methods for measuring iodine in urine. Comparison with HPLC and Technicon Autoanalyzer II. Exp Clin Endocrinol Diabetes. 1998;106(suppl 3):S27–S31.
29. Delange F. Neonatal screening for congenital hypothyroidism: results and perspectives. Horm Res. 1997;48:51–61.
30. World Health Organization/International Council for the Control of the Iodine Deficiency Disorders/ United Nations Childrens Fund. *Indicators for assessing Iodine Deficiency Disorders and Their Control through Salt Iodization. WHO/NUT/94.6.* Geneva: WHO; 1994.
31. Zimmermann MB, Aeberli I, Torresani T, Burgi H. Increasing the iodine concentration in the Swiss iodized salt program markedly improved iodine status in pregnant women and children: a 5-y prospective national study. Am J Clin Nutr. 2005;82:388–392.
32. Knudsen N, Bülow I, Jorgenson T, et al. Serum thyroglobulin-a sensitive marker of thyroid abnormalities and iodine deficiency in epidemiologic studies. J Clin Endocrinol Metab. 2001;86:3599–3603.
33. Zimmermann MB, Moretti D, Chaouki N, Torresani T. Development of a dried whole blood spot thyroglobulin assay and its evaluation as an indicator of thyroid status in goitrous children receiving iodized salt. Am J Clin Nutr. 2003;77:1453–1458.
34. Diosady LL, Alberti JO, Mannar MGV, FitzGerald S. Stability of iodine in iodized salt used for correction of iodine-deficiency disorders, II. Food Nutr Bull. 1998;19:240–250.
35. Jooste PL, Weight MJ, Lombard CJ. Iodine concentration in household salt in South Africa. Bull World Health Org. 2001;79:534–540.
36. Dunn JT. Complacency: the most dangerous enemy in the war against iodine deficiency. Thyroid. 2000; 10:681–683.
37. Zimmermann MB, Wegmüller R, Zeder C, et al. Rapid relapse of thyroid dysfunction and goiter in school age children after withdrawal of salt iodization. Am J Clin Nutr. 2004;79:642–645.
38. Benmiloud M, Chaouki ML, Gutekunst R, et al. Oral iodized oil for correcting iodine deficiency: optimal dosing and outcome indicator selection. J Clin Endocrinol Metab. 1994;79:20–24.
39. Squatrito S, Vigneri R, Runello F, et al. Prevention and treatment of endemic iodine-deficiency goiter by iodination of a municipal water supply. J Clin Endocrinol Metab. 1986;63:368–375.
40. Zimmermann MB, Delange F. Iodine supplementation in pregnant women in Europe: a review and recommendations. Eur J Clin Nutr. 2004;58:979–984
41. Pennington JA. A review of iodine toxicity reports. J Am Diet Assoc. 1990;90:1571–1581.
42. Parsad D, Saini R. Acneform eruption with iodized salt. Int J Dermatol. 1998;37:478.
43. Chow CC, Phillips DI, Lazarus JH, Parkes AB. Effect of low dose iodide supplementation on thyroid function in potentially susceptible subjects: Are dietary iodide levels in Britain acceptable? Clin Endocrinol. 1991;34:413–416.
44. Zimmermann MB, Ito Y, Hess SY, et al. High thyroid volume in children with excess dietary iodine intakes. Am J Clin Nutr. 2005;81:840–844.
45. Wolff J. Iodide goiter and the pharmacologic effects of excess iodide. Am J Med. 1969;47:101–124.
46. Nishiyama S, Mikeda T, Okada T, et al. Transient hypothyroidism or persistent hyperthyrotropinemia in neonates born to mothers with excessive iodine intake. Thyroid. 2004;14:1077–1083.
47. Franceschi S. Iodine intake and thyroid carcinoma—A potential risk factor. Exp Clin Endocrinol Diabetes. 1998;106:S38–S44.
48. Kahaly G, Dienes HP, Beyer J, Hommel G. Randomized, double blind, placebo-controlled trial of low dose iodide in endemic goiter. J Clin Endocrinol Metab. 1997;82:4049–4053.
49. Delange F, de Benoist B, Alnwick D. Risks of iodine-induced hyperthyroidism after correction of iodine deficiency by iodized salt. Thyroid. 1999;9: 545–556.
50. Corvilain B, Van Sande J, Dumont JE, et al. Autonomy in endemic goiter. Thyroid. 1998;8:107–113.

# 38 Selenium

Roger A. Sunde

## Introduction

The nutrient selenium possesses many attributes that excite the public and the research community. These include anticarcinogenic activity, a role in reproduction, toxicity, its apparent activity to protect against oxidant damage or aging, protection in animals against nutritional forms of muscular dystrophy, and even as a nutrient to be considered in treatment strategies for AIDS. Selenium also possesses many unique and novel nutritional, biochemical, and molecular biology properties that continue to make it an exciting target for nutrition research. This research increasingly provides molecular details that help explain the role of selenium in promoting health and preventing disease. This chapter will review the current status of our present knowledge of selenium both in areas of public interest and in topics of research interest. Additional information can be obtained from other symposia and reviews.[1-3]

Selenium essentiality was first discovered in 1957 when Schwarz and Foltz[4] showed that traces of dietary selenium prevented liver necrosis in rats fed a diet also deficient in vitamin E. This led to the demonstration that selenium is a nutritionally essential trace element for animals. Widespread use of selenium supplementation in animal feeds eliminated a number of animal diseases attributable to selenium or vitamin E deficiency.[5] In the 1960s and 1970s, epidemiological data and animal research began to demonstrate that selenium also possesses anticarcinogenic activity.[6] Using biochemistry, the first selenium-containing enzyme, glutathione peroxidase-1 (GPX1), was discovered in 1973[7]; 30 years later, bioinformatics and molecular biology have revealed that the human genome encodes 25 selenoproteins.[3] These recent discoveries have the promise to uncover the full range of roles for selenium in health and disease, and in the process, perhaps reveal key new players in long-term health.

## Deficiency Diseases

### *Selenium Deficiency in Animals*

The foundation for our knowledge of selenium nutrition lies in animal experiments. In the laboratory, rats fed selenium-deficient diets develop liver necrosis if these diets are also deficient in vitamin E and sulfur amino acids.[5] This degenerative liver disease is distinct from fatty liver and liver cirrhosis, and in the past resulted in death within 21 to 28 days. In 1969, selenium was shown to be unconditionally essential for rats and chickens in diets containing adequate levels of vitamin E and the sulfur amino acids. The specific disease associated with selenium deficiency depends on the species; in contrast to rats, which develop primarily liver necrosis during combined selenium and vitamin E deficiency, the mouse develops a multiple necrotic degeneration of skeletal muscle, heart, kidney, liver, and pancreas. Reproductive failure also occurs in males of both rodent species due to defective sperm production. New mouse knockout models with deleted selenoprotein genes are now revealing critical roles for Se in neural function[8] and in gastrointestinal disease.[9]

The nature of selenium deficiency in production animals provides examples of selenium deficiency diseases that might be useful in characterizing selenium's full role in human health.[5] Swine develop a cardiac condition called mulberry heart, lambs develop a nutritional muscular dystrophy called white muscle disease, and turkeys develop a gizzard myopathy. Cattle also develop a nutritional myopathy affecting skeletal and heart muscle. Reproductive problems associated with dietary selenium deficiency in cattle also include retained placenta in cows and reproductive failure in bulls. These conditions usually require concomitant vitamin E deficiency. Chickens develop one of several deficiency diseases depending on dietary selenium, vitamin E, and the sulfur amino acids. A degeneration of capillary beds called exudative diathesis is prevented either by selenium or vitamin E, but a pancreatic atrophy is only prevented by dietary selenium when vitamin E is at normal levels. Super levels of vitamin E and other antioxidants, however, will prevent pancreatic atrophy.[10] These laboratory animal diseases can also develop in animals fed practical rations produced from selenium-deficient areas.

Several additional observations emerge from these animal studies. The laboratory selenium deficiency diseases reported in the 1950s and 1960s, however, cannot be reproduced today, probably because commercially produced animals now have adequate selenium stores. Second-generation selenium-deficient animals, however, still grow at half the rate of their selenium-supplemented littermates,[11] clearly indicating that selenium deficiency in a diet otherwise adequate in nutrients has impact. These animals now often thrive into old age, suggesting that something else is different in the laboratory setting of the past versus what exists today; one such factor may be disease. Second, the differences in disease signs in different species elicited by selenium deficiency indicate that there is species-to-species variation in selenium's protective role relative to other protective mechanisms. A fuller understanding of these alternative mechanisms (e.g., why capillary beds are exclusively sensitive in the chicken but well protected in the rat) may provide clues for disease resistance in humans. Last, the minimum dietary selenium requirements necessary to prevent selenium deficiency disease is remarkably constant across a wide range of species, suggesting that common molecular regulatory mechanisms are shared between these species.[12]

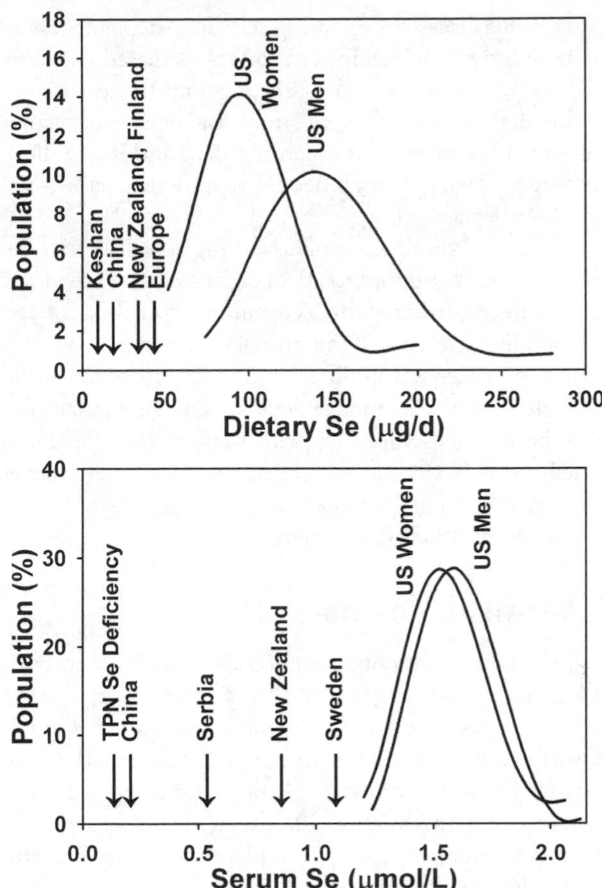


Figure 1. U.S. Dietary Selenium Intakes and Serum Concentrations. The distribution of U.S. selenium dietary intakes (top) and serum selenium concentrations (bottom) for adults (31–50 years old). Arrows show reported levels in other countries, as discussed in the text. (Data from Food and Nutrition Board, Institute of Medicine, 2000.[2])

## *Selenium Deficiency in Humans*

Selenium deficiency in humans, known as Keshan disease, still occurs naturally in China as an endemic cardiomyopathy that is localized primarily in peasant populations in certain hilly and mountainous regions in China with low soil selenium.[13] This disease was eliminated in the 1970s by an aggressive selenium supplementation program after a large study involving over 46,000 subjects clearly demonstrated that selenium supplementation would protect against the disease. The average daily unsupplemented selenium intake for women in these affected areas of China was estimated to be 12 μg Se/d (see Figure 1). This disease does not occur in the United States, where Se intakes are 5 to 15 times higher, and it is also unknown in New Zealand, another world area with low soil selenium, where intakes are approximately 30 μg Se/d.[14]

Human selenium deficiency can also occur clinically. The first report in 1979 was in a New Zealand patient undergoing total parental nutrition (TPN).[15] The patient lived in a rural area with low-selenium soils in which endemic white muscle disease in sheep was controlled by selenium dosing. Following surgery and TPN, she developed dry flaky skin and bilateral muscular discomfort and muscle pain. Plasma selenium had dropped to 0.11 μmol Se/L (9 μg Se/L) versus 0.32 μmol Se/L (25 μg Se/L) immediately before the start of TPN (Figure 1). The patient was then infused intravenously with a 100 μg Se/d. Within the next week, muscle pain disappeared and she returned to full mobility. Similar TPN-induced cases of muscle pain and cardiomyopathy leading to death have been reported in the United States. These cases are associated with very low plasma and red blood cell selenium and GPX1 activity, with elevated plasma marker enzymes indicative of tissue damage, and often with white nail beds.

Selenium deficiency in humans is often associated with other conditions. With Keshan disease, selenium supplementation is but one factor. An accompanying infection, perhaps viral, is associated with the development of actual Keshan disease.[13] Coxsackie virus has been isolated from Keshan disease patients, and recent animal experiments (see below) suggest that the virulence of a viral infection may be a influenced by selenium status. Selenium and iodine deficiency also exacerbate each other. In Zaire, a combined selenium and iodine deficiency contributes to the etiology of endemic myxedematous cretinism characterized by both thyroid enlargement and reduced intelligence. Administration of selenium alone appears to aggravate this disease by restoring selenium-dependent deiodinase activity, which in turn fosters increased synthesis and use of thyroxine and iodine, leading to exacerbated iodine deficiency.[16] This illustrates the danger of restoring one nutrient but not the entire diet, and it also illustrates the impact of combined nutrient deficiencies at the organism level.

A regional disease of unknown origin, called Kashin-Beck disease, continues to affect eight million individuals in regions of northern China consuming corn-based diets. This endemic disease of the cartilage occurs in preadolescent and adolescent children and is hypothesized to be associated with selenium deficiency. Unlike Keshan disease, however, selenium supplementation does not eliminate Kashin-Beck disease. Alternative hypotheses include mycotoxins, mineral imbalances, contamination of drinking water, and iodine deficiency.[17]

# Chemical Forms

Selenium is present in food and in the body in both inorganic and organic forms. Plants absorb inorganic selenium from the soil and metabolize selenium as though it was sulfur to form the amino acid selenomethionine (Figure 2), which has the selenium atom replacing the sulfur atom in methionine. Plants readily incorporate selenomethionine into proteins in place of methionine, and thus selenomethionine is the major form of selenium found in most plants.[18] A few species of plants specifically accumulate selenium as analogs of intermediates in sulfur amino acid metabolism, such as selenocystathionine and methylselenocysteine.

Inorganic forms of selenium, selenite ($SeO_3^{2-}$) and selenate ($SeO_4^{2-}$), are often used to supplement animal feed, and these forms of selenium are used in food supplements as well. Alternatively, selenium supplements from health food stores and some vitamin pills can contain selenium as selenized yeast; selenomethionine is the major form of selenium in selenized yeast. Most importantly, humans, animals, and many microorganisms also possess a unique metabolic pathway (see below) that specifically synthesizes selenocysteine, the selenium-containing analog of cysteine, for incorporation into selenoproteins. Selenocysteine is sometimes called the 21$^{st}$ amino acid, "Sec" is the three-letter code commonly used for selenocysteine, and "U" is the one-letter code for selenocysteine in protein sequences. Catabolism of selenomethionine or selenocysteine releases reduced inorganic selenium (as selenide, $HSe^-$), which can be reincorporated into selenoproteins, or can be methylated to form the excretory forms methyl selenol, or $CH_3SeH$; dimethyl selenide, or $(CH_3)_2Se$; trimethyl selenonium ion, or $(CH_3)_3Se^+$; and 1β-methylseleno-N-acetyl-D-galactosamine ($CH_3Se$-GalN).

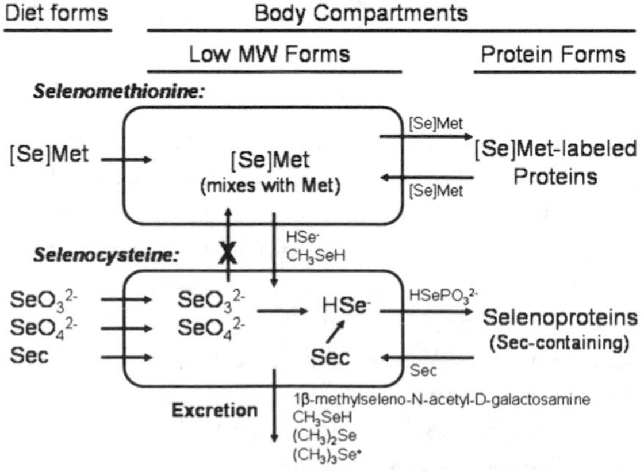


Figure 2. Two compartments of selenium metabolism. Entry points for dietary forms of selenium and the low molecular weight (MW) and protein forms of selenium are shown for the selenomethionine (top) and selenocysteine (bottom) compartments. Common compounds in these pools include selenomethionine ([Se]Met), selenocysteine (Sec), selenite ($SeO_3^{2-}$), selenate ($SeO_4^{2-}$), selenide ($HSe^-$) and selenophosphate ($HSePO_3^{2-}$). Excretory forms are 1β-methylseleno-N-acetyl-galactosamine, methyl selenol ($CH_3SeH$), dimethyl selenide ($(CH_3)_2Se$) and trimethyl selenonium ion ($(CH_3)_3Se^+$).

# Analytical Methods

Analytical methods commonly used today for selenium are precise and accurate, largely because of refined instrumentation, and technical expertise is required. The apparent large spread in published tissue and food selenium concentrations, in contrast, arises because of wide differences in selenium status due to geographical differences in soil selenium. Four methods are commonly used for selenium analysis. Fluorometric determination of selenium requires exacting chemical separations,[19] whereas neutron activation analysis is limited to collaboration with scientists at research reactors.[20] Atomic absorption spectroscopy using either hydride generation[21] or graphite furnace[22] is now the most common method for routine analysis. Improved instrumentation and availability suggests that inductively coupled plasma-mass spectroscopy[23] will increasingly provide reliable analysis of selenium in combination with analysis of other elements.

# Body Selenium

Estimates of total selenium content of humans, determined from cadavers, range between 13.0 and 20.3 mg. Metabolic stable isotope methodology models using US subjects predict that total body selenium asymptotically approaches 30 mg.[24] Individuals living in New Zealand or China with considerably lower selenium intakes thus will have a much lower total body burden of selenium. Muscle, liver, blood, and kidneys contain 61% of the estimated total body selenium in humans; if skeleton is included, this increases to 91.5%.[25]

The NHANES III survey found the mean serum selenium concentration of young adults (19–30 years of age) in the United States is 1.61 and 1.57 μmol Se/L

(127 and 124 μg/L) for males and females, respectively.[2] These values are quite similar to most earlier reports for North America. Tabulations of adult European serum or plasma selenium concentrations determined since 1990 range from 1.09 μmol Se/L (86 μg/L) in Sweden, France, and Italy, to 0.55 μmol Se/L (43 μg/L) in Serbia.[26] Adult concentrations in New Zealand in a recent group of subjects were reported to be 0.79 to 0.88 μmol Se/L (62–69 μg/L).[27] In contrast, subjects in low-selenium areas in China have plasma selenium concentrations of 0.14 to 0.20 μmol Se/L (11–16 μg/L).[13,28] A new tabulation of milk selenium concentrations indicates that human milk from mothers in Canada and the United States averages 0.19 to 0.25 μmol Se/L (15–20 μg/L), with selenium content in colostrum more than double, ranging from 0.42 to 1.02 μmol Se/L (33–80 μg Se/L).[2]

## Selenium Metabolism

### *Body Compartments*

The two major selenium compartments in the body are the unregulated selenomethionine compartment and the well-regulated selenocysteine/inorganic selenium compartment (Figure 2). These compartments reflect underlying metabolism and storage of selenium, and profoundly influence the selenium we find in food and measure in tissues. The key difference between these two compartments is that the selenocysteine compartment is homeostatically regulated by selenium status, whereas the selenomethionine compartment is not.

The selenomethionine compartment expands and contracts in proportion to selenomethionine intake. This is because selenomethionine cannot be synthesized from inorganic selenium by higher animals. In addition, mammalian enzymes do not differentiate between selenomethionine and methionine.[12] Dietary selenomethionine originating from plants, from animals fed selenomethionine, and from supplements such as selenized yeast mixes with the methionine pool and is incorporated into protein as a methionine analog according to protein needs, which are unrelated to selenium status.[29] The selenium in these selenomethionine-labeled proteins (Figure 2) is unavailable until the proteins turn over. Thus, individuals consuming foods with high selenomethionine content will have elevated tissue selenium levels that reflect elevated dietary selenomethionine. Tourists from New Zealand visiting the United States have profoundly increased levels of tissue selenium but not selenium-dependent enzymes, and these levels of selenium return to New Zealand levels upon their returned to their homeland.[14]

The selenocysteine compartment consists of the selenium in selenoproteins plus low molecular weight, inorganic forms of selenium (Figure 2). The selenium in mammalian selenoproteins is always present as selenocysteine. This compartment constitutes the biochemically active pool of selenium in the body, and regulation of the selenoproteins in this compartment appears to account for selenium homeostasis across a wide range of selenium intakes.

Exchange between these two compartments is only one-way. Catabolism of selenomethionine releases selenide via the transulfuration pathway or methyl selenol via the decarboxylase pathway.[12] These low-molecular-weight species then become part of the selenocysteine compartment.

### *Absorption*

Selenium homeostasis is clearly not regulated by absorption. Animals and humans readily digest proteins containing selenomethionine, and absorb the selenomethionine intact. Selenite, selenate, and selenomethionine are highly available, and selenium from selenocysteine-containing selenoproteins is also highly available. Numerous studies demonstrate absorption rates well above 50%; in one recent series of studies with large doses,[24] selenite and selenomethionine absorption from 200 μg selenium doses was 84% and 98%, respectively, illustrating that these high rates are real. Differences in availability of selenomethionine versus selenite have generally been reported to be small compared with day-to-day and individual-to-individual intake, but a recent study reported that selenomethionine was twice as available as selenite when given as daily single-tablet supplements to treat extremely selenium-deficient Chinese subjects.[30] Exceptionally low selenium availability (<10%) has been found for selenium in high-mercury tuna and in mushrooms, apparently due to complexed forms that are not available.

The enzymes/transporters responsible for absorption or movement of selenium across membranes are unknown. Selenomethionine is actively transported by the same systems that transport methionine.

### *Metabolism*

The intracellular metabolism of selenium is unique relative to other mineral nutrients because this trace "metal" bonds covalently to carbon. In addition, novel metabolic pathways are necessary to convert simple dietary forms of selenium into the selenocysteine moiety found in selenoproteins.

The central metabolism of selenium occurs within the selenocysteine compartment.[12] The conversion of dietary selenate and selenite to selenide ($HSe^-$) proceeds via a reductive pathway that now appears to be catalyzed by the selenoenzyme thioredoxin reductase.[1] Glutathione and glutathione reductase may also possibly catalyze this reduction. This reduction usually occurs in intestinal cells or in red blood cells, but also is readily accomplished in other tissues. Selenium released from selenomethionine catabolism also enters this pool as selenide (Figure 2).

Synthesis of selenocysteine occurs during protein synthesis, involves several unusual intermediates, and requires at least five unique gene products (four proteins/

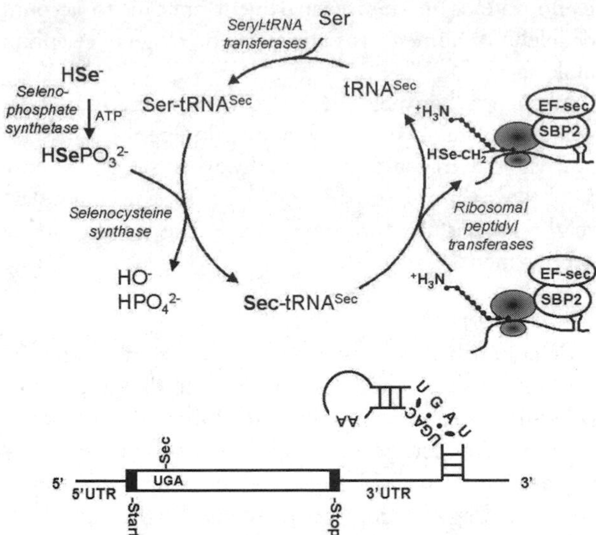


Figure 3. Selenocysteine (Sec) synthesis and incorporation during protein synthesis (top) and diagram of a typical selenoprotein gene (bottom). Top: Sec is synthesized co-translationally from serine (Ser) and selenide ($HSe^-$) while esterified to $tRNA^{sec}$ by the indicated enzyme activities. Bottom: diagram of typical selenoprotein mRNA showing the UGA codon in the coding region (open box) and the SECIS in the 3′UTR. Also shown are the consensus sequences in the SECIS stem-loop, including the loop AA and a typical non-Watson-Crick base-pair motif (UGAC/UGAU) that causes a 90-degree bend in the stem.

enzymes and a unique tRNA, $tRNA^{Sec}{}_{UCA}$) (Figure 3). In addition, each selenoprotein mRNA must contain two specific mRNA elements (a novel use of the UGA codon plus a unique SECIS element) for selenium incorporation to occur.[31] Selenoproteins are found in all three kingdoms (prokaryotic, eukaryotic, and archaea), and the mechanism of selenocysteine synthesis and incorporation is generally the same in all three kingdoms.[32] Much of what we know about mammalian selenoprotein synthesis was first characterized in bacteria.[33]

Synthesis of selenocysteine (Figure 3 ) starts with selenide and the formation of selenophosphate ($HSePO_3{}^{2-}$), which is the activated selenium compound used in the synthesis of selenoproteins. This reaction is catalyzed by selenophosphate synthetase using ATP.[34] Intact selenocysteine from the diet or from selenomethionine catabolism is not used for synthesis of selenoproteins. Instead, the amino acid serine provides the carbon skeleton for selenocysteine.[35] Serine, from the same cellular pool used for protein synthesis, is esterified to the 3′ terminal adenosine of $tRNA^{Sec}{}_{UCA}$ to form Ser-$tRNA^{Sec}{}_{UCA}$,[36] in a reaction catalyzed by the regular seryl-tRNA synthases. Next, the unique enzyme, selenocysteine synthase,[37] replaces the serine-OH with -SeH from selenophosphate to form selenocysteine-$tRNA^{Sec}{}_{UCA}$. Thus the synthesis of all selenocysteine occurs while the serine is esterified to the $tRNA^{Sec}{}_{UCA}$.

Selenocysteine is degraded by a selenium-specific enzyme, selenocysteine lyase,[38] which directly releases elemental selenium. This selenium is then reduced nonenzymatically to selenide by glutathione or other thiols. There is recent evidence that selenocysteine lyase may directly transfer selenium to selenophosphate synthase to facilitate reutilization.[38] This may enhance homeostatic selenium retention in selenium deficiency.

## *Excretion*

In rats, selenide is converted in liver to a selenosugar, 1β-methylseleno-N-acetyl-D-galactosamine ($CH_3$Se-GalN), which is the major urinary form under low to adequate selenium conditions.[39] Selenide can also be methylated using S-adenosylmethionine (SAM) by either microsomal or cytosolic methyl transferases to form methyl selenol, trimethyl selenonium ion, and dimethyl selenide.[12] Both the size of the dose and the selenium status of an animal influence the form and amount of urinary selenium excretion. Trimethyl selenonium constitutes only a small fraction of urinary selenium in rats with low selenium status, whereas it is the major urinary selenium form in animals ingesting super-nutritional levels of selenium.[25] When pharmacological doses of selenium are injected into rats, selenium is expired in the breath as dimethyl selenide; 50% of selenite selenium and 35% of selenomethionine selenium are expired as dimethyl selenide in the first 24 hours after rats are injected with 5 mg Se/kg body weight.

In humans, $CH_3$Se-GalN is likely to be the major urinary form of selenium under deficient and adequate conditions.[39] Following the administration of 200 μg of selenium to selenium-adequate adult humans, 17% and 11% of the selenium from tracer selenite and tracer selenomethionine, respectively, appears in the urine over the following 12 days; between 7% and 17% of urinary selenium is present as trimethyl selenonium ion.[24] Dimethyl selenide with a garlic-like odor may be detected in the breath of people ingesting high levels of selenium. Thus, under physiological conditions, selenium homeostasis is clearly not regulated by absorption, but, rather, urinary excretion is likely to be important for homeostasis.

## *Molecular Biology*

In all three kingdoms, the genes for selenoproteins employ a novel use of TGA, usually a termination codon, to encode selenocysteine.[40] These TGA codons reside within exons of the gene DNA, and thus result in in-frame UGA codons in the selenoprotein mRNA (Figure 3). Because UGA in mRNA routinely and unambiguously serves as a termination codon for many proteins, an additional RNA element in the 3′ untranslated region (3′UTR) of eukaryotic mRNAs is necessary for UGA-encoded selenocysteine incorporation. This element is called a eukaryotic SECIS element (for selenocysteine insertion sequence).[31] A single SECIS is used in most selenoproteins, but two SECIS elements are present in the 3′UTR of plasma selenoprotein P (SELP). The consensus SECIS element is a stem-loop structure with 10 to 19 unpaired bases including an AA sequence in the loop and a quartet of non-Watson and Crick base pairs, which results in over a 90-degree kink in the stem-loop.[41] Two additional forms of SECIS loops have been identified, and the specific secondary structure of the SECIS elements found in different selenoproteins may affect the rate of selenocysteine insertion.[42]

Two unique selenocysteine-specific elongation factors—SBP2 and EFSec—are also necessary for incorporation of UGA-encoded selenocysteine. EFSec is very specific for selenocysteine-$tRNA^{Sec}$,[43] and SBP2 binds the SECIS on the mRNA as well as EFSec and GTP.[44] These factors are thought to increase the concentration of the selenocysteine-tRNA on the mRNA.

These components assemble in a complex on the ribosome for co-translational selenocysteine incorporation (Figure 3 ). The SECIS is tethered via the 3′UTR to the mRNA, and the SBP2-GTP-EFSec-Sec-$tRNA^{Sec}$-mRNA complex is hypothesized to orient the selenocysteine at just the correct position to position the tRNA anti-codon to interact with the approaching UGA.[31] Peptide bond formation is then catalyzed by the ribosomal peptidyltransferase, resulting in the formation of a peptide bond between selenocysteine and the growing polypeptide chain. The location of the SECIS in the 3′UTR provides necessary spacing for orientation of the selenocysteine insertion complex; too short a distance between the UGA and the SECIS reduces or blocks efficient incorporation of selenocysteine.[31]

## Biochemical Functions

The logical role for selenium as a trace element is as a catalytic component in enzymes or proteins, and thus biochemical roles of selenium should arise as a consequence of the biological functions of these proteins. Almost all selenoproteins contain the selenocysteine in a variant of the CxxC redox motif, such as UxxT.[45] Knocking out the $tRNA^{Sec}{}_{UCA}$ gene is fatal, demonstrating that one or more selenoproteins are essential.[46] A newly discovered role for a selenoprotein in sperm is the only known structural role.

The absolute requirement of the molecular biology components (described above) for encoding and synthesizing selenoproteins has now been used to screen the human genome and other genomes for selenoproteins. A bioinformatics-based program called the SECIS-search protocol was developed and used by Vadim Gladyshev[3] to screen genomes for conserved SECIS elements. The newly identified SECIS elements were then compared with known SECIS elements in orthologous selenoprotein genes in rodents to refine the list. Next, upstream genomic sequences were screened for open reading frames that contained in-frame TGA codons. Lastly, these predicted human selenoprotein genes were further screened for homologs in other species that contained cysteine rather than selenocysteine. The result is that the entire human "selenoproteome" has now been identified[3] (Table 1). This is the first complete proteome to be identified for any nutrient, and it illustrates the powerful implications of genome science and bioinformatics.

**Table 1.** Human Selenoproteins in the Selenoproteome

| Abbr. | Selenoprotein |
|---|---|
| GPX1 | Classical glutathione peroxidase (GSH-Px) Chambers[47] |
| GPX2 | Gastrointestinal glutathione peroxidase (GPX-GI) Chu[52] |
| GPX3 | Plasma glutathione peroxidase (plasma GPX) Yoshimura[53] |
| GPX4 | Phospholipid hydroperoxide GPX (PHGPX) Pushpa-Rekha[54] |
| GPX6 | Glutathione peroxidase-6 Kryukov[3] |
| DI1 | Iodothyronine 5′-deiodinase-1 (Type I DI) Berry[55] |
| DI2 | Iodothyronine 5′-deiodinase-2 (Type II DI) St Germain[56] |
| DI3 | Iodothyronine 5-deiodination-3 (Type III DI) St. Germain[56] |
| TRR1 | Thioredoxin reductase-1 Gladyshev[57] |
| TRR2 | Thioredoxin reductase-2 Sun[58] |
| TRR3 | Thioredoxin reductase-3 Sun[58] |
| SPS2 | Selenophosphate synthetase-2 Guimaraes[59] |
| SELP | Plasma selenoprotein P Hill[60] |
| SELW | Muscle selenoprotein W Gu[61] |
| SELV | Selenoprotein V (paralog of SELW) Kryukov[3] |
| SEP15 | 15 kD selenoprotein Hatfield[1] |
| SELR | Methionine-R-sulfoxide reductase (MsrB1) Kim[62] |
| SELT | Selenoprotein T (18.8 kD, globular) Kryukov[63] |
| SELM | Selenoprotein M (localized to golgi, ER) Korotkov[64] |
| SELN | Selenoprotein N (47.5 kD) Lescure[65] |
| SELH | Selenoprotein H (globular) Kryukov[3] |
| SELI | Selenoprotein I (phosphotransferase) Kryukov[3] |
| SELK | Selenoprotein K (plasma membrane protein) Kryukov[3] |
| SELO | Selenoprotein O (globular) Kryukov[3] |
| SELS | Selenoprotein S (plasma membrane protein) Kryukov[3] |

### *Glutathione Peroxidase-1*

GPX was discovered in 1957 by Mills[47] in his search for factors that protect against oxidative damage to erythrocytes.[48] GPX was also the first protein shown to contain selenium[7] and the first cloned selenoprotein. There are now five identified selenium-containing GPXs, all with the UxxT redox motif. Classical GPX (GPX1) is the major form of selenium in the body, found in all tissues, and is estimated to account typically for more than 50% of total body selenium. Mitochondrial GPX arises from the GPX1 gene.[49] The selenocysteine is located at residue 47 of the 201 amino acid (23-kD) polypeptide chain, and selenocysteine is the active moiety in the enzyme reaction. GPX1 is potentially important because it not only destroys hydrogen peroxide, but also works on a number of hydroperoxides that might be produced during oxidant damage in the body. In the past decade, however, GPX1-knockout mice have been produced and have been found to display no effects on growth, reproduction, resistance to disease, etc.,[50] thus indicating that GPX1 does not have a critical role under normal conditions. It has been postulated that GPX1 functions as a biological selenium buffer that can be used to expand and store selenium before excretion mechanisms are activated.[12,51]

The work with the GPX1-knockout mouse has demonstrated two laboratory conditions where GPX1 activity is still important. GPX1-knockout mice are far more susceptible to acute paraquat toxicity, demonstrating that GPX1 activity can protect against the peroxides generated from this deleterious chemical.[66] Secondly a Coxsackie virus is more virulent in GPX1-knockout mice than in wild-type mice, just as in selenium-deficient versus selenium-adequate mice,[67] indicating a role for peroxidases or peroxides in this process (see below).

### *Glutathione Peroxidase-2*

GPX2 or GPX-GI was initially identified from a human liver cDNA library, but now is found to be the predominant GPX species in rat intestine.[52] This peroxidase is thought to be important in the protection of the intestine against external peroxides. GPX2-knock out mice are viable, indicating that both GPX1 and GPX2 functions appear redundant under normal conditions,[68] but double-knockout mice lacking GPX1 and GPX2 develop ileocolitis.[9]

### *Glutathione Peroxidase-3*

Plasma GPX3 arises from a distinct GPX3 gene,[53] and is predominantly secreted by human kidney. GPX3 normally accounts for 20% of plasma selenoproteins.[69] This secreted GPX3 is also the major form of selenium in milk,[70] and the role of GPX3 in milk may be to ensure that milk has adequate selenium levels. The function of GPX3 in plasma is unclear because of the low levels of circulating plasma GSH; it has been hypothesized that the major protective role of GPX3 may be in the intracellular spaces, especially in the kidney.[71]

### *Glutathione Peroxidase-4*

Phospholipid hydroperoxide GPX or GPX4 is unique in several aspects. This enzyme is active as a monomer rather than as a tetramer.[72] In addition, its more open, active site allows it to react with bulky hydroperoxides that are not substrates for the other peroxidases. GPX4 is also lipophilic and is postulated to roll along membranes and destroy peroxides.

GPX4 has been shown to account for the high concentration of selenium present in sperm and testis.[73] This GPX apparently is deposited as precipitated selenoenzyme during spermatogenesis, perhaps in response to elevated hydroperoxide production in the absence of sufficient glutathione to keep it reduced. The impact is that the enzyme GPX4 becomes a critical structural protein necessary for the integrity of sperm mid-piece. This may be the first case where we can identify a specific biochemical lesion that causes a selenium-deficiency disease, in this case sperm mid-piece breakage and male infertility. Knocking out GPX4 in mice is embryonically lethal.[74]

### *Glutathione Peroxidase-6*

GPX6 is an odorant-metabolizing protein, with about 40% amino acid sequence identity to GPX1, and appears to be expressed only in Bowman's gland of the rodent olfactory system. The screening of the human genome found that GPX6 in humans and swine is a selenoprotein, whereas orthologs in mice and rats contain Cys in place of selenocysteine.[3]

GPX7 is another member of the GPX family that so far has only been found as a Cys homolog. The function of these GPX homologs is especially unclear, as enzymatic activity of Cys as opposed to selenocysteine homologs are expected to differ dramatically.

### *Non-Selenium GPXs*

Several members of the GPX family with unknown function have been cloned and found to have a cysteine codon replacing the UGA codon,[12] including GPX5 in humans, which is androgen-regulated epididymal secretory protein that lacks a functional SECIS. The non-selenium dependent GPX activity found in the liver of selenium-deficient humans and animals is due to several of the glutathione-S-transferases.[75] Levels of this enzyme increase two-fold in selenium-deficient liver when GPX1 is fully depleted.

### *Iodothyronine Deiodinases*

Activation and metabolism of thyroid hormone requires a family of three selenoenzymes, the iodothyronine deiodinases (Table 1). Thyroxine 5′-deiodinase-1 (DI1) in liver is the major enzyme that converts thyroxine ($T_4$) to triiodothyronine ($T_3$), and is responsible for the majority of circulating plasma $T_3$ levels. In selenium deficiency, decreased DI1 activity results in lower $T_3$ levels, but compensatory feedback raises circulating $T_4$ levels such that hypothyroidism does not typically occur.[76] DI1 is a 249-amino acid (27-kD) polypeptide with a UGA encoding selenocysteine at residue 126 in a SxxU motif, and functions as a homodimer with a molecular weight of 55 kD.[55] Two additional selenium-dependent deiodinases, type II (DI2) and type-III (DI3), are also found in more specialized tissues.[56] DI2 is found in brain, pituitary, brown adipose tissue, placenta, and skin, and its principal physiological role is local, intracellular production of $T_3$. DI3 catalyzes the deiodination of the inner ring of $T_4$ and $T_3$.

DI3 activity levels are highest in adult brain, skin, and placenta, and in fetal liver, muscle, brain, and central nervous system. The role of DI3 is thought to protect against high levels of $T_4$ and $T_3$ by converting them to the inactive $rT_3$ and $T_2$, respectively.[31]

### Thioredoxin Reductases

Mammalian thioredoxin reductases (TRRs) are a family of three selenium-dependent enzymes that reduce small intracellular molecules, that regulate intracellular redox state, and that may have important roles in antioxidant defense and in control of cell cycling.[58] Only mammalian TRRs are selenoenzymes. These enzymes transfer reducing equivalents from NADPH through tightly bound FAD to disulfide in the enzyme, and then reduce thioredoxin or other species including selenite. TRRs are 57 kD-subunit (499-amino acid) selenoproteins that contain selenocysteine as the penultimate amino acid in a CU motif.[57] TRR1 is found in the cytosol and nucleus, whereas TRR2 is found in mitochondria. Selenium deficiency studies in rats have indicated that TRR activity is less affected by selenium deficiency than GPX1 activity, but more affected than plasma selenoprotein-P levels. Loss of TRR activity may be important in the development of the signs and symptoms of selenium deficiency. The discovery that TRR will reduce dehydroascorbate, ascorbate radical, and perhaps vitamin E offers a new potential antioxidant role for selenium.[77] In addition, TRRs offer a potential biochemical role to explain selenium's anticarcinogenic activity.[58]

### Plasma Selenoprotein P

Plasma selenoprotein P (SELP) is the major plasma selenoprotein and normally accounts for about 40% of plasma selenium.[8] Mature human SELP, secreted primarily from liver, contains 381 amino acids and is glycosylated, resulting in a molecular weight of approximately 57 kD.[60] Levels of SELP decrease in patients with liver disease, thus accounting for decreased plasma selenium in diseases with reduced liver function. SELP mRNA has 10 open reading frame UGAs and two SECIS stem loops. When selenium is limiting, early termination at the second UGA reduces the selenium content of SELP and results in a smaller circulating protein.

The SELP gene has now been knocked out in mice,[8] resulting in dramatic decreases in brain and testis selenium concentrations and increases in urinary selenium excretion, which is consistent with the role of SELP as a critical selenium transport protein. Mice lacking SELP develop a lack of coordination leading to paralysis and then death, indicating a critical role for selenium in neurological tissues, and further indicating the importance of delivering selenium to these tissues. Dietary administration of high levels of selenium will prevent these conditions. Knockout mice also have low fertility, and the males cannot be used for breeding even when they are supplemented with high-selenium diets. These studies with knockout mice thus make it clear that the function of SELP is to deliver selenium to important tissues. In addition, these animals provide models to study critical new roles for selenium in neurological function.

### Selenoprotein W

Selenoprotein W (SELW) is small (9.8-kD) selenoprotein found in muscle, which is also postulated to have antioxidant function.[61] The 87-amino acid polypeptide has a UGA-encoded selenocysteine at residue 13, but also can use UGA as a stop codon because the stop-UGA is too close to the SECIS to allow selenocysteine insertion.[31] The protein was definitively identified after a more than two-decade search for the selenium-dependent factor that would explain white muscle disease in selenium-deficient sheep.[5] mRNA levels indicate that SELW is abundant in muscle and brain of primate and sheep but not rodents. The role of SELW is unknown, but may involve the tightly bound GSH often isolated with purified SELW, and/or involve the CxU motif in a catalytic role.[1]

### Selenoprotein V

Selenoprotein V (SELV) is a paralog of SELW that was discovered in the SECIS search of the human genome. Expression of SELV mRNA is restricted to testis, where it occurs in the seminiferous tubules of mouse testis.

### Selenoprotein R or Methionine-R-Sulfoxide Reductase

Methionine sulfoxide is produced during oxidative attack of proteins, so methionine-sulfoxide reductases are an essential component in coping with oxidative stress. SELR encoded a small (12-kD) selenoprotein that contains zinc and reduces methionine-R-sulfoxide but not methionine-S-sulfoxide. SELR is now designated MsrB1.[62] Two other MsrB genes are present in mammalian genomes, but these MsrB genes contain cysteine rather than selenocysteine. An additional human gene, MsrA, encodes a cysteine-containing enzyme that is specific for methionine-S-sulfoxide.

### SEP15

A 15-kD selenoprotein, SEP15, was initially purified from human T-cells as a $^{75}$Se-labeled protein.[1] The gene for SEP15 is apparently universally expressed in mammalian cells, and may be involved in protein folding. The protein is differentially expressed in tumor cells, and single nucleotide polymorphisms in the SEP15 gene suggest that the allylic frequency may vary with susceptibility to cancer.

### Selenophosphate Synthetase-2

As discussed above, one of the mammalian selenophosphate synthetases, SPS2, is a selenocysteine-containing selenoprotein. SPS2 may use selenium from selenite reduction, whereas SPS1 appears to be associated with recycling selenium from selenocysteine.[78]

### *Selenoprotein T*

Selenoprotein T, discovered using the SECIS-search program, is a 182-amino acid globular selenoprotein with no known function.[63]

### *Selenoprotein M*

The discovery of SELM in a mammalian EST database led to the discovery in the 3'UTR of a second SECIS form with an AUGA...CC...GA motif. The N-terminal protein contains a signal peptide that locates the selenoprotein to the Golgi and endoplasmic reticulum, and SELM mRNA is present in multiple organs, especially in brain, kidney, and uterus.[64]

### *Selenoprotein N*

Selenoprotein N is a selenoprotein with no homology to any known protein.[65]

### *Selenoprotein H*

Selenoprotein (SELH) is a new globular selenoprotein with no known function. SELH was shown to be a selenoprotein by transfecting the gene into mammalian cells and demonstrating $^{75}$Se labeling of the expressed selenoprotein.[3]

### *Selenoprotein O*

Selenoprotein O (SELO) is another globular selenoprotein identified the using the SECIS search program. SELO is the largest human selenoprotein (669 residues), with a selenocysteine located three residues from the C terminus in a CxxU motif. The SECIS also has the AUGA...CC...GA motif.[3]

### *Selenoprotein I*

Selenoprotein I is another new selenoprotein identified by a SECIS search. SELI is homologous to human and yeast choline/ethanolamine phospho transferases, and has seven putative transmembrane domains.[3]

### *Membrane Selenoproteins K and S*

Selenoprotein K (SELK) and selenoprotein S (SELS) are newly identified selenoproteins that are unique because the amino acid sequence predicts that they are membrane proteins. GFP fusion constructs of SELK and SELS expressed in mammalian cells localize to the plasma membrane, indicating that these are the first demonstrated membrane selenoproteins. SELK and SELS mRNAs are found in a variety of mouse tissues.[3]

Selenoprotein S gene expression is increased by glucose deprivation and/or disturbances in the endoplasmic reticulum that generally cause the accumulation of misfolded proteins. Thus, SELS appears to be a novel member of the glucose-regulated protein family. Overexpression of SELS can significantly increase cell tolerance to oxidative stress, suggesting that it may have a role in regulating reactive oxygen species.[79]

The picture emerging from the evaluation of various genomes for selenoproteins reveals that the selenoproteins have a scattered phylogenetic distribution. Methionine-S-sulfoxide reductase (MsrA) occurs as a selenoprotein in *Chlamydomonas reinhardtii*, a green algae, but contains cysteine in vertebrates. A novel selenoprotein family, named SELU, was recently identified in the puffer fish, but mammals, worms, and land plants contain the cysteine homolog. Humans contain three separate genes in the SELU family, each encoding a cysteine-containing protein.[80] No selenoproteins have yet been found in yeast and land plants, but at least three selenoproteins have been found in insects.[81]

A new survey of bacterial genomes found in the Sargasso Sea identified 310 selenoprotein genes in 25 families, including 101 new selenoproteins. The sporadic distribution suggests that the many selenoproteins evolved recently from cysteine-containing homologs. In addition, eukaryotic and bacterial selenoprotein sets partially overlap, suggesting that lateral transfer of selenoprotein genes occurs across wide phylogenetic distances.[82]

## *Biochemical Role in Protection Against Viral Infection*

A series of exciting studies by Beck[83] have demonstrated that a virulent Coxsackie virus B3 (CVB3/20) that induces myocardial lesions in the hearts of mice is more virulent in selenium-deficient than in selenium-supplemented mice. Infection of mice with a benign amyocarditic Coxsackie virus B3 (CVB3/0), which causes no pathology in the hearts of selenium-adequate mice, induces extensive cardiac pathology in selenium-deficient mice. Most interestingly, the virus recovered from the hearts of selenium-deficient mice and inoculated into selenium-adequate mice induces significant heart damage. Characterization of the isolated virus indicates that the avirulent virus has mutated back to the wild-type genotype. The GPX1-knockout mouse also shows increased susceptibility to viral infection.[84] Notably, the same susceptibility to an avirulent Coxsackie virus also occurs in vitamin E-deficient mice, suggesting that protection is not limited to selenium-dependent proteins. Recent work suggests that selenium-deficient mice will also have increased susceptibility to other viral infections.[67] Along with Keshan disease, these studies add an anti-viral component to selenium's roles in preventing human disease.

A note of caution is warranted here. A number of reports show decreased levels of plasma selenium in patients with AIDS, and the suggestion has been made that nutritional selenium supplementation may be helpful.[26] Shisler et al.[85] found a human skin poxvirus, *Molluscum contagiosum*, that acquired in its genome a cDNA sequence for mammalian GPX1. The discoverers propose that the poxvirus expresses the captured mammalian GPX1 as a counter-measure against the host's anti-virus mechanisms, which include peroxidative stimulation of programmed cell death. This scenario thus suggests that indiscriminate supplementation of AIDS patients with selenium may aid the virus during infection by providing excess selenium for this pox GPX1, which in turn could block full activation of anti-virus mechanisms.

## Mechanism of Selenium Regulation

The 25 selenoproteins are all part of the well-regulated selenocysteine compartment and constitute a high percentage of total body selenium. The underlying mechanisms responsible for tight regulation of this compartment and thus responsible for the uniformity of dietary selenium requirements across species, are emerging in molecular biology studies conducted in laboratory animals and in cultured cells.[86] The effect of selenium status on multiple biochemical and molecular biology parameters in a single model is best characterized in detail in the rat. Selected response curves (Figure 4) illustrate the differential regulation of selenoprotein expression likely to also underlie human response to selenium status. These curves illustrate where changes in a biomarker such as plasma GPX3 reside in this hierarchy of responses.

In selenium-deficient male rats, liver GPX1 activities and mRNA levels can decrease to 1% and 7% of that of selenium-adequate animals.[87] In progressive selenium deficiency in rats, there is a coordinated exponential drop in GPX1 mRNA ($t_{1/2}$ = 3.2 d), GPX1 activity ($t_{1/2}$ = 3.3 d), and GPX1 protein ($t_{1/2}$ = 5.0 d).[88] When young, rapidly growing weanling rats are fed a selenium-deficient diet and supplemented with graded levels of selenium as $Na_2SeO_3$ for 28 days, liver GPX1 activity and mRNA levels respond sigmoidally to increasing dietary selenium concentration,[87,89] with GPX1 activity and mRNA reaching plateaus at 0.1 and 0.05 μg Se/g diet, respectively (Figure 4 ). At concentrations greater than 0.1 μg Se/g diet, selenium status no longer regulates either GPX1 mRNA or GPX1 activity. In contrast, liver GPX4 activity only decreases to 41% of selenium adequate levels and reaches a plateau at 0.05 μg Se/g diet; liver GPX4 mRNA is not significantly affected by dietary selenium. Plasma GPX3 activity in selenium-deficient rats is 7% to 8% of the levels found in selenium-adequate animals, and reaches a plateau at 0.07 μg Se/g diet,[89] such that when liver GPX1 mRNA is at the plateau, plasma GPX3 activity is about 75% of its plateau. In other studies, rat liver DI1, SELP, and TRR1 activities all decrease to 5% to 10% of selenium-adequate levels, but the corresponding mRNA levels are only modestly affected.[90-93] These experiments clearly show the tight regulation of selenoproteins by selenium status in mammalian species, and also illustrate clear differences in the regulation of individual selenoproteins.

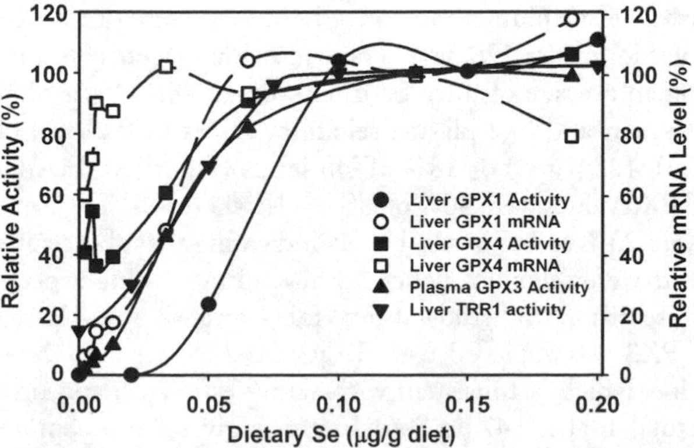


Figure 4. Response curves for GPX1, GPX4, GPX3 and TRR1 in rats. Weanling rats were fed the indicated levels of dietary selenium for 4 weeks. Shown are relative liver GPX1 activity and mRNA, liver GPX4 activity and mRNA, plasma GPX3 activity, and liver TRR1 activity (87,89,93). The hierarchy in terms of dietary selenium necessary to reach plateau levels (lowest to highest) is: GPX4 mRNA<GPX1 mRNA,GPX4 activity, TRR1 activity<GPX3 activity<GPX1 activity.

The novel changes in GPX1 mRNA occur because GPX1 mRNA concentration is regulated by mRNA stability; in selenium deficiency, GPX1 mRNA is specifically degraded by a process called non-sense-mediated decay.[94,95] Decreases in the levels of all selenoproteins in selenium deficiency appear to arise because of reduced protein synthesis when insufficient selenium and thus selenocysteine is available.[86] In addition, potential effects of age, pregnancy, lactation, and gender may affect selenoprotein transcription unrelated to selenium status,[92] and should be considered when evaluating selenoprotein markers for the assessment of selenium status. With the sequencing of the human genome and the development of array approaches, mRNA-based evaluation of nutrient status will likely become a common approach, so selenoprotein mRNA levels will likely become useful parameters for assessing human selenium status in the future.

## Requirements

The earlier sections in this chapter have discussed a number of direct and indirect measures that could be used to determine selenium status and requirements. Tissue concentration, a measure often used for other nutrients, is particularly unsuitable for selenium because the unregulated selenomethionine compartment reflects selenomethionine intake, not selenium status. In contrast, early studies using biochemical assays in laboratory animals suggest that selenoenzyme expression is highly regulated by selenium status and is very useful for assessing status and requirements.

The current Recommended Dietary Allowance (RDA) requirement for selenium is one of two human dietary requirements for mineral elements that is based on a biochemical parameter[2] as opposed to diet assessment, balance studies, tissue mineral content, etc. This illustrates the importance of selenium regulation of GPX expression. In 1980, an initial estimated safe and adequate daily dietary intake for humans of 50 to 200 μg Se/d was proposed, based upon extrapolation from animal experiments that used GPX activity to assess selenium status.[96]

Balance studies to determine selenium requirements are of little help, because selenium's homeostatic mechanisms permit human subjects to come to balance between 9 and 200 μg Se/d[24,97] by adjusting urinary excretion to match intakes. In 1989, the Food and Nutrition Board of the US Institute of Medicine (FNB) set an RDA of 70 and 55 μg Se/d for North-American males and females, respectively.[98]

## *2000 RDA*

The FNB in 2000[2] reevaluated plasma GPX3 activity data from a study in Chinese men with very low basal selenium intakes (about 10 μg Se/d) who were supplemented with graded levels of selenium. Groups supplemented with 30 μg Se/d or higher (a total of 40 μg Se/d) reached plateau levels of plasma GPX3 activity, indicating that 40 μg Se/d was the minimum requirement. Adjusting this value for the standard weight of North-American males, the Board estimated a minimal selenium requirement for maximal plasma GPX3 of 52 μg Se/d.[2]

The FNB also reevaluated a second study from New Zealand[27] that used 52 subjects consuming an average of 28 μg Se/d and supplemented with 0 to 40 μg Se as selenomethionine. The authors concluded that the plateau in plasma GPX3 activity was reached at a total intake (diet plus supplement) of 58 or 68 μg Se/d, but the Board's independent analysis of the data[2] found that plasma GPX3 activity increased for nearly every individual supplemented with selenium. Furthermore, differences between groups in plasma GPX3 activity were small relative to the variations between individual values within the same supplementation group, such that the increase in the lowest supplementation group (38 μg total Se/d) was not statistically different from that of the highest supplementation group (68 μg Se/d). Thus, the FNB conservatively concluded that these data could only support an Estimated Average Requirement (EAR) of 38 μg Se/d. The FNB used an average of the these two studies to choose an EAR of 45 μg Se/d for men. Because Keshan disease suggests that women have a greater susceptibility to selenium deficiency, an EAR of 45 μg Se/d was retained for women in spite of smaller body weight. The RDA, based on this average EAR, was calculated to be 55 μg Se/d for North-American men and women. An Adequate Intake (AI) was estimated to be 15 and 20 μg Se/d for babies under 6 and 12 months, respectively, based on typical human milk selenium levels. Estimates for children of other ages were extrapolated from the adult values. Human EAR and RDA during pregnancy were estimated to be 49 and 60 μg Se/d, based on calculated fetal selenium deposition of 4 μg Se/d, and human EAR and RDA during pregnancy were estimated to be 59 and 70 μg Se/d, based on an estimated additional need of 14 μg Se/d for selenium deposition in milk.[2]

The RDA for selenium in the United States, however, may be high. Comparison of dietary selenium intakes in adult Chinese populations in areas susceptible to Keshan disease versus areas seemingly protected, suggests a protective level of 21 μg Se/d for 65-kg males and 16 μg/d for 55-kg females.[99] New Zealand estimates of daily selenium intakes that are not associated with any selenium deficiency symptoms suggest that 33 and 23 μg/d for men and woman, respectively, are adequate.[14] In addition, it is clear that daily selenium consumption in the rest of the world is well below the 2000 RDA recommendations without apparent adverse impact on health.

## *World Health Organization Requirement*

The World Health Organization (WHO) proposed a new approach to evaluate selenium requirements, again based on plasma GPX3 activity as the biochemical parameter, by selecting a normative requirement for selenium calculated by estimating the dietary intake needed to achieve two-thirds of the maximum attainable activity of GPX3[99]: 26 μg Se/d for a 65-kg male. Further adjustment for 16% interindividual variation results in a calculated 40 μg Se/d for adult males and 30 μg Se/d for adult females as lower limits of the safe range of population mean intakes.[99]

These WHO requirements are still below the 2000 RDA recommendations, but are far more in line with typical selenium consumption worldwide. When the authors of the New Zealand study[27] used a criterion of 67% of maximal GPX3 activity to establish a requirement, this approach yielded a normative requirement of 39 μg Se/d, almost identical to the WHO normative requirement. Additional studies to determine the nature of human selenium response curves, similar to those in Figure 4, should help to link selenium requirements more closely to the underlying homeostatic mechanisms.

## *Human Requirements Based on SELP*

A new study has further carefully evaluated the human selenium requirement in selenium-deficient subjects in China[30]; 120 subjects were supplemented with graded levels of selenium up to 66 μg Se/d as selenite or selenomethionine for 120 days. These individuals were consuming an average of 9 μg Se/d for women and 11 μg Se/d for men and had plasma selenium values of 0.28 μmol Se/L (22 μg/L) or 18% of US levels (Figure 3). Plasma GPX3 values were 40% of US levels, whereas SELP levels were 23% of US levels, clearly indicating that these subjects were selenium deficient. Several interesting aspects arose from this study. First, full expression of plasma GPX3 was achieved with 37 μg Se/d as selenomethionine, which is consistent with earlier estimates, and thus a total intake of 47 μg Se/d. Interestingly, selenite supplementation in this study required 66 μg Se/d to achieve plateau levels, clearly indicating a dramatic difference in the bioavailability of inorganic selenite selenium compared with selenomethionine selenium in these subjects when provided in as a single dietary pill per day. Plasma SELP levels were also very low, but continued to increase with increasing dietary selenium at all levels of Se, indicating that apparent US plateau levels could not be achieved for plasma SELP.

Because SELP appears to be a transport form of selenium, it is not clear whether this indicates that selenium supplementation as high as 66 μg Se/d is suboptimal in these subjects, or that these initially selenium-deficient subjects were still not at steady-state, or that the SELP transport protein cannot be saturated at these levels. Whatever the case, it is clear that supplementation in acutely selenium-deficient individuals over 120 days is not sufficient to raise selenium parameters up to those seen in Americans consuming 98 to 145 μg Se/d.

## Dietary Sources

There is a wide range in selenium content in soils, and thus the selenium content in foods of plant origin varies widely. Cereals and grains range from <0.1 to >0.8 μg Se/g, and fruits and vegetables are typically <0.1 μg Se/g.[99] Corn, rice, and soybeans grown in a areas of China where Keshan disease is prevalent had 0.005, 0.007, and 0.010 μg Se/g, respectively, whereas in a seleniferous area in China they had 8.1, 4.0, and 11.9 μg Se/g, respectively.[100] Selenium content of livestock animals will similarly be affected. Organ meats and seafood can range 0.4 to 1.5 μg Se/g, muscle meats 0.1 to 0.4 μg Se/g, and dairy products <0.1 to 0.3 μg Se/g.[99] Thus, handbook values for selenium in foods reflecting average content should be considered unreliable unless confirmed by actual analysis.[2] As livestock in the United States are typically supplemented with inorganic selenium, animal products will usually contain substantial selenium as selenoproteins and thus as selenocysteine. Thus, the range in selenium content of animal products reflects variations in selenomethionine content of the feedstuffs.

Dietary supplements and foods today are often supplemented with selenium. Inorganic selenium, generally selenite and sometimes selenate, is used most commonly, but selenized yeast or selenomethionine is also used. Supplementation levels are typically under 100 μg Se/pill, such that total selenium intakes will still be <250 μg Se/d based on reported average US intakes. The impact of supplements on daily dietary selenium intake was <3% in the NHANES III study.[2]

Drinking water usually has negligible selenium content. Well waters in seleniferous areas in Wyoming and South Dakota can contain much higher levels.[101]

## Vitamin E

Vitamin E and selenium have been inexorably linked since of the discovery that selenium would prevent liver necrosis. Interest remains high because of the links between reactive oxygen species and aging. The overlapping roles of these two nutrients are illustrated by seminal studies comparing the efficacy of selenium and vitamin E in preventing lipid peroxidation, as measured by volatile gas evolution and formation of F2-isoprostanes, and in modulating Coxsackie virus virulence (see above). Unfortunately, direct evidence linking vitamin E and selenium to aging remains tenuous. As discussed above, selenium-dependent TRR may be important in vitamin E recycling.[77]

Early studies showed that combined selenium and vitamin E deficiency (double deficiency) results in elevated levels of tissue malondialdehyde, which arises from the free radical attack on polyunsaturated fatty acids. More specific indicators of peroxidation, ethane and pentane evolution in the breath, are due to peroxidative breakdown of Ω-3 or Ω-6 unsaturated fatty acids, respectively. Ethane and pentane evolution is minimized by vitamin E alone, and partially reduced by 0.2 μg Se/g diet alone to 40% of the rate in doubly-deficient rats.[102]

$F_2$-isoprostanes are an exciting new marker of in vivo peroxidation. These prostaglandin $F_2$-like compounds result from the free radical-catalyzed peroxidation of arachidonic acid in vivo. These $F_2$-isoprostanes are found esterified to phospholipids in tissues and are also found as free $F_2$-isoprostanes in plasma. Plasma $F_2$-isoprostanes in rats fed a double vitamin E/selenium-deficient diet are 5-fold higher than animals fed the control diet. Selenium deficiency alone is not associated with the production of $F_2$-isoprostanes, but the plasma $F_2$-isoprostane level is twice that of control rats in the vitamin E-deficient alone group. $F_2$-isoprostanes present in phospholipids in various tissues also show similar results, with selenium deficiency exacerbating vitamin E deficiency in most tissues, whereas selenium deficiency alone is without effect compared with rats adequate in vitamin E and selenium.[103]

## Toxicity

Selenium was first known as a toxic element, due to high soil levels resulting in the accumulation of selenium in plants, which then caused chronic and acute toxicity in livestock.[5] The range of dietary selenium concentrations that are adequate and yet not toxic is very narrow. In rats, while the minimum dietary requirement is 0.1 μg Se/g diet, dietary levels above 2 μg Se/g diet are chronically toxic, resulting in a factor of 20 between the requirement and the onset of toxicity. Inorganic selenium and amino acid forms are readily available and toxic, whereas methylated forms such as trimethyl selenonium chloride and dimethyl selenide are one to three orders of magnitude, respectively, less toxic. The gas hydrogen selenide is the most toxic form of selenium. There is no evidence for the existence of homeostatic mechanisms to decrease selenium uptake under toxic dietary conditions.[12]

The biochemical mechanism underlying selenium toxicity is unknown. In one known case, inorganic selenium inactivates eukaryotic initiation factor-2α,[104] but further details are not known.

In humans, modest selenium intakes (<800 μg Se/d) are clearly not toxic.[105] In seleniferous regions of the

United States (South Dakota and Wyoming), a study evaluating 142 subjects consuming as much as 724 μg Se/d found no evidence of selenium toxicity. Consumption of well water, with inorganic selenium levels as much as 50 times the US drinking water standard of 10 μg Se/L, results in increased urinary selenium but without increased blood selenium content, illustrating that blood selenium cannot be used as a good marker for high selenium intakes.[101]

There are only a few reports in the literature of fatal or near-fatal acute selenium poisoning, and these are associated with ingestion of gun blueing or sheep drench solutions.[2] Ingestion of gram quantities of selenium, for which there is no ready antidote, can result in severe gastrointestinal and neurological disturbance, acute respiratory distress syndrome, myocardial infarction, and renal failure. Selenosis, or chronic selenium toxicity, is associated most commonly in humans with changes in nail structure and loss of nails and hair.[2] With continuous intakes and higher doses of excess selenium, symptoms can include lesions of the skin and nervous system, nausea, weakness and diarrhea, and mottling of the teeth. These toxicity symptoms are present with selenium intakes ranging from 3200 to 6700 μg Se/d. Milder morphological changes in the fingernails also will occur in individuals consuming an average of 1260 μg Se/d.[105,106]

A study conducted in a seleniferous region of China continues to be used to calculate the no-observed-adverse-effect level (NOAEL) for selenium, using nail morphology as the endpoint. Mildly prolonged prothrombin times and reduced glutathione concentrations were observed in these Chinese subjects, but were not found to be reliable indicators of selenosis. A lowest observed adverse effect was found at 913 μg Se/d, with 853 μg Se/d being the level calculated to not be accompanied by adverse effects.[106] Based on these studies, the FNB has recently selected a NOAEL of 800 μg Se/d.[2] Using an uncertainty factor of two, this results in a tolerable upper intake level (UL) of 400 μg Se/d for adults, including pregnant and lactating women.

Selenium intoxication due to misformulation of supplements can also occur. In the early 1980s, 13 people were identified who had been taking over-the-counter dietary selenium supplements containing 27.3 mg Se/tablet (182 times higher than the amount specified on the label). One individual took one pill a day for a 2.5-month period in spite of symptoms of selenium toxicity.[107]

Selenium is especially toxic to waterfowl. The Kesterson Reservoir, located in the San Joaquin Valley, gained considerable notoriety in the 1980s for environmental selenium toxicity. A high incidence of dead and deformed newborn and adult waterfowl was observed at the reservoir, and selenium was identified as the probable cause. The origin of the selenium was the high-selenium soils that led to an average concentration of 350 μg Se/L in the runoff, and further concentrated in the reservoir.[108] This toxicity is specific to birds, apparently because embryos in the egg have limited ability to excrete the selenium.

# Cancer

The association between dietary selenium and cancer protection began in the 1960s and 1970s[6] with the observation that country-by-country selenium intakes were inversely associated with cancer incidence. There is considerable evidence that selenium supplementation at levels that are chronically toxic (2–5 μg Se/g diet) will decrease the tumor incidence in several animal models.

Excitement about selenium's anti-carcinogenic role rose in the 1980s were due to a retrospective study using prediagnostic serum selenium concentrations.[109] Subjects in the lowest quintile of serum selenium concentration had a cancer risk that was twice as high as those in the highest quintile. Biologically, however, there was little difference in the average serum selenium values in cancer versus non-cancer subjects (129 vs. 136 μg Se/L). A number of additional studies have since also concluded that low selenium status is associated with increased cancer incidence,[26] although at least six case-controlled, prospective studies using tissue selenium and breast cancer incidence have provided no evidence for a protective effect of selenium.[110] A clear impact of selenium, however, was observed in a prospective study of 33,700 men on selenium status and prostate cancer incidence, with men in the lowest quintile of selenium status (as assessed by toenail selenium) having three times the risk of developing advanced prostate cancer as those in the highest selenium status quintile.[111] Collectively, these studies suggest that subjects who self-select foods with lower selenium content have a higher risk of developing cancer.

Two recent intervention trials have further drawn attention to selenium and cancer. A randomized trial with 1312 patients with histories of basal cell or squamous cell carcinomas of the skin were supplemented with either an oral supplement of 200 μg Se/d or a placebo.[112] Selenium supplementation did not significantly reduce the primary endpoints of incidence of new basal or squamous cell carcinoma of the skin, and actually significantly increased the risk of squamous cell carcinoma (25%) and total non-melanoma skin cancer (17%).[113] In the initial analysis,[112] however, selenium treatment was associated with a statistically significant reduction in several secondary endpoints that were not the focus of the study (total and lung cancer mortality, total cancer incidence, colon rectal cancer, and prostate cancer incidence); total cancer incidence was 42% lower in the selenium group ($P < 0.001$).[112] Analysis of the complete study,[114] however, found that selenium supplementation reduced total cancer and prostate cancer risk but not lung and colorectal cancer incidence, and the cancer-protective effect was confined to males. Furthermore, only subjects with plasma selenium levels in the lowest two tertiles at entry into the trial (<1.54 μmol Se/L or <121.6 μg/L) experienced total reduction in cancer incidence, whereas those in the highest tertile showed an elevated incidence.[114]

Randomized nutrition intervention trials involving

nearly 30,000 participants over 5 years were conducted in a rural county in north central China. These studies found a small but significant reduction in total mortality in subjects receiving a combination of 15 mg β-carotene, 50 μg Se as selenized yeast, and 30 mg α-tocopherol, whereas no appreciable effects were found for other supplements, which included retinol, zinc, riboflavin, niacin, ascorbate, and molybdenum.[115]

Collectively, these studies in humans and animals indicate an overall inverse relationship between cancer risk and selenium status. US prospective studies using supplementation of 200 μg Se/d support a hypothesis that supplemental selenium above the levels needed to maximize selenoprotein levels is beneficial in reducing cancer risk, especially for prostate cancer. This hypothesis is especially intriguing for residents of countries with selenium intakes that will not maximize selenium incorporation into all selenoproteins.[26] However, at this time, small sample sizes, other confounding factors, and potential for excess selenium supplementation to raise cancer risk collectively do not allow use of these studies as the basis to set a higher RDA.[2]

## Future Directions

The identification of the complete selenoproteome in humans using molecular biology and bioinformatics approaches shows that a full understanding of selenium's role in health and disease is just around the corner. Continued use of knockout animals and genome-based discovery of inborn errors of selenium metabolism have promise in identifying the specific roles of selenium in protection against human and animal diseases. Identification of the transporters involved in selenium absorption and excretion, and characterization of the regulation of selenium excretion are needed to more fully understand selenium homeostasis. A complete characterization of patterns of regulation of selenoprotein expression in humans by selenium status, including regulation of mRNA levels, is needed to better identify the optimum parameter(s) for use as biomarkers for establishing human selenium requirements and for use in individualized medicine. Similarly, fuller characterization of the pathways activated in selenium toxicity are needed so that good biomarkers of selenium toxicity can be identified. The impact of selenium deficiency and selenium supplementation on viral infection, including AIDS, should be assessed. Lastly, results from ongoing large trials are needed, both in the United States and in other countries, to directly answer the question about cancer and higher levels of selenium supplementation.

## References


1. Hatfield DL. *Selenium: Its Molecular Biology and Role in Human Health.* Norwood, MA: Kluwer Academic Publishers; 2001.
2. Food and Nutrition Board, Institute of Medicine. *Selenium. Dietary Reference Intakes for Vitamin C, Vitamin E, Selenium and Carotenoids.*Washington, DC: National Academies Press; 2000:284–324.
3. Kryukov GV, Castellano S, Novoselov SV, et al. Characterization of mammalian selenoproteins. Science. 2003;300:1439–1443.
4. Schwarz K, Foltz CM. Selenium as an integral part of factor 3 against dietary necrotic liver degeneration. J Am Chem Soc. 1957;79:3292–3293.
5. National Research Council. *Selenium in Nutrition.* Washington, DC: National Academies Press; 1983.
6. National Research Council. *Diet, Nutrition, and Cancer.* Washington, DC: 1982.
7. Rotruck JT, Pope AL, Ganther HE, Swanson AB, Hafeman DG, Hoekstra WG. Selenium: biochemical role as a component of glutathione peroxidase. Science. 1973;179:588–590.
8. Burk RF, Hill KE. Selenoprotein P: An extracellular protein with unique physical characteristcs and a role in selenium homeostasis. Annu Rev Nutr. 2005;25:215–235.
9. Esworthy RS, Yang L, Frankel P, Chu F. The role of epithelium-specific glutathione peroxidase, GPX2, in prevention of intestinal inflammation in selenium-deficient mice. J Nutr. 2005;135:740–745.
10. Whitacre ME, Combs GF, Combs SB, Parker RS. Influence of dietary vitamin E on nutritional pancreatic atrophy in selenium-deficient chicks. J Nutr. 1987;117:460–467.
11. Thompson KM, Haibach H, Sunde RA. Growth and plasma triiodothyronine concentrations are modified by selenium deficiency and repletion in second-generation selenium-deficient rats. J Nutr. 1995;125:864–873.
12. Sunde RA. Selenium. In: O'Dell BL, Sunde RA, eds. *Handbook of Nutritionally Essential Mineral Elements.* New York: Marcel Dekker; 1997: 493–556.
13. Chen X, Yang G, Chen J, Wen Z, Ge K. Studies on the relations of selenium and Keshan Disease. Biol Tr Elem Res. 1980;2:91–107.
14. Robinson MF, Thomson CD. The role of selenium in the diet. Nutr Abst Rev. 1983;53:3–26.
15. van Rij AM, Thomson CD, McKenzie JM, Robinson MF. Selenium deficiency in total parenteral nutrition. Am J Clin Nutr. 1979;32:2076–2085.
16. Vanderpas JB, Contemprë B, Duale NL, et al. Selenium deficiency mitigates hypothyroxinemia in iodine-deficient subjects. Am J Clin Nutr. 1993;57: 271S–275S.
17. Moreno-Reyes R, Mathieu F, Boelaert M, et al. Selenium and iodine supplementation of rural Tibetan children affected by Kashin-Beck osteoarthropathy. Am J Clin Nutr. 2003;78:137–144.
18. Beilstein MA, Whanger PD. Deposition of dietary

organic and inorganic selenium in rat erythrocyte proteins. J Nutr. 1986;116:1701–1710.

19. Watkinson JH. Fluorometric determination of selenium in biological material with 2,3-diaminonaphthalene. Anal Chem. 1966;38:92–6.
20. McKown DM, Morris JS. Rapid measurement of selenium in biological samples using instrumental neutron activation analysis. J Radioanal Chem. 1978;43:409–418.
21. Hahn MH, Kuennen RW, Caruso JA, Fricke FL. Determination of trace amounts of selenium in corn, lettuce, potatoes, soybeans, and wheat by hydride generation of condensation and flame atomic absorption spectrometry. J Agric Food Chem. 1981; 29:792–796.
22. Henn EL. Determination of selenium in water and industrial effluents by flameless atomic absorption. Anal Chem. 1975;47:428.
23. Chan S, Gerson B, Reitz RE, Sadjadi SA. Technical and clinical aspects of spectrometric analysis of trace elements in clinical samples. Clin Lab Med. 1998;18:615–629.
24. Swanson AB, Patterson BH, Levander OA, et al. Human selenomethionine metabolism: a kinetic model. Amer J Clin Nutr. 1991;54:917–926.
25. Sunde RA. Selenium. In: Stipanuk MH, ed. Biochemical and Physiological Aspects of Human Nutrition. New York: W.B. Sanders; 2000:782–809.
26. Rayman MP. The importance of selenium to human health. Lancet. 2000;356:233–241.
27. Duffield AJ, Thomson CD, Hill KE, Williams S. An estimation of selenium requirements for New Zealanders. Am J Clin Nutr. 1999;70:896–903.
28. Sunde RA, Gutzke GE, Hoekstra WG. Effect of dietary methionine on the biopotency of selenite and selenomethionine in the rat. J Nutr. 1981;111: 76–86.
29. Waschulewski IH, Sunde RA. Effect of dietary methionine on tissue selenium and glutathione peroxidase activity in rats fed selenomethionine. Br J Nutr. 1988;60:57–68.
30. Xia Y, Hill KE, Byrne DW, Xu J, Burk RF. Effectiveness of selenium supplements in a low-selenium area of China. Am J Clin Nutr. 2005;81:829–834.
31. Low SC, Berry MJ. Knowing when not to stop: selenocysteine incorporation in eukaryotes. Trends Biochem Sci. 1996;21:203–208.
32. Wilting R, Schorling S, Persson BC, Böck A. Selenoprotein synthesis in archaea: identification of an mRNA element of Methanococcus jannaschii probably directing selenocysteine insertion. J Mol Bio. 1997;266:637–641.
33. Stadtman TC. Selenocysteine. Annu Rev Biochem. 1996;65:83–100.
34. Low SC, Harney JW, Berry MJ. Cloning and functional characterization of human selenophosphate synthetase, an essential component of selenoprotein synthesis. J Biol Chem. 1995;270:21659–21664.
35. Sunde RA, Evenson JK. Serine incorporation into the selenocysteine moiety of glutathione peroxidase. J Biol Chem. 1987;262:933–937.
36. Hatfield DL, Choi IS, Ohama T, Jung J-E, Diamond AM. Selenocysteine $tRNA^{[Ser]Sec}$ isoacceptors as central components in selenoprotein biosynthesis in eukaryotes. In: Burk RF, ed. *Selenium in Biology and Human Health*. New York: Springer-Verlag New York, Inc.; 1994:25–44.
37. Tormay P, Wilting R, Lottspeich F, Mehta PK, Christen P, Böck A. Bacterial selenocysteine synthase—structural and functional properties. Eur J Biochem. 1998;254:655–661.
38. Mihara H, Kurihara T, Watanabe T, Yoshimura T, Esaki N. cDNA cloning, purification, and characterization of mouse liver selenocysteine lyase. Candidate for selenium delivery protein in selenoprotein synthesis. J Biol Chem. 2000;275:6195–6200.
39. Kobayashi Y, Ogra Y, Ishiwata K, Takayama H, Aimi N, Suzuki KT. Selenosugars are key and urinary metabolites for selenium excretion within the required to low-toxic range. Proc Natl Acad Sci. 2002;99:15932–15936.
40. Kryukov GV, Gladyshev VN. The prokaryotic selenoproteome. EMBO Rep. 2004;5:538–543.
41. Walczak R, Carbon P, Krol A. An essential non-Watson-Crick base pair motif in 3'UTR to mediate selenoprotein translation. RNA. 1998;4:74–84.
42. Grundner-Culemann E, Martin GW III, Harney JW, Berry MJ. Two distinct SECIS structures capable of directing selenocysteine incorporation in eukaryotes. RNA. 1999;5:625–635.
43. Tujebajeva RM, Copeland PR, Xu XM, et al. Decoding apparatus for eukaryotic selenocysteine insertion. EMBO Rpts. 2000;1:158–163.
44. Copeland PR, Fletcher JE, Carlson BA, Hatfield DL, Driscoll DM. A novel RNA binding protein, SBP2, is required for the translation of mammalian selenoprotein mRNAs. EMBO J. 2000;19:306–314.
45. Fomenko DE, Gladyshev VN. Identity and functions of CxxC-derived motifs. Biochem. 2003;42: 11214–11225.
46. Bosl MR, Takaku K, Oshima M, Nishimura S, Taketo MM. Early embryonic lethality caused by targeted disruption of the mouse selenocysteine tRNA gene (*Trsp*). Proc Natl Acad Sci USA. 1997;94: 5531–5534.
47. Chambers I, Frampton J, Goldfarb PS, Affara N, McBain W, Harrison PR. The structure of the mouse glutathione peroxidase gene: the selenocysteine in the active site is encoded by the 'termination' codon, TGA. EMBO J. 1986;5:1221–1227.
48. Mills GC. Hemoglobin catabolism. I. Glutathione

peroxidase, an erythrocyte enzyme which protects hemoglobin from oxidative breakdown. J Biol Chem. 1957;229:189–197.
49. Esworthy RS, Ho YS, Chu FF. The *Gpx1* gene encodes mitochondrial glutathione peroxidase in the mouse liver. Arch Biochem Biophys. 1997;340: 59–63.
50. Ho YS, Magnenat JL, Bronson RT, et al. Mice deficient in cellular glutathione peroxidase develop normally and show no increased sensitivity to hyperoxia. J Biol Chem. 1997;272:16644–16651.
51. Sunde RA. Intracellular glutathione peroxidases - structure, regulation and function. In: Burk RF, ed. *Selenium in Biology and Human Health, 5 ed.* New York, NY: Springer-Verlag; 1994:45–77.
52. Chu F-F, Doroshaw JH, Esworthy RS. Expression, characterization, and tissue distribution of a new cellular selenium-dependent glutathione peroxidase, GSH-Px-GI. J Biol Chem. 1993;268:2571–2576.
53. Yoshimura S, Suemizu H, Taniguchi Y, Arimori K, Kawabe N, Moriuchi T. The human plasma glutathione peroxidase-encoding gene: organization, sequence and localization to chromosome 5q32. *Gene.* 1994;145:293–297.
54. Pushpa-Rekha TR, Burdsall AL, Oleksa LM, Chisolm GM, Driscoll DM. Rat phospholipid-hydroperoxide glutathione peroxidase: cDNA cloning and identification of multiple transcription and translation start sites. J Biol Chem. 1995;270: 26993–26999.
55. Berry MJ, Banu L, Larsen PR. Type I iodothyronine deiodinase is a selenocysteine-containing enzyme. Nature. 1991;349:438–440.
56. St.Germain DL, Galton VA. The deiodinase family of selenoproteins. Thyroid. 1997;7:655–668.
57. Gladyshev VN, Jeang KT, Stadtman TC. Selenocysteine, identified as the penultimate C-terminal residue in human T-cell thioredoxin reductase, corresponds to TGA in the human placental gene. Proc Natl Acad Sci USA. 1996;93:6146–6151.
58. Sun QA, Zappacosta F, Jeang KT, Lee BJ, Hatfield D, Gladyshev VN. Redox regulation of cell signaling by selenocysteine in mammalian thioredoxin reductases. J Biol Chem. 1999;274:24522–24530.
59. Guimaraes MJ, Peterson D, Vicari A, et al. Identification of a novel *selD* homolog from eukaryotes, bacteria, and archaea: Is there an autoregulatory mechanism in selenocysteine metabolism? Proc Natl Acad Sci USA. 1996;93:15086–15091.
60. Hill KE, Lloyd RS, Yang JG, Read R, Burk RF. The cDNA for rat selenoprotein P contains 10 TGA codons in the open reading frame. J Biol Chem. 1991;266:10050–10053.
61. Gu QP, Beilstein MA, Vendeland SC, Lugade A, Ream W, Whanger PD. Conserved features of selenocysteine insertion sequences (SECIS) elements in selenoprotein W cDNAs from five species. Gene. 1997;193:187–196.
62. Kim HY, Gladyshev VN. Methionine sulfoxide reduction in mammals: characterization of methionine-R-sulfoxide reductased. Mol Bio Cell. 2004; 15:1055–1064.
63. Kryukov GV, Kryukvo VM, Gladyshev VN. New mammalian selenocysteine-containing proteins identified with an algorithm that searches for selenocysteine insertion sequence elements. J Biol Chem. 1999;274:33888–33897.
64. Korotkov KV, Novoselov SV, Hatfield DL, Gladyshev VN. Mammalian selenoprotein in which selenocysteine (Sec) incorporation is supported by a new form of Sec insertion sequence element. Mol Cell Biol. 2002;22:1402–1411.
65. Lescure A, Gautheret D, Carbon P, Krol A. Novel selenoproteins identified in silico and in vivo by using a conserved RNA structural motif. J Biol Chem. 1999;274:38147–38154.
66. Cheng WH, Ho YS, Valentine BA, Ross DA, Combs GF, Lei XG. Cellular glutathione peroxidase is the mediator of body selenium to protect against paraquat lethality in transgenic mice. J Nutr. 1998;128:1070–1076.
67. Beck MA, Handy J, Levander OA. Host nutritional status: the neglected virulence factor. Trends Microbio. 2004;12:417–423.
68. Esworthy RS, Mann JR, Sam M, Chu F-F. Low glutathione peroxidase activity in Gpx1 knockout mice protects jejunum crypts from gamma-irradiation damage. Am J Physiol. 2000;279:G426–G436.
69. Burk RF, Hill KE, Boeglin ME, Ebner FF, Chittum HS. Plasma selenium in patients with cirrhosis. *Hepatology.* 1998;27:794–798.
70. Avissar N, Slemmon JR, Palmer IS, Cohen HJ. Partial sequence of human plasma glutathione peroxidase and immunologic identification of milk glutathione peroxidase as the plasma enzyme. J Nutr. 1991;121:1243–1249.
71. Cohen HJ, Avissar N. Extracellular glutathione peroxidase: a distinct selenoprotein. In: Burk RF, ed. *Selenium in Biology and Human Health, 1 ed.* New York: Springer-Verlag; 1994:81–91.
72. Maiorino M, Gregolin C, Ursini F. Phospholipid hydroperoxide glutathione peroxidase. Meth Enzymol. 1990;186:448–457.
73. Ursini F, Heim S, Kiess M, et al. Dual function of the selenoprotein PHGPx during sperm maturation. *Science.* 1999;285:1393–1396.
74. Yant LJ, Ran Q, Rao L, et al. The selenoprotein GPX4 is essential for mouse development and protects from radiation and oxidative damage insults. Free Radic Biol Med. 2003;34:496–502.
75. Lawrence RA, Parkhill LK, Burk RF. Hepatic cytosolic non selenium-dependent glutathione peroxi-

dase activity: its nature and the effect of selenium deficiency. J Nutr. 1978;108:981–987.

76. Larsen PR, Berry MJ. Nutritional and hormonal regulation of thyroid hormone diodinases. Annu Rev Nutr. 1995;15:323–352.
77. May JM, Qu Z-C, Mendiratta S. Protection and recycling of α-tocopherol in human erythrocytes by intracellular ascorbic acid. Arch Biochem Biophys. 1998;349:281–289.
78. Tamura T, Yamamoto S, Takahata M, et al. Selenophosphate synthetase genes from lung adenocarcinoma cells: Sps1 for recycling L-selenocysteine and Sps2 for selenite assimilation. Proc Natl Acad Sci. 2004;101:16162–16167.
79. Gao Y, Feng H, Walder K, et al. Regulation of the selenoprotein SelS by glucose deprivation and endoplasmic reticulum stress - SelS is a novel glucose-regulated protein. FEBS Letters. 2004;563: 185–190.
80. Castellano S, Novoselov SV, Kryukov GV, et al. Reconsidering the evolution of eukaryotic selenoproteins: a novel nonmammalian family with scattered phylogenetic distribution. EMBO Rpts. 2004; 5:71–77.
81. Kwon SY, Badenhorst P, Martin-Romero FJ, et al. The Drosophila selenoprotein BthD is required for survival and has a role in salivary gland development. Mol Cell Biol. 2003;23:8495–8504.
82. Zhang Y, Fomenko DE, Gladyshev VN. The microbial selenoproteome of the Sargasso Sea. Genome Biol. 2005;6:R37.
83. Beck MA, Kolbeck PC, Shi Q, Rohr LH, Morris VC, Levander OA. Increased virulence of a human enterovirus (Coxsackievirus B3) in selenium-deficient mice. J Infect Dis. 1994;170:351–357.
84. Beck MA, Esworthy RS, Ho YS, Chu F-F. Glutathione peroxidase protects mice from viral-induced myocarditis. FASEB J. 1998;12:1143–1149.
85. Shisler JL, Senkevich TG, Berry MJ, Moss B. Ultraviolet-induced cell death blocked by a selenoprotein from a human dematotropic poxvirus. Science. 1998;279:102–105.
86. Sunde RA, Evenson JK. Control of gene expression of glutathione peroxidase-1 and other selenoproteins in rats and cultured cells. In: Roussel AM, Anderson RA, Favier AE, eds. *Trace Elements in Man and Animals, 10th ed.* New York: Plenum Publishers; 2000:21–27.
87. Lei XG, Evenson JK, Thompson KM, Sunde RA. Glutathione peroxidase and phospholipid hydroperoxide glutathione peroxidase are differentially regulated in rats by dietary selenium. J Nutr. 1995; 125:1438–1446.
88. Sunde RA, Saedi MS, Knight SAB, Smith CG, Evenson JK. Regulation of expression of glutathione peroxidase by selenium. In: Wendel A, ed. *Selenium in Biology and Medicine, 4th ed.* Heidelberg, Germany: Springer-Verlag; 1989:8–13.
89. Weiss SL, Evenson JK, Thompson KM, Sunde RA. Dietary selenium regulation of glutathione peroxidase mRNA and other selenium-dependent parameters in male rats. J Nutr Biochem. 1997;8: 85–91.
90. Bermano G, Nicol F, Dyer JA, et al. Tissue-specific regulation of selenoenzyme gene expression during selenium deficiency in rats. Biochem J. 1995;311: 425–430.
91. Hill KE, Lyons PR, Burk RF. Differential regulation of rat liver selenoprotein mRNAs in selenium deficiency. Biochem Biophys Res Commun. 1992; 185:260–263.
92. Sunde RA, Evenson JK, Thompson KM, Sachdev SW. Dietary selenium requirements based on glutathione peroxidase-1 activity and mRNA levels and other selenium parameters are not increased by pregnancy and lactation in rats. J Nutr. 2005;135: 2144–2150.
93. Hadley KB, Sunde RA. Selenium regulation of thioredoxin reductase activity and mRNA levels in rat liver. J Nutr Biochem. 2001;12:693–702.
94. Weiss SL, Sunde RA. Cis-acting elements are required for selenium regulation of glutathione peroxidase-1 mRNA levels. RNA. 1998;4:816–827.
95. Moriarty PM, Reddy CC, Maquat LE. Selenium deficiency reduces the abundance of mRNA for Se-dependent glutathione peroxidase 1 by a UGA-dependent mechanism likely to be nonsense codon-mediated decay of cytoplasmic mRNA. Mol Cell Biol. 1998;18:2932–2939.
96. National Research Council. *Recommended Dietary Allowances, 9th ed.* Washington, DC: National Academy of Sciences; 1980.
97. Levander OA. Considerations on the assessment of selenium status. FASEB J. 1985;44:2579–2583.
98. National Research Council. *Recommended Dietary Allowances, 10th ed.* Washington, DC: National Academy Press; 1989.
99. World Health Organization. *Selenium. Trace Elements in Human Nutrition and Health.* Geneva, Switzerland: World Health Organization; 1996: 105–122.
100. Yang G, Wang S, Zhou R, Sun S. Endemic selenium intoxication of humans in China. Am J Clin Nutr. 1983;37:872–881.
101. Valentine JL, Faraji B, Kang HK. Human glutathione peroxidase activity in cases of high selenium exposures. Environ Res. 1988;45:16–27.
102. Hafeman DG, Hoekstra WG. Protection against carbon tetrachloride-induced lipid peroxidation in the rat by dietary vitamin E, selenium, and methionine as measured by ethane evolution. J Nutr. 1977; 107:656–665.
103. Awad JA, Morrow JD, Hill KE, Roberts LJ, Burk

RF. Detection and localization of lipid peroxidation in selenium-and vitamin E-deficient rats using F2-isoprostanes. J Nutr. 1994;124:810–816.

104. Safer B, Jagus B, Crouch D. Indirect inactivation of eukaryotic initiation factor 2 in reticulocyte lysate by selenite. J Biol Chem. 1980;255:6913–6917.

105. Abernathy CO, Cantilli R, Du JT, Levander OA. Essentiality versus toxicity: some considerations in the risk assessment of essential trace elements. In: Saxena J, ed. *Hazard Assessment of Chemicals, 1st ed.* Washington, D.C.: Taylor and Francis; 1993: 81–113.

106. Yang G-Q, Wang SZ. Further observations on the human maximum safe dietary intake in a seleniferous area of China. J Trace Elem Electrolytes Health Dis. 1994;8:159–165.

107. Helzlsouer K, Jacobs R, Morris S. *Acute Selenium Intoxication in the United States, 44th ed.* 1985:1670.

108. Davis EA, Maier KJ, Knight AW. The biological consequences of selenium in aquatic ecosystems. California Agriculture. 1988;18–29.

109. Willett WC, Polk BF, Morris JS. Prediagnostic serum selenium and risk of cancer. Lancet. 1983;ii: 130–134.

110. Hunter DJ, Willett WC. Diet, body build, and breast cancer. Annu Rev Nutr. 1994;14:393–418.

111. Yoshizawa K, Willett WC, Morris JS, et al. Study of prediagnostic selenium level in toenails and the risk of advances prostate cancer. J Natl Cancer Inst. 1998;90:1219–1224.

112. Clark LC, Combs GF, Turnbull BW, et al. Effects of selenium supplementation for cancer prevention in patients with carcinoma of the skin. JAMA. 1996;276:1957–1963.

113. Duffield-Lillico AJ, Slate EH, Reid ME, et al. Selenium supplementation and secondary prevention of nonmelanoma skin cancer in a randomized trial. J Natl Cancer Inst. 2003;95:1477–1481.

114. Duffield-Lillico AJ, Reid ME, Turnbull BW, et al. Baseline characteristics and the effect of selenium supplementation on cancer incidence in a randomized clinical trial: a summary report of the Nutritional Prevention of Cancer Trial. Cancer Epidemiol Biomarkers Prev. 2002;11:630–639.

115. Taylor PR, Wang GQ, Dawsey SM, et al. Effect of nutrition intervention on intermediate endpoints in esophageal and gastric carcinogensis. Amer J Clin Nutr. 1995;62:1420S–1423S.

# 39 Chromium

Barbara J. Stoecker

## Introduction

In 1957, Schwarz and Mertz[1] reported that a compound extracted from porcine kidney restored impaired glucose tolerance in rats, and this compound, chromium, was identified as the essential element that potentiated insulin action. In the next decade, malnourished children with impaired glucose tolerance were given oral supplements of 250 μg chromium as $CrCl_3{\cdot}6H_2O$, and improvement in glucose removal rate was noted in children presumed to be chromium deficient.[2] Subsequently, chromium supplementation was reported to correct chromium depletion in a patient receiving total parenteral nutrition[3] and was confirmed in others. Comprehensive reviews of chromium metabolism have been compiled by several investigators.[4-8]

Chromium is present in biological tissues at very low concentrations, making it crucial to avoid contamination of samples and complicating the collection of specimens in a clinical setting.[9] Over the years, the reported concentration of chromium in serum and urine has decreased by more than 1000-fold.[5,9] These lower values reflect improvements in analytical instrumentation and greater attention to the many sources of chromium contamination in sample collection and analysis.[9]

## Chemistry

Chromium is a transition element that can occur in a number of valence states, with $Cr^{3+}$, and $Cr^{6+}$ being the most common.[10] $Cr^{3+}$ is the most stable form in biological systems.[4,10,11] $Cr^{6+}$ is a strong oxidizing agent that comes primarily from industrial sources.[10,11] $Cr^{6+}$ consumed in small amounts is reduced to $Cr^{3+}$ in the acidic environment of the stomach.[4,11] Solubilities of chromium compounds in aqueous solution differ substantially and affect their absorption.[10,12] Various organic complexes help to prevent formation of biologically inert chromium oxides and increase solubility at the pH of intestinal contents.[4,10,12]

## Absorption, Transport, Storage, and Turnover

### *Absorption*

Intestinal absorption of $Cr^{3+}$ is low, with estimates of absorption ranging from <0.5% to 2%. Most chromium from an oral dose remains unabsorbed in the intestinal tract and is excreted in the feces.[4-7] In a 12-day metabolic balance study, two men consuming an average of 36.8 μg/d of chromium had a mean apparent net absorption of chromium of 1.8%.[6]

Because of the analytical problems associated with the measurement of actual chromium absorption, several researchers have used urinary excretion as an indicator of absorption. Normal subjects given a dose of $^{51}CrCl_3$ had a mean of 0.69% (range = 0.3%–1.3%) of the dose in the urine within 72 hours.[13] In adults receiving 200-μg chromium supplements daily, urinary excretion was approximately 0.4%.[5] Prior chromium status and amount of chromium present in the diet apparently affect chromium absorption in animals and humans.[5,14] When dietary chromium intake was 10 μg, approximately 2% of that amount was absorbed (estimated as urinary excretion), whereas at chromium intakes of 40 μg, only 0.4% to 0.5% of the chromium was recovered in urine.[5]

Various dietary components such as ascorbic acid also alter chromium absorption.[6,7] In three women who consumed 1 mg chromium as chromium chloride with or without 100 mg ascorbic acid, plasma chromium concentrations were consistently higher after the chromium given in conjunction with ascorbic acid.[6]

Chelation of a mineral may increase or decrease its availability depending on the absorption characteristics of the compound formed. Some of the most widely marketed chromium supplements are chelates of chromium, with various amino acids or their derivatives.[15]

Common medications apparently enhance or impair the absorption of chromium. Chelation and changes in cytoprotective factors in the gastrointestinal tract may contribute to these effects. Gastric intubation of rats with aspirin markedly enhanced orally administered $^{51}Cr$ from $^{51}CrCl_3$ in blood, tissues, and urine compared with controls.[16] Intraperitoneal injection of rats with indomethacin at 5 mg/kg body weight before oral dosing with $^{51}CrCl_3$ significantly increased $^{51}Cr$ in blood, tissues, and urine, indicating that blocking the synthesis of gastrointestinal prostaglandins enhanced chromium absorption. Intubating rats with an analog of prostaglandin $E_2$ reduced $^{51}Cr$ in blood and tissues significantly below that of the control group.[17] A single oral dose of several antacids also significantly reduced $^{51}Cr$ in blood and tissues of rats compared with controls dosed with $^{51}CrCl_3$ but no antacid.[7,16] The low concentration of chromium in blood and its low rate of absorption have precluded a systematic evaluation of the effects of medications on chromium absorption in humans.

### *Transport*

When transferrin was precipitated from $^{51}Cr$-labeled human serum, 80% of the isotope was present in the precipitate. Iron added to the serum before the addition of $^{51}Cr$ resulted in a dose-responsive reduction in $^{51}Cr$ bound to transferrin.[18] Clodfelder et al.[19] demonstrated in rats that transferrin served as the major transport protein for chromium, and that chromium transport to the tissues was stimulated by insulin. In Earle's medium, human apotransferrin bound chromium in the presence of citric acid, and iron uptake by apotransferrin was reduced by either aluminum or chromium. The addition of iron to the medium reduced binding of aluminum or chromium to apotransferrin.[20] It has been hypothesized that iron interferes with the transport of chromium in hemochromatosis.[21]

### *Storage*

After either injection or oral dosing of $^{51}CrCl_3$ in rats, $^{51}Cr$ accumulated in liver, kidney, testis, bone, and spleen.[6,16,22] In humans, $^{51}Cr$ accumulated in the liver, spleen, soft tissue, and bone,[23] but concentrations were still in the picomolar range.[6]

### *Turnover*

Studies using $^{51}Cr$ showed that chromium circulating in the blood does not appear to be in equilibrium with tissue chromium stores.[4,18] Several models for chromium turnover have been developed in rats and humans, and are summarized in several comprehensive reviews of chromium metabolism.[4,6,7,12] Do Canto et al.[24] injected $^{51}Cr$ as chromium chloride intravenously into seven adults with type 2 diabetes and compared their data with data from three normal subjects. The average half-life for urinary excretion was 0.97 days for the diabetic group and 1.51 days for normal subjects. A four-compartment model was formulated containing a central compartment, a compartment within the blood pool, and slow-exchange and fast-exchange tissue compartments. The fast-exchange tissue compartment showed the most difference between groups; half-life values were 19 hours for normal subjects, but only 5 hours for the diabetic subjects ($P < 0.005$). The investigators suggested that this fast-exchange tissue pool is the best candidate for chromium used in glucose metabolism.[24]

Dietary factors may also impact chromium turnover. For example, of 37 subjects who consumed high-sugar diets (35% of total energy from simple sugars) for 6 weeks, 27 had increased urinary chromium excretion compared with the period when they consumed only 15% of total energy from simple sugars.[25]

## Physiologic Functions

Chromium potentiates insulin action. The addition of chromium to epididymal fat tissue from chromium-deficient rats stimulated glucose uptake in the presence of added insulin.[4] In the early studies of chromium, a factor was extracted from brewer's yeast that improved glucose tolerance of chromium-deficient rats.[1,4] This factor, which appeared to contain nicotinic acid, glutamic acid, glycine, and a sulfur-containing amino acid, was called glucose tolerance factor. Chromium, as found in brewer's yeast and in some other naturally occurring and synthetic complexes, was more effective in stimulating glucose use by animals and by cells than was chromium chloride or chromium found in torula yeast.[5,6]

Yamamoto et al.[26] and Davis and Vincent[27] characterized a low-molecular-weight chromium-binding substance containing glutamate, aspartate, glycine, and cysteine. This oligopeptide has a molecular weight of approximately 1500 and has been isolated from the tissues of a number of different species[8] and from bovine colostrum.[26] Vincent[27] suggested the name "chromodulin" for this substance on the basis of his data on activation of the tyrosine kinase activity of the insulin receptor and the resultant amplification of insulin signaling. The proposed mechanism of action for this low-molecular-weight chromium-binding substance is outlined in Figure 1.

### *Chromium Effects on Growth*

A significantly increased rate of growth was observed in a group of malnourished children given a chromium supplement compared with a similar group who received no chromium supplementation.[6] The weight loss associated with receiving a chromium-deficient total parenteral nutrition solution was restored with chromium supplementation.[3]

Chromium supplements have been widely marketed as effective in enhancing lean body mass, but most studies have not supported this hypothesis.[15] For example, supplementation with chromium as chromium picolinate at 924 μg/d for 12 weeks. along with a twice-weekly resistance training program were evaluated in 23 men 50 to 75

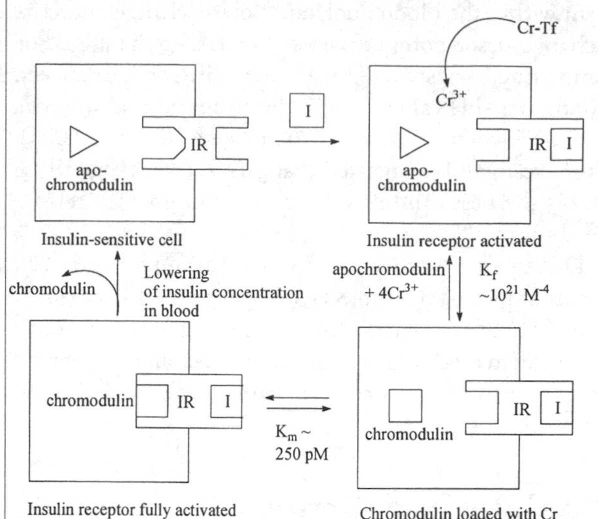


Figure 1. Proposed mechanism for the activation of insulin receptor kinase activity by chromodulin in response to insulin. The inactive form of the insulin receptor (IR) is converted to the active form by binding insulin (I). This triggers a movement of chromium, presumably in the form of Cr-transferrin (Cr-Tf) from the blood into insulin-dependent cells, which in turn results in the binding of chromium to apochromodulin (triangle). The holochromodulin (square) then binds to the insulin receptor, further activating the receptor kinase activity. (Used with permission from Vincent 2000.[8])

years of age. The chromium supplements did not enhance muscle size or strength or lean body mass accretion in older men. but resistance training did have significant, independent effects on these variables.[28] Dietary chromium intake of these men was not reported, but if adequate dietary chromium was already being consumed, no effect of a chromium supplement would be expected.

Several studies cited by Mertz[4] reported increases in growth and survival of chromium-supplemented rats and mice. Growth also was impaired in guinea pigs that were fed diets containing chromium at levels of less than 60 μg/kg diet.[29]

The potential effects of chromium on feed efficiency and muscle area have been of interest to the livestock industry, but results have been inconsistent. Page et al.[30] noted increased daily gain in weight and percent of muscle in pigs when diets were supplemented with 200 μg chromium as chromium picolinate. However, pigs whose diets were supplemented with porcine pituitary somatotropin, chromium at 300 μg/kg diet (as picolinate), or both in a 2 × 2 factorial design had improved growth performance with somatotropin, but chromium supplementation did not produce a significant effect.[31] A recent study supplementing gilts with 200 μg/kg chromium as chromium propionate likewise found no effects on growth performance or carcass traits.[32]

## *Chromium Effects on Glucose Tolerance*

The effects of chromium supplementation in humans have been reviewed previously.[5-7,33,34] Mertz[33] noted that in 12 of 15 controlled studies, chromium supplementation improved the efficiency of insulin or the blood lipid profiles of subjects. Subjects with some degree of impaired glucose tolerance were more responsive to chromium supplementation than other subjects.[33] However, authors of a systematic meta-analysis of effects of chromium on glucose and insulin found no effects of chromium on glucose or insulin concentrations in non-diabetic subjects.[34]

One study controlled dietary chromium intake for several weeks. Subjects were provided with diets that contained chromium at 5 μg/1000 kcal (1.2 μg/MJ) for 14 weeks. Glucose and insulin in response to a glucose load of 1 g/kg body weight were evaluated at baseline, 4 weeks, 9 weeks, and 14 weeks. Blood was sampled at 0, 30, 60, 90, 120, 180, and 240 minutes. Values were summed over 0 to 90 minutes and over 0 to 240 minutes for the evaluation of chromium depletion or supplementation on glucose and insulin. After adapting to the diet for 4 weeks, subjects were assigned to placebo or chromium supplementation groups for 5 weeks, followed by a crossover without washout for another 5 weeks. After 4 weeks on the diet containing 5 μg/1000 kcal, there were no significant changes in variables measured. However, in the 8 subjects who consumed 5 μg/1000 kcal for 9 consecutive weeks, significant increases from baseline in sums of glucose and in glucose at 90 minutes after the glucose load were observed. Sums of insulin and of glucose over 90 minutes tended ($P < 0.10$) to be reduced when these subjects were supplemented with 200 μg chromium as chromium chloride daily for 5 weeks. Subjects with initially impaired glucose tolerance appeared to deteriorate further during the placebo period and improve during chromium supplementation. Chromium supplementation in subjects with normal glucose tolerance had no effect, suggesting that chromium at under 20 μg/d for several weeks was sufficient to prevent impaired glucose tolerance in selected subjects.[35] How long normal glucose tolerance could be maintained on such a low chromium intake is unknown.

Early studies of chromium supplementation on type 2 diabetes were generally unremarkable. However, in China 180 individuals with type 2 diabetes took placebo or a total of 200 or 1000 μg of chromium as chromium picolinate in divided doses twice per day for 4 months.[36] After 2 months, fasting and 2-hour insulin concentrations were decreased significantly at both supplementation levels. At that time, glycosylated hemoglobin in the higher dose group was 7.4 ± 0.2% compared with 8.6 ± 0.2% in the group receiving placebo. Fasting and 2-hour glucose concentrations decreased significantly after 2 months in the higher-dose group but not in the lower-dose group. After 4 months of supplementation, the amount of glycosylated hemoglobin was significantly reduced in the lower- and higher-dose groups (7.5 ± 0.2% and 6.6 ± 0.1%, respectively) compared with the placebo group (8.5 ± 0.2%). The authors reported that supplemental chromium had no effect on body mass index, suggesting that the beneficial effects of chromium were not mediated by weight loss.[36] No data are available on the basal dietary intake of chromium in these diabetic subjects. Additional strengths and limitations of this study have been summarized by Hellerstein.[37]

Cefalu et al.[38] evaluted the effects of 1000 μg Cr/d as chromium picolinate in an 8-month, double-blind, placebo-controlled trial of 29 individuals at high risk for type 2 diabetes. Insulin sensitivity of the controls did not change, but the group supplemented with chromium picolinate had significantly improved insulin sensitivity at the mid point ($P < 0.05$) and end ($P < 0.005$) of the study compared with the control group.[38] Subsequently, they used the hyperinsulinemic (JCR-LA Corpulent) rat, a model for the insulin resistance syndrome and found that the obese rats given chromium picolinate had significantly lower fasting insulin concentrations and improved glucose disappearance compared with obese controls. Membrane-associated Glut-4 was significantly increased in chromium-supplemented obese rats after insulin stimulation compared with obese controls. Supplementation with chromium picolinate did not alter plasma glucose or insulin or membrane-associated Glut-4 in lean rats.[39]

### *Chromium Effects on Lipid Metabolism*

Data on effects of chromium on serum cholesterol in experimental animals and humans are equivocal and have been reviewed in several papers.[4-6] Some studies reported decreased total serum cholesterol and increased high-density lipoprotein cholesterol and apolipoprotein A concentrations with chromium supplementation; others showed no effects of chromium supplementation. One contributor to this variability is the inability to determine initial chromium status of the subjects.

In JCR-LA corpulent rats, Cefalu et al.[39] reported lower plasma total cholesterol in obese rats supplemented with chromium picolinate than in obese controls. However, there were no effects of chromium supplementation in lean rats.[39]

### *Chromium Effects on Immune Response*

A number of reports have suggested benefits of chromium supplementation in diets of stressed cattle.[40] For example, after market-transit stress, steer calves receiving chromium supplements of 0.4 mg/kg diet had significantly decreased serum cortisol and increased serum immunoglobulin.

### *Chromium Needs of the Elderly*

Bunker[41] conducted 5-day metabolic balance studies with 22 apparently healthy elderly subjects aged 69 to 86 years. They had mean chromium intakes of 24.5 μg/d (12.8 μg/1000 kcal, or 3.06 μg/MJ), with a range of 13.6 to 47.7 μg/d. At these intakes, 16 were in equilibrium, 3 were in positive balance, and 3 were in negative balance. Davies et al.[42] noted highly significant age-related decreases in chromium in hair, sweat, and serum samples from patients in England. However, Offenbacher[6] has suggested that age per se does not cause chromium depletion even though some cases of glucose intolerance observed in elderly people responded to chromium supplementation.

### *Chromium Needs in Special Cases*

Trauma patients and persons who exercised strenuously have been shown to have elevated urinary excretion of chromium.[43,44] Ravina et al.[45] reported that chromium supplementation improved glucose control in steroid-induced diabetes.

## Effects of Chromium Deficiency

Chromium was designated an essential element because of its role in restoring glucose tolerance in rats.[4] However, because chromium is ubiquitous in the environment, it is difficult to produce a clear chromium deficiency in laboratory animals. No chromium-dependent enzyme has been identified. Chromium concentrations in serum and plasma are near the detection limits of currently available instruments.[9] Investigators have not been able to predict response to chromium supplementation on the basis of plasma or serum chromium measurements.[5,6] Therefore, studies that seek to reverse a possible chromium deficiency symptom by supplementation are hampered by inadequate means to assess the initial chromium status of the subjects. Nonetheless, understanding of the physiological functions of chromium is increasing. Metabolic stress may exacerbate the deficient state.[6,43,45]

### *Cellular Level*

In cell culture, mouse myotubes were differentiated in chromium-adequate or chromium-poor media. In the chromium-poor media, insulin-stimulated uptake of radiolabeled glucose was reduced by almost 50% compared with that in myotubes in chromium-replete media. Physiological concentrations of inorganic chromium restored the uptake of glucose. Sensitivity of the cells to insulin was lessened by a reduction in the chromium content of the media and was increased when chromium was returned to the media.[46]

### *Animal Studies*

Decreased weight gain was reported for rats, mice, and guinea pigs whose diets were depleted of chromium.[4,29] Rats given chromium chloride supplements had significantly lower fasting glucose than rats fed chromium-depleted diets.[4]

### *Human Studies*

In studies of patients whose total parental nutrition solutions contained no chromium or were supplemented with inadequate amounts of chromium, insulin requirements were reduced and glucose intolerance was reversed with chromium chloride supplementation.[3] In addition, chromium supplementation restored lost weight and reversed peripheral neuropathy.[3,6]

## Recommended Dietary Allowance

Data were not available on which to base an average chromium requirement for any age group. Therefore, an Adequate Intake (AI) estimate has been provided in the latest report released by the National Academy of Sciences.[47] The AI for men 19 to 50 years of age is 35 μg/d and for women of the same age is 25 μg/d. The mean chromium intake of 10 adult men was 33 μg/d (range = 22–48 μg/d) and chromium intake for 22 women was 25 μg/d (range = 13–36 μg/d).[48]

Adequate intakes for other adult age groups were set by multiplying 13.4 μg/1000 kcal by an energy intake estimate for the age. For children, the AI was estimated by extrapolating down from adult values on the basis of body weight to the 3/4 power and adding a factor for growth.[47] Because no enzyme has been identified as an indicator of chromium status and because of the very low concentrations of chromium in accessible tissues, it has not been possible to monitor a large group of subjects with variable chromium intakes, which is what is needed to make dietary recommendations with confidence.

The AI for infants 0 to 6 months of age is 0.2 μg/d based on the chromium content of human milk. An infant consuming 750 mL of human milk receives <1 μg/d of chromium.[49,50] For infants 7 to 12 months of age, the AI is 5.5 μg/d. The increase in the AI for this age group is due to the higher concentration of chromium in weaning foods than in human milk.

## Food and Other Sources

In the United States, meat, poultry, fish, and especially dairy products tend to be low in chromium. Many foods provide substantially less than 1 μg/serving. Fruits and vegetables and grain products have variable chromium concentrations, with whole grains tending to provide more chromium than refined products. Processed meats also appear to gain chromium during manufacture.[51]

Loss of chromium in the process of refining sugar has been noted[5]; however, processing also may add chromium to the food supply. In one study, chromium was leached from stainless steel containers, particularly when contents were acidic.[52] Some brands of beer contain significant amounts of chromium, some of which is presumably exogenous.[51]

## Excess and Toxicity

The safety of 200 μg chromium supplements given as chromium chloride has been established in studies lasting several months.[33] Because chromium chloride is poorly absorbed, high oral intakes would be necessary to attain toxic levels.

Using Chinese hamster ovary cells, Stearns et al.[53] raised the question of mutagenicity associated with chromium picolinate; however, the high concentations of chromium picolinate added to the culture media make the results difficult to interpret. Therefore, another group tested commercially available chromium picolinate in similar assays and found it to be non-mutagenic.[54] Vincent[8] has suggested that the release of chromium from chromium picolinate is a process that can potentially lead to the production of harmful hydroxyl radicals. These hypotheses need to be explored more thoroughly in animal models.

Toxic effects of industrial exposure have been attributed primarily to airborne $Cr^{6+}$ compounds.[55-57] Toxicity symptoms included allergic dermatitis, skin lesions, and increased incidence of lung cancer.[11,58] A key to the toxicity of $Cr^{6+}$ compounds may be the products of its cellular reduction to $Cr^{3+}$.[11,58] Welding of stainless steel generates $Cr^{6+}$. In a meta-analysis for lung cancer that accounted for asbestos exposure and smoking, a pooled relative risk of 1.94 was found for the welders.[55,57,59]

## Future Directions

Chromium analysis remains challenging because of the low levels of chromium in biological tissues and the potential for sample contamination.[9] Furthermore, chromium concentrations in accessible tissues apparently do not reflect metabolically active chromium pools in the body.[6] The essentiality of chromium has been demonstrated, but further research is necessary to clarify its physiological functions. The work indicating that a low-molecular-weight chromium-binding substance may amplify insulin receptor tyrosine kinase activity in response to insulin offers an exciting mechanistic explanation for the role of chromium in biological systems. However, the inability to accurately assess chromium status hampers study design and interpretation. Most people in the United States consume between 12 and16 μg/1000 kcal (2.9 and 3.8 μg/MD) of chromium.[6,48,51] Long-term consequences of low dietary intakes of chromium and of factors that may increase the chromium requirement need to be determined. Clinical tests that identify chromium-deficient individuals clearly are needed.

Appropriate chromium supplementation for patients on total parenteral nutrition (TPN) should be carefully evaluated. On the basis of signs of chromium deficiency, an expert panel of the American Medical Association has recommended 10 to 15 μg/d of chromium for adults on TPN whose disease condition has stabilized. Initial supplementation with at least 20 μg/d chromium was suggested.[60] There are indications that trauma patients have increased urinary chromium losses; however, if chromium administered orally and intravenously is utilized similarly, an intravenous dose of 15 μg/d chromium is equivalent to an oral intake of 3000 or 1500 μg/d at absorption rates of 0.5% and 1%, respectively.

Another area to be investigated in terms of both safety and efficacy is the widespread practice of self-supplementation with chromium. Some studies have suggested chromium has an effect on muscle and fat distribution, but chromium supplementation should not have a nutritional effect unless a deficiency exists. Most studies have not supported beneficial effects of chromium supplementation on body composition in humans.[15]

The value of chromium supplementation in type 2 diabetes needs systematic investigation, including documentation of dietary intakes and minimal effective doses. A method to prospectively identify chromium status of subjects would greatly enhance the potential to conduct the needed clinical trials in various population groups.

## References


1. Schwarz K, Mertz W. Chromium(III) and the glucose tolerance factor. Arch Biochem Biophys. 1959; 85:292–295.
2. Hopkins LL, Jr., Ransome-Kuti O, Majaj AS. Improvement of impaired carbohydrate metabolism by chromium(III) in malnourished infants. Am J Clin Nutr. 1968;21:203–211.
3. Jeejeebhoy KN, Chu RC, Marliss EB, Greenberg GR, Bruce-Robertson A. Chromium deficiency, glucose intolerance, and neuropathy reversed by chromium supplementation, in a patient receiving long-term total parenteral nutrition. Am J Clin Nutr. 1977;30:531–538.
4. Mertz W. Chromium occurrence and function in biological systems. Physiol Rev. 1969;49:163–239.
5. Anderson RA. Chromium. In: Mertz W, ed. *Trace Elements in Human and Animal Nutrition*. New York: Academic Press; 1987; 225–244.
6. Offenbacher EG, Pi-Sunyer FX, Stoecker BJ. Chromium. In: O'Dell BL, Sunde RA, eds. *Handbook of Nutritionally Essential Mineral Elements*. New York: Marcel Dekker; 1997; 389–411.
7. Stoecker BJ. Chromium. In: Merian E, Anke M, Ihnat M, Stoeppler M, eds. *Elements and their Compounds in the Environment*. Weinheim: Wiley-VCH Verlag GmbH; 2004; 709–729.
8. Vincent JB. The biochemistry of chromium. J Nutr. 2000;130:715–718.
9. Veillon C, Patterson KY. Analytical issues in nutritional chromium research. J Trace Elem Exper Med. 1999;12:99–109.
10. Losi ME, Amrhein C, Frankenberger WT Jr. Environmental biochemistry of chromium. Rev Environ Contam Toxicol. 1994;136:91–121.
11. Cohen MD, Kargacin B, Klein CB, Costa M. Mechanisms of chromium carcinogenicity and toxicity. Crit Rev Toxicol. 1993;23:255–281.
12. O'Flaherty EJ, Kerger BD, Hays SM, Paustenbach DJ. A physiologically based model for the ingestion of chromium(III) and chromium(VI) by humans. Toxicol Sci. 2001;60:196–213.
13. Doisy RJ, Streeten DHP, Souma ML, Kalafer ME, Rekant SI, Dalakos TG. Metabolism of chromium-51 in human subjects. In: Mertz W, Cornatzer WE, eds. *Newer Trace Elements in Nutrition*. New York: Marcel Dekker; 1971; 155–168.
14. Seaborn CD, Stoecker BJ. Effects of ascorbic acid depletion and chromium status on retention and urinary excretion of 51chromium. Nutr Res. 1992;12: 1229–1234.
15. Lukaski HC. Chromium as a supplement. Annu Rev Nutr. 1999;19:279–302.
16. Davis ML, Seaborn CD, Stoecker BJ. Effects of over-the-counter drugs on 51chromium retention and urinary excretion in rats. Nutr Res. 1995;15: 201–210.
17. Kamath SM, Stoecker BJ, Davis-Whitenack ML, Smith MM, Adeleye BO, Sangiah S. Absorption, retention and urinary excretion of chromium-51 in rats pretreated with indomethacin and dosed with dimethylprostaglandin E2, misoprostol or prostacyclin. J Nutr. 1997;127:478–482.
18. Hopkins LL Jr, Schwarz K. Chromium (III) binding to serum proteins, specifically siderophilin. Biochim Biophys Acta. 1964;90:484–491.
19. Clodfelder BJ, Emamaullee J, Hepburn DDD, Chakov NE, Nettles HS, Vincent JB. The trail of chromium(III) in vivo from the blood to the urine: the roles of transferrin and chromodulin. J Biol Inorg Chem. 2001;6:608–617.
20. Moshtaghie AA, Ani M, Bazrafshan MR. Comparative binding study of aluminum and chromium to human transferrin: Effect of iron. Biol Trace Elem Res. 1992;32:39–46.
21. Sargent T, III, Lim TH, Jenson RL. Reduced chromium retention in patients with hemochromatosis, a possible basis of hemochromatotic diabetes. Metabolism. 1979;28:70–79.
22. Hopkins LLJ. Distribution in the rat of physiological amounts of injected Cr-51(III) with time. Am J Physiol. 1965;209:731–735.
23. Lim TH, Sargent T, III, Kusubov N. Kinetics of trace element chromium(III) in the human body. Am J Physiol. 1983;244:R445–R454.
24. Do Canto OM, Sargent T, III, Liehn JC. Chromium (III) metabolism in diabetic patients. In: Sive Subrananian KN, Wastney ME, eds. *Kinetic Models of Trace Element and Mineral Metabolism*. Boca Raton, FL: CRC Press; 1995; 416.
25. Kozlovsky AS, Moser PB, Reiser S, Anderson RA. Effects of diets high in simple sugars on urinary chromium losses. Metabolism. 1986;35:515–518.
26. Yamamoto A, Wada O, Suzuki H. Purification and properties of biologically active chromium complex from bovine colostrum. J Nutr. 1988;118:39–45.
27. Davis CM, Vincent JB. Chromium oligopeptide activates insulin receptor tyrosine kinase activity. Biochemistry. 1997;36:4382–4385.
28. Campbell WW, Joseph LJO, Davey SL, Cyr-Campbell D, Anderson RA, Evans WJ. Effects of resis-

tance training and chromium picolinate on body composition and skeletal muscle in older men. J Appl Physiol. 1999;86:29–39.

29. Seaborn CD, Cheng NZ, Adeleye B, Owens F, Stoecker BJ. Chromium and chronic ascorbic acid depletion effects on tissue ascorbate, manganese and $^{14}C$ retention from $^{14}C$-ascorbate in guinea pigs. Biol Trace Elem Res. 1994;41:279–294.
30. Page TG, Southern LL, Ward TL, Thompson DLJ. Effect of chromium picolinate on growth and serum and carcass traits of growing-finishing pigs. J Anim Sci. 1993;71:656–662.
31. Evock-Clover CM, Polansky MM, Anderson RA, Steele NC. Dietary chromium supplementation with or without somatotropin treatment alters serum hormones and metabolites in growing pigs without affecting growth performance. J Nutr. 1993;123:1504–1512.
32. Matthews JO, Guzik AC, Lemieux FM, Southern LL, Bidner TD. Effects of chromium propionate on growth, carcass traits, and pork quality of growing-finishing pigs. J Anim Sci. 2005;83:858–862.
33. Mertz W. Chromium in human nutrition: A review. J Nutr. 1993;123:626–633.
34. Althuis MD, Jordan NE, Ludington EA, Wittes JT. Glucose and insulin responses to dietary chromium supplements: a meta-analysis. Am J Clin Nutr. 2002;76:148–155.
35. Anderson RA, Polansky MM, Bryden NA, Canary JJ. Supplemental-chromium effects on glucose, insulin, glucagon, and urinary chromium losses in subjects consuming controlled low-chromium diets. Am J Clin Nutr. 1991;54:909–916.
36. Anderson RA, Cheng NZ, Bryden NA et al. Elevated intakes of supplemental chromium improve glucose and insulin variables in individuals with type 2 diabetes. Diabetes. 1997;46:1786–1791.
37. Hellerstein MK. Is chromium supplementation effective in managing type II diabetes? Nutr Rev. 1998;56:302–306.
38. Cefalu WT, Bell-Farrow AD, Stegner J et al. Effect of chromium picolinate on insulin sensitivity in vivo. J Trace Elem Exper Med. 1999;12:71–83.
39. Cefalu WT, Wang ZQ, Zhang XH, Baldor LC, Russell JC. Oral chromium picolinate improves carbohydrate and lipid metabolism and enhances skeletal muscle glut-4 translocation in obese, hyperinsulinemic (JCR-LA corpulent) rats. J Nutr. 2002;132:1107–1114.
40. Borgs P, Mallard BA. Immune-endocrine interactions in agricultural species: Chromium and its effect on health and performance. Domestic Animal Endocrinology. 1998;15:431–438.
41. Bunker VW, Lawson MS, Delves HT, Clayton B. The uptake and excretion of chromium by the elderly. Am J Clin Nutr. 1984;39:797–802.
42. Davies S, Howard JM, Hunnisett A, Howard M. Age-related decreases in chromium levels in 51,665 hair, sweat, and serum samples from 40,872 patients: Implications for the prevention of cardiovascular disease and type II diabetes mellitus. Metabolism. 1997;46:469–473.
43. Borel JS, Majerus TC, Polansky MM, Moser PB, Anderson RA. Chromium intake and urinary chromium excretion of trauma patients. Biol Trace Elem Res. 1984;6:317–326.
44. Rubin MA, Miller JP, Ryan AS et al. Acute and chronic resistive exercise increase urinary chromium excretion in men as measured with an enriched chromium stable isotope. J Nutr. 1998;128:73–78.
45. Ravina A, Slezak L, Mirsky N, Anderson RA. Control of steroid-induced diabetes with supplemental chromium. J Trace Elem Exper Med. 1999;12:375–378.
46. Morris B, Gray T, MacNeil S. Evidence for chromium acting as an essential trace element in insulin-dependent glucose uptake in cultured mouse myotubes. J Endocrinol. 1995;144:135–141.
47. Food and Nutrition Board, Institute of Medicine. Dietary Reference Intakes for Vitamin A, Vitamin K, Arsenic, Boron, Chromium, Copper, Iodine, Iron, Manganese, Molybdenum, Nickel, Silicon, Vanadium, and Zinc. Washington, DC: National Academies Press; 2001. Available online at: http://www.nap.edu/books/0309072794/html/.
48. Anderson RA, Kozlovsky AS. Chromium intake, absorption and excretion of subjects consuming self-selected diets. Am J Clin Nutr. 1985;41:1177–1183.
49. Anderson RA, Bryden NA, Patterson KY, Veillon C, Andon MB, Moser-Veillon PB. Breast milk chromium and its association with chromium intake, chromium excretion, and serum chromium. Am J Clin Nutr. 1993;57:519–523.
50. Mohamedshah FY, Moser-Veillon PB, Yamini S, Douglass LW, Anderson RA, Veillon C. Distribution of a stable isotope of chromium ($Cr^{53}$) in serum, urine, and breast milk in lactating women. Am J Clin Nutr. 1998;67:1250–1255.
51. Anderson RA, Bryden NA, Polansky MM. Dietary chromium intake: Freely chosen diets, institutional diets, and individual foods. Biol Trace Elem Res. 1992;32:117–121.
52. Offenbacher EG, Pi-Sunyer FX. Temperature and pH effects on the release of chromium from stainless steel into water and fruit juices. J Agric Food Chem. 1983;31:89–92.
53. Stearns DM, Wise JP, Sr., Patierno SR, Wetterhahn KE. Chromium(III) picolinate produces chromosome damage in Chinese hamster ovary cells. FASEB J. 1995;9:1643–1649.
54. Slesinski RS, Clarke JJ, RH CS, Gudi R. Lack of mutagenicity of chromium picolinate in the hypoxan-

thine phosphoribosyltransferase gene mutation assay in Chinese hamster ovary cells. Mut Res. 2005;585: 86–95.

55. Beyersmann D. Effects of carcinogenic metals on gene expression. Toxicol Lett. 2002;127:63–68.
56. International Programme on Chemical Safety. *Chromium. Environmental Health Criteria 61.* Geneva: World Health Organization; 1988.
57. Barceloux DG. Chromium. Clin Toxicol. 1999;37: 173–194.
58. O'Flaherty EJ. Comparison of reference dose with estimated safe and adequate daily dietary intake for chromium. In: Mertz W, Abernathy CO, eds. *Risk Assessment of Essential Elements.* Washington, DC: ILSI Press; 1994; 213–218.
59. Sjogren B, Hansen KS, Kjuus H, Persson P-G. Exposure to stainless steel welding fumes and lung cancer: a meta-analysis. Occup Environ Med. 1994;51: 335–336.
60. Frankel DA. Supplementation of trace elements in parenteral nutrition: rationale and recommendations. Nutr Res. 1993;13:583–596.

# 40

# Boron, Manganese, Molybdenum, and Other Trace Elements

Forrest H. Nielsen

## Introduction

If the lack of a mineral element cannot be shown to cause death or interrupt the life cycle, then that element is not generally considered essential unless it has a defined biochemical function. On this basis, three elements discussed in this chapter can be considered essential for higher animals: manganese and molybdenum, which are known enzyme cofactors, and boron, the dietary lack of which interrupts the life cycle of some vertebrates. Numerous other elements have been suggested to be of nutritional importance because of some promising physiological or clinical finding, most often in an animal model or special human situation. These elements include aluminum, arsenic, bromine, cadmium, fluorine, germanium, lead, lithium, nickel, rubidium, silicon, strontium, tin, and vanadium. Of these elements, arsenic, fluorine, nickel, silicon, and vanadium have received the most research attention focused on the determination of their nutritional and biochemical properties; thus, these elements will be discussed in some detail here. Only brief summaries of findings of possible nutritional importance will be presented for the other elements. (Note: To limit the number of references, review articles instead of original reports are often cited in this chapter.)

## Essential Trace Elements

### *Boron*

**Basis for Essentiality or Biochemical Function.** The foremost evidence for the nutritional essentiality of boron is that it is required by some animals to complete the life cycle (i.e., deficiency causes impaired growth, development, or maturation such that procreation is prevented). The lack of boron was shown to adversely affect reproduction and embryo development in both the African clawed frog (*Xenopus laevis*) and zebrafish.[1,2] In the *Xenopus* model, dietary boron deprivation induced a marked increase in necrotic eggs and a high frequency of abnormal gastrulation in the embryo characterized by bleeding yolk and exogastrulation.[1] Boron deprivation of zebrafish resulted in a high rate of death during the zygote and cleavage periods before the formation of a blastula.[2] Pathological changes in the embryo before death included extensive blebbing and the extrusion of cytoplasm.

Studies with mammals have not been as definitive as those with the frog and zebrafish in showing that the life cycle can be interrupted by boron deprivation. In one study, however, the pre-implantation development of two-cell embryos from both boron-deprived and boron-supplemented female mice was significantly impaired by culturing in boron-deficient medium; the impairment in reaching the morula stage by day 1 and blastocyte stage by day 3 was more marked with embryos from boron-deficient females.[3] The proportion of embryonic degenerates formed after 72 hours of culture in a boron-deficient medium was 57% for embryos from boron-deprived mice, and 20% for embryos from boron-supplemented mice.

Two hypotheses have been advanced for the biochemical function of boron in higher animals. It is emphasized that these are speculated, not confirmed, functions of boron. The hypotheses accommodate a large and varied response to boron deprivation and the known biochemistry of boron. One hypothesis is that boron has a role in cell membrane function or stability such that it influences the response to hormone activity, transmembrane signaling, or transmembrane movement of regulatory cations or anions. This hypothesis is supported by the frog and zebrafish findings described above and the identification of boron-containing biomolecules associated with cell signaling. Recently, a bacterial quorum-sensing signal molecule was characterized as a furanosyl borate ester.[4] Quorum sensing is the cell-to-cell communication in bacteria that is accomplished through the exchange of extracellular signaling molecules called auto-inducers. One such auto-inducer, AI-2, is synthesized from adenosylmethionine, which supplies the 2′-3′-*cis*-diol of a ribose moiety that binds boron well.

Another group of biomolecules that contain ribose moieties, the diadenosine phosphates, have been characterized as novel boron binders.[5] Diadenosine phosphates function as signal nucleotides associated with platelet aggregation and neuronal response.[5] The finding that boron deprivation affects the aggregation of platelets obtained from rats[6] supports the hypothesis that boron may play a role in diadenosine phosphate signaling in platelet aggregation. Also supporting the membrane role hypothesis for boron is a report describing a possible mechanism through which boron affected frog egg development.[1] Culturing stage 1 and stage 2 oocytes from boron-adequate frogs in medium containing progesterone resulted in successful maturation to stage 5 or 6 oocytes. In contrast, oocytes from boron-deprived frogs did not respond to progesterone and did not mature in vitro. The boron-deprived oocytes were capable of producing progesterone and maturation-promoting factor (involved in binding progesterone to its receptor on the plasma membrane), and responding to this factor. It was hypothesized that the impaired maturation process was caused by progesterone not being bound efficiently to the membrane receptor because of changes in its structural homology. Numerous findings suggest that boron has an essential role in cell membranes of plants.[7] In boron-deficient plants, cell membranes are highly leaky and lose their functional integrity; substantial changes occur in ion fluxes and proton pumping.

The second biochemical function hypothesized for boron is based upon knowledge that two classes of enzymes are competitively inhibited in vitro by borate or its derivatives and that dietary boron can alter the activity of a number of these enzymes in vivo. The hypothesis is that boron acts as a metabolic regulator through controlling a number of metabolic pathways by competitively inhibiting some key enzyme reactions. The reactions inhibited may include oxidoreductases that require the boron-binding *cis*-hydroxyl-containing pyridine of flavin nucleotides as a cofactor. For example, it has been suggested that boron regulates the inflammatory process by dampening the activity of NADP-requiring oxidoreductase, which is involved in the generation of reactive oxygen species during the respiratory burst in activated leukocytes.[5] Evidence that boron affects the metabolism of reactive oxygen species includes increased erythrocyte catalase activity in rats,[8] increased plasma 8-iso-prostaglandin $F_{2\alpha}$ in rats,[9] and decreased erythrocyte superoxide dismutase activity in men and postmenopausal women[10] in response to dietary boron restriction.

**Boron Deficiency Signs and Beneficial Actions.** Although it has not been definitively established that boron deficiency interrupts the life cycle, nor has a biochemical function been identified in mammals, substantial evidence exists for boron being a bioactive food component that is beneficial, if not required, for higher animals and humans.

The beneficial action of boron may be the result of ensuring the optimal function of a hormone or some other nutrient. In the *Xenopus* model, the supplementation of thyroxine, a known enhancer of tail resorption, and, to a lesser extent, iodine reversed the delayed tail absorption in boron-deprived larvae.[1] This finding indicates that boron promotes optimal thyroid hormone metabolism or utilization during metamorphosis of the frog. In humans, estrogen therapy to maintain bones increases serum 17β-estradiol, and this increase is depressed when dietary boron intake is low (0.25–0.35 mg/d).[11] Boron has been shown to enhance the beneficial effects of 17β-estradiol on trabecular bone volume and plate density in tibias of ovariectomized rats.[12] Although neither boron nor estradiol supplementation alone affect calcium, phosphorus, or magnesium balance, a combined boron and estradiol supplementation improves the apparent absorption of calcium, magnesium, and phosphorus, and retention and serum concentrations of calcium and magnesium in ovariectomized rats.[13] These findings suggest that boron complements the action of estrogen. In 1981, one of the first studies suggesting that boron is essential[10] found that boron improved bone calcification in chicks fed a diet deficient but not completely lacking in vitamin D. At the microscopic level, boron deprivation was found to exacerbate the distortion of marrow sprouts (location of calcified cartilage erosion and new bone formation) caused by vitamin D deficiency and to delay the initiation of cartilage calcification.[10,14] Boron deprivation also decreased serum 25-hydroxycholecalciferol and ionized calcium when chicks were fed marginal vitamin D, but not when they were fed diets devoid of or luxuriant in vitamin D. These findings suggest that boron is needed for the optimal utilization of, but does not substitute for, vitamin D.

In addition to affecting the utilization of vitamin D and enhancing the action of estrogen, findings have been obtained that indicate boron is beneficial to bone calcification and metabolism in otherwise nutritionally adequate animals. In chicks, boron deprivation (0.18 mg/kg diet compared with a 1.5 mg/kg diet) decreased femoral calcium, phosphorus, magnesium, and copper concentrations and diminished the maturation of the growth plate.[14] Boron deprivation reduced bone strength in pigs[15] and rats[16] and induced abnormal limb development in frogs.[1]

Findings indicate that boron may be a modulator of the inflammatory or immune response in higher animals. When injected with an antigen to induce arthritis, boron-supplemented (2.0 mg/kg diet) rats had less swelling of the paws, lower circulating neutrophil concentrations, and higher circulating concentrations of natural killer cells and $CD8a^+/CD4^-$ cells than did boron-deficient rats (0.1 mg/kg diet).[8] In pigs, low dietary boron increased inflammation caused by the intradermal injection of phytohemagglutinin[17] and decreased the production of some cytokines (e.g., tumor necrosis factor-α and interferon-γ) following an inflammatory stress.[18] Also among the immune or inflammatory parameters affected by a change in boron intake are altered distributions and numbers of circulating immune cells. Perimenopausal women excreting an average of 1.1 and 3.0 mg boron/d during placebo and boron supplementation periods, respectively, had increased white blood cell numbers, an increased percentage of polymorphonuclear neutrophils, and a decreased percentage of lymphocytes during the boron supplementation period.[19] Compared with safflower oil, fish oil increased white blood cell number, with most of the increase in the lymphocyte fraction, in boron-adequate but not in boron-deficient rats, but increased monocyte and basophil numbers in boron-deficient but not in boron-adequate rats.[9]

Boron status apparently has an impact on the utilization of energy from carbohydrate. In humans, boron deprivation increased serum glucose and decreased serum triglyceride concentrations.[11] In chicks, boron deprivation decreased the hepatic concentrations of fructose-1,6-biphosphate, glycerate-2-phosphate and dihydroxyacetone phosphate and exacerbated the cholecalciferol deficiency-induced elevation in plasma glucose and decrease in serum triglycerides.[20] The effect of boron deficiency on carbohydrate metabolism may involve insulin sensitivity or production. Boron deprivation increased plasma insulin concentrations in rats.[20] Also, peak insulin secretion was higher from pancreas isolated from boron-deprived than boron-supplemented chicks.[21]

Both brain function and composition are affected by dietary boron.[11] In rats, boron deprivation results in decreased brain electrical activity similar to that observed in non-specific malnutrition. In humans, boron supplementation after boron deprivation yielded changes in encephalograms that suggested improved behavior activation (e.g., less drowsiness) and mental alertness, improved psychomotor skills of motor speed and dexterity, and elicited improvements in the cognitive processes of attention and short-term memory. Increased copper and calcium concentrations in total brain and increased phosphorus in the cerebellum have been found in boron-deprived rats. In zebrafish, boron deficiency induced photoreceptor dystrophy; the photoreceptor cells were shortened because of reduction in the myoid and outer segment regions.[2] These changes apparently were the reason boron-deficient zebrafish developed photophobia.

**Boron Absorption, Transport, Storage, and Turnover.** Because there is no usable radioisotope of boron, the study of its metabolism has been difficult. It is likely that most ingested boron is converted into boric acid, the normal hydrolysis end product of most boron compounds and the dominant inorganic species at the pH of the gastrointestinal tract. About 85% of ingested boron is absorbed and then efficiently excreted via the urine mainly as boric acid.[19,22,23] During transport in the body, boric acid most likely is weakly attached to organic molecules containing *cis*-hydroxyl groups. Recently, a borate transporter was identified that should give a better understanding of boron transport and homeostasis in animal cells. NaBC1 was found to be a ubiquitous electrogenic, voltage-regulated, $Na^+$-coupled $B(OH)_4^-$ transporter essential for boron homeostasis, growth, and proliferation of the mammalian HEK293 cells.[24] This transporter may explain the finding that RAW264.7 and HL60 cells accumulate boron against a concentration gradient.[25] A boron transporter may be involved in the excretion of boron via the kidney because the concentration of boron in urine can be higher than in blood, and the plasma boron concentration is resistant to change,[19,23] facts suggesting that the mechanism involved in boron excretion is more than just the movement down a concentration gradient.

Boron is distributed throughout the soft tissues at concentrations mostly between 1.39 and 185 μmol/kg fresh tissue (0.015 and 2.0 μg/g).[26] Based on studies with postmenopausal women, fasting plasma boron concentrations range from 3.14 to 8.79 mmol/L (34–95 ng/mL).[19,23] The concentration of boron in human milk was found to be relatively stable over a 12-week period, with mean concentrations ranging from 2.50 to 3.42 μmol/kg (27–37 μg/kg).[27] Individual values did not exceed 9.25 μmol/kg (100 μg/kg) nor decrease below 0.93 μmol/kg (10 μg/kg). As with other mineral elements, overcoming homeostatic mechanisms by high boron intakes will elevate tissue and blood boron concentrations.

**Dietary Guidance for Boron.** The Food and Nutrition Board of the National Academy of Sciences[28] set no Recommended Dietary Allowance (RDA) for boron, but did set Tolerable Upper Intake Levels (UL), which are shown in Table 1. Developmental and reproductive defects in animals induced by high dietary boron were used to estimate the ULs. In human depletion-repletion experiments, subjects responded to a boron supplement after consuming a diet supplying about 0.25 to 0.35 mg/d for 63 days.[10,11] Thus, humans benefit from intakes higher than this. An analysis of both human and animal data have suggested that an acceptable safe range of population mean intakes for boron for adults could be 1 to 13 mg/d.[29]Many people apparently have boron intakes of less than 1 mg/d. The Continuing Survey of Food Intakes by Individuals (CSFII), 1994–1996, indicated that boron intakes ranged from a low of about 0.33 mg/d to a high of about 3.0 mg/d for adults. The median boron intakes

**Table 1.** Dietary Reference Intakes (DRIs): Recommended Dietary Allowances (RDAs), Adequate Intakes (AIs) and Tolerable Upper Levels (ULs) for Boron, Manganese, Molybedenum, and Other Trace Elements

| Life Stage Group | Boron UL | Fluoride AI | Fluoride UL | Manganese AI | Manganese UL | Molybdenum RDA | Molybdenum UL | Nickel UL | Vanadium UL |
|---|---|---|---|---|---|---|---|---|---|
| | mg/d | | | | | | | | |
| Infants | | | | | | | | | |
| 0–6 mo | ND[b] | 0.01 | 0.7 | 0.003 | ND | 0.002(AI) | ND | ND | ND |
| 7–12 mo | ND | 0.5 | 0.9 | 0.6 | ND | 0.003(AI) | ND | ND | ND |
| Children | | | | | | | | | |
| 1–3 yr | 3 | 0.7 | 1.3 | 1.2 | 2 | 0.017 | 0.3 | 0.2 | ND |
| 4–8 yr | 6 | 1 | 2.2 | 1.5 | 3 | 0.022 | 0.6 | 0.3 | ND |
| Males | | | | | | | | | |
| 9–13 yr | 11 | 2 | 10 | 1.9 | 6 | 0.034 | 1.1 | 0.6 | ND |
| 14–18 yr | 17 | 3 | 10 | 2.2 | 9 | 0.043 | 1.7 | 1.0 | ND |
| >18 yr | 20 | 4 | 10 | 2.3 | 11 | 0.045 | 2.0 | 1.0 | 1.8 |
| Females | | | | | | | | | |
| 9–13 yr | 11 | 2 | 10 | 1.6 | 6 | 0.034 | 1.1 | 0.6 | ND |
| 14–18 yr | 17 | 3 | 10 | 1.6 | 9 | 0.043 | 1.7 | 1.0 | ND |
| >18 yr | 20 | 3 | 10 | 1.8 | 11 | 0.045 | 2.0 | 1.0 | 1.8 |
| Pregnant Females | | | | | | | | | |
| ≤18 yr | 17 | 3 | 10 | 2.0 | 9 | 0.050 | 1.7 | 1.0 | ND |
| 19–50 yr | 20 | 3 | 10 | 2.0 | 11 | 0.050 | 2.0 | 1.0 | ND |
| Lactating Females | | | | | | | | | |
| ≤18 yr | 17 | 3 | 10 | 2.6 | 9 | 0.050 | 1.7 | 1.0 | ND |
| 19–50 yr | 20 | 3 | 10 | 2.6 | 11 | 0.050 | 2.0 | 1.0 | ND |

[b]ND = Not determined.

Data from Food and Nutrition Board, Institute of Medicine, 2001.[28]

for various age groups of adults ranged from 0.81 to 1.22 mg/d. Food sources of boron are indicated in Table 2.

## Manganese

**Basis for Essentiality or Biochemical Function.** The essentiality of manganese has been known for over 50 years. Manganese deficiency has been induced in many animal species.[30] However, manganese deficiency has been difficult to induce or identify in humans, and is generally not considered to be of nutritional concern. Nonetheless, manganese is considered an essential nutrient for humans because it is known to function as an enzyme activator and to be a constituent of several metalloenzymes.[31] The numerous enzymes that can be activated by manganese include oxidoreductases, lyases, ligases, hydrolases, kinases, decarboxylases, and transferases. Most enzymes activated by manganese in higher animals and humans can also be activated by other metals, especially magnesium; exceptions are the manganese-specific activation of glycosyltransferases, glutamine synthetase, farnesyl pyrophosphate synthetase, and phosphoenolpyruvate carboxykinase.[31] The few manganese metalloenzymes in higher animals and humans include arginase, pyruvate carboxylase, and manganese superoxide dismutase.[31]

**Manganese Deficiency Signs.** Manganese deficiency causes a variety of effects depending on the animal species.[30] Deficiency causes depressed growth, testicular degeneration, seizures (rats), slipped tendons or perosis (chicks), osteodystrophy, severe glucose intolerance (guinea pigs), and ataxia (mice and mink). Signs of manganese deficiency have not been firmly established because most reports describing human manganese deficiency have shortcomings. In one study,[30] men were fed

**Table 2.** Dietary Sources of Boron, Manganese, Molybdenum, and Other Trace Elements

| Element | Rich Dietary Sources |
|---|---|
| Aluminum (Al) | Processed cheese, baking powder, grains, vegetables, herbs, tea, antacids |
| Arsenic (As) | Fish, seafood, grains, cereal products |
| Boron (B) | Foods of plant origin, especially fruits, leafy vegetables, nuts, legumes, pulses, wine |
| Bromine (Br) | Grains, nuts, fish |
| Cadmium (Cd) | Shellfish, grains grown in high Cd soils |
| Fluorine (F) | Marine fish with bones, tea, fluoridated water |
| Germanium (Ge) | Wheat bran, vegetables, pulses |
| Lead (Pb) | Seafood, food grown on high Pb soils |
| Lithium (Li) | Eggs, meat, fish, milk, potatoes, vegetables (content varies with geological origin) |
| Manganese (Mn) | Unrefined grains, nuts, leafy vegetables, tea |
| Molybdenum (Mo) | Milk and milk products, pulses, organ meats (liver and kidney), cereals |
| Nickel (Ni) | Chocolate, nuts, pulses, grains |
| Rubidium (Rb) | Fruits, vegetables, poultry, fish, tea, coffee |
| Silicon (Si) | Unrefined grains, cereal products |
| Tin (Sn) | Canned foods |
| Vanadium (V) | Shellfish, mushrooms, parsley |

Used with permission from Nielsen 1996[55] and Nielsen 1998.[58]

a purified diet supplying only 0.11 mg/d of manganese for 39 days. The men developed a finely scaling, minimally erythematous rash and decreased cholesterol concentrations, and increased serum alkaline phosphatase activity. Short-term (10 days) manganese supplementation, however, did not reverse these changes; this suggests that a longer repletion period should have been used. In two studies where the manganese intake was 0.8 or 1.0 mg/d from conventional Western-type diets for several weeks, minimal responses were found when the diet was supplemented with manganese. In one study, 14 young women consumed a diet providing about 1.0 mg/d manganese for 39 days, and were then supplemented with manganese to provide about 5.6 mg/d.[32] The only reported responses to the low manganese intake were slightly increased plasma glucose concentrations during an intravenous glucose tolerance test and increased menstrual losses of manganese, calcium, iron, and total hemoglobin. Whether these responses were signs of manganese deficiency may be questioned, because the women did not exhibit negative manganese balance during the low-manganese period, nor were the changes very marked. In the other study, 17 young women were fed diets that provided 0.8 mg or were supplemented to provide 20 mg/d of manganese for 8 weeks in a cross-over design.[33] The dietary manganese intake did not affect any clinical or neuropsychological measures, and only minimally affected psychological variables (e.g., self-confidence). These two studies indicate that intakes of less than 0.8 mg/d of manganese for an extended period of time are necessary to see significant signs of manganese deficiency in humans. The most convincing case of manganese deficiency is that of a child on long-term parenteral nutrition who exhibited diffuse bone demineralization and poor growth that were corrected by manganese supplementation.[34]

Manganese deficiency may contribute to disease processes. Low dietary manganese has been associated with osteoporosis, diabetes, epilepsy, atherosclerosis, impaired wound healing, and cataracts.[35] Animal findings described below have provided some support for these associations.

Manganese apparently affects carbohydrate metabolism.[36,37] Offspring of manganese-deficient guinea pigs that were weaned to manganese-deficient diets exhibited impaired glucose tolerance and utilization. Insulin release from isolated perfused pancreas from manganese-deficient rats is less than that found with manganese adequacy. Increased insulin degradation was also found in manganese-deficient rats. In both the guinea pig and rat, manganese deficiency causes pancreatic pathology characterized by hypoplasia of all cellular components. Decreased pre-proinsulin mRNA may be contributing to decreased insulinogenesis in the manganese-deficient rat. Manganese deficiency also apparently causes a defect in the response to insulin in peripheral tissues, because adipocytes isolated from manganese-deficient rats had decreased in vitro insulin-stimulated glucose transport, oxidation, and conversion to fatty acids. The biochemical bases for the changes in insulin metabolism and action induced by manganese deficiency have not been clearly defined.

Manganese superoxide dismutase (SOD-2) is the major antioxidant in mitochondria. The importance of this enzyme was demonstrated by the finding that the deletion mutation of the SOD-2 gene in mice resulted in death within 5 to 21 days of birth.[38] Severe mitochondrial damage occurred that was attributed to the increased concentration of reactive oxygen species in these mice. The importance of this enzyme for protection against oxidant stress has also been demonstrated by studies with animals or cells that overexpress SOD-2. For example, this overexpression has been shown to prevent alcohol-induced liver injury in rats[39] and attenuate myocardial injury following ischemia and reperfusion.[40] Additionally, high dietary manganese protected against heart lipid peroxidation in rats fed high amounts of polyunsaturated fatty acids.[41] Protection against oxidant stress may be the basis for the association between manganese and atherosclerosis and cataracts.

When imposed in utero or in young, growing animals, manganese deficiency has marked adverse effects on the skeleton; these effects include shortening of the limbs, enlargement of the joints, twisting of the legs, stiffness, and lameness.[31] These skeletal abnormalities have been largely ascribed to a reduction in proteoglycan synthesis secondary to a reduction in the activities of manganese-dependent glycosyltransferases.[31] However, manganese deficiency also has been found to impair osteoblast and osteoclast activities. This impairment may lead to altered bone growth and remodeling that contributes to bone deformities or weakness.[42] Manganese deficiency also may decrease circulating insulin-like growth factor, which has osteotrophic actions.[43] The bone findings suggest that manganese may be important in maintaining strong bones and healthy joints.

**Manganese Absorption, Transport, Storage, and Turnover.** For the adult human, absorption of manganese from the diet has often been stated to be no higher than 5%. Arriving at this value was problematic because endogenous manganese is almost totally excreted through biliary, pancreatic, and intestinal secretions into the gut. If manganese status is adequate, endogenous excretion of absorbed manganese into the gut is so rapid that it is difficult to determine the portion of fecal manganese not absorbed from the diet and the portion endogenously excreted. With this in mind, true absorption of manganese has been estimated to be 8% in young rats.[43] Manganese absorption decreases as manganese intake increases and increases with low manganese status.[44] Endogenous excretion of manganese apparently is not markedly influenced by dietary intake or status.[44] Thus, variable absorption apparently is a significant factor, with excretion contributing, in the regulation of manganese homeostasis.

Absorption of manganese apparently occurs equally well throughout the small intestine. There are indications that manganese is absorbed through a rapidly saturable, active transport mechanism that involves a high-affinity, low-capacity system. Diffusion also has been implicated in manganese absorption. Perhaps both processes are involved in manganese movement across the gut. This suggestion is supported by the finding that apical to basolateral manganese uptake and transport by Caco-2 cell cultures were strictly concentration dependent, but basolateral to apical uptake and transport were saturable.[45] Other Caco-2 cell studies indicate that transepithelial movement of iron and manganese are regulated by the same mechanism at the basolateral membrane,[46] that the metal transporters DMT-1 and Fpn are down-regulated in response to a high manganese intake,[47] and that manganese transport is regulated more by Fpn than by DMT-1.[47] Because iron competes with manganese for binding sites during movement across the gut, one of these metals, if present in high amounts, can exert an inhibitory effect on the absorption of the other.

Both $Mn^{2+}$ bound to plasma α-2-macroglobulin[31] and $Mn^{2+}$ bound to albumin[44] have been suggested to be the form of manganese entering the portal blood from the gastrointestinal tract. Regardless of form, manganese is rapidly removed from the blood by the liver. A fraction is oxidized to $Mn^{3+}$ and is transported in plasma bound to transferrin[31] or possibly to a specific transmanganin protein. Transferrin-bound manganese is taken up by extrahepatic tissue.

Within cells, manganese is found predominantly in mitochondria, so liver, kidney, and pancreas have relatively high manganese concentrations. In contrast, manganese is present in extremely low concentrations in the plasma and urine of humans.

**Dietary Guidance for Manganese.** The Food and Nutrition Board[28] has set Adequate Intakes (AIs) and ULs for manganese, which are shown in Table 1. The Total Diet Study of 1991–1997 indicated that the manganese intake of adults ranged from 0.31 to 8.31 mg/d. The range of median intake of manganese for various age and sex groups of adults ranged from 1.64 to 2.31 mg/d. Food sources of manganese are indicated in Table 2.

Neurotoxicity was the adverse effect on which the ULs were set. In the past, manganese was considered to be one of the least toxic of the essential mineral elements. Very high amounts of manganese (2000–7000 mg/kg diet) were required to induce the most commonly reported signs (depressed growth and iron and hematological variables). Recently, however, magnetic resonance imaging has shown that signals for manganese in brain are strongly associated with neurological symptoms (e.g., sleep disturbances) exhibited by patients with chronic liver disease.[48] Findings such as this have resulted in the suggestion that high intakes of manganese are ill-advised because of potential neurotoxicological effects, especially in people with compromised homeostatic mechanisms or infants whose homeostatic control of manganese is not fully developed. High intakes of manganese also may be of concern for people not consuming adequate amounts of magnesium. Pigs fed diets providing inadequate magnesium (about 25% of the dietary recommendation) died suddenly and showed heart changes when the diet was made rich in manganese (52 mg/kg).[49]

## *Molybdenum*

**Basis for Essentiality or Biochemical Function.** Molybdenum is an established essential element based on its need for the synthesis of a molybdenum cofactor containing a pterin nucleus that is required for the activity of sulfite oxidase, xanthine dehydrogenase, and aldehyde oxidase in mammals.[50] These enzymes catalyze the conversion of sulfite to sulfate, the transformation of hypoxanthine to xanthine, and oxidation and detoxification of various pyrimidines, purines and pteridines. The identification of inborn errors of metabolism that affected the molybdenum cofactor synthesis has provided the bulk of the evidence for classifying molybdenum essential for humans. This synthesis defect, however, is not reversed by molybdenum supplementation. Nutritional molybdenum deficiency has not been unequivocally identified in humans other than in one individual nourished by total parenteral nutrition. Thus, molybdenum generally is considered to be of no practical nutritional concern for humans.

**Molybdenum Deficiency Signs.** The signs of molybdenum deficiency in animals have been reviewed previously.[40] In rats and chickens, molybdenum deficiency aggravated by excessive dietary tungsten results in the depression of molybdenum enzymes, disturbances in uric acid metabolism, and increased susceptibility to sulfite toxicity. Deficiency uncomplicated by high dietary tungsten or copper in goats resulted in depressed food consumption and growth, and impaired reproduction characterized by infertility and elevated mortality in both mothers and offspring.

Knowledge of the signs and symptoms of human molybdenum deficiency has come from a patient receiving prolonged total parenteral nutrition, and from individuals with the genetic disease that results in molybdoenzyme deficiencies. The patient on total parenteral nutrition developed hypermethioninemia, hypouricemia, hyperoxypurinemia, hypouricosuria, and very low sulfate excretion; these changes were exacerbated by methionine administration.[52] In addition, the patient suffered mental disturbances that progressed to coma. The findings indicated defects in the oxidation of sulfite to sulfate and in uric acid production. Supplementation of the patient with ammonium molybdate improved the clinical condition, reversed the sulfur-handling defect, and normalized uric acid production.

Molybdenum cofactor deficiency is a rare inborn error of metabolism.[50] Diagnosis of the deficiency is usually made shortly after birth because of a failure to thrive and neonatal seizures that are often unresponsive to therapy. Biochemical changes include abnormal sulfur and purine metabolites in urine, such as elevated urinary sulfite and S-sulfocysteine, hypouricemia, and the detection of molybeoenzyme activity deficiency in fibroblasts. The disease is associated with a pronounced and progressive loss of white matter in the brain. There currently is no effective therapy for the genetic disorder. Most individuals with the genetic disorder die in early childhood and some survive only a few days.

**Molybdenum Absorption, Transport, Retention, and Turnover.** Molybdenum in foods and in soluble complexes is readily absorbed. Humans absorbed 88% to 93% of the molybdenum fed as ammonium molybdate in a liquid-formula diet.[53] In another study, about 57% of intrinsically labeled molybdenum in soy and about 88% in kale were absorbed.[54] Molybdenum absorption occurs rapidly in the stomach and throughout the small intestine, with the rate of absorption being higher in the proximal than in the distal parts. Molybdate may be transported across the gastrointestinal tract by both diffusion and active transport, but at high concentrations, the relative contribution of active transport to molybdenum flux is small.[55] The absorption and retention of molybdenum are influenced strongly by interactions between molybdenum and various forms of sulfur.[51]

Molybdate is transported loosely attached to erythrocytes in blood.[50] Organs that retain the highest amounts of molybdenum are liver and kidney.[51] The molybdenum in liver is entirely present in macromolecular association, partly as known molybdoenzymes and the remainder as the molybdenum cofactor.

After absorption, most molybdenum is turned over rapidly and eliminated as molybdate through the kidney[50,55]; this elimination is increased as dietary intake is increased. Thus, excretion rather than regulated absorption is the major homeostatic mechanism for molybdenum. Some of this excretion occurs through the bile.[56]

**Dietary Guidance for Molybdenum.** The Food and Nutrition Board[28] has set AIs for infants, RDAs for adults and ULs for molybdenum, which are listed in Table 1. Based on balance studies done by Turnland et al.,[56] which indicated that molybdenum balance could be achieved on an intake of 22 μg/d, the requirement of adults was estimated to be 25 μg/d (22 μg/d plus 3 μg to allow for miscellaneous losses not measured). Because some foods have lower bioavailability than those in the balance studies, an average bioavailability of 75% was used to set an estimated average requirement (EAR) of 34 μg/d for adults (25 μg/0.75). The RDA was set as the EAR plus 30%, or 45 μg/d for adults. Detrimental effects of molybdenum on reproduction and fetal development in animals were used to set the ULs.

Many people do not achieve the RDA for molybdenum according to NHANES III (1988–1994) data. The median molybdenum intakes found for adult females and males were 22.7 and 23.9 μg/d, respectively. This suggests that a search for molybdenum-responsive syndromes in humans may be warranted. The molybdenum hydroxylases may help in metabolizing drugs and foreign compounds. Thus, low dietary molybdenum may be detrimental to human health because of an inability to effectively detoxify some xenobiotic compounds. Food sources of molybdenum are given in Table 2.

## Possibly Essential or Beneficial Bioactive Trace Elements

### *Arsenic*

**Deficiency Signs, Beneficial Actions, and Possible Biochemical Function.** Arsenic is unquestionably a bioactive element in higher animals and humans. However, the concept that arsenic has beneficial or essential activity at physiological intakes is not well accepted. Nonetheless, the large number of responses to apparent arsenic deprivation (e.g., <12 μg/kg diet for rats and chicks; <35 μg/kg diet for goats) reported for a variety of animal species by more than one research group suggests that it may have an essential or beneficial function in ultra trace amounts.[57-59] In the goat, pig and rat, the most consistent signs of apparent arsenic deprivation have been depressed growth and abnormal reproduction characterized by impaired fertility and increased perinatal mortality. Other notable signs include depressed serum triglyceride concentrations and death, with myocardial damage during lactation in goats.[57] Arsenic deficiency in rats depressed S-adenosylmethionine and resulted in hypomethylation of DNA in liver.[59] In addition, feeding methyl depleters, including high dietary arginine, exacerbates the signs of arsenic deficiency in animals.[59] The responses to arsenic deprivation suggest that arsenic affects the utilization of labile methyl groups arising from methionine in higher animals. Thus, arsenic may affect the methylation of metabolically or genetically important molecules, whose functions are dependent on or influenced by methyl incorporation.

Correlation-type and in vitro findings also suggest that arsenic has beneficial actions in low amounts. For example, subtoxic amounts of arsenite induced a multicomponent protective response against oxidative stress in cultured human keratinocytes and fibroblasts.[60] Decreased serum arsenic concentrations in people undergoing hemodialysis treatment were correlated to injuries of the central nervous system, vascular diseases, and cancer.[61]

Some forms of arsenic have beneficial effects in supranutritional amounts. High doses of arsenic trioxide recently have been found to be an effective treatment for acute promyelocytic leukemia through apoptotic, not necrotic, mechanisms.[62]

**Arsenic Absorption, Transport, Storage, and Turnover.** The form of arsenic influences its absorption by the gastrointestinal tract.[55] In humans and most laboratory animals, more than 90% of inorganic arsenate and arsenite in a water solution is absorbed. About 60% to 75% of inorganic arsenic ingested with food is absorbed. When orally dosed, over 90% of arsenobetaine was recovered in the urine of hamsters; 70% to 80% of arsenocholine was recovered in the urine of mice, rats, and rabbits; and 45% of dimethylarsinic acid was recovered in the urine of hamsters.[55] Arsenosugars as found in seaweed are poorly absorbed[63]; they must be metabolized to another form before the arsenic can be absorbed.

There apparently are two components to the absorption of arsenic.[64] Initially, arsenate becomes sequestered primarily in or on the mucosal tissue. Eventually, the sites of sequestration become filled, with concomitant movement down a concentration gradient into the body. In rats, some forms of organic arsenic are absorbed at rates directly proportional to their intestinal concentration over a 100-fold range.[65] This finding suggests that organic arsenicals are absorbed mainly by simple diffusion. The absorption and metabolism of arsenic may be influenced by intestinal bacteria that can methylate arsenic or metabolize methylated arsenic.

Once absorbed, inorganic arsenic is transferred to various tissues, including the liver and testis, where arsenic is methylated with S-adenosylmethionine as the methyl donor.[66] Before arsenate is methylated, it is reduced to arsenite, and this reduction is facilitated by glutathione.[67] Arsenite methyltransferase methylates arsenite to form monomethylarsonic acid, which is then reduced to monomethylarsonous acid [$CH_3As(OH)_2$]. Monomethylarsonous acid, a relatively toxic form of arsenic, is rapidly methylated by a methyltransferase to form dimethylarsinic acid; in humans, monomethylarsonous acid is found in the urine only when excessive inorganic arsenic is consumed.[68] Dimethylarsinic acid can be reduced to dimethyarsinous acid [$(CH_3)_2AsOH$], which is a relatively toxic form of arsenic. However, the formation of dimethylarsinic acid usually is the final step in the metabolism of arsenic in humans and most animals, and thus is the major form of arsenic in urine. Pregnancy increases arsenic methylation, especially late in gestation; dimethyarsinic acid is the main form of arsenic transferred to the fetus.[69]

In addition to the methylated forms, inorganic arsenic bound to transferrin is found in plasma.[70] Trimethylated organic forms of arsenic stay trimethylated after absorption. Arsenobetaine passes through the body into the urine without biotransformation. Some orally ingested arsenocholine appears in the urine, and some can be incorporated into body phospholipids in a manner similar to choline; however, most is transformed into arsenobetaine before being excreted in the urine. Absorbed tetramethylarsonium also is not biotransformed before excretion. Unlike arsenobetaine and tetramethylarsonium, arsenosugars are transformed to many different arsenic species before excretion. Francesconi et al.[71] found at least 12 arsenic metabolites in the urine of humans after they ingested an oral dose of a synthetic arsenosugar. The metabolism of arsenic in some animal species is quite unusual. For example, unlike other mammals, rats concentrate arsenic in their erythrocytes. Chimpanzees, marmosets, squirrel monkeys, tamarins, and guinea pigs are unable to methylate arsenic. These species apparently have other mechanisms for facilitating arsenic excretion.[66,67,69]

Because homeostatic mechanisms exist for arsenic, no tissue significantly accumulates this element if low amounts are ingested. The highest amounts of arsenic are usually found in skin, hair, and nails, probably because inorganic arsenic binds SH groups of proteins that are relatively plentiful in these tissues.

Excretion of ingested arsenic is rapid, principally in the urine. In some species, significant amounts of arsenic are excreted in the bile in association with glutathione.[67,72] The usual proportions of the forms of arsenic in human urine are about 20% inorganic arsenic, 15% monomethylarsonic acid, and 65% dimethylarsinic acid.[69] The proportions are quite different, however, with the consumption of organic arsenic in forms found in seafood (mostly trimethylated arsenic, e.g., arsenobetaine).

**Dietary Guidance for Arsenic.** The Food and Nutrition Board set no Dietary Reference Intakes (DRIs) for arsenic.[28] Although no UL was set, high intakes of inorganic arsenic are clearly toxic. Although food is generally the major source of orally ingested arsenic, most adverse effects associated with arsenic occur upon ingestion of arsenic present in drinking water. Most arsenic in foods occurs in organic forms that are much less toxic than inorganic arsenic that can occur in relatively high amounts in some drinking waters. Countries with water used for drinking in specific areas that is high in inorganic arsenic and associated with human disorders include Taiwan, Chile, Hungary, Bangladesh, India, Thailand, China, Argentina, Mexico, Peru, United States of America, Bolivia, Vietnam, Romania, and Nepal.[73] The classical symptoms of arsenic toxicosis include numbness, tingling, and "pins and needles" sensations in the extremities; decreased touch, pain, and temperature sensation; and muscular tenderness. Chronic consumption of high amounts of inorganic arsenic in drinking water results in hyperkeratosis of the hands and feet, symmetrical pigmentation, conjunctivitis, tracheitis, acrocyanosis, and polyneuritis (Stoeppler, 2004).

Based on the estimated requirements for experimental animals, if humans need arsenic, the requirement most likely would be near 12 to 25 μg/d.[58] Based on the Total Diet Study (1991–1997), the median intake of arsenic from foods is less than this: 2.0 and 2.6 μg/d for women and men 19 to 70 years of age, respectively. Other surveys, however, indicate higher intakes of arsenic. For example, in the United States, the individual mean total arsenic intake from all food, excluding shellfish, has been estimated to be 30 μg/d.[58] Food sources of arsenic are given in Table 2.

## *Nickel*

**Deficiency Signs, Beneficial Actions, and Possible Biochemical Function.** Nickel is essential for some lower forms of life, where it participates in hydrolysis and redox reactions, regulates gene expression, and stabilizes certain structures. In these roles, nickel forms ligands with sulfur, nitrogen, and oxygen, and exists in the oxidation states $Ni^{3+}$, $Ni^{2+}$, and $Ni^{1+}$. In lower forms of life, nickel has been identified as an essential component of seven different enzymes: urease, hydrogenase, carbon monoxide dehydrogenase, methyl-coenzyme M reductase, Ni-superoxide dismutase, glyoxylase I, and acireductone dioxygenase.[58,74] Interestingly, the substrates or products for all of these enzymes are dissolved gases: hydrogen, carbon monoxide, carbon dioxide, methane, oxygen, and ammonia.

Nickel is generally not accepted as an essential nutrient for higher animals and humans, apparently because of the lack of a clearly defined specific biochemical function. However, nickel deprivation studies show that it is a bioactive element with beneficial, if not essential, actions in higher animals.[75]

Nickel deprivation detrimentally affects reproductive function in goats and rats. In breeding goats, success of first insemination and conception rate was decreased, and the number of breeding attempts to achieve pregnancy was increased.[75] In rats, sperm production and motility were decreased.[76]

There is considerable evidence that nickel deprivation changes carbohydrate and lipid metabolism in experimental animals.[75] One of the first reports suggesting that nickel may be essential described findings indicating that nickel deprivation depressed activities of enzymes that degrade glucose to pyruvate and enzymes that produce energy through the citric acid cycle. Also, glucose and glycogen were reduced in liver, and ATP and glucose were reduced in serum of rats fed low dietary nickel. The amount of nickel fed to the supplemented controls was quite high relative to the suggested nickel requirement of rats of 0.15 to 0.20 mg/kg diet. Because this high dietary concentration of nickel can affect iron metabolism in an apparent pharmacologic manner,[77] uncertainty existed about whether the changes in carbohydrate and lipid metabolism variables were caused by a nickel deprivation or pharmacologic action. Subsequent studies using more nutritionally balanced diets and a lower amount of nickel supplementation for controls showed that some of the differences were probably caused by nickel deprivation. Compared with rats fed a diet supplemented with 1 mg of nickel/kg, rats fed 0.013 mg of nickel/kg diet had decreased activities of the lipogenic enzymes glucose-6-phosphate dehydrogenase, 6-phosphogluconate dehydrogenase, malic enzyme, and fatty acid synthase.[78]

Nickel deprivation also resulted in increased concentrations of triacylglycerol concentrations in liver and serum. Because the enzymes affected by nickel deprivation are not nickel-requiring enzymes, the mechanism through which nickel affects glucose and lipid metabolism is not clear. However, because nickel apparently can affect iron metabolism through physiologic as well as pharmacologic mechanisms,[77,78] and iron status can affect energy metabolism, some of the changes induced by nickel deprivation may have been caused by a depressed iron status or utilization. Also, the effects of nickel deprivation may have been partly caused by a change in thyroid hormone metabolism, because nickel deprivation has been shown to decrease the concentrations of circulating thyroxine, triiodothyronine, and free thyroxine in rats.[79] The mechanism through which nickel affects thyroid hormone metabolism is also unknown.

There is evidence that nickel has beneficial effects in bone. Early findings[75] suggesting such an effect include nickel deprivation decreasing femur calcium and phosphorus content in rats, and decreasing the calcium concentration in ribs, carpal bones, and skeleton in miniature pigs. More recently, it was found that nickel deprivation decreased the bone-breaking variables maximum force and moment of inertia (which indicate decreased bone strength) in rats.[80] Mechanisms through which nickel affects bone strength and composition have not been defined. Nickel deprivation most likely has an effect on the organic matrix of bone because nickel was incorporated mostly in the organic phase of mouse calvaria in vitro,[81] and nickel can bind to cartilage oligomeric matrix protein and bring about the binding of this protein with collagen I/II and procollagen I/II (82). In high amounts, nickel may be affecting bone composition through activating the osteoclast calcium "receptor," which results in an increase intracellular $Ca^{2+}$.[83] This increase is a signal for the osteoclasts to resorb less bone.

Nickel might have a function that is associated with vitamin $B_{12}$, because lack of this vitamin inhibits the response to nickel supplementation when dietary nickel is low,[84] and nickel can alleviate vitamin $B_{12}$ deficiency in higher animals.[85]

**Nickel Absorption, Transport, Storage, and Turnover.** It is generally accepted that less than 10% of nickel ingested with food by humans or animals is absorbed.[55] When soluble nickel in water is ingested after an overnight fast, as much as 50%, but usually closer to 20% to 25% of the dose is absorbed.[55] Nickel absorption is heightened by iron deficiency, pregnancy, and lactation.[55] The mechanisms involved in the transport of nickel through the gut are not conclusively established, but there apparently is no specific nickel carrier in the brush-border membrane.[86] It has been suggested that some nickel is transported through an iron-transport system.[86] Nickel homeostasis may be partially regulated by absorption from the gut. The rate of nickel transfer was greater in everted jejunal sacs from nickel-deprived than nickel-adequate rats.[87]

Nickel is transported in blood principally bound to serum albumin. Small amounts of nickel in serum are associated with the amino acids histidine and aspartic acid, and with $\alpha_2$-macroglobulin (nickeloplasmin).[55] Uptake of soluble nickel from serum into tissues is believed to be governed by ligand exchange reactions.[88] It has been suggested that histidine removes nickel from serum albumin and mediates its entry into cells. The transfer of nickel across plasma membranes apparently involves both active and diffusion mechanisms, which have not been defined. Nickel may share a common transport system with magnesium and/or iron (e.g., transported into the cell bound to transferrin) and some nickel probably enters cells via calcium channels.[88]

In humans, the thyroid and adrenal glands have been found to contain relatively high nickel concentrations of 2.40 and 2.25 μmol/kg (141 and 132 μg/kg) dry weight, respectively.[89] Most organs contain $<$0.85 μmol/kg ($<$50 μg/kg) dry weight.

Although fecal nickel excretion (mostly unabsorbed nickel) is 10 to 100 times higher than urinary excretion, most of the small fraction of absorbed nickel is rapidly and efficiently excreted through the kidney as urinary low-molecular-weight complexes.[55] In healthy humans, urinary nickel concentrations generally range from 0.1 to 13.3 μg/L.[88] The nickel content of sweat of humans is high (about 70 μg/L), which points to active secretion of nickel by the sweat glands.[55] Based on isotopic studies in which nickel was administered intravenously, the excretion of exogenous nickel through the bile or gut is insignificant.[90,91]

**Dietary Guidance for Nickel.** The Food and Nutrition Board set no RDA or AI for nickel, but did set ULs,[28] which are shown in Table 1. Extrapolations from animal studies showing detrimental effects on reproduction were used to set the ULs. Except for the possibility that individuals with a nickel allergy may be sensitive to high intakes of soluble nickel after fasting, there are no reports that associate a high intake of nickel through the consumption of a normal diet containing nickel-rich foods with adverse effects in humans. If a dietary requirement is found for humans, based upon animal studies, it most likely will be less than 100 μg/d.[58] Typical daily dietary intakes for nickel are 70 to 260 μg/d.[58] Food sources of nickel are shown in Table 2.

## *Silicon*

**Deficiency Signs, Beneficial Actions, and Possible Biochemical Function.** Silicon is nutritionally essential for some lower forms of life.[86] Silicon has a structural role in diatoms, radiolarians, and some sponges. It may be essential for some higher plants (e.g., rice). Diatoms, which are unicellular microscopic plants, have an absolute requirement for silicon as monomeric silicic acid for normal cell growth. The diatom *Cylindrotheca fusiformis* has five silicon transporter genes that tightly control silicon uptake and use in cell wall formation.

For over 35 years, the nutritional interest in silicon for higher animals and humans has focused on its beneficial effects on collagen and glycosaminoglycan formation or function, which could influence bone formation and maintenance, cardiovascular health, and wound healing. Shortly after the discovery of silicon changes in bone during events leading to calcification, it was reported that silicon was required for the normal development of bones.[92] Leg bones of silicon-deficient chicks (less than 3 mg/kg diet) were shorter and had smaller circumferences and thinner cortexes than those of silicon-supplemented chicks (100 mg silicon/kg diet as sodium metasilicate). Femurs and tibias fractured more easily under pressure and the cranial bones appeared somewhat flatter.

Compared with rats fed 500 mg silicon/kg diet (as sodium metasilicate), those fed a diet containing less than 5 mg silicon/kg diet had skulls that were shorter, with distorted bone structure around the eye socket. In both of these experiments, the animals were not growing optimally. Subsequent to these findings, it was reported that when chicks were exposed to the dietary treatments shown above, silicon deficiency decreased articular cartilage and water in long bones, and decreased the hexosamine content of articular cartilage. Bone and cartilage abnormalities still were found in chicks fed improved diets resulting in near optimal growth. Compared with chicks fed 250 mg silicon/kg diet as sodium metasilicate, chicks fed diets containing 1 mg silicon/kg diet had tibias with a lower percentage and total amount of hexosamine, a greater percentage of collagen, and a smaller proliferation zone in the epiphyseal cartilage. The skulls of silicon-deficient chicks had stunted parietal, occipital, and temporal bone areas, and the bone matrix lacked the normal striated trabecular pattern. The nodular pattern of the bone arrangement in silicon-deficient skulls indicated a more primitive type of bone. Additionally it was found that collagen was decreased and non-collagenous protein was increased in skull bones from 14-day-old chick embryos grown in silicon-deficient culture; these bones also had decreased prolylhydroxylase activity.

Although these early studies suggested that silicon may be essential for higher animals, the suboptimal growth of some experimental animals and the high silicon supplementation of controls could be interpreted that some of the responses to silicon were possibly pharmacologic and thus were overcoming a dietary shortcoming of something other than silicon. Nonetheless, the studies showed that silicon is a bioactive element that has beneficial effects when consumed in relatively high amounts in the relatively soluble metasilicate form.

Because the early animal and organ culture studies were clouded by the use of high, possibly pharmacological, amounts of fairly soluble silicon for supplemented controls, the effects of silicon deprivation in rats were reexamined by Seaborn and Nielsen.[58,93] In these studies, supplemented control rats were fed a diet containing 4.5 to 35 mg silicon/kg as sodium metasilicate and compared with rats fed diets containing $\leq$2 mg silicon/kg. These studies confirmed that silicon deprivation affects bone, hexosamine, and collagen metabolism. Silicon deprivation decreased femur acid and alkaline phosphatase, humerus hydroxyproline, and plasma ornithine aminotransferase (a key enzyme in collagen synthesis). A recent study[94] found that silicon deprivation decreased plasma osteopontin concentration, increased plasma sialic acid concentration, and increased urinary excretion of helical peptide, a bone collagen breakdown product. Also, the response of bone metabolism indicators to ovariectomy in young growing rats was generally lower in silicon-deprived than in silicon-supplemented rats. Also, it has been reported that orthosilicic acid at physiological concentrations stimulates collagen type I synthesis in human osteoblast-like cells and enhances osteoblastic differentiation in culture.[95] These findings support the hypothesis that silicon affects bone growth processes before bone crystal formation, and this effect influences bone collagen turnover and circulating concentrations of sialic acid-containing extracellular matrix proteins such as osteopontin. The osteopontin finding also suggests that silicon influences the presence of cytokines in tissues and fluids other than bone, which could be the basis for silicon being beneficial to immune function[96] and wound healing.[97]

Although numerous apparent silicon-deficiency signs have been described, silicon is still not generally accepted as an essential nutrient for higher animals, apparently because of the lack of a clearly defined specific biochemical function. In 1978, Schwarz[98] described the difficulty in defining a biochemical function for silicon. He first suggested that silicon as an ether- or ester-like derivative of silicic acid had a cross-linking role in connective tissue. However, based on improved silicon analysis of connective tissue, Schwarz indicated that his suggestion needed to be redefined. His subsequent suggestion was, because of the stability of the O-Si-O bond, silicon is involved in binding structures such as cell surfaces or macromolecules to each other. If this is found true, silicon may be involved in the interaction between an extracellular matrix macromolecule and osteotrophic cells such that it affects cartilage composition and ultimately cartilage calcification.

It also has been suggested that the role of silicon in higher animals is to interact (as silicic acid) with aluminum species (e.g., $Al[OH]^{2+}$) to form an aluminosilicate that prevents aluminum from competing for iron-binding sites (e.g, in prolyl hydroxylase), which results in decreased function.[99] Thus, in the absence of silicon (or in the presence of excess aluminum) collagen synthesis and structure are adversely affected and this would be the basis for the observed effects of apparent silicon deficiency (e.g., bone organic matrix changes, impaired wound healing). There are experimental and epidemiological findings indicating that some of the beneficial actions of high intakes of silicon may be occurring through this mechanism.[92,100] In addition to alleviating the toxicity of aluminum, high intakes of silicon apparently can be beneficial through facilitating the absorption or utilization of some essential minerals, including copper[101] and magnesium.[102]

Whether it is by affecting the formation and structure of collagen, the binding of macromolecules to cell receptor sites, or the utilization or absorption of some mineral affecting bone formation, there is evidence that increased silicon consumption is beneficial to bone health. Jugdaohsingh et al.[103] reported that in a cross-sectional, population-based study (2847 participants), dietary silicon correlated positively and significantly with bone mineral density at all hip sites in men and premenopausal women, which suggests that increased silicon intake is associated with increased cortical bone density in these populations.

**Silicon Absorption, Transport, Storage, and Turnover.** The form of dietary silicon has a major influence on its absorption. For example, silicon was found to be absorbed better from stabilized orthosilicic acid than from herbal silica (*Equisetum arvense* extract) or colloidal silicic acid.[104]

Early balance studies with animals indicated that almost all ingested silicon is unabsorbed. The finding of low absorption probably resulted from the intake of highly unavailable silicon and the intake of silicon that exceeded the amount needed to achieve maximal absorption. Thus, these studies may be misleading about the bioavailabilty of silicon when consumed in low or milligram quantities in various foods. Recently, it was found that an average of 41% of dietary silicon was excreted in the urine (an indicator of absorption).[105] Silicon in grains and grain products was readily absorbed, as indicated by a mean urinary excretion of 49 ± 34% of intake. Silicon was as available in several of the grain products as from mineral waters. For example, urinary silicon excretion was 41% to 86% from corn flakes, white rice, and brown rice, and 50% to 86% from mineral waters. Silicon in fruits and vegetables, except green beans and raisins, was readily absorbed, with a mean urinary excretion of 21 ± 29% of intake. The mechanisms involved in the intestinal absorption of silicon are unknown.

Within 2 hours of ingestion of a tracer dose of $^{32}Si$, uptake was complete in a healthy male.[106] Within 48 hours, 36% of the dose was excreted in the urine, and the elimination was nearly complete. Elimination occurred by two simultaneous first-order processes with half-lives of 2.7 and 11.3 hours, representing about 90% and 10%, respectively, of the total output. It was suggested that the rapidly eliminated silicon was probably retained in the extracellular fluid volume, while the slower component may have represented intracellular uptake and release. In another study of silicon kinetics,[107] silicon peaked in blood about one hour after the intake of 27 to 55 mg orthosilicic acid/L of water in eight healthy adults. A relatively high renal clearance of 82 to 90 mL/min suggests that the majority of silicon in serum is filterable by the kidney, and that re-absorption of silicon by the nephron is low.

Silicon is not protein-bound in plasma, where it is believed to exist almost entirely as undissociated monomeric silicic acid.[55,86] Further evidence that silicon entering the bloodstream is transferred rapidly to tissues and urine is that the silicon concentration in blood remains relatively constant over a range of dietary intakes. Recent analyses indicate that human serum contains 11 to 25 μg/dL.[108] Connective tissues, including aorta, bone, skin, tendon, and trachea, contain much of the silicon that is retained in the body.[92] As indicated above, absorbed silicon is mainly eliminated via the urine, where it probably exists as orthosilicic acid and/or magnesium orthosilicate.[55,86] The upper limits of urinary excretion apparently are set by the rate and extent of silicon absorption and not by the excretory ability of the kidney, because peritoneal injection of silicon can elevate urinary excretion above the upper limit achieved by dietary intake.[55] This suggests that silicon homeostasis is controlled by absorption mechanisms in addition to excretory mechanisms.

**Dietary Guidance for Silicon.** The Food and Nutrition Board[28] judged that animal and human data were too limited for the setting of any DRIs for silicon. On the basis of weak balance data, a recommended silicon intake of 30 to 35 mg/d was suggested for athletes, a recommendation 5 to 10 mg higher than for non-athletes.[109] Based on extrapolations from animal data, Seaborn and Nielsen[93] speculated that a recommended intake may be between 5 and 10 mg/d. Carlisle[92] suggested that a daily minimum requirement might be near 10 to 25 mg based on the amount excreted in urine in 24 hours. High-fiber diets, aging, and high dietary molybdenum may increase the need for silicon. An antagonistic relationship between dietary molybdenum markedly decreased the retention of these two elements in chicks.[92] In the United Kingdom, a Safe Upper Level of 12 mg/kg body weight/d has been suggested for humans. However, based on findings with rats and chicks, intakes of relatively bioavailable silicon in the range of 35 to 45 mg/kg body weight/d can be beneficial. Thus, a safe intake for a 70-kg man may be greater than 2 g/d. Based on the Total Diet Study (1991–1997), the median daily intakes of silicon were 15 and 22 mg/d for women and men (19–70 years of age), respectively. The range of intakes (1st and 99th percentile for all individuals) was 3.5 to 80 mg/d. Food sources of silicon are indicated in table 2.

## *Vanadium*

**Deficiency Signs, Beneficial Actions, and Possible Biochemical Function.** Vanadium is essential for some lower forms of life, where it is required for some enzymes.[110] Vanadium-dependent bromoperoxidases have been found in marine brown algae, marine red algae, and a terrestrial lichen. Vanadium-dependent iodoperoxidases have been detected in brown seaweeds, and a vanadium-dependent chloroperoxidase has been identified in the fungus *Curvularia inaequalis*. These haloperoxidases catalyze the oxidation of halide ions by hydrogen peroxide, thus facilitating the formation of a carbon-halogen bond. The enzymatic roles for vanadium in lower forms of life suggest the possibility that vanadium has a similar role in higher forms of life.

At present, vanadium is generally not accepted as an essential nutrient, because a specific biochemical function has not been defined for vanadium at physiological intakes. However, there is no question that vanadium is a bioactive element. Its ability to selectively inhibit protein tyrosine phosphatases at submicromolar concentrations probably explains the broad range of effects that high intakes causing elevated tissue vanadium concentrations have on cellular regulatory cascades.[111] Protein tyrosine phosphatase inhibition is thought to be the basis for vanadium having insulin-like actions at the cellular level and stimulating cellular proliferation and differentiation. The insulin-mimetic action of vanadium has resulted in an effort to develop vanadium compounds that could be therapeutic agents for diabetes.[112] In addition to having effects at pharmacological intakes, vanadium may affect phosphorylation/dephosphorylation at physiological or nutritional intakes such that a regulatory cascade is altered. This may be the basis for observations that vanadium deprivation altered thyroid hormone metabolism, impaired reproduction, and altered bone morphology.[110,113]

The insulin-like actions of vanadium have been well reviewed.[112] The potential of vanadium for use as an orally active insulin-mimetic agent was stimulated by reports beginning in 1985. Since then, studies with animal models of type 1 diabetes showed that chronic treatment with vanadium salts lowered plasma glucose concentration, increased peripheral glucose utilization, and normalized hepatic glucose output, but had no effect on plasma insulin concentration. Treatment of human patients with type 1 diabetes reduced insulin requirements. Several organic vanadium compounds have been developed and, in addition to inorganic vanadium compounds, have been examined as potential therapeutic agents for type 2 diabetes. The vanadium compounds significantly decreased plasma insulin concentrations and improved insulin sensitivity in several animal models of insulin resistance and type 2 diabetes. Oral treatment of type 2 diabetic humans with vanadium reduced fasting plasma glucose concentrations, suppressed hepatic glucose production, and improved insulin sensitivity in skeletal muscle. Treatment with vanadyl sulfate had no effect on insulin sensitivity and fasting plasma glucose and insulin concentrations in healthy adults, an observation made for several animal models. The mechanisms through which vanadium has insulin-mimetic actions are not completely understood. Suggested mechanisms include inhibition of key gluconeogenic enzymes and the inhibition of protein tyrosine phospatases. Vanadium inhibition of protein dephosphorylation would indirectly enhance insulin receptor and/or insulin receptor substrate phosphorylation and thus its action.

The amounts of vanadium used in animals to show insulin-mimetic actions were extremely high relative to normal intakes. In some cases, the intakes were toxic and caused poor growth and diarrhea. The vanadium doses in human experiments were about 100-fold lower than those used for most studies of diabetic animal models. Nevertheless, the doses used (e.g., 100 mg vanadyl sulfate or 125 mg sodium metavanadate/d) were an order of magnitude greater than possible nutritional needs (described below).

Vanadium may be beneficial for bone or connective tissue formation or function. Bone abnormalities were found in vanadium-deprived goats.[110,113] Compared with goats fed 0.5 to 2 mg vanadium/kg diet, goats fed less than 10 μg/kg diet exhibited pain in the extremities, swollen forefoot tarsal joints, and skeletal deformations in the forelegs. Other findings suggesting that vanadium may have beneficial effects on bone include that of orthovanadate stimulating bone cell proliferation and collagen synthesis,[114] increasing phosphotyrosine levels, and inhibiting collagenase production by chondrocytes in vitro.[115]

In the experiments showing that vanadium has a beneficial effect on bone, the amount of vanadium provided to supplemented animals and cells was high relative to those that may be needed nutritionally. Thus, one cannot dismiss the possibility that the high vanadium supplementation was acting pharmacologically to overcome bone changes induced by something other than a simple vanadium deficiency. Further study is required to establish whether low dietary vanadium intakes increase the susceptibility to bone abnormalities and whether supranutritional intakes of vanadium are beneficial to bone and joint health.

In the goat experiments, there was an increased death rate in kids from vanadium-deficient mothers. Some of the deaths were preceded by convulsions. Because the supplemented controls were fed relatively high dietary vanadium, these suggested signs of vanadium deficiency also need confirmation.

**Vanadium Absorption, Transport, Storage, and Turnover.** Most ingested vanadium is unabsorbed and is excreted in the feces.[116] Because very low concentrations of vanadium, generally $<0.8$ μg/L, are found in urine (compared with estimated daily intakes of 12 to 30 μg) and the high fecal content of vanadium, apparently $<5\%$ of vanadium ingested normally is absorbed. Animal studies generally support the concept that vanadium is poorly absorbed. However, some results from rats indicate that vanadium absorption can exceed 10% under some conditions, a finding that suggests caution in assuming that ingested vanadium is always poorly absorbed from the gastrointestinal tract.[116,117]

Most vanadium that is absorbed is probably transformed in the stomach to the vanadyl ion and remains in this form as it passes into the duodenum.[116] The mechanisms involved in the absorption of vanadium in the cationic or vanadyl ($VO^{2+}$) form are unknown.[116] In vitro studies suggest that vanadium in the anionic or vanadate ($HVO_4^{2-}$) form can enter cells through phosphate or other anion transport systems. Vanadate is absorbed 3 to 5 times more effectively than vanadyl. Apparently, the different absorbability rates for vanadate and vanadyl, the effect of other dietary components on the binding and forms of vanadium in the stomach, and the rate at which vanadate is transformed into vanadyl markedly affect the percentage of ingested vanadium absorbed. Other dietary substances that apparently affect the binding and forms of vanadium in the stomach include chromium, protein, ferrous ion, chloride, and aluminum hydroxide.[116]

When vanadate appears in the blood, it is quickly converted into the vanadyl cation.[116] However, as a result of oxygen tension, vanadate still exists in blood. Vanadyl, the most prevalent form of vanadium in blood, is bound and transported by transferrin and albumin.[116] Vanadate is transported by transferrin only. Vanadyl also forms complexes with ferritin in plasma and body fluids.[116] It remains to be determined whether vanadyl-transferrin can transfer vanadium into cells through the transferrin receptor or whether ferritin is a storage vehicle for vanadium. Vanadium is rapidly removed from plasma and is generally retained in tissues under normal conditions at concentrations less than 10 ng/g fresh weight.[116] Bone apparently is a major sink for excessive retained vanadium.

Excretion patterns after parenteral administration indicate that urine is the major excretory route for absorbed vanadium.[116] However, a significant portion of absorbed vanadium may be excreted through the bile.

**Dietary Guidance for Vanadium.** No RDA or AI was set for vanadium by the Food and Nutrition Board.[28] Based on animal experiments, any requirement for vanadium would be small; a daily dietary intake of 10 μg probably would meet any postulated requirement.[113] Based on renal toxicity in animals, ULs were set for vanadium, which are shown in Table 1. Typical intakes of vanadium from foods are 6 to 18 μg/d for adults.[118] Table 2 shows food sources of vanadium.

## *Fluorine*

**Deficiency Signs, Beneficial Actions, and Possible Biochemical Function.** Fluoride is an element with a well-established beneficial function in humans; it protects against pathological demineralization of calcified tissues. Fluoride is especially important in the prevention of dental caries. The effect of fluoride on teeth and bones is not an essential function in the true sense, but is a pharmacological action.

Unequivocal or specific signs of fluoride deficiency have not been described for higher animals or humans.[58] In the early 1970s, it was reported that mice fed low fluoride (5 μg/kg diet) exhibited anemia and infertility compared with mice supplemented with fluoride (50 mg/L water). Subsequently, it was determined that the diets of these mice were low in iron and that high dietary fluoride, similar to that fed to supplemented controls, improved iron absorption or use. Mice fed low-fluoride diets containing sufficient iron exhibited neither anemia nor infertility. Relatively high fluoride supplementation (2.5–7.5 mg/kg diet) slightly improved growth of suboptimally growing rats fed 0.04 to 0.46 mg/kg fluoride/kg diet. A fluoride supplement of 25 mg/kg diet enhanced the growth of chicks. The high-fluoride supplements indicate that these growth-promoting effects were probably pharmacologic. High or pharmacologic amounts of fluoride have also been found to depress lipid absorption and to alleviate nephrocalcinosis induced by phosphorus feeding and to alter soft tissue calcification caused by magnesium deprivation. It has been reported that a fluoride deficiency in goats decreased life expectancy and caused pathological histology in the kidney and endocrine organs. These findings need to be confirmed before they will be accepted as signs of fluoride deficiency in higher animals.

**Fluorine Absorption, Transport, Storage, and Turnover.** A review of fluoride metabolism[119] stated that essentially 100% of fluoride ingested in the fasted state as fluoridated water, and 50% to 80% of fluoride ingested with food is absorbed from the gastrointestinal tract. Absorption of fluoride is rapid: about 50% of a moderate dose of soluble fluoride is absorbed in 30 minutes, and complete absorption occurs in 90 minutes. The rapidity of absorption indicates that a significant portion of ingested fluoride is absorbed from the stomach. Absorption also occurs throughout the small intestine.

Fluoride absorption is generally considered to occur by passive diffusion and to be inversely related to pH. Thus, factors that promote gastric acid secretion increase the rate of absorption. The pH dependence of absorption is consistent with the generally accepted view that hydrogen fluoride ($pK_a$ 3.4), and not ionic fluoride, is the form that is absorbed from the stomach. Diffusion of hydrogen fluoride in the small intestine because of its high pH is less likely. In the small intestine, the hydrogen fluoride concentration would be very low and the gradient small. In contrast, the concentration and gradient of fluoride ion would be high.

Removal of fluoride from the circulation occurs principally through two mechanisms: renal excretion and calcified tissue deposition. Approximately 50% of fluoride absorbed each day is deposited in calcified tissue (bone and developing teeth), which results in about 99% of the body burden of fluoride being associated with these tissues. The rate of uptake by bone is affected by the stage of skeletal development. About 50% of the daily intake of fluoride is cleared by the kidney. Urinary excretion of fluoride is directly related to urinary pH. Thus, factors that affect urinary pH, such as diet, drugs, metabolic or respiratory disorders, and altitude of residence, can affect how much absorbed fluoride is excreted.

**Dietary Guidance for Fluorine.** The Food and Nutrition Board[120] set AIs and ULs for fluoride, which are given in Table 1. The ULs were set on the basis of dental fluorosis in children and skeletal fluorosis in adults. The AIs are based on amounts that protect against dental caries and generally do not result in any mottling of teeth.

The major source of dietary fluoride in the United States is drinking water: over 50% of the population uses water with a fluoride concentration adjusted to between 37 and 63 nmol/L (0.7–1.2 mg/L). Food sources of fluoride are shown in Table 2. Fluoride is ubiquitous in foods, but similar products can vary greatly with source; thus, estimating fluoride intakes is difficult. Estimated daily fluoride intakes range from 1.4 to 3.4 mg/d for an adult male residing in a community with fluoridated water. This range is reduced to 0.3 to 1.0 mg/d in areas without fluoridation.[120]

# Other Elements

Because suggested deficiency signs need confirmation, or reports of beneficial actions are limited, only brief statements will be made for the following elements. For all of these elements, the typical daily dietary intakes indicated should provide an adequate amount for any postulated essential or beneficial actions. Except for the findings referenced, references for the information presented are given in two reviews.[55,58]

## *Aluminum*

A dietary deficiency of aluminum in goats reportedly results in increased abortions, incoordination and weakness in hind legs, and decreased life expectancy. Aluminum deficiency also has been reported to depress growth in chicks. Aluminum in vitro has been shown to stimulate osteoblasts to form bone through activating a putative G-protein-coupled sensing system, and is described as being required for the activation of a guanine nucleotide-binding regulatory component of adenylate cyclase by fluoride. The typical daily dietary intake of aluminum is 2 to 25 mg.

## *Bromine*

A dietary deficiency of bromide has been reported to result in depressed growth, fertility, hematocrit, hemoglobin, and life expectancy, and in increased abortions in goats. Insomnia exhibited by some hemodialysis patients has been suggested to be caused by a bromide deficiency. Bromide has been found to alleviate growth retardation caused by hyperthyroidism in mice and chicks, and to be able to substitute for part of the chloride requirement of chicks. A bromine-containing compound has been isolated from human cerebrospinal fluid with properties corresponding to 1-methyl heptyl-$\gamma$-bromoacetoacetate; this compound has been shown to provoke paradoxical sleep when administered intravenously to cats. The typical daily intake of bromide is 2 to 5 mg.

## *Cadmium*

Cadmium deficiency has been reported to depress the growth of goats and rats. Cadmium is mostly of toxicological concern because it has a long half-life in the body and thus it does not take much of an elevation in intake to result in an accumulation that could lead to damage to some organs, especially the kidney. In addition to renal dysfunction, high cadmium intakes have been associated with hypertension, some types of cancer, and osteomalacia. The World Health Organization has set 70 µg/d for a 70-kg person as a safe upper intake for cadmium. The typical daily dietary intake of cadmium is 10 to 20 µg.

## *Germanium*

Low dietary germanium compared with more normal intakes alters bone and liver mineral composition and decreases tibial DNA in rats. Compared with a diet supplemented with 1 mg germanium/kg, a diet with 10 mg/kg germanium dioxide stimulated growth in rats[121] and chickens.[122] Pharmacological amounts of some organic germanium compounds have anti-tumor activity in animals. The suggested mechanism behind tumor inhibition is that germanium enhances immune function. This has resulted in the promotion of over-the-counter supplements containing germanium (e.g., germanium-132 or carboxyethyl germanium sesquioxide; lactate-citrate-germanate) as anticancer agents and for the treatment of rheumatoid arthritis, osteoarthritis, and chronic viral infections. Recently, it was reported that germanium-132 supplementation (18 mg/kg diet) improved transverse bone strength and bone mineral density in rats with experimental osteoporosis.[123] It should be noted that high intakes of inorganic germanium, which is more toxic than organic forms of germanium, cause kidney damage. Some individuals consuming high amounts of organic germanium supplements contaminated with inorganic germanium have died from kidney failure.[124] The typical daily dietary intake of germanium is 0.4 to 1.5 mg.

## *Lead*

A large number of findings have come from one research group that found that a low dietary intake of lead had adverse effects in pigs and rats. Apparent deficiency signs found included depressed growth; anemia; elevated serum cholesterol, phospholipids, and bile acids; disturbed iron metabolism; decreased liver glucose, triglycerides, LDL-cholesterol, and phospholipids concentrations; increased liver cholesterol; and altered blood and liver enzymes. Others have found that lead supplementation improved the development of suboptimally growing rats and alleviated iron deficiency in young rats; these findings have been suggested to be pharmacological in nature. Any requirement for lead is likely to be small and covered by the typical daily intake of lead with a balanced diet; such intakes are in the range of 5 to 50 µg/d.

In clinical nutrition, lead intakes that are too high are the major concern. Although environmental lead exposure has been significantly reduced by the removal of lead from gasoline, the elimination of lead-based paints and plumbing materials, and the reduction of solder used in food and soft drink cans, lead exposure from contaminated soil and dust, dishware containing lead glazes, old paint and plumbing, and bone-containing supplements still exists. The toxicity of lead apparently is not dependent upon the route of exposure and is readily predicted by blood lead levels. Correlation and regression analyses indicate that when blood concentrations reach 10 to 15 µg/dL, toxic effects on bone development, mental development, and blood pressure occur, and anemia, nephrotoxicity and more overt neurological impairments occur when concentrations exceed 30 µg/dL.[125] Recently, however, it has been stated that a blood concentration of 10 ug/dL is no longer a safe threshold because it was reported that with each 1.0 µg/dL increase, there is a decrease in IQ in children with the greatest effect below 10 µg/dL.[126]

### *Lithium*

There is no question that lithium is a pharmacologically beneficial element because of its antimanic properties. Its ability to affect mental function perhaps may relate to observations that the incidence of violent crimes is higher in areas with low-lithium drinking water concentrations. Rats on a lithium-deficient diet exhibited diminished wheel-running activity, decreased response to handling, and decreased aggression in social interaction with other rats.[127] Lithium deficiency reportedly results in depressed fertility, birth weight, life span, liver monoamine oxidase activity, and serum isocitrate dehydrogenase, malate dehydrogenase, aldolase and glutamate dehydrogenase acitivities, and increased serum creatine kinase activity. In rats, lithium deficiency was found to depress fertility, birth weight, litter size, and weaning weight. Another pharmacologic action of lithium is that it has insulin-mimetic properties. These findings suggest that having some lithium in the diet is beneficial. The typical daily dietary intake of lithium of 0.2 to 0.6 mg probably is close to amounts that are beneficial but yet safe. Usual pharmacologic intakes of lithium range between 140 to 210 mg/d and have to be monitored to ensure that they are not toxic.

### *Rubidium*

Rubidium deficiency in goats has been reported to result in depressed food intake, milk production, growth, and life expectancy, and increased spontaneous abortions. In the rat, rubidium deprivation altered tissue mineral concentrations in a manner suggesting that rubidium intake can affect potassium, phosphorus, calcium, and magnesium metabolism. The typical daily dietary intake of rubidium is 1 to 5 mg.

### *Strontium*

In 1949, it was reported that strontium deprivation depressed growth, impaired the calcification of bones and teeth, and increased dental caries incidence in rats and guinea pigs,[128] but these findings have not been confirmed. Recently, interest in strontium has been heightened by its ability, especially in the form of strontium ranelate (a compound containing the organic acid, ranelic acid, and two atoms of strontium), to increase bone formation and uncouple bone formation from bone resorption.[129,130] Strontium ranelate is a promising pharmaceutical for the treatment of postmenopausal osteoporosis. The typical daily dietary intake of strontium is 1.5 to 3 mg.

### *Tin*

A dietary deficiency of tin has been reported to cause hair loss, and to depress growth, response to sound, feed efficiency, heart zinc and copper, tibial copper and manganese, muscle iron and manganese, spleen iron, kidney iron, and lung magnesium. The typical daily dietary intake of tin is 1 to 40 mg.

## Summary and Future Research Directions

Although the nutritional importance of each of the elements covered in this chapter is limited, unclear, or speculative, many of them have been or will be brought to the attention of the general public as being of possible importance in the prevention of disease with nutritional roots or for the enhancement of health and longevity. Thus, health and nutrition professionals need to be prepared to answer inquiries about these elements. The information in this chapter should help in providing current knowledge about the nutritional importance of elements that are often considered unimportant. Moreover, the information presented indicates that some of these elements (e.g., boron and silicon), apparently have beneficial properties in nutritional or supra-nutritional amounts, and thus may be of more nutritional importance than currently acknowledged. Therefore, future studies are needed to determine the mechanisms behind the beneficial effects, whether some effects reflect an essential function, and dietary intakes that give optimal response. Future research studies that may provide information that promotes health and well-being include:

- Identifying the mechanisms of action and establish intakes of boron that are beneficial to immune function, bone and joint health, and cognitive function.
- Determining whether a dietary intake of manganese less than the AI is a nutritional concern under circumstances (e.g. oxidant stress) that would require increased utilization of its essential function.
- Determining whether high dietary intakes of manganese may cause neurotoxicological manifestations in persons with a low iron status or may affect heart health in persons with a low magnesium status.
- Confirming that dietary silicon is associated with bone mineral density and determine the basis for this association.
- Investigating whether nutritional intakes of arsenic influence the susceptibility to cancer and whether nickel influences calcium and lipid metabolism.
- Determine whether there are dietary intakes (not pharmacologic amounts) of vanadium that are beneficial to glucose metabolism and of strontium that are beneficial to bone health.

These studies may find that some elements considered relatively unimportant in nutrition may be of more health importance than currently acknowledged.

## References

1. Fort DJ, Rogers RL, McLaughlin DW, et al. Impact of boron deficiency on *Xenopus laevis.* Biol Trace Elem Res. 2002;90:117–142.
2. Eckhert CD. Rowe RI. Embryonic dysplasia and adult retinal dystrophy in boron-deficient zebrafish. J Trace Elem Exp Med. 1999;12:213–219.

3. Lanoue L, Strong PL, Keen CL. Adverse effects of a low boron environment on the preimplantation development of mouse embryos in vitro. J Trace Elem Exp Med. 1999:12:235–250.
4. Chen X, Schauder S, Potier N, et al. Structural identification of a bacterial quorum-sensing signal containing boron. Nature. 2002;415:545–549.
5. Hunt CD. Boron-binding-biosubstances: a key to understanding the beneficial physiologic effects of dietary boron from prokaryotes to humans. In: Goldbach HE, Rerkasem B, Wimmer MA, et al, eds. *Boron in Plant and Animal Nutrition.* New York: Kluwer Academic/Plenum Publishers; 2002:21–36.
6. Nielsen FH. Does boron have an essential function similar to an omega-3 fatty acid function? In: Anke M, Muller R, Schafer U, et al., eds. *Macro and Trace Elements* (Mengen- und Spurenelemente). Leipzig: Schubert-Verlag; 2002:1238–1250.
7. Goldbach HE, Wimmer MA, Chaumont F, et al. Rapid responses of plants to boron deprivation. In: Goldbach HE, Rerkasem B, Wimmer MA, et al., eds. *Boron in Plant and Animal Nutrition.* New York: Kluwer Academic/Plenum Publishers; 2002: 167–180.
8. Hunt CD, Idso JP. Dietary boron as a physiological regulator of the normal inflammatory response: a review and current research progress. J Trace Elem Exp Med. 1999;12:221–233.
9. Nielsen FH, Poellot R. Boron status affects differences in blood immune cell populations in rats fed diets containing fish oil or safflower oil. In: Anke, M, Flachowsky, G, Kisters K, et al., eds. *Macro and Trace Elements* (Mengen- und Spurenelemente), vol 2. Leipzig: Schubert-Verlag; 2004:959–964.
10. Nielsen FH. Boron in human and animal nutrition. Plant Soil. 1997;193:199–208.
11. Nielsen FH. Evidence for the nutritional essentiality of boron. J Trace Elem Exp Med. 1996;9: 215–229.
12. Sheng MH-C, Taper LJ, Veit H, et al. Dietary boron supplementation enhanced the action of estrogen, but not that of parathyroid hormone, to improve trabecular bone quality in ovariectomized rats. Biol Trace Elem Res. 2001;82:109–123.
13. Sheng MH-C, Taper LJ, Veit H, et al. Dietary boron supplementation enhances the effects of estrogen on bone mineral balance in ovariectomized rats. Biol Trace Elem Res. 2001;81:29–45.
14. Hunt CD, Herbel JL, Idso JP. Dietary boron modifies the effects of vitamin $D_3$ nutriture on indices of energy substrate utilization and mineral metabolism in the chick. J Bone Miner Res. 1994;9: 171–181.
15. Armstrong TA, Spears JW, Crenshaw TD, Nielsen FH. Boron supplementation of a semipurified diet for weanling pigs improves feed efficiency and bone strength characteristics and alters plasma lipid metabolites. J Nutr. 2000;130:2575–2581.
16. Nielsen FH. Dietary fat composition modifies the effect of boron on bone characteristics and plasma lipids in rats. Biofactors. 2004;20:161–171.
17. Armstrong TA, Spears JW, Lloyd KE. Inflammatory response, growth, and thyroid hormone concentrations are affected by long-term boron supplementation in gilts. J Anim Sci. 2001;79:1549–1556.
18. Armstrong TA, Spears JW. Effect of boron supplementation of pig diets on the production of tumor necrosis factor-α and interferon-γ. J Anim Sci. 2003;81:2552–2561.
19. Nielsen FH, Penland JG. Boron supplementation of peri-menopausal women affects boron metabolism and indices associated with macromineral metabolism, hormonal status and immune function. J Trace Elem Exp Med. 1999;12:251–261.
20. Hunt CD. Biochemical effects of physiological amounts of dietary boron. J Trace Elem Exp Med. 1996;9:185–213.
21. Bakken NA, Hunt CD. Dietary boron decreases peak pancreatic in situ insulin release in chicks and plasma insulin concentrations in rats regardless of vitamin D or magnesium status. J Nutr. 2003;133: 3577–3583.
22. Sutherland B, Woodhouse LR, Strong P, King JC. Boron balance in humans. J Trace Elem Exp Med. 1999;12:271–284.
23. Hunt CD, Herbel JL, Nielsen FH. Metabolic responses of postmenopausal women to supplemental dietary boron and aluminum during usual and low magnesium intake: boron, calcium, and magnesium absorption and retention and blood mineral concentrations. Am J Clin Nutr. 1997;65:803–813.
24. Park M, Li Q, Shcheynikov N, et al. NaBC1 is a ubiquitous electrogenic $Na^+$-coupled borate transporter essential for cellular boron homeostasis and cell growth and proliferation. Mol Cell. 2004;16: 331–341.
25. Ralston NVC, Hunt CD. Transmembrane partitioning of boron and other elements in RAW 264.7 and HL60 cell cultures. Biol Trace Elem Res. 2004; 98:181–192.
26. World Health Organization, International Programme on Chemical Safety. Boron Environmental Health Criteria *204.* Geneva: WHO; 1998.
27. Hunt CD, Friel JK, Johnson LK. Boron concentrations in milk from mothers of full-term and premature infants. Am J Clin Nutr. 2004;80:1327–1333.
28. Food and Nutrition Board, Institute of Medicine. *Dietary Reference Intakes for Vitamin A, Vitamin K, Arsenic, Boron, Chromium, Copper, Iodine, Iron, Manganese, Molybdenum, Nickel, Silicon, Vanadium, and Zinc.* Washington, DC: National Academies Press; 2001. Available online at: http://www.nap.edu/books/0309072794/html/.

29. World Health Organization. *Trace Elements in Human Nutrition and Health*. Geneva: WHO; 1996:175–179.
30. Freeland-Graves J, Llanes C. Models to study manganese deficiency. In: Klimis-Tavantzis DJ, ed. *Manganese in Health and Disease*. Boca Raton: CRC Press; 1994:59–86.
31. Leach RM Jr, Harris ED. Manganese. In: O'Dell BL, Sunde RA, eds. *Handbook of Nutritionally Essential Minerals*. New York: Marcel Dekker; 1997: 335–355.
32. Johnson PE, Lykken GI. Manganese and calcium absorption and balance in young women fed diets with varying amounts of manganese and calcium. J Trace Elem Exp Med. 1991; 4:19–35.
33. Finley JW, Penland JG, Pettit RE, Davis CD. Dietary manganese intake and type of lipid do not affect clinical or neuropsychological measures in healthy young women. J Nutr. 2003;133:2849–2856.
34. Norose N, Arai K. Manganese deficiency due to long-term total parenteral nutrition in an infant. Jap J Parent Ent Nutr. 1987;9:978–981.
35. Klimis-Tavantzis DJ, ed. *Manganese in Health and Disease*. Boca Raton: CRC Press; 1994.
36. Baly DL, Walter RM Jr, Keen CL. Manganese metabolism and diabetes. In: Klimis-Tavantzis DJ, ed. *Manganese in Health and Disease*. Boca Raton: CRC Press; 1994:101–113.
37. Keen CL, Ensunsa JL, Watson MH, et al. Nutritional aspects of manganese from experimental studies. NeuroToxicol. 1999;20:213–224.
38. Li Y, Huang T-T, Carlson EJ, et al. Dilated cardiomyopathy and neonatal lethality in mutant mice lacking manganese superoxide dismutase. Nature Genetics. 1995;11:376–381.
39. Wheeler MD, Nakagami M, Bradford BU, et al. Overexpression of manganese superoxide dismutase prevents alcohol-induced liver injury in the rat. J Biol Chem. 2001;276:36664–36672.
40. Malecki EA, Greger JL. Manganese protects against heart mitochondrial lipid peroxidation in rats fed high levels of polyunsaturated fatty acids. J Nutr. 1996;126:27–33.
41. Strause L, Saltman P, Glowacki J. The effect of deficiencies of manganese and copper on osteoinduction and on resorption of bone particles in rats. Calcif Tissue Int. 1987;41:145–150.
42. Clegg MS, Donovan SM, Monaco MH, et al. The influence of manganese deficiency on serum IGF-1 and IGF binding proteins in the male rat. Proc Soc Exp Biol Med. 1998;219:41–47.
43. Davis CD, Zech L, Greger JL. Manganese metabolism in rats: an improved methodology for assessing gut endogenous losses. Proc Soc Exp Biol Med. 1993;202:103–108.
44. Davis CD, Wolf TL, Greger JL. Varying levels of manganese and iron affect absorption and gut endogenous losses of manganese by rats. J Nutr. 1992; 122:1300–1308.
45. Finley JW, Monroe P. Mn absorption: the use of Caco-2 cells as a model of the intestinal epithelium. Nutr Biochem. 1997;8:92–101.
46. Tallkvist J, Bowlus CL, Lönnerdal B. Functional and molecular responses of human intestinal Caco-2 cells to iron treatment. Am J Clin Nutr. 2000;72: 770–775.
47. Kelleher S, Lonnerdal B. Effects of Mn intake and Fe status on Mn and Fe metabolism, metal transporters, dopamine levels and behavior.FASEB J. 2003;17:A1130.
48. Lucchini R, Albini E, Cortesi I, et al. Brain magnetic resonance imaging and manganese exposure. NeuroToxicol. 2000;21:769–776.
49. Miller KB, Caton JS, Schafer DM, et al. High dietary manganese lowers heart magnesium in pigs fed a low-magnesium diet. J Nutr. 2000;130: 2032–2035.
50. Johnson JL. Molybdenum. In: O'Dell BL, Sunde RA, eds. *Handbook of Nutritionally Essential Mineral Elements*. New York: Marcel Dekker; 1997: 413–438.
51. Mills CF, Davis GK. Molybdenum. In: Mertz W, ed. *Trace Elements in Human and Animal Nutrition, vol 1*. San Diego: Academic Press; 1987:429–463.
52. Abumrad NN, Schneider AJ, Steel D, Rogers LS. Amino acid intolerance during prolonged total parenteral nutrition reversed by molybdate therapy. Am J Clin Nutr. 1981;34:2551–2559.
53. Tunrland JR, Keyes WR, Peiffer GL. Molybdenum absorption, excretion, and retention studied with stable isotopes in young men at five intakes of dietary molybdenum. Am J Clin Nutr. 1995;62: 790–796.
54. Turnland JR, Weaver CM, Kim SK, et al. Molybdenum absorption and utilization in humans from soy and kale intrinsically labeled with stable isotopes of molybdenum. Am J Clin Nutr. 1999;69: 1217–1223.
55. Nielsen FH. Other trace elements. In: Ziegler EE, Filer LJ Jr, eds. *Present Knowledge in Nutrition, 7th ed*. Washington DC: ILSI Press; 1996:352–377.
56. Turnland JR, Keyes WR, Peiffer GL, Chiang G. Molybdenum absorption, excretion, and retention studied with stable isotopes in young men during depletion and repletion. Am J Clin Nutr. 1995;61: 1002–1109.
57. Anke M. Arsenic. In: Mertz W, ed. *Trace Elements in Human and Animal Nutrition, vol 2*. Orlando: Academic Press; 1986:347–372.
58. Nielsen FH. Ultratrace elements in nutrition: current knowledge and speculation. J Trace Elem Exp Med. 1998;11:251–274.
59. Uthus EO. Arsenic essentiality: a role affecting me-

thionine metabolism. J Trace Elem Exp Med. 2003; 16:345–355.

60. Snow ET, Schuliga M, Chouchane S, Hu Y. Subtoxic arsenite induces a multi-component protective response against oxidative stress in human cells. In: Chappell WR, Abernathy CO, Calderon RL, eds. *Arsenic Exposure and Health Effects IV*. Oxford: Elsevier Science; 2001:265–275.
61. Mayer DR, Kosmus W, Pogglitsch H, et al. Essential trace elements in humans. Serum arsenic concentrations in hemodialysis patients in comparison to healthy controls. Biol Trace Elem Res. 1993;37: 27–38.
62. Chen Z, Chen G-Q, Shen Z-X, et al. Treatment of acute promyelocytic leukemia with arsenic compounds: in vitro and in vivo studies. Semin Hematol. 2001;38:26–36.
63. Shiomi K. Arsenic in marine organisms: chemical forms and toxicological aspects. In: Nriagu JO, ed. *Arsenic in the Environment, Part II: Human Health and Ecosystem Effects*. New York: Wiley;1994: 261–282.
64. Fullmer CS, Wasserman RH. Intestinal absorption of arsenate in the chick. Environ Res. 1985;36: 206–217.
65. Hwang SW, Schanker LS. Absorption of organic arsenical compounds from the rat small intestine. Xenobiotica. 1973;3:351–355.
66. Healy SM, Wildfang E, Zakharyan RA, Aposhian HV. Diversity of inorganic arsenite transformation. Biol Trace Elem Res. 1999;68:249–266.
67. Vahter M. Species differences in the metabolism of arsenic. In: Chappell WR, Abernathy CO, Cothern CR, eds. *Arsenic. Exposure and Health*. Northwood: Science and Toxicology Letters; 1994:171–179.
68. Aposhian HV, Gurzau ES, Le XC, et al. The discovery, importance and significance of monomethylarsonous acid ($MMA^{III}$) in urine of humans exposed to inorganic arsenic. In: Chappell WR, Abernathy CO, Calderon RL, eds. *Arsenic Exposure and Health Effects IV*. Oxford: Elsevier Science; 2001:305–313.
69. Vahter M, Concha G, Nermell B. Factors influencing arsenic methylation in humans. J Trace Elem Exp Med. 2000;13:173–184.
70. Zhang X, Cornelis R, DeKimpe J, et al. Study of arsenic-protein binding in serum of patients on continuous ambulatory peritoneal dialysis. Clin Chem. 1998;44:141–147.
71. Francesconi KA, Tanggaard R, McKenzie CJ, Goessler W. Arsenic metabolites in human urine after ingestion of an arsenosugar. Clin Chem. 2002; 48:92–101.
72. Stoeppler M. Arsenic. In: Merian E, Anke M, Ihnat M, Stoeppler M, eds. *Elements and Their Compounds in the Environment, Occurrence, Analysis, and Biological Relevance, Vol 3, Nonmetals, Particular Aspects, 2nd ed.* Weinheim: Wiley-VCH; 2004: 1321–1364.
73. Kala SV, Neely MW, Kala G, et al. The MRP2/cMOAT transporter and arsenic-glutathione complex formation are required for bilary excretion of arsenic. J Biol Chem. 2000;275:33404–33408.
74. Pochapsky TC, Pochapsky S, Ju T, et al. Modeling and experiment yields the structure of acireductone dioxygenase from *Klebsiella pneumoniae*. Nature Struc Biol. 2002;9:966–972.
75. Nielsen FH. Nickel. In: Mertz W, ed. *Trace Elements in Human and Animal Nutrition, vol 1*. San Diego: Academic Press; 1987:245–273.
76. Yokoi K, Uthus EO, Nielsen FH. Nickel deficiency diminishes sperm quantity and movement in rats. Biol Trace Elem Res. 2003;93:141–153.
77. Nielsen FH, Shuler TR, McLeod TG, Zimmerman TJ. Nickel influences iron metabolism through physiologic, pharmacologic and toxicologic mechanisms in the rat. J Nutr. 1984;114:1280–1288.
78. Stangl GI, Kirchgessner M. Nickel deficiency alters liver lipid metabolism in rats. J Nutr. 1996:126: 2466–2473.
79. Stangl GI, Kirchgessner M. Comparative effects of nickel and iron depletion on circulating thyroid hormone concentrations in rats. J Anim Physiol Anim Nutr. 1998;79:18–26.
80. Nielsen FH. The effect of nickel deprivation on bone strength and shape and urinary phosphorus excretion is not enhanced by a mild magnesium deprivation in rats. In: Anke M, Flachowsky M, Kisters K, et al., eds. *Macro and Trace Elements* [Mengen- und Spurenelemente], *vol 2*. Leipzig: Schubert-Verlag; 2004:965–970.
81. Jacobsen N, Jonsen J. Strontium, lead and nickel incorporation into mouse calvaria *in vitro*. Path Europ. 1975;10:115–121.
82. Rosenberg K, Olsson H, Mörgelin M, Heinegärd D. Cartilage oligomeric matrix protein shows high affinity zinc-dependent interaction with triple helical collagen. J Biol Chem. 1998;273:20397–20403.
83. Shankar V, Bax CMR, Bax BE, et al. Activation of the $Ca^{2+}$ "receptor" on the osteoclast by $Ni^{2+}$ elicits cytosolic $Ca^{2+}$ signals: evidence for receptor activation and inactivation, intracellular $Ca^{2+}$ redistribution, and divalent cation modulation. J Cell Physiol. 1993;155:120–129.
84. Nielsen FH, Zimmerman TJ, Shuler TR, et al. Evidence for a cooperative relationship between nickel and vitamin $B_{12}$ in rats. J Trace Elem Exp Med. 1989;2:21–29.
85. Stangl GI, Roth-Maier DA, Kirchgessner M. Vitamin B-12 deficiency and hyperhomocysteinemia are partly ameliorated by cobalt and nickel supplementation in pigs. J Nutr. 2000;130:3038–3044.
86. Nielsen FH. Boron, manganese, molybdenum, and other trace elements. In: Bowman BA, Russell RM,

eds. *Present Knowledge in Nutritioin, 8th ed.* Washington DC: ILSI Press; 2001:384–400.

87. Stangl GI, Eidelsburger U, Kirchgessner M. Nickel deficiency alters nickel flux in rat everted intestinal sacs. Biol Trace Elem Res. 1998;61:253–262.
88. Sutherland JE, Costa M. Nickel. In: Sarkar B, ed. *Heavy Metals in the Environment*. New York: Marcel Dekker; 2002:349–407.
89. Rezuke WN, Knight JA, Sunderman FW Jr. Reference values for nickel concentrations in human tissue and bile. Am J Ind Med. 1987;11:419–426.
90. Marzouk A, Sunderman FW Jr. Biliary excretion of nickel in rats. Toxicol Lett. 1985;27:65–71.
91. Patriarca M, Lyon TDB, Fell GS. Nickel metabolism in humans investigated with an oral stable isotope. Am J Clin Nutr. 1997;66:616–621.
92. Carlisle EM. Silicon. In: O'Dell BL, Sunde RA, eds. *Handbook of Nutritionally Essential Minerals*. New York: Marcel Dekker; 1997:603–618.
93. Seaborn CD, Nielsen FH. Silicon: a nutritional beneficence for bones, brains, and blood vessels? Nutr Today. 1993;28:13–18.
94. Nielsen, FH, Poellot R. Dietary silicon affects bone turnover differently in ovariectomized and sham-operated growing rats. J Trace Elem Exp Med. 2004;17:137–149.
95. Reffitt DM, Ogston N, Jugdaohsingh R, et al. Orthosilicic acid stimulates collagen type I synthesis and osteoblastic differentiation in human osteoblast-like cells in vitro. Bone. 2003;32:127–135.
96. Seaborn CD, Nielsen FH. An interaction between dietary silicon and arginine affects immune function indicated by Con-A-induced DNA synthesis of rat splenic T-lymphocytes. Biol Trace Elem Res. 2002; 87:133–142.
97. Seaborn CD, Nielsen FH. Silicon deprivation decreases collagen formation in wounds and bone, and ornithine transaminase enzyme activity in liver. Biol Trace Elem Res. 2002;89:251–261.
98. Schwarz K. Significance and function of silicon in warm-blooded animals. Review and outlook. In: *Biochemistry of Silicon and Related Problems*. Bendz G, Lindquist I, eds. New York: Plenum Press; 1978: 207–230.
99. Birchall JD, Espie AW. Biological implications of the interaction (via silanol groups) of silicon with metal ions. In: Evered D, O'Connor M, eds. *Silicon Biochemistry, Ciba Foundation Symposium 121*. Chichester: John Wiley & Sons; 1986:140–159.
100. Forbes WF, Agwani N, Lachmaniuk P. Geochemical risk factors for mental functioning, based on the Ontario Longitudinal Study of Aging (LSA) IV. The role of silicon-containing compounds. Can J Aging. 1995;14:630–641.
101. Emerick R, Kayongo-Male H. Silicon facilitation of copper utilization in the rat. J Nutr Biochem. 1990;1:487–492.
102. Kikunaga S, Kitano T, Kikukawa T, Takahashi M. Effects of fluoride and silicon on distribution of minerals in the magnesium-deficient rat. Magunes-humu. 1991;10:181–191.
103. Jugdaohsingh R, Tucker KL, Qiao N, et al. Dietary silicon intake is positively associated with bone mineral density in men and premenopausal women of the Framingham offspring cohort. J Bone Min Res. 19:297–307.
104. Calomme MR, Cos P, D'Haese PC, et al. Absorption of silicon in healthy subjects. In: Collery Ph, Brätter P, Negretti de Brätter V, et al, eds. *Metal Ions in Biology and Medicine, vol 5*. Paris: John Libbey Eurotext; 1998:228–232.
105. Jugdaohsingh R, Anderson SHC, Tucker KL, et al. Dietary silicon intake and absorption. Am J Clin Nutr. 2002;75:887–893.
106. Popplewell JF, King SJ, Day JP, et al. Kinetics of uptake and elimination of silicic acid by a human subject: a novel application of $^{32}Si$ and accelerator mass spectrometry. J Inorg Biochem. 1998;69: 177–180.
107. Reffitt DM, Jugdaohsingh R, Thompson RP, Powell JJ. Silicic acid: its gastrointestinal uptake and urinary excretion in man and effects on aluminum excretion. J Inorg Biochem. 1999;76:141–147.
108. Van Dyck K, Robberecht H, Van Cauwenbergh R, et al. Indication of silicon essentiality in humans. Serum concentrations in Belgian children and adults, including pregnant women. Biol Trace Elem Res. 2000;77:25–32.
109. Nasolodin VV, Rusin VY, Vorob'ev VA. Zinc and silicon metabolism in highly trained athletes under hard physical stress (In Russian). Vopr Pitan. 1987; 37–39.
110. Nielsen FH. Vanadium. In: O'Dell BL, Sunde RA, eds. *Handbook of Nutritionally Essential Mineral Elements*. New York: Marcel Dekker; 1997: 619–630.
111. Hulley P, Davison A. Regulation of tyrosine phosphorylation cascades by phosphatases: what the actions of vanadium teach us. J Trace Elem Exp Med. 2003;16:281–290.
112. Marzban L, McNeill JH. Insulin-like actions of vanadium: potential as a therapeutic agent. J Trace Elem Exp Med. 2003;16:253–267.
113. Nielsen FH. The nutritional essentiality and physiological metabolism of vanadium in higher animals. In: Tracey AS, Crans DC, eds. *Vanadium Compounds. Chemistry, Biochemistry, and Therapeutic Applications*. ACS Symp Ser 711. Washington DC: American Chemical Society; 1998:297–307.
114. Lau K-HW, Tanimoto H, Baylink DJ. Vanadate stimulates bone cell proliferation and bone collagen synthesis in vitro. Endocrinology. 1988;123:2858–2867.
115. Cruz T, Mills G, Pritzker KPH, Kandel RA. Inverse correlation between tyrosine phosphorylation

and collagenase production in chondrocytes. Biochem J. 1990;269:717–721.

116. Nielsen FH. Vanadium in mammalian physiology and nutrition. In; Sigel H, Sigel A, eds. *Metal Ions in Biological Systems, vol 31*. Vanadium and Its Role in Life. New York: Marcel Dekker; 1995:543–573.
117. Setyawati IA, Thompson KH, Yuen VG, et al. Kinetic analysis and comparison of uptake, distribution, and excretion of $^{48}$V-labeled compounds in rats. J Appl Physiol. 1998;84:569–575.
118. Pennington JA, Jones JW. Molybdenum, Nickel, Cobalt, Vanadium, and Strontium in total diets. J Am Diet Assoc. 1987;87:1644–1650.
119. Cerklewski FL. Fluorine. In: O'Dell BL, Sunde RA, eds. *Handbook of Nutritionally Essential Mineral Elements*. New York: Academic Press; 1997: 583–602.
120. Food and Nutrition Board. *Dietary Reference Intakes for Calcium, Phosphorus, Magnesium, Vitamin D, and Fluoride*. Washington DC: National Academy Press; 1997.
121. Venugopal B, Luckey TD. *Metal Toxicity in Mammals. Chemical Toxicity of Metals and Metalloids, vol 2*. New York: Plenum Press; 1978:175–180.
122. Li JF, Kirchgessner M, Steinruck U. Growth promoting effect and toxicity of germanium in chickens. Arch Geflugelk. 1993;57:205–210.
123. Matsumoto H, Jiang G-Z, Hashimoto T, et al. Effect of organic germanium compound (Ge-132) on experimental osteoporosis in rats: the relationship between transverse strength and bone mineral density (BMD) or bone mineral content (BMC). Int J Oral-Med Sci. 2002;1:10–16.
124. Tao S-H, Bolger PM. Hazard assessment of germanium supplements. Reg Toxicol Pharmacol. 1997; 25:211–219.
125. Agency for Toxic Substances and Disease Registry. Toxicological profile for Lead. Available online at [www.atsdr.cdc.gov], Accessed July 17, 2006.
126. Canfield RL, Henderson CR Jr, Cory-Slechta DA, Cox C, Jusko TA, Lanphear BP. Intellectual impairment in children with blood lead concentrations below 10 microg per deciliter. N Engl J Med. 2003; 348:1517–1526.
127. Schrauzer GN. Lithium: occurrence, dietary intakes, nutritional essentiality. J Amer Coll Nutr. 2002;21:14–21.
128. Rygh O. Recherches sur les oligo-éléments. I. De l'importance du strontium, du barium et du zinc. Bull Sté Chim Biol. 1949;31:1052–1061.
129. Marie PJ, Hott M, Modrowski D, et al. An uncoupling agent containing strontium prevents bone loss by depressing bone resorption and maintaining bone formation in estrogen-deficient rats. J Bone Miner Res. 1993;8:607–615.
130. Marie PJ, Ammann P, Boivin G, Rey C. Mechanisms of action and therapeutic potential of strontium in bone. Calcif Tissue Int. 2001;69:121–129.

PRESENT KNOWLEDGE IN
**NUTRITION**

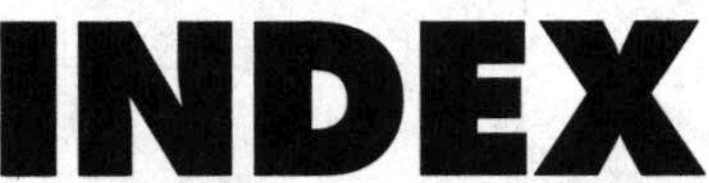

Page numbers followed by a t indicate a table, those followed by f indicate a figure.

## A

## B

## C

## D

## E

# F

## G



## H

## O



## P

## Q



## R

## S

# V

## W

# X



# Z